SRB's

Volume 2

Surgical Operations

Text and Atlas

SRB's Surgical Operations
Text and Atlas

Volume 2

Third Edition

Sriram Bhat M MS (General Surgery) FRCS (Glasgow)
Professor and Unit Head
Department of Surgery
Kasturba Medical College
Mangaluru, Karnataka, India

Honorary Medical Officer
Government District Wenlock Hospital, Mangaluru
Dakshina Kannada, Karnataka, India
e-mail: meera_sriram2003@yahoo.com

Forewords
K Ganesh Pai
Ashok Pandit

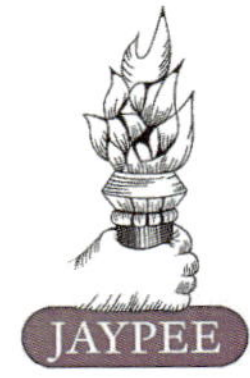

JAYPEE BROTHERS MEDICAL PUBLISHERS
The Health Sciences Publisher
New Delhi | London

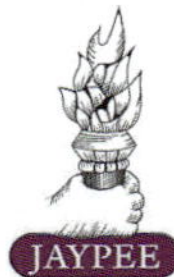

Jaypee Brothers Medical Publishers (P) Ltd

Headquarters
Jaypee Brothers Medical Publishers (P) Ltd
EMCA House, 23/23-B
Ansari Road, Daryaganj
New Delhi 110 002, India
Landline: +91-11-23272143, +91-11-23272703
+91-11-23282021, +91-11-23245672
Email: jaypee@jaypeebrothers.com

Corporate Office
Jaypee Brothers Medical Publishers (P) Ltd
4838/24, Ansari Road, Daryaganj
New Delhi 110 002, India
Phone: +91-11-43574357
Fax: +91-11-43574314
Email: jaypee@jaypeebrothers.com

Overseas Office
JP Medical Ltd.
83, Victoria Street, London
SW1H 0HW (UK)
Phone: +44 20 3170 8910
Fax: +44 (0)20 3008 6180
Email: info@jpmedpub.com

Website: www.jaypeebrothers.com
Website: www.jaypeedigital.com

Inquiries for bulk sales may be solicited at: jaypee@jaypeebrothers.com

SRB's Surgical Operations: Text and Atlas (2 Volumes)

First Edition: 2014

Second Edition: 2018

Revised Reprint: 2024

Third Edition: **2025**

ISBN: 978-93-5696-956-8

Printed at: Samrat Offset Pvt. Ltd

Contents

VOLUME 1

VOLUME 2

20

CHAPTER

Surgery of Oesophagus

SURGICAL ANATOMY

Oesophagus is a hollow muscular tube which begins at the lower edge of the cricoid cartilage (C6 vertebra) and ends at oesophagogastric junction (T12 vertebra). It is 25 cm in length. Upper end is closed by cricopharyngeus muscle which is 18 cm from upper incisors. Lower end is 40 cm from the upper incisors (Upper jaw is fixed and so is used as the landmark to measure, but not the lower jaw which is mobile). It lies anterior to vertebral column and posterior to the trachea. It lacks serosal layer but is surrounded by a layer of loose fibroareolar adventitia.

Anatomical specialities

- Lacks serosa (other structure without serosa is rectum).
- Contains 2 different types of muscles (striated and smooth at proximal 1/3 and distal 2/3, respectively)
- Contains 2 different types of epithelium.
- Segmental blood supply.
- Only part of GIT which shows *very thinly scattered* Meissner's plexus.
- Longitudinal arrangement of veins and lymphatics.

It is lined by non-keratinising stratified squamous epithelium throughout the length except the last 3 cm (oesophagogastric junction) which is lined by columnar epithelium. Submucosa of the oesophagus is thick and strongest part.

Mucosa → basement membrane → lamina propria → muscularis mucosa (causes wrinkling/folding of mucosa) → submucosa containing mucous secreting glands with thin Meissner's plexus of nerves → two layers of muscles inner thick circular and outer thin longitudinal muscles (in between two layers lies the Auerbach's myenteric nerve plexus) → outermost loose adventitial coverings (no serosa; no mesentery). Endoscopic ultrasound is very useful tool to identify and evaluate different layers of the oesophagus. During anastomosis bites from submucosa and lamina propria should be adequate. Transection of the oesophagus at hiatal level causes retraction of the proximal cut end into the posterior mediastinum due to contraction of the longitudinal layer as it is fixed superiorly.

Muscles are striated in proximal 1/3rd of oesophagus; smooth muscles in distal 1/3rd and mixture of two in middle 1/3rd. This is mainly observed in circular muscle fibres.

Parts

1. ***Cervical oesophagus:*** It extends from cricopharyngeus which is the horizontal part of inferior constrictor muscle. Upper oblique part is called as thyropharyngeus. Gap between the two is called as *Killian's dehiscence* which is a *site of occurrence of pharyngeal pouch.* Cricopharyngeus originates from thyroid and cricoid cartilages. Cervical oesophagus is related to trachea and recurrent laryngeal nerve. It is 6 cm in length extends from C6 to T1. It deviates towards left of trachea and it is easier to approach the oesophagus on left side than right. Its lower end is 15 cm from upper incisor extends from hypopharynx to the level of sternal notch. *Laimer's triangle* is formed with base above by cricopharyngeus and on either side divergent longitudinal oesophageal muscles. Laimer's triangle lies in the posterior part of the oesophagus in midline **(Fig. 20-1)**.

2. ***Thoracic oesophagus:*** It lies initially towards the right side. It extends from T1 to T11 vertebrae. It is located in superior and posterior mediastinum. In lower third it deviates towards the left

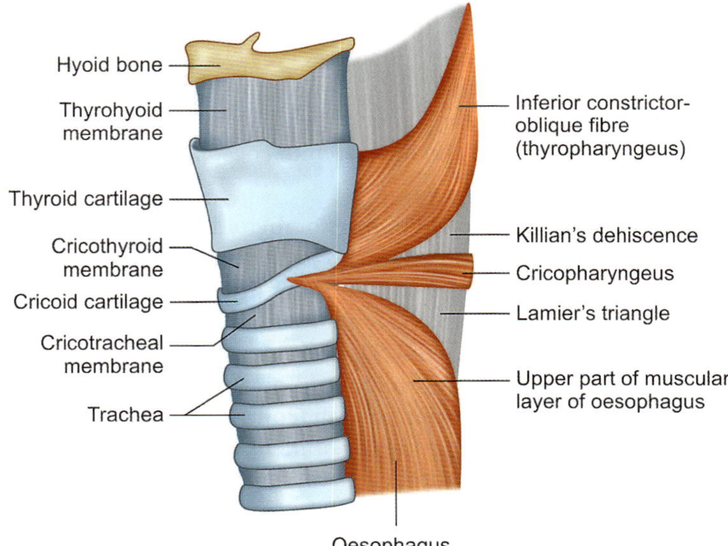

Fig. 20-1: *Killian's dehiscence* which is a *site of occurrence of pharyngeal pouch. Laimer's triangle* is formed with base above by cricopharyngeus and on either side divergent longitudinal oesophageal muscles. Laimer's triangle lies in the posterior part of the oesophagus midline.

and continues as abdominal oesophagus. It is related to azygos vein, thoracic duct (which crosses the oesophagus posteriorly from right to left), aorta, pleura and pericardium.

3. ***Abdominal oesophagus*** is 2.5 cm long and grooves behind the left lobe of the liver. It lies over T11 and T12 vertebral level. Oesophageal hiatus is at T10 level. Anteriorly it is related to left lobe of the liver, left vagus and oesophageal plexus; posteriorly crura of diaphragm, left inferior phrenic artery and aorta; to the right related to caudate lobe of liver; to the left to fundus of stomach. Abdominal oesophagus is more or less retroperitoneal with peritoneum covering its anterior and towards left only. In the hiatus oesophagus lies on the left/deep pillar of the right crus of the diaphragm. Angle of entry of oesophagus to stomach is called as *angle of His* which is 30° to 70°. Fundus of stomach is that part of the stomach which lies above an imaginary line drawn horizontally through angle of His. Gastro-oesophageal junction is called as cardia.

***AJCC has classified oesophagus as cervical; upper thoracic; middle* thoracic; lower thoracic.**

Cervical—same as original anatomical nomenclature.

Upper thoracic oesophagus extends from level of sternal notch (thoracic inlet) to lower border of azygos vein.

Middle thoracic oesophagus extends from lower border of azygos vein to the level of inferior pulmonary veins below.

Lower thoracic oesophagus extends from inferior pulmonary veins to stomach. It is older abdominal oesophagus. It includes OG junction.

Three areas of anatomic narrowing

Cervical constriction—occurs at the level of cricopharyngeal sphincter—*narrowest point of GIT*—15 cm from upper incisor—site of foreign body impaction.

Bronchoaortic constriction—located at the level of T4–25 cm from upper incisor—site of endoscopic perforation. Here left main bronchus (T5) and arch of aorta (T4) crosses it in front. Even though it is considered anatomically as one it has got two components—aortic at T4 and bronchial at T5 level.

Diaphragmatic constriction—occurs where oesophagus traverses the diaphragm (Level of T10)—40 cm from upper incisor.

There are minor constrictions also—retrosternal between cervical and bronchoaortic constrictions; cardiac behind the pericardium; supradiaphragmatic by tortuous aorta.

In the neck it initially deviates towards the left side; then at the level of 5th thoracic vertebra it deviates towards midline; then again it deviates towards left to end as abdominal oesophagus.

Arterial supply of oesophagus

It is segmental and is supplied by inferior thyroid artery, oesophageal branches of the aorta, gastric arteries and inferior phrenic arteries. Cervical part is mainly supplied by inferior thyroid artery and partly by pharyngeal, subclavian, vertebral, common carotid, superior thyroid, and costocervical trunk. Upper part of thoracic oesophagus is supplied by mainly inferior thyroid artery (mainly right side artery) and partly by anterior oesophagotracheal branch. Middle oesophagus is supplied by superior branchial artery and branches directly from aorta. Lower thoracic oesophagus is supplied by single broncho-oesophageal artery arising from aorta. Left gastric and left inferior phrenic artery also supplies abdominal oesophagus. These vessels are *small* and form a rich network in submucosa. Communicating branch between inferior phrenic artery and left gastric artery is called as *Belsey's artery* which should be preserved in Belsey Mark IV surgery **(Fig. 20-2)**.

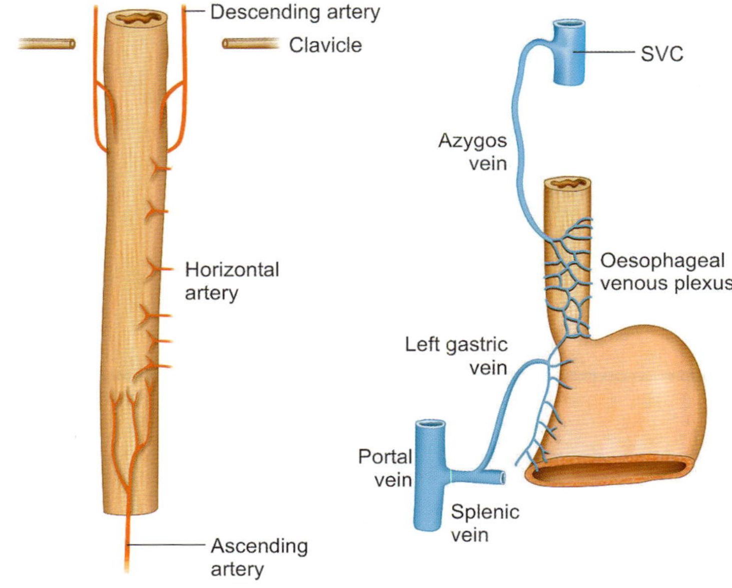

Fig. 20-2: Blood supply of the oesophagus.

Venous drainage of oesophagus

It is by both longitudinal and segmental veins into inferior thyroid vein, brachiocephalic vein, and hemiazygos vein, azygos vein, coronary vein, bronchial, posterior intercostal, splenic vein and inferior phrenic vein. Veins are longitudinal and they lie in submucosal plane in lower third and in muscular plane above. Subepithelial longitudinal venous plexus in lamina propria → submucous intrinsic venous plexus → extrinsic venous plexus → larger veins. Venous plexus in lower oesophagus communicates with portal venous system **(Fig. 20-3)**.

Lymphatic drainage

Lymphatic arrangement in oesophagus is longitudinal and so spread of carcinoma to distant lymph nodes occurs early. Longitudinal lymphatics are 6 times more than transverse one. There are *more lymph vessels* in submucosa than blood vessels **(Fig. 20-4)**.

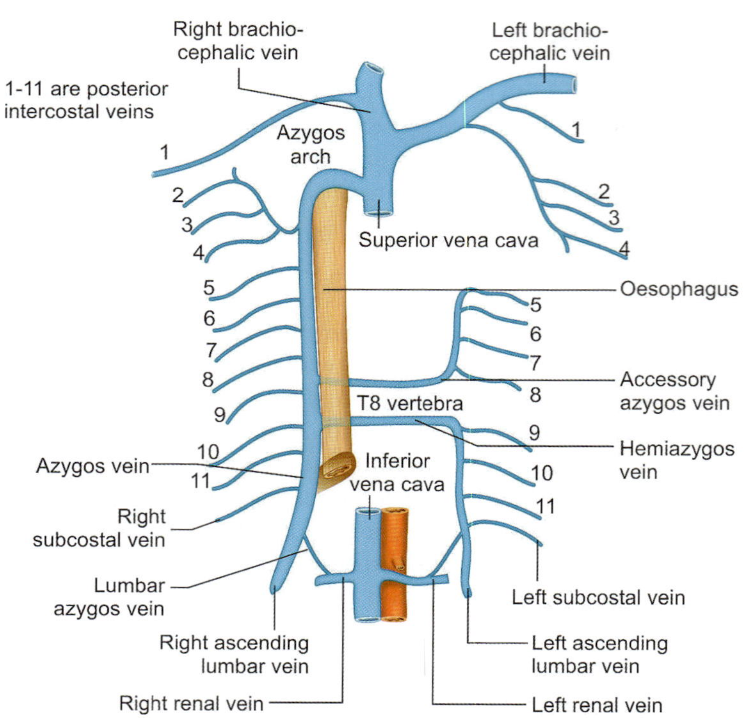

Fig. 20-3: Venous drainage of oesophagus.

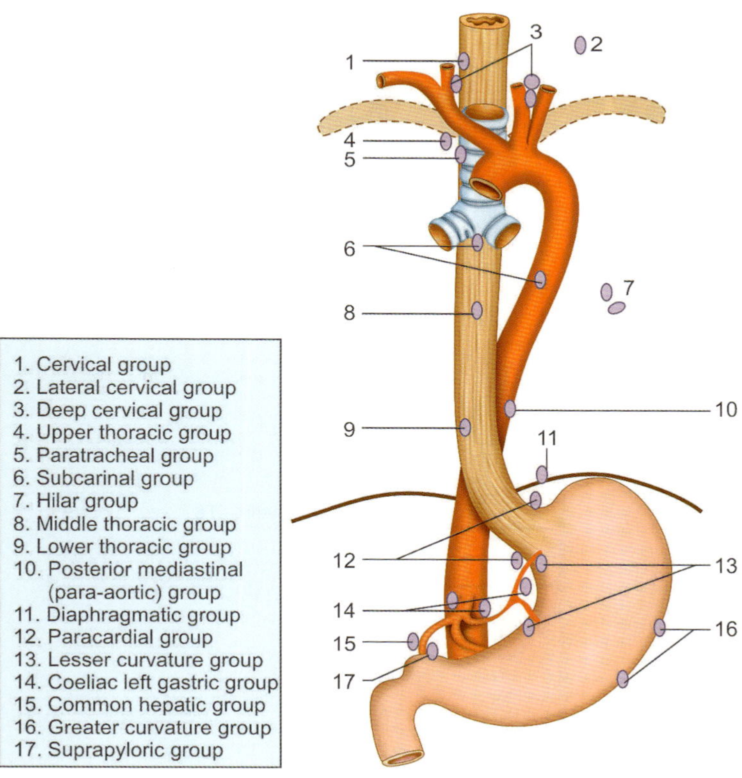

Fig. 20-4: Lymph nodes draining the oesophagus.

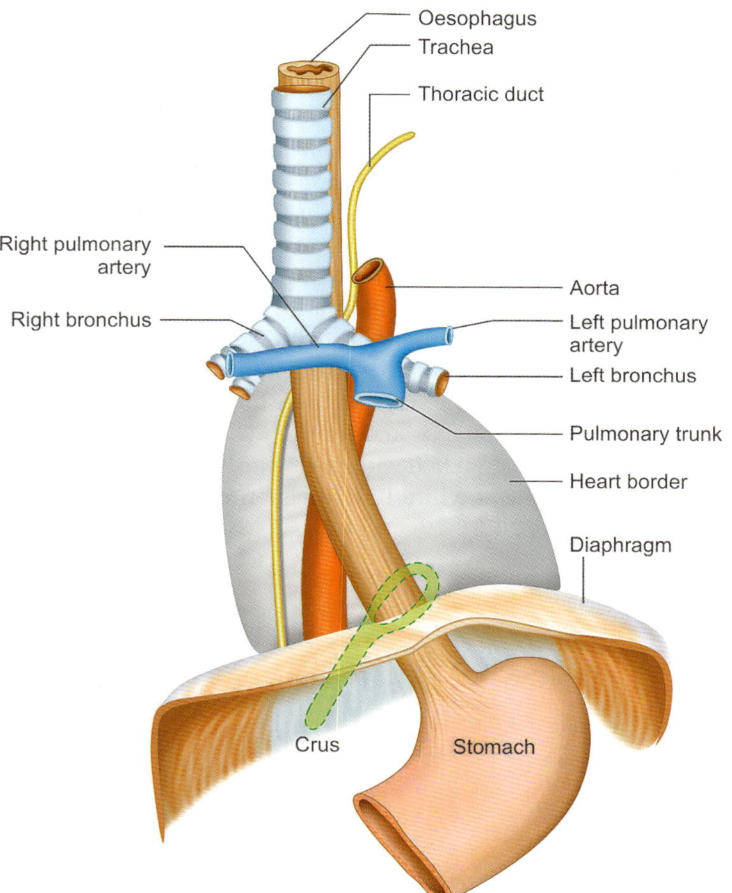

Fig. 20-5: Oesophageal relations in thorax.

Lymph nodes are:
Paraoesophageal groups located in the wall of the oesophagus and are cervical, thoracic, paraoesophageal and paracardial nodes.

Perioesophageal groups located immediately adjacent to oesophageal wall. They are deep cervical, scalene, paratracheal, mediastinal, diaphragmatic, gastric and coeliac lymph nodes.

Lateral oesophageal groups receive lymph from para- and perioesophageal lymph nodes.

Upper oesophagus drains into supraclavicular nodes. Thoracic oesophagus drains into paraoesophageal and tracheobronchial nodes in thorax. Abdominal oesophagus drains into coeliac nodes.

However due to longitudinal arrangement of lymphatic plexus in the wall of oesophagus, any group of (neck/thorax/coeliac) lymph nodes can get involved in diseases at any level. In T1a only mucosa is involved by carcinoma and so metastasis is rare. In T1b submucosa is involved by tumour and so nodal metastases is up to 30–50%. AJCC has adapted different lymph node stations for oesophageal carcinoma (1–19).

Anatomical Relations of Oesophagus

Oesophagus begins at lower edge of cricoid cartilage at C6 vertebral level and ends at oesophagogastric junction at T11 vertebral level. OG junction is at the level of 7th intercostal space anteriorly. Above it lies the cricopharyngeal sphincter which is 18 cm from upper incisor. Lower oesophageal sphincter is 40 cm from upper incisor.

Relation in the neck
Oesophagus along with trachea is covered with pretracheal fascia which also encloses the thyroid gland. So anterior relations are larynx and trachea. Posteriorly buccopharyngeal fascia separates it from prevertebral space and this fascia extends laterally as carotid sheath. Recurrent laryngeal nerve lies in tracheooesophageal groove. Left RLN is closer to oesophagus than right. Thoracic duct is towards left of the oesophagus and its upper end is 4 cm above clavicle. Lateral relations from lateral to medial end are—carotid sheath, inferior thyroid artery, lateral lobe of thyroid gland, recurrent laryngeal nerve **(Fig. 20-5)**.

Retropharyngeal space continues below towards posterior mediastinum and so infection can cause mediastinitis. Cervical oesophagus is closely related to trachea through *tracheal pars membranacea* and so during transhiatal dissection injury to this membranacea can cause tracheal perforation. Oesophageal perforation within the pretracheal fascia may extend into mediastinum causing mediastinitis.

Relation in the thorax
Thoracic oesophagus is related in front from above downwards to: trachea; aortic arch; right pulmonary artery; left main bronchus; pericardium and left atrium; anterior vagus; oesophageal hiatus. Posterior relations are: vertebral column; longus coli muscles; right posterior intercostal arteries; thoracic duct (crosses it from behind); right pleura; azygos, hemiazygos and accessory azygos vein; aorta; posterior vagus. Laterally - on right side are: mediastinal pleura, azygos vein, right main bronchus, root of right lung, right vagus nerve; on left side are: aortic arch, left subclavian artery, left recurrent laryngeal nerve, thoracic duct from T4 to C7, pleura, descending thoracic aorta. Arch of azygos vein (azygos arch) crosses the right main bronchus.

In thorax oesophagus descends posterior and medial to the aortic and azygos arches and left main bronchus. Right and left mediastinal pleura are on both sides. Left recurrent laryngeal nerve is lateral and thoracic duct is posteromedial. At the carinal level, oesophagus is separated from tracheal carina by subcarinal nodes, and thoracic duct crosses it from behind. Below oesophagus is behind the fibrous pericardium and right of the descending aorta. Both vagi run longitudinally on the surface of the oesophagus in front and behind (left anterior; right posterior).

Phrenooesophageal ligament or membrane is condensation of pleura, endothoracic fascia, phrenooesophageal fascia of Lamier, transversalis fascia and peritoneum into two sheaths; upper one is attached to the outer muscular layer of oesophagus; lower one into cardia extending into gastric serosa and gastrohepatic and gastrosplenic ligaments. Pleura and peritoneum maintains airtightness; other components provide strength and flexibility. Membrane is well developed in front than behind. Superficial layer is peritoneum; deeper layer is thick fibrous tissue. It provides barrier between oesophagus and thorax. When the peritoneum in front of the hiatus is stretched with downward traction, the ligament becomes obvious as a white line; division of it allows access to mediastinum **(Fig. 20-6)**.

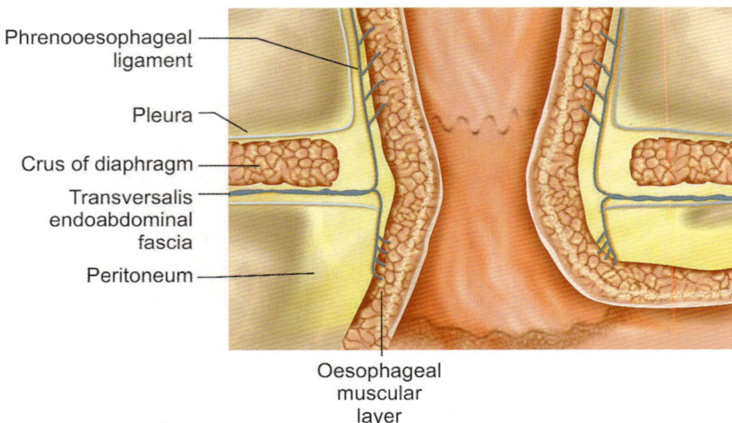

Fig. 20-6: Phrenooesophageal membrane.

Gastrohepatic ligament is the peritoneal reflections on the right side enclosing the oesophagus. It contains left gastric artery and vein, left vagus with branches and lymph nodes. Occasionally it can contain branches of right gastric artery, left hepatic artery when it is arising from left gastric artery (20%).

Gastrosplenic/gastrolienal ligament is formed by peritoneal reflections on the left side **(Fig. 20-7)**.

Relations in abdomen

Right crus of diaphragm arises from the first 3-4 lumbar vertebrae running upwards and divides into superficial and deep slings to enclose the oesophagus. Superficial right pillar of the right crus gets attached to central tendon of the diaphragm; deeper left pillar encircles the oesophagus and joins the right pillar. Left crus arises left of the upper 2-3 lumbar vertebrae, runs vertically upwards to the diaphragm without any divisions. Left crus runs left of the aorta and is actually not in direct relation to the oesophagus even though variations are common. Right crus is longer than left. Right is supplied by right phrenic nerve and left is supplied by left phrenic nerve. Median arcuate ligament is tough 2 mm wide condensed medial fibrous margins of the both right and left crura of the diaphragm. It is just proximal to the origin of coeliac artery encircling the descending aorta; but origin of coeliac artery may vary in 30% of individuals either at or above the median arcuate ligament **(Fig. 20-8)**.

Angle of His is angle between fundus of the stomach and oesophagus. Tendinous tissue binds between right and left crus inferior and posterior to oesophagus to form median arcuate ligament. This tissue is important in hiatus hernia repair while placing anchoring sutures. Both pillars of the right crura have got muscular and tendinous parts. Tendinous part is more posterior than muscular part which is in front. It is important to take bites deep enough to include tendinous parts in anchorage stitches. Tendinous parts, which are posterior, are better visible through thoracotomy incision.

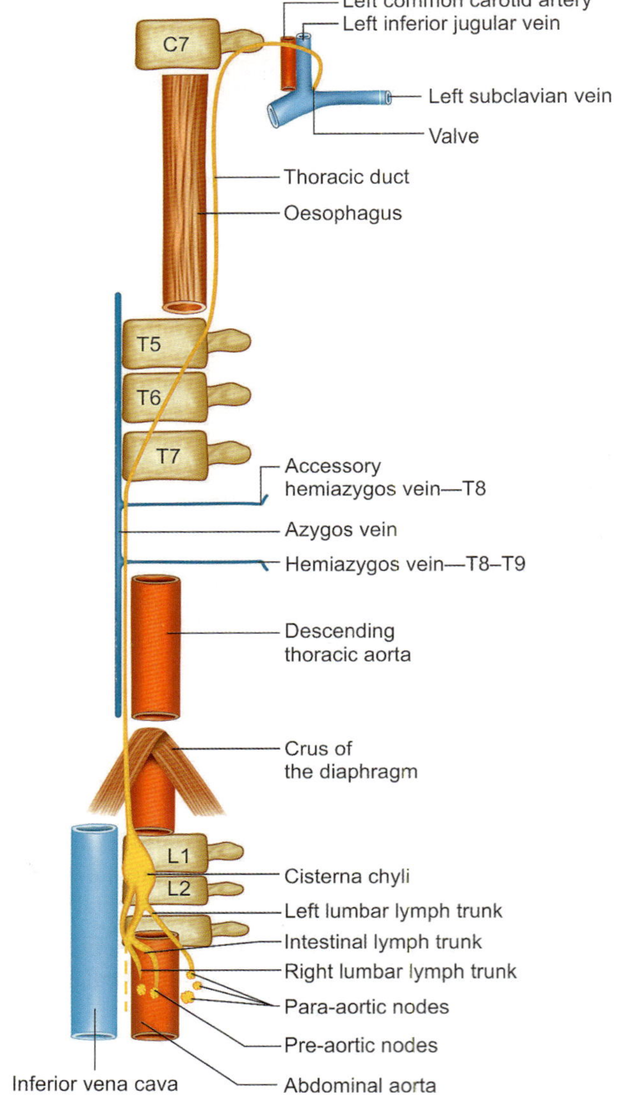

Fig. 20-7: Relations of the oesophagus.

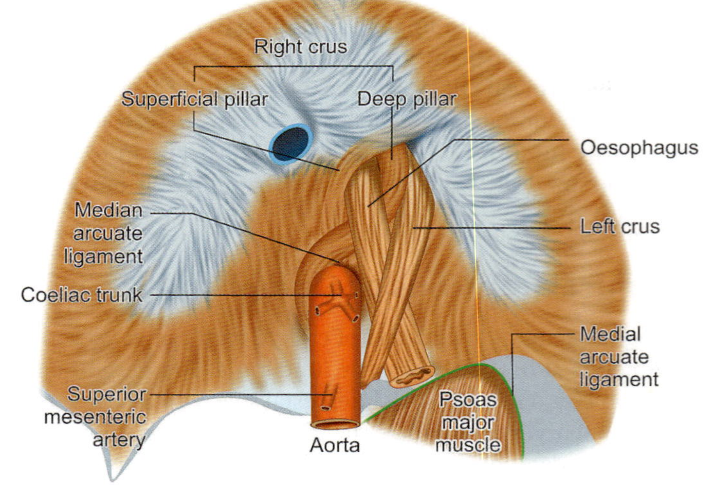

Fig. 20-8: Oesophageal hiatus—anatomy.

Antireflux mechanism is both anatomical and physiological. LOS mechanism at terminal oesophagus as a high pressure zone is physiological. Anatomical are—thickening of gastric oblique fibres; Rosette like gastric mucosal folds; angle of His; phrenooesophageal membrane and pinching action of crura.

Principles in Oesophageal Surgery

Upper half of the thoracic oesophagus is approached through right thoracotomy as aortic arch is present on left side. Lower half can be approached by right or left thoracotomy incision. Azygos vein should be double *ligated at arching of the oesophagus to reach* superior vena cava. Azygos vein enters the SVC on its posterior surface. Injury to SVC should be avoided and SVC cannot be ligated.

Left side *oesophageal triangle* (only on left side) is present on the left upper mediastinum which is formed by descending aorta, left subclavian artery and vertebral column. Floor of the triangle is mediastinal pleura under which, part of oesophagus is located.

Triangle of Truesdale is formed by diaphragm below, pericardium above and in front, descending thoracic aorta behind **(Fig. 20-9)**.

Two pleura both right and left approximates behind (posterior approximation) oesophagus and aorta as mesooesophagus in the lower part of the thorax. Anterior approximation of both pleura occurs at sternal angle level.

Right pleura is very closely related to lower oesophagus up to the oesophageal hiatus. During hiatal dissection, right pleura may get torn to cause pneumothorax **(Fig. 20-10)**.

Mobilisation of distal oesophagus: Adequate exposure of the OG junction (cardia) is done. Stomach is retracted downwards and towards left using hand. Usually clean mop is used under the fingers to achieve proper grip and prevent injury to stomach. Assistant retracts the stomach. Left triangular ligament is cut by folding the left of the liver which is retracted towards right and down. Peritoneum over the phrenooesophageal ligament is held using long non-toothed dissecting forceps; using long curved scissor peritoneum and phrenooesophageal ligament is cut horizontally across the full length of the anterior aspect of the oesophagus. Ligament with peritoneum is reflected upwards to expose the cardia. Cautery can be used for dissection but should avoid injuring the bowel wall. Anterior vagus can be felt by running the index finger horizontally on the lower oesophagus maintaining the traction on the stomach. Often anterior vagus lies very closely to oesophageal wall or often embedded in the wall. Anterior vagus is dissected along the length of the lower oesophagus. Right index finger is passed behind the oesophagus gently and loose areolar tissue is separated with blunt finger dissection to reach right of the oesophagus to create a window. A scissor cut may be needed while entering the right index finger towards right from left, from behind. Posterior right vagus is little away from the oesophageal tube and usually will not come into the hooked index finger. To feel the posterior vagus index finger should be rolled with traction on the stomach. Usually posterior vagus which is thicker is dissected using finger. Often perioesophageal scarring may be present behind due to hiatal disease like reflux. In such situation sharp scissor dissection under vision is better to avoid tear in the muscle or mucosa of the oesophagus. Mobilisation further can be obtained by cutting the hiatus either anteriorly or posteriorly (*median phrenicotomy*). Care should be taken not to injure the pericardium and anterior branch of inferior phrenic vein which crosses the hiatus in front to reach IVC or hepatic vein. This vein should be ligated during phrenicotomy. But most of the time it is not necessary. Distal end of the cardia is mobilised downwards but it is limited by *gastric trinity - left gastric artery and vein (coronary vein) and coeliac branch of the posterior vagus nerve.* Dissection is done from lesser curve side of the stomach. Lesser omentum over the proximal 3 cm of lesser curve (3 cm distal to OG junction) is incised; left index finger is passed obliquely directing towards the angle of His (cardia notch) with blunt gentle careful finger dissection. Oesophageal hiatus is located left of the midline at T10 vertebral level. Hiatus is formed by pillars of right crus of diaphragm. It is obliquely placed opening 1 cm behind the central tendon of the diaphragm. Oesophageal hiatus is separated from aorta by median arcuate ligament **(Fig. 20-11)**.

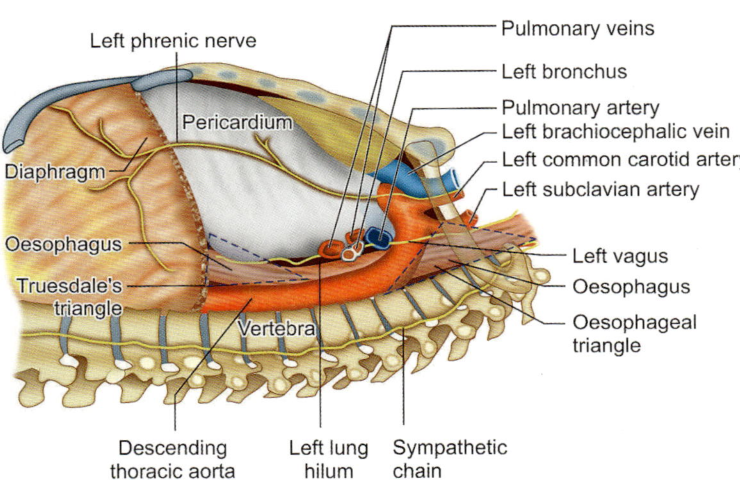

Fig. 20-9: Left side mediastinum—surgical anatomy.

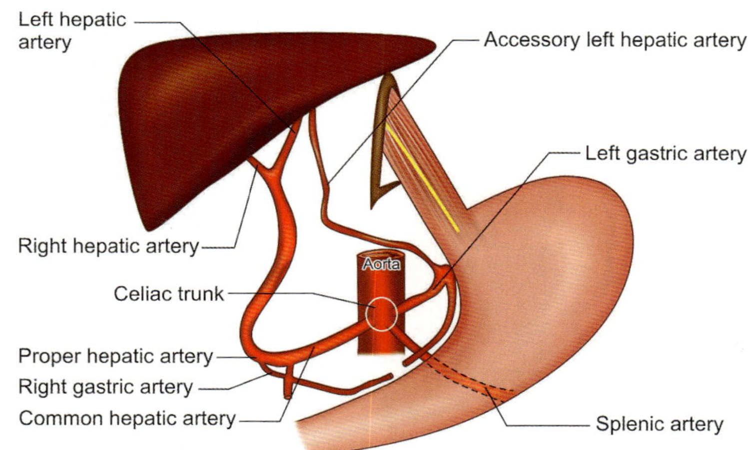

Fig. 20-10: Accessory left hepatic artery when present should be preserved. It is arising from the left gastric artery.

Adequate exposure is important in oesophageal surgery. Proper retraction, adequate exposure and lighting, slow careful meticulous anatomical dissection is ideal. Both sharp and finger dissections are used. Bipolar cautery or harmonic scalpel are ideal energy sources in oesophageal surgery.

Anastomosis is done using 2- or 3-zero silk interrupted sutures. Two layers are commonly used. Taking bites from mucosa is very important. Traction tear or ischaemia due to holding on the wall of the oesophagus should be avoided. Gentle firm holding is important. Often horizontal mattress (box) may be used to prevent tear at suture bite. Inner layer often sutured with 2 zero vicryl; outer layer with 2 zero silk; both should be interrupted. Adequate vascularity should be maintained at the anastomotic site. Oesophageal end anastomosis should be always as **end to side, to the side** (anterior wall)

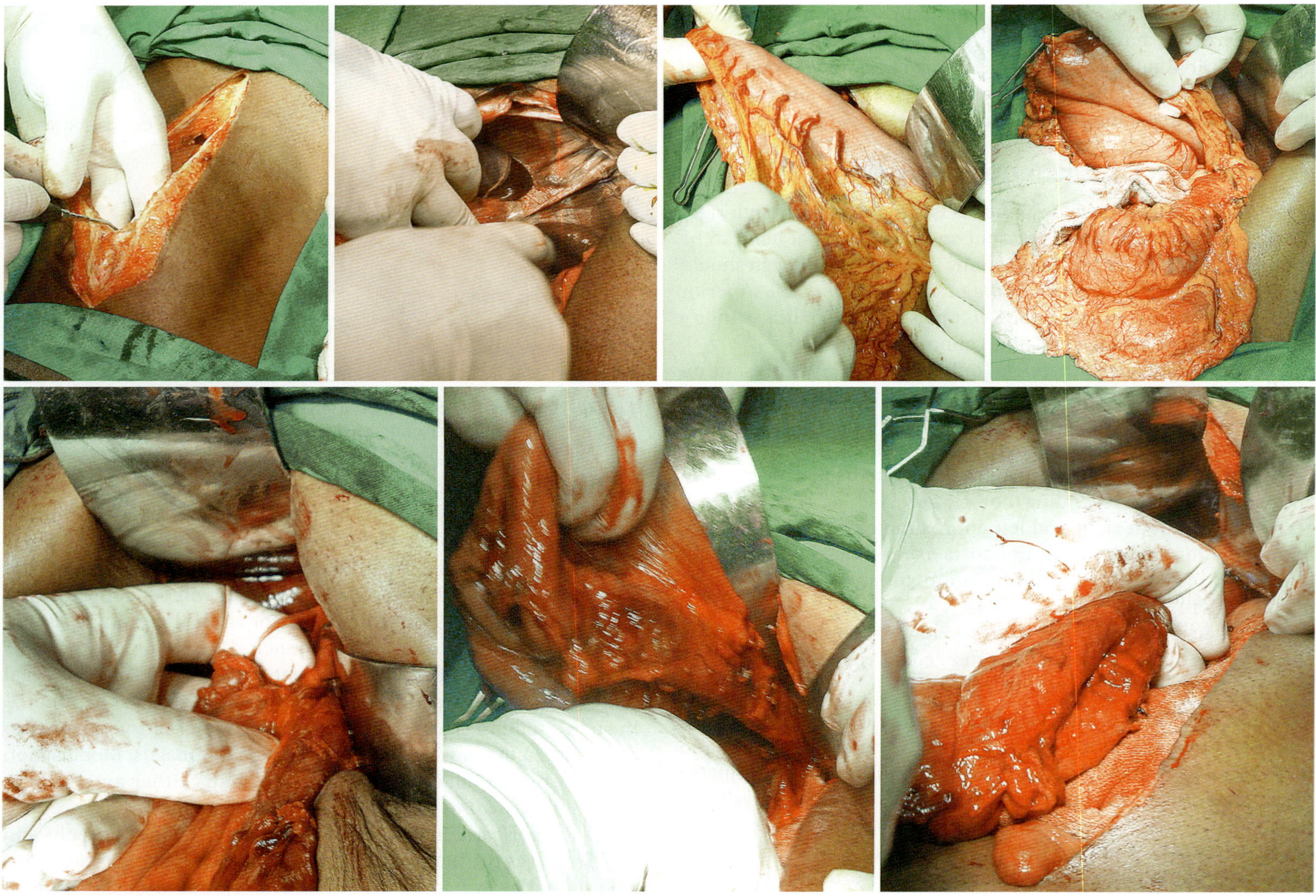

Fig. 20-11: Hiatal dissection in oesophageal surgeries.

of the stomach. *End to end oesophagogastric anastomosis is not preferred* as—disparity between lumens of oesophagus and stomach; technical difficulty in performing end to end anastomosis; lesser blood supply near the proximal cut open end of the gastric pouch; there is no protection from posterior leak from the anastomotic site; postoperative reflux is more. In end to side anastomosis, better blood supply is maintained in the stoma; buttressing effect of the stomach pouch behind prevents posterior leak; technically easier; lesser chance of postoperative reflux and hence it is preferred. Even stapler anastomosis (28 mm/31 mm) should be ideally end to side of the stomach. One should avoid using unnecessary clamp on the oesophageal side; if at all gentle soft occlusion clamp can be used to avoid crushing effect and compromise the viability. *No tension and accurate apposition are essential basis in oesophageal anastomosis.* Knots of inner layer should be inside to prevent the mucosal hernia and to achieve the mucosal inversion which prevents leak. Omental wrap around the anastomosis should be placed. Before starting the anterior inner layer (3rd layer) nasogastric tube should be positioned or ideally at least before placing final stitch of inner anterior layer. But many prefer to negotiate the tube after completion of the anastomosis in view of avoiding the contamination. Anterior cut edge of oesophagus should be 1 cm lengthier than posterior edge.

Kocherisation for duodenal mobilisation; mobilisation of stomach; retaining right gastroepiploic vessels (mainly) and right gastric artery; ligating left gastric and left gastroepiploic arteries; adequate widening of the hiatus (to prevent venous congestion of pulled up stomach/colon); absolute haemostasis are main technical needs in oesophageal surgeries.

Spillage of the gastric contents should be avoided to prevent sepsis as in oesophagectomy stomach is pulled upwards into the thorax; sepsis in thorax is really risky.

Three field lymphadenectomy is often added with clearing the abdominal, thoracic and neck lymph nodes (bilateral). Here anastomosis is done in the neck. McKeown approach may be suitable here.

Feeding jejunostomy is commonly used in oesophageal resection surgeries. Few advocate passage of nasogastric tube across the stoma and fix it to the nostril securely. It acts as a stent across the stoma; keeps the stoma patent; allows nasogastric feeding also even though there is no clear cut evidence for this.

Blood should be kept ready in case there is bleeding during thoracic dissection. Intraarterial catheter is required. CVP line is better to keep always.

SURGICAL TREATMENT FOR ACHALASIA CARDIA

Heller's cardiomyotomy is done for achalasia cardia. Extended myotomy is done when there is diffuse oesophageal spasm.

In 14th April 1913 Ernest Heller, a German surgeon did first cardiomyotomy based on Gottstein's idea through abdominal approach. He did myotomies at both anterior and posterior walls. It is an extramucosal oesophagomyotomy. Later many modifications were tried on this procedure. Original Heller's myotomy was double myotomies. In 1918 Groeneveldt from Holland modified it as only anterior myotomy which was popularised by Zaaijer (1923). Myotomy facilitates gravity induced swallowing. Incidence of reflux and oesophagitis is very high (20%) and so partial or often total Nissen's fundoplication is added to prevent reflux. Pressure of the lower oesophageal sphincter (LES) is completely reduced but not eliminated by myotomy. Relief of dysphagia occurs *immediately after* recover from anaesthesia.

Vigorous achalasia and with severe suspected metaplasia confirmed by endoscopic biopsy needs resection of the lower oesophagus and oesophagogastric anastomosis. In megaoesophagus/ sigmoid oesophagus results of myotomy is not good. Hence resection is better option **(Fig. 20-12)**.

Preparation

Contrast oesophageal study, oesophagoscopy oesophageal manometry should be done. Manometry shows absence of peristalsis in lower oesophagus with incomplete relaxation of LES. Contrast CT scan is better option to see extent and dilatation. Chest X-ray to see the lungs for pneumonia, double mediastinal strip of oesophagus is also important. Barium swallow shows *bird beak appearance*. Fluoroscopy may be useful to see elongation, sigmoid oesophagus. Endoscopy shows dilated proximal oesophagus, closed puckered LES which will not open freely. Biopsy should be done to check mucosal changes and malignant transformation (adenocarcinoma).

Oesophagus is lavaged with normal saline on previous day and same day morning to prevent aspiration during induction of anaesthesia. Preoperative antibiotic is not necessary.

Nasogastric tube into the oesophagus is helpful especially while dissecting the lower oesophagus.

Approaches

Laparoscopy is an excellent approach for modified Heller's cardiomyotomy. *Toupet's posterior partial fundoplication* is added usually. It has become standard now. It is not useful in diffuse oesophageal spasm, vigorous achalasia and failure/recurrence.

Open thoracotomy through left sided thoracotomy approach is also better as it avoids laparotomy, retains integrity of the phreno-oesophageal ligament thereby reducing the chances of reflux. Lengthy myotomy for diffuse oesophageal spasm is possible by thoracotomy approach. Disadvantages are morbidities of thoracotomy; if unidentified mucosal leak occurs it will cause empyema which is dangerous and needs drainage. Belsey Mark IV antireflux procedure can be done safely through this approach if needed. Thoracotomy is better in obese patients or in patients where adhesions at hiatus are anticipated through abdominal approach or failed abdominal myotomy. *Thoracoscopic approach* even though is practiced is not readily accepted.

Laparotomy—open abdominal approach (described by Ellis et al in 1958)—Heller's original approach was also abdominal. It is technically easier; general surgeons are more comfortable with laparotomy approach. But reflux is more common through this approach. Toupet's partial posterior fundoplication is done in this approach.

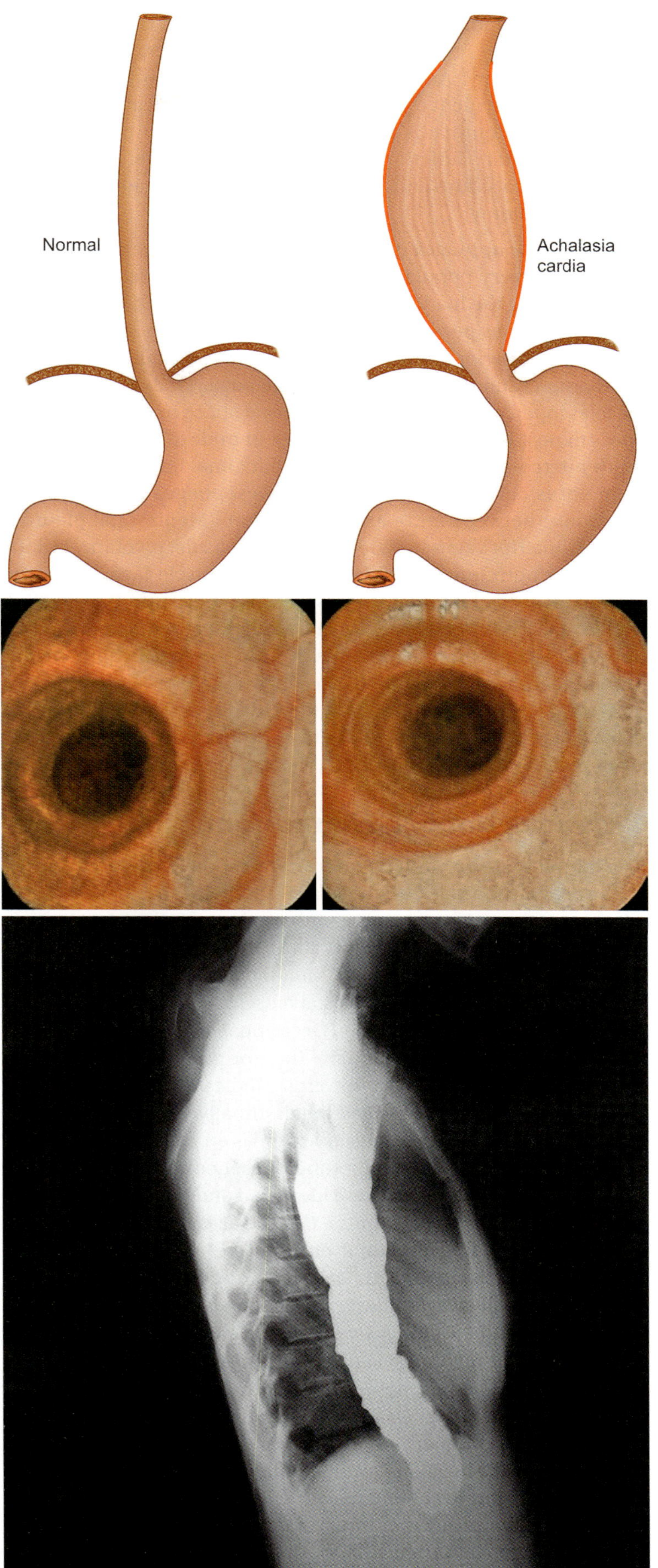

Fig. 20-12: Achalasia cardia—diagram; endoscopic view; barium study view.

Nissen's total fundoplication is also done but it may cause dysphagia and *gas bloating syndrome* and it is obstructive wrap which is not ideal in myotomy. Anterior partial fundoplication is also useful and is non-obstructive wrap. Respiratory complications are less here. Transabdominal is preferred in patients with compromised cardiopulmonary function and in patients who need additional abdominal procedure and in patients who have already undergone prior thoracotomy.

Thoracoscopic approach is similar to thoracotomy technique. It has not become very popular due to technical difficulties in reaching and dissecting the hiatus. Right lateral decubitus with left thorax up is the position as per left thoracotomy. 1st port is in 3rd intercostal space 2 cm anterior to the posterior axillary line. 2nd 10 mm port is in 7th intercostal space 4 cm behind the posterior axillary line used for telescope; 3rd port is in 6th intercostal space in anterior axillary line; 4th port is in 7th intercostal space in midaxillary line; 5th port is 8th intercostal space in anterior axillary line. Inferior pulmonary ligament is cut; left lung is retraced. Oesophagus is identified in the groove between aorta and pericardium. Mediastinal pleura is incised; anterior vagus is dissected and kept aside; myotomy is done by cutting both longitudinal and circular muscle layers for 8 cm proximally. Distal myotomy across OG junction onto the stomach wall for 1 cm is done. This is the most difficult part of the procedure in thoracoscopy approach. Reflux is common in this approach as fundoplication is not possible. Belsey Mark IV procedure can be done to prevent reflux; but it is technically difficult. *Right sided thoracoscopic approach* is also used for myotomy in case laparoscopy is not possible or failure of previous laparoscopy.

Technique through Thoracotomy

Procedure is done under general anaesthesia. Double lumen endotracheal tube may be beneficial. Position of the patient is for full left thoracotomy. After cleaning and draping, skin incision is made along left 7th intercostal space just above the 8th rib. Latissimus dorsi and serratus anterior are divided. Monopolar cautery is used. Pleura is opened after cutting the intercostal muscles. *Finochietto retractor* is placed and widened adequately. Occasionally rib resection may be needed if approach is inadequate. Inferior pulmonary ligament is divided. Left lung is retracted upwards. Mediastinal pleura overlying the lower oesophagus is incised longitudinally. Oesophagus gently dissected using finger at its lower part and is encircled using Penrose or latex drain or infant feeding tube. Presence of nasogastric tube facilitates the dissection. Vagi are identified and safeguarded.

Index finger is placed under the lower oesophagus. Narrow segment and dilated proximal part can be easily seen and felt. Longitudinal incision is made over left anterolateral aspect of the oesophageal wall away and anterior to left vagus using number 15 blade gently and carefully. Cranially incision is slowly extended for 7-8 cm until myotomy is extended into dilated segment also. Myotomy above should be extended into 2 cm over the proximal dilated segment. Distal extent of incision up to oesophagogastric junction may be maximum 10 mm over the stomach. But it is sufficient to make incision around 3 mm downwards over stomach. Lengthier incision over stomach should be avoided. Stomach wall is identified by presence of transverse small veins traversing over the mucosa deep to muscular layer. Outlook of gastric muscle differs from oesophageal musculature. Edge of the cut musculature is held using dissecting forceps and using fine scissor it is raised from the deeper mucosal plane for half the circumference. It prevents from

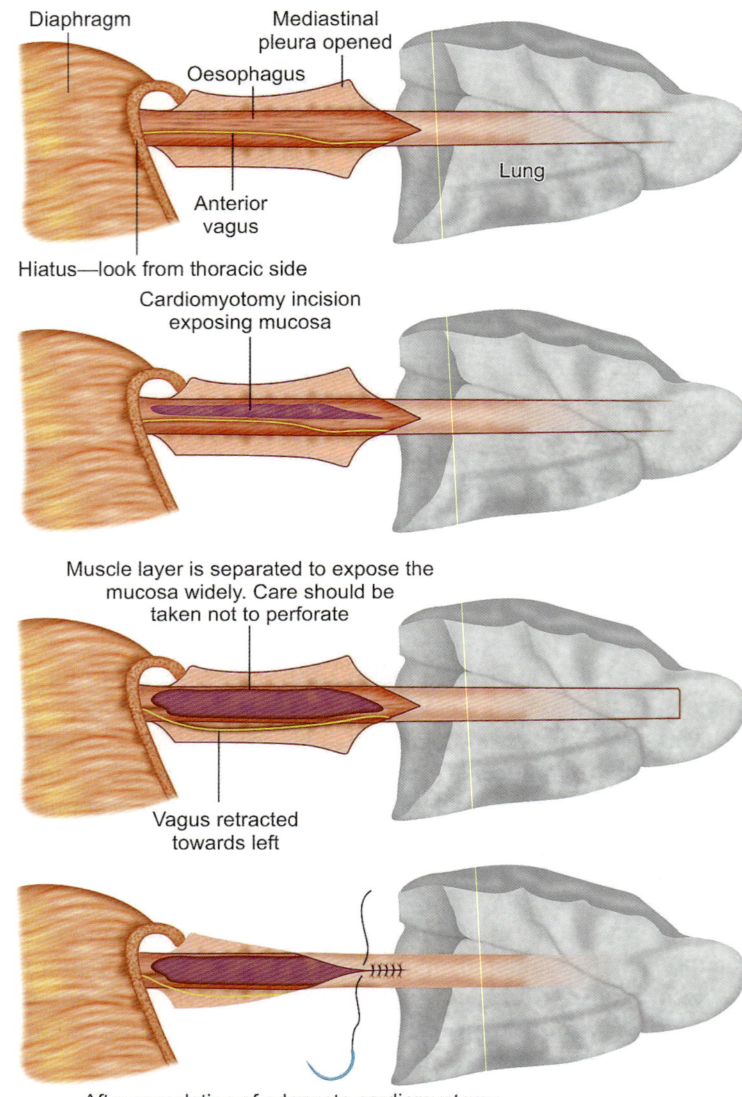

Fig. 20-13: Cardiomyotomy through thoracotomy (left) approach.

muscle reuniting again leading into stenosis. Raising of the muscle is done on both edges. Bulging of the mucosa onto the myotomy gap is clearly evident **(Fig. 20-13)**.

Anaesthetist is asked to infuse 200 mL of methylene blue into the oesophagus from above to see any leak from the mucosa. On table oesophagoscopy (flexible) is also often done. Saline infusion from above also can be done. If there is a leak mucosa is sutured using 3- or 4-zero silk or vicryl interrupted sutures.

Extended myotomy is done in diffuse oesophageal spasm. Extension is done proximally above adequately until entire spasmodic segment is released.

Intercostal tube (30 French no.) is placed. Lung is inflated. Thoracotomy wound is closed in layers.

Postoperative Care

Intravenous fluids and nasogastric aspiration is done. Nasogastric tube can be removed in 24–48 hours. Oral liquids started in 48 hours. Chest tube is removed in 4 days once drain reduces to minimum and chest X-ray confirms lung expansion.

Postoperative endoscopy and manometry may be done if needed to confirm the efficacy of the procedure.

Complications and Problems

Respiratory infection, empyema if there is leak postoperatively.

Recurrent dysphagia after initial symptomatic response or persistent dysphagia can occur. An *incomplete myotomy* that does not adequately lower the LES pressure will cause persistent or recurrent dysphagia. Here dilatation can be tried. Otherwise laparoscopic myotomy is done. Alternatively resection of lower oesophagus with oesophagogastric anastomosis is done.

Reflux oesophagitis is one of the complications even though it is less common and less severe in thoracotomy approach compared to abdominal approach. Antireflux procedure is needed. Few undertake modified Belsey Mark IV procedure while doing initial myotomy through thoracotomy approach itself. A non-obstructive wrap is always better.

Oesophageal perforation can occur but incidence is less.

Diaphragmatic hernia is another complication which can occur.

Technique through Abdominal Approach

Incision: Upper midline incision extending down beside the left side of the umbilicus. Xiphoid process may need to be excised. Patient is in head up (reverse Trendelenburg) position.

A self-retaining retractor is placed. Sternal self-retaining chain retractor is better if available. Left lobe is mobilised by placing surgeon's left hand over the left lobe retracting it below and towards right. Left triangular ligament is divided using cautery and scissor. Thus left lobe is mobilised and retraced by folding it inwards to expose hiatus fairly adequately. Wet mop should be placed under the retractor to avoid injury to left lobe of liver during retraction. Stomach is displaced below by downward traction by first assistant using fingers or Babcocks. Peritoneal reflection over the OG junction is lifted using long dissecting forceps and using long curved scissor it is cut horizontally to push it upwards towards hiatus. Anterior left vagus should be safeguarded, gently dissected and kept aside using smooth sling. Entire abdominal oesophagus is mobilised using right index finger with blunt dissection. Dissection facilitates separation of the abdominal oesophagus from behind away from aorta. Mobilised lower oesophagus is hooked with right index finger and long gauze or tape or infant feeding tube or Penrose drain is passed around. Phrenooesophageal membrane is divided to allow the dissection into the peritoneum. Right pleura may get injured while dividing this membrane/ligament and so care should be taken to avoid it. Oesophagus is dissected by blunt and sharp dissection further upwards across the hiatus.

Oesophagus is held under tension by giving traction on the sling. Constriction part can be felt with this method. Using left index finger lower oesophagus is encircled; longitudinal incision is made on the anterior left lateral aspect of the oesophagus over the muscle; both longitudinal and circular muscles are cut; mucosa can be visualised. Both muscles are cut even though only circular muscle is hypertrophied and thickened due to the disease. Care should be taken not to injure it. Using right angles Mixter forceps dissection between mucosa and muscular layers is carried out upwards creating separation; separated muscle is cut using curved scissor; bipolar cautery can be used for small bleeder with care to avoid injury to mucosa. Energy sources like harmonic may be useful. Such *separation/adequate lifting/cutting of the muscle* are done sequentially with each time around 1 cm only. One should not take longer segment in a hurry as it will cause injury to mucosa by lifting of the mucosa. Cranially myotomy is done 8–10 cm. Often a metal clip is placed at this point for future identification of uppermost point of myotomy. Upper myotomy should go to the proximal 2 cm dilated segment of oesophagus. Myotomy is also done downwards over the stomach wall for less than 1 cm. It should never exceed more than 1 cm. Small veins traverse horizontally in submucosa of the stomach which are the identification markers of stomach wall. Edge of the cut musculature is held using dissecting forceps and using fine scissor it is raised from the deeper mucosal plane for half the circumference. It prevents from muscle reuniting again leading to stenosis. Raising of the muscle is done on both edges. Metal clip is also placed over the lowermost cut edge for identification. 200 mL methylene blue instillation is done to check for perforation **(Figs. 20-14A to K)**.

It is usual to add on to Toupet's partial fundoplication along with closure of the oesophageal hiatus. Crural pillars/crura of the diaphragm behind are identified and approximated using interrupted 3-4 2 zero silk or polypropylene sutures. It should be only adequate apposition; should not be too tight; should able to pass finger through it. Gastric fundus is mobilised by dividing few gastric veins along the fundus. Cut muscle edges of the myotomy are sutured to the mobilised stomach which has wrapped from behind to complete the posterior partial fundoplication. Interrupted 3 zero polypropylene or silk sutures are used. Wound is closed without drain usually. Drain is kept if there is perforation or more bleeding **(Figs. 20-15A to C)**.

Modifications

Often *anterior partial fundoplication* (*Dor's*) is also done instead of posterior fundoplication. In anterior fundoplication, after fundal mobilisation, it is placed back in normal position. Left sided cut edge of the myotomy is sutured to the medial aspect of the fundus from below upwards for about 4 cm as 3 zero silk or polypropylene continuous seromuscular suture; last bite is taken from the left crus of the diaphragm fixing it to the hiatus. Gastric fundus flap is rotated in front towards right medially on to the right cut edge of the myotomy **(Fig. 20-16)**.

After taking the bite from the right cut edge of the myotomy wound seromuscular bites are taken from the anterior stomach wall close to greater curvature from below upwards. Again upper most suture is taken from the right crus of the diaphragm. This keeps the cut edges of the muscle in separation preventing reunion and stenosis and it also protects exposed mucosa by covering it. But incidence of reflux is more with Dor's anterior wrap than Toupet's posterior wrap. So Toupet's posterior fundoplication is preferred commonly **(Figs. 20-17A to D)**.

Often initial myotomy is guided by passing a *balloon* which is inflated across. Anterior gastrotomy is done. Foley's catheter is inserted into the stomach and gently negotiated across the stenotic segment. Balloon is inflated slowly to stretch the muscle fibres which can be cut easily and mucosa can be identified easily. Later Foley's catheter is removed and gastrotomy is closed. Specialised balloon for the purpose is also can be used similarly **(Figs. 20-18A to C)**.

Postoperative care

Nasogastric tube is removed in 24 hours. If there was perforation it is kept for 5 days. Drain if kept when indicated is removed in 5 days. Oral fluids started in 24 hours; later gradually semisolid and solid diet. Patient needs postoperative follow up with gastroscopy and manometry study in few months to confirm the adequacy of the cardiomyotomy.

Results and complications

Results of myotomy are very good. It is 90%.

Mucosal perforation, mediastinitis are rare complications. If there is mucosal perforation it is closed using interrupted sutures.

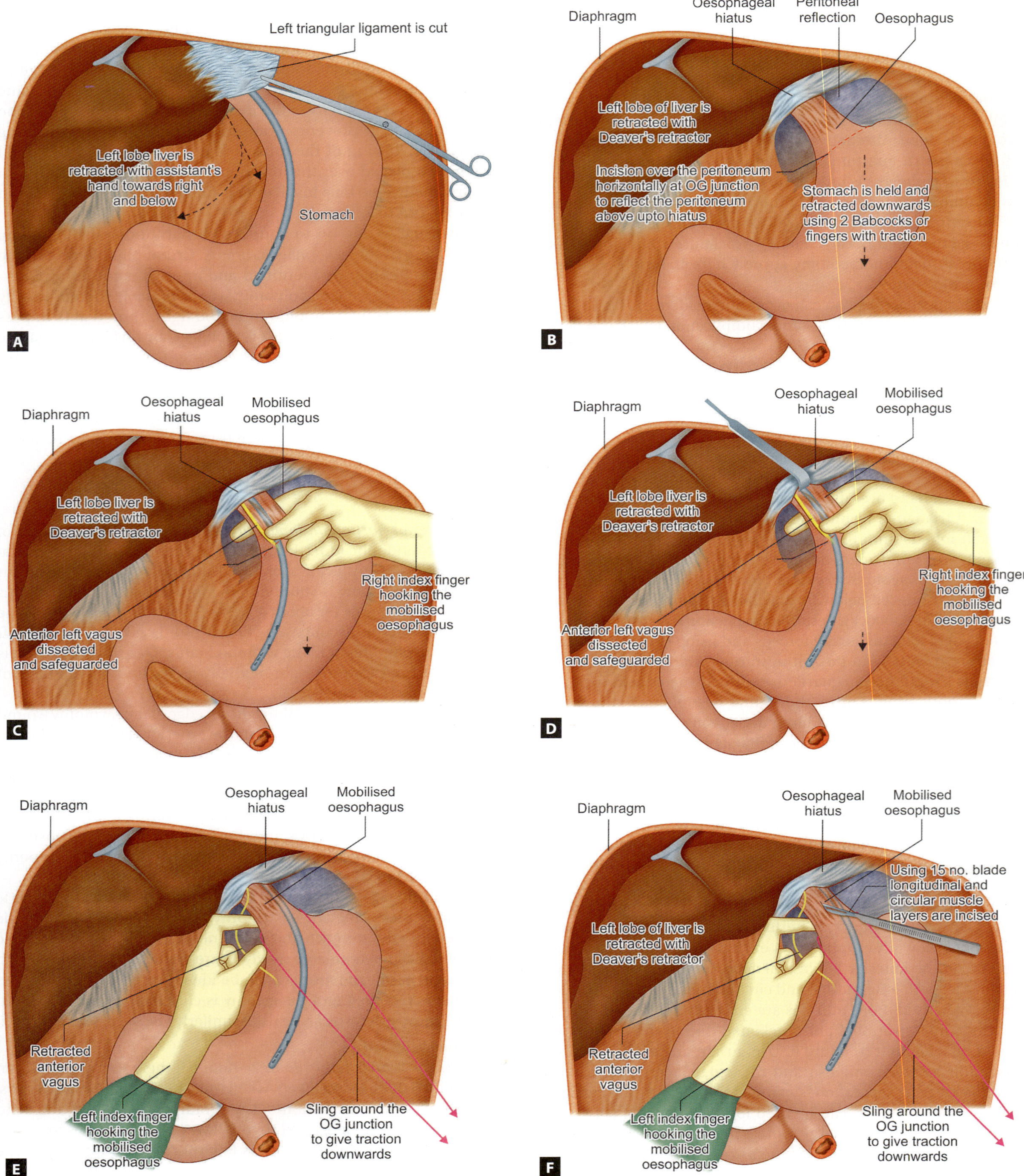

Figs. 20-14A to F

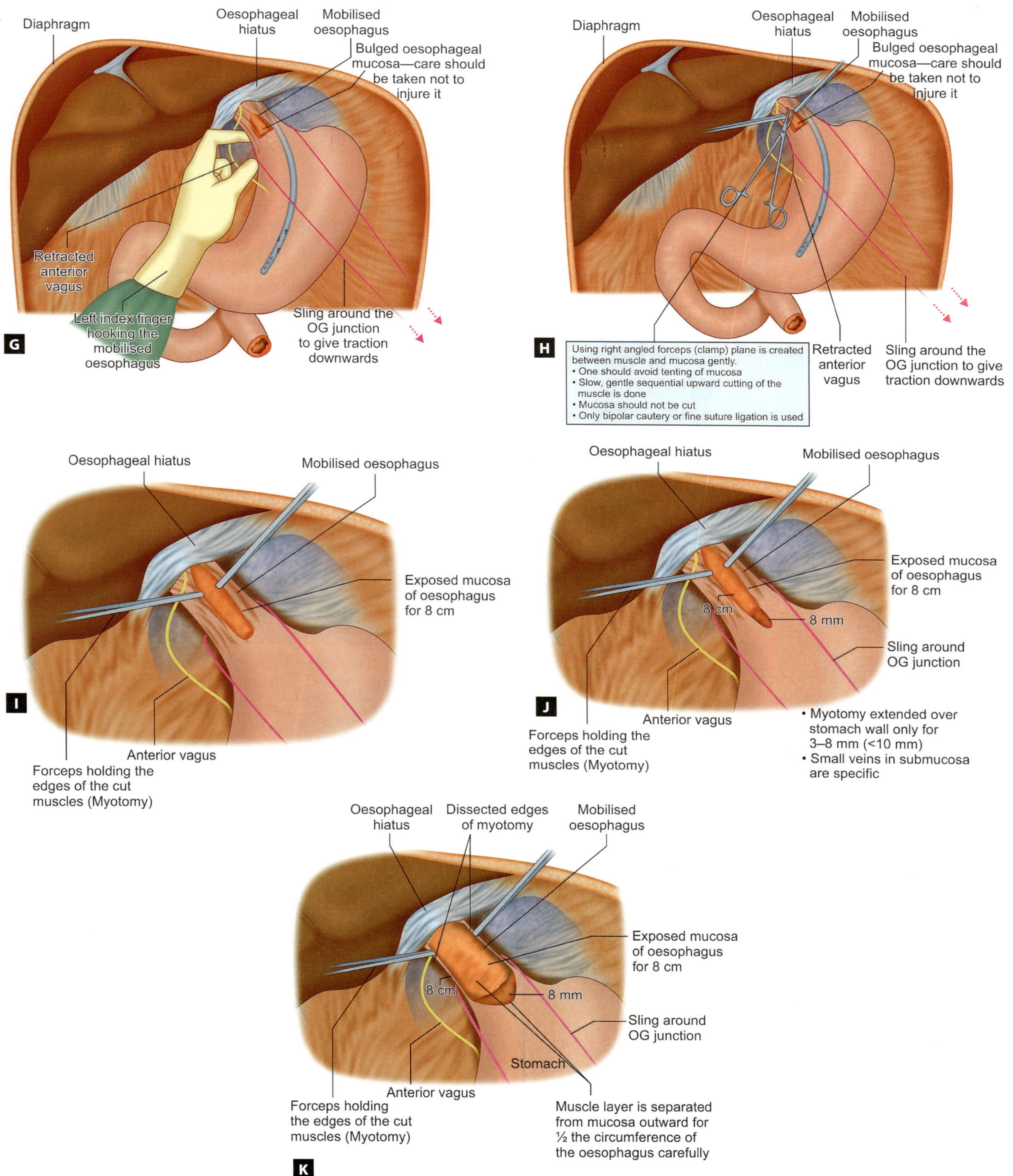

Figs. 20-14G to K

Figs. 20-14A to K: Achalasia cardia—modified Heller's cardiomyotomy open method through abdominal approach.

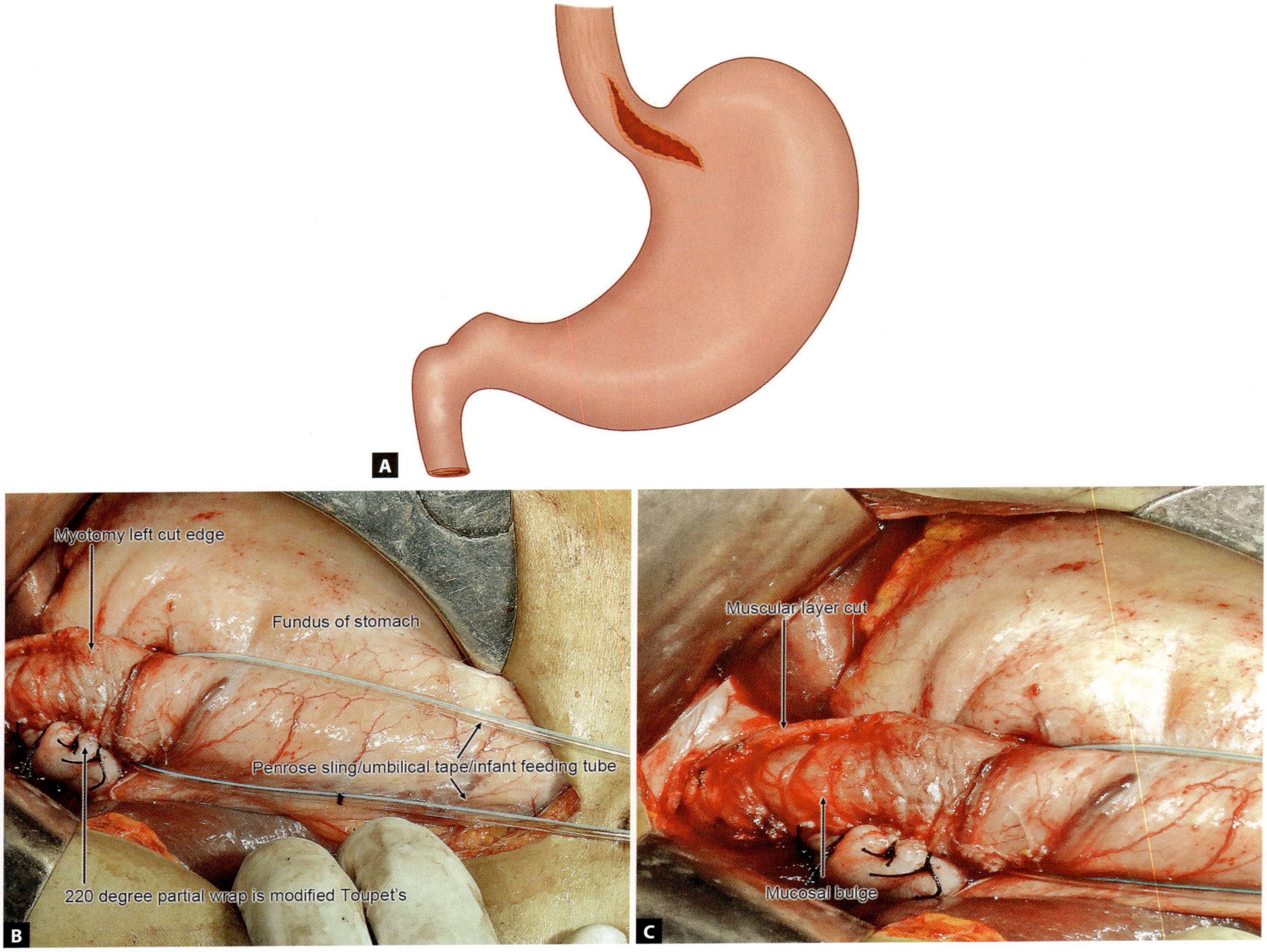

A
Myotomy left cut edge
Fundus of stomach
Penrose sling/umbilical tape/infant feeding tube
220 degree partial wrap is modified Toupet's
B
Muscular layer cut
Mucosal bulge
C

Figs. 20-15A to C: Heller's cardiomyotomy.

I row
II row
First row behind
Second row front, also to right crus

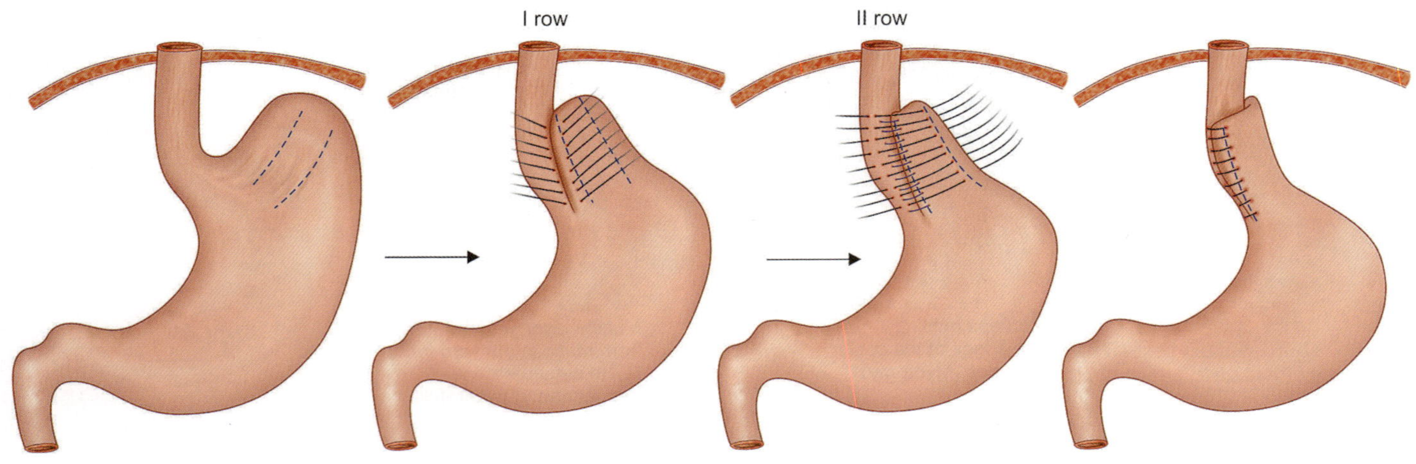

Fig. 20-16: Dor's anterior fundoplication.

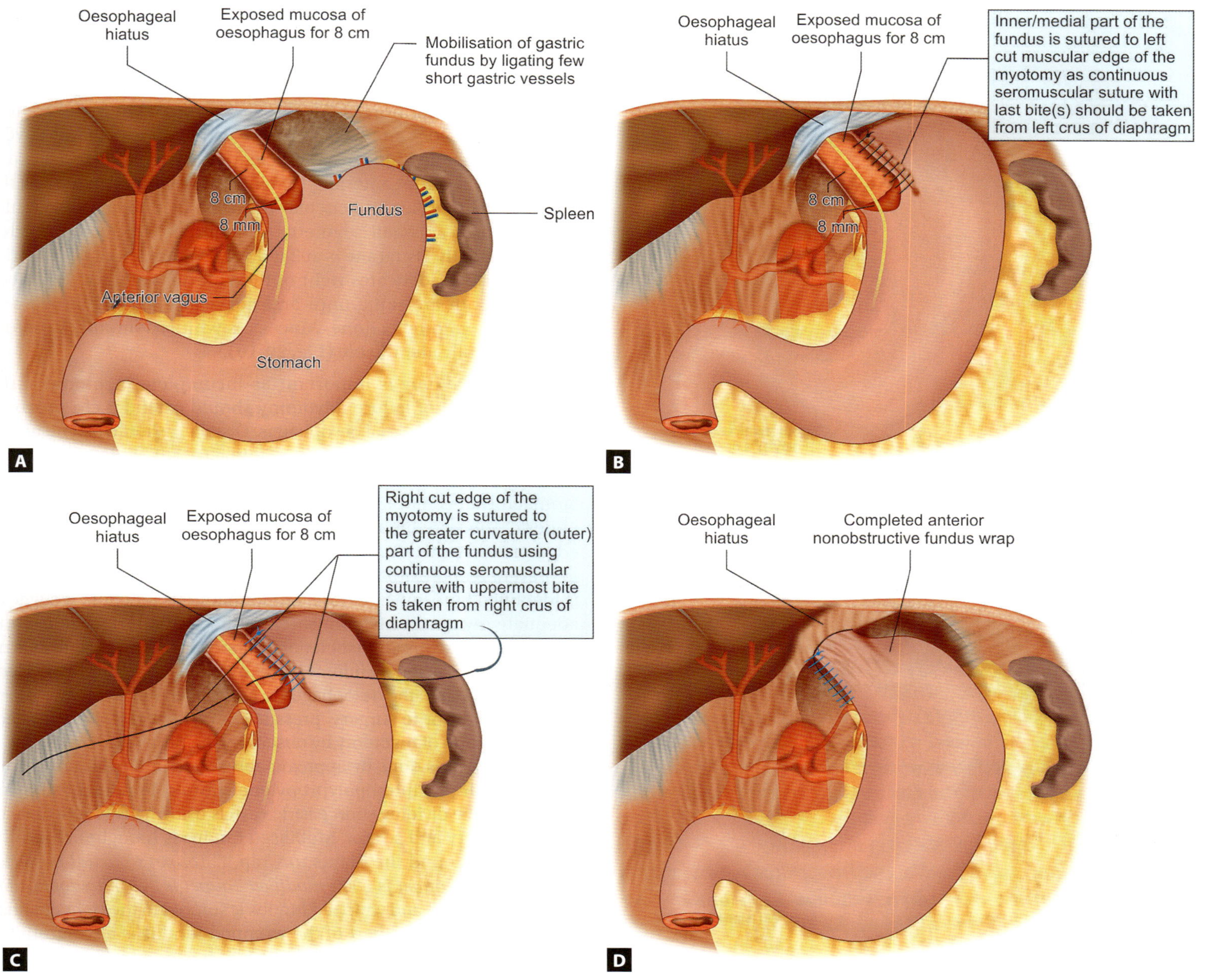

Figs. 20-17A to D: Anterior fundoplication (Dor's) for achalasia cardia.

Rarely splenic injury may occur. Pleural effusion, pneumothorax or empyema are rare known complications.

Dysphagia and gas bloating syndrome is the problem, but it is less in partial fundoplication.

Laparoscopic Cardiomyotomy

Shimi and colleague (UK) in 1991 did first Heller's cardiomyotomy laparoscopically. Cuschieri described proper technique of laparoscopic cardiomyotomy.

Procedure is done under general anaesthesia. Nasogastric tube should be placed prior to surgery. Often orogastric tube is passed until procedure is over. Patient is in supine position with abducted and flexed legs with head up position 40° (reverse Trendelenburg). Surgeon stands in between legs. Camera surgeon on the right side of the patient; assisting surgeon on the right side proximally; scrub nurse on the right side distally left of the left leg of the patient. Manometry and endoscopy needed should be kept in place to assess the completion and pressure before and after myotomy.

Supraumbilical incision in the epigastrium is made at 5 cm above the umbilicus (15 cm below the xiphoid). This 10 mm port site is used for 30° telescope with camera. Peritoneal access is done either by open method or by Veress needle. 10 mm trocar is passed. Other trocars at 5 mm left anterior axillary; 5 mm just below the xiphoid; 5 mm left midclavicular; 10 mm left midclavicular.

Left lobe of the liver is retracted through 5 mm subxiphoid port. Stomach is held with bowel holding forceps and retracted downwards and outwards by assistant through left anterior axillary 5 mm port. Gastrohepatic ligament is divided. After identifying right crus, behind the oesophagus dissection is done to create a window. Deep pillar of right crus and left crus are identified. Anteriorly phrenooesophageal ligament and peritoneum is divided transversely. Oesophagus is mobilised adequately proximally as well as at OG junction distally for 3 cm. Anterior left vagus is identified, dissected and safeguarded. Oesophagus is held with a tape or 0.62 cm width and 15 cm length Penrose drain and pulled down towards left lower abdomen. It facilitates further easy dissection.

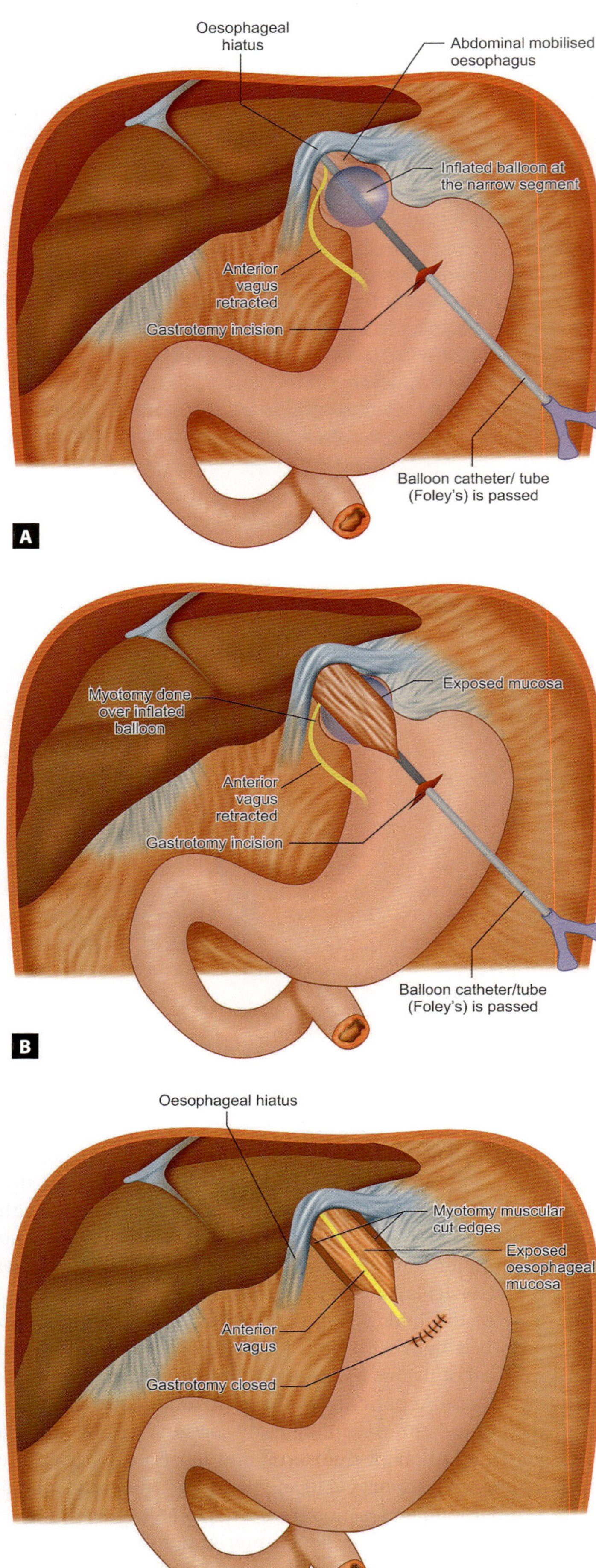

Figs. 20-18A to C: Cardiomyotomy balloon is often used.

Myotomy is done on the anterolateral surface of the oesophagus left of anterior vagus as longitudinal incision starting at cardia extending upwards for 6–8 cm. After dissecting longitudinal muscle circular muscle should be cut up to mucosa. Fine laparoscopic scissor is used. Harmonic scalpel is very useful. Monopolar cautery may injure mucosa and so better to be avoided. As bleeding is very less if at all needed bipolar is sufficient. In harmonic scalpel active blade should be kept anteriorly. Technique is splitting, elevating the longitudinal muscles and circular muscles; then to cut the circular muscle fibres as small segments sequentially up to the needed proximal length. Usual site is at 2 o'clock position left of the anterior vagus. But few advocates right of the anterior vagus at 11 o'clock position. Both are same until anterior vagus is safeguarded and adequate myotomy is done. Mucosa is whitish, smooth structure which is readily identifiable **(Fig. 20-19)**.

Adequate myotomy is important as incomplete myotomy is the common cause of failure. Myotomy should extend 3 cm proximal over the dilated proximal oesophagus. Distally it should extend across stomach only for less than 1 cm. Stomach wall is identified by its pattern of veins which is submucosal and transverse (*bridging veins*). Stomach wall is more vascular and difficult to dissect and chances of perforation are higher during this dissection. After myotomy cut edges are dissected for half the circumference of oesophagus (50%) to prevent reapproximation. Ideally gastroscopy is done. OG junction is identified by Z line and observed for patulous junction; it suggests adequate myotomy. Myotomy area is filled with normal saline and through gastroscopy air insufflation is done to confirm that there is no air leak bubble seen per abdomen over myotomy site. Often methylene blue is infused into the oesophagus to confirm leak. Manometry if kept in place just prior to surgery, pressure can be checked for adequacy and completion of myotomy by observing the drop in pressure.

Hiatal repair is done by approximating the crural pillar using non-absorbable interrupted polypropylene sutures. Fundus of stomach is mobilised by dividing short gastric vessels using harmonic scalpel or bipolar cautery and scissor. Mobilised fundus is brought behind the OG junction round the hiatus to wrap it. *Toupet's partial posterior 220° (original Toupet is 180°; modified Toupet is 270°) fundoplication* is done. Mobilised and wrapped fundus is sutured to the right cut edge of the myotomy. This part of the wrapped fundus is also sutured to the right crus in its upper part. Left cut edge is sutured to the left part of the mobilised fundus with interrupted sutures with its uppermost bite taken from the left crus. It prevents reflux and recurrent dysphagia by keeping the cut edges separate. *Dor's anterior partial fundoplication* is often advocated by many as it does not require posterior dissection and it covers the mucosa and may seal small injury which is unnoticed. But reflux incidence is more in anterior Dor's fundoplication. Left cut edge of the myotomy is sutured to the inner part of the fundus of the stomach with seromuscular sutures (2-zero silk/polypropylene). After that right cut edge of the myotomy is sutured on to the greater curvature (outer side) part of the stomach to pull and rollback the fundus over anterior surface of the myotomy area. Anterior fundoplication is used if there was mucosal injury (perforation) which is sutured on table; as it seals sutured site securely.

Intraoperative gastroscopy is very useful to identify the completion of the myotomy. Manometry on table is also very useful.

Robotic-assisted laparoscopic cardiomyotomy is very useful which reduces the hand tremors increasing the precision.

Postoperative care

Nasogastric tube/orogastric tube is removed after 24 hours. Oral fluids are started. Normal diet is started in 10 days. Straining is avoided for one month to prevent herniation of fundal wrap across the hiatus into the mediastinum.

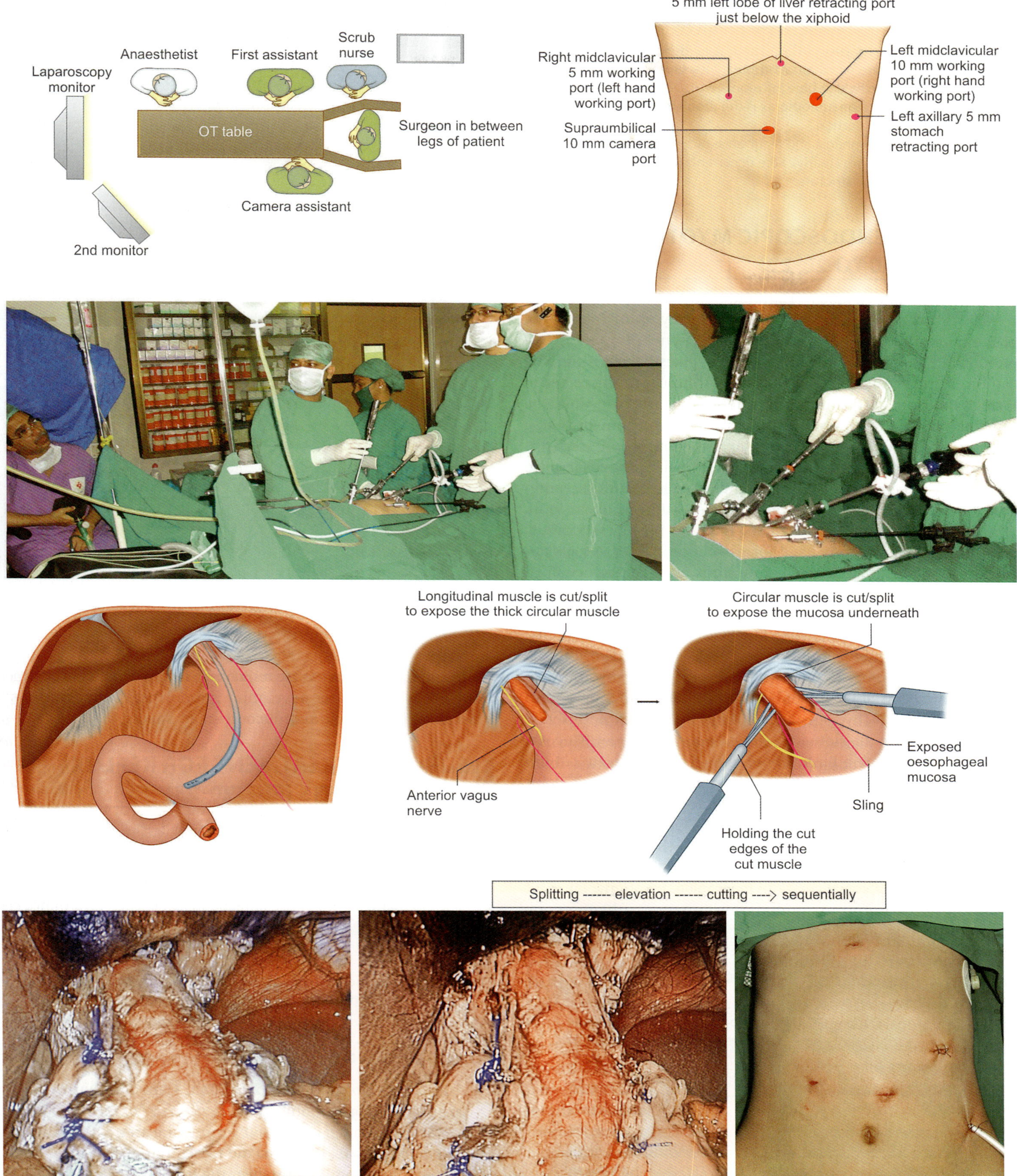

Fig. 20-19: Technique of laparoscopic cardiomyotomy.

Complications

Oesophageal perforation (4%)—once it is identified it should be sutured using 4-zero vicryl intracorporeal interrupted sutures. Closure is confirmed by methylene blue infusion.

Pleural injury and pneumothorax is the problem. It may occasionally need a chest tube insertion.

Postoperative dysphagia and recurrence of symptoms is usually due to incomplete myotomy (early). Late occurrence of dysphagia is due to reflux induced peptic stricture.

PER ORAL ENDOSCOPIC MYOTOMY (POEM) (FIGS. 20-20 TO 20-22)

POEM is new invention (2008—Haruhiro Inoue, Japan) as a palliative therapy for achalasia cardia wherein cardiomyotomy (cutting of circular muscle fibres of lower oesophagus) is done using endoscopy per orally. Procedure is done under general anaesthesia with supine position. 10 mL of saline with 0.3% indigo carmine stain is injected at 2 o'clock and 5 o'clock positions to create submucosal plane initially. 2 cm longitudinal incision is made in the oesophageal mucosa using endocautery dry cut mode. Submucosal tunnelling is done depends on the situation as decided by endoscopist. Initial submucosal space is created by injecting the saline into the plane and fine dissection using knife; few people advocate blunt dissection using balloon. CO_2 insufflation is used to keep space open for precise technique. Spray mode coagulation is used for dissection; larger vessels are cauterised individually. Circular muscle is cut using specialised devices; again with spray mode coagulator from proximal to distal, beginning at 2–3 cm distal to the mucosal incision. Triangular tip knife (Inoue) or T type hybrid knife can be used for myotomy. Repeated endoscopy towards the stomach is needed to identify possible mucosal injury and to confirm extent of the myotomy up to entire lower end of the oesophagogastric (OG) junction and to guide the dissection (by transillumination) by another endoscopy which is passed into the stomach (*double scope technique*). Mucosal incision is closed using endoscopic clips. Usually up to 2–4 cm beyond OG junction across the stomach circular muscle is cut. Point of entry and myotomy site is either 2 o'clock or 5 o'clock position. Hybrid POEM is combining oesophageal POEM endoscopically with laparoscopic antireflux fundoplication which avoids the taking of lifelong PPIs. *Complications are*—perforation of the oesophagus; bleeding; inadequate space creation; incomplete myotomy; mucosal disruption; Pneumothorax, pneumoperitoneum, subcutaneous emphysema, Empyema, peritonitis.

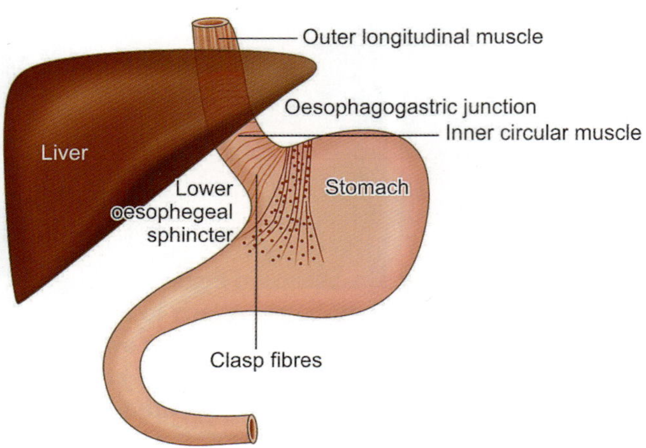

Fig. 20-20: Lower oesophageal sphincter anatomy.

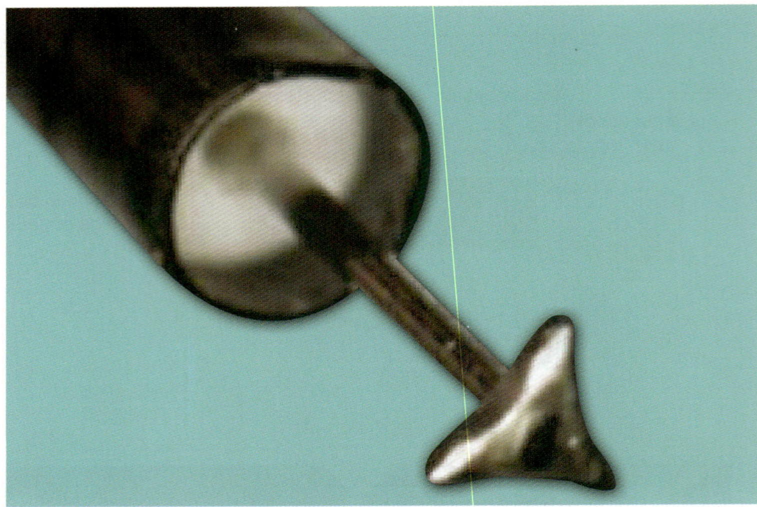

Fig. 20-21: Triangular tip knife (Inoue) for POEM.

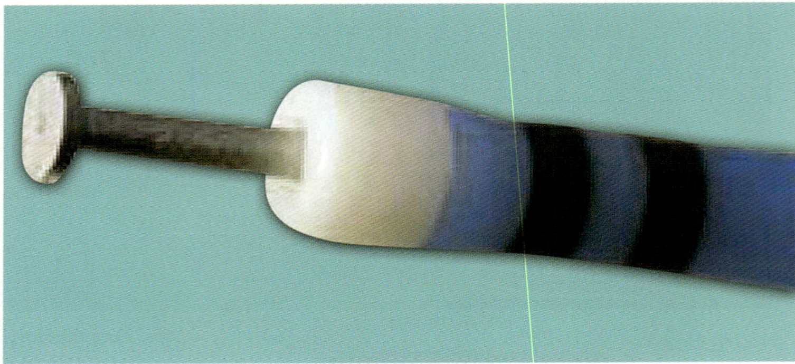

Fig. 20-22: T type (hybrid) knife used for POEM.

Submucosal tunnel endoscopic resection (STER) is further development of POEM wherein after developing submucosal tunnel lesions in muscularis propria and submucosal are removed.

SURGICAL TREATMENT FOR REFLUX OESOPHAGITIS (FIG. 20-23)

Principles of antireflux surgeries

- Operation should restore the LES pressure twice the resting gastric pressure
- The adequate length of the intraabdominal oesophagus should be maintained
- Apposition of diaphragmatic crurae, reduction of hiatus hernia when present
- Repaired OG junction should relax during swallowing adequately
- Tension free fundoplication should be done.

Fundoplication

- *Nissen's posterior total fundoplication:* Here after narrowing the crus of diaphragm, mobilised *posterior part of the fundus* of the stomach is wrapped totally 360° around the area of OG junction.
  - *Rudolph Nissen* (1959) first did total fundoplication.
  - Opening the peritoneum over the oesophagus to mobilise the lower oesophagus.
  - Dissection of the diaphragmatic crura of the oesophagus.
  - Mobilisation of entire fundus by ligating short gastric vessels.
  - Vagi are preserved.

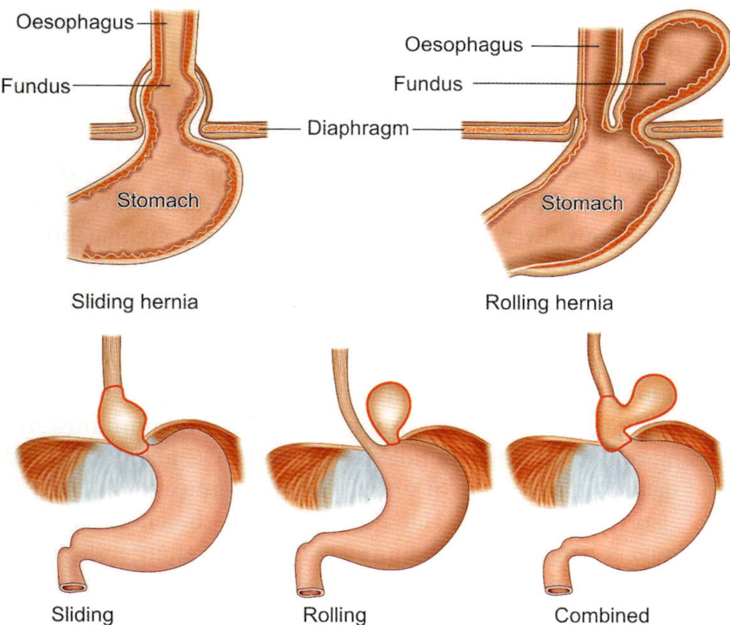

Fig. 20-23: Types of hiatus hernia—sliding, rolling, combined.

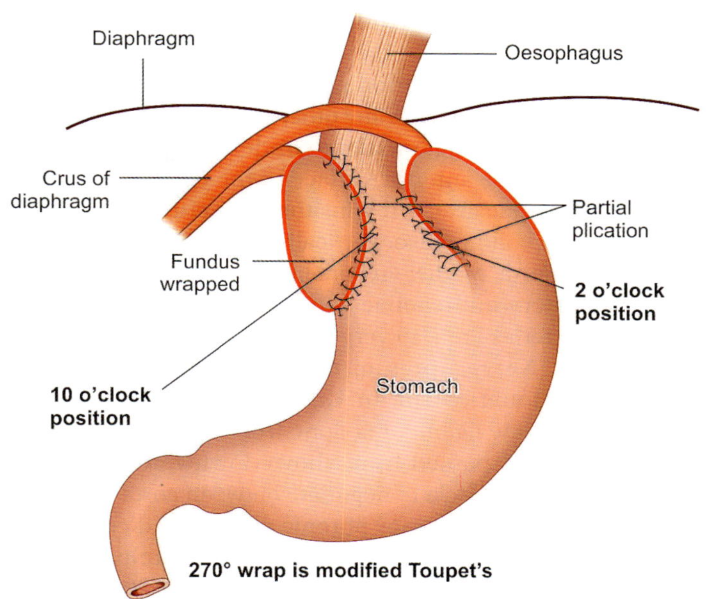

Fig. 20-24: Toupet's partial fundoplication.

- In Nissen's, 60 French bougie wrap is ideal; after complete mobilisation, only *posterior part of the fundus* is wrapped around after crural repair (otherwise fundoplication may displace into thorax causing paraoesophageal hernia); intraabdominal length of 2 cm oesophagus is created (not more); fundus of the stomach is known to relax in concert with oesophageal sphincter so only fundus should be used to buttress the sphincter; wrapping should be done only around sphincter of oesophagus not around the body of stomach; fundoplication should be kept in abdomen without any tension and without displacing into thorax. Non-absorbable polypropylene sutures are used.
- Crural repair is done using interrupted polypropylene sutures.
- Fundoplication should prevent sphincter shortening/unfolding during gastric distension, should preserve normal swallowing ability, allow proper belching and allow vomiting whenever needed.
- Bougie; on table and postoperative manometry to assess the pressure of new LOS; on table and postoperative gastroscopy—are commonly used in fundoplication.
- Mortality of procedure is very less; other parts of the abdomen can be assessed and addressed like gall stones.
- *Complications* are—*Gas bloat syndrome* (inability to belch); dysphagia; inability to vomit; slippage, proximal migration; paraoesophageal hernia, splenic injury. Floppy Nissen's fundoplication reduces the incidence of gas bloat syndrome.
- *Laparoscopic Nissen's fundoplication* is ideal and equally successful.
- *Transthoracic approach* is used for Nissen's fundoplication in patients who has had hiatus hernia repair earlier; who has had short oesophagus; in patients who has sliding hiatal hernia that does not reduce below the diaphragm, associated pulmonary disease, in obese, in patients who have narrow subcostal angle or barrel-shaped chest.

- *Toupet's partial 180° posterior fundoplication:* It is similar to Nissen's posterior fundoplication; it controls reflux alike Nissen's but gas bloat is very less. It is commonly done procedure now. Short gastric vessels are divided completely or partially. Modified 270° type is better placing sutures at 10 o'clock and 2 o'clock positions **(Fig. 20-24)**.
- *Dor anterior fundoplication:* Here right margin of the fundus is sutured to left margin of the oesophagus; front part of fundus is sutured to right margin of the oesophagus; 2nd row is also sutured to right crus. It is useful after Heller's cardiomyotomy if perforation of oesophagus has occurred. It will cover the sutured mucosal injury safely.
- *Rosetti Hell anterior fundoplication:* Here *anterior part of fundus* of stomach is used. Superomedial part of the fundus is brought around oesophagus to suture to anterior part of fundus. Here *short gastric vessels are not ligated* and much less fundus need to be mobilised.
- *Watson's anterolateral fundoplication:* 5 cm intraabdominal oesophagus is created with blunt transhiatal dissection. 120° anterolateral fundoplication augments the LOS function during stomach distension. Bougie insertion, division of short gastric vessels is not needed here.
- *Lind both anterior and posterior fundoplication* of 300° with 60° anteriorly uncovered area is not routinely practiced now.
- *Partial fundoplication with mesh wrap* around is also used. But complications of mesh like erosion, stricture and adhesions are so many.

Fundoplications

- Nissen's—total 360° posterior fundoplication
- Toupet's—partial 180° posterior fundal/posterolateral
- Rosette Hell—total anterior fundal
- Dor—anterior partial
- Watson's—anterolateral 120° partial
- Lind—posterior and anterior

Other Procedures

- *Hill's operation* (Dr Lucius Hill, USA, 1959):
  - Intra-abdominal fixation of OG junction (cardia) into median arcuate ligament to augment the effect LOS, to enable the effective oesophageal peristalsis. Procedure is done through

transabdominal approach which is assessed by intraoperative manometry. But it is technically difficult, may damage celiac plexus.

- Oesophagogastric junction and crura of the diaphragm are dissected properly like in any other procedure in this location. Median arcuate ligament is condensed preaortic fascia arching over the anterior surface of the aorta just above the origin of coeliac artery. It joins the right crus and is attached to vertebral column also. Vertically, it extends for about 3 cm along the aorta. Medial arcuate ligament is dissected off from coeliac artery and coeliac ganglion; right and left inferior phrenic arteries are also very close which should be carefully dissected. Nerve fibres of coeliac ganglion close to the ligament should be cut. In *Vasanth's method*, dissection at median arcuate ligament is done from upper margin; gently index finger is passed from above downwards underneath dense preaortic fascia to negotiate between aorta and median arcuate ligament. Inferior phrenic arteries and coeliac trunk and coeliac ganglion which lie in close proximity should not be injured. Using no. 1-zero polypropylene, suture bites are taken between pillars of right crus and left crus to repair the oesophageal hiatus **(Fig. 20-25)**.
- Three suture bites are taken which are not tied but held with haemostats. Then either finger or flat instrument is placed underneath the median arcuate ligament to safeguard aorta and other structures; 1-zero polypropylene suture bites are taken; first from anterior phrenooesophageal bundle (near gastric fundus) from left towards right; next bite from lower oesophagus, posterior phrenooesophageal bundle with part of the lesser curve of the stomach; last bite is from the median arcuate ligament. Anterior phrenooesophageal bundle is left and lateral to anterior vagus at the base of the angle of His distal to oesophago-fundic junction; posterior phrenooesophageal bundle is behind the OG junction towards right of posterior (right) vagus. Remaining two lower bites are also taken similarly. Haemostasis should be checked at this stage. Crural fibres are sutured to do hiatal repair; index finger should be able to pass through the sutured oesophageal hiatus.

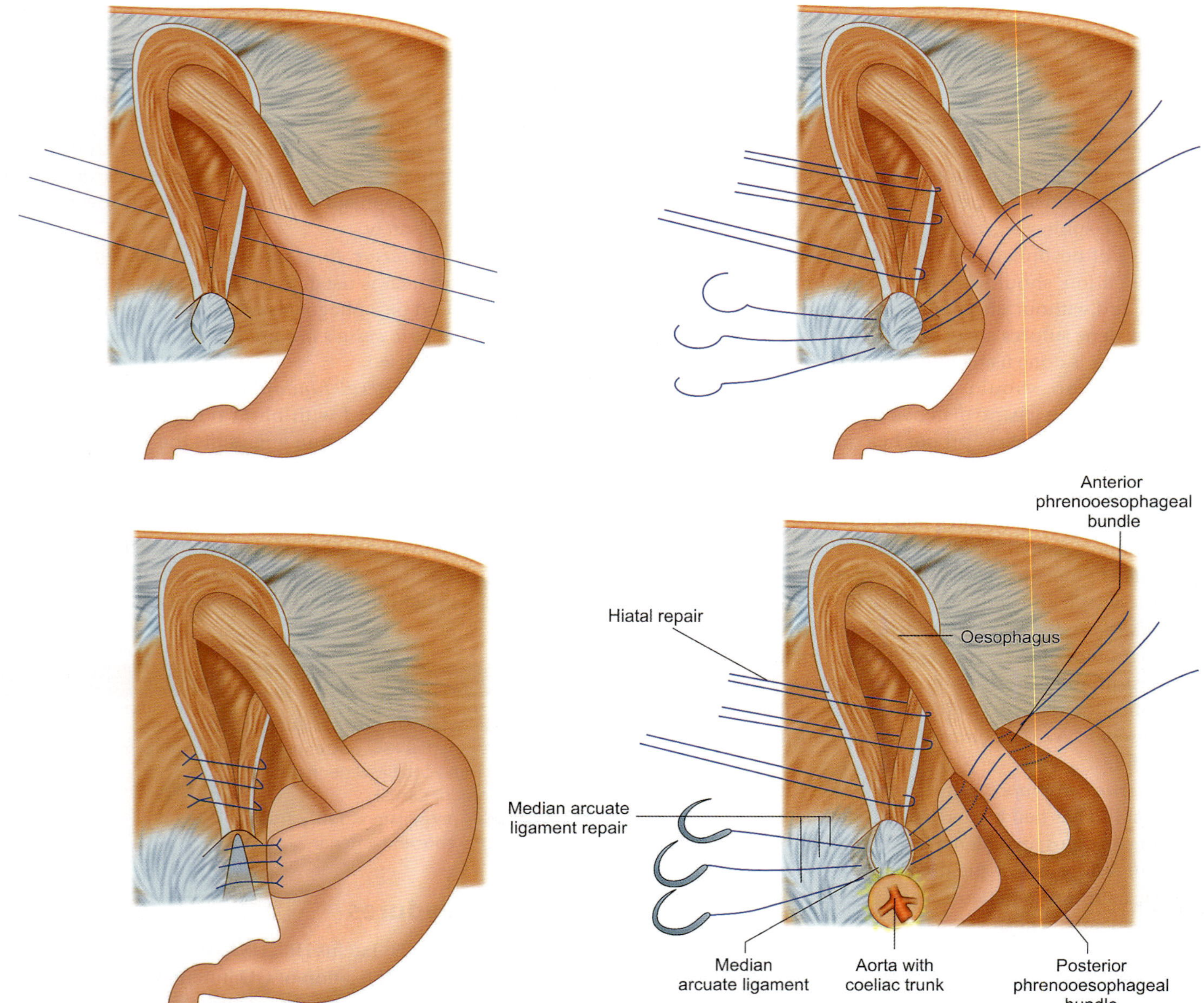

Fig. 20-25: Hill's repair of hiatus hernia.

Then arcuate ligament repair sutures are tied to complete Hill's posterior gastropexy. Often Teflon pledgets are used into the arcuate ligament sutures but it is not mandatory. Antireflux adequacy is confirmed using saline.

- *Belsey Mark IV operation* (Ronald Belsey, Britain, 1967):
  - It is plication of oesophagus to the diaphragm through many interrupted mattress sutures so as to push the oesophagus downwards to make it intraabdominal with adequate length. It is done through left transthoracic approach. 240° fundoplication, creation of intraabdominal oesophagus, crural sling repair are the techniques. It corrects GERD and also maintains normal eructation and physiological reflux. But long hospital stay and respiratory complications are distressing problems **(Fig. 20-26)**.
  - Left posterolateral thoracotomy is done through 6th intercostal space. Oesophagus is mobilised from diaphragm to aortic arch. Left superior and inferior bronchial arteries are ligated. Direct oesophageal arteries are also ligated. Adequate mobilisation is essential. Vagi should be preserved carefully. Phrenooesophageal membrane is divided to enter into the peritoneal cavity. With the left hand fingers the OG junction and gastric fundus is mobilised and retracted and, with the right hand scissor dissection is done under vision. Short gastric vessels are divided. All attachments between stomach and hiatus are divided. Fundus and abdominal oesophagus are drawn into thoracic cavity by holding with Babcock's clamps.
  - Hiatal repair sutures are placed using 1 zero polypropylene sutures from below upwards. All sutures are placed (3-4) first (tied together later only after completing the fundoplication).
  - Gastric fundus is plicated around the anterior 2/3rd of the lower 4 cm of oesophagus. First row of sutures are 1.5 cm above the cardia. 3-zero or 2-zero polypropylene suture material is used. Left anterolateral position of the oesophagus used for plication as view over right side is inadequate. Bite taken from the gastric fundus (seromuscular) then from the muscular wall of the oesophagus horizontally then again on to the gastric fundus adjacent to first bite with a 5 mm gap. All first row plication sutures are placed; then they are tied to pull up the fundus **(Figs. 20-27A to H)**.
  - Second row of sutures are placed 2 cm above the first row using 2-zero or 3-zero polypropylene suture or silk. From gastric fundus as seromuscular to the oesophagus as muscular then back to the gastric fundus as seromuscular with a 5 mm gap. All sutures are placed and then tied; ends are not cut but held with haemostats. Now each free ends of the suture are passed through (after passing needles to each tails) the diaphragm from abdominal side towards thoracic side. Once all ends are passed like that; knotting is done securely. Fundus with the oesophagus is pushed down into the abdominal cavity.
  - Hiatal sutures which were taken earlier (previously placed) are tied now securely to complete the hiatal repair.

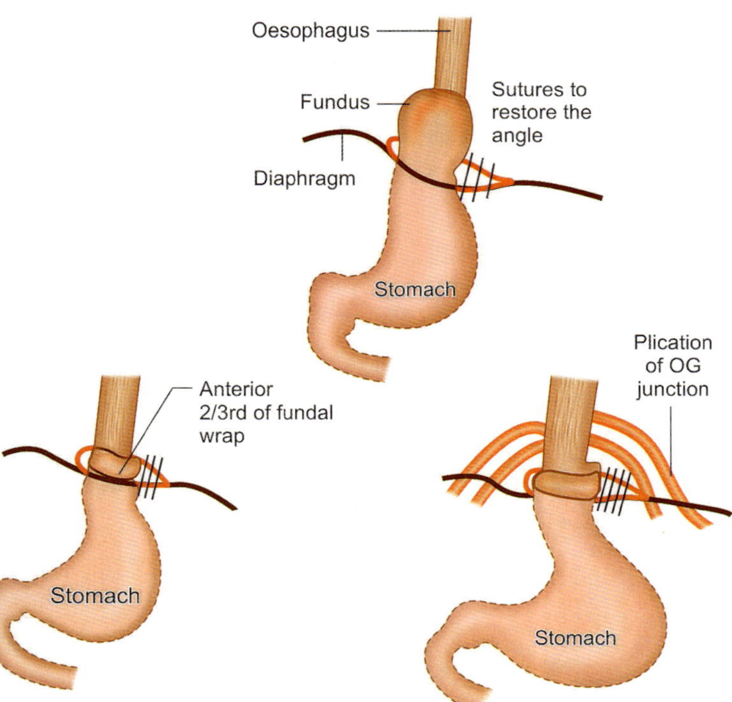

Fig. 20-26: Belsey Mark IV operation.

- *Placement of Angelchik prosthesis:* Annular silicone gel filled angelchik prosthesis with a tape on either end. After insertion around OG junction ends are tied around.
- *Collis' vertical gastroplasty* is done using fundus stomach. A vertical cut along the line of oesophagus is made on the fundus which is sutured to create extra length of oesophagus and new lesser curvature. It is done whenever oesophagus cannot be mobilised due to oesophageal shortening by a stricture developed as a complication of GORD. Partial fundoplication is added to this usually. Previous gastrectomy is contraindication to this **(Fig. 20-28)**.
- *Transthoracic Collis–Nissen's gastroplasty:*
  - It is used in short oesophagus with stricture and recurrence after an earlier antireflux procedure. Open mind should be also kept for need of bowel (colon) interposition in such patients. New oesophagus is created by lengthening it. Then antireflux procedure is done. Entire procedure is done through thoracotomy **(Fig. 20-29)**.
  - Double lumen endotracheal lumen tube is placed. One lung anaesthesia is given. Nasogastric tube should be passed. Lateral left side up position is used for 6th intercostal space thoracotomy. Latissimus dorsi and serratus anterior muscles are cut. Incision posteriorly should extend up to the lateral margin of the spinal muscles. Pleura is opened. Often 7th rib excision posteriorly is needed to have a better access with ligation of intercostal vessels running under 7th rib at its lower margin. If needed conversion into thoracoabdominal by anterior extension of the thoracotomy should be done to facilitate the better dissection of the hiatus.
  - Inferior pulmonary ligament and then mediastinal pleura has to be incised medial to the thoracic aorta. With blunt and sharp dissection and nasogastric tube as a guide, oesophagus with anterior vagus is encircled using sling (umbilical/Penrose drain). Proximally dissection is extended up to the inferior pulmonary vein. Lower part of the incision is extended in front along the pericardiophrenic sulcus to facilitate the hiatal dissection.
  - Phrenooesophageal ligament and peritoneum is incised. Hiatus is dissected circumferentially. Hernial sac if existing is identified. Hernial sac is dissected by holding the oesophagus with traction. A branch of inferior phrenic artery is ligated. Gastrohepatic ligament is incised and opened towards right with adequate traction. An accessory left hepatic artery is commonly seen in this ligament which should be ligated.

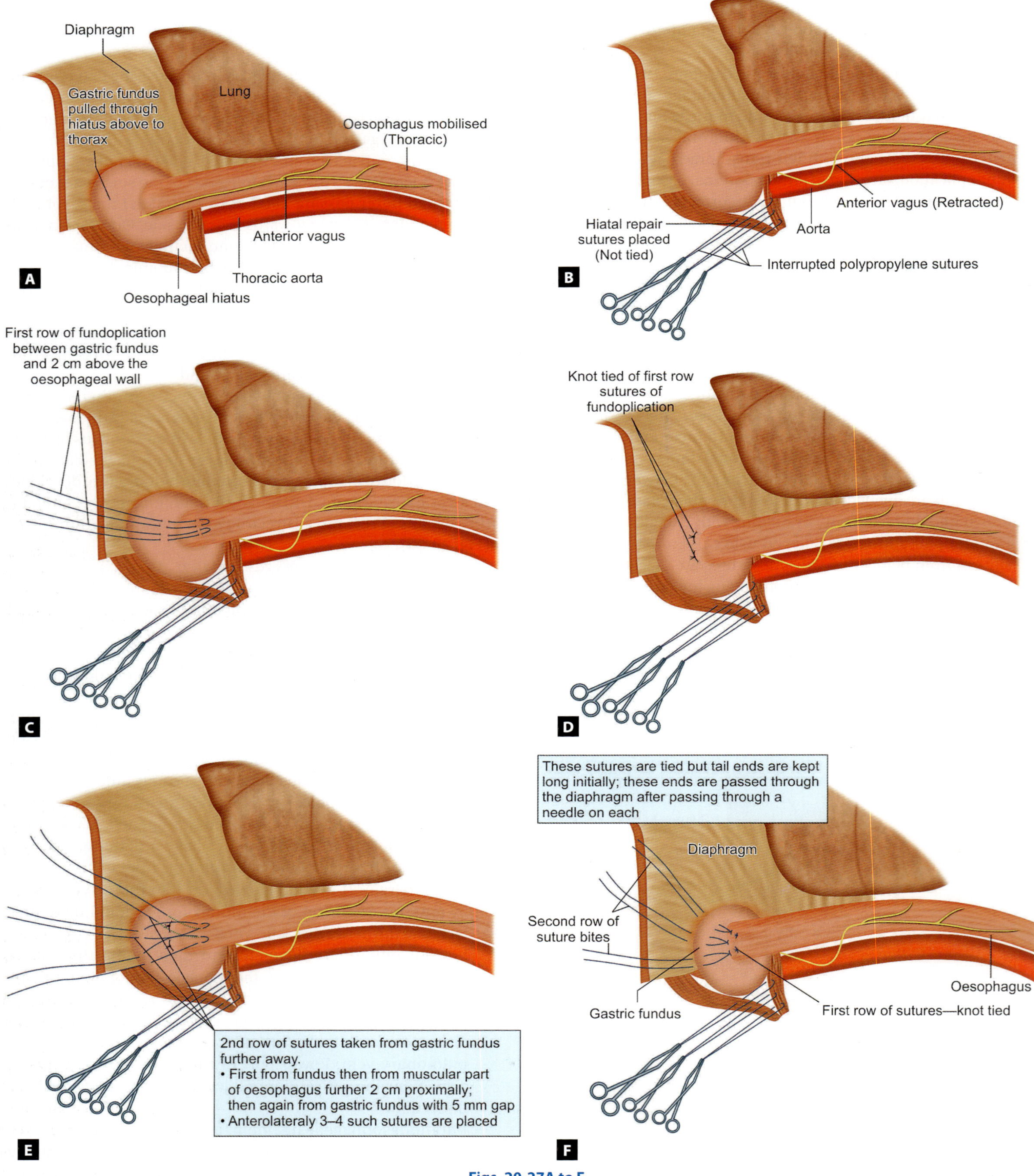

Figs. 20-27A to F

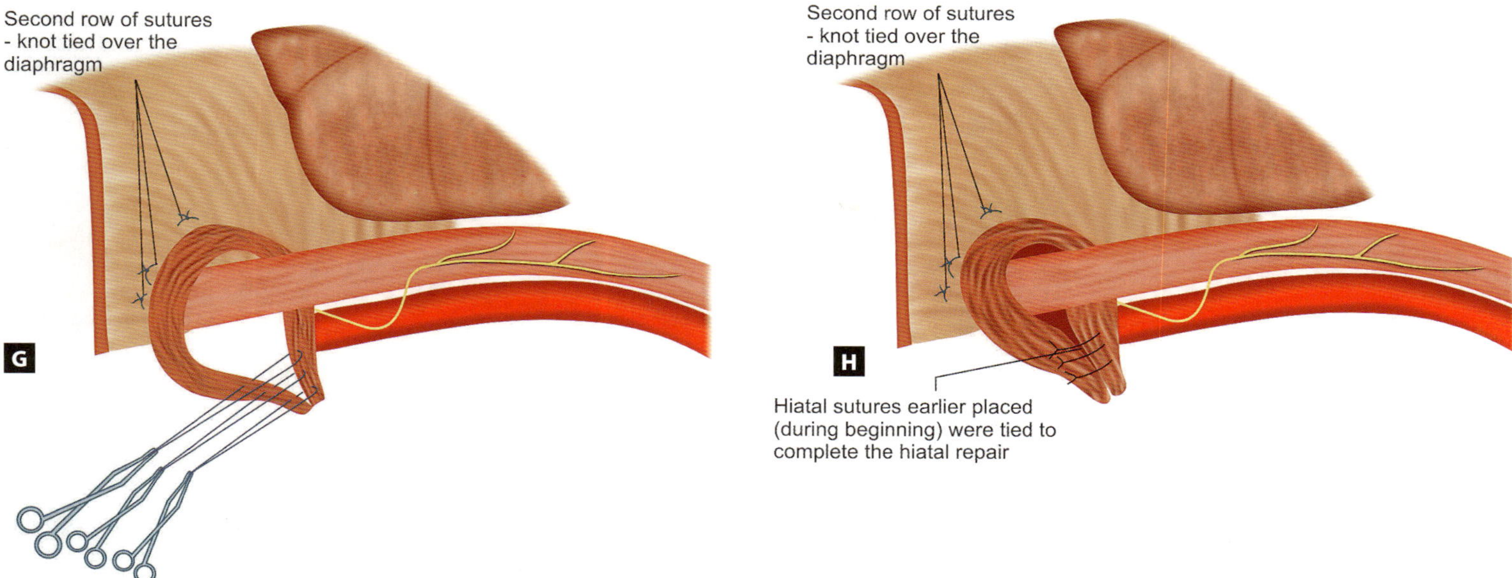

Figs. 20-27G and H

Figs. 20-27A to H: Technique of Belsey mark IV operation.

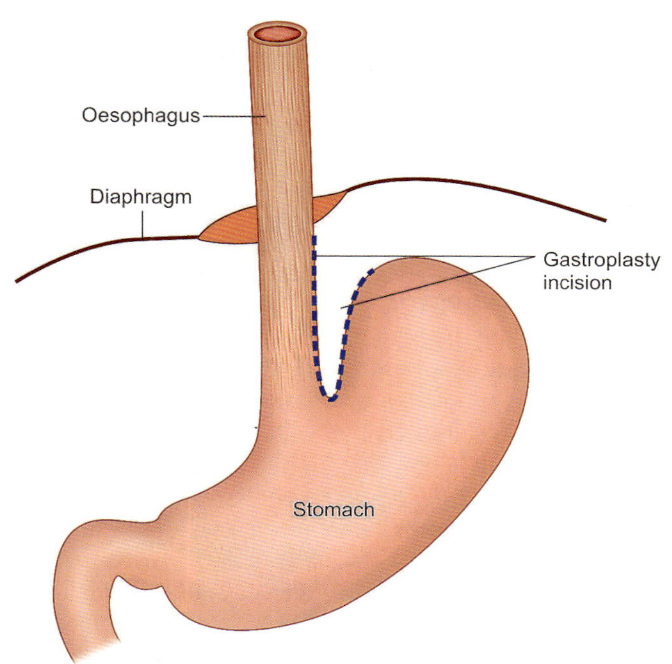

Fig. 20-28: Gastroplasty technique.

Other attachments between hiatus and proximal stomach are divided using bipolar cautery or harmonic scalpel.

- Oesophageal stricture should be dilated using series of Maloney dilators. Peritoneum of the hernial sac is excised. Short gastric vessels along the greater curvature are ligated and divided or using harmonic scalpel for about 15 cm of greater curvature. Pad of fat around the OG junction is dissected and removed. 60 no. French Maloney dilator is passed across the hiatus. Lineal stapler is fired along the fundus left of the oesophagus to create a new fundus and neooesophagus of 7–8 cm (lengthened oesophagus). Stapled lines along the neooesophagus and gastric fundus are often inverted using continuous seromuscular sutures using 3 zero PDS or vicryl. Metal clip is applied at the junction of neooesophagus and stomach as a marker.
- New fundus is brought under the neooesophagus to create a wrap; it is sutured to the greater curvature with interrupted 2-zero polypropylene sutures to complete the wrap. Usually 3 sutures for 3 cm length are placed. Bite also should be taken from the neooesophagus. Wrap should accommodate index finger to prove it as floppy. After that hiatal repair is done by apposing the right and left crura using interrupted polypropylene sutures. Mediastinal pleura may or may not be sutured. Intercostal tube is placed (36 F). Thoracotomy wound is closed.
- Complications are—gastroplasty tube necrosis; recurrence; leak; empyema; obstruction.

- *Thal's patch procedure:* It is done for localised non-dilatable stricture oesophagus. Stricture is incised full thickness longitudinally. Mobilised fundus of stomach is placed and sutured as a serosal patch technique over the defect **(Fig. 20-30)**.
- *Narbona's ligamentum teres cardiopexy* (commonly done in Spain): Ligamentum teres is mobilised from falciform ligament with its blood supply from left lobe of liver; it is detached from umbilicus and brought around the mobilised lower oesophagus with traction until LOS pressure becomes 15–20 mmHg with manometry; flap end is sutured to left of OG junction and anterior wall of stomach. It is more physiological and division of short gastric vessels is not required.
- *Boerema operation:* It is fixing OG junction in front into anterior abdominal wall. It is not practiced now.
- *Oesophagogastrectomy* is required whenever there is *failure of antireflux procedure/metaplasia* is present/*non-dilatable stricture* is present. Lower end of oesophagus and proximal stomach is resected with oesophagogastric anastomosis done through thoracoabdominal approach.
- *Transhiatal oesophagectomy* with anastomosis between cervical oesophagus and stomach in the neck is an alternate procedure which can be used in severe extensive disease and stricture.

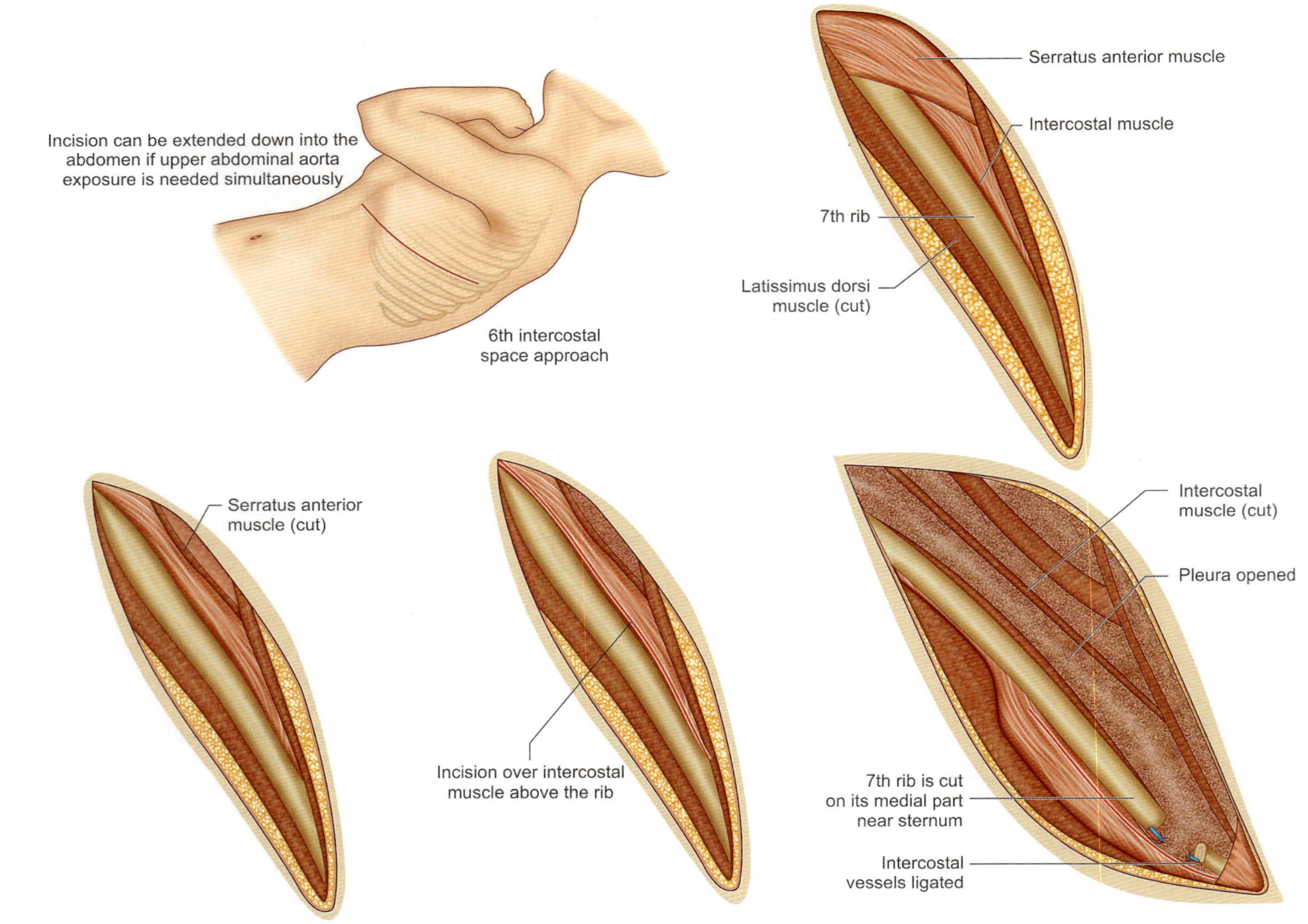

Fig. 20-29: Transthoracic Collis-Nissen's gastroplasty.

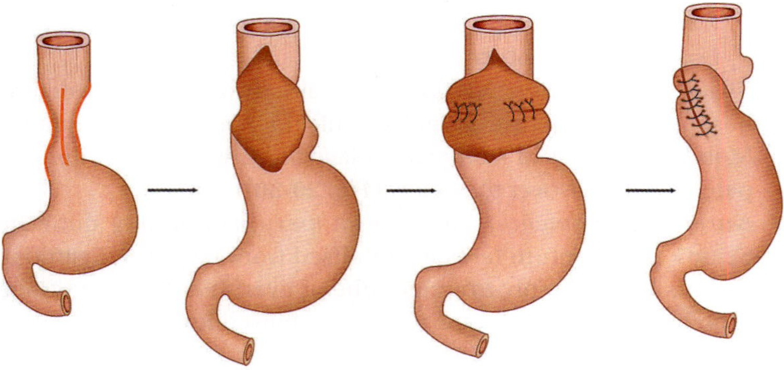

Fig. 20-30: Thal's patch.

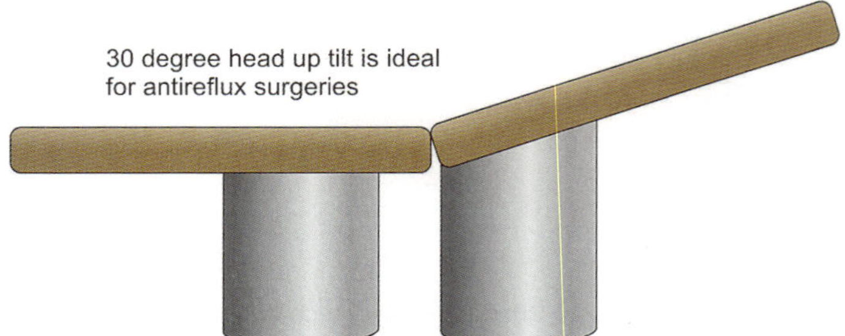

Fig. 20-31: Operation table position in fundal wrap procedure with patient is in reverse Trendelenburg position with head up (15–0°).

Nissen's Fundoplication (Nissen–Rosetti)

It is done either through laparotomy/laparoscopy or through thoracotomy.

Preparation

Preoperative gastroscopy, pH studies, oesophageal manometry, contrast CT chest are needed as investigations. Nasogastric tube should be passed. Often oesophageal bougie or orogastric tube is also used as a guide for mobilisation.

Procedure

Patient is in reverse Trendelenburg position with head up (15-30°); general anaesthesia is used always. Upper midline incision is put from xiphoid process often extending to left of the umbilicus below. Self retaining retractor is essential. After laparotomy, abdominal cavity is quickly explored **(Fig. 20-31)**.

Mobilisation: Stomach is held downward and left by assistant. This stretches the tissue around the oesophagus to facilitate dissection and also reduces any hiatal hernial component. Left triangular ligament is cut to mobilise the left lobe of liver which is retracted down and towards right. Care should be taken not to injure left hepatic vein or IVC. Gastrohepatic ligament is divided. Accessory left hepatic artery may be present in the ligament which is usually saved. It is a branch of left gastric artery. It is now found that ligation of accessory hepatic artery is safer and so if needed can be ligated. Phrenooesophageal ligament and peritoneum is incised circumferentially in the hiatus to visualise the crura of diaphragm from behind. Mobilisation is done like mobilisation of the distal oesophagus as described above. Blunt, peanut and sharp dissections are used. Energy sources can be used carefully. Three fingers should be passed easily, freely through post-oesophageal window. Anterior and posterior vagi nerve trunks should be preserved dissected carefully and safeguarded. Penrose drain or sling is passed around the hiatus which is used as traction for further dissection.

Gastrophrenic ligament is identified and divided. Short gastric vessels are divided from the fundus to mobilise it adequately to create a wrap. Short gastric vessels are short, thin walled and stout. Tear of these vessels cause torrential haemorrhage. Often tear may extend into the splenic capsule creating further damage. Traction over the spleen should be gentle and minimal to prevent this; vessels should be ligated using 3 zero silk or vicryl and divided with bipolar cautery. Harmonic energy source is better. Sling over the hiatus is used for continuous traction over the fundus. Two Babcock clamps are passed underneath the oesophagus from right towards left to hold the mobilised fundus; fundus is brought underneath and to the front of oesophagus. Babcock clamps are relaxed to check any tension on the mobilised fundus. Mobilised fundus should stay there comfortably without any tendency to return back to its original position. If it is not so, further mobilisation of fundus is needed.

Hiatal repair is a must to prevent fundoplication to slip into the thoracic cavity (mediastinum). Distal slippage of wrap does not occur as gastric trinity prevents that. Using zero polypropylene sutures, deep bites are taken from peritoneum → right crus including tendinous portion then of left crus and peritoneum over it. From below upwards 3 interrupted sutures are placed. Sutures are tied sequentially from below upwards. It should not be too tight or too loose. Index finger should be able to pass through the repair and oesophagus comfortably **(Fig. 20-32)**.

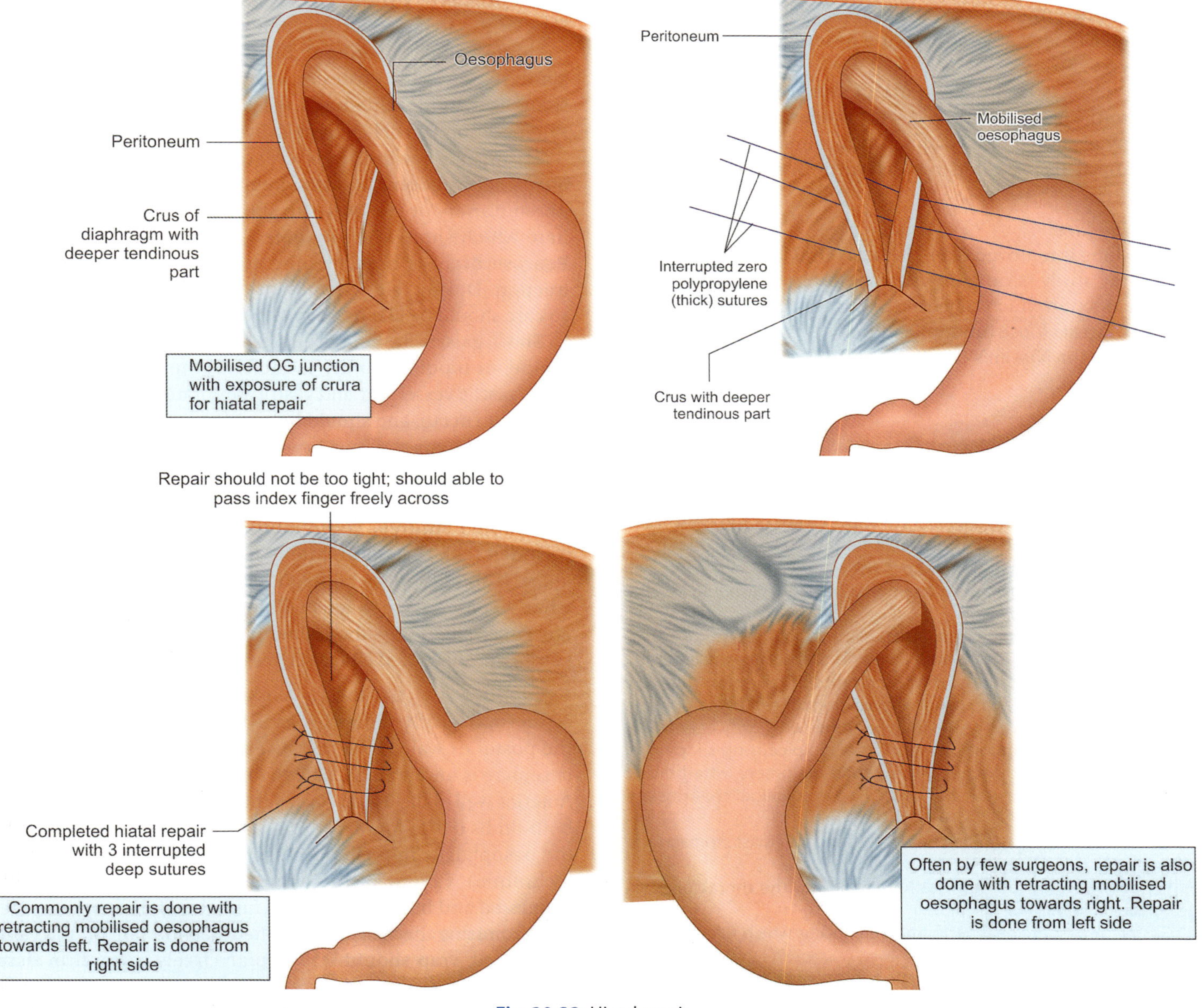

Fig. 20-32: Hiatal repair.

Fundoplication: Adequate mobilisation of the hiatus, distal oesophagus (6–8 cm) and fundus is essential. *Wrap* can be done with vagi within or outside. Vagi are kept outside the wrap often. But many advocate wrap with keeping both vagi in position. Often *posterior vagus is kept outside the wrap and anterior vagus is within* the wrap. It does not make any difference until wrap is loose, free (*Floppy*) and suturing bites should not pass through the vagi. No. 2-zero polypropylene interrupted sutures are placed between wrapped part of the fundus through oesophageal muscle wall to the left part of the mobilised fundus to complete 360° plication. First three sutures each at 0.5–1.0 cm apart are placed from below upwards; then sutures are tied. First bite should be from mobilised fundus of the right of oesophagus of patient; through the lesser curve; then from the fundus at left of the oesophagus. Thickness of bite should be around 5 mm; but should not enter the lumen. Interrupted sutures are placed at 1 cm gap. Maximum 3 cm wrap is created not more than that. After completion of the wrap, two fingers should able to pass under the wrap to confirm that fundoplication is not too tight. Suture is also often placed from the wrapped fundus to the hiatal wall (right crus) to stabilise the fundoplication; but it is not necessary **(Figs. 20-33 to 20-35)**.

Single suture 360° wrap with Teflon pledget buttress is also often done. Even though many advocate mesh usage for hiatal repair it is not advisable as mesh erosion into the oesophagus is threatening and dangerous.

Through nasogastric tube 400 mL of saline is infused into the stomach. Stomach is compressed with moderate pressure to see if there is any expelling of the saline from stomach to oesophagus. If saline cannot be expelled means antireflux valve created is competent.

Postoperative care

Nasogastric tube is removed after 48 hours. Oral fluid is started. Oral contrast X-ray study is done to visualise progressively narrowing tapered OG junction which suggests the successful surgery. Absence of tapering suggests loose fundoplication.

Success rate for Nissen's fundoplication is 90%. Recurrence or failure rate is 10%.

Complications

Dysphagia is common after Nissen's fundoplication. It is usually temporary lasting for 3 weeks due to mucosal oedema. If dysphagia persists it is due to tight/wide (>3 cm width) wrap or too tight hiatal repair or missed other causes like achalasia, motility disorders. Indwelling bougie placement across the hiatus during surgery will prevent fundal wrap becoming too tight. Two fingers should be able to pass under the wrap.

Gas bloat syndrome is inability to belch causing tightness in the upper abdomen. It is due to too tight wrap. Floppy fundoplication prevents this. Fundoplication can disrupt causing recurrence or failure. So it is ideal to use monofilament non-absorbable 2 zero sutures. Polypropylene is commonly used. Vicryl or silk may get digested slowly eventually. Failure is due to disruption of wrap; loose wrap causing slipping of fundoplication; sliding hernia with wrap in abdomen; intrathoracic migration of fundoplication can occur. Barium swallow confirms the diagnosis.

Fundoplication may slip downward causing hour glass stomach and obstruction.

Fundoplication wrap may get herniated into the thorax or para-oesophageal hernia may occur.

Gastric or oesophageal perforation can occur which needs proper suturing.

Injury to spleen (1–5%), vagi, pneumothorax, and subphrenic abscess are rare complications.

Laparoscopic Nissen's Fundoplication

Laparoscopic approach has become ***standard*** since 1992 for fundoplication. Preoperative preparation is same as open method. Contrast study; gastroscopy, 24-hour pH monitoring, oesophageal manometry, chest X-ray are needed. Severity of the reflux; presence of oesophagitis, Barrett's oesophagus, stricture, shortening are to be evaluated properly before planning the surgery. Patients who are intolerant or poorly responding to proton pump inhibitors; patients with large hiatal hernia; presence of complications are the indications for surgical intervention.

Technique: Under general anaesthesia, patient is lied down in reverse Trendelenburg (30°)/head up with semilithotomy position. Surgeon stands in between legs. Three 10 mm trocars and two 5 mm trocars are placed. Supraumbilical port is 5 cm above towards left (to avoid falciform ligament) which is used for 30° laparoscope. Pneumoperitoneum is created. Camera assistant is on the right of the patient; assistant on the left; scrub nurse either right or left distally.

Hiatal mobilisation is done like in Heller's cardiomyotomy. Gastrohepatic ligament (hepatogastric omentum) is incised. Hepatic branch of left gastric artery is divided; there may be aberrant left hepatic artery which may be the only branch supplying the left lobe of the liver (15%). It is safeguarded. Peritoneum is divided circumferentially all around. Right crus is identified and dissected; similarly left crus. Posterior vagus which is in the loose areolar tissue is also identified and dissected carefully for preservation. Phrenooesophageal ligament is divided all around.

Retrogastric window is created by incising the peritoneal attachment adjacent to gastric fundus near angle of His. Left inferior phrenic artery or few posterior short gastric vessels may be present here which should be fulgurated and divided. Umbilical tape or Penrose drain is used to sling around the OG junction and for traction. During left side mobilisation left pleura may get injured so care should be taken to avoid it.

Short gastric vessels are divided adequately using harmonic scalpel or bipolar cautery to mobilise the fundus. Splenic injury, short gastric vessel tear and gastric perforation are the complications which can occur, and should be avoided.

Hiatal repair is done by retracting the sling at OG junction towards left by approximating both pillars of right crus with left crus with their tendinous attachments using thick no. zero polypropylene interrupted sutures. Peritoneum overlying the crura should be included with the suture bites. Usually 3 sutures are placed 1 cm apart. It should not be too tight or too loose. Sling at OG junction when released oesophagus will retract and fill the hiatus without any constriction or without entering through the hiatus. Additional suture may be added if need arises.

Fundoplication: Grasper is passed from right side across the retroesophageal window towards left side of OG junction to hold the posterior wall of the mobilised fundus; it is pulled behind the oesophagus towards right side to form right limb of the fundic wrap. Anterior wall of the fundus forms the left limb of the wrap. By holding both limbs of the fundus/proposed wrap it is glided gently behind the oesophagus to position it properly (John Hunter's shoe shine technique). Colour of the wrap should be noted. If it becomes congested and bluish that means fundal mobilisation is inadequate compromising the vascularity. When traction pull on the right limb is released wrap should stay in place freely to confirm that wrap is adequately mobilised. 2-zero polypropylene suture is used for fundoplication. 60 French oesophageal bougie/dilator is passed

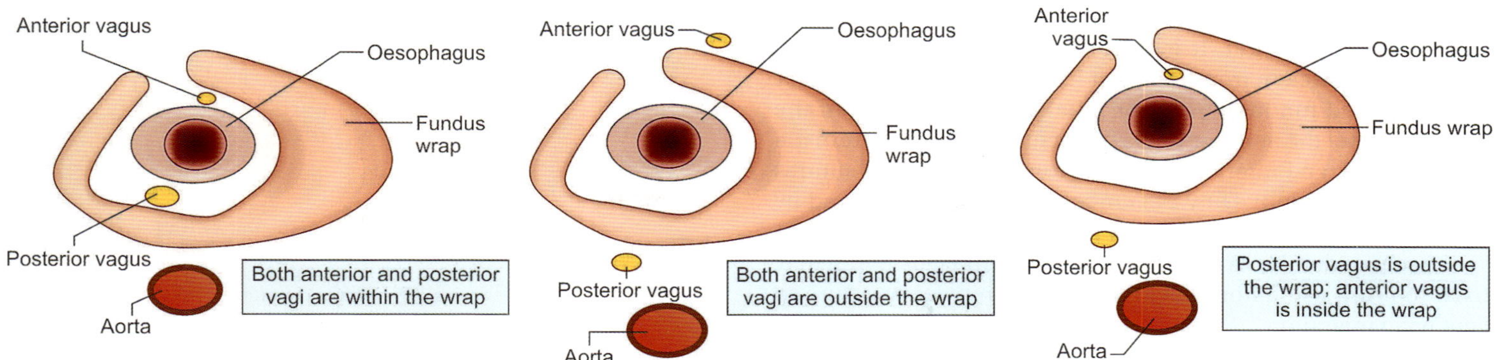

Fig. 20-33: During fundal wrap vagi are kept in different positions depending on the choice.

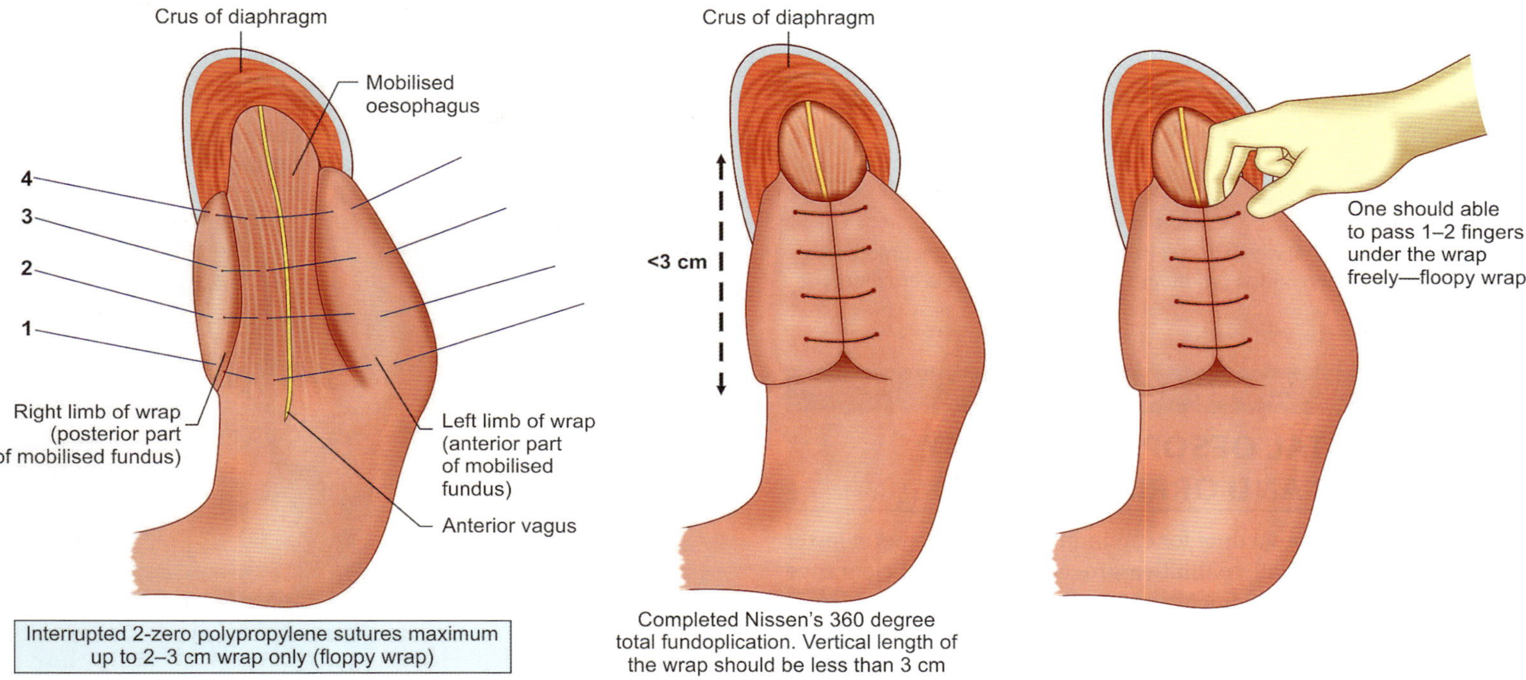

Fig. 20-34: 360° wrapping of the fundus in Nissen's fundoplication.

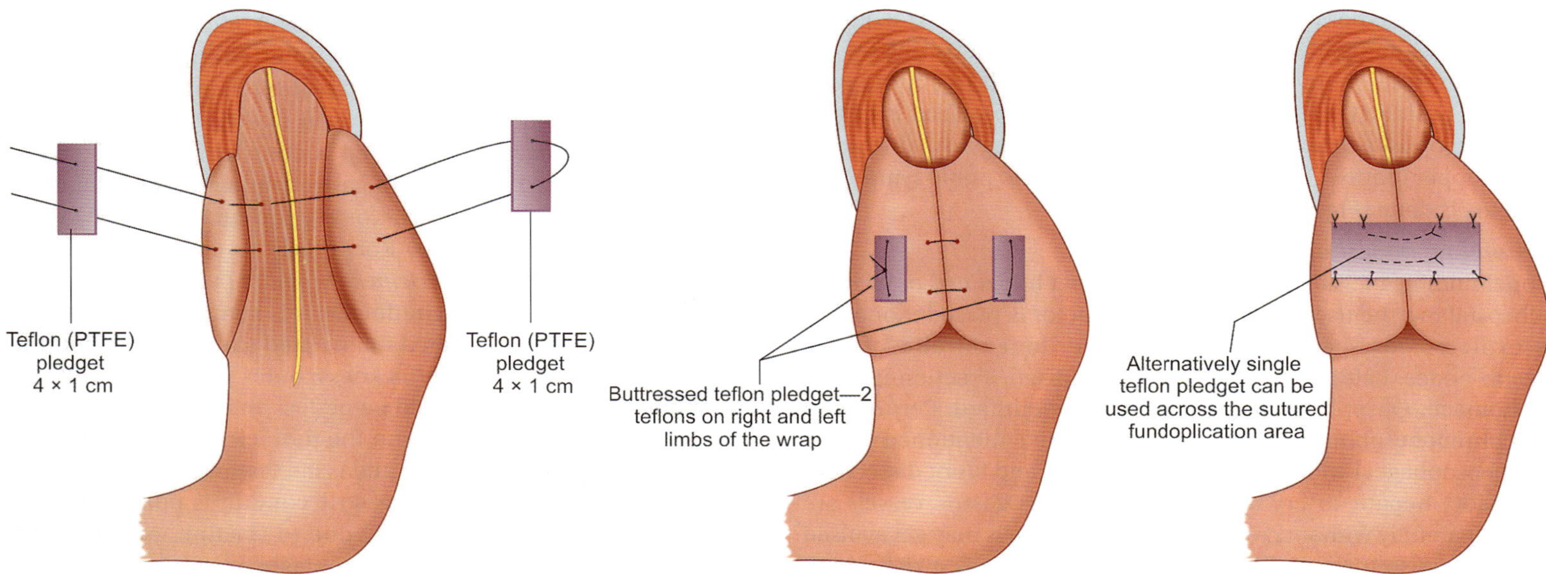

Fig. 20-35: Teflon pledget buttressing in fundoplication.

per orally by anaesthetist to reach the OG junction which facilitates the floppy fundoplication. It is not necessary but optional. Bite (seromuscular) is taken from the right limb of the wrap (posterior wall of mobilised fundus); next bite is taken from the wall of the oesophagus left of the anterior vagus (muscular); last bite is from the left limb of the wrap (anterior wall of the fundus). Usually 3 sutures are placed but not more. Only 2–3 cm length should be covered by the wrap to make it floppy. Floppiness is checked by passing 5 m grasper freely under the wrap in front of the oesophagus. Wrap may be fixed to crura using non-absorbable (polypropylene) suture to prevent wrap migration.

Modified Toupet's partial posterior fundoplication is also done to prevent gas bloat syndrome by suturing the right limb of the wrap to oesophageal muscular wall at 10 o'clock position using interrupted polypropylene sutures; left limb of the wrap is sutured to the left wall of the oesophagus similarly at 2 o'clock position to complete the 270° wrap.

Postoperative care

Nasogastric tube is removed in 24–48 hours. Oral sips are started. Gastroscopy is done during follow up period.

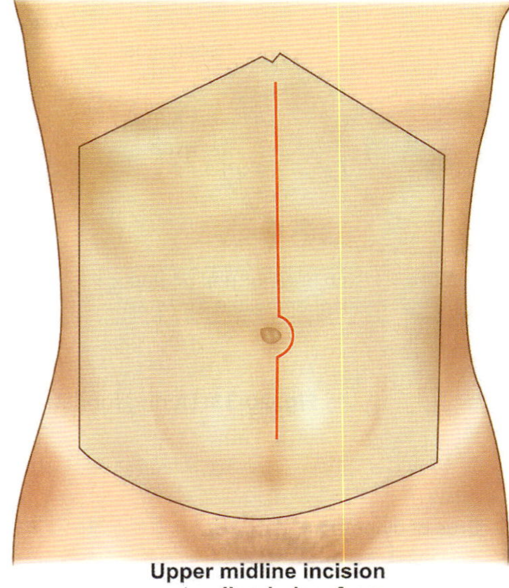

Fig. 20-36: Midline laparotomy incision is commonly used. Often upper horizontal or bilateral subcostal may be used.

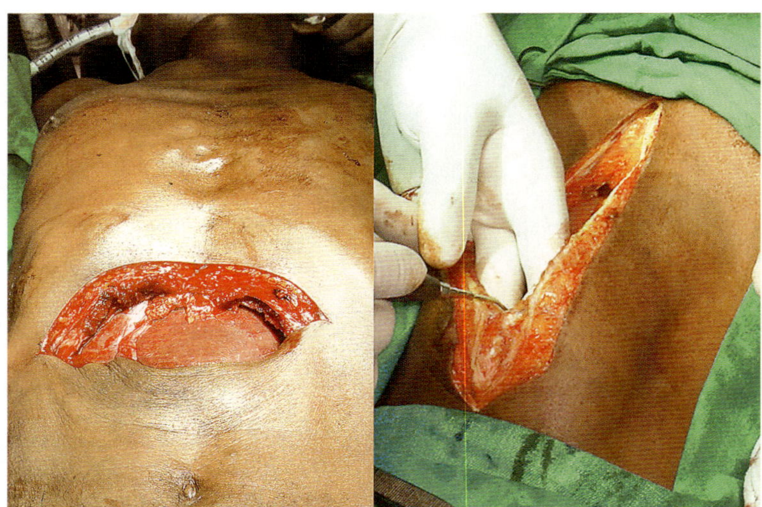

Fig. 20-37: Midline or bilateral subcostal incision can be used.

Complications

Wrap herniation (1%) which occurs in 48 hours; left sided pneumothorax; perforation; spleen injury; gas bloat syndrome; dysphagia are different complications.

OESOPHAGECTOMY

TRANSHIATAL OESOPHAGECTOMY (ORRINGER AND ORRINGER, 1983)

It is commonly done procedure for carcinoma of oesophagus at lower third region. It is basically palliative procedure as nodal clearance not addressed. It is also logically a blind and blunt procedure as thoracic mobilisation of the oesophagus is not under vision. But it avoids the thoracotomy and its problems. Pulmonary complications are less and also duration of hospital stay compared to Ivor Lewis approach. It is also done for benign stricture of the oesophagus.

Procedure is done under general anaesthesia. Nasogastric tube should be in place. Blood should be kept ready in case there is bleeding during thoracic dissection. Intraarterial catheter is required. CVP line has to be ideally placed always. Intravenous line on the left upper limb should be avoided. Position lied in supine with head up position (reverse Trendelenburg position). Head is turned towards opposite side. Neck is extended by placing a small blanket under upper thorax. Cleaning is done from chin to pubic symphysis. Draping is done **(Figs. 20-36 and 20-37)**.

Abdominal dissection

Upper midline incision is placed. Often upper horizontal or bilateral subcostal may be used. Self-retaining retractor is placed. Abdomen is explored for secondaries in liver, peritoneum and coeliac lymph nodes. Left lobe of the liver is mobilised. Traction is given to stomach. Oesophagogastric junction is identified. Peritoneum and phrenooesophageal ligament is incised like mentioned above. Retrooesophageal window is created by sharp and blunt dissection. Accessory hepatic artery may be ligated. Short gastric vessels are ligated carefully without creating traction as vessels may get avulsed and can cause torrential bleeding. Splenic injury is a risk which should be avoided. Handling and traction over the spleen should be gentle with care. Left gastric vessels are doubly ligated securely. Energy sources like harmonic are very useful. But it is ideal to ligate left gastric artery. Vascular clips are other alternative used. Left gastroepiploic vessels are ligated. Greater omentum is cut using harmonic or be sequential ligations to free greater curvature of the stomach. Retrogastric dissection is done by finger and scissor dissection. Right gastric and right gastroepiploic vessels should be retained. Both anterior and posterior vagi are cut **(Fig. 20-38)**.

Duodenum is mobilised by Kocherisation. Pyloromyotomy or pyloroplasty is done. Usually *Heineke Mikulicz* pyloroplasty is done. Pyloroduodenum is cut longitudinally; it is sutured transversely to widen the pylorus. Two layered interrupted sutures are commonly used. Inner 2 zero vicryl full thickness; outer seromuscular 2 zero silk sutures. Pyloroplasty should be perfect and properly done with care as after pull up it will stay in the thoracic cavity and any bile leak will enter the pleural cavity and is life threatening. Many prefer pyloromyotomy because while gastric conduit is pulled upwards pyloroplasty suture may give way due to traction. Metallic clips are placed at the edges of the pyloroplasty or pyloromyotomy as identification radiologic markers **(Fig. 20-39)**.

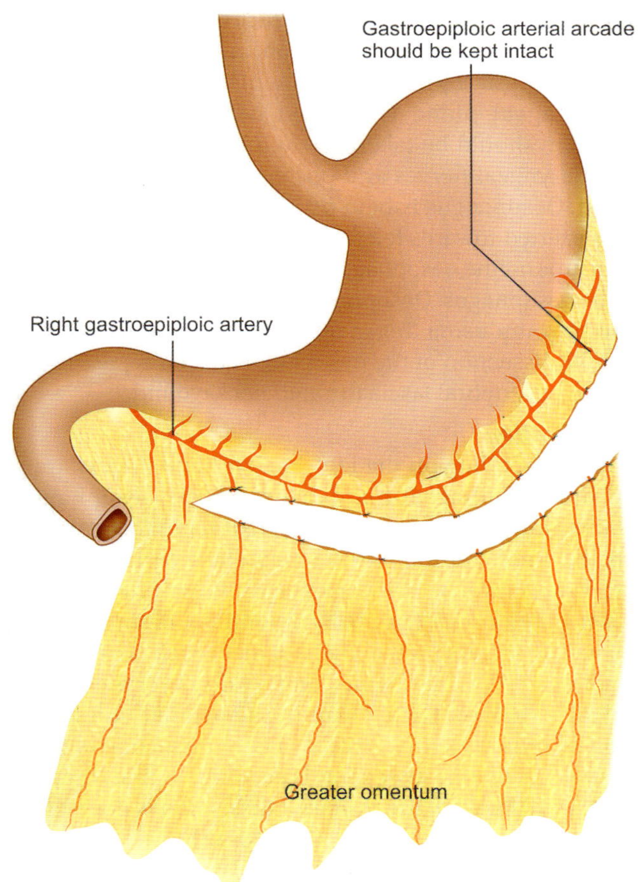

Fig. 20-38: Gastroepiploic arcade should be kept intact in gastric pull up procedures when stomach is used as conduit.

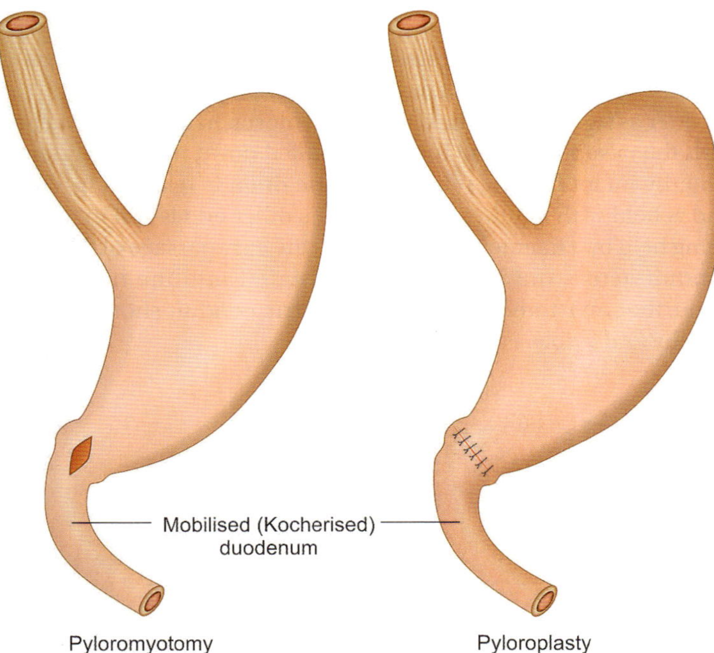

Fig. 20-39: Kocherisation is done; pylorus is widened usually by pyloromyotomy; often pyloroplasty is done.

Hiatus is gently dissected to free oesophagus; often a cut in the crus may be needed. Transverse phrenic vein which is present there needs ligation. This also facilitates the adequate accommodation of the pulled up stomach; if hiatus is not widened, congestion of the stomach can occur which is risky. Penrose drain or umbilical tape or any type of slings is passed around the OG junction, which helps in providing traction and further dissection. Hiatus should be widened about 3 fingers. Fingers are passed across the hiatus to feel the tumour and if it is adherent to aorta or vertebra transhiatal procedure is contraindicated. Pericardium can be gently reflected forward. Both side pleura are retracted laterally. Index and middle fingers are passed across the hiatus close to the oesophageal wall to dissect the perioesophageal loose areolar tissue. If fingers are kept adjacent to oesophageal wall it is less likely to injure the azygos veins even though there is small risk as procedure is blind. Fingers can be reached easily up to the carina of trachea. One should be very careful here as membranous trachea may be closer to oesophageal wall which may get injured. Injury to trachea membranacea is very difficult to manage and is near life threatening even though immediate right sided thoracotomy and suturing of the carina at its membrane is done but most of the time it is futile and patient succumbs. Dissection often still is possible to do under direct vision up to the arch of aorta; it is done with gentle traction, clipping of perioesophageal vessels and cutting the tissue; further traction and clipping like that sequentially. This is better facilitated by using a head lamp by the surgeon **(Fig. 20-40)**.

Dissection in the neck

Cervical oesophagus is approached usually through left side as in the neck oesophagus more towards left side. Surgeon stands on the left side of the patient. But if patient has undergone any surgery of the neck earlier then right side approach is used **(Figs. 20-41A to C)**.

Incision is usually oblique vertical along the anterior border of the sternocleidomastoid muscle from sternal notch to mandibular level. Cosmetic low horizontal incision also can be used. Sternocleidomastoid muscle is retracted laterally; *omohyoid* and often sternothyoid are divided. Carotid sheath with vessels is retracted laterally. Strap muscles are retracted medially to expose the thyroid and middle thyroid vein. Middle thyroid vein is ligated. Inferior thyroid artery is dissected and usually requires ligation but often preserved. Recurrent laryngeal nerve is identified and safeguarded. It is not always necessary to identify the recurrent laryngeal nerve. It is better to use *assistant's finger as retractor* on the medial aspect over trachea to prevent injury to recurrent laryngeal nerve by a metal retractor.

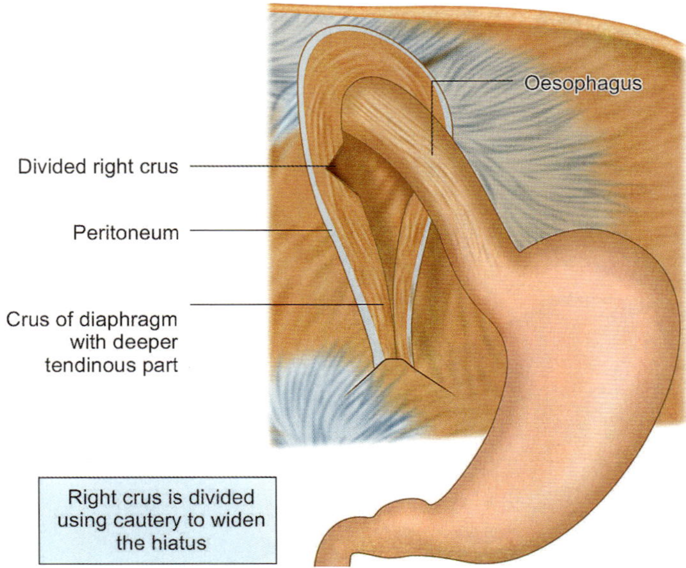

Fig. 20-40: To widen the hiatus right crus may be cut when needed.

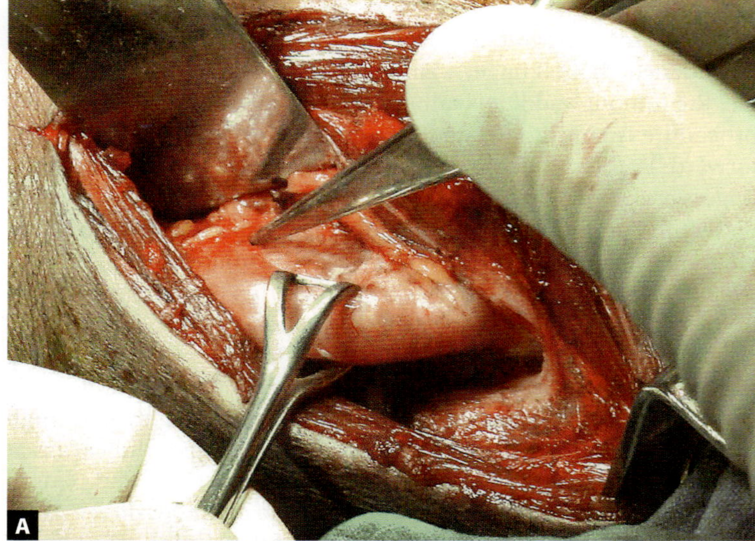

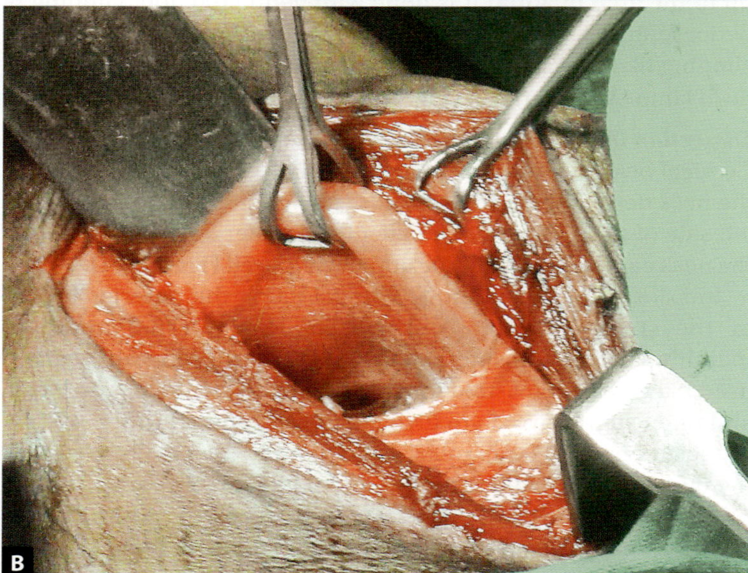

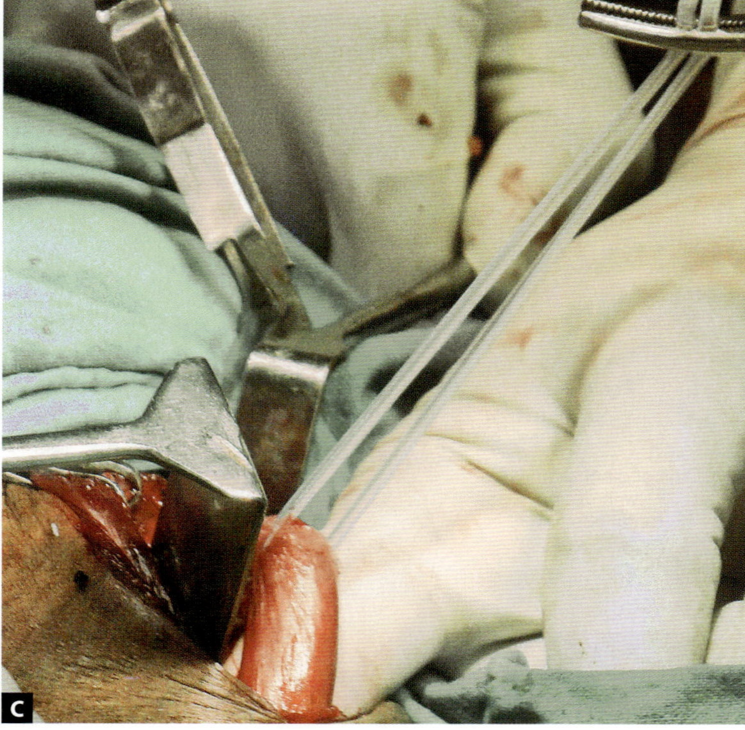

Figs. 20-41A to C: Neck dissection to mobilise cervical oesophagus.

Oesophagus is visualised behind trachea as a vertical muscular tube. Lateral lobe of the thyroid is in front and lateral to it. Nasogastric tube can be felt easily by fingers. By careful blunt and sharp dissection retrooesophageal plane is created between oesophagus and vertebra. Care should be taken not to injure the oesophageal wall. Recurrent laryngeal nerves and posterior wall of trachea also may get injured. Oesophagus is held using a Babcock clamp and gentle traction is exerted towards left side to complete the finger and sharp dissection around the oesophagus. A Penrose drain or sling is passed around the oesophagus. Oesophagus is further mobilised in the neck up to the sternum using finger. *Sponge on a stick* also can be used for posterior dissection of the oesophagus which is passed gently in front of the prevertebral fascia through neck wound.

Final mobilisation

With surgeon standing on the left side left hand fingers are passed through the oesophageal hiatus close to the oesophageal wall along the posterior mediastinum and right hand fingers are passed through the neck behind the trachea close to the oesophagus. Slight traction is given to the oesophagus. Blunt finger dissection is carried out gently circumferentially around the oesophagus. Fingers from below and fingers from above will meet each other to complete the dissection and mobilisation. Compression over the heart should be avoided; if there is any change in the arterial pressure fingers should be withdrawn temporarily and later dissection is completed again. Usually posterior dissection is carried out first; then anterior dissection. Upper part of the posterior dissection is done often from upper part using a *sponge on stick* **(Fig. 20-42)**.

Oesophagus is transected 5 cm distal to the cricopharyngeus between two occlusion clamps. Stay sutures are placed on to the proximal cut end of the oesophagus including the mucosa to prevent mucosal retraction. Linear stapler can also be used. A roller gauze or Penrose drain is tied around the distal cut of the oesophagus in the neck.

Oesophagus is pulled down into the abdomen across the posterior mediastinum and hiatus. Long Penrose drain or infant feeding tube is better as its free end is held with a haemostat in the neck; other end with the oesophagus and tumour is pulled down into the abdomen. Lengthy infant feeding tube or Penrose drain is released by cutting and is held with another haemostat; its other end is still in the neck being held by a haemostat. This allows the easy passage of the gastric conduit across the posterior mediastinum into the neck wound for further anastomosis. Tip of the gastric conduit should be pink, healthy and viable.

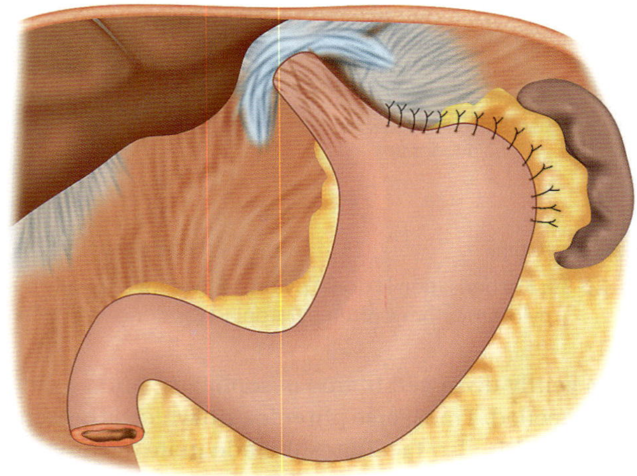

Fig. 20-42: fundal mobilisation.

Gastric conduit (Neooesophagus) creation

In the abdomen stomach is transected just distal to the OG junction using stapler. Stomach along the greater curvature is longitudinally transected distal to the OG junction for 6 cm. Stomach wall is sutured securely using 2-zero sutures in two layers. If stapler is used stapler line may be supported with seromuscular sutures. Entire oesophagus with tumour is removed. Gastric conduit is passed across the posterior mediastinum towards the neck wound. Often stay suture/s is/are placed on the wall/s of the gastric conduit to confirm that twist/rotation of stomach wall has not occurred. Often posterior part of the gastric conduit is fixed to the longus coli muscle in the neck with few serosal interrupted sutures. These *suspension sutures* are no longer said to be essential. Hiatus should be three finger width to prevent venous congestion over the pulled up gastric conduit. Extra width of the hiatus is narrowed by placing 2-3 interrupted silk sutures to the hiatus which prevents intestinal herniation. Often at the hiatus one or two interrupted sutures are placed between hiatus and anterior gastric wall (adjacent to hiatus). Pyloromyotomy/pyloroplasty usually stays 2–3 cm below the hiatus after gastric conduit pull through **(Fig. 20-43)**.

Anastomosis

Proximal cut end of the oesophagus is anastomosed to the anterior wall of the pulled up gastric conduit as end to side anastomosis. Adequate bleeding from the cut edges of both oesophagus and gastric conduit should be ensured. Oesophageal cut end should be made oblique (anterior flap/part of the oesophagus should be 1 cm longer than posterior flap). Anterior wall of the stomach is incised 3 cm lower to the tip of the gastric conduit. Usually vertical or transverse incision is made and is of 2.5 cm in size; often same sized elliptical piece of the stomach wall may be excised but it is not mandatory. Inner all layer full thickness/mucosa and submucosal layer 3-zero vicryl interrupted sutures are used; outer layer seromuscular/muscular 2- or 3-zero silk sutures are used to complete the anastomosis. Often posterior inner layer interrupted all sutures are placed first and held with different haemostats; knots are tied at the end one by one to achieve proper apposition and inversion. After posterior layer it is better to pass a nasogastric tube across the stoma into the gastric conduit and fix it. But many surgeons pass the nasogastric tube after the completion of the anastomosis by gentle milking of the tube tip. Anastomosis should stay above the level of the clavicle. It should be tension free also **(Fig. 20-44)**.

Suction drain is placed in the neck wound; drain is brought out through a separate wound and fixed to skin. Abdomen is inspected again for any blood trickling from the posterior mediastinum. Position of the gastric conduit gently felt and confirmed. Hiatus should able to accommodate three fingers. If it is widened more than 3 fingers then extra gap can be sutured with few interrupted sutures; this prevents bowel herniation across the hiatus. Feeding jejunostomy is done 15 cm distal to ligament of Treitz for post-operative care **(Figs. 20-45 and 20-46)**.

Abdomen wound is closed in layers. Usually abdomen cavity is not drained; but oozing if expected tube drain is kept in the abdominal cavity. Neck is also closed in layers after placing a suction drain.

If pleural breach is suspected intercostal tube is placed in the thoracic cavity (in 75% of cases ICT is needed). Tube is removed in 72 hours once check chest X-ray shows adequate lung expansion and if there is no air leak or if pleural drain is less than 100 mL **(Fig. 20-47)**.

- Wide gastric conduit is important to preserve the submucosal collateral circulation.
- Adequate/extended Kocherisation is essential to avoid tension on the tip of the gastric conduit.
- Trauma should be avoided on the gastric conduit tip.
- Adequate (3 fingers) hiatal passage to prevent congestion of the gastric conduit.
- Twist/torsion/rotation of the gastric conduit should be avoided.
- Anastomosis should be above the level of clavicle (cervical oesophago-gastric anastomosis; CEGA); it should be tension free; it should have good blood supply.
- Safe pyloromyotomy/pyloroplasty
- Preserve right gastroepiploic and right gastric arterial supply.

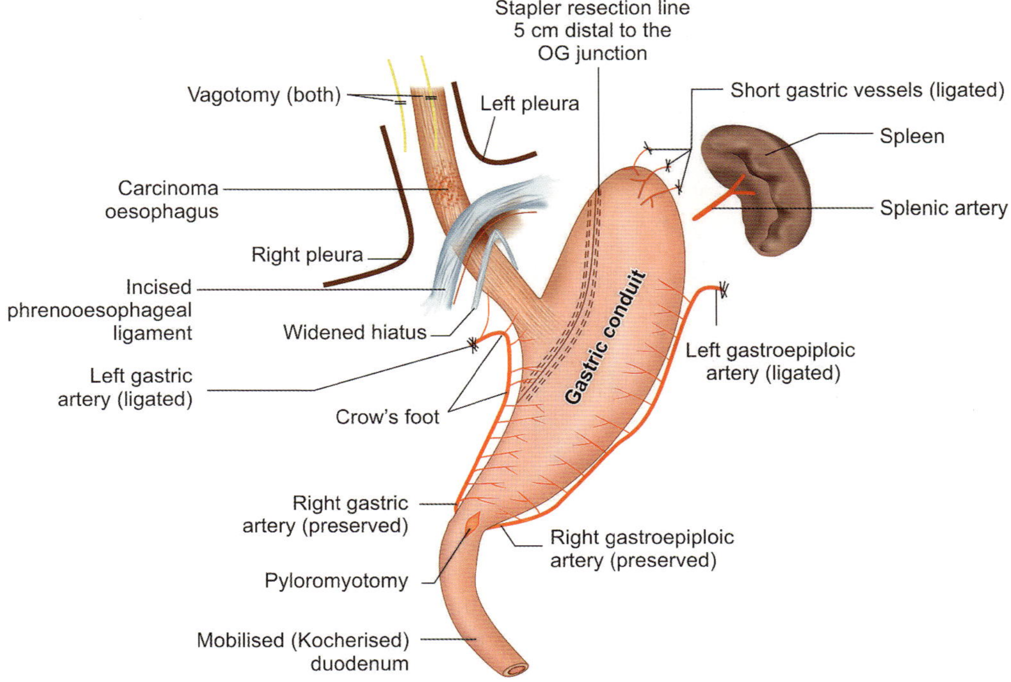

Fig. 20-43: Mobilisation and creation of conduit in transthoracic oesophagectomy.

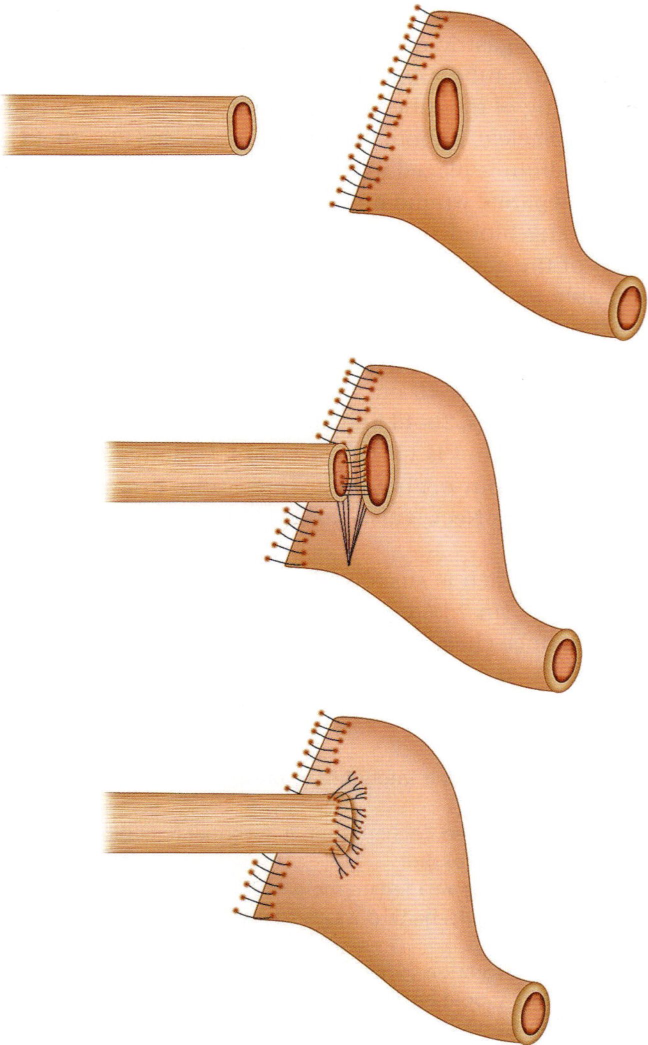
Fig. 20-44: End to side oesophagogastric anastomosis.

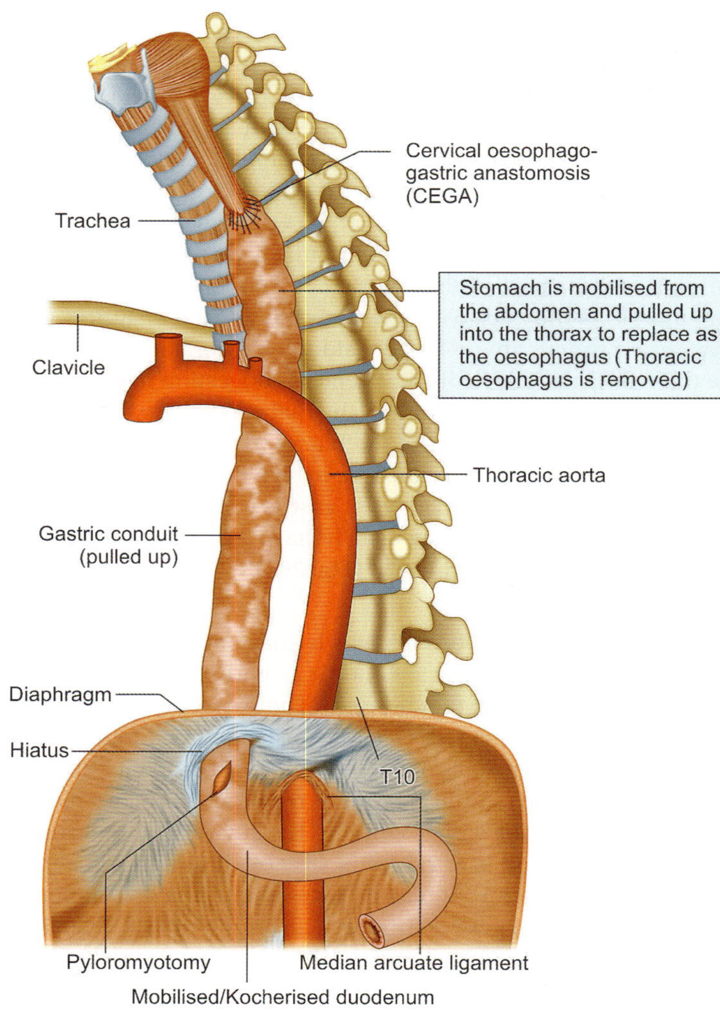

Fig. 20-45: Final look of oesophagogastric anastomosis.

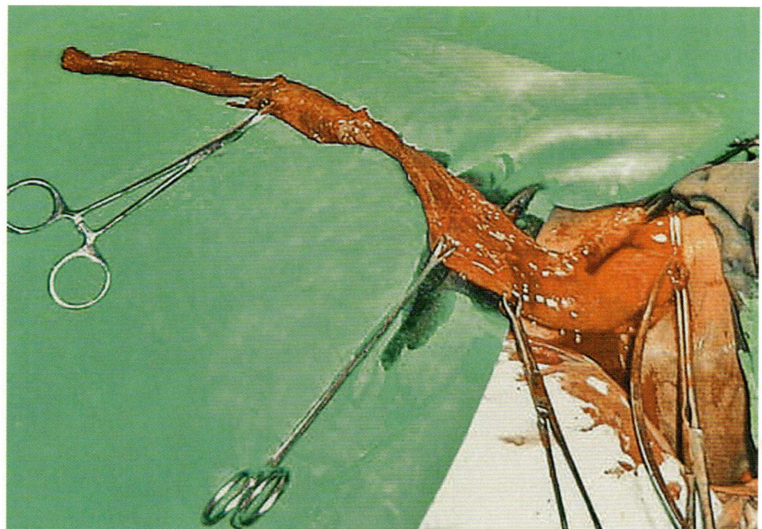
Fig. 20-46: Transhiatal oesophagectomy.

Postoperative care

Nasogastric tube is removed in 5–8 days once bowel sound is heard. Water soluble contrast study may be done after removal of the nasogastric tube (7th day) to confirm that—there is no anastomotic leak; stomach empties adequately; there is no obstruction. Oral sips are started initially later to switch over to semisolid and solid diet.

Complications and problems

Injury to azygos vein and tracheal membrane (less than 1%) at carina even though rare are most dangerous complications. It needs immediate thoracotomy. In case of azygos vein injury, immediate right sided thoracotomy is done; azygos vein is ligated at azgos arch where it enters to superior vena cava. Massive bleeding can occur from avulsion of oesophageal arterial branches from aorta. Whatever the reason, immediate packing through the hiatus and thoracotomy should be done to deal these problems under direct vision. Small linear tear in membranous trachea can be repaired; but avulsion of this part is life threatening. Mortality in transhiatal oesophagectomy is less than 1%.

Injury to spleen may warrant splenectomy (3%). Gastric wall oedema, congestion and necrosis may occur. In such situation if gastric viability is doubtful reexploration is done. Gastric conduit is resected. Colonic conduit is used for maintaining the continuity.

Bile leak, leak through the pleural cavity is again risky, and is difficult to manage. It needs reexploration through thoracotomy and suturing or conversion as colonic conduit. Mortality is very high if there is bile leak into the thoracic cavity. Leak may be from gastric conduit suture line or from pyloroplasty suture site.

Anastomotic leak from oesophagogastric anastomosis site (<10%) is even though not uncommon is less risky as leak is into the neck. Further it is less usually partial and will heal spontaneously. It is better in such situation to keep the nasogastric tube in situ until leak subsides. Rarely it needs surgical reexploration at neck and resuturing.

Thoracic duct injury and lymph ooze can occur. Chylothorax (1%) is suspected when drain persists more than 800 mL/day after 4th postoperative day. Cream is infused through the jejunostomy to observe an opalescent colour in the intercostal tube drain. Thoracic duct injury needs reexploration and duct ligation.

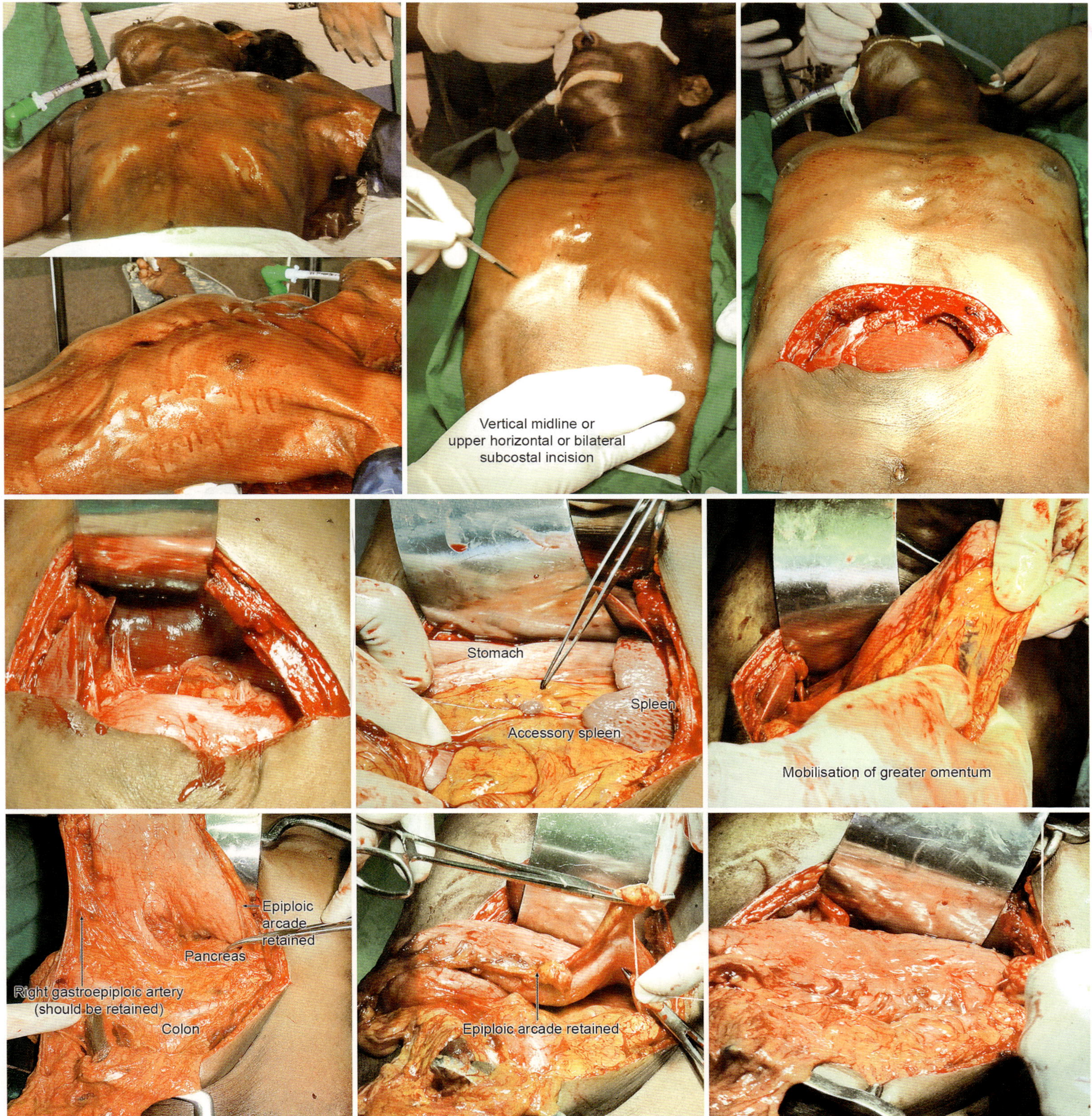

Figs. 20-47(1)

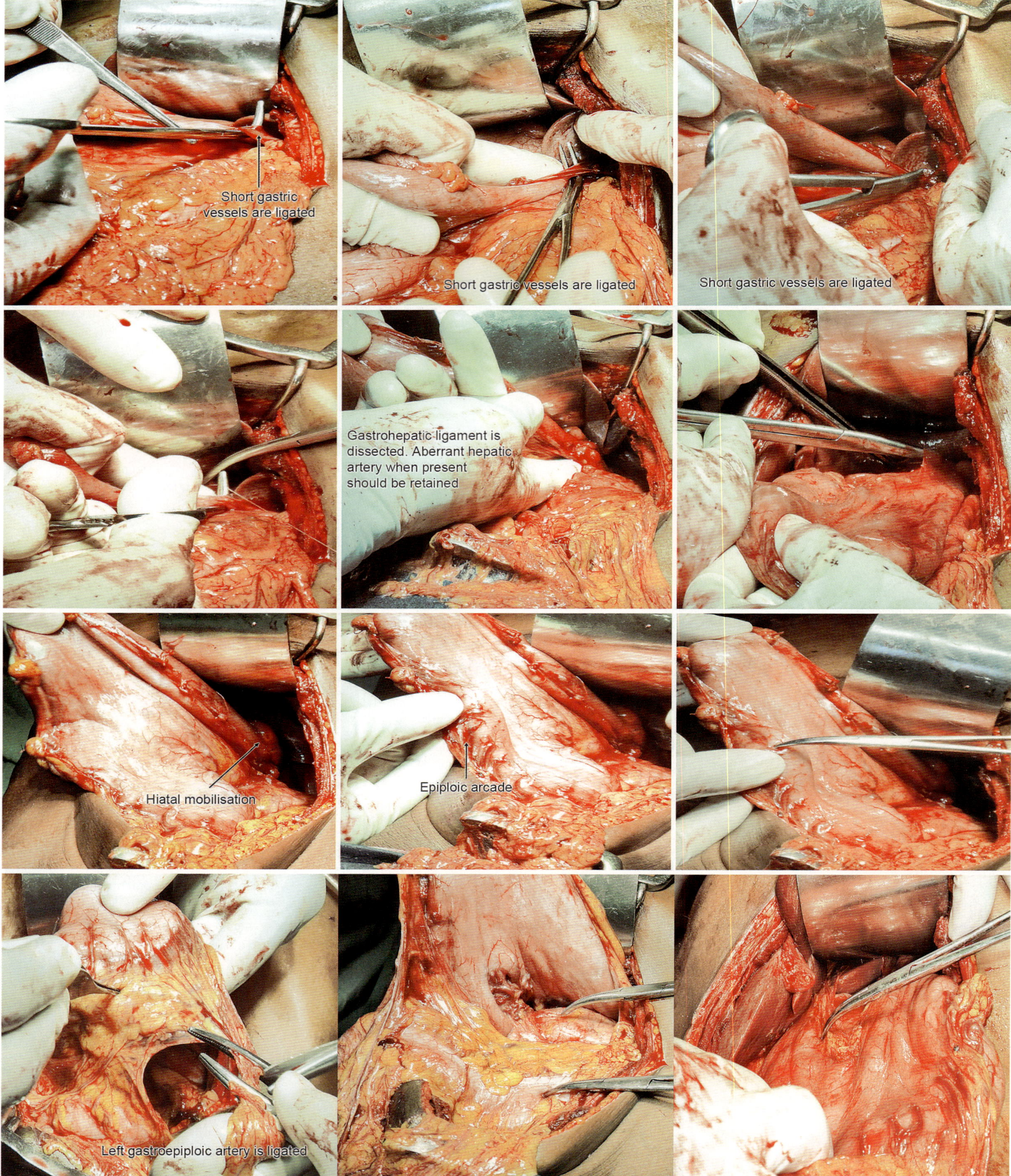
Short gastric vessels are ligated
Short gastric vessels are ligated
Short gastric vessels are ligated
Gastrohepatic ligament is dissected. Aberrant hepatic artery when present should be retained
Hiatal mobilisation
Epiploic arcade
Left gastroepiploic artery is ligated

Figs. 20-47(2)

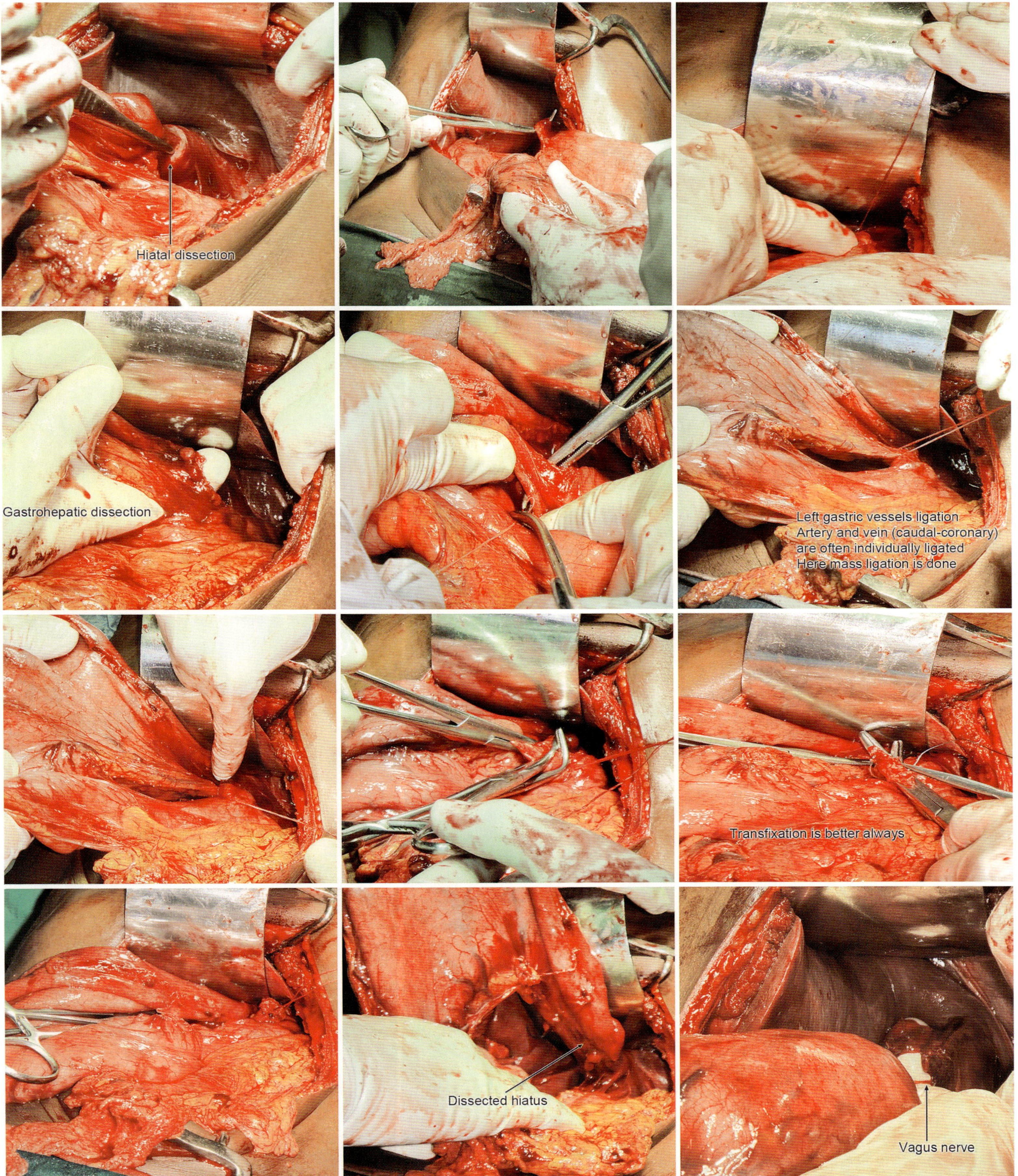
Hiatal dissection
Gastrohepatic dissection
Left gastric vessels ligation
Artery and vein (caudal-coronary)
are often individually ligated
Here mass ligation is done
Transfixation is better always
Dissected hiatus
Vagus nerve

Figs. 20-47(3)

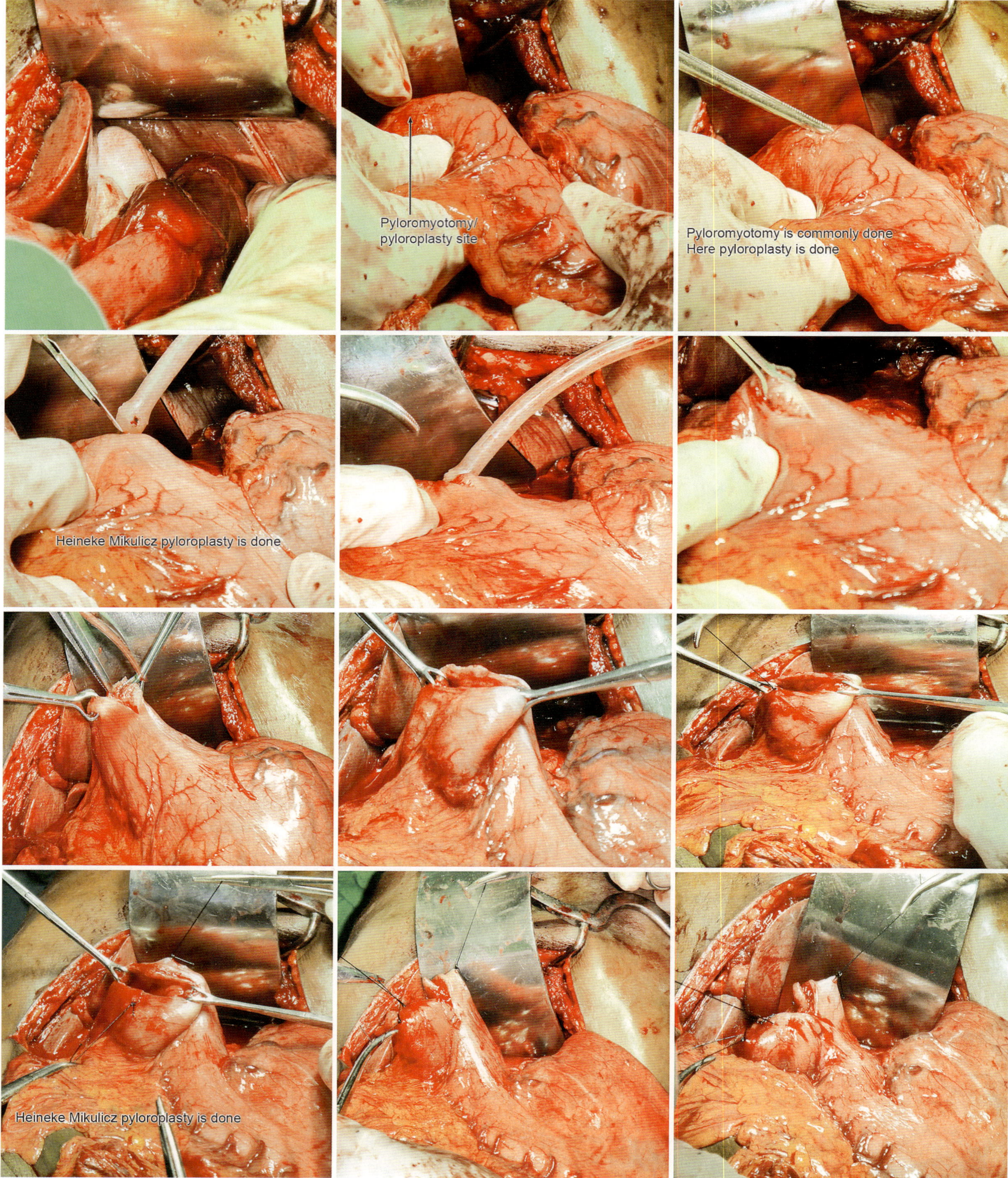
Pyloromyotomy/
pyloroplasty site
Pyloromyotomy is commonly done
Here pyloroplasty is done
Heineke Mikulicz pyloroplasty is done
Heineke Mikulicz pyloroplasty is done

Figs. 20-47(4)

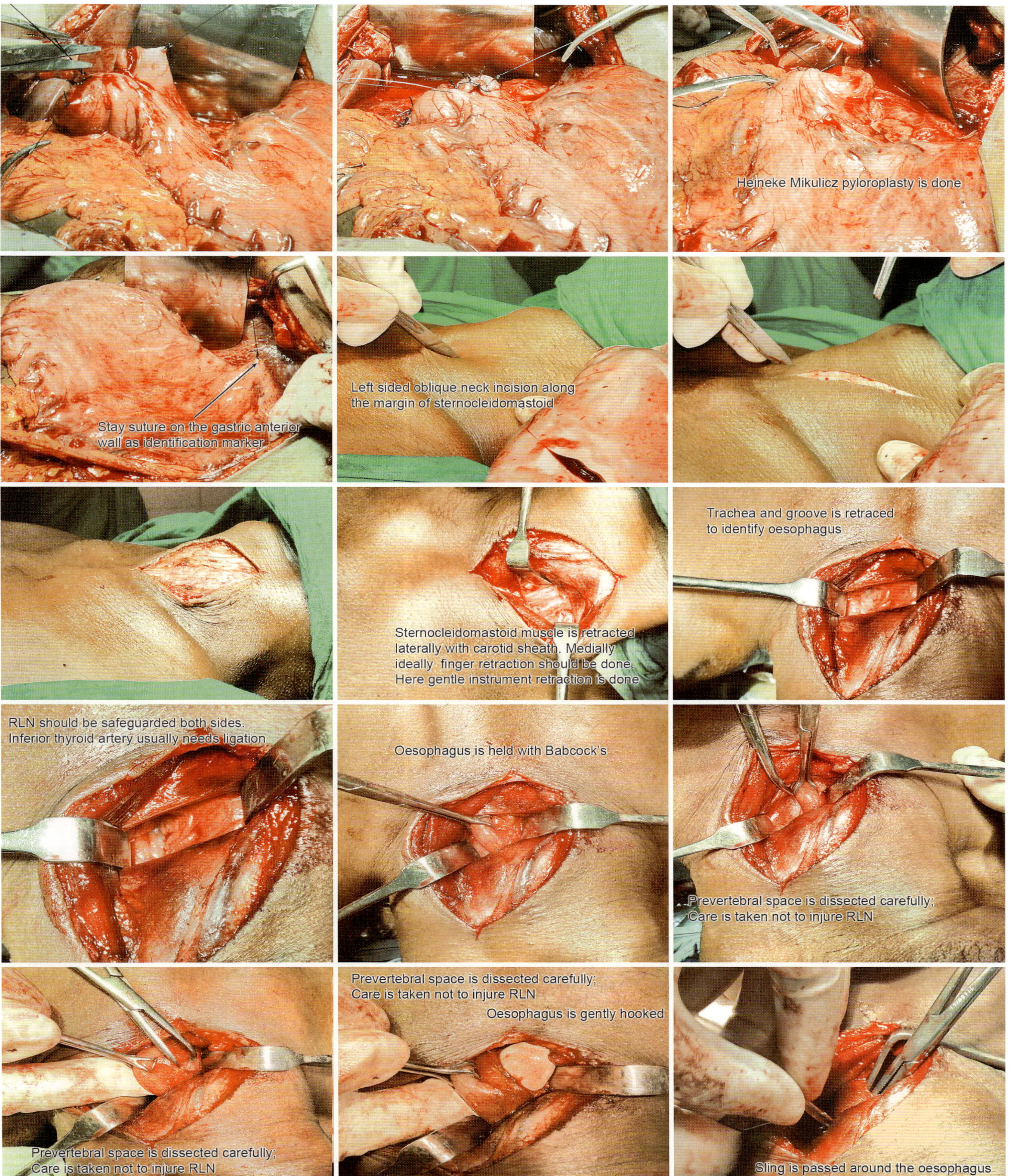
Heineke Mikulicz pyloroplasty is done
Stay suture on the gastric anterior wall as identification marker
Left sided oblique neck incision along the margin of sternocleidomastoid
Sternocleidomastoid muscle is retracted laterally with carotid sheath. Medially ideally finger retraction should be done. Here gentle instrument retraction is done
Trachea and groove is retraced to identify oesophagus
RLN should be safeguarded both sides. Inferior thyroid artery usually needs ligation
Oesophagus is held with Babcock's
Prevertebral space is dissected carefully; Care is taken not to injure RLN
Prevertebral space is dissected carefully; Care is taken not to injure RLN
Prevertebral space is dissected carefully; Care is taken not to injure RLN
Oesophagus is gently hooked
Sling is passed around the oesophagus

Figs. 20-47(5)

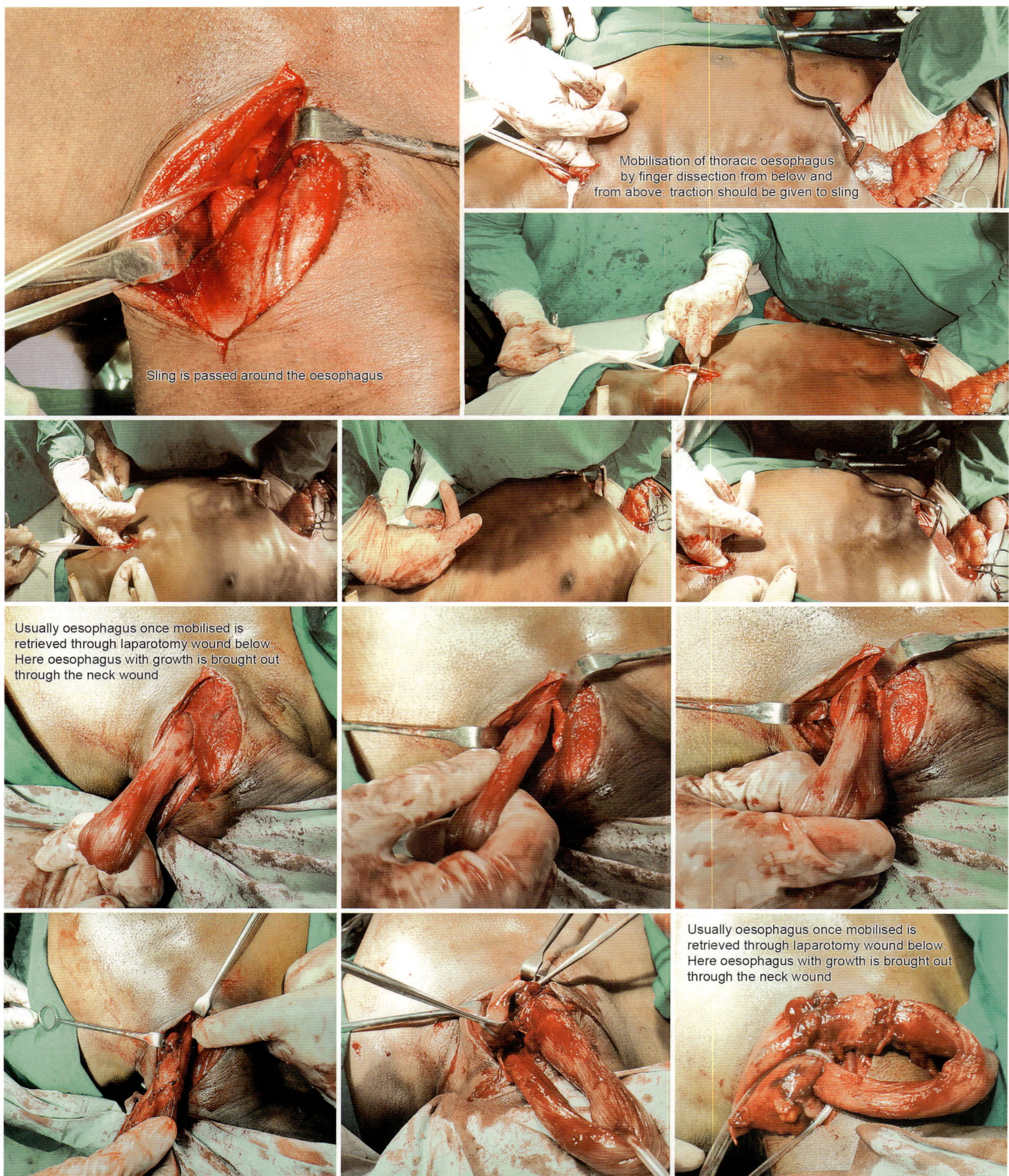
Sling is passed around the oesophagus
Mobilisation of thoracic oesophagus
by finger dissection from below and
from above; traction should be given to sling
Usually oesophagus once mobilised is
retrieved through laparotomy wound below.
Here oesophagus with growth is brought out
through the neck wound
Usually oesophagus once mobilised is
retrieved through laparotomy wound below.
Here oesophagus with growth is brought out
through the neck wound

Figs. 20-47(6)

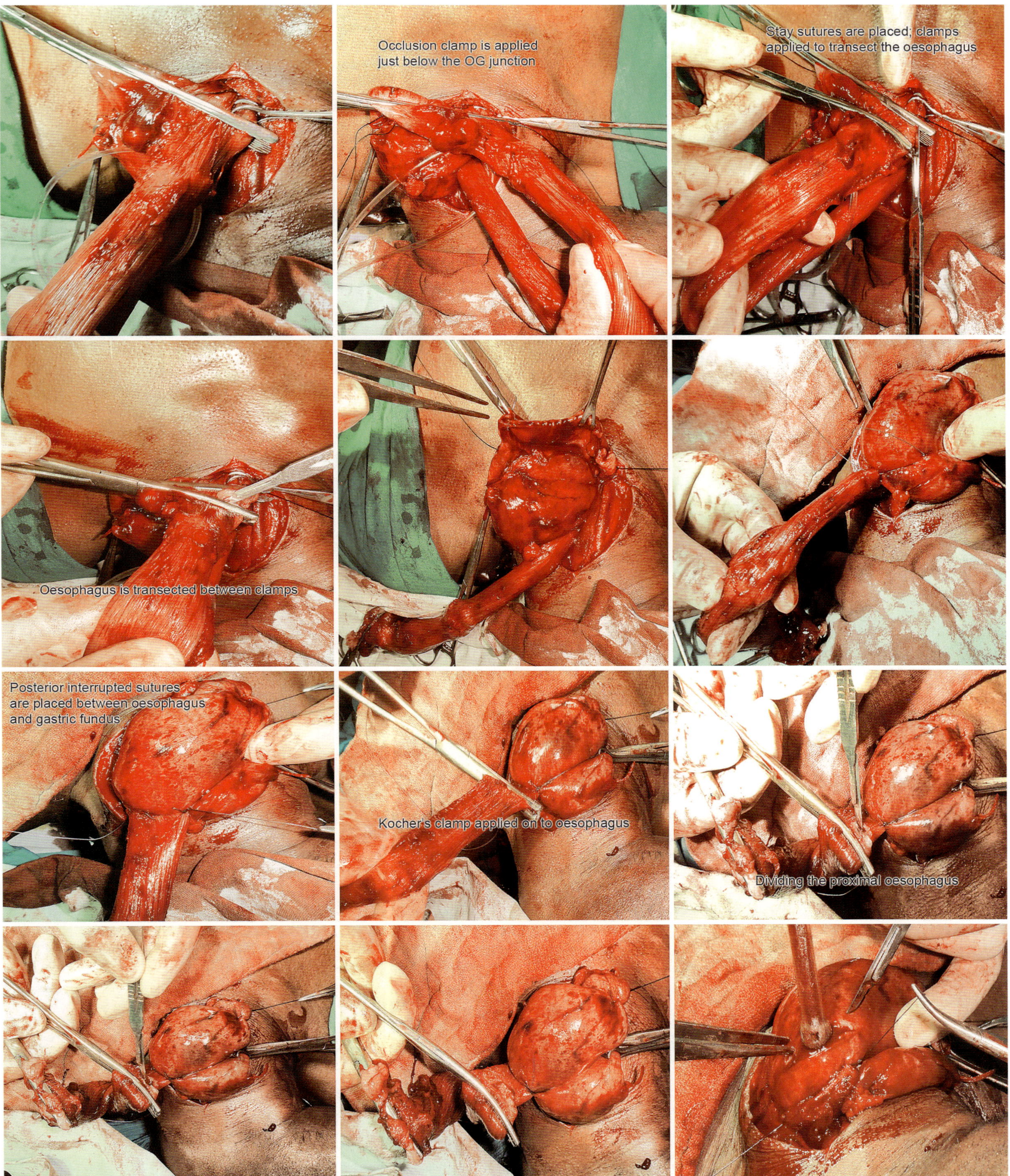
Occlusion clamp is applied
just below the OG junction
Stay sutures are placed; clamps
applied to transect the oesophagus
Oesophagus is transected between clamps
Posterior interrupted sutures
are placed between oesophagus
and gastric fundus
Kocher's clamp applied on to oesophagus
Dividing the proximal oesophagus

Figs. 20-47(7)

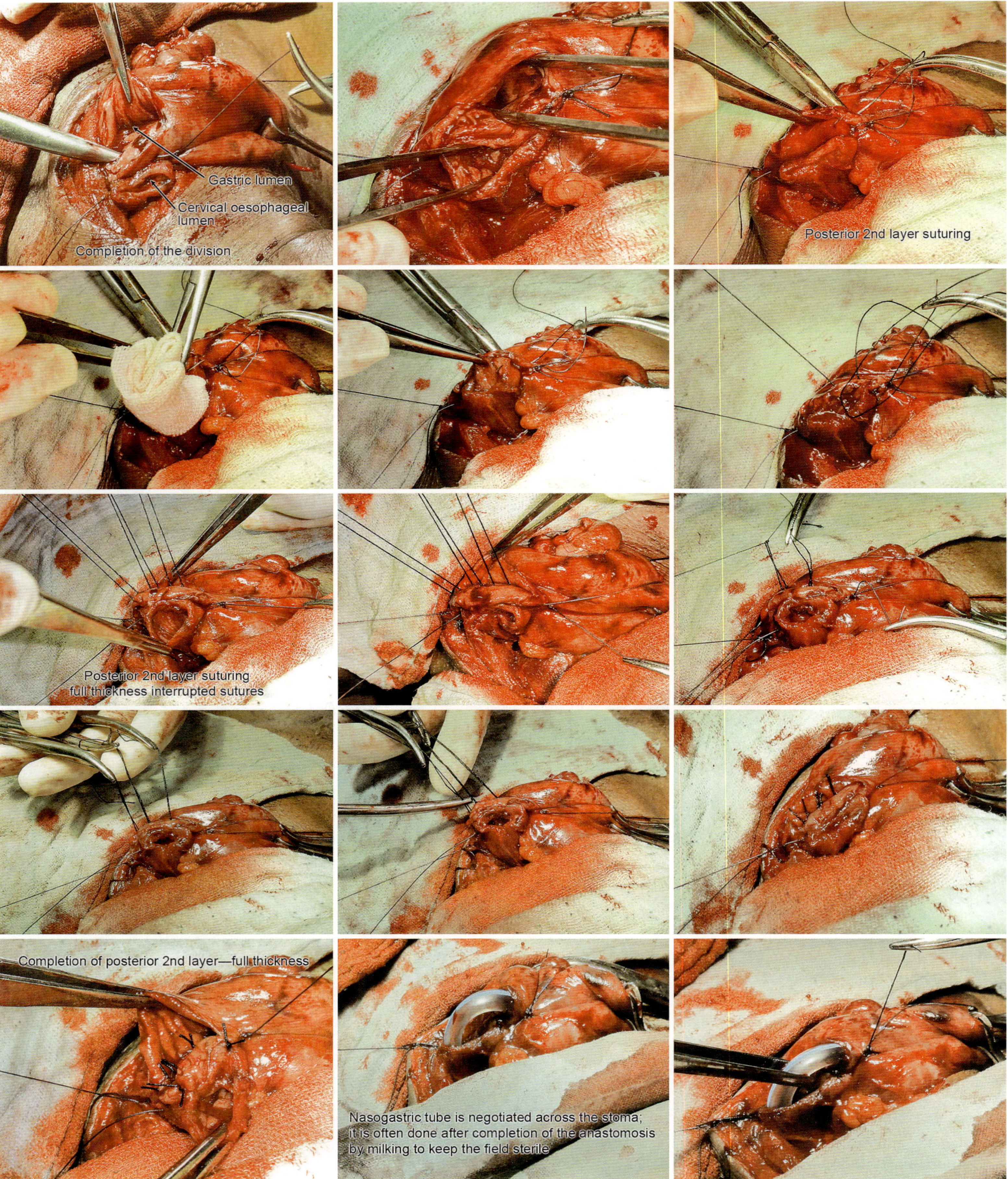
Gastric lumen
Cervical oesophageal lumen
Completion of the division
Posterior 2nd layer suturing
Posterior 2nd layer suturing
full thickness interrupted sutures
Completion of posterior 2nd layer—full thickness
Nasogastric tube is negotiated across the stoma;
it is often done after completion of the anastomosis
by milking to keep the field sterile

Figs. 20-47(8)

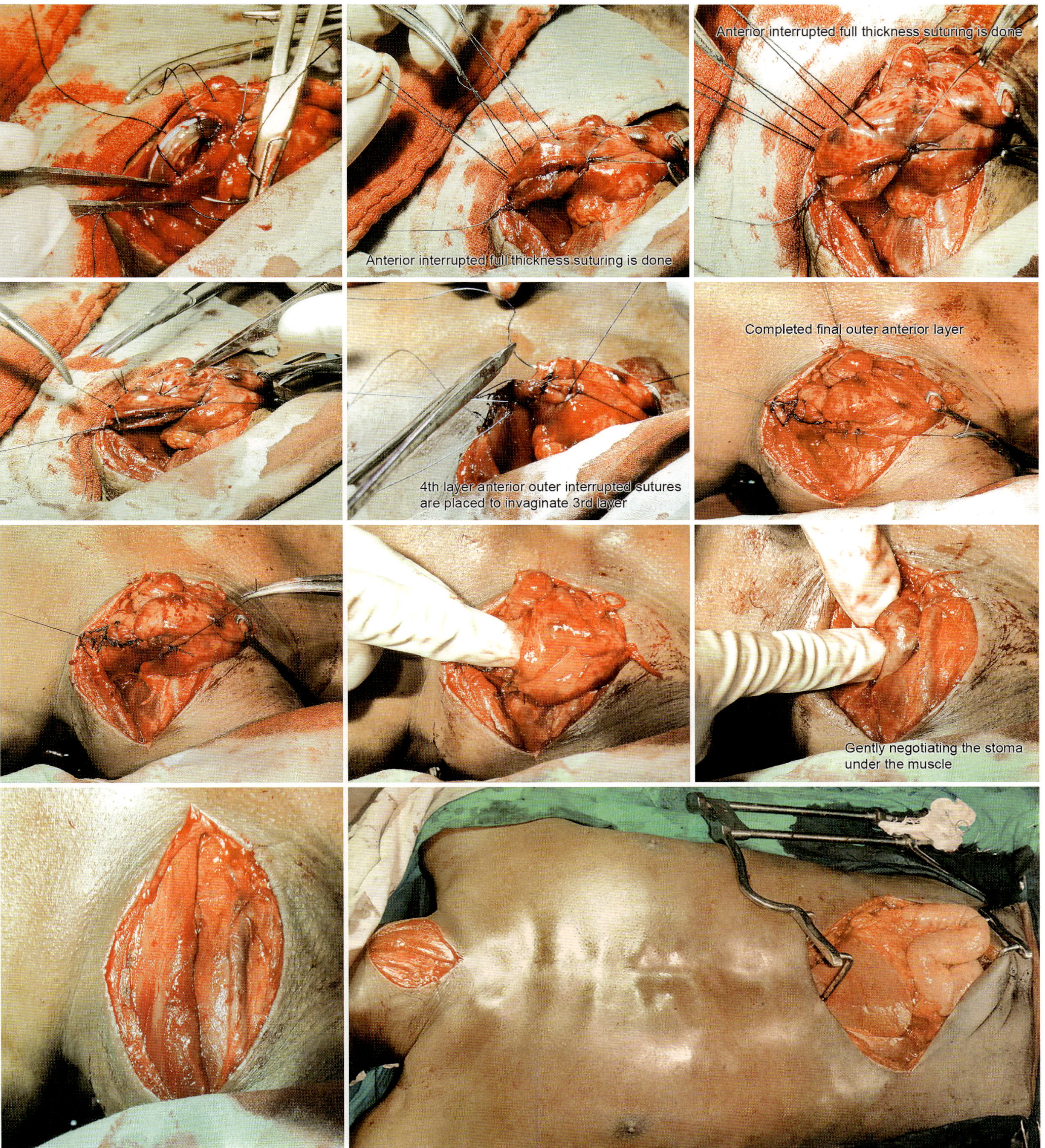
Anterior interrupted full thickness suturing is done
Anterior interrupted full thickness suturing is done
Completed final outer anterior layer
4th layer anterior outer interrupted sutures
are placed to invaginate 3rd layer
Gently negotiating the stoma
under the muscle

Figs. 20-47(9)

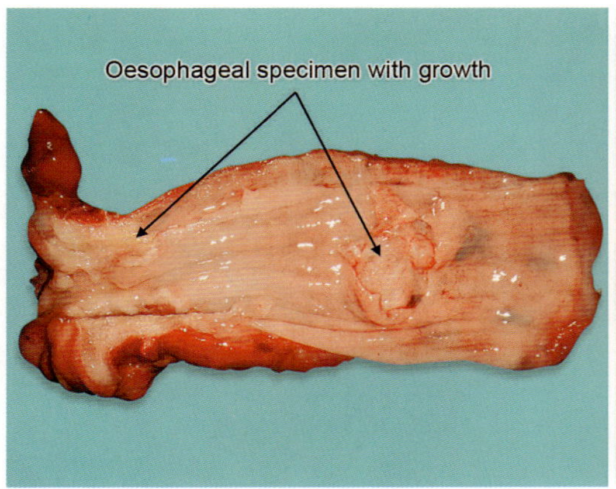

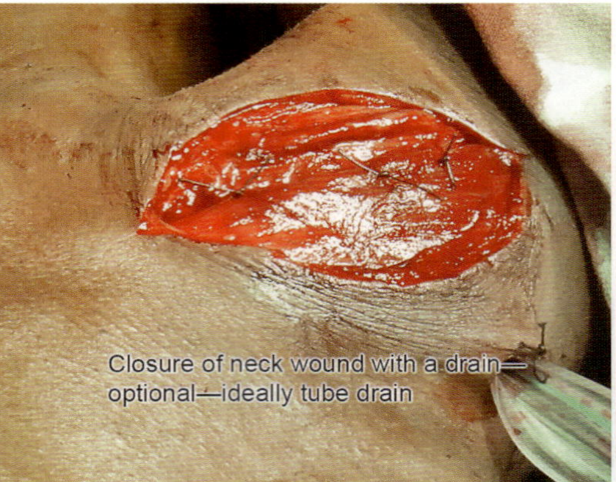

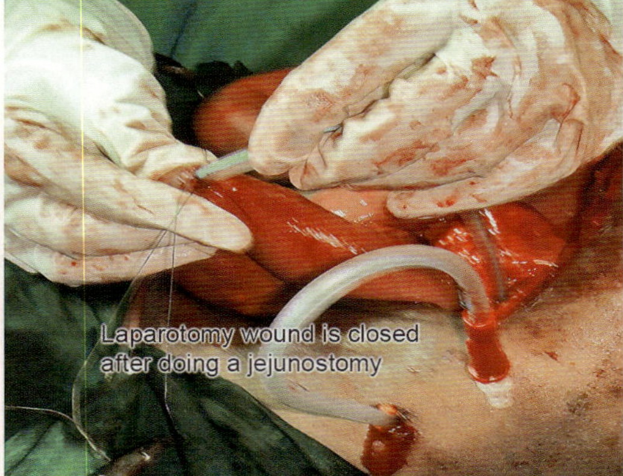

Figs. 20-47(10)

Figs. 20-47 (1 to 10): Technique of transthoracic blunt oesophagectomy with cervical oesophagogastric anastomosis.

Recurrent laryngeal nerve injury (5%) can occur while dissecting in the neck. Metallic retractor medially over the tracheooesophageal groove should be better avoided. Finger retraction is better.

Sepsis, empyema, mediastinitis, bronchopneumonia, ARDS are other complications.

Anastomotic stricture (3%) is not uncommon. It needs regular dilatation. Regurgitation, dumping, post-vagotomy diarrhoea are also common (17%). More frequent food of less quantity, sleeping in upright position, prokinetic drugs are beneficial.

Delayed gastric emptying may be due to pyloric obstruction, obstruction at hiatal level or redundant intrathoracic stomach (retort-shaped stomach into right thorax) lying in the posterior costophrenic gutter. Proper on table pyloromyotomy, 3 fingers hiatal width can prevents this. Additionally prokinetic drugs and often dilatations are beneficial.

Survival rate for carcinoma after transhiatal oesophagectomy is 51% in 2 years and 29% in 5 years. It is comparable with the results of radical oesophagectomy and lymph node dissection.

IVOR LEWIS OPERATION (LEWIS-TANNER)

In 1946, Ivor Lewis (Tanner, 1947) described this procedure. Laparotomy is done. Tumour staging is done to mobilise stomach and stage the disease; right thoracotomy is done; tumour with part of oesophagus and stomach is resected; oesophagogastric anastomosis is done in the thorax. Technique involves coeliac node as well as adjacent thoracic node clearance. Original Ivor Lewis approach is initial laparotomy in supine position; repositioning into right thoracotomy position for thoracic dissection. Now commonly, it is modified as synchronous combined abdominothoracic oesophagectomy without altering the position to approach abdomen and thorax. But finally it is surgeon's comfort and preference.

Patient is placed in semidecubitous position with right side upwards; it makes both abdominal and right posterolateral thoracotomy feasible without changing the position in the middle of the operation. Often midline incision is made in supine position; once initial abdominal part is over patient is positioned in right up position.

General anaesthesia with double lumen endotracheal tube is placed. Cleaning is done from neck along the right chest wall area up to pubic symphysis including entire abdomen. Draping is done.

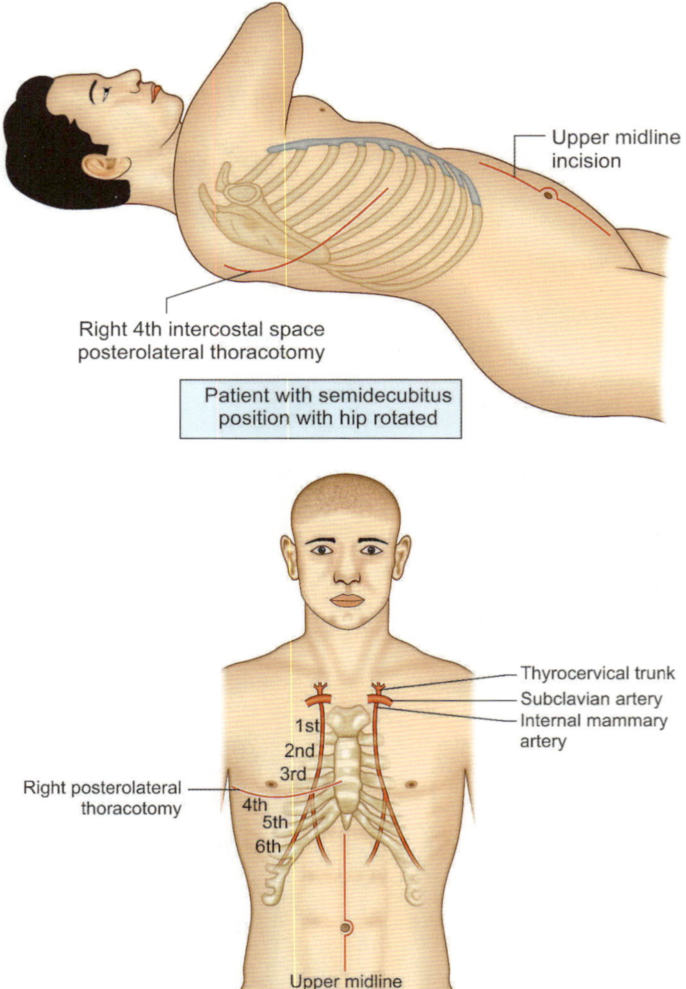

Fig. 20-48: Incision for Ivor Lewis operation.

Head should be turned towards opposite side and right side neck should also be prepared so when need arises anastomosis can be done in the right side neck.

Once exploration through upper midline incision confirms the operability per abdomen thoracotomy is done in right posterolateral 4th intercostal space. Then abdominal mobilisation and thoracic mobilisation of the oesophagus is done **(Fig. 20-48)**.

Abdominal Mobilisation

Self-retaining retractor is placed. Abdomen is explored for secondaries in liver and lymph nodes. Once operability is confirmed, left triangular ligament is divided to retract left lobe of the liver. Phrenooesophageal ligament and peritoneum is incised horizontally and OG junction is mobilised circumferentially with creation of retrooesophagus window. Gastrohepatic ligament is incised; accessory hepatic artery is ligated and divided. Left aberrant hepatic artery which originates from left gastric artery should be suspected if artery is wider than 5 mm and as it may be supplying exclusively left lobe of the liver; if suspected it should be isolated, dissected and preserved. Greater omentum is divided. Short gastric vessels are ligated and divided. Energy sources are better for this. Left gastric artery is ligated at its origin to include the fat and lymph nodes. It is double ligated securely. Left gastric vein is also ligated separately (it is coronary vein and is caudal to artery). Right gastroepiploic and right gastric vessels should be preserved carefully. Bilateral truncal vagotomy is done. Dissection along the greater curvature should be done outside the gastroepiploic arcade and arcade should not get injured. Duodenum is mobilised up to its 3rd part by Kocherisation. Duodenal ligament between the posterior part of the duodenum to Gerota's fascia laterally is a ligamentous structure needs to be divided during Kocherisation. Care should be taken not to injure the superior mesenteric vein while mobilising the 3rd part of the duodenum as traction injury can occur. Heineke Mikulicz pyloroplasty or pyloromyotomy (circular muscle is cut using no. 15 blade) is done. Often stay suture is placed on the anterior part of the stomach to avoid rotation while pulling the stomach into the thorax. Hiatus may be widened by cutting it transversely using cautery.

Thoracic Mobilisation

Right posterolateral thoracotomy is done through 4th or 5th intercostal space. In females incision is made through inframammary crease. Pectoralis major and serratus anterior muscles are cut using cautery along the 4th space. Intercostal muscles are cut adjacent to upper border of 5th rib in the lower part of 4th space to avoid injury to intercostal vessels. Internal mammary artery near the sternal margin is identified, doubly ligated and divided. Pleura is opened. 4th rib near its sternal end is cut using bone cutter. Intercostal vessels at its lower margin is ligated and divided. Finochietto retractor is used to retract the ribs and so to expose the thoracic cavity. Usually wet mops are placed under the blades of the retractor. If further retraction is needed 5th rib can be cut like 4th rib. Incision if needed can be extended posteriorly up to the paraspinal muscles. Thoracic cavity is explored for secondaries in the lung and nodes. Mediastinal pleura is incised longitudinally on the surface of the oesophagus. Nasogastric tube facilitates identification of the oesophagus. On table, endoscopy may be useful to identify the oesophagus or to improve the dissection. At one point oesophagus is mobilised circumferentially with sharp and blunt dissection; it is encircled with a sling (or umbilical tape or infant feeding tube). Sling is used for traction to proceed with further mobilisation of the oesophagus. Oesophagus is mobilised below up to the hiatus through which finger can be passed easily as hiatus below is already dissected. Upwards dissection is done behind the tracheal carina. Small arterial branches entering are divided between ligatures or haemoclips or harmonic scalpel can be used. Monopolar cautery is usually avoided; but bipolar cautery is quite useful. Azygos vein is visible on the right side which is arching above towards the superior vena cava. Azygos vein is doubly ligated (two on each side) at the beginning where it arches. Double ligation is needed. Care should be taken not to injure the superior vena cava. Vascular stapler can be used for the same. Often azygos vein is ligated at the level of hemiazygos vein (T8) especially if oesophageal transection is being done at lower level. If possible it is better to ligate the thoracic duct at this level to avoid its injury and leak. Fat, lymph nodes and adjacent tissues are dissected which should be included in the oesophageal specimen. Oesophagus is mobilised from thoracic aorta. All small vessels are ligated or fulgarated using bipolar or by harmonic scalpel. Proximal mobilisation should be 10 cm from the upper margin of the gross tumour. Mobilised stomach is passed through the widened hiatus into the thoracic cavity. Rotation of the stomach should be avoided by identifying the stay suture. Stomach just beyond the OG junction along the lesser curve is divided using stapler. Otherwise transection is done in between two occlusion clamps and stomach side is closed with two layer sutures (inner continuous 2-zero vicryl sutures; outer interrupted 2-zero silk sutures). 10 cm proximal to the tumour oesophagus is transected between clamps; specimen is removed. Proximal margin should be sent for frozen section biopsy.

Oesophagogastric Anastomosis

On the anterior wall of the mobilised stomach just distal to the sutured/stapled line 1.5 cm wide circular stomach wall is excised; alternatively just 1.5 cm horizontal/vertical incision is also sufficient instead of circular tissue. It is said that removal of circular piece of stomach wall prevents anastomotic stricture formation but that is not proved; so it is of surgeon's preference. Oesophageal cut end is made oblique for anastomosis. Outer layer suturing is done using interrupted 2 or 3 zero silk sutures taking bite from seromuscular layers of stomach and muscular layer of oesophagus (Once posterior outer layer suturing is over if stomach is not yet incised or circular piece is not removed, then an incision is made over the anterior wall of the stomach 2 cm below the transected part of the stomach). Inner all layer full thickness bite taken from the stomach wall; bite is taken from the mucosa and submucosa of the oesophagus (often muscular layer bite is also taken) using 2- or 3-zero silk or vicryl. Knots can be placed inside. Similarly anterior inner layer interrupted sutures are placed with knots inside. Sutures should be placed for every 3 mm width with bite point at 3 mm from the cut edge. After that anterior outer layer sutures are placed as interrupted seromuscular sutures. As oesophagus is cut obliquely with anterior edge lengthier (1 cm) than posterior edge, anastomosis becomes tension free **(Fig. 20-49)**.

In another method: OG junction is transected using stapler or between clamps and sutured. Stomach is pulled upwards into the right thoracic cavity across the widened hiatus. Mobilised oesophagus with tumour is held upwards; two stay sutures using 3-zero silk are placed between oesophagus 10 cm proximal to the upper margin of the tumour and 5–6 cm below uppermost part of the mobilised anterior wall of the stomach. Posterior interrupted sutures are placed between seromuscular stomach wall and muscular oesophageal wall. Posterior wall of the oesophagus is cut 5–6 mm distal to the sutured layer using 15 no. blade to identify nasogastric tube and mucosa. Incision (full thickness) over the stomach is made similarly distal to posterior layer; bleeding edges can be suture ligated or cauterised using bipolar cautery. Posterior mucosal layers of the oesophagus and stomach taking proper bites including submucosa at 3 mm intervals and 3 mm distant from the cut edges of stomach and oesophagus. Knots are tied inside the lumen.

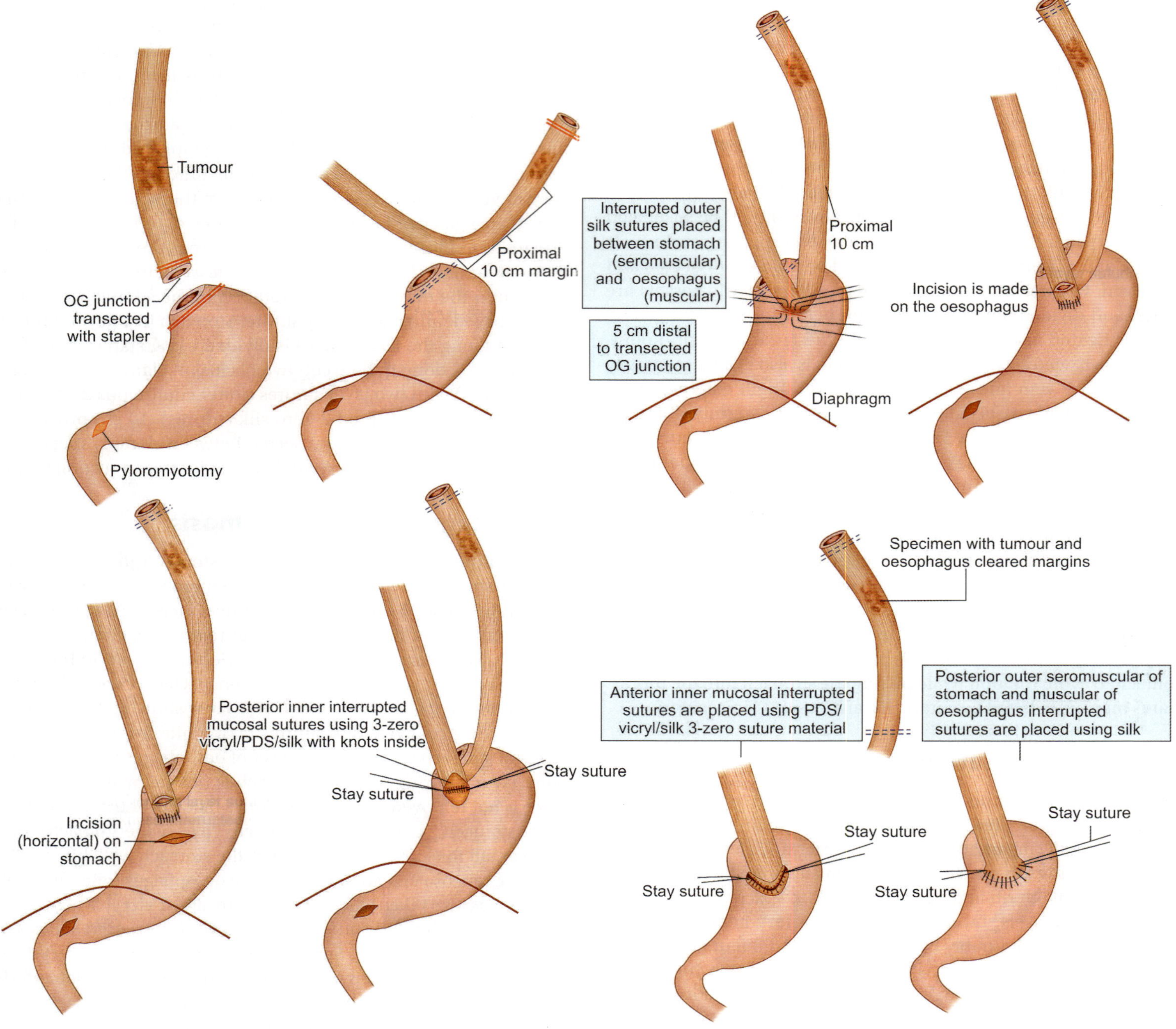

Fig. 20-49: Oesophagogastric anastomosis in thorax in Ivor Lewis operation.

This layer is usually of interrupted sutures but continuous suture also can be placed. Anterior wall of the oesophagus is cut 1 cm distal to the level of posterior wall to retrieve the specimen. Anterior mucosal layers are sutured similarly with knots tied inside the lumen. Anterior layers (seromuscular) of stomach and of oesophagus (muscular) are finally sutured with interrupted sutures.

Note: Anastomosis can also be done using stapler.

Stomach is fixed to prevertebral fascia with interrupted sutures to prevent tension over the anastomosis. Omentum may be tagged over the anastomotic site. Hiatus should be 3 fingers wide. Hiatus is fixed to the stomach using few interrupted silk sutures. Jejunostomy is done 15 cm from the ligament of Treitz.

Intercostal tube is placed into the thoracic cavity. Thoracotomy is closed in layers. Abdomen is also closed in layers with or without tube drain **(Fig. 20-50)**.

Postoperative Care

Nasogastric tube should be kept in situ for 5–7 days. Chest tube is removed once adequate lung expansion has occurred which is confirmed by chest X-ray and pleural drain is less than 100 mL/day.

Complications

Anastomotic leak is dangerous as anastomosis is in the thorax.
Bleeding can occur; but usually subsides.
Respiratory distress, pneumonia, cardiac arrhythmias, DVT are other problems.
Stenosis of the anastomosis can occur which often needs repeated oesophageal dilatation using bougies (Maloney's).
Subphrenic abscess can occur which is diagnosed by CT scan. Guided tube drainage or open drainage may be needed.

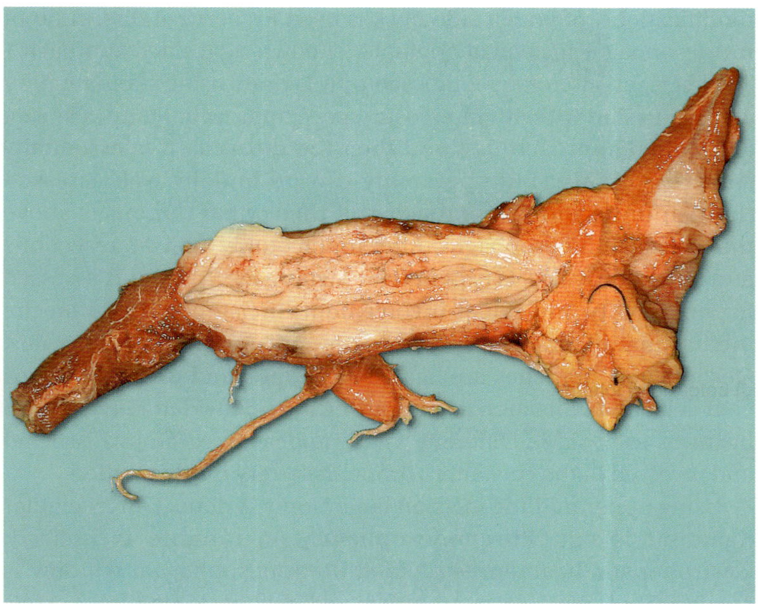

Fig. 20-50: Oesophagectomy specimen after resection.

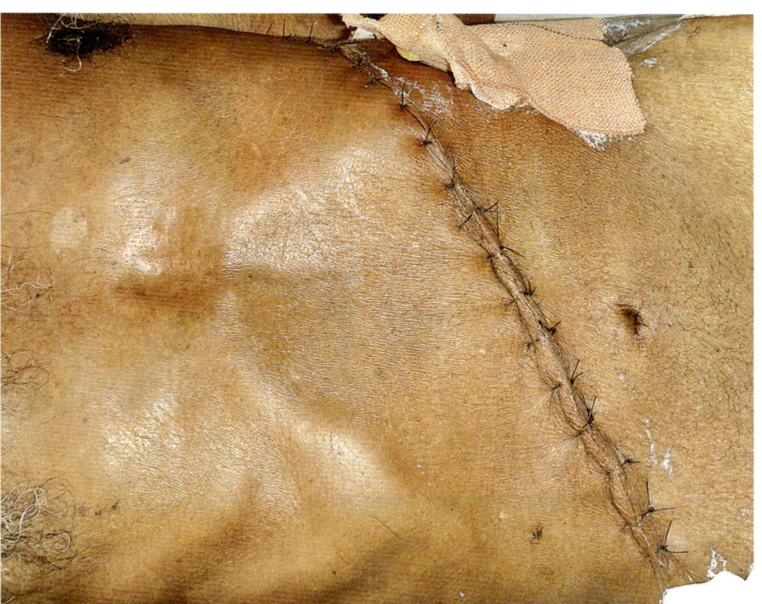

Fig. 20-52: Abdominothoracic (left) approach for OG junction or lowermost oesophageal carcinoma.

Respiratory physiotherapy, prevention of deep vein thrombosis and sepsis control should be done. Oral sips started once nasogastric tube is removed. Normal diet is started in 10–14 days.

LEFT THORACOABDOMINAL APPROACH OESOPHAGOGASTRECTOMY (CHURCHILL AND SWEET, 1942)

It is done only if growth is in OG junction. Much proximal tumour is difficult approach through this as access is difficult. Phrenic nerve injury is a possible complication when diaphragm is cut radially and it may lead into diaphragmatic paralysis.

Double lumen endotracheal tube is used for general anaesthesia. Left side of the patient is upwards 60°–90° with right arm is straight in the arm board and left arm is suspended above towards head away from surgical field. Patient is supported with sandbags or supportive frames **(Figs. 20-51 and 20-52)**.

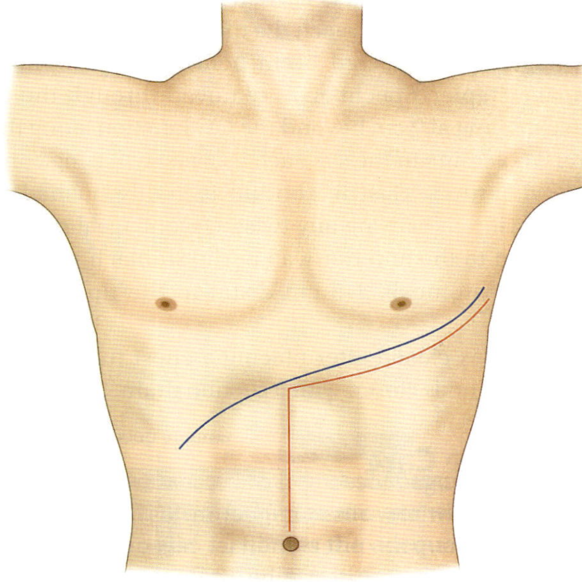

Fig. 20-51: Incision for left thoracoabdominal approach.

Technique

Incision can be either upper midline incision which is extended over the thorax or oblique incision between xiphoid and umbilicus extending towards left into the thoracic cage. First abdomen is opened; explored for operability/secondaries/lymph node and peritoneal status. Once decided to be operable, incision is extended across the 6th intercostal space upwards and posteriorly towards scapula and erector spinae. Latissimus dorsi and serratus anterior are cut. Scapula is retracted upwards. Intercostal muscles are cut on the upper part of 7th rib. Pleura is opened. Costal margins are divided using heavy scissor or bone cutter or 22 no. blade. Internal mammary artery may require to be ligated. Diaphragm should not be incised radially even though it is technically looks easier as phrenic nerve may get injured. It should be incised circumferentially (*Merendino and associates safe zones*, 1956). Incision is made in a line 3 cm from the rib margin parallel to it for 15 cm length **(Fig. 20-53)**.

Inferior pulmonary ligament is cut using long scissor or cautery; above up to inferior pulmonary vein. Mediastinal pleura is incised longitudinally from the thoracic descending aorta. Both vagi are cut

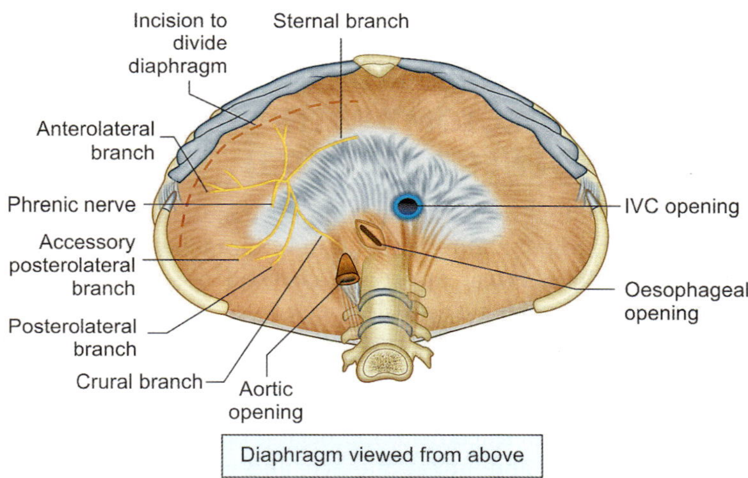

Fig. 20-53: Incision placed in diaphragm—safe zones (*Merendino and associates safe zones*)

high up below the level of lung hilum. Arterial branches entering the oesophagus are fulgarated using harmonic or bipolar cautery or ligated or occluded with haemoclips.

OG junction along the hiatus, lower oesophagus, stomach is mobilised through the abdominal wound same way like for other oesophagectomy (refer above). Gastroepiploic arcade should be retained along the greater curvature of the stomach while dividing the greater omentum; around 5 cm of redundant omentum should be attached to the stomach towards duodenal side. Right gastric and right gastroepiploic vessels are preserved. Kocherisation, hiatal dissection, ligation of left gastric vein (coronary vein—it is caudal to left gastric artery), left gastric artery, left gastroepiploic artery, accessory left hepatic artery are ligated securely to mobilise proximal stomach behind. Left gastric artery needs double ligation. Lymph nodes, fat should be cleared. Splenectomy may be done if needed. Pyloromyotomy is done. Oesophagus is transected using stapler 10 cm proximal to tumour; stomach is also transected 5 cm distal to the OG junction or the tumour (if tumour is extending into the stomach). Specimen is removed through the abdominal wound.

Crus of the diaphragm is cut if needed to widen the hiatus to prevent venous congestion of the pulled up mobilised stomach. Stomach is pulled across the hiatus up into the thoracic cavity. Anastomosis is done between the end of the oesophagus and anterior wall of the stomach as two layers. Posterior wall of the stomach may be fixed to the prevertebral fascia and hiatus using interrupted non-absorbable sutures to stabilise the gastric pouch.

Abdomen is closed in layers. Intercostal tube is placed. Diaphragm is closed using interrupted horizontal mattress 1 zero polypropylene sutures. Second continuous suture layer may be added to this. Thoracotomy is also closed in layers.

Postoperative Care

Intercostal tube is removed once lung has expanded fully in 5–7 days. Respiratory physiotherapy, antibiotics, observation are done regularly. Nasogastric tube is removed in 7 days. Oral sips started later. Often contrast study is done to confirm the adequacy of the stoma.

Complications

Respiratory complications, anastomotic leak, infection, subphrenic abscess formation, stenosis of the stoma, paralysis of the diaphragm are the complications.

MCKEOWN THREE PHASE OESOPHAGECTOMY WITH LYMPHADENECTOMY (1972)

McKeown modified Ivor Lewis technique by mobilising the entire oesophagus through abdominal and right thoracotomy approach and with right cervical approach cervical oesophagogastric anastomosis is done in the right side neck.

Procedure is done under general anaesthesia with double lumen endotracheal intubation. Original McKeown procedure was abdominal/thoracic one after another with change of positions each time; then right sided neck approach is done for anastomosis. Now synchronised abdominal, thoracic and neck approaches are used even though technique is of three phases. Cleaning and draping is done exposing abdomen, thorax and right sided neck. In further modifications, often left side neck is used for cervical dissection of the oesophagus instead of original McKeown right sided approach.

First right anterolateral thoracotomy is done using submammary crease incision with 4th intercostal space approach. Many advocate abdominal approach first and then the thoracic. It is essentially surgeon's choice. But operability can be initially well assessed through thoracotomy approach and then when tumour is above the lower 1/3rd oesophagus. After thoracotomy with rib resections and retraction, cavity is explored for metastases. Tumour is assessed for operability and nodal involvement. Incision is made on the mediastinal pleura. Oesophagus is mobilised with lymph nodes. Oesophageal branches are ligated or clipped and divided. Azygos vein is ligated at its arch level (four ligatures; divided between two ligatures each side). Different lymph nodes are carefully dissected and involved in the specimen. Bronchial artery is safeguarded.

Using upper midline incision laparotomy is done. Left triangular ligament is cut. Phrenooesophageal membrane is incised. Gastrohepatic ligament is divided. Retrooesophageal window is created. Short gastric vessels are ligated. Left gastroepiploic vessels are ligated and divided. Left gastric artery is ligated near its origin. Left gastric vein is ligated separately and divided which is caudal to artery (coronary vein). Nodes at this level are cleared. Right gastric and right gastroepiploic vessels are safeguarded. Gastroepiploic arcade is retained without traumatising it. Kocherisation is done to mobilise the duodenum. Pyloromyotomy is done. Oesophageal hiatus is widened adequately and hiatal dissection is done to communicate towards already dissected thoracic oesophagus.

Cervical dissection is carried out with oblique incision along the anterior border of the sternocleidomastoid muscle. Cosmetic horizontal incision also can be used. Deep fascia is incised. Carotid sheath is identified. Sternomastoid with carotid is retracted laterally. Omohyoid is divided using cautery. Thyroid with trachea is retracted medially using finger as retractor (assistant's finger). Inferior thyroid artery may require to be ligated. Oesophagus is identified by feeling the nasogastric tube inside. Oesophagus is dissected off from the prevertebral fascia using finger dissection. In front care should be taken not to injure recurrent laryngeal nerves of both sides while hooking the oesophagus using finger. Oesophagus is slinged with infant feeding tube or umbilical tape or Penrose drain. Dissection is carried towards mediastinum with sharp and blunt methods to reach the thoracic dissection.

Oesophagus is transected 5 cm below the cricopharyngeus muscle using stapler. Specimen is removed through the thoracic cavity after stapling at 2 cm beyond the OG junction along the lesser curvature. Stapler line in the stomach is oversewn using continuous 3-zero vicryl sutures. Gastric conduit is gently pushed towards neck wound without causing any twist. Oesophageal proximal end is anastomosed to the anterior wall of the stomach with two layer interrupted anastomosis 3–5 cm distal to the tip of the gastric conduit.

Thoracotomy is closed after placing a chest tube. Abdomen is closed. Neck wound is closed with a suction drain.

Postoperative Care

It is same as in other oesophagectomies—chest tube care, nasogastric tube care, and observation for bleeding, leak and sepsis and respiratory problems. Chest tube, drain and nasogastric tubes are removed in 5–7 days.

Complications

Bleeding, leak, thoracic duct injury, gastric conduit problems, recurrent laryngeal injuries, tracheal injury, anastomotic stenosis—can occur.

EN BLOC RESECTION OF OESOPHAGUS (SKINNER, 1983)

It is en bloc resection of oesophageal carcinoma (radical oesophagectomy) with 10 cm proximal and distal clearance along with removal of perioesophageal tissues, lymphatics, vessels of the oesophagus, azygos vein, bilateral pleural surfaces, pericardium anteriorly (partial removal), thoracic duct, cuff of the diaphragm, upper mediastinal and abdominal lymphadenectomy.

Laparotomy and right or left (for lower oesophagus) 6th intercostal space thoracotomy is done. Diaphragm is incised in safe area as phrenotomy. Abdominal oesophagus and coeliac nodal areas can be approached by large semilunar diaphragmatic division without doing laparotomy. All retroperitoneal tissues cephalad to pancreas including splenic and hepatic lymph nodes along with gastric nodes are dissected. OG junction is mobilised like usual oesophagectomy. Cuff of the diaphragmatic muscle is included in the oesophageal specimen. After en bloc resection, for lower oesophageal carcinoma, anastomosis is done above the aortic arch level. Thoracic duct is ligated just above the aortic hiatus through which it emerges from the abdomen.

In proximal (middle and upper) tumours, pleura is incised in superior mediastinum in front along the tracheooesophageal groove. Recurrent laryngeal nerves should be preserved. Oesophagus is dissected off the membranous trachea from thoracic inlet to carina. Azygos vein is ligated flush with the superior vena cava. Subcarinal lymph nodes are dissected. Posterior part of the pericardium is exposed. Pericardium is incised from superior pulmonary vein sleeve to inferior pulmonary vein sleeve. Pericardium is incised transversely to remove oval part of it. Broncho-oesophageal arteries are ligated. Incision is extended in front of the aorta onto the left pleural cavity. Left pleura is incised and included in the specimen.

In lower oesophageal tumour anastomosis is done in thoracic cavity in the pleural space or posterior mediastinum. In upper and middle tumours anastomosis is done in the right or left side of the neck. Approach and technique is similar as mentioned earlier. Neck nodes are cleared usually in en bloc dissection.

Patient often requires blood transfusions.

Postoperative care and complications

Respiratory care, intensive care is needed for 72 hours. Chest tube is removed once fluid quantity reduces less than 100 mL/day. Leak, pneumonia, mediastinitis lymph leak and cardiac arrhythmias are to be anticipated. Usual hospitalisation period is 14 days.

THREE FIELD LYMPHADENECTOMY FOR OESOPHAGEAL CARCINOMA

Forty per cent of upper 1/3rd tumours, 20% of lower 1/3rd tumours involve cervical nodes. Mucosal lesion has got 30% chances of nodal spread; submucosal has 50%; muscularis propria 60%; muscular and perioesophageal involvement has got 80% chances of nodal disease. Commonly nodes along the recurrent laryngeal nerves and behind the internal jugular vein are involved. Supraclavicular nodes when involved has got worse outcome. Its benefit over two field lymphadenectomy is controversial **(Fig. 20-54)**.

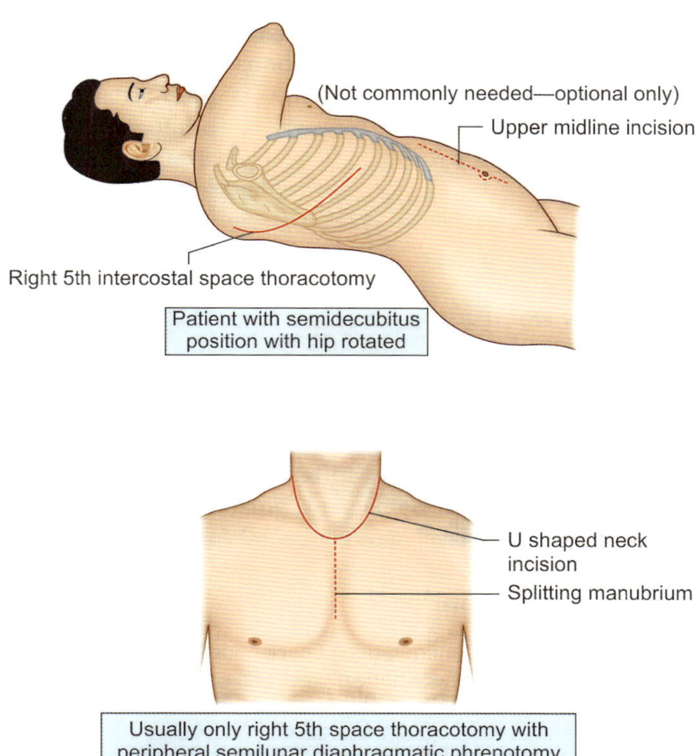

Fig. 20-54: Incision for three field dissection.

Thorax and abdomen can be approached by right 6th space thoracotomy with large semilunar incision over the diaphragm. It is only optional not a mandatory to do laparotomy as once phrenotomy is done, abdomen can be approached comfortably through thorax.

First field: In the abdomen, coeliac, renal, superior mesenteric, hepatic, splenic, gastric nodes are dissected along with the mobilisation of the abdominal oesophagus, and ligation of left gastric and left gastroepiploic vessels retaining gastroepiploic arcade. Parahiatal nodes are also cleared. Lesser curve is transected using stapler 2 cm distal to OG junction and stapler line is buried using continuous vicryl/silk seromuscular sutures. Kocherisation, pyloromyotomy is added. Gastric conduit is pushed into the thorax.

Second field: In the chest, posterior mediastinectomy is done to clear perioesophageal nodes, subcarinal nodes, nodes along the main bronchus, thoracic duct and azygos vein. Prevertebral and retrotracheal dissection is done to include further paratracheal nodes. Left recurrent laryngeal nerve is identified near its origin at the level of the aortic arch and dissected towards the neck; right recurrent laryngeal nerve is dissected at a place where it loops around the right subclavian artery with clearing the recurrent nodes adjacent to its superior mediastinal component (even though recurrent nodes are continuous chain nodes along the course recurrent laryngeal nerve in the mediastinum and neck, it is often classified as cervical and superior mediastinal components). Gastric conduit is pushed towards the thoracic inlet to reach neck for cervical oesophagogastric anastomosis.

Third field: U shaped neck incision is made with manubrium split to facilitate lower neck and superior mediastinal nodes properly. Brachiocephalic nodes, nodes lateral and posterior to carotid sheath, supraclavicular nodes and cervical recurrent nodes bilaterally are cleared with this approach **(Fig. 20-55)**.

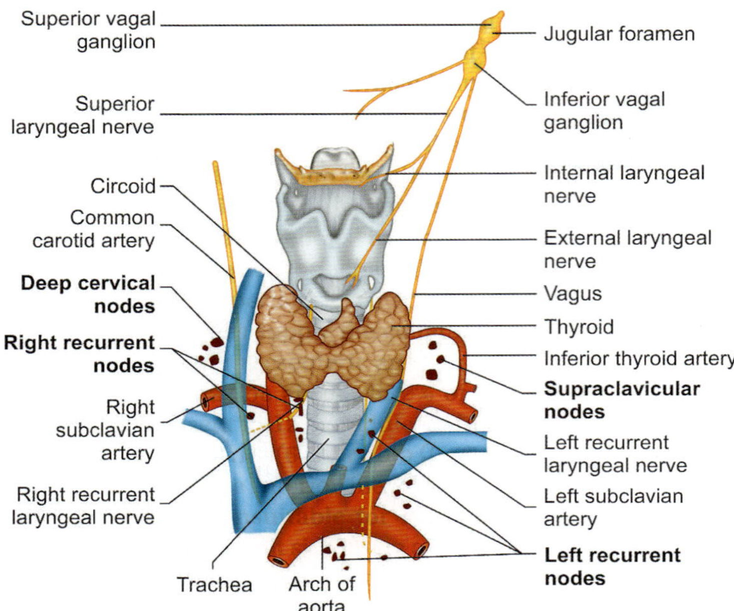

Fig. 20-55: Configuration of neck nodes in 3 field neck node dissection.

Anastomosis is done in the neck. Diaphragm is sutured using non-absorbable horizontal interrupted mattress sutures often with two layers. Thoracotomy is closed after placing bilateral chest tubes.

Problems

Delayed postoperative recovery, long hospital stay, sepsis, respiratory complications, recurrent laryngeal nerve palsy (10–50%), need for tracheostomy often, leak and lymph ooze are the problems. Mortality is 1–10%.

MINIMALLY INVASIVE SURGERY FOR CARCINOMA OF OESOPHAGUS (VIDEO-ASSISTED APPROACHES)

In 1996 DePaula did laparoscopic transhiatal oesophagectomy and reported a series of 48 patients. Later Luketich and Cuschieri described thoracolaparoscopic oesophagectomy.

Procedure is done in different positions. Initially thoracoscopic procedure is done to mobilise the oesophagus and to complete lymphadenectomy in the mediastinum. This is done in lateral decubitus position or in prone position also. Infracarinal and supracarinal lymph nodes are included in the specimen as part of lymphadenectomy—paraoesophageal, bronchopulmonary, subcarinal, tracheobronchial, recurrent and paratracheal nodes are dissected carefully. Later in supine position, laparoscopic mobilisation of the stomach and abdominal oesophagus is done. Gastric conduit is created using endostapler. Gastric tube is pulled into the cervical incision after placing a nasogastric tube into the peritoneal cavity and fixing to gastric conduit through a minilaparotomy. Specimen is removed through the minilaparotomy; gastric conduit is pulled up. Cervical oesophagogastric anastomosis is done.

Laparoscopic and thoracoscopic intrathoracic oesophagogastric anastomosis also can be done in lower oesophageal carcinomas.

Problems and complications are similar to open surgery. *Advantages are*—better visualisation and dissection, avoiding thoracotomy, faster recovery. *Disadvantages are*—technical expertise, learning curve, availability, cost, prolonged anaesthesia.

COMPLICATIONS AFTER OESOPHAGEAL RESECTION

Complications after resection of the oesophagus for carcinoma (commonly) are intraoperative, early or delayed/late (after 30 days) postoperative. It can be major or minor complications.

Intraoperative	*Early*	*Delayed/late*
Injury to lungs, pericardium Azygos vein bleeding Injury to spleen, coeliac artery Injury to thoracic duct Injury to tracheal membrane	Abdominal bleeding—intra-abdominal Gastrointestinal bleeding Respiratory complications like ARDS, pneumonia, collapse of lung Chylothorax, haemothorax, empyema Mediastinitis Cardiac complications Bowel ischaemia, bowel obstruction Anastomotic leak Recurrent laryngeal nerve palsy Subphrenic/intrathoracic abscess DVT, pulmonary embolism Wound infections	Anastomotic stricture Delayed gastric emptying Internal diaphragmatic herniation through the hiatus

Anastomotic leak

It is the most problematic complication. It is around 14%. Leak may be into the neck wound or into the thorax. Leak into neck wound is safer and usually resolves by conservative therapy. Leak into the thoracic cavity is life threatening. It needs immediate thoracotomy. Small leak can be closed. Gastric conduit can be drained by placing a T tube. Large leak needs repositioning of the gastric conduit into the abdominal cavity. Temporary oesophageal diversion is done in the neck as oesophagostomy. Later if patient recovers from acute shock and its problems, elective diversion using colon can be done. Leak often may be from the staple line placed along the lesser curvature. It is usually into the thorax. Management is similar to anastomotic leak. Leak also can occur from pyloroplasty or pyloromyotomy. It is usually into the abdominal cavity. It needs redoing of the pyloroplasty through relaparotomy. Site of leak is confirmed by water contrast dye study. Contrast CT is also helpful.

Tracheal membrane tear

Tracheal membrane tear is another complication which is often very difficult to manage with high mortality. Small tear is sutured using non-absorbable interrupted sutures (polypropylene). Large tear is difficult to tackle. It is managed by anterior mediastinal tracheostomy with resection of clavicle and manubrium and half of first rib (anterior breast plate resection). Supportive pectoralis major muscle flap or intercostal muscle flap is also needed around tracheostomy.

Major complications	*Minor complications*
Anastomotic leak Tracheal membrane tear Cardiac complications Gastric conduit necrosis Recurrent laryngeal nerve injury Delayed gastric emptying Respiratory complications Chylothorax Pancreatitis, mediastinitis, septicaemia Intracavitary abscess formation Deep vein thrombosis Renal failure	Atelectasis of lung Problems of feeding jejunostomy Wound infection Urinary retention Paralytic ileus

OESOPHAGEAL SUBSTITUTES

Oesophageal substitute is the one which is used as an interposed functioning bowel tube between the proximal normal oesophagus in the neck or thorax and stomach in the abdomen. It can be used after removal of thoracic oesophagus in its entirety or partly ***(oesophageal replacement)***; in this type, oesophagus is placed in the same or similar place after oesophagectomy. Often diseased oesophagus is retained as in advanced carcinoma oesophagus or in adherent multiple strictures where it is difficult to dissect safely; in this type it is used as ***oesophageal bypass*** through different routes commonly retrosternal. Usually stomach, colon, jejunum are used. Occasionally local flaps (myocutaneous or free flaps) may be used for cervical oesophagus along with pharynx.

When oesophagus is excluded and gastric conduit is used as bypass, oesophagus should be drained to prevent abscess or mucocele formation or blow out of the distended oesophagus. It is done by doing oesophagojejunostomy or proximal end of the excluded oesophagus is brought out as tube oesophagostomy. If there is a broncho or tracheooesophageal fistula (in malignancy or other causes), then excluded oesophagus can be left alone as fistula drains into the respiratory tract functioning as pseudodiverticulum.

Transposition Routes

Transposition is done through posterior mediastinum (*shortest route*), right pleural space (transpleural), retrosternal or subcutaneous route.

Posterior mediastinal route is ideal if oesophagectomy has been done prior to transposition. Otherwise it is not useful as a bypass route for cancer cases with inoperable tumour or in strictured oesophagus. It has got shortest distance between neck and abdomen.

Transpleural route is easier; but can cause gastric or colonic distension due to negative thoracic pressure. It is often used after thoracic oesophagectomy. It is not ideal for bypass substitute as thoracotomy is required.

Retrosternal route is through anterior mediastinum behind the sternum across its entire length. Length of this route is longer than posterior mediastinal route; but gastric or colonic conduits can be bridged across without any tension in this route. This is commonly used bypass route when oesophagus is not removed. It is anatomically separated from the oesophageal tumour and so bypass conduit will not get involved by tumour. Oesophagus in the neck is mobilised like other similar procedure. Anterior fibres of the diaphragm are detached from the xiphoid process to access the retrosternal plane. Tunnel is created by passing fingers from below and from above by blunt dissection. It is avascular plane and hence bleeding is not common.

Approaches for Different Level Tumours

Postcricoid tumour (Squamous cell carcinoma):
Treated mainly by radiotherapy. Radical radiotherapy—5000–6000 rads. Often pharyngolaryngectomy is done along with gastric or colonic transposition. But complications are more in this procedure. Free jejunal transfer is the other option.

Upper third growth (Squamous cell carcinoma):
It is treated mainly by radiotherapy. Commonly it is advanced with left recurrent laryngeal nerve palsy and bronchial invasion. If it is early and operable, *McKeown three phased oesophagectomy* and anastomosis is done in the neck. Initially thoracotomy through right 5th space is done and oesophagus is mobilised. Then laparotomy is done to mobilise the stomach. Through right side neck approach, oesophagus with growth is removed. Anastomosis between pharynx and stomach is done in the neck.

Split sternum approach oesophagectomy is also practiced.

Middle third growth (Squamous cell carcinoma):
Ivor Lewis operation (Lewis-Tanner two-phased oesophagectomy): After laparotomy stomach is mobilised. Pyloroplasty is done. Through right 5th space thoracotomy is done and growth with tumour is mobilised. Partial oesophagectomy and oesophagogastric anastomosis is done in the thorax. Intercostal tube drainage is placed during closure. Right gastro-epiploic vessels/epiploic arcade should be retained safely (essential). Azygos vein should be ligated securely. Mediastinal nodes should be dissected. Thoracic duct should be ligated if needed just above the aortic hiatus where it enters the thorax. Feeding jejunostomy is better to maintain nutrition. If the growth is inoperable, palliative radiotherapy is given.

Lower third growth (Squamous cell carcinoma + adenocarcinoma):
Here through left thoracoabdominal approach, partial oesophago-gastrectomy is done with oesophagogastric anastomosis. Often jejunal Roux-en-Y loop anastomosis is done. *Orringer approach,* i.e. *transhiatal blind/blunt total oesophagectomy* with anastomosis in the left side of the neck. Through laparotomy, stomach and lower part of the oesophagus are mobilised. Through left sided neck approach, upper part of the oesophagus is mobilised using finger. Blind dissection is completed by meeting both fingers above and below in the thorax. Later oesophagus is pulled up out above through the neck wound and removed. Continuity is maintained in the neck. It is a *palliative* surgery.

Other Approaches
Thoracoscopic-laparoscopic oesophagectomy and lymphadenectomy is becoming popular, safer and effective.

Radical oesophagectomy with 3-field clearance of abdominal/thoracic and cervical nodes is also practiced in many centres. 3-field clearance (coeliac, thoracic and neck) is done for mainly squamous cell carcinoma as spread here is upwards. In adenocarcinoma 2-field clearance is sufficient (abdominal—coeliac and thoracic) as spread is downwards.

Skinner en bloc resection used to be of practice in olden days in which tumour with oesophagus is resected along with thoracic duct, azygos vein, intercostal vessels crossing the vertebral bodies, pericardium and mediastinal pleura. There is no survival benefit with this procedure.

Vagal sparing oesophagectomy with HSV is tried to preserve pylorus functioning avoiding pyloroplasty to reduce the chances of postprandial fullness. But it is technically tedious.

Lymphadenectomy in carcinoma oesophagus: *Standard*: Nodes removed are—paratracheal, parabronchial, carinal, paraoesophageal, posterior mediastinal, paracardial, left gastric, along lesser curve of stomach. *Extended/three field/ultraradical:* As like standard above, with bilateral cervical lymphadenectomy, removal of upper mediastinal, coeliac, retroperitoneal, subhepatic nodes is done.

Conduit is pushed gently upwards using hand and fingers; instrument pull should be avoided as it will damage the conduit. Often head of the clavicle, first rib and part of the manubrium is removed to widen the thoracic inlet. This reduces the compression over the conduit and maintains its blood supply optimally.

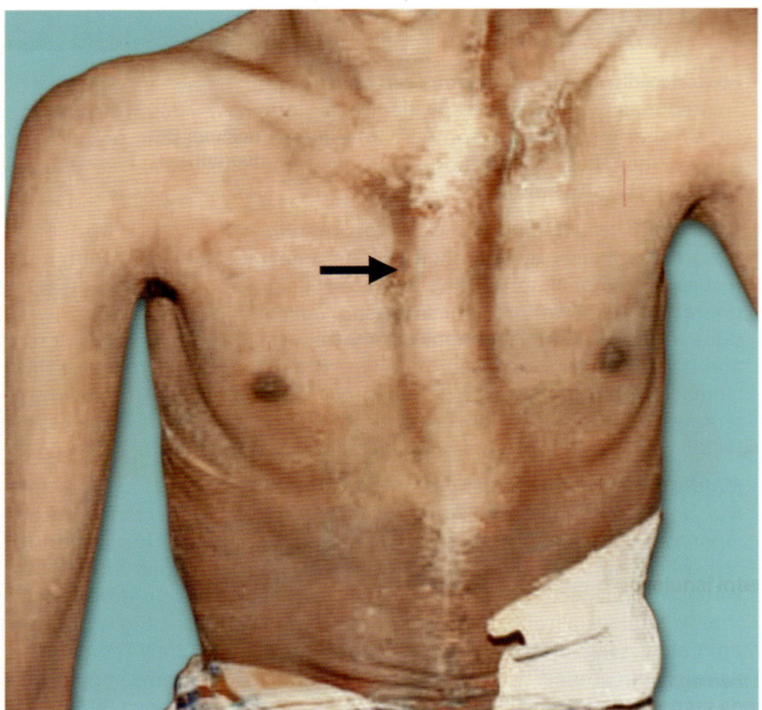

Fig. 20-56: Subcutaneous route—colon transposition.

Subcutaneous route is done when all other routes are not possible to utilise. If patient has undergone prior open cardiac surgery then retrosternal route is not possible and subcutaneous route is used. It is technically easier but lengthier conduit is needed. It is antesternal route. Anastomosis takes up well; but conduit is visible on the chest wall **(Fig. 20-56)**.

Stomach (Gastric Conduit)

It is preferred one and is based on right gastric and right gastroepiploic arteries. It is the most commonly used oesophageal substitute at present. It needs only one anastomosis and take up is well due to good vascularity. But it can cause postprandial fullness with bile or acid regurgitation (>50%). It also needs a pyloromyotomy/pyloroplasty for gastric drainage as vagotomy is done to prevent delayed gastric emptying. Entire stomach or tubed part or reverse tubed part can be transposed. Stomach has got lengthier gastroepiploic arcade closer to greater curvature which straightens when stomach becomes straight; it does not kink when moved/transposed unlike colon or jejunum (here fan-shaped mesentery kinks and get tensed when transposed). Colon after years gets dilated and becomes redundant leading to stasis and improper emptying. Prior gastrostomy is not a contraindication for using stomach as conduit; gastrostomy feeding more with fluid dilates the stomach significantly making it as a better conduit. Site of the gastrostomy even though is not very important but preferred to place towards lesser curvature side. Presence of gastric outlet obstruction or gastric resection or previous gastrojejunostomy makes it a relative *contraindication* for preparing it as a suitable conduit.

For bypass in an advanced carcinoma entire stomach is used without making tubes. Here OG junction is transected and entire stomach is mobilised as usual with retaining the gastroepiploic arcade with its blood supply from right gastroepiploic artery. Kocherisation, pyloromyotomy, ligation of left gastric and left gastroepiploic pedicle and short gastric vessels are done. Mobilised stomach is pushed upwards towards neck for anastomosis with the cervical oesophagus. **(Fig. 20-57)**

For replacement tubed stomach is commonly used. It may be reversed gastric tube based on left gastroepiploic artery or non-reversed gastric tube based on right gastroepiploic artery. Greater omentum is dissected off from the transverse colon and from both flexures. Middle colic artery should be safeguarded. Short gastric vessels are ligated and divided. Splenectomy is usually not necessary. Left gastric vessels are ligated. OG junction is mobilised.

In reversed gastric tube, right gastroepiploic artery is ligated 4 cm from the pylorus. Double row stapling along the greater curvature at this point is applied transversely for 2.5 cm. Proximal stapling row is held and few staples adjacent to greater curvature is removed and 40 French rubber catheter is passed through this proximally along the greater curvature up to the fundus. Multiple staplers are fired parallel to the tube towards the fundus to create reversed gastric tube. Staple line is oversewn using continuous 3 zero silk sutures to bury the staple line. Tube placed should be loosely accommodated there. Omentum is wrapped around the gastric tube. Tube based on the left gastroepiploic artery is tunneled through posterior mediastinum if oesophagectomy is undertaken; otherwise passed under the xiphoid through retrosternal space if oesophagus is not removed (as bypass, where entire stomach is used without tube usually) and anastomosed in the neck to cervical oesophagus **(Fig. 20-58)**.

In non-reversed gastric tube, right gastroepiploic artery is used as base; here left gastroepiploic vessels, short gastric vessels and left gastric vessels are ligated. Pyloromyotomy is done; extended Kocherisation is needed. Circular stapler is fired 4 cm proximal to the pylorus to facilitate the passage of the consecutive series of stapler lines until the outer aspect of the fundus to create 2.5 cm diameter vascularised tube based on right gastroepiploic artery. Staple line is inverted with continuous seromuscular sutures. Omentum is wrapped around the gastric tube **(Fig. 20-59)**.

Advantages of gastric conduit—adequate length is available; good blood supply; good anastomotic take up; easier to mobilise.

Disadvantages of gastric conduit—need for pyloromyotomy/pyloroplasty; gastric conduit tip necrosis; anastomotic stricture; delayed gastric emptying.

Colon

Technique is more with the need of three anastomoses. Right colon is used with middle colic artery based as antiperistaltic loop. Left colon is used with ascending branch of left colic artery as isoperistaltic loop. Postprandial problems are less in colonic conduit compared to stomach. Colon is used as right/left/transverse segment depending on need and vasculature and preference. It can be isoperistaltic or antiperistaltic. When a short segment of colon is used it is called as *short segment colon in interposition (probably used as bridge gap in localised benign diseases)*; total or subtotal oesophageal replacement is called as *long segment colon interposition* (in multiple strictures, carcinoma oesophagus). Colon behaves more or less as a passive conduit **(Fig. 20-60)**.

Left colon is preferred with easier technique; with smaller diameter compared to right side; reliable vascularity; excellent length; easier mobilisation; it is isoperistaltic. *Preoperative* superior and/or inferior mesenteric angiogram and colonoscopy is a must as a prerequisite. Vascular identification is done by on table transillumination; temporary vascular isolation is done by placing bulldog clamps and waiting or 10–15 minutes for signs of ischaemia. Length of the conduit needed should be measured using tape and marked; length required

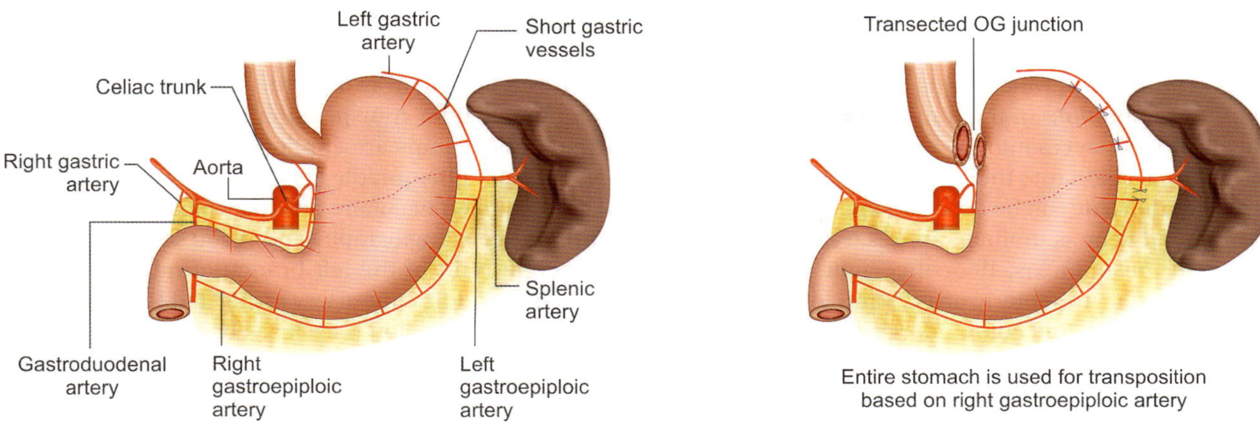

Fig. 20-57: Gastric conduit using entire stomach.

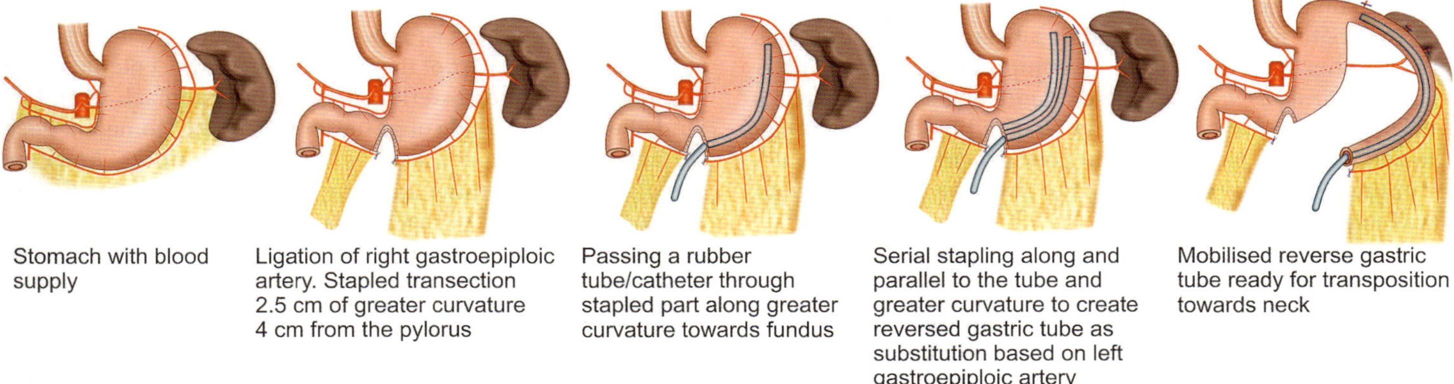

Fig. 20-58: Gastric conduit—reversed type.

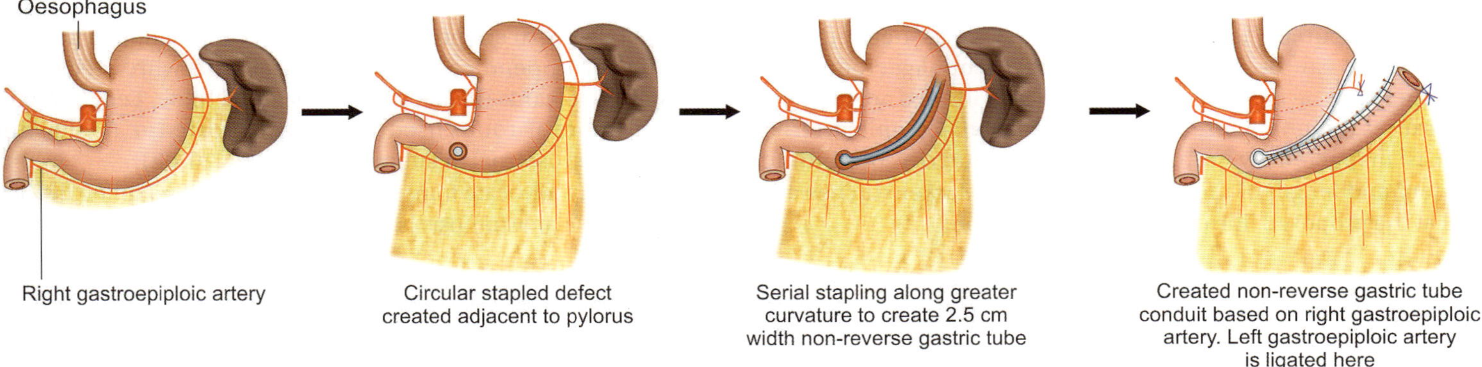

Fig. 20-59: Gastric conduit—non-reversed type.

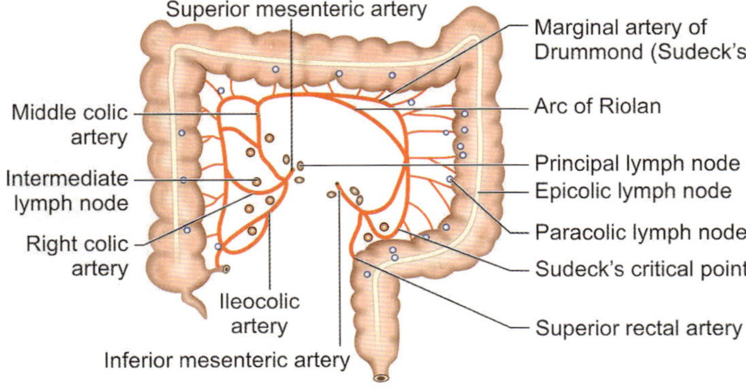

Fig. 20-60: Blood supply of colon.

is approximately from the jaw to 5 cm below the xiphoid process for posterior route; for anterior retrosternal route more lengthier conduit is needed and measurement is taken from ear lobule to 5 cm below the xiphoid process. Greater omentum is separated; colon is mobilised from its lateral peritoneal and mesenteric attachment. After mesenteric dissection with vascular isolation carefully, penrose drain or chest tube can be placed into the conduit to facilitate the delivery of the conduit into the neck without any twist or kink or compression. Adequate space should be created in the proposed/decided route towards the neck in the thorax/mediastinum. Lower end is anastomosed first to stomach or duodenum or jejunum depending on the stomach is intact (usually normal) or resected (like in severe chemical injury). Next anastomosis is done in the neck—upper end.

Colon functions as a passive conduit and empties much slower than oesophagus. Motility of the colon is of three types—*right sided retrograde annular contractions* which helps in fluid and electrolyte absorption; *annular contractions* of the transverse and descending colon which slowly propels faeces into the rectum; *strong propulsive contractions* of the distal colon into the rectum. So right side can be used as antiperistaltic; left side can be used as isoperistaltic. Arterial supply of the colon and venous drainage makes it more proficient to use as conduit for oesophagus. Ileocolic, right colic, middle colic (branches of superior mesenteric artery) and left colic artery and sigmoid branches supply the colon. Marginal artery connects branches of superior mesenteric and inferior mesenteric arteries. Marginal artery may be absent in 2% of individuals. Right colic artery may be absent in 12%; middle colic in 4% cases. Right (8%) and middle colic arteries (6%) or both (0.5%) may be multiple often. Atherosclerosis of the inferior mesenteric artery makes marginal artery poorer and unsuitable for colonic conduit. There is no marginal vein on the right side colon and it is said that anastomotic leak in 25% of right sided colonic conduit substitute is due to venous congestion rather than arterial. More commonly preferred one is left side colon. *Reasons are*—smaller diameter of left colon matches relatively to oesophagus; constant and reliable blood supply of the left side colon; ability to propel solid content—make left colon is the first option. Right side colon is used as a reserve if left side colon is not available or cannot be used.

Indications: Colon is used when stomach is not available or not suitable for replacement. It can be used as bypass in advanced carcinoma oesophagus. It is useful in multiple oesophageal strictures, oesophageal atresia if stomach is not adequate for replacement. It is also used in patients for resurgery with failed gastric conduits of any reasons.

Contraindications: Primary colonic disease; inadequate blood supply to the colon; short/fibrosed colonic mesentery. Prior colonoscopy may be a need.

Technique: Adequate large bowel preparation is needed. For replacement it can be combined with the oesophagectomy and same upper midline incision is used. Colon is mobilised adequately. Both flexures, colonic mesentery are mobilised. Colonic arterial arcade is inspected by transillumination. Integrity of colonic mesentery and length of the colon is assessed. Marker stitches are placed at the proposed line of the colonic resection.

For left sided isoperistaltic colonic conduit, descending branch of left colonic artery which is communicating into the sigmoid arteries is ligated away from the main left colic trunk. Length of the colon needed for transposition is measured using umbilical tape. Atraumatic clamps are applied to the marginal artery right of the left branch of the middle colic artery and middle colic artery itself. If left side colon maintains adequate blood supply which is confirmed by fluorescein angiography and Wood's light examination, marginal branch at right of the left branch of middle colic artery and left branch of middle colic artery are ligated **(Fig. 20-61)**.

Now left side colon is exclusively supplied by the left colic artery. Colon is transected at proposed level with retaining the marginal arterial arcade and left colic artery. Right side part of the conduit is passed behind the colon and stomach; then across the thorax by suitable decided route to reach the neck. If only bypass is done without prior oesophagectomy, similar neck incision is done to reach the oesophagus. Oesophagus is transected and anastomosed to the colonic conduit at proximal right side colon. Proximal cut end of the oesophagus is anastomosed to side of the colon in the neck as end to side. Distal part of the left side end of the colonic conduit is anastomosed to the posterior surface of the stomach as end to side (end of the colon to side of posterior wall of the stomach). Posterior surface of the stomach acts as antireflux support. Anastomosis can also be done on the anterior surface of the stomach. Vertical gastrotomy is done for anastomosis. Colonic continuity is maintained by colocolic anastomosis. Feeding jejunostomy is usually done.

In right sided antiperistaltic colonic transposition, right colon is made to perfuse by middle colic artery. After deciding the line of and length of the needed right sided colon, atraumatic clamps are placed on to the marginal arteries, ileocolic, right colic, terminal ileal vessels to confirm the adequacy of perfusion of the proposed conduit through the middle colic artery. Once perfusion is confirmed, these vessels are ligated, middle colic artery is safely and carefully retained to maintain the perfusion. Isolated colon is transected distally, terminal ileum 10 cm proximal to ileocaecal junction is transected proximally. Appendicectomy is done. Ileum with caecal end is transposed towards the neck in the specified route. Length required is 4 cm more if route used other than posterior mediastinum especially retrosternal or subcutaneous **(Fig. 20-62)**.

Now many advocate transection at caecal level retaining the ileum. Ileotransverse anastomosis is done to maintain the bowel continuity.

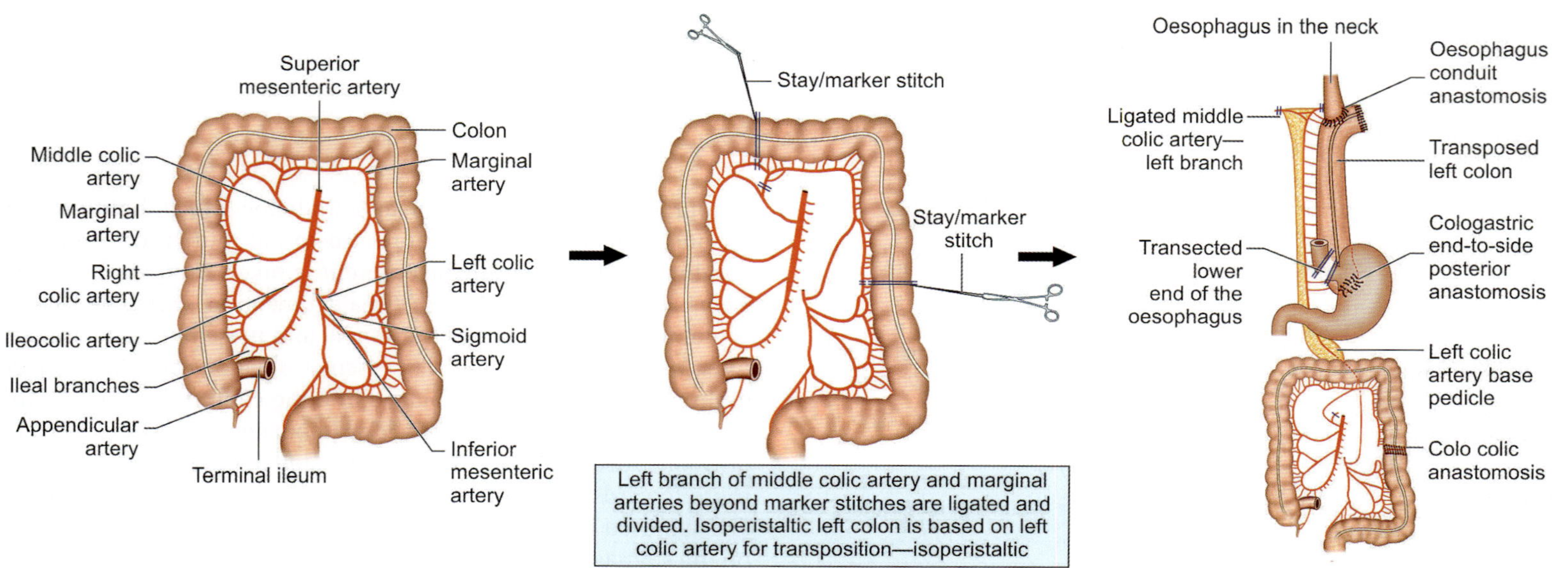

Fig. 20-61: Left sided colon transposition.

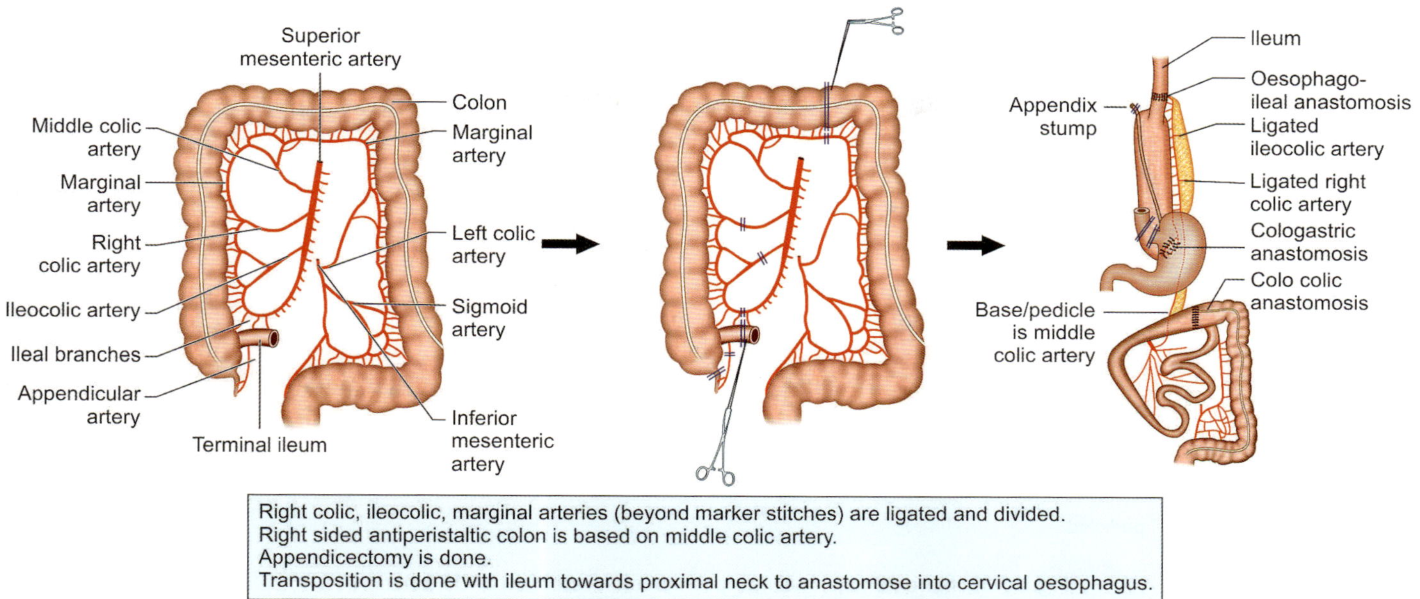

Fig. 20-62: Right sided colon transposition.

Oesophagoileal/colic anastomosis is done in the neck between the end of the oesophagus to side of the colon/ileum. Below colon is anastomosed behind or front of the stomach.

Problems with colon substitute

Preoperative preparation of colon is more complex and demanding. Multiple anastomoses (3) are required; it is more risky as far as colon is considered. Necrosis and leak is potentially life threatening in colon. Colon has got poor acid resistance unlike jejunum. Tendency to dilate gradually and causing redundancy is a problem. Extremely slow emptying time is another problem. Food is retained in the colon conduit for long time without emptying into the stomach.

Complications

Complications of colonic substitute depends on the length of the segment and indication for colonic substitute. Complications may be mechanical or functional. It may be immediate, late and long term. Immediate complications are, haemorrhage, chylothorax, pulmonary complications, pericardial tamponade, myocardial infarction, oesophageal conduit necrosis. Anastomotic disruption, leak, septicaemia, empyema, and mediastinitis. Late and long term complications are many. They are—transhiatal herniation, colocutaneous/colobronchial fistulas, stricture at oesophagogastric or oesophagocolic sites, pouching effects of the localised part or entire colonic conduit causing redundancy at cervical or thoracic inlet or supraaortic or supradiaphragmatic or infradiaphragmatic portions of the conduit leading into mechanical delay in emptying; cologastric adenocarcinoma; peptic ulceration of the redundant colon and bleeding; post vagotomy syndrome. Many of these complications need revision surgeries but with poor results.

Jejunum

Isolated required length of pedicled jejunum is transposed. Jejunal free transfer is also tried; vessels are anastomosed to internal mammary vessels or to the vessels available in the neck (linguofacial trunk or superior thyroid artery). Pedicled jejunum is also *supercharged (boosting)* with microvascular anastomoses with internal mammary vessels. It is used as a last option even though it is ideal. Segment of the 2nd/3rd/4th loop of the jejunum (distal to ligament of Treitz) is harvested with its mesenteric arcade to transplant in the neck with microvascular anastomosis. Jejunum caliber approximates proximal oesophagus. Free jejunal transfer can be used as isolated reconstructive flap for pharyngooesophagus. Function of the remaining large part of the small bowel is not disturbed. Segment of the jejunum should be supplied by a single vascular arcade of adequate dimension. Anastomosis is done proximally to pharynx and distally to oesophagus with microvascular anastomosis. Jejunum retains its effective peristalsis when transposed. Jejunal mesentery limits pedicled transfer of the jejunum; it can reach only up to the inferior pulmonary vein. Free jejunal transfer is ideal and suitable. Pedicled jejunum can be transplanted for 20 cm length; can be increased by supercharging. Otherwise free transfer is the only possibility. Pyloromyotomy is required; gastrostomy is done in case of pedicled jejunal transfer to lower oesophagus. Approach for pedicled jejunal transfer to lower oesophagus is by left sided thoracoabdominal.

Recipient vessels are evaluated for diameter, patency, length, flow and associated vein by CT/MR angiogram. Linguofacial trunk or superior thyroid artery is used. Arterial anastomosis is done superficial to hypoglossal nerve. External jugular vein or tributary of internal jugular vein is used as recipient vein. Anastomosis is done using interrupted or continuous 9-zero polypropylene sutures using microscopy. Tension should be avoided in vascular anastomosis site.

Jejunal conduit is the third choice for oesophageal replacement. It is resistant to acid and bile. It gives adequate length. Problem is mobilisation; preservation of blood supply; in free jejunal transfer, graft take up after vascular microanastomosis and supercharging. *Indicator graft* is harvested often 4–6 cm of the jejunal pedicled graft; it is exteriorised as indicator graft with jejunal loop with its mesenteric pedicle coming out through the one end of the main wound as indicator. It indicates the patency of main graft indirectly; indicator graft is removed in 7 days after ligating the pedicle.

Merendino jejunal interposition is used when short segment distal oesophagus needs resection for conditions like corrosive non-dilatable stricture, failed reflux surgery, early adenocarcinoma of gastro-oesophageal junction (OGJ) and benign tumours of distal oesophagus **(Fig. 20-63)**.

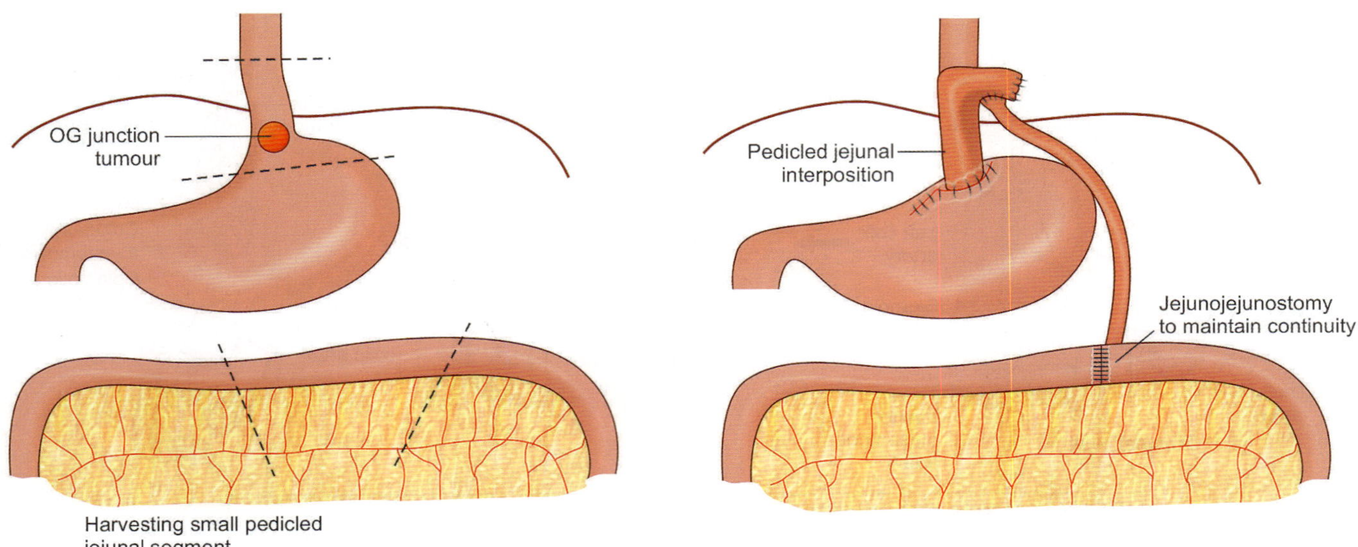

Fig. 20-63: Merendino jejunal interposition after resection of OG junction.

Other Substitutes Used

Radial forearm free flap based at radial artery is used similarly using microvascular anastomosis. Lateral thigh free flap is also often used based on 3rd perforator of the profunda femoris artery along with the accompanied vein. These are mainly used to reconstruct pharyngooesophagus in the neck with microvascular anastomosis.

CRICOPHARYNGEAL MYOTOMY WITH PHARYNGEAL DIVERTICULECTOMY (REFER ALSO CHAPTER 14—SURGERY OF FACE, HEAD AND NECK)

It is done in pharyngeal diverticulum. It is usually towards left side. If diverticulum is less than 3 cm, just myotomy is sufficient. If it is more than 3 cm then diverticulectomy is needed. *Belsey diverticulopexy* with fixing the most dependent portion of the diverticulum to the prevertebral fascia of upper cervical region with non-absorbable interrupted sutures is often done; but not very acceptable. Anatomical upper sphincter cricopharyngeus muscle is 2.5 cm in length but physiologic upper oesophageal sphincter is 4 cm in length. So myotomy should be more than 4 cm extending beyond the anatomic cricopharyngeus proximally (2 cm) **(Figs. 20-64 and 20-65)**.

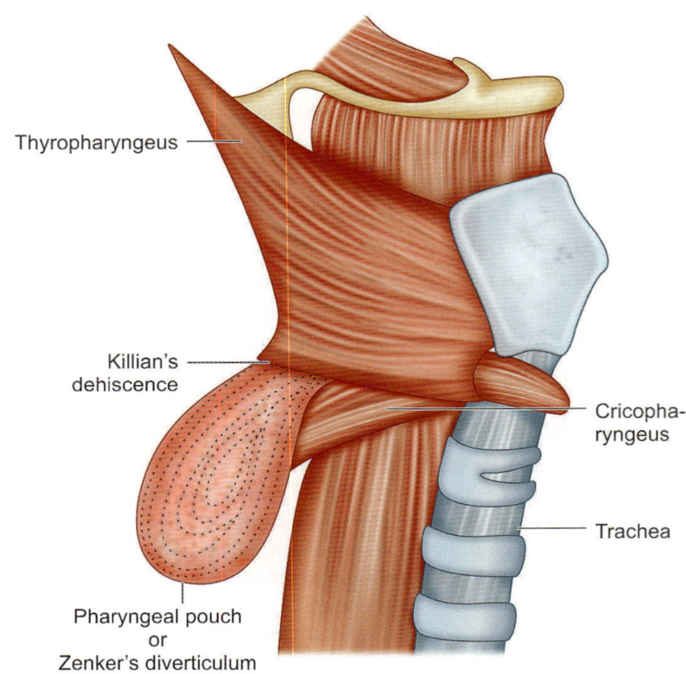

Fig. 20-64: Anatomy of pharyngeal pouch.

Incision

Under general anaesthesia with nasogastric tube in place left lower horizontal or oblique incision along the inner margin of the sternocleidomastoid muscle is used **(Fig. 20-66)**.

Dissection

Skin, platysma, deep fascia is incised; sternocleidomastoid muscle is retracted; omohyoid muscle is divided; carotid sheath is retracted laterally; strap muscles are retracted medially along with thyroid gland. Middle thyroid vein is ligated. Inferior thyroid artery is ligated; recurrent laryngeal nerve is identified and safeguarded which is in front of the diverticulum. Diverticulum is identified between inferior constrictor of the pharynx (thyropharyngeus) and cricopharyngeus (Killian's dehiscence). Fundus of the diverticulum is held with Babcock's forceps and diverticulum is dissected from surrounding tissues using peanut blunt dissection and scissor and bipolar cautery. Care should be taken not to injure recurrent laryngeal nerve and oesophageal mucosa.

Myotomy

Right angled haemostat/clamp is passed between the mucosa and transverse fibres of the cricopharyngeus without opening the mucosa. Instrument is elevated and fibres are incised for 5 cm below; later similarly upper fibres are also incised for few (2–3) cm **(Fig. 20-67)**.

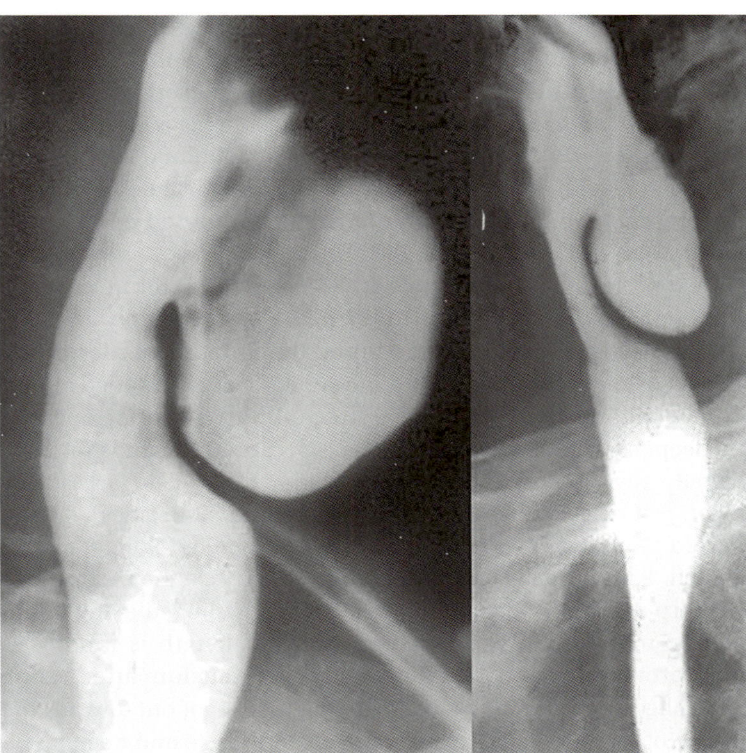

Fig. 20-65: Contrast X-ray look of oesophagus in pharyngeal pouch.

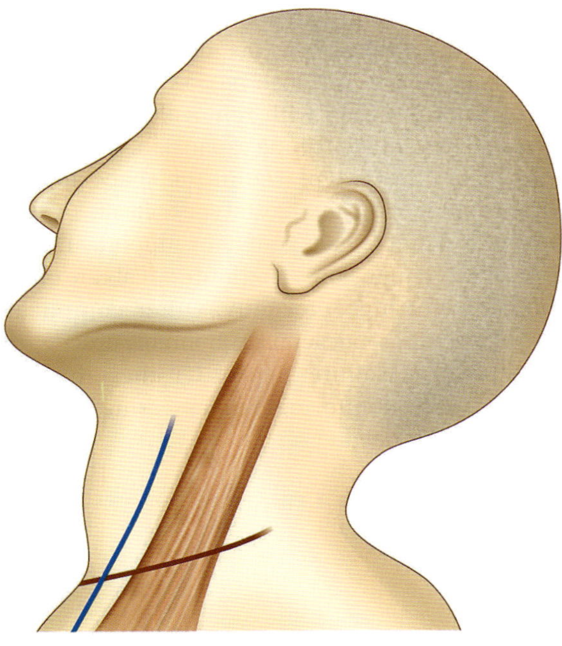

Fig. 20-66: Incision for excision of pharyngeal pouch.

Diverticulectomy

40 French Maloney's bougie is passed through the mouth into the oesophagus to identify the neck and opening of the diverticulum. Diverticulum is transected using 30 or 55 mm TA stapler. It also can be transected and hand suturing can be done using inner interrupted 3-zero vicryl and outer interrupted 3-zero silk sutures.

Drain is placed; wound is closed in layers. Maloney's bougie is removed. Nasogastric tube is kept for 48 hours and removed. Soft diet is started. Drain is removed in 4 days.

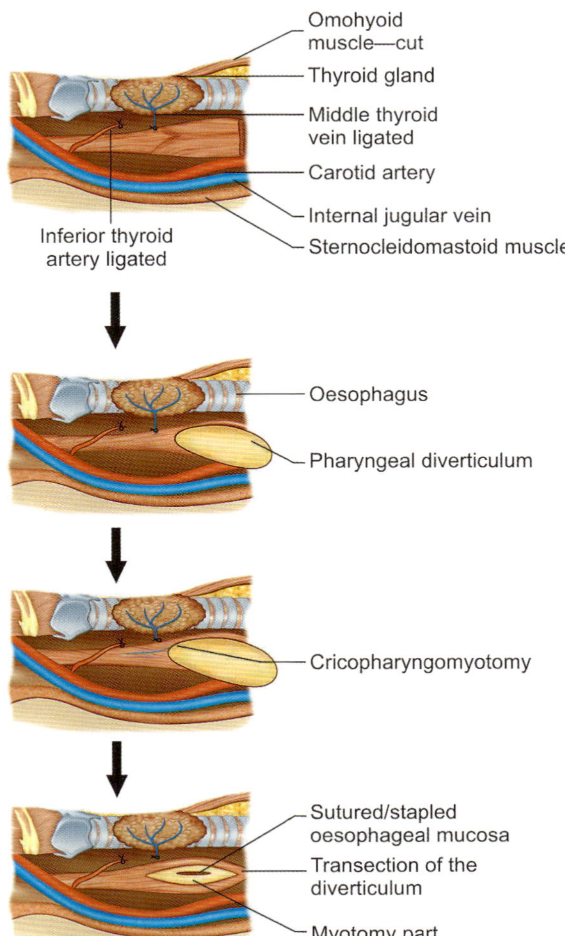

Fig. 20-67: Surgical technique for pharyngeal pouch.

Complications

Leak from sutured site; infection; abscess formation; stricture formation. Complications like fistula formation, empyema, pneumonia and mediastinitis can occur whenever there is dense adhesion, sepsis, and large diverticulum extending into the thorax.

MANAGEMENT OF OESOPHAGEAL PERFORATION

Oesophageal perforation may be due to instrumentation or vomiting induced like in Boerhaave's syndrome or postoperative leak. For cervical oesophageal perforation lateral film with neck extension X-ray is taken. Contrast CT scan is diagnostic. Patient needs higher generation antibiotics, nasogastric tube at proximal part, intercostal tube, blood, CVP line, urinary cauterisation.

Perforation may be bigger than what is thought of usually. Large perforation is difficult to close and in such situation, muscle or pleural or pericardial flap is needed to cover the defect. Resection and diversion to exclude the thoracic oesophagus are other options.

Right or left thoracotomy is done depending on the location of the perforation whether upper or lower part. Perforation may be clearly seen or may not be clear. In such situation, instillation of air or methylene blue per orally into the oesophagus by anaesthetist will help to identify the site of perforation. Often there will be necrotic material, sepsis, pus due to severe mediastinal infection.

In early cases (within 8 hours), perforation can be still closed in layers—inner mucosal interrupted 3-zero vicryl; outer muscular 3-zero silk sutures; adjacent pleural flap is elevated; covered over the suture line and sutured beyond using interrupted non-absorbable sutures. Stapler closure can be tried but it is often difficult.

Perforation after 8 hours will have marked inflammatory oedema and is often difficult to close the defect with sutures. Here direct pleural flap or intercostal muscle flap is raised and covered over the defect directly. *Rectangular pleural flap* is dissected and raised from behind forward with base in front; elevated pleura is wrapped around the perforation fully and sutured to the oesophageal mucosa in depth using multiple interrupted 3-zero non-absorbable sutures. *In intercostal muscle flap*, adjacent intercostal muscle is elevated from inside posteriorly adjacent to aorta with intact blood supply with its base at medial end; this vascularised flap is conveniently rotated forward encircling as a wrap around the perforated oesophagus and is sutured **(Figs. 20-68 to 20-71)**.

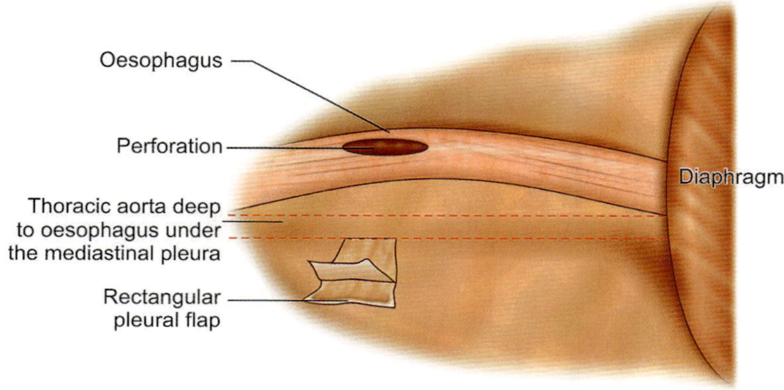

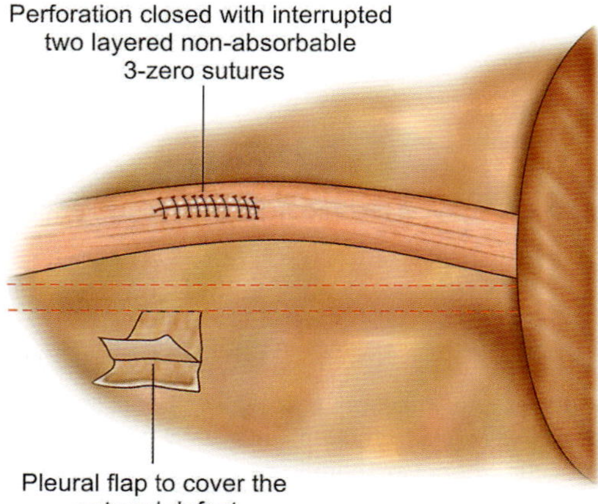

Fig. 20-68: Primary closure of oesophageal perforation with pleural flap switch.

Oesophagus is often *excluded/diverted* by doing cervical proximal oesophagostomy. *Cervical oesophagostomy* is done through left side neck incision along the anterior border of the sternomastoid. Mobilisation is done similarly as mentioned above. Sternocleidomastoid muscle is retracted outward after opening the deep fascia; omohyoid muscle is cut; carotid sheath is retraced laterally; thyroid and trachea is retracted medially using assistant's finger; recurrent laryngeal nerve is safeguarded (both sides). Middle thyroid vein and inferior thyroid artery if needed is ligated and divided. Prevertebral fascia is dissected to encircle the oesophagus by sharp and blunt dissection. Oesophagus is slinged using infant feeding tube or umbilical tape; significant length is mobilised both proximally and distally to prevent tension after doing oesophagostomy. Oesophagus with sling is brought out towards the middle of the wound. Sternocleidomastoid muscle and deep fascia are sutured using 3-zero vicryl. Platysma and skin is sutured in the wound leaving middle of about 4 cm length for oesophagostomy. Transverse incision on the half circumference of the brought out oesophagus is done; one should confirm that there is no tension. Partially opened up cervical oesophagus is sutured to skin using interrupted subcuticular 3 zero absorbable sutures.

Decortication of the lung with removal of both parietal and visceral pleura allows adequate lung expansion.

Two intercostal tubes are placed in the space adjacent to the perforation site; other in the intercostal space itself.

Postoperatively patient needs ventilator support, antibiotics, total parenteral nutrition, jejunostomy feed and critical care management.

Condition has got high mortality. Other complications are empyema, mediastinitis, septicaemia, subphrenic abscess, respiratory failure and acute renal failure. Repeat CT chest, blood or blood product transfusions, monitoring by reassessing the patient with biochemical analysis is needed.

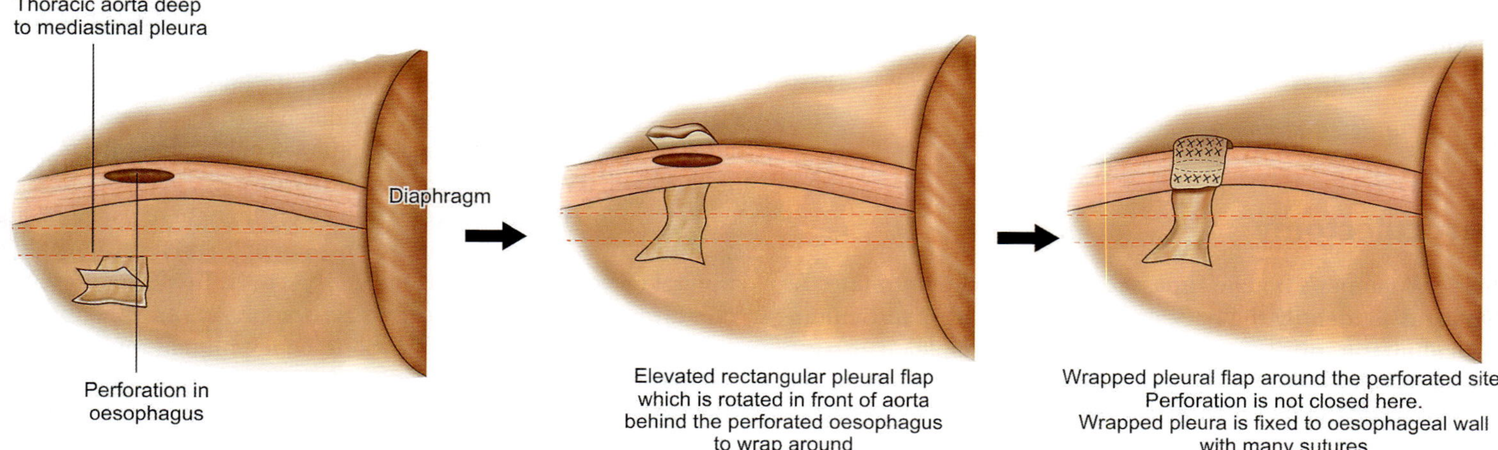

Fig. 20-69: Oesophageal perforation is not closed here; instead rectangular pleural flap is mobilised to cover the defect and suture on the oesophageal wall away from the perforation defect.

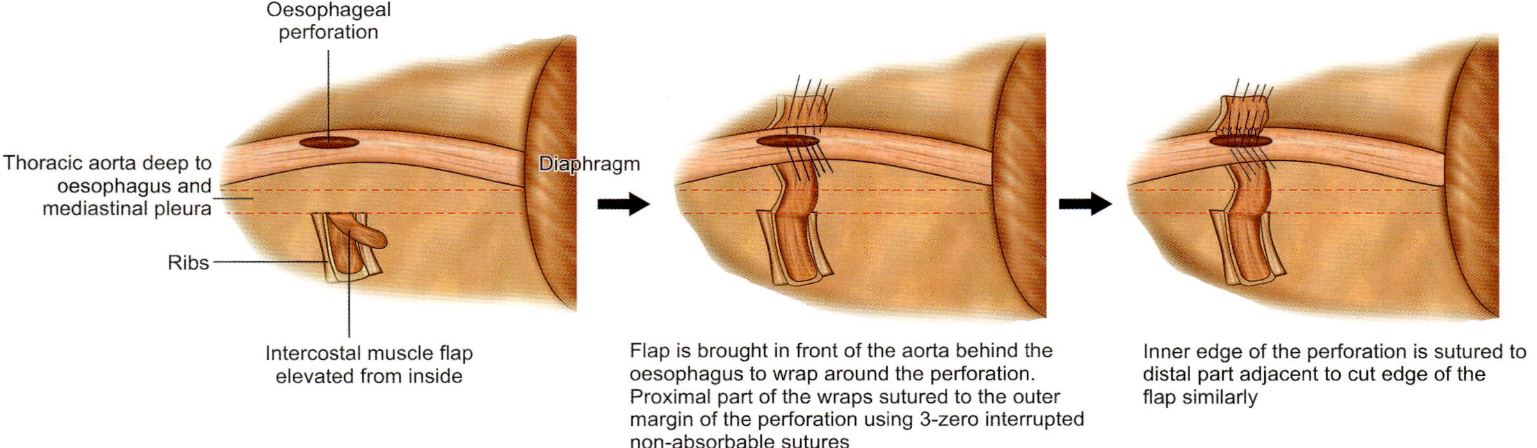

Fig. 20-70: Closure of the oesophageal perforation with intercostal muscle flap.

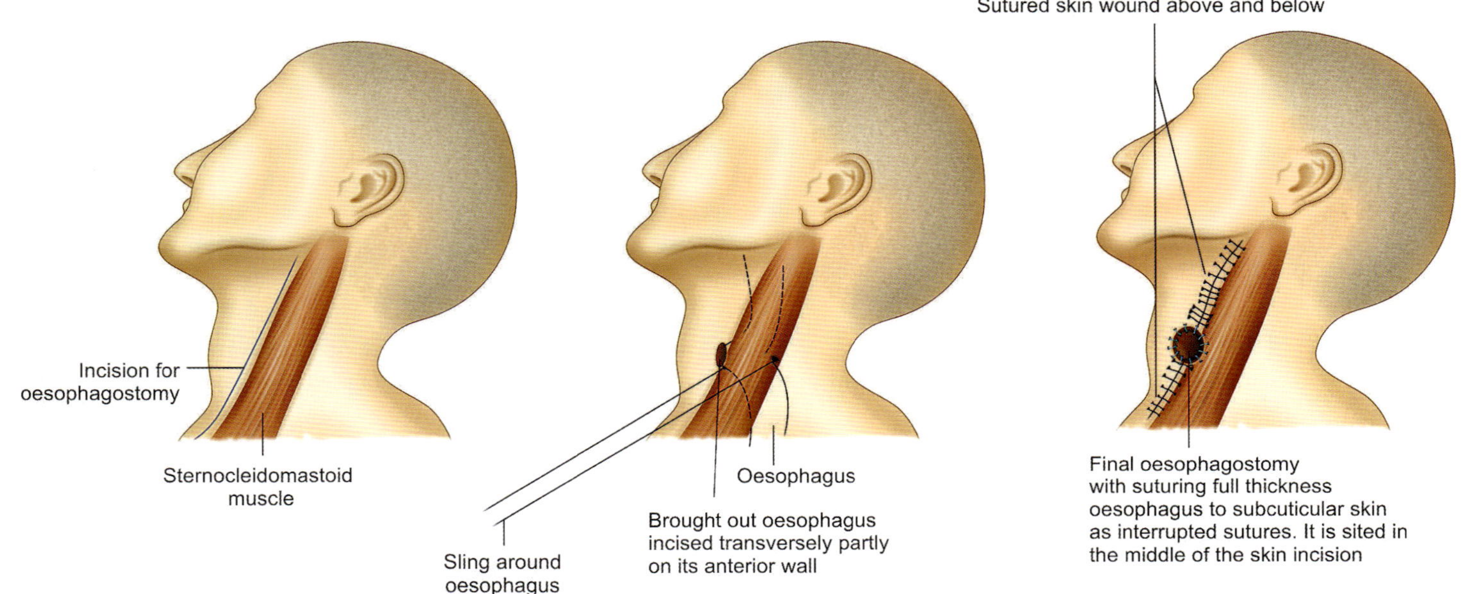

Fig. 20-71: Cervical oesophagostomy for severe oesophageal perforation.

INTUBATION SURGERIES FOR ADVANCED CARCINOMA OF OESOPHAGUS

Intubation of oesophagus across the growth was practiced earlier as a palliative technique to relieve dysphagia is no longer commonly done. Now it is a surgical legacy. Atkinson tube, Celestin tube, Souttar tube, Mousseau-Barbin tube were used. Now endoscopic self-expanding metal stents (SEMS) are commonly used and ideal.

Celestin tube (armoured tube with a long tail): It is a flexible polythene tube which is wider proximally with a barrel shaped funnel. It is 25 cm in length. It is 9 and 14 mm in diameter at luminal level. It is oval on cross section. There is a fine pilot bougie of 60 cm length made up of solid polythene. It is passed through endoscopy and laparotomy. Through an oesophagoscope pilot tube is passed across the growth into the stomach; oesophagoscope is removed; Celestin tube is anchored after plugging into the proximal end of the pilot bougie using a stitch through holes in both. Mini upper midline laparotomy is done. Anterior gastrotomy is done on the proximal part of the anterior wall of the stomach; end of the pilot bougie is identified and withdrawn through gastrotomy wound to pull down the anchored Celestin tube until proximal funnel impacts against the narrowed segment of the oesophagus. Excess end in the stomach is trimmed. Gastrotomy and laparotomy is closed. It is traction tube **(Fig. 20-72)**.

Souttar tube (coiled German silver wire): Block is first dilated with bougies; tube is passed over small sized bougie and pushed across the block. It is mainly useful for lower oesophagus. Its introduction does not require laparotomy. It is a pulsion tube.

Mousseau-Barbin tube: Cheaper but needs laparotomy. After laparotomy anterior wall of the stomach is opened.

MB tube is passed from mouth with the help of anaesthetist by stitching its tip to nasogastric tube and pulled down into the stomach. Tip is cut near the cone part. It is sutured to anterior wall of the stomach. Gastrotomy is closed. It is a traction tube **(Fig. 20-73)**.

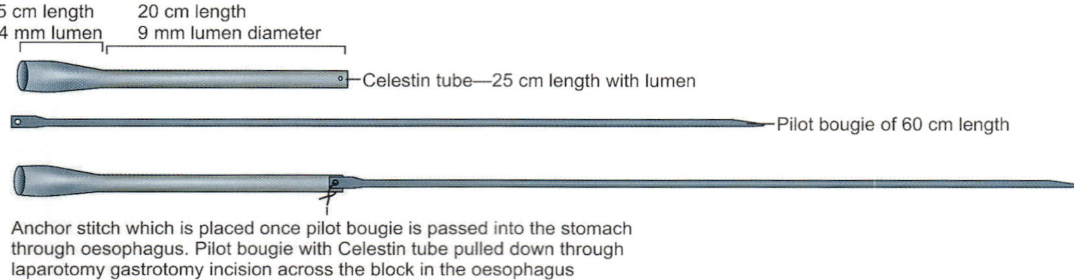

Fig. 20-72: Celestin tube used for oesophageal intubation.

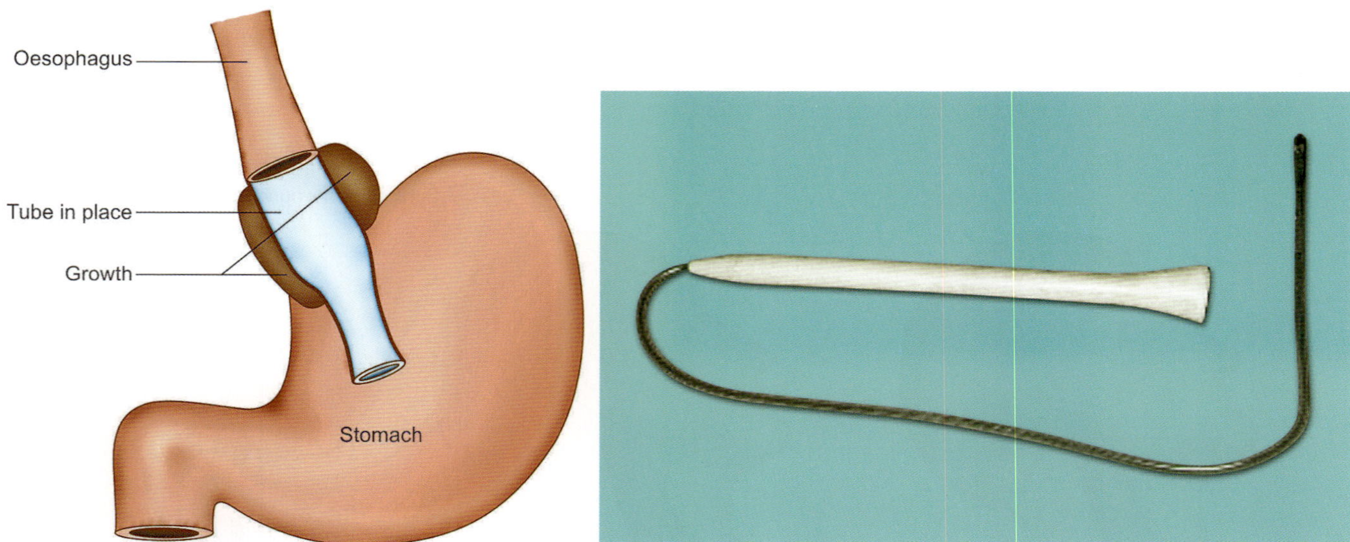

Fig. 20-73: *Mousseau-Barbin tube*—placement in advanced carcinoma of oesophagus. It is not used nowadays.

21

CHAPTER

Surgery of Stomach and Duodenum

SURGICAL ANATOMY OF STOMACH AND DUODENUM

The stomach lies obliquely in the upper left part of the abdomen occupying epigastric, umbilical and left hypochondriac regions. Most of it lies under left costal margin and ribs. Cardiac orifice on surface marking is located 2.5 cm left of the midline in the left 7th costal cartilage. Pyloric orifice is located in the transpyloric line 1.2 cm right of the midline. Fundus extends upwards from a line along the left of the cardiac orifice to a point up to the left 5th intercostal space just below the nipple. Stomach is J-shaped when empty; pyriform-shaped when distended. Stomach is 25 cm in length. It has got capacity of 30 mL at birth; 1 litre at puberty; 2 litres in adult.

The stomach contains four anatomic regions **(Fig. 21-1)**:

1. Fundus.
2. Cardia.
3. Body.
4. Pylorus—pyloric antrum and pyloric canal.

Angle of His is angle of entry of oesophagus into the stomach which is 30°–70°. In cadaver, it reduces to 20°. This oesophagogastric junction is often termed as cardia. Fundus is the segment of the stomach above an arbitrary horizontal line drawn from the angle of His. Fundus of the stomach is covered by the peritoneum anteriorly; posteriorly, it is covered in most parts except a crescent-shaped part along the upper right part of the fundus and posterior lesser curvature and this area is called as bare area of stomach. Occasionally, it is wide enough to cause difficulty in mobilising the stomach. Behind fundus of the stomach is related to the diaphragm **(Fig. 21-2)**.

Stomach per se anatomically is a very mobile organ which is easier to understand. But while doing surgical procedures like gastrectomies, it is mandatory to mobilise the proximal or distal stomach and so stomach is often considered as *two gastric units* - proximal and distal **(Fig. 21-3)**.

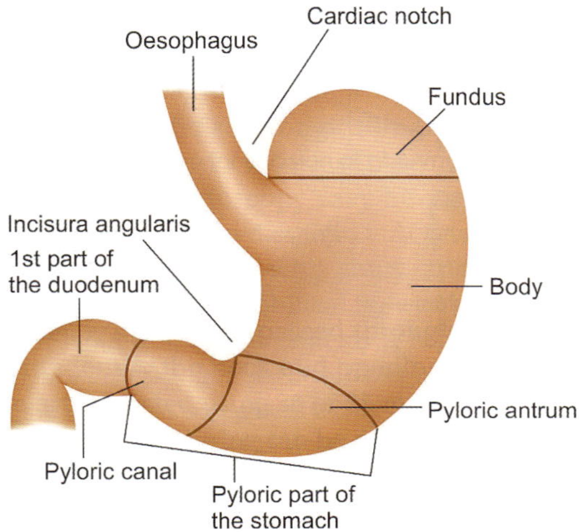

Fig. 21-1: Parts of the stomach.

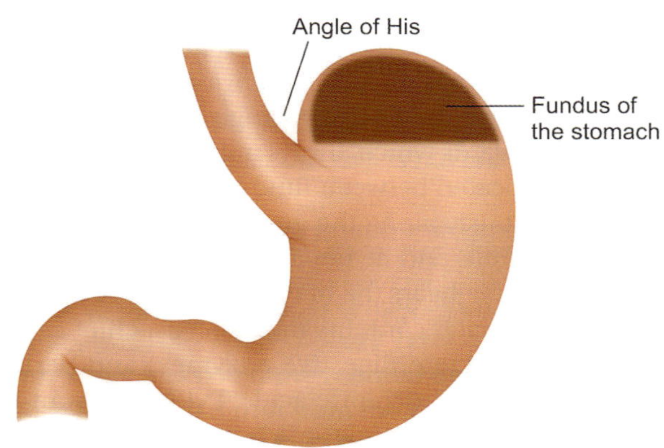

Fig. 21-2: Angle of His.

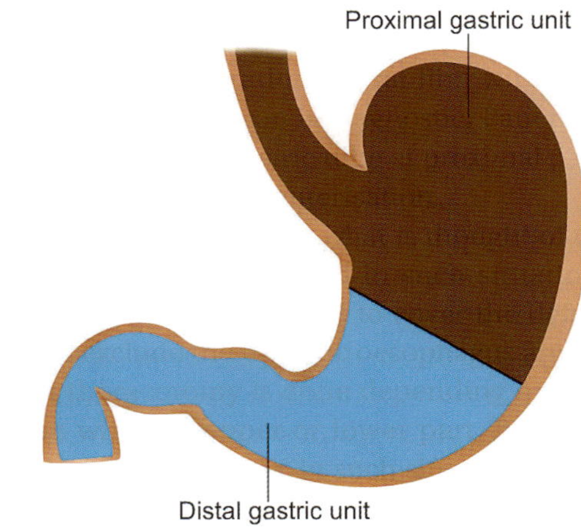

Fig. 21-3: Stomach is considered as two units—proximal and distal. It is relevant while doing gastrectomies.

Proximal gastric unit contains proximal stomach with fundus, oesophagogastric junction, oesophageal hiatus and distal oesophagus. *Distal gastric unit* contains gastric antrum, pylorus and 1st part of the duodenum. It is related in front to the posterior surface of the left lobe of the liver; behind to right crus of the diaphragm, right side to caudate lobe of the liver, left side to the splenic inner surface. Antral mucosa is flat without rugae. It is often demarcated from outside from incisura angularis along the lesser curve, even though it is very much variable. Line is usually located 4 cm proximal to the *'crow's foot'* of the descending part of the anterior vagus nerve; 10 cm proximal to pylorus. Antrum ends at pyloric canal as pylorus. Pylorus ends to thin walled duodenum as pyloric ring (pylorus means *gate guard*). Pyloric ring is formed by a septum from submucosal connective tissue at pyloroduodenal junction; circular muscle proximal to this ring is thickened, acting as pyloric sphincter; distal to this forms thin circular muscle layer of the duodenum. First part of the duodenum is 2.5 cm in length. Pyloric orifice is located at the level of lower border of L1 vertebra in transpyloric plane. Pylorus on the surface feels like a circular groove/constriction due to pyloric sphincter. Pylorus feels like a firm nodule with prepyloric vein located in front of the pyloric constriction. Distal gastric unit is related behind to floor of the lesser sac, transverse mesocolon, head and neck of pancreas, aorta and celiac trunk with branches, gastroduodenal unit, common bile duct, portal vein and hepatic artery. In front, it is related to left and right lobes of the liver, transverse mesocolon, gallbladder with its neck often, anterior abdominal wall.

Oesophageal hiatus is formed by the two pillars of the right crus of the diaphragm. Phrenooesophageal membrane is present in front.

Stomach is often divided into two parts by a line drawn downwards and towards left from incisura angularis. Proximal part is called as cardia which is larger and is divided into fundus and body. Smaller distal pyloric part is again divided into pyloric antrum and pyloric canal. Fundus is above the line from angle of His, which is dome-shaped directed upwards which always normally contains gas. Body of the stomach is located between fundus and pyloric antrum and can distend enormously along the greater curvature. Lesser curve is very less distensible and at much posterior level than greater curvature. Lesser curve bears the maximum insult of the swallowed liquids. Body of stomach contains mucus cells, chief cells (peptic or zymogenic cells secrete digestive enzymes) and parietal cells (oxyntic cells secrete hydrochloric acid). Pyloric antrum is 7.5 cm in length which contains mainly mucous glands. Narrow tubular pyloric canal is 2.5 cm long **(Fig. 21-4)**.

Greater omentum is present along the greater curvature which extends downwards as a free apron on the abdomen; reflects back towards transverse colon where it is attached with avascular tissue. Within it exists the *omental bursa* which is of surgical importance, especially in radical gastrectomies. Omental bursa extends from the upper margin of the transverse colon along the superior leaf of the transverse mesocolon towards front of the pancreas, reflecting back in front to the greater omentum. Two layers of the greater omentum meet near the fundus in its upper part as gastrosplenic ligament.

Peritoneum on the posterior surface of the stomach near upper part reflects on the diaphragm as gastrophrenic ligament. Its upper part is avascular and through which a window can be created in vagotomy or during mobilisation of the oesophageal hiatus. Its lower part contains short gastric vessels and lymph nodes.

Gastrocolic ligament is part of greater omentum extending from the greater curvature of the stomach and first part of the duodenum to the transverse colon. Mobilisation of this ligament is essential in many gastric and pancreatic surgeries.

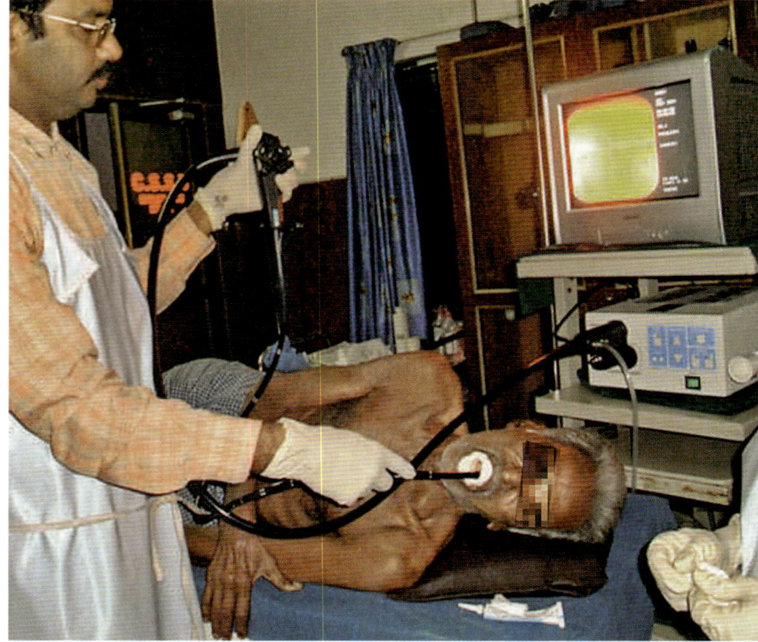

Fig. 21-4: Gastroscopy reveals the demarcation between the body and pyloric antrum. Antrum does not have rugosity.

Lesser omentum is much thinner and extends from lesser curvature towards the liver. Hepatogastric ligament is the proximal part of lesser omentum extends from porta hepatis and lesser curvature of the stomach; above it extends as ventral mesentery of abdominal oesophagus. Hepatogastric ligament contains left gastric vessels, hepatic branch of anterior vagus, posterior gastric divisions of the vagus and lymph nodes. In 23% of individuals an aberrant left hepatic artery may be present in this ligament which may be exclusive supply of the left lobe of the liver.

Hepatoduodenal ligament is distal part of the lesser omentum extending from the liver to 1st 2.5 cm of the duodenum. Its free edge contains hepatic triad and lymph nodes **(Fig. 21-5)**.

Diaphragm separates the stomach from left pleura, pericardium and lower ribs (6th to 9th). Posteriorly stomach is related to diaphragm, left kidney, left adrenal gland, splenic flexure of colon, transverse mesocolon and splenic artery. Gastrosplenic ligament is spread between greater curvature of the stomach and spleen.

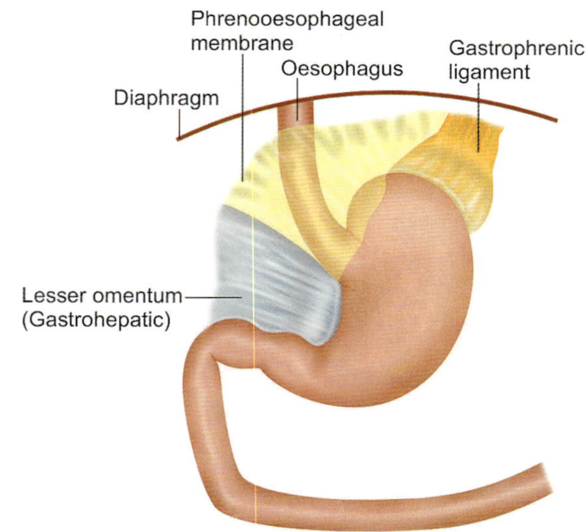

Fig. 21-5: Oesophagogastric junction and ligaments of stomach.

Arterial Supply of Stomach

Stomach is supplied by left gastric artery, a branch of coeliac artery (smallest branch of coeliac axis); right gastric artery, a branch of proper hepatic artery; right gastroepiploic artery, a branch of gastroduodenal artery (a largest branch of common hepatic artery); left gastroepiploic artery, a branch of splenic artery; short gastric arteries, branches of splenic artery; left inferior phrenic artery, a branch of aorta; posterior gastric artery, a branch of left gastric/splenic artery or from coeliac trunk which supplies distal oesophagus, fundus and OG junction. Gastroepiploic arteries are also called as gastroomental arteries. Vessels in the omentum form an arcade called as *arc of Barkow* **(Figs. 21-6A and B)**.

Left gastric artery after originating from coeliac trunk (90%) runs retroperitoneally upwards and left giving oesophageal branches. Then it runs downwards to reach the proximal lesser curve to continue along lesser curvature of stomach to anastomose with the right gastric artery. When it enters the lesser curve, it gives cardiooesophageal branch, often called as ascending branch which runs upwards. Left gastric artery then runs downwards as descending branch which eventually gives into anterior and posterior branches. Numerous gastric branches enter the stomach to supply it. As a variation, left gastric artery may originate from common hepatic artery, splenic artery, aorta, superior mesenteric artery; or as gastrosplenic trunk or hepatogastric trunk. Rarely it can originate directly from aorta. Aberrant left hepatic artery may arise (24%) from left gastric artery, and in such situation, artery will be much wider than usual.

Right gastric artery commonly arises from proper hepatic artery (65%); but can arise from left hepatic artery (25%) or common hepatic artery (3%). It runs along the lesser curvature of stomach for 6 cm, 0.5 cm from lesser curve margin to join left gastric artery. Supraduodenal artery which usually arises from proper hepatic artery just proximal to right gastric artery can arise from right gastric artery (13%).

Common hepatic artery arises from coeliac trunk that runs behind the lesser sac towards right reaching the upper border of the duodenum. Here it gives large branch, gastroduodenal artery which descends vertically downwards from 1st part of the duodenum behind to divide as *right gastroepiploic artery* and superior pancreaticoduodenal artery (which often divides into anterior and posterior branches running along the pancreaticoduodenal groove to communicate with inferior pancreaticoduodenal artery which is a branch of superior mesenteric artery). Common hepatic artery continues as proper hepatic artery which later gives supraduodenal artery and right gastric artery enters and runs along the free border of the lesser omentum in front of the portal vein and left of the common bile duct to reach porta hepatis. Here it divides into right and left branches.

Left gastroepiploic artery arises from the splenic artery distally close to greater curvature. Posterior gastric artery arises from splenic artery proximal to the origin of the left gastroepiploic artery. Often this is the only blood supply which is left in subtotal gastrectomy wherein left gastric artery is ligated at its origin and many short gastric vessels are also ligated.

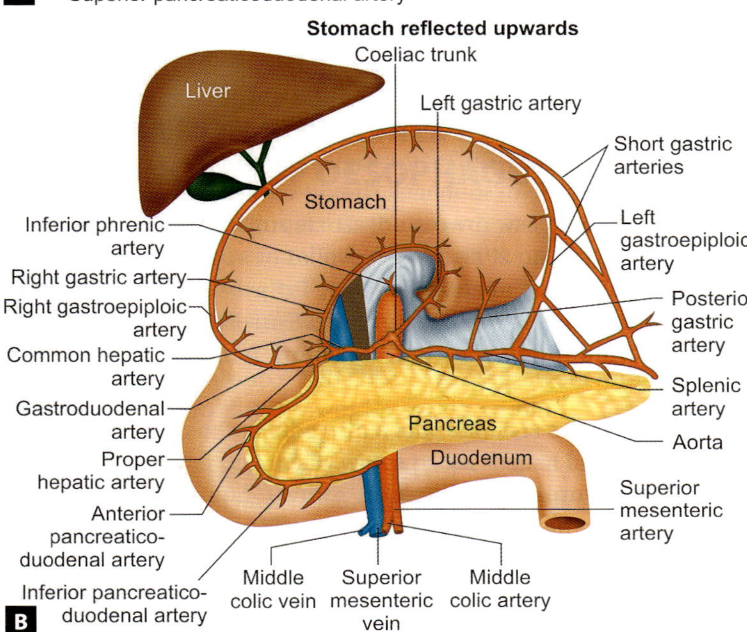

Figs. 21-6A and B: Arterial supply of stomach. View also shown after reflecting the stomach upwards.

Venous Drainage of Stomach (Fig. 21-7)

Right and left gastric veins drain into portal vein. Left gastric vein is caudal to left gastric artery and also called as coronary vein. Left gastric vein receives tributaries from oesophageal hiatus and oesophagus; runs downwards and towards right to join commonly to portal vein (70%) or splenic vein near its junction to portal vein (30%). Left gastric vein communicates with azygos vein which will lead into the varices when there is portal hypertension. Left gastroepiploic and short gastric veins drain into splenic vein. Splenic vein block causes extensive varices in the proximal gastric unit. Right gastroepiploic vein drains into superior mesenteric vein. It receives anterior

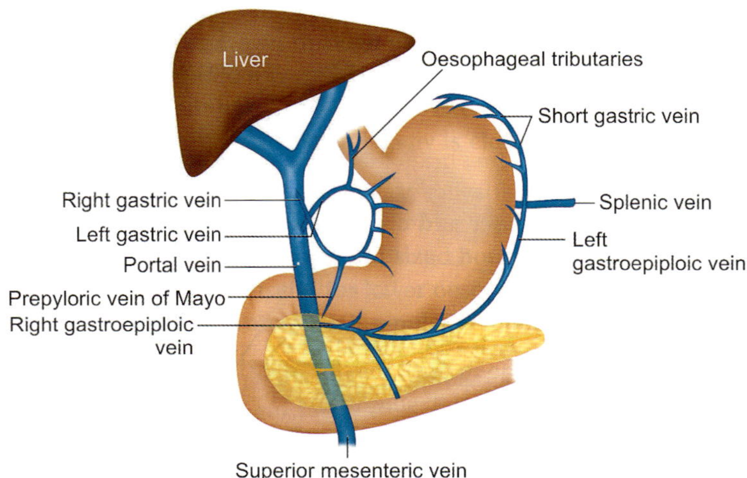

Fig. 21-7: Venous drainage of the stomach.

superior pancreaticoduodenal vein and middle colic vein in front of pancreatic head. Blockage of right gastroepiploic vein can cause duodenal varices. In portal hypertension, congestion of veins and varices can develop between right and left gastroepiploic vessels. Right gastric vein runs close to right gastric artery towards right along distal gastric unit to drain into the portal or superior mesenteric or splenic vein. Often *Henle's gastrocolic vein* may be present (70%) formed by right gastroomental vein and right colic vein; it is short run along the root of the transverse mesocolon and anterior surface of the head of the pancreas. Prepyloric vein of *Mayo* distinguishes pyloric canal from the first part of duodenum. It drains into the right gastric vein.

Nerve Supply of Stomach

Intrinsic innervation occurs through myenteric plexus of *Auerbach* and submucous plexus of *Meissner.*

Right vagus is posterior and left vagus is anterior. Right posterior vagus is away from oesophagus closer to aorta, unlike left vagus. Both right and left vagi are usually right of the midline in 80% of cases; but anterior vagus is more left compared to posterior vagus. Hence, it is better to name them as posterior and anterior even though right and left vagi are commonly used terminologies. Posterior vagus gives *criminal nerve of Grassi* (Professor Grassi, Rome), which supply lower oesophagus and fundus of stomach, which, if not cut properly during vagotomy, may lead to recurrent ulcer. It is a single nerve arising from posterior vagus that runs behind the cardia to supply part of fundus and proximal stomach. Vagus also gives splanchnic branches (*hepatic and coeliac branches),* ends as *nerve of Latarjet* (Latarjet - French surgeon, 1921) which supplies the antrum and maintains the antral pump. Each vagus gives divisions—splanchnic and gastric. Anterior gastric nerve from anterior trunk after running along the anterior surface of the lesser curvature ends as anterior nerve of Latarjet (greater anterior nerve of Mitchell) supplying the antral pump. Similarly posterior gastric nerve arises from posterior vagus. Anterior vagus gives hepatic branch (frequently multiple); posterior vagus gives a single stout coeliac branch to coeliac ganglion. Hepatic branch of the anterior vagus often gives a direct branch to the pylorus. Nerve of Latarjet arising from posterior trunk is much smaller and ends much proximal than that of anterior vagus. Parietal branches help in HCl secretion, which is an important concept in vagotomy that is done as a treatment in duodenal ulcer. *Truncal vagotomy* with posterior gastrojejunostomy is done for chronic duodenal ulcer with pyloric stenosis. Right vagus is thicker than left vagus; left vagus is embedded in the anterior oesophageal wall **(Fig. 21-8)**.

Among hepatic, anterior/posterior gastric and celiac divisions, coeliac division is the largest one. Coeliac division lies on the gastropancreatic peritoneal fold. It is a single trunk arising from the posterior vagus which supplies coeliac plexus.

Anterior vagus gives hepatic, gastric and antral branch. Hepatic branches originate as first branches of the anterior vagus below the diaphragm runs in the layers of the lesser omentum reaching liver; it gives branches to liver and continues as plexus around hepatic artery giving branches to gallbladder, bile duct and pancreas. A pyloric branch begins here runs along the right gastric artery downwards to supply pylorus and part of the stomach. One more branch runs along the gastroduodenal artery and right gastroepiploic artery to supply greater curvature of the stomach. About 5–10 gastric branches arise from anterior vagus supplying anterior portion of the proximal stomach and fundus. It runs closely associated with vessels of the lesser curvature entering the serosal layer of the stomach to run in the subserosal plane for 2 cm; then it enters the submucosal and mucosal planes. They supply parietal cells and smooth muscle cells

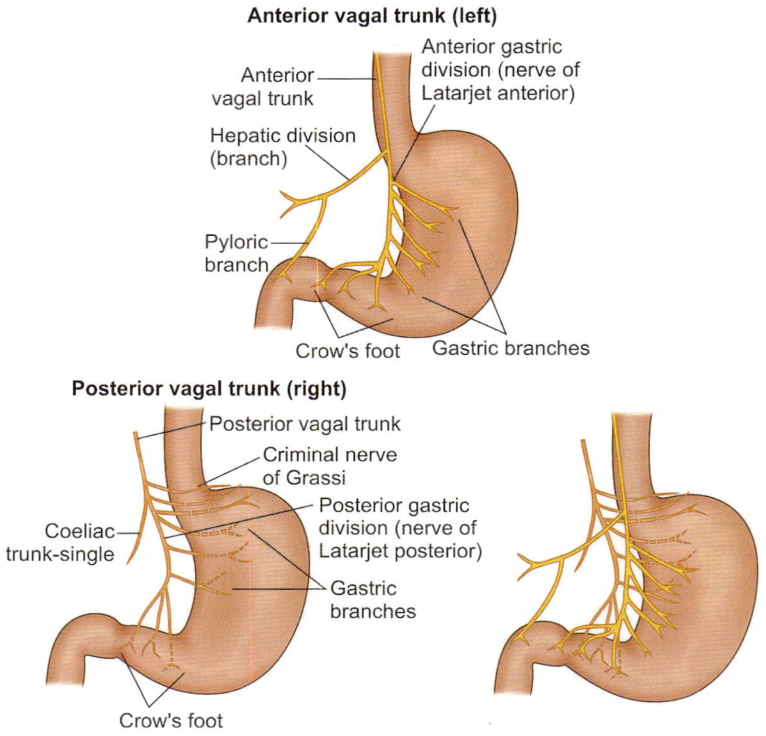

Fig. 21-8: Distribution of vagal trunks in the abdomen.

of the body and fundus of the stomach. Often branch/branches may present at higher level at or beyond angle of His. *Anterior nerve of Latarjet* is the final continuation of the anterior vagus towards pylorus; near incisura angularis, it fans out many branches over the gastric antrum as 'crow's foot' (this word is coined by Goligher). Anterior and posterior nerves of Latarjet supply antropyloric mechanism. This nerve has to be preserved in highly selective vagotomy to retain antral pump function.

Posterior vagus gives single coeliac branch which joins coeliac plexus. It often receives a communicating branch from anterior vagus. Around 5–6 gastric branches descend and enter the posterior wall of the stomach to supply similar to gastric branches of the anterior vagus. Posterior vagus continues downwards as posterior nerve of Latarjet to supply antrum and pylorus. *Posterior nerve of Latarjet* ends at more proximal level than anterior nerve of Latarjet. *Criminal nerve of Grassi arises* from the posterior vagus running behind OG junction to supply fundus and proximal stomach.

Vagus in the distal 6–8 cm of oesophagus also supplies the stomach by different fibres through distal oesophageal plexus. So distal 8 cm of the oesophagus should be skeletonised to achieve optimum results of the vagotomy. The proximal most branch of '*crow's foot*' is 7 cm from pyloroduodenal junction. Junction of antrum and body is 4 cm proximal to this. Antrum does not have parietal and chief cells. So in highly selective vagotomy, dissection is done proximal to 'crow's foot'. In the OG junction, vagal fibers are located within the peritoneal fold left of the oesophagus. So all loose areolar tissue should be dissected towards left of the oesophagus and angle of His to achieve complete vagotomy.

Highly selective vagotomy (HSV) is done in case of uncomplicated chronic duodenal ulcer (refractile ulcer) which is not responding to available medical line of treatment. In HSV, nerve of Latarjet is retained so as to retain antral pump and no drainage is required. Here only the fibres entering the stomach are ligated close to the lesser curve to reduce the acid secretion. Usually vessels accompanying nerves are also ligated together. In *selective vagotomy,* splanchnic branches are retained but it is presently not done.

Gastroduodenal pain is sensed via sympathetic fibres (T5-T10). Term *extended proximal gastric vagotomy* means additional division of the recurrent branch of hepatic vagal branches distributed to greater curvature along gastroduodenal and right gastroepiploic arteries.

Histology

The fundus and body contain parietal (acid producing) and chief cells. *Parietal cells* secrete acid and intrinsic factor. *Chief cells* produce pepsinogen. There are two types of pepsinogen secreted by chief cells—I and II. Pepsinogen I is produced only in stomach. In gastric atrophy, pepsinogen I is decreased. In the antrum, *endocrine cells* produce *gastrin* (G cells) and somatostatin (D cells). 12% of epithelial cells of stomach are parietal (oxyntic) cells; 45% chief (zymogenic cells); 40% mucous cells; 3% endocrine cells. Submucosa is strongest, collagen rich layer of gastric mucosa. Gastric mucus is a mucosal barrier containing mucopolysaccharides which maintains the integrity of gastric mucosa. Muscles of the stomach wall are outer longitudinal; middle circular and inner oblique. Middle circular and innermost oblique muscles blend in angle of His forming collar of *Helvetius*.

Lymphatic Drainage of Stomach

Lymphatics of proximal half of stomach drain into left gastric, splenic, and superior pancreatic lymph nodes. From antrum, it drains into right gastric, right gastroepiploic and subpyloric lymph nodes. From pylorus, it drains into right gastric and subpyloric lymph nodes. Efferent lymphatics from suprapyloric region drain into para-aortic lymph nodes and so into left supraclavicular lymph nodes. Efferent lymphatics from subpyloric lymph nodes drain into superior mesenteric lymph nodes. Lymphatics near *oesophagogastric* (OG) junction communicate with oesophageal lymphatics. In carcinoma stomach if upper lymphatics are blocked, retrograde spread through lower lymphatics can occur. Presently in carcinoma stomach, different resections are classified as R0, R1, R2, R3, or D1, D2 (dissection) based on levels of lymph nodes in the abdomen in relation to the stomach. R0 is no residual disease; R1 is microscopic residual disease; R2 is macroscopic residual disease; R3 is inoperable **(Fig. 21-9)**.

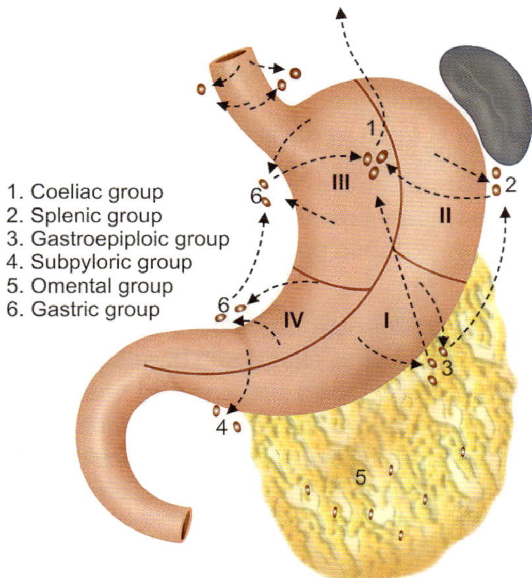

Fig. 21-9: Lymphatic drainage of stomach.

Zones of lymphatic drainage in stomach: Four zones.

Zone 1-inferior gastric: It lies in gastrocolic omentum along the right gastroepiploic vessels, draining pyloric portion of the greater curve to pyloric, coeliac and aortic lymph nodes.

Zone 2-splenic: It lies in gastrocolic and gastrosplenic omentum along the left gastroepiploic vessels draining from upper half of greater curve to pancreaticosplenic and aortic lymph nodes.

Zone 3-superior gastric: There is drainage from proximal two-thirds of the stomach and the upper lesser curve along the left gastric artery. Zone 3 drains into perioesophageal lymph nodes.

Zone 4-hepatic: It is from distal portion of lesser curve and pylorus along hepatic artery into para-aortic nodes.

Lymph node groups

Group I: Perigastric nodes
Group II: Along the root of major vessels
Group III: At the root of superior mesenteric artery and hepatoduodenal ligament
Group IV: Distant lymph nodes.

SURGERY FOR DUODENAL ULCER PERFORATION

It is an emergency surgery. Preoperatively X-ray abdomen in erect or lateral decubitus confirms the diagnosis. Additionally ultrasound abdomen may be useful. Electrolyte estimation, renal functions should be confirmed. Initial resuscitation with proper fluid therapy, antibiotics, CVP line, nasogastric aspiration and urinary catheterisation should be done **(Figs. 21-10 to 21-12)**.

Occasionally when stomach is empty, perforation may get sealed-off automatically or may form localised abscess in the lesser sac, subphrenic space or paracolic gutter. Mikulicz (1887) and Dean (1894) did first successful closure of perforation by suturing edges of the perforation. Later Cellan Jones (1929) and Graham (1937) popularised the omental plugging and suturing the perforation which was originally thought by Bennett (1899).

Technique (Fig. 21-13)

Emergency laparotomy through upper midline incision is done. All infected fluid is sucked out. Perforation is identified.

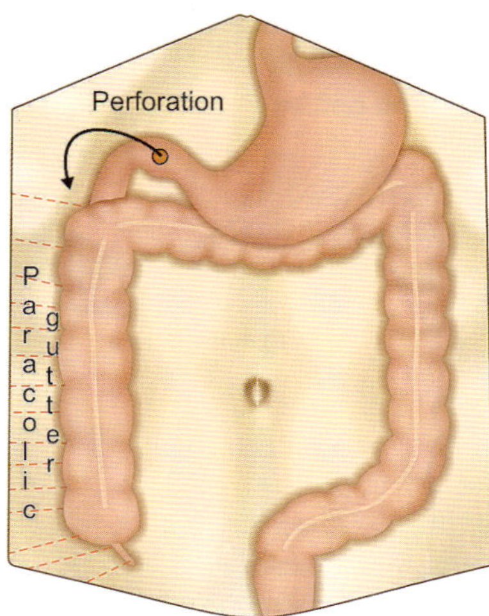

Fig. 21-10: Duodenal ulcer perforation. Here fluid from perforated site travels along the right paracolic gutter.

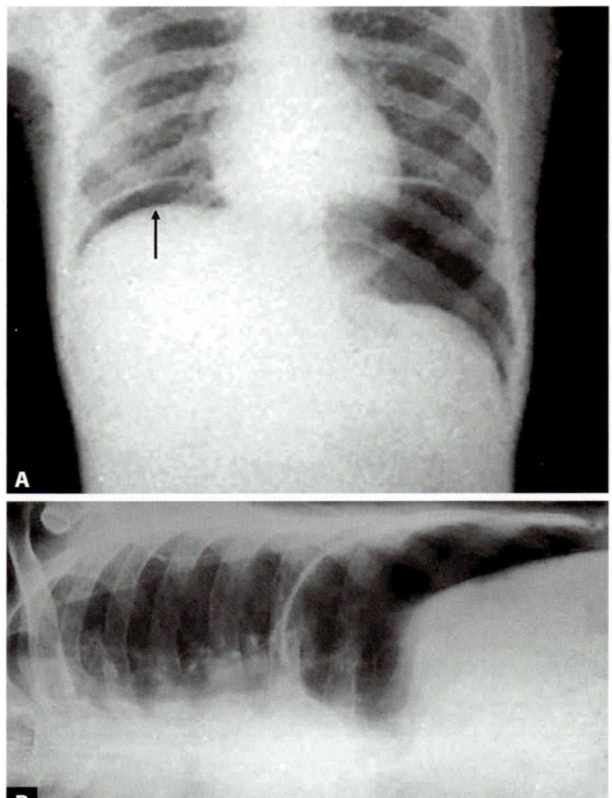

Figs. 21-11A and B: X-ray chest and upper abdomen or lateral decubitus showing gas under diaphragm.

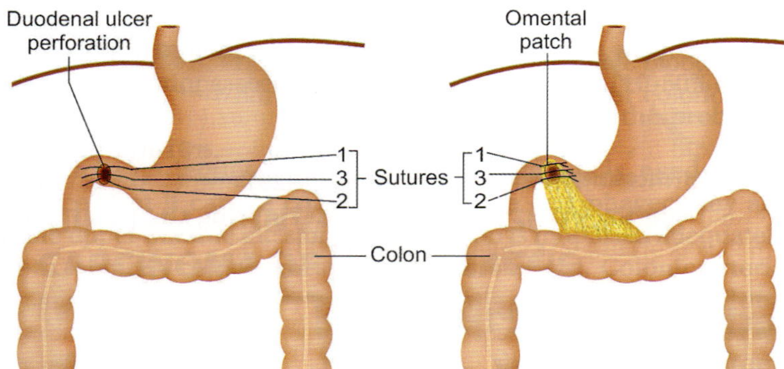

Fig. 21-12: Closure of duodenal ulcer perforation using Graham's omental patch.

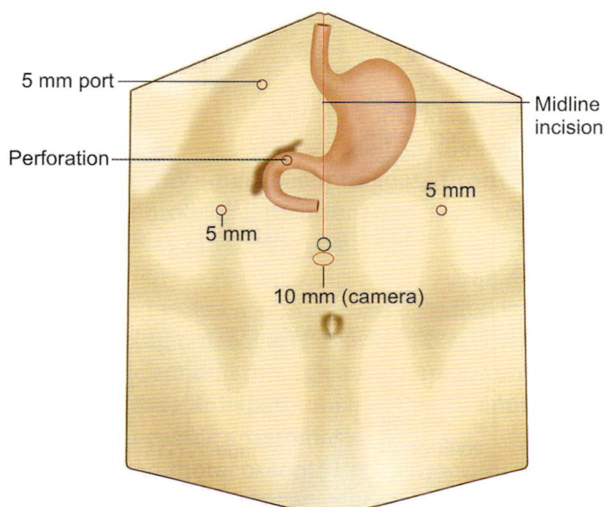

Fig. 21-13: Incision for closure of perforated duodenum for open and laparoscopic approach.

Usually duodenal ulcer perforation is less than 1 cm in size. Giant ulcer is more than 2 cm in size. Omentum will be adherent to the site of perforation. It is gently separated. If duodenum is not perforated then stomach, posterior wall of stomach (lesser sac), small bowel and colon are thoroughly checked for possible sites.

Once perforation is identified, surrounding area is sucked out with suction. Liver, colon and proximal stomach are retracted. Suture material used for perforation is 3-0 vicryl or PDS or silk. As perforation edge is friable and oedematous, needle bites should be very gentle. Bite from each edge (5 mm from the edge) is taken separately. Each suture is kept away using haemostats on either side untied. Three stitches are taken at equal distances. Omental pedicle is used like a patch. Viable segment of omentum should be used. Often it needs placing few ligatures to get adequate length of the omental pedicle. Omentum is placed on the perforation site to seal it. Knots are placed on it. Initially side sutures are tied on omentum; then centre one to avoid tearing of the friable edge of perforated site. First suture towards the upper part, i.e. apex of the omental pedicle is tied. All sutures should be interrupted horizontal one. Omental patch is placed *before suturing*—it is called as ***Graham Operation***. Because of its *adhesion property,* it seals perforation; good vascularity and lymphatics promote the healing effectively **(Figs. 21-14 to 21-16)**.

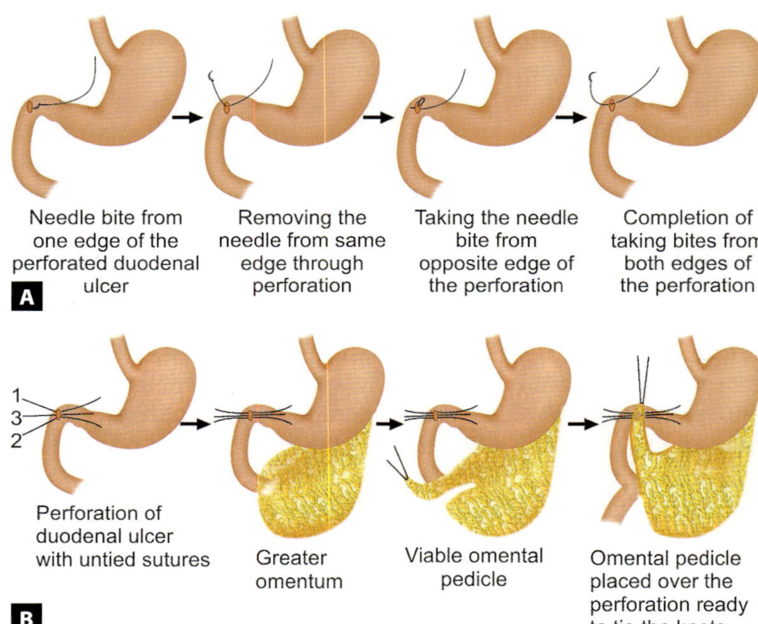

Figs. 21-14A and B: Closure of duodenal perforation—technique.

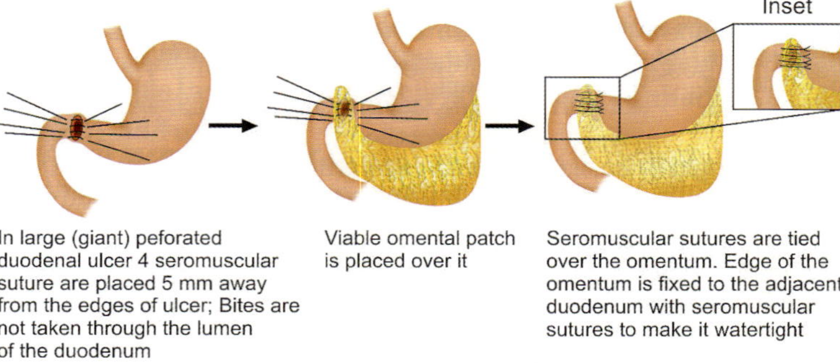

Fig. 21-15: Perforated giant duodenal ulcer is closed by taking only seromuscular bites to hold omental patch; here bites are not taken through the mucosal layer across the lumen.

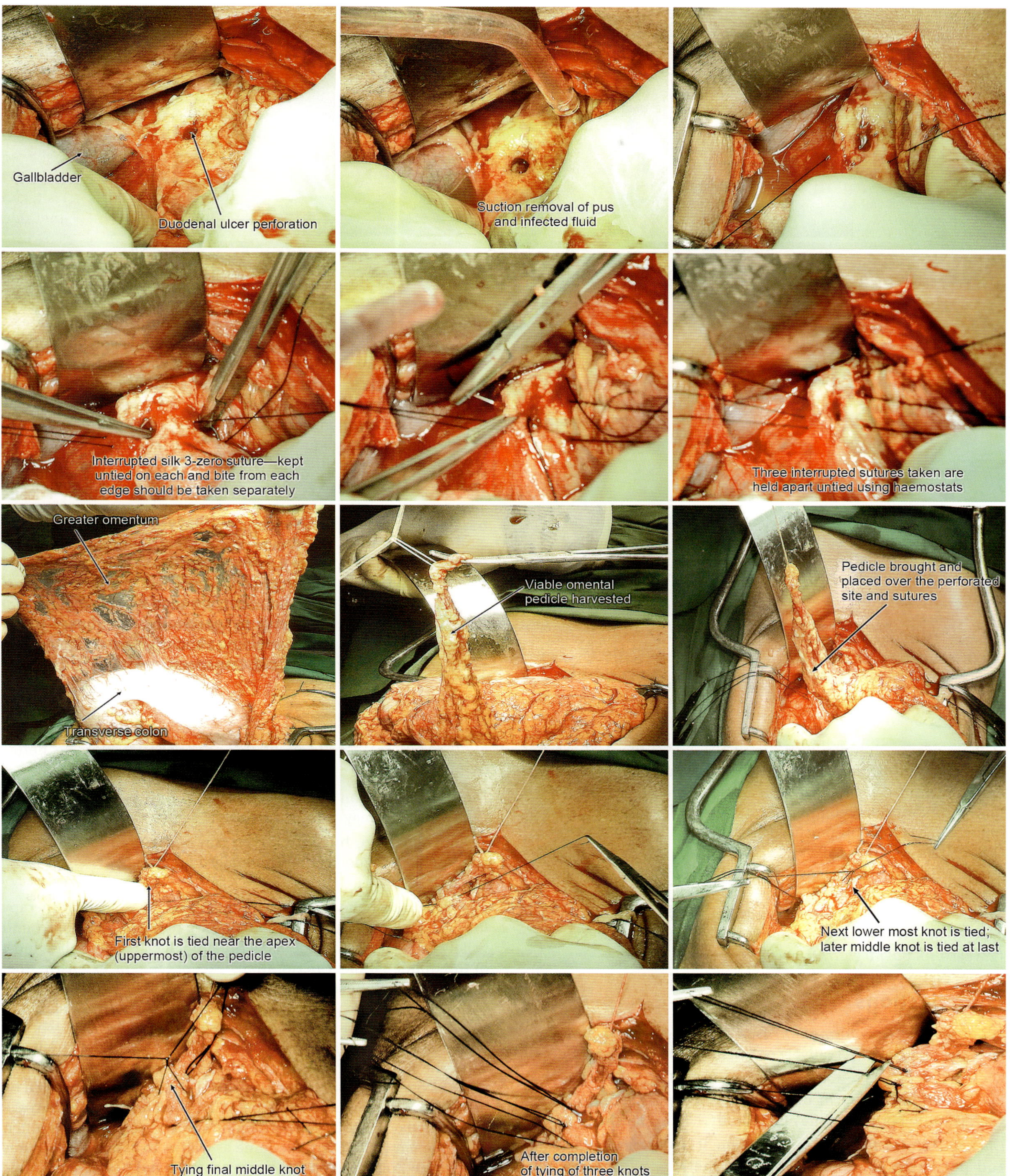
Gallbladder
Duodenal ulcer perforation
Suction removal of pus and infected fluid
Interrupted silk 3-zero suture—kept untied on each and bite from each edge should be taken separately
Three interrupted sutures taken are held apart untied using haemostats
Greater omentum
Transverse colon
Viable omental pedicle harvested
Pedicle brought and placed over the perforated site and sutures
First knot is tied near the apex (uppermost) of the pedicle
Next lower most knot is tied; later middle knot is tied at last
Tying final middle knot
After completion of tying of three knots

Figs. 21-16(1)

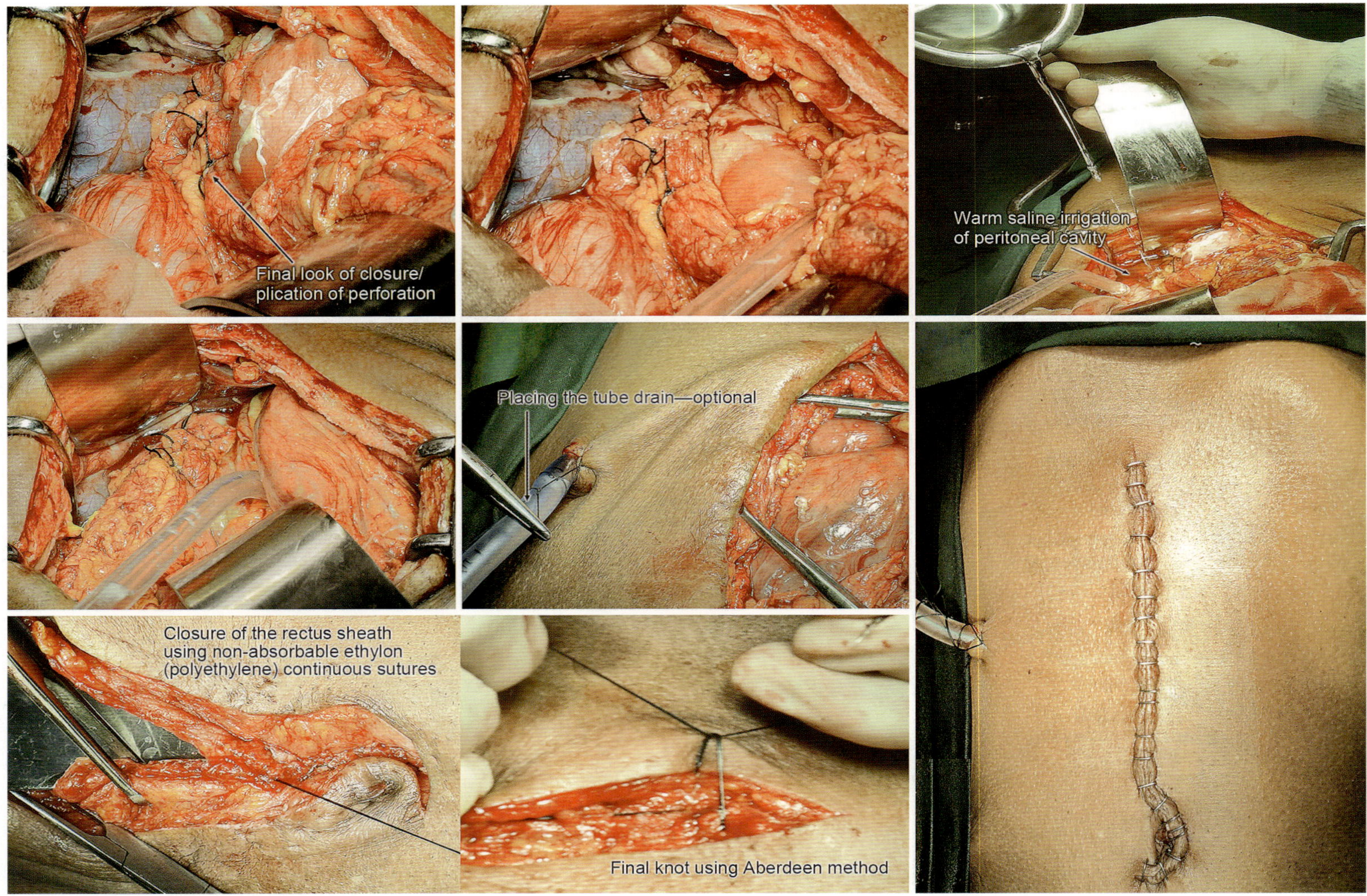

Figs. 21-16(2)

Figs. 21-16(1 and 2): Closure of duodenal ulcer perforation.

Peritoneal wash (toilet) using 5–10 litres of warm saline is given. Drain is only optional. Drain is placed and abdomen is closed with modified Smead Jones technique (often if required using *tension sutures*. But tension/retention sutures are not recommended now, even though commonly practiced by significant number of surgeons). Drain is removed in 3–5 days. Nasogastric tube is removed in 5 days. Oral fluid is started once bowel sounds are heard adequately; patient passes flatus; no abdominal pain.

During discharge, patient is advised to avoid alcohol and to take H2 blockers or proton pump inhibitors for 6–12 weeks. After 12 weeks, *follow-up gastroscopy must be done.*

Complications

Subphrenic abscess formation: It is confirmed by CT abdomen. It can be treated conservatively or by guided tube drainage or open drainage.

Reperforation rarely can occur which needs resection of distal stomach with perforated site and Billroth II anastomosis.

Duodenal obstruction is not uncommon. It causes gastric dilatation and persistent vomiting. With fluid therapy, nasogastric tube aspiration, it may subside. If not then oral contrast study of the gastroduodenum is needed. Relaparotomy and gastrojejunostomy is needed. Vagotomy to reduce the acid load is added depending on the general condition of the patient. HSV may be better option.

Duodenal fistula can occur occasionally. It may stop spontaneously. Occasionally, it may require a diversion, serosal patch at the site.

Wound infection, burst abdomen can occur if patient's general condition is not good and nutritionally deprived.

Note:

Laparoscopy is beneficial for both diagnoses, as well as for therapy for perforation closure using omental patch. It is proposed and widely used for early duodenal perforation. It can be useful for most of the duodenal ulcer perforations except large or extensive one. If it is problematic, conversion options should always be kept in mind. Patient is in supine with head up position (reverse Trendelenburg position); surgeon stands in between legs or on the left side. Monitor is on the head end right side. Camera holding person should be on the left of the surgeon. Trocar is placed as in the diagram. Technique is same as open method. Often integrity of omental patch is tested by insufflation of stomach with air, and air bubble is checked on the saline filled near the closed perforation site. Gastroscopy is also often used by many to confirm the same as well as to assure that sutures placed are not too deep. Mouret et al. 1989 did first laparoscopic perforation closure. Nathanson et al. later did laparoscopic closure of perforation. Intracorporeal knots are commonly used. Other methods are extracorporeal knots, fibrin glue fixation of omental patch, gelatin sponge sealing, stapled patch closure, placement of ligamentum teres onto the perforation. *Advantages are*—better visualisation, less postoperative pain and early recovery. *Drawbacks are*—difficulty in suturing, and inadequate peritoneal toilet which takes long time. *Contraindications are*—elderly, cirrhotic, cardiac patients, obesity and coagulopathy.

Large perforated duodenal ulcer is often difficult to close. Here instead of taking bites directly through the edges of the perforated ulcer across the lumen, seromuscular bites are taken 5 mm away from the edges of the ulcer on either side. Usually 4 such interrupted sutures are placed and viable omental patch is placed over it to tie. After that omentum again is sutured to the duodenum on its margin with seromuscular stitches to make it watertight.

Once perforation is closed, either by open or laparoscopic method, patient should be advised *anti-Helicobacter pylori* therapy (triple regime for 14 days) with PPI for 3 months after recovery. It reduces rate of reperforation and ulcer recurrence in duodenal ulcer.

In patients with severe peritonitis and critically ill, it is better to insert a nasojejunal tube or feeding jejunostomy for nutrition in postoperative recovery period after closure of perforation. Even if patient develops a temporary duodenal leak, this supports nutrition well until the leak stops.

Occasional *large perforated duodenal ulcer* with oedema which cannot be closed should be managed by serosal patch/duodenal drainage followed by pyloric exclusion/gastrostomy, duodenostomy and jejunostomy/Roux-en-Y jejunal patch over the perforation. Vagotomy with pyloroplasty; vagotomy with antrectomy are all other options used with care.

Definitive procedure can be done or not is a matter of debate. But if contamination is less and ulcer is chronic, highly selective vagotomy can be added in selected patients.

Gastric Ulcer Perforation

It is difficult to manage gastric ulcer perforation as plication may not hold properly. Gastric ulcer perforation causes large amount of gas leak showing gas under the diaphragm on both sides in erect X-ray film. Partial gastrectomy and gastrojejunostomy or gastro-duodenostomy is preferred one.

GASTROSTOMY

It is the communication of the anterior wall of the stomach to the abdominal wall skin mainly for feeding purpose whenever oral or nasogastric feeding is not possible or there is fear of reflux and aspiration pneumonia and in oesophageal stricture due to long-term nasogastric feeding.

Indications

It is used for feeding purpose in multiple strictures of oesophagus, in congenital oesophageal conditions as an initial stage of surgery during radiotherapy in head and neck cancers. It improves the nutrition; medications can be given through this tube as well. It keeps the small bowel function active. It is also done in major trauma, sepsis, major surgeries, burns and severe malnutrition.

Types

Gastrostomy can be *temporary* wherein gastrostomy tube is removed later to allow the gastrostomy to close spontaneously; or *permanent* where gastrostomy is kept permanently for life-long for feeding purpose **(Fig. 21-17)**.

Gastrostomy can be serosa/*serous lined*; it is temporary and easier to do. It can be *mucus lined* which is permanent and is technically difficult. Stamm (1894), Kader-Senn (1896), Witzel (1891) are temporary types. Depage-Janeway (1913), Spivack, Beck Carrell-Jeau (1905, 1912), Tavel are permanent types **(Figs. 21-18 to 21-22)**.

Gastrostomy can be done by *open* method; *endoscopic* [Percutaneous Endoscopic Gastrostomy (PEG)]; or *laparoscopic-assisted endoscopic* method. PEG has become more popular nowadays. Stamm and Janeway gastrostomies can be done laparoscopically also.

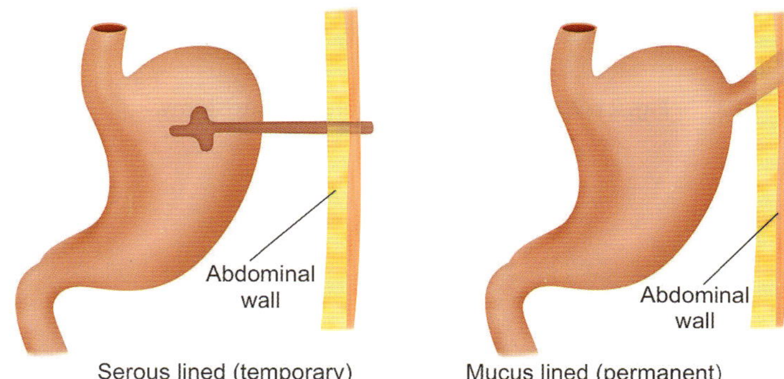

Fig. 21-17: Types of gastrostomies—serous-lined (temporary); mucus-lined (permanent).

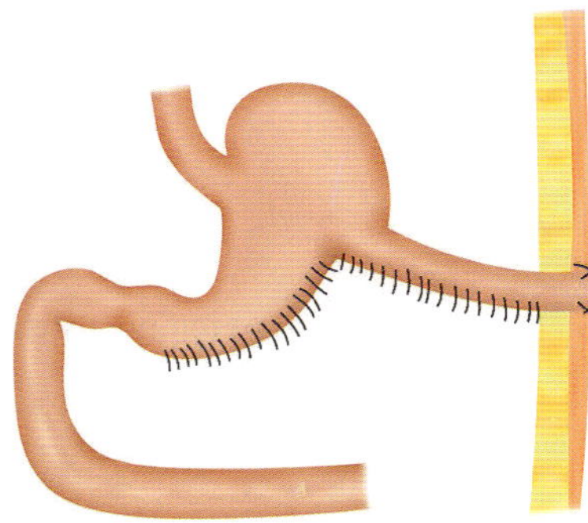

Fig. 21-18: Beck Carrell Jean gastrostomy. It is a mucus lined permanent gastrostomy.

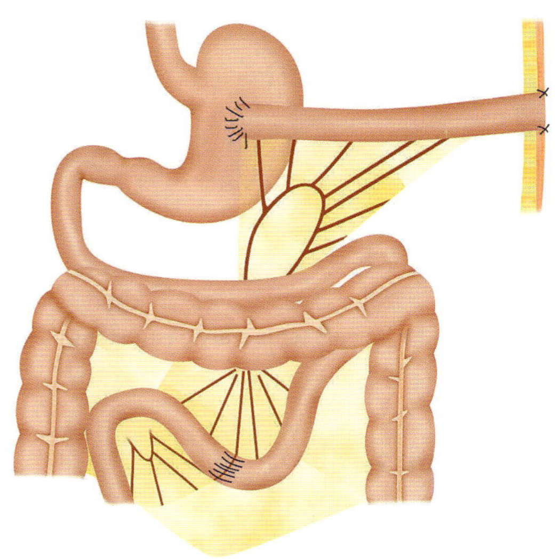

Fig. 21-19: Tavel permanent gastrostomy.

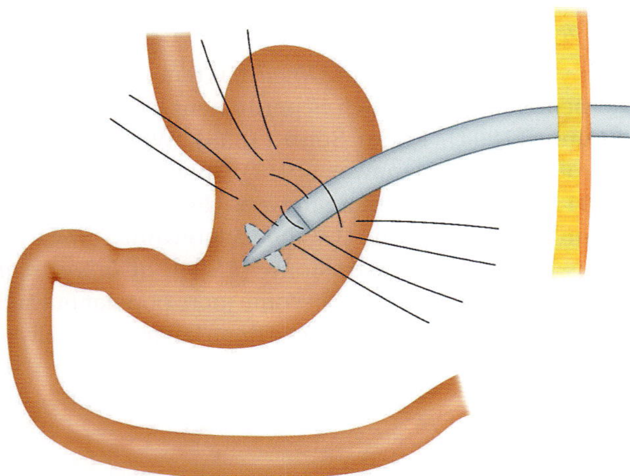

Fig. 21-20: Kader Senn temporary gastrostomy.

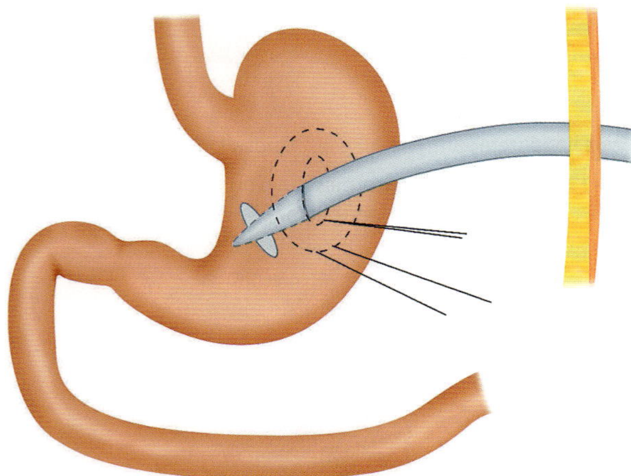

Fig. 21-21: Stamm gastrostomy is a temporary gastrostomy.

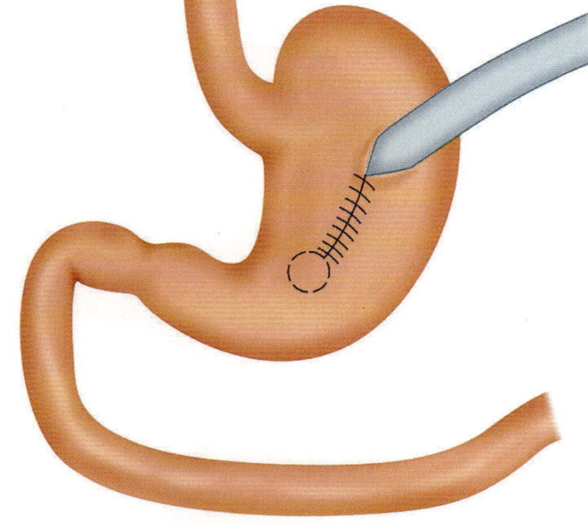

Fig. 21-22: Witzel's temporary gastrostomy.

Contraindications

Previous gastric surgeries, intestinal obstruction, gastric outlet obstruction, gastric diseases with impaired gastric emptying are contraindications.

Problems in Gastrostomy

Leak—gastric fistula is very dangerous one. Gastrostomy is the commonest cause of gastric fistula. Infection can occur which can cause skin excoriation. Aspiration, pneumonia, diarrhoea is common—30%, bloating, abdominal cramps, displacement, blockage of the tube, trauma to other organs like colon.

Technique of Temporary (Stamm's) Gastrostomy

Commonly done type is Stamm's gastrostomy. It is serous-lined temporary gastrostomy. Upper midline incision is done. Stomach is held upwards towards wound using two Babcocks forceps applied at lesser and greater curvatures near middle of the stomach. In the midpoint of the stomach closer to greater curvature, marker stitch is placed. Seromuscular purse string sutures are placed with 2 cm diameter using 2-0 silk or vicryl. Using two Allis tissue holders, left edge of the cut linea alba is held apart; 2 cm vertical or horizontal incision is made on the skin over the middle of the rectus muscle; anterior rectus sheath is incised; rectus muscle is split; posterior rectus sheath and peritoneum is incised. Alternatively same can be achieved by a stab incision from skin towards the peritoneum under vision. Haemostat (medium sized or large) is passed from inside (peritoneum) out (towards skin) to grasp the selected gastrostomy tube (20 French Malecot/Foley's catheter/mushroom catheter) which is pulled into the peritoneal cavity. Incision is made within the purse string, suture placed (gastrotomy) using 15 number blade or cautery; tip of the gastrostomy tube is passed into the gastric lumen. Tip is usually directed downwards. If Foley's catheter is used, it is inflated with distilled water. Purse string suture is tied with knot to create inversion of serosa snugly on to the tube. It is supported by 2nd layer of purse string suture using 2-0 silk. This also ensures rapid closure of the stomach opening after removal of gastrostomy tube. Tube should be anchored to abdominal wall to prevent leak and spillage of the gastric contents. It is achieved by taking seromuscular bites from the stomach and to the peritoneal (or peritoneum with posterior rectus sheath) layer of the abdominal wall; 4 interrupted 2-0 silk or vicryl sutures are placed and kept untied initially. Once all four sutures are placed, they are tied and cut to anchor the tube to abdominal wall. Tube is fixed outside to the skin. Linea alba is sutured using polypropylene continuous sutures; skin is closed using stapler or non-absorbable interrupted sutures **(Figs. 21-23 and 21-24)**.

Temporary gastrostomy can be used for function in 48 hours. It should not be removed earlier than 3 weeks until proper sealing and track has formed.

Technique of Permanent (Depage Janeway) Gastrostomy

Permanent gastrostomy is mucus lined; it prevents regurgitation of gastric contents and avoids placing of a tube; it remains patent without any tendency to close. It is actually a permanent fistula **(Figs. 21-25A and B)**.

Abdomen is opened with upper midline incision. Stomach is held with two Babcock forceps adjacent to greater and lesser curvature. Occlusion clamps can be applied to upper and lower part of the stomach to prevent spillage of the gastric content and bleeding from the cut edges. Rectangular flap from the gastric anterior wall is taken. It can be horizontal with apex of the flap towards lesser curve and base towards greater curve; or as a rectangular flap along the middle of the anterior wall of the stomach more towards the greater curvature with base directed either below or above. Flap should be

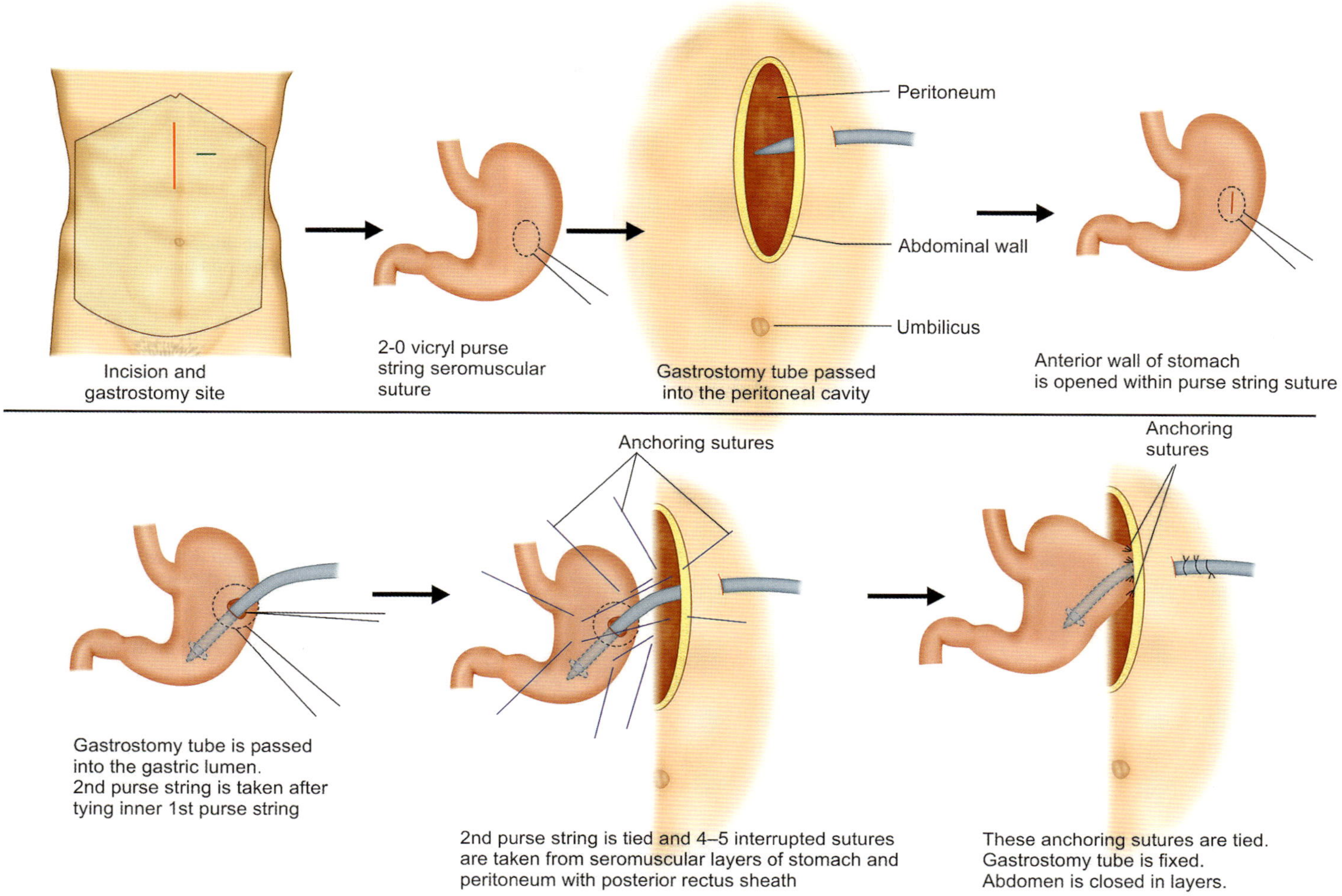

Peritoneum

Abdominal wall

Umbilicus

Incision and gastrostomy site

2-0 vicryl purse string seromuscular suture

Gastrostomy tube passed into the peritoneal cavity

Anterior wall of stomach is opened within purse string suture

Anchoring sutures

Anchoring sutures

Gastrostomy tube is passed into the gastric lumen.
2nd purse string is taken after tying inner 1st purse string

2nd purse string is tied and 4–5 interrupted sutures are taken from seromuscular layers of stomach and peritoneum with posterior rectus sheath

These anchoring sutures are tied.
Gastrostomy tube is fixed.
Abdomen is closed in layers.

Fig. 21-23: Stamm temporary gastrostomy—technique.

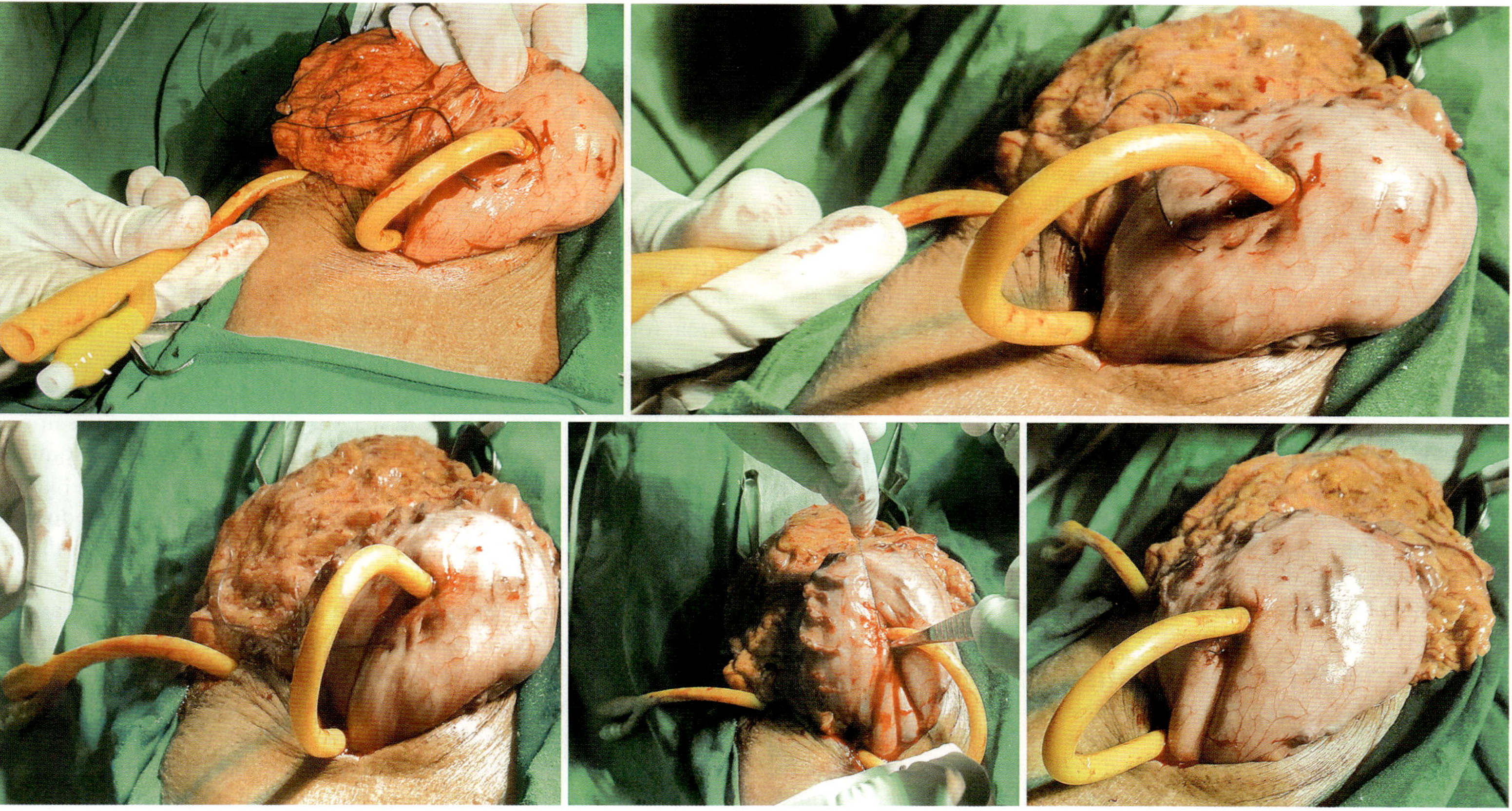

Fig. 21-24: Technique of temporary gastrostomy.

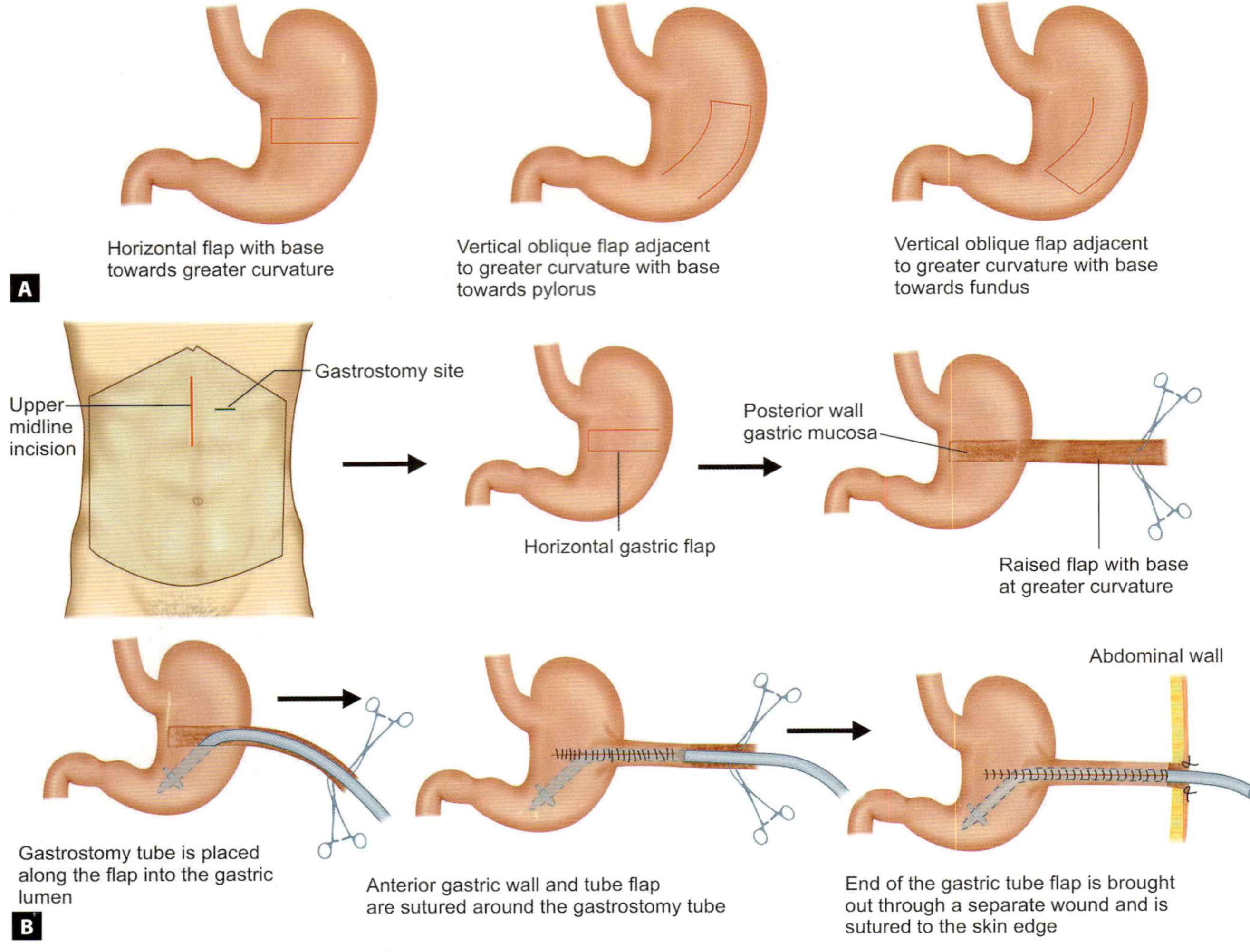

Figs. 21-25A and B: Janeway's permanent gastrostomy.

adequately wide and lengthy as after harvesting, it shrinks significantly. Once flap is elevated adequately, no 20 Foley's catheter is placed across the inner part of the flap into the stomach. Flap is sutured like a tube around the catheter using inner interrupted 2-or 3-zero vicryl and outer interrupted 3-0 silk sutures. Similar sutures are placed along the stomach wound from the base in two layers. Anterior wall is fixed to peritoneum using 2 or 3 interrupted sutures. Such permanent gastric tube can also be created comfortably using stapler device. A stab wound or layer by layer opening of the abdominal wound of 1.5 to 2.0 cm in length along the middle of the rectus muscle using a horizontal incision is used to bring the gastric tube outside for exteriorization and gastric mucosa is fixed to the skin (usually skin is incised horizontally; anterior rectus sheath is incised horizontally; rectus muscle is split; posterior rectus sheath and peritoneum are incised). Abdomen is closed in layers.

Fluid therapy can be started with catheter in situ in 48 hours. Catheter can be removed in 7 days. But tube (any tube of adequate size) should be reapplied and kept **(Fig. 21-26)**.

Technique of Percutaneous Endoscopic Gastrostomy (PEG)

It is done using gastroscope without doing laparotomy. It is useful in children and adult for feeding and decompression. Stomach should be amenable for distension through endoscope; transillumination should be visible across the abdominal wall to do PEG. Dr Jeffrey Ponsky developed this method in 1980.

Ascites, coagulopathy, gastric outlet obstruction, gastroparesis, previous abdominal surgeries, gastrectomies, obesity are contraindications for PEG **(Figs. 21-27A and B)**.

Patient should be kept nil oral like for gastroscopy. Sedation, intravenous line and fluid are started. Patient is placed in supine head up position. Local anaesthetic spray or gargle is instilled to the throat (oropharynx). Gastroscope is passed. Stomach is distended by air insufflation sufficiently so as to make anterior wall of the stomach abut onto the abdominal wall. Room is made dark by switching off the bright lights to make transillumination visible better along the upper abdomen. Position is confirmed by finger indentation of abdominal wall in the upper midline which is seen in endoscope image. Local anaesthetic agent is infiltrated (xylocaine 2%) in the upper abdomen in the suitable place for about 2 cm area. One cm skin incision is made. 16 gauge IV cannula with needle is passed under endoscopic vision per abdomen across the skin incision into the anterior stomach wall. Safe tract method is used while passing the needle. Cannula needle is connected to syringe with xylocaine and passed forward progressively with suctioning in the syringe; when needle enters the lumen (confirmed by endoscopic view), air bubble can be seen; if air bubble is seen but needle has not entered the gastric lumen then it is presumed that bowel is interposed, and needle is immediately withdrawn. Needle is removed; cannula is kept in place;

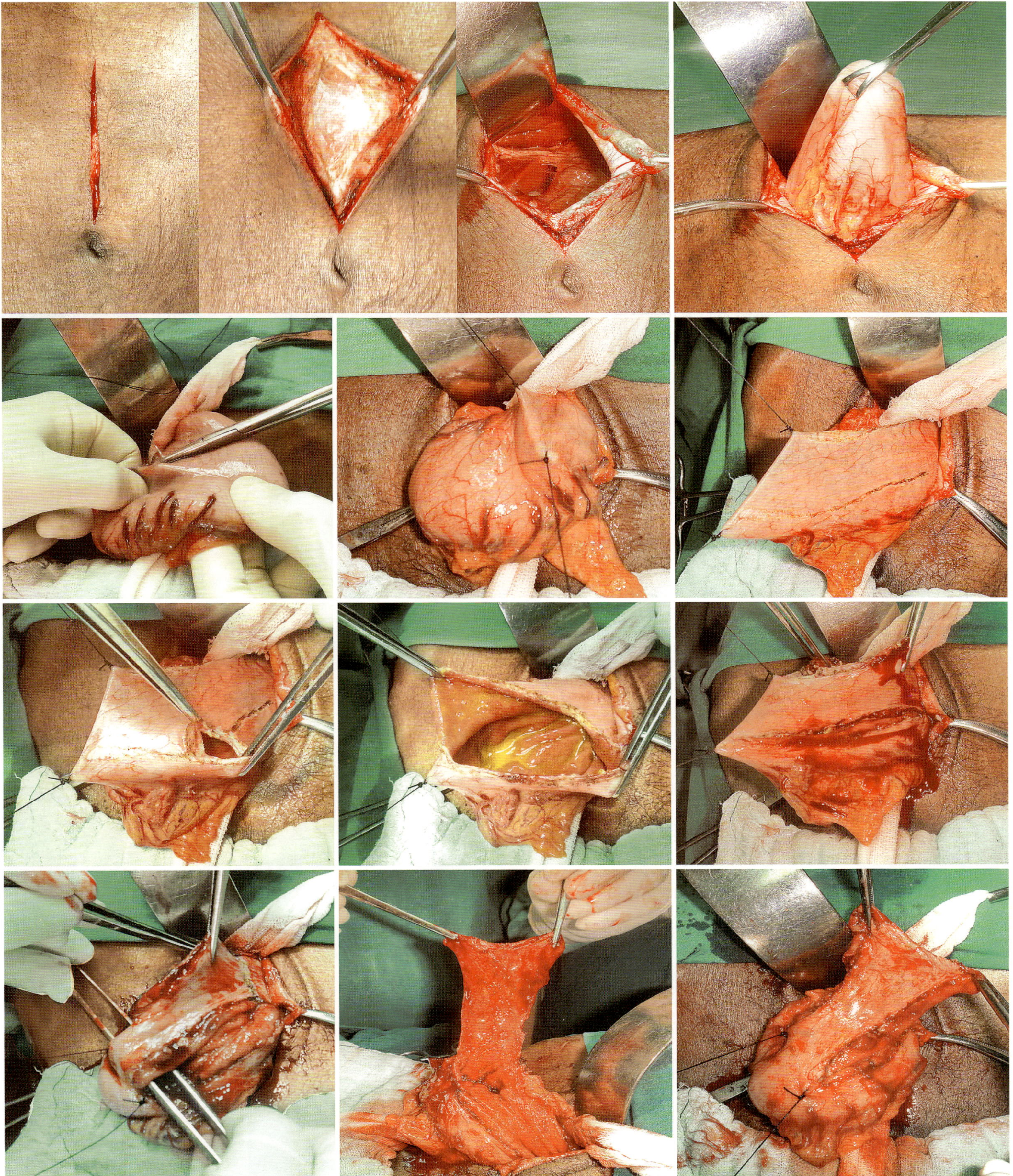

Figs. 21-26(1)

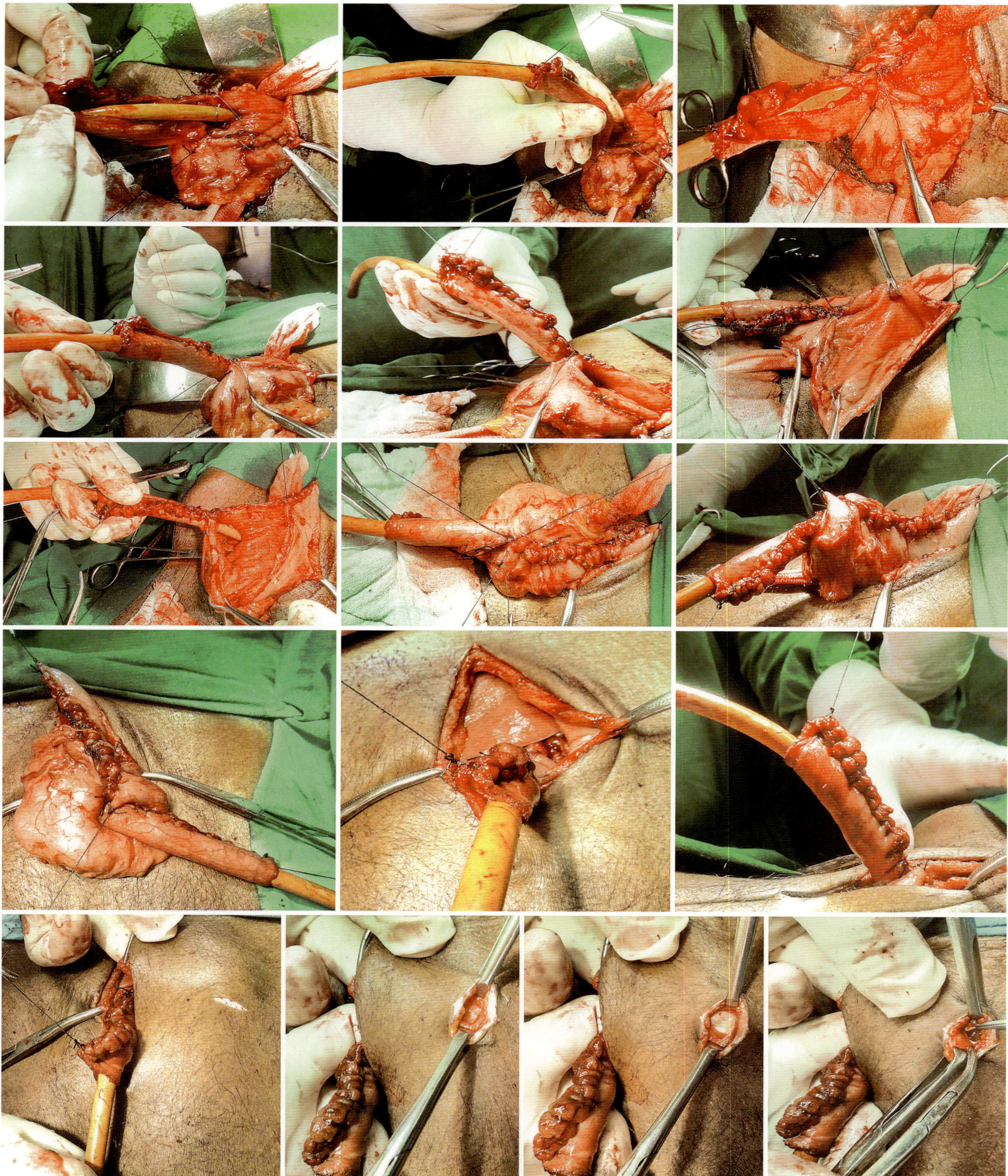

Figs. 21-26(2)

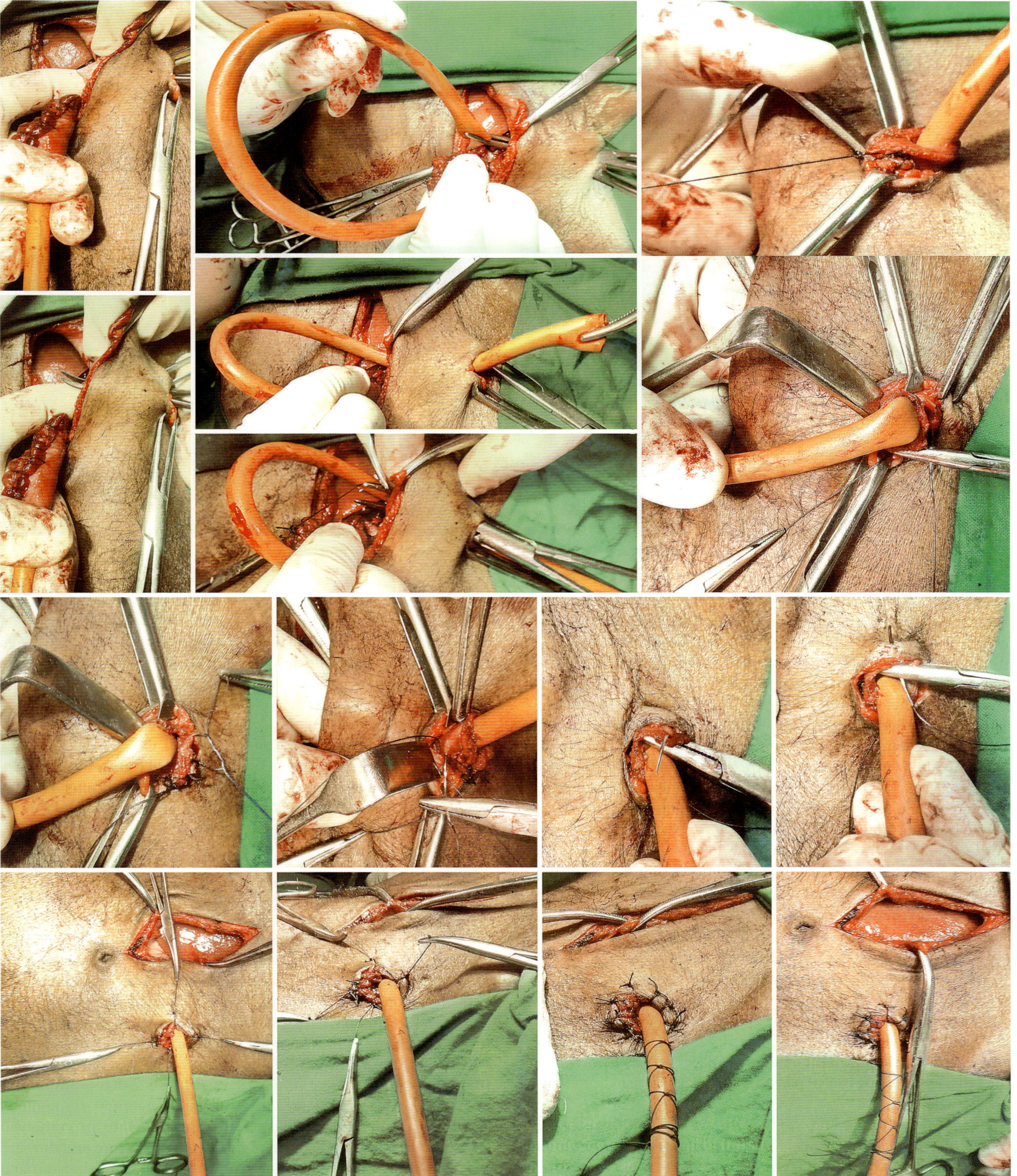

Figs. 21-26(3)

Figs. 21-26(1 to 3): Janeway's permanent gastrostomy.

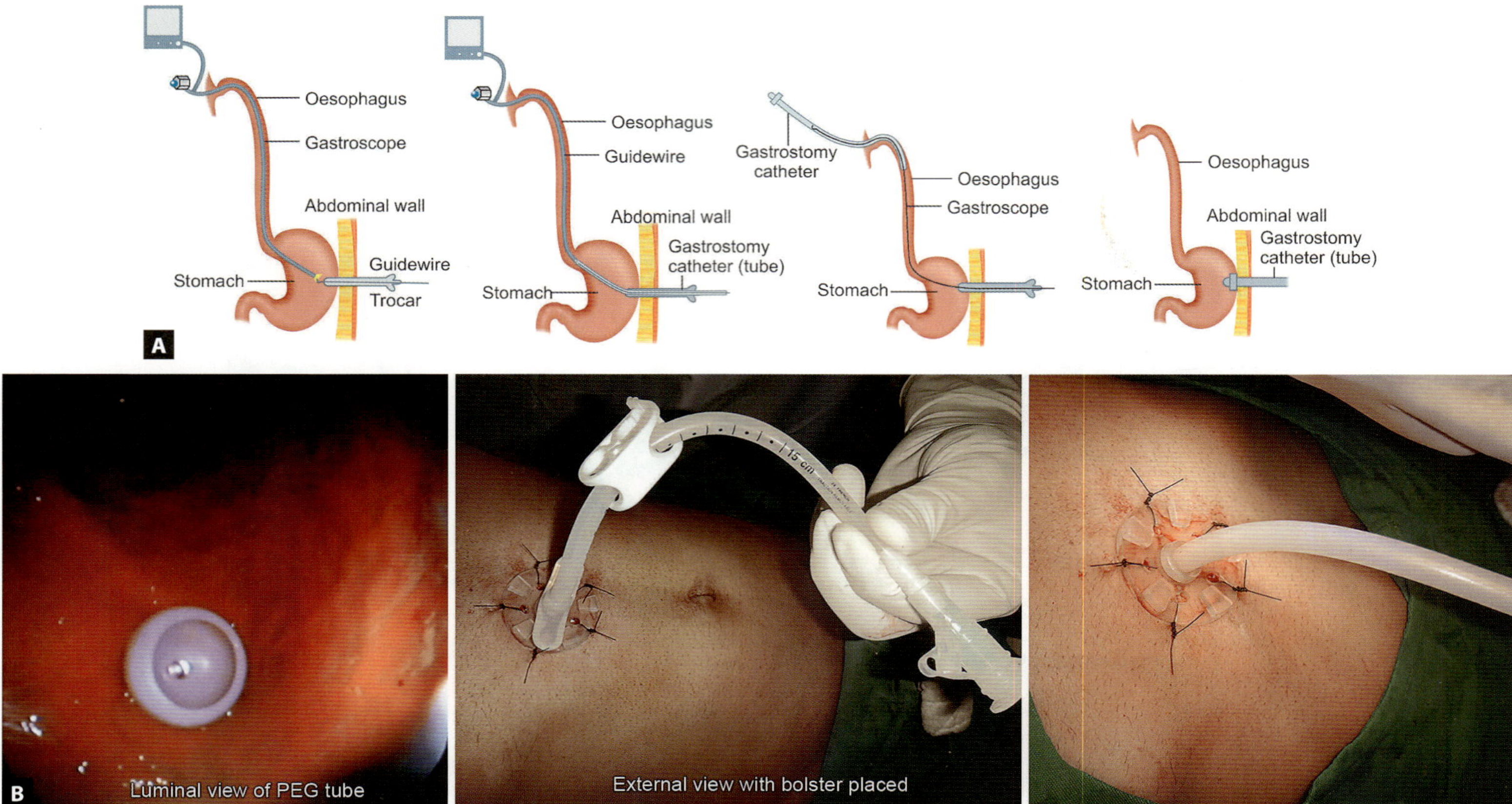

Figs. 21-27A and B: Percutaneous endoscopic gastrostomy procedure.

a long thick (number 1) nylon or polyethylene or silk or guide wire is passed across the cannula into the stomach which is visualised through gastroscope. An endoscopic snare is passed through the working channel of the gastroscope into the stomach through which guidewire or nylon is held and pulled out along with endoscope. This causes guidewire or nylon to pass across the abdominal wall, stomach, oesophagus and mouth with one end in the abdominal wall and other end coming out through the mouth. Specialised PEG tube or de Pezzer catheter is tied to the guidewire or nylon at its oral end; nylon or guidewire at abdominal wall is pulled out with gentle traction until the PEG catheter or de Pezzer catheter comes and stays across the stomach and abdominal wall. Tube is fixed to the abdominal skin. Inside position of catheter is confirmed by gastroscopy. An external bolster is kept on the tube to prevent migration. It is kept few mm away from the skin, usually by keeping sterile dressing pads or sponge underneath. Migration of PEG tube downwards may cause pylorus obstruction.

When one end of the guidewire/nylon brought out it is tied to the end of the PEG catheter and other end of the guidewire in the abdominal wall is pulled out to reach the PEG tube into the stomach and across the abdominal wall, this is called as "pull technique" which is the original method that is still popular. While pulling the tube, gastroscope is also passed from above to visualise the tube placement.

Instead of tying the end of guidewire in the mouth to the PEG tube, PEG tube itself is pushed on to the guidewire across the mouth and is pushed by holding the guidewire ends at oral cavity, and at abdominal wall it is held taut to reach the stomach and across the abdominal wall. Later gastroscopy is done to confirm the position, and guidewire is removed. It is called as "push technique".

Bowel interposition between stomach and abdominal wall is a real risk in PEG. Either small bowel or colon may get interposed. 'Safe tract' method (Foutch et al.) can identify the bowel interposition. Here while passing the needle through the illuminated abdominal wall, continuous aspiration at the skin incision is created; if air gets aspirated before entering the endoscopically visible gastric lumen, it confirms the bowel interposition.

Feeding can be started in 48 hours. If needed catheter tube can be changed with a new one by railroad technique but only after 4 weeks. Complications like skin infection, gastric wall necrosis, gastric leak, colon injury can occur occasionally.

Complications of PEG—Abdominal wall infection; migration of the gastrostomy tube; interposition of bowel (small or large) between stomach and abdominal wall while doing the technique and getting injured is a real risk which may cause fatal peritonitis or external faecal fistula or gastrocolic fistula; separation of stomach wall from abdominal wall causing leak; inadvertent early pulling and extraction of the PEG tube which may settle spontaneously but occasionally may need a laparotomy however observation of all such patients is a must.

Laparoscopic-assisted endoscopic gastrostomy is probably technically comfortable to a laparoscopic surgeon. Laparoscope is passed through an umbilical crease incision. With 15 mm Hg pneumoperitoneum, peritoneal cavity is inspected and proper site on anterior wall of the stomach is selected; pneumoperitoneum is reduced to 7 mm Hg. Four T fasteners are inserted into the peritoneal cavity to form a square pattern in the greater curvature and they are held together with traction to bring anterior wall of the stomach close to the abdominal wall; 16 gauge needle and guidewire or nylon is passed percutaneously through the abdominal wall into the stomach lumen. By doing gastroscopy, position of the guidewire may be confirmed and procedure may be continued by passing the PEG tube per orally across guidewire which has been brought to mouth through gastroscope into anterior abdominal wall. Alternatively through a J guidewire across the needle into the gastric lumen and dilatation, PEG tube can be directly facilitated into the gastric lumen across the abdominal wall.

GASTROJEJUNOSTOMY

Gastrojejunostomy can be anterior or posterior or Roux-en-Y types. It can be antecolic or retrocolic. In palliative procedures, gastrectomies and antecolic anterior gastrojejunostomy are done. In chronic duodenal ulcer with pyloric stenosis after truncal vagotomy, posterior retrocolic gastrojejunostomy is done. Roux-en-Y gastrojejunostomy is done after subtotal high gastrectomy or in recurrent diseases or whenever there are complications after initial drainage procedures **(Fig. 21-28)**.

Anterior Gastrojejunostomy

Anterior gastrojejunostomy is done only as a palliative procedure for gastric outlet obstruction due to advanced distal gastric tumour wherein patient presents with vomiting (by Wolfer). It is often done in advanced unresectable carcinoma of pancreas or duodenum with obstruction. Gastrojejunostomy along with gastric resection for malignancy is usually of antecolic type as mesocolon may get involved by the tumour or might have already be involved.

Patient is kept with nasogastric tube. Often stomach wash using normal saline may be needed. Stomach wash is better given using a gastric tube like Ewald's. Electrolyte estimation, anaemia should be assessed. Adequate hydration with normal saline should be done.

Procedure is done under general anaesthesia, with upper midline incision. Abdomen is explored for secondaries in liver, peritoneum and ascites. Primary tumour is assessed for resectability. Advanced carcinoma can be resectable as palliation even though it is not operable with lymph node clearance. In fact, when possible resection is better palliation than gastrojejunostomy. Usually anterior gastrojejunostomy is done as a palliation. Posterior gastrojejunostomy is not possible in advanced carcinoma of stomach as posterior surface is not accessible and also often fixed. As anterior gastrojejunostomy is non-dependent and takes more time to start functioning, it is better to add on enteroenterostomy between afferent and efferent loops (jejunojejunostomy—Braun's) **(Fig. 21-29)**.

Stomach, proximal to the growth/obstruction is selected. It should be mobile and more towards greater curvature. Two Babcock's forceps are used to hold the part of the anterior wall of the stomach for about 8 cm in between at greater curvature proximally and distally. Often lower end may be slightly deviated towards the lesser curvature, but it is not mandatory. It is better to separate the greater omentum adjacent to the proposed gastrojejunostomy anastomotic site by ligating the branches of the gastroepiploic arcade for 8 cm.

Ligament of Treitz is identified at duodenojejunal junction; inferior mesenteric vein that runs underneath very closely is also a marker to identify the duodenojejunal junction. This step is essential to avoid inadvertent selection of ileal loop leading to disastrous wrong gastroileostomy. After opening, mucosal pattern also confirms the jejunum (valvulae conniventes mucosal folds). Thirty cm length of the jejunum is brought towards the selected part of the stomach as antecolic.

The segment of the jejunum is held parallel to the part of the stomach held with Babcock's forceps. Antimesenteric part of the jejunum is used for anastomosis. Stay sutures are placed using 3-0 silk or vicryl at the corners of the selected parts of the stomach and jejunum taking seromuscular bites from both stomach and jejunal corners. Two occlusion clamps are placed proximal to the selected parts of the stomach and jejunum. Clamps prevent bleeding from the cut edges, prevent spillage of the bowel contents into the peritoneal cavity and also to steady the bowel. (Presently many surgeons feel that occlusion clamps are not necessary as when cautery is used bleeding will not occur; spillage can be controlled by using good suction device; this is more true probably while doing retrocolic gastrojejunostomy, as applying occlusion clamp towards gastric side is more cumbersome; however in olden days, occlusion clamps like Carwardine's or Lane's twin clamps were used for the same). Wet gauze is often placed in between two bowel segments as a sausage to absorb the spilled contents posteriorly; but one should remember to remove it at the end **(Figs. 21-30A and B)**.

Presently, it is proved that single layer interrupted (both edges two layers) or continuous 2- or 3-zero vicryl all layer sutures are sufficient. However whenever gastric wall oedema is present and nutrition is inadequate, two layers (both edges four layers) anastomosis is done. Here again, outer layer may be placed as continuous or interrupted seromuscular (Lembert in interrupted) sutures.

In four layer anastomosis, posterior seromuscular suture is placed as continuous or interrupted using silk sutures. In continuous type, sutures are placed from one end to other end for about 5–6 cm length each bite is taken at 5 mm interval; from the jejunal side, it is of practice to take bite 5 mm posterior to the antimesenteric border so that later incision on the jejunum will run on the antimesenteric line; once it reaches the other end, suture material with needle is kept in wet gauze which is again used at a later period for anterior seromuscular layer. During continuous suturing, one or two knots may be placed in between to prevent loosening. Posterior seromuscular layer ideally should involve submucosa also, even though depth assessment is blind. In interrupted posterior seromuscular suturing, 3 zero silk is used in same place as continuous suture line; ideally all sutures are placed first and kept long; knots of each is tied later; ends of tied sutures are not cut immediately instead are held upwards to give traction so that gastrotomy and enterotomy is done easily. Once opening is done in the stomach and jejunum, ends of these sutures are cut. Stomach is incised first; and then jejunum is incised; jejunal opening should be smaller than gastric opening as jejunal wall stretches and enlarges significantly.

Anterior wall of the stomach is opened (gastrotomy) using number 15 blade or cautery for 5 cm; it runs 5 mm from the posterior seromuscular suture line. Ends of the cuts in gastric and jejunal side should be 1 cm shorter than posterior seromuscular suture line. It is often practiced to ligate small but definitive bleeders from the cut edges of the stomach using 4-zero vicryl (von Haberer submucosal sutures); however bipolar cauterisation is more than sufficient for that. Mucosal pattern of gastric rugae may be identified. Jejunum is opened using number 15 blade for corresponding length. First seromuscular layer is incised at full length; then mucosa is opened at one point; bile will exude out to confirm that lumen is exposed; non-toothed dissecting forceps placed into the lumen along the line of incision; using curved scissor rest of the jejunum part is incised. Jejunum also can be opened using cautery. Jejunal mucosa bulges out.

Second posterior all layer sutures are placed using 2-0 or 3-0 vicryl or silk. At the left angle, needle bites are taken from outside in of the gastric cut edge and inside out from jejunal cut edge which are tied with knots. Suture material is passed again into the lumen at the left angle; continuous sutures are taken as through and through all layers towards right side. Bites are taken at 2–5 mm intervals and 2–5 mm from the edges. Care should be taken that all layers are

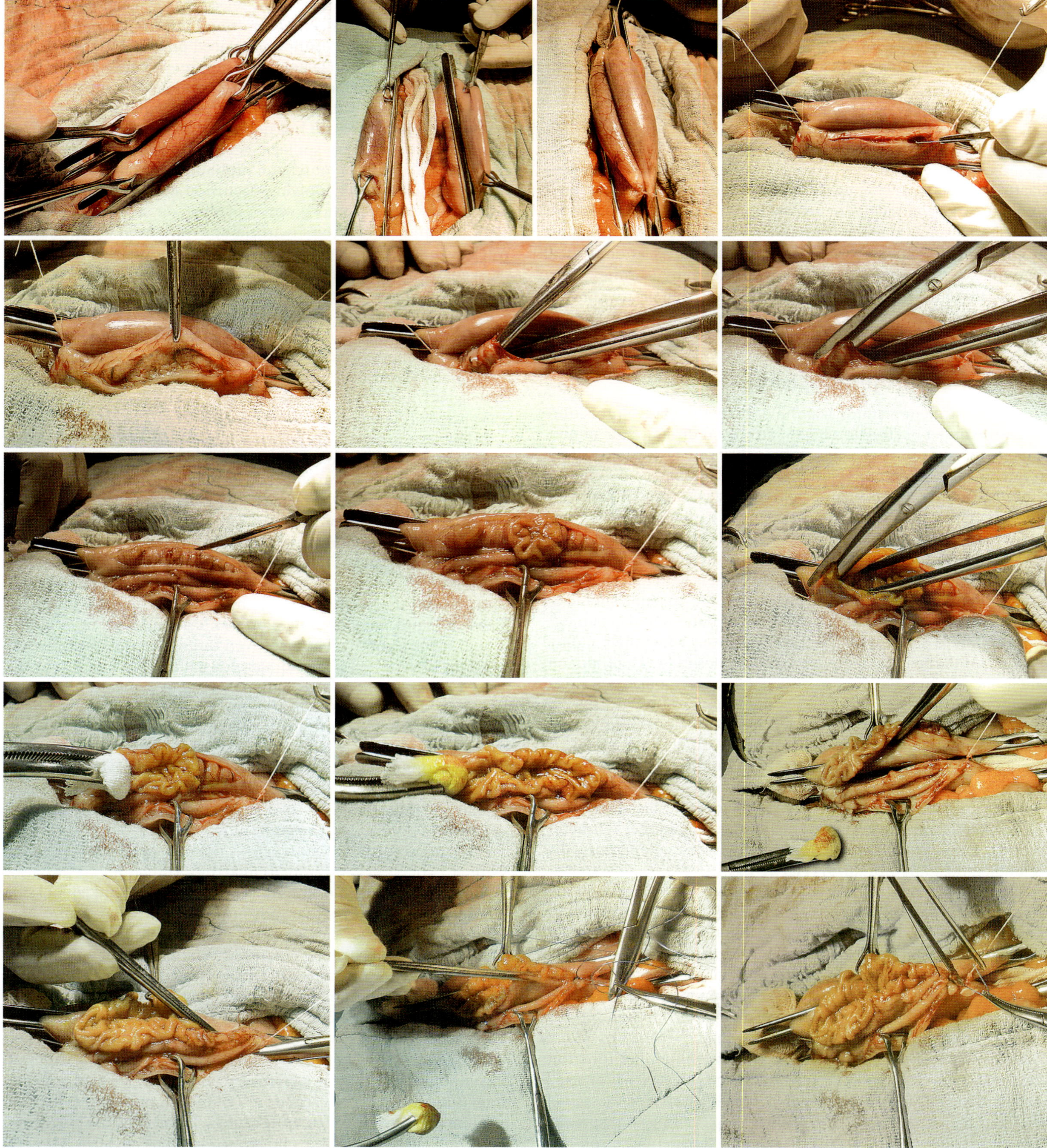

Figs. 21-28(1)

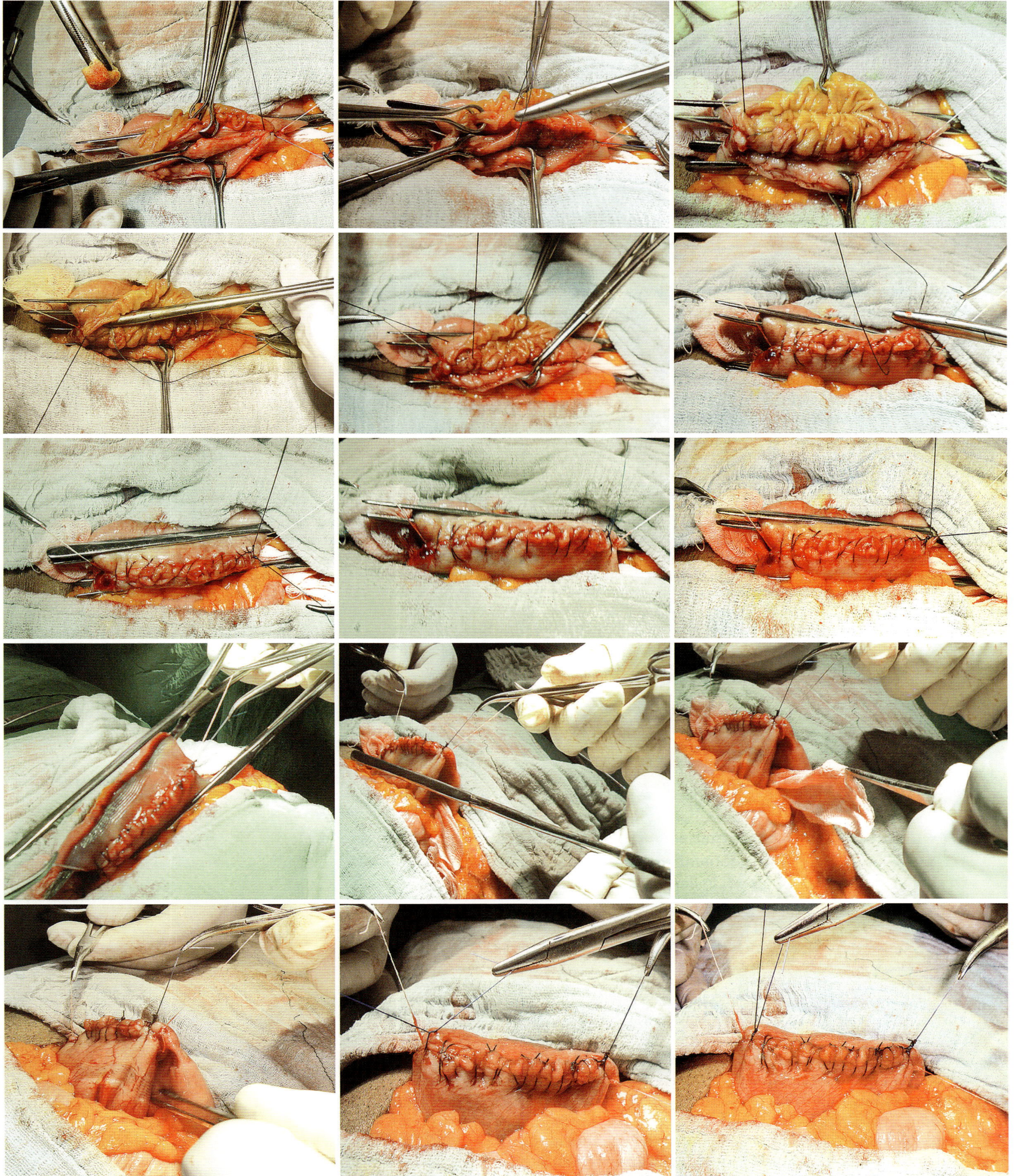

Figs. 21-28(2)

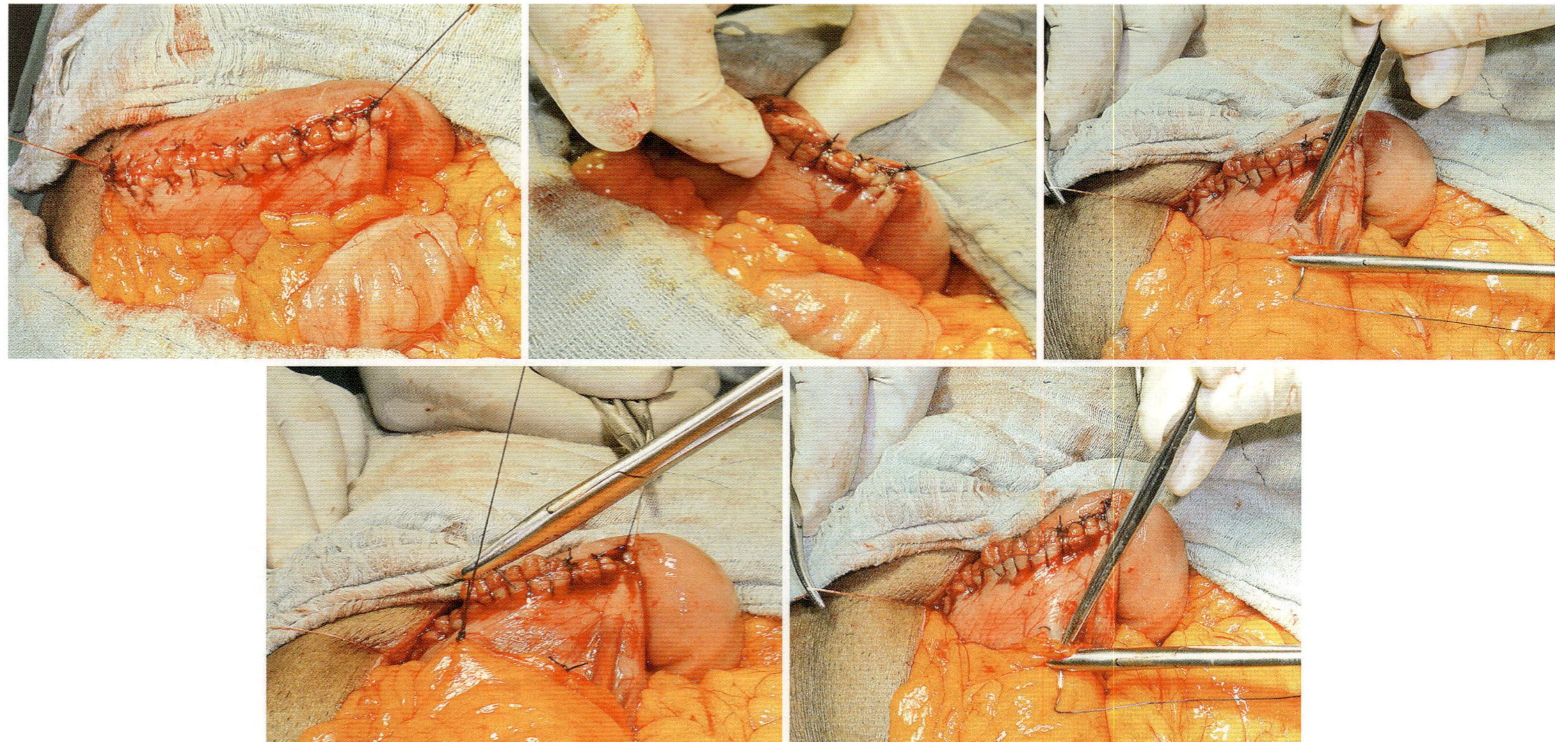

Figs. 21-28(3)

Figs. 21-28(1 to 3): Gastrojejunostomy (GJ) technique. Note the isolation of the both gastric and jejunal parts; stay sutures; doing first gastrotomy and then jejunotomy; opening in the jejunum should be shorter than the gastric side; note the mucosal look and pattern of both gastric and jejunal wall; note the vessels in the cut edge of the gastric wall which can be ligated with 4-zero silk (von Haberer); note the posterior layer continuous suture and anterior inverting suture; clamps used are occlusion type ideally elliptical one; twin clamps can be used; stoma should be checked for patency; in posterior gastrojejunostomy, gastric wall should be fixed with interrupted seromuscular sutures to make stoma infracolic.

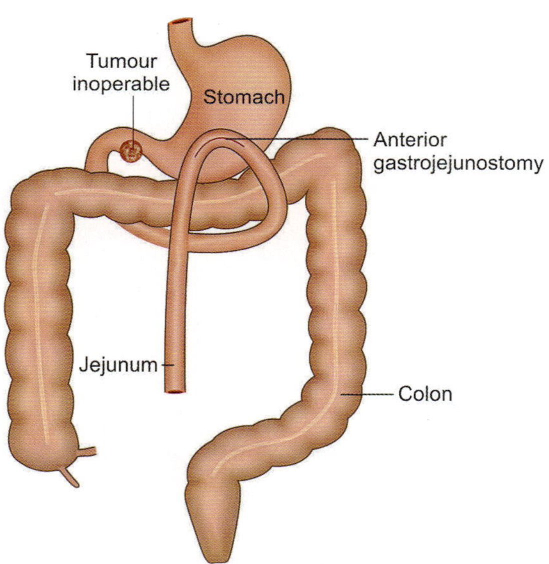

Fig. 21-29: Anterior gastrojejunostomy is done for advanced carcinoma of stomach.

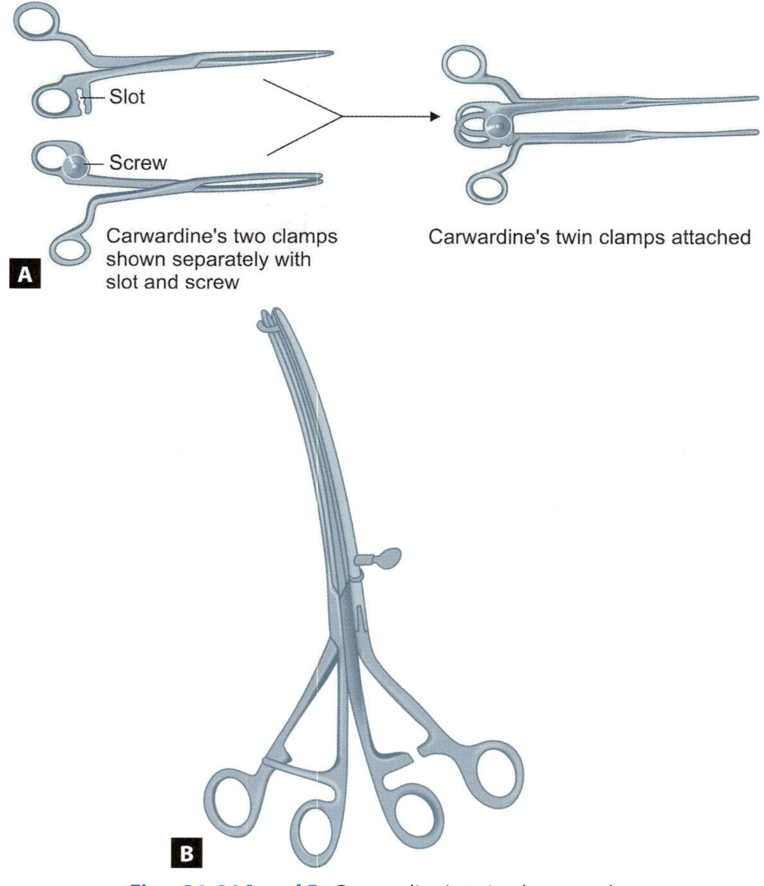

Figs. 21-30A and B: Carwardine's twin clamp and or Lane's gastrojejunostomy clamp used for gastrojejunostomy.

included in the suture bites; less mucosa with more serosa is taken to avoid eversion but to create inversion. Once in 3–4 bites, locking of the suture is done to prevent purse string effect on the stoma. It is reached to the right edge.

Here needle bite is taken from inside-out of the jejunum at the angle and outside in of the stomach side to reach anterior wall and continue as anterior all layer (3rd layer) sutures. Continuous sutures of inside-out and outside-in can be taken. Connell stitch can be used here—with outside in of the stomach edge and inside out of the stomach edge again; then looping across the wound edge towards jejunal side to pass again outside-in and inside-out at jejunal edge which is again looped across towards stomach edge of the wound. This 3rd layer passes from right towards left. Prior to completion of the 3rd layer, it is often advisable to pass the nasogastric tube across the efferent loop. Near the left angle during ending, the suturing continues as through and through sutures. Last bite should pass beyond the beginning bite to avoid gap as a possible site of leak. Suture is tied to the end of the first bite suture. Second layer is also can be placed as interrupted all layer vicryl sutures.

Final 4th anterior seromuscular layer is placed, using already kept silk suture in the wet gauze after completion of the 1st layer. Bites as seromuscular inverting sutures are taken towards left end and are tied to the original end.

Corner sutures additionally may be placed, if needed. Stoma should admit two fingers to confirm adequacy. Patency and integrity of the stoma should be checked. Omentum can be wrapped around the stoma.

Often afferent and efferent loops are communicated with short enteroenterostomy (jejunojejunostomy) to avoid alkali reflux. It is done usually 20 cm from the gastrojejunostomy site. Patency and integrity of the stoma should be checked. Jejunojejunostomy is also done using stapler **(Fig. 21-31)**.

Gastrojejunostomy can also be done using stapling device. Stay suture is placed on the right side ends of the selected part of the stomach and jejunum. Stomach and jejunum loop are brought together. Small gastrotomy and enterotomy are done in the left side of gastric and jejunal side. One fork of the linear cutting stapler device is inserted into the stomach side and other onto the gastric wall side. Both walls are adjusted properly with proper placing of the antimesenteric border of the jejunum. Device is locked; interpositions of other tissues are avoided by careful look; stapler is fired and removed accordingly. Staple line is observed for bleeding; such specific points are reinforced with 3-zero or 4-zero vicryl sutures. Gastrotomy and enterotomy wounds are closed using 3-zero vicryl continuous sutures. These both openings can also be closed using 55 mm linear stapler. Abdomen is closed in layers without keeping drain.

Posterior Gastrojejunostomy

It is done in case of duodenal ulcer after truncal vagotomy as a drainage procedure, especially whenever there is scarring and stenosis with gastric outlet obstruction. It is posterior, retrocolic, short afferent loop (5–8 cm), oblique or vertical gastrojejunostomy (of Mayo) with completed anastomosis lying in infracolic compartment. It is not commonly advocated in malignancy as tumour invasion of mesocolon may obstruct the gastrojejunostomy loop.

Preparation

Stomach wash is required using saline in case of gastric outlet obstruction. Electrolyte estimation, daily preoperative intravenous normal saline infusion, correction of alkalosis, and magnesium deficiency are needed. Nasogastric tube is passed.

Technique

Upper midline incision is placed. Once truncal vagotomy is done, mop is kept in the vagotomy site which should be removed at the end prior to closure. Gastrocolic omentum is opened, through lesser sac posterior surface of the stomach is exposed **(Fig. 21-32)**.

Transverse colon is held forward through the laparotomy wound to expose transverse mesocolon. Through transillumination, middle colic vessels are identified. Avascular plane usually towards left of middle colic (but can be on either side) is identified; held with haemostat and opened (for 6–8 cm) to reach the posterior surface of the stomach which is brought through this rent in the mesocolon. Posterior surface of the gastric wall is held with Babcock's forceps on two sides—one at greater curvature (towards right), another at lesser curvature (towards left). (Greater curvature towards greater surgeon; lesser curvature towards lesser surgeon). Many advocate fixing the mesocolon edge to the stomach wall with interrupted 3-zero silk sutures 2 cm from the proposed gastrojejunostomy site to keep it infracolic. But it is usual practice to do this once anastomosis is over which allows the placement of occlusion clamps comfortably on the gastric wall side. First loop of the jejunum is identified by recognising duodenojejunal junction using ligament of Treitz and inferior mesenteric vein. Afferent loop should be only around 8 cm, unlike in anterior antecolic type. Occlusion clamps are placed on gastric and jejunal side. Sausage gauze can be kept between stomach and jejunal segments. Stay sutures are placed from corners of the selected parts of the stomach and jejunal wall using seromuscular 3-zero silk suture; Babcock's forceps can be removed. Posterior seromuscular continuous or interrupted 3-zero silk sutures are placed with each bites at 5 mm interval. (In single layer anastomosis, this step is not necessary) Gastric wall is opened using cautery or no. 15 blade and curved scissor. Jejunum is opened on the antimesenteric margin similarly. Jejunal opening should be less than gastric opening. Posterior all layer anastomosis is done using continuous 3-zero or 2-zero vicryl sutures with in between, locking; haemostasis achieved becomes secure and prevents purse string effect on the stoma. It is continued as anterior all layer suturing using Connell suture or continuous sutures; it is tied to the original end of the vicryl. Then anterior seromuscular suture is placed as continuous or interrupted silk sutures. Clamps are removed; any bleeding points are controlled by suture. Stoma should allow two fingers through it. Mesocolon is sutured to stomach wall 1–2 cm away from the suture line (both anteriorly and posteriorly). It is done to prevent herniation of the small bowel through mesocolon (Stammers).

Variations in Technique

Traditional method is outer seromuscular using silk continuous sutures and inner all layer vicryl sutures. Outer seromuscular layer can be interrupted sutures. Inner layer is usually continuous.

Single all layer sutures using interrupted or continuous silk or vicryl can also be used for gastrojejunostomy.

Roux-en-Y gastrojejunostomy can be done in case of complications after gastrojejunostomy.

Stapler gastrojejunostomy reduces the operating time.

Postoperative Care

Nasogastric tube aspiration is continued for 3–5 days. Once nasogastric tube aspiration reduces to minimum, it is removed. Oral sips are started.

Intravenous fluid is given for first 5 days. Antibiotics may be needed.

Complications

Anastomotic bleeding (1.5%) can occur which is confirmed by blood in the nasogastric tube. It usually subsides in 24 hours. Rarely, it may require reopening and placing additional suture at the bleeding point. Leak from the site may occur which again may need reexploration.

Initial delayed gastric emptying is due to stomal oedema or suture line haematoma which resolves spontaneously. Haematoma

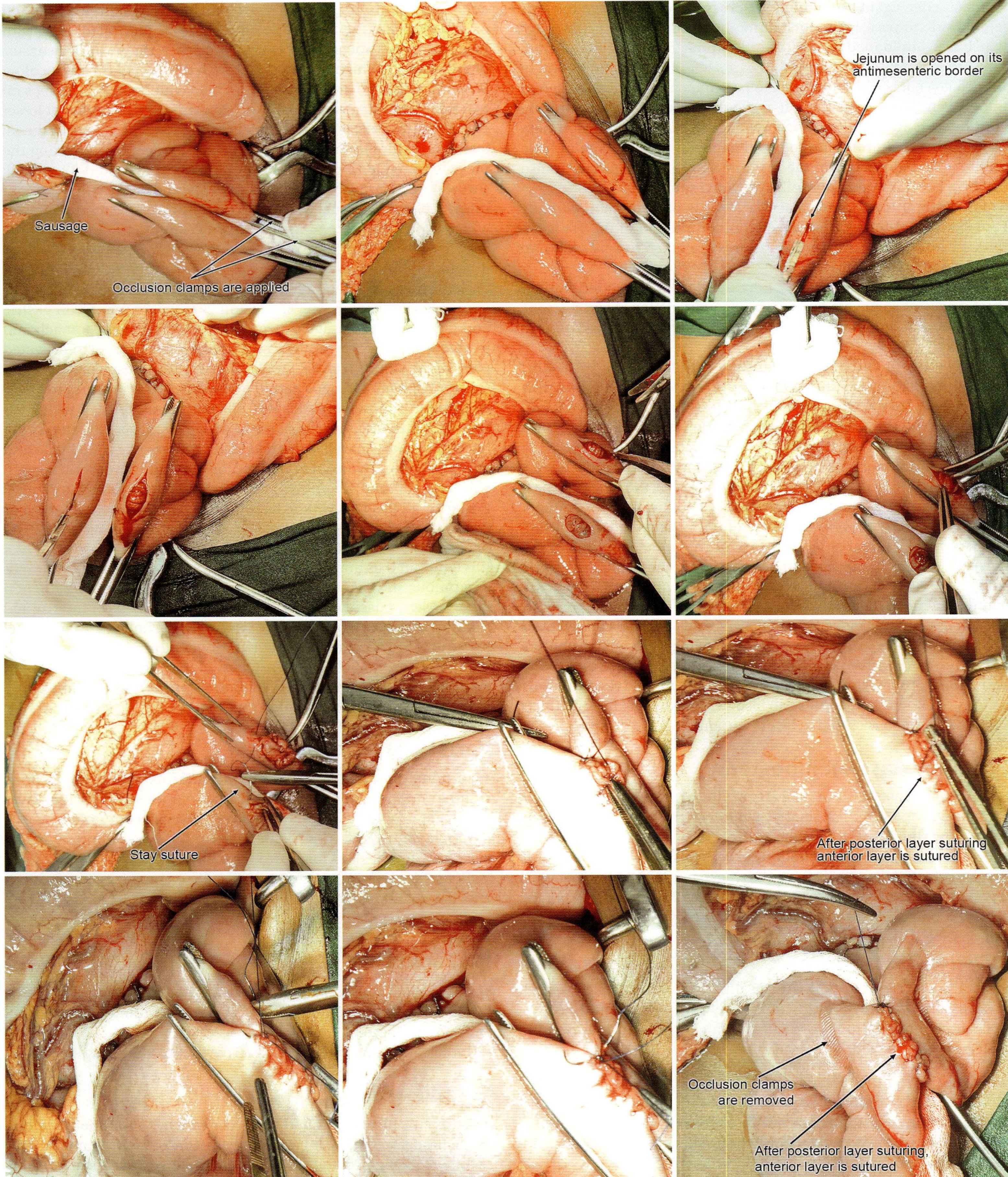
Sausage
Occlusion clamps are applied
Jejunum is opened on its antimesenteric border
Stay suture
After posterior layer suturing anterior layer is sutured
Occlusion clamps are removed
After posterior layer suturing, anterior layer is sutured

Figs. 21-31(1)

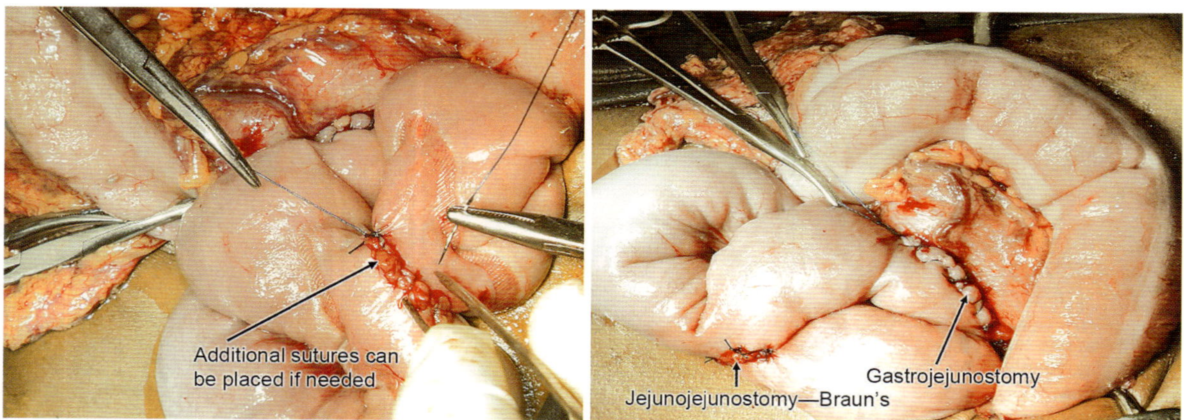

Figs. 21-31(2)

Figs. 21-31(1 and 2): Jejunojejunostomy between afferent and efferent loop.

is more common in stapled anastomosis as stapler is not entirely haemostatic.

Efferent loop obstruction can cause persistent vomiting. Delayed gastric emptying in spite of adequate anatomical stomal opening is often difficult to manage.

Twist in the mesentery can cause afferent loop obstruction. Afferent limb syndrome can occur if the afferent limb becomes larger than needed; it is due to accumulation of large quantity of bile in the lengthy afferent limb making it as a reservoir which impairs its motility leading to poor afferent loop emptying. This false reservoir empties at time together into the stomach causing bilious vomiting in the morning time.

Antecolic gastroenterostomy shows poorer gastric emptying; causes afferent loop syndrome and volvulus compared to retrocolic type.

Jejunogastric intussusception is rare but definitive complication which occurs in loop (omega) gastrojejunostomy only; not in Roux-en-Y type. In 80% cases efferent limb intussusception occurs; 20% cases afferent; rarely both. It causes acute abdomen pain, haematemesis, tender mass on left side of the umbilicus. Contrast X-ray shows coiled spring appearance; gastroscopy is diagnostic. Treatment is surgical resection, doing gastrectomy and Roux-en-Y anastomosis.

VAGOTOMY

Dragstedt in 1940–1942 started vagotomy through thoracic approach. He also later in 1951 postulated that just vagotomy is not sufficient; drainage procedure is essential and truncal vagotomy should be combined with either pyloroplasty or gastrojejunostomy. It used to be the standard surgical therapy for peptic ulcer disease for around 40–50 years. Later selective and highly selective vagotomies became popular. However presently because of the availability of good drugs, surgical therapy is specified mostly for refractory duodenal ulcers, and complications like bleeding and pyloric stenosis. Truncal vagotomy and posterior gastrojejunostomy is more suitable for pyloric stenosis (gastric outlet obstruction) due to chronic duodenal ulcer. Proximal gastric vagotomy/PGV (highly selective vagotomy) is the procedure of choice with refractory ulcers. Grinding, propulsive and retropulsive action of antral mill (antral motility) mainly depend on vagal nerves through their nerves of Latarjet. It is essential to empty the solid food by grinding food into chyme then propelling across the pylorus. Liquid emptying is basically by pressure in the body and fundus of the stomach. Antral mill is weakened permanently by truncal vagotomy. Pyloroplasty is probably done whenever there is bleeding.

H2 receptor antagonist like ranitidine, should be discontinued 24 hours prior to surgery; Proton pump inhibitors (PPIs) should be discontinued 7 days prior to surgery. It restores the acidity of the gastric lumen which reverses the bacterial colonisation of the stomach which is important especially when drainage procedure is undertaken to prevent sepsis.

Truncal Vagotomy

General anaesthesia is used. Nasogastric tube should be placed. Patient is placed in supine head up (reverse Trendelenburg) position. Upper midline incision is placed; often it is necessary to extend 3 cm proximal to xiphoid process and across the umbilicus. Occasionally, excision of the xiphoid process may be needed. In olden days, surgeons were using left upper paramedian incision. Now it is not practiced. Routine exploration is done after laparotomy. Duodenal ulcer is identified with scarring, deformed duodenum and dilated stomach. Cayenne pepper look may be evident on the surface. Head of the pancreas should be examined for possible presence of the gastrinoma, of course it is often difficult to feel on table as lesion may be small. If gastrinoma is suspected, it is better to do specific evaluation like serum gastrin estimation and multidetector CT (MDCT) abdomen.

Left triangular ligament is divided if needed, even though it is not necessary always. Inferior phrenic vein which is on the extreme right extent of the ligament should not be injured. Left lobe of the liver is folded towards right to expose the hiatus properly. Self-retaining retractor is placed. Assistant is asked to hold the greater curvature of the stomach with wet mop to give traction downwards and towards left gently. This makes vagus taut to feel like a string. Peritoneum on front of the hiatus is incised and opened horizontally to expose the anterior surface of the oesophagus. Dissection begins on the left side of the hiatus. Index finger is passed gently from left side behind the oesophagus towards right side by breaking the loose areolar tissue; any small vessels if encountered are fulgurated with bipolar cautery. Nasogastric tube inside oesophagus guides the dissection as well. Posteriorly aortic pulsation can be felt. Gently hepatogastric ligament is incised on the right side to allow index finger to pass and encircle the hiatus; with further blunt, sharp and cautery dissection hiatus is dissected properly. Infant feeding tube or Penrose drain is encircled around the hiatus to facilitate the traction. With traction towards left and downwards, hiatus is further dissected posteriorly.

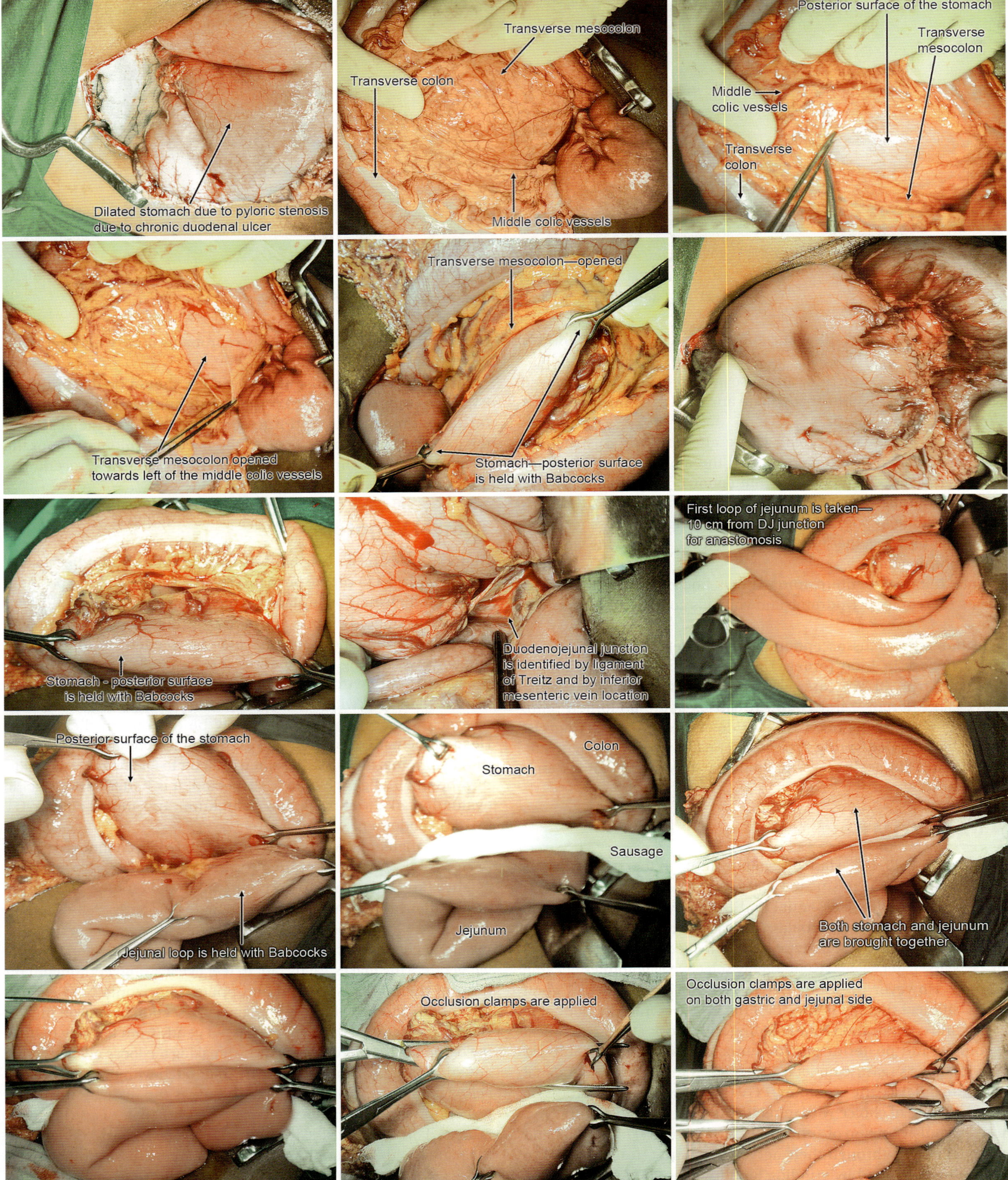
Dilated stomach due to pyloric stenosis due to chronic duodenal ulcer
Transverse mesocolon
Transverse colon
Middle colic vessels
Posterior surface of the stomach
Transverse mesocolon
Middle colic vessels
Transverse colon
Transverse mesocolon opened towards left of the middle colic vessels
Transverse mesocolon—opened
Stomach—posterior surface is held with Babcocks
Stomach - posterior surface is held with Babcocks
Duodenojejunal junction is identified by ligament of Treitz and by inferior mesenteric vein location
First loop of jejunum is taken—10 cm from DJ junction for anastomosis
Posterior surface of the stomach
Jejunal loop is held with Babcocks
Colon
Stomach
Sausage
Jejunum
Both stomach and jejunum are brought together
Occlusion clamps are applied
Occlusion clamps are applied on both gastric and jejunal side

Figs. 21-32(1)

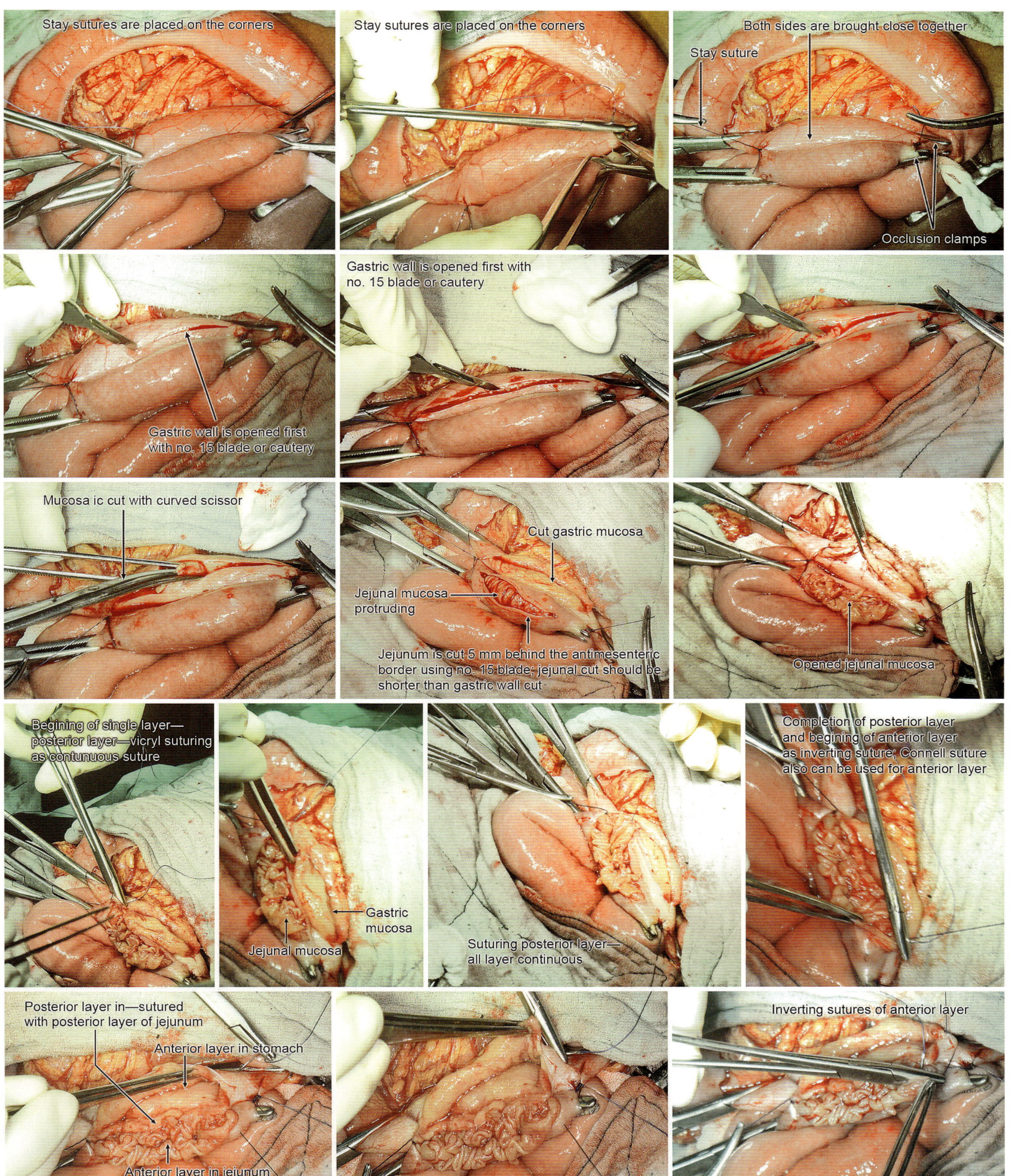

Stay sutures are placed on the corners
Stay sutures are placed on the corners
Both sides are brought close together
Stay suture
Occlusion clamps
Gastric wall is opened first with no. 15 blade or cautery
Gastric wall is opened first with no. 15 blade or cautery
Mucosa ic cut with curved scissor
Cut gastric mucosa
Jejunal mucosa protruding
Jejunum is cut 5 mm behind the antimesenteric border using no. 15 blade; jejunal cut should be shorter than gastric wall cut
Opened jejunal mucosa
Begining of single layer—posterior layer—vicryl suturing as continuous suture
Gastric mucosa
Jejunal mucosa
Suturing posterior layer—all layer continuous
Completion of posterior layer and begining of anterior layer as inverting suture; Connell suture also can be used for anterior layer
Posterior layer in—sutured with posterior layer of jejunum
Anterior layer in stomach
Anterior layer in jejunum
Inverting sutures of anterior layer

Figs. 21-32(2)

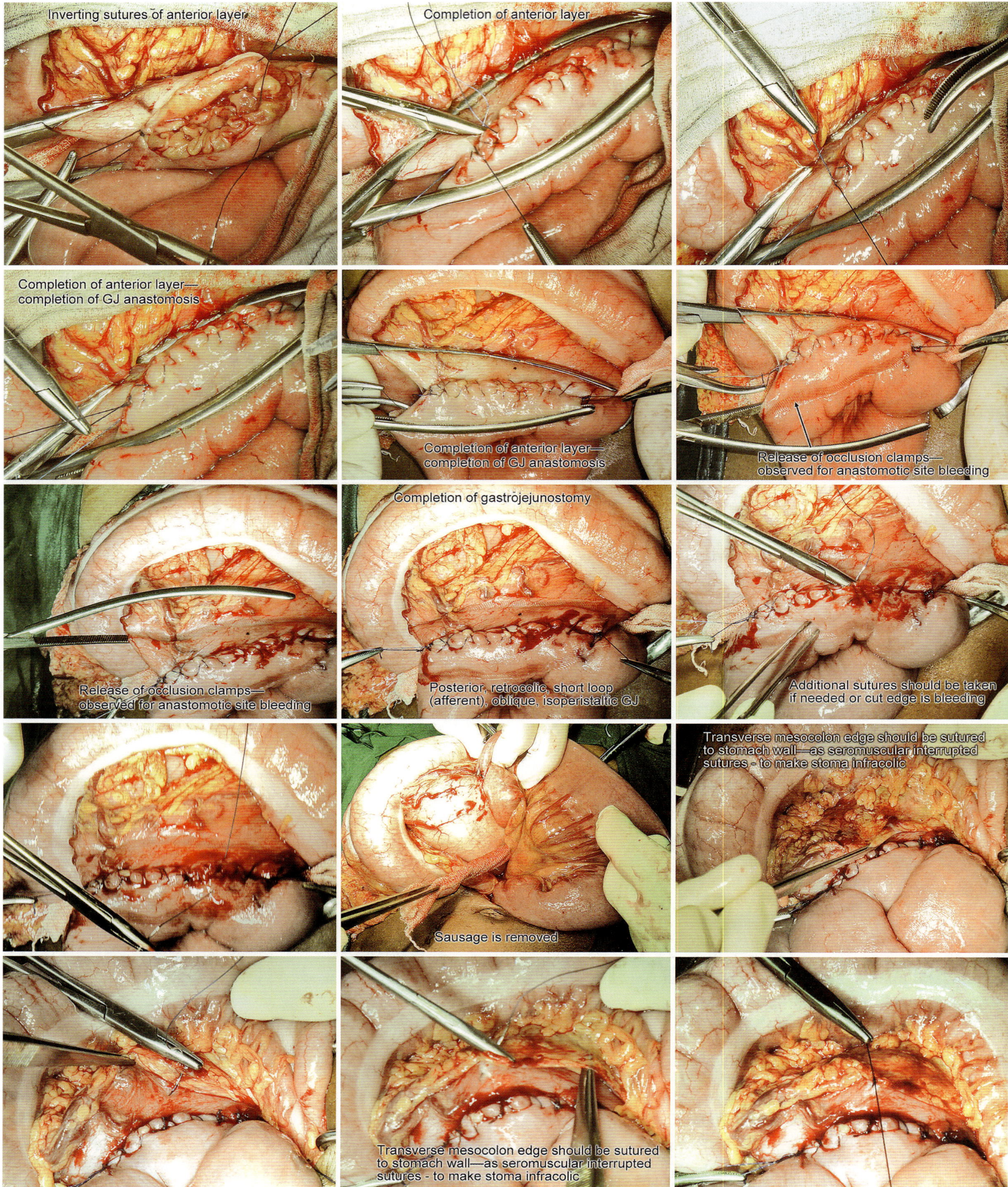
Inverting sutures of anterior layer
Completion of anterior layer
Completion of anterior layer—
completion of GJ anastomosis
Completion of anterior layer—
completion of GJ anastomosis
Release of occlusion clamps—
observed for anastomotic site bleeding
Completion of gastrojejunostomy
Release of occlusion clamps—
observed for anastomotic site bleeding
Posterior, retrocolic, short loop
(afferent), oblique, isoperistaltic GJ
Additional sutures should be taken
if needed or cut edge is bleeding
Transverse mesocolon edge should be sutured
to stomach wall—as seromuscular interrupted
sutures - to make stoma infracolic
Sausage is removed
Transverse mesocolon edge should be sutured
to stomach wall—as seromuscular interrupted
sutures - to make stoma infracolic

Figs. 21-32(3)

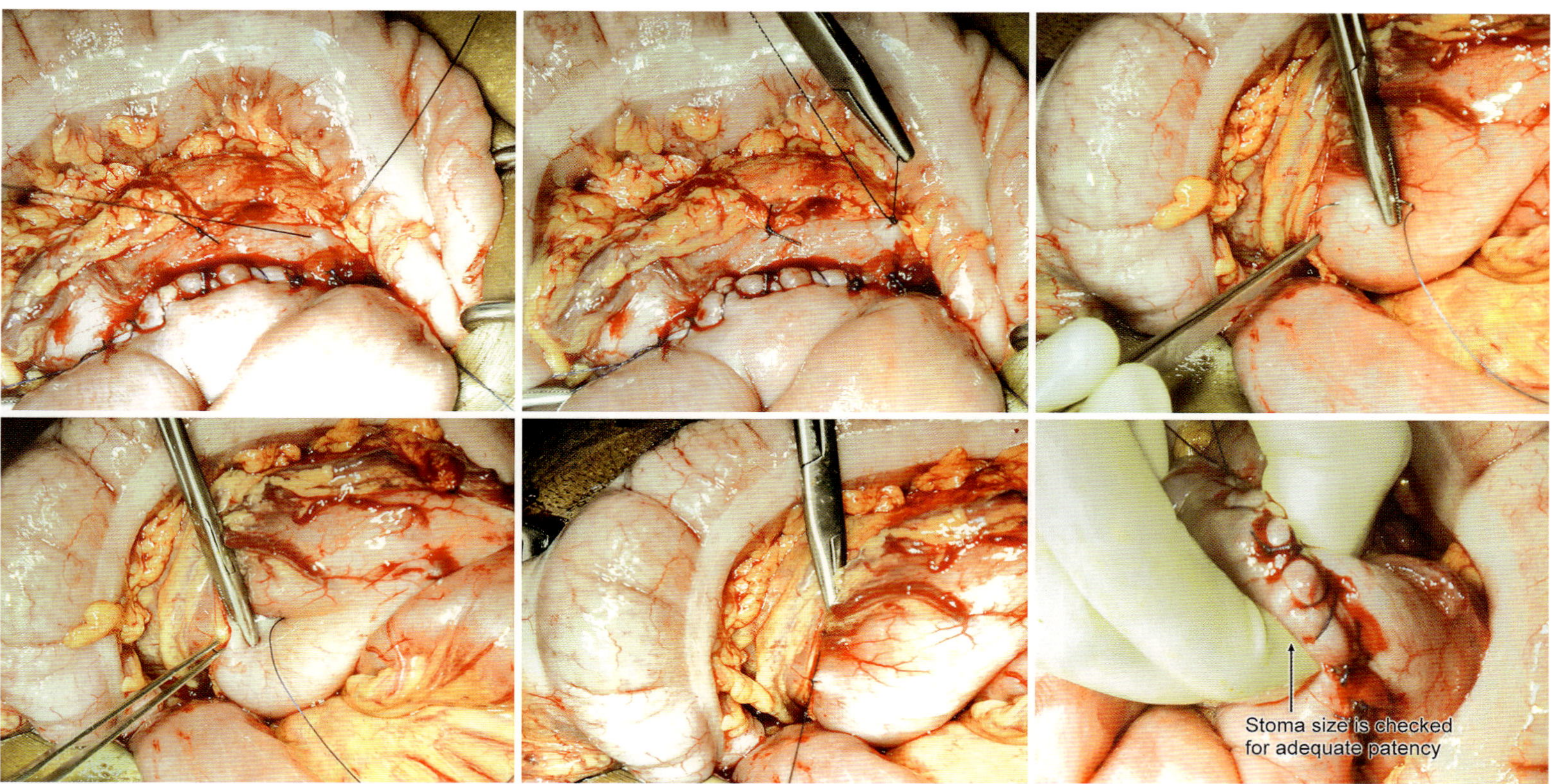

Figs. 21-32(4)

Figs. 21-32(1 to 4): Posterior gastrojejunostomy—technique.

First anterior vagotomy is done. Anterior vagal trunk is felt like string while running finger in front of the oesophagus. Traction on stomach below is continued. Vagus is dissected off the oesophagus using right angled forceps; any small bleeders should be fulgurated with bipolar forceps. Nerve hook may be used for dissection. About 2–3 cm length of the nerve is dissected. Two long curved haemostats are placed on the dissected nerve. Nerve segment (1 cm) is excised between clamps. It should be placed in a bottle for biopsy with anterior vagus as label. Vagal ends are ligated with 2 zero silk suture. Long suture is needed to pass the ligature around. Additional anterior vagal trunks may be present in 40% of individuals and they should be dissected and cut. Small nerve fibres should also be divided. It is done by giving traction to the greater curvature **(Fig. 21-33)**.

Posterior vagotomy is done next. This nerve is more away from the oesophageal wall, unlike anterior trunk. Often it may be on the right crus of diaphragm. Oesophagus is held towards left; on the hiatus towards right, gentle dissection helps to identify it. It is thicker than anterior vagus. It is also similarly clamped, divided and excised (1 cm) and cut ends are ligated with silk. Posterior vagus often is associated with a significant sized vein which if get disrupted can cause bleeding. It is again sent for biopsy in separate bottle. Lower oesophagus for 7 cm is dissected meticulously and all nerve branches are identified and divided. Criminal nerve of Grassi is behind the hiatus; it also should be divided. Nerve fibres along the fundus and angle of His are also dissected and divided. Entire OG junction and lower oesophagus should be cleared of the nerve branches to avoid incomplete vagotomy and so recurrence of ulcer. Posterior vagus is commonly a single trunk unlike anterior vagus. Incidence of additional posterior vagal trunk is only 5%. Communicating trunk to anterior vagus is often present which should also be divided. Missing of posterior vagus is common and intact posterior vagus is one of the common causes of incomplete vagotomy. Posterior vagotomy is done often by different methods. First index finger is passed left of the hiatus behind the OG junction and with traction on the stomach, posterior vagus can be felt as a string like thick structure which is hooked with index finger from left to delineate left side and forward; it is clamped, 1 cm of it is excised and ligated by surgeon or assistant similarly. In another modification, entire hiatal dissection is not necessary. Only right side is dissected to identify the posterior vagus to complete the vagotomy. Coeliac branch is in a constant position as a constant single trunk which is identified close to the left gastric artery; if this branch is traced upwards, posterior vagal trunk is identified. This avoids extensive dissection and prevents complication. Truncal vagotomy should be completed with a drainage procedure like posterior gastrojejunostomy **(Figs. 21-34 and 21-35)**.

Note:

Truncal vagotomy can be done through laparoscopy also. Vagotomy with antrectomy also can be done which reduces the ulcer forming area of the stomach and also reduces the gastrin release (gastrin is released from G cells of the antrum).

Proximal Gastric Vagotomy (PGV)

It is also called as parietal cell vagotomy (PCV) or highly selective vagotomy (HSV) or superselective vagotomy. It denervates the supply of cells in fundus and body specifically. Meantime, it preserves antropyloric gastric emptying function. PGV reduces both acid and pepsin secretion. PGV was first described by Amdrup and Johnston in 1969.

Indications

PGV is useful in refractory/intractable duodenal ulcer; repeated recurrences by drug therapy, perforated duodenal ulcer when presents within 24 hours; selected bleeding duodenal ulcers in females. PGV is not useful in gastric outlet obstruction due to duodenal ulcer.

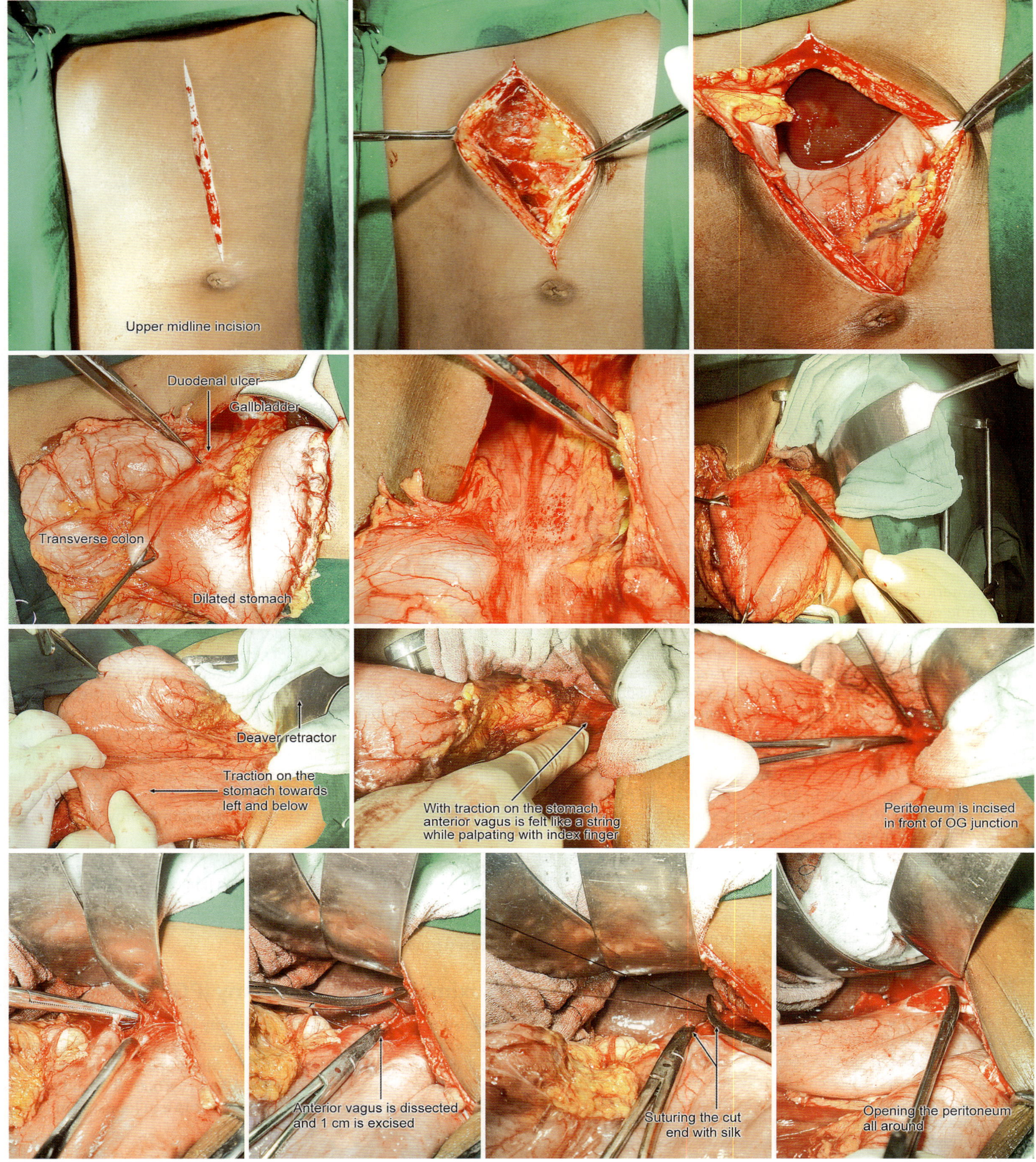
Upper midline incision
Duodenal ulcer
Gallbladder
Transverse colon
Dilated stomach
Deaver retractor
Traction on the stomach towards left and below
With traction on the stomach anterior vagus is felt like a string while palpating with index finger
Peritoneum is incised in front of OG junction
Anterior vagus is dissected and 1 cm is excised
Suturing the cut end with silk
Opening the peritoneum all around

Figs. 21-33(1)

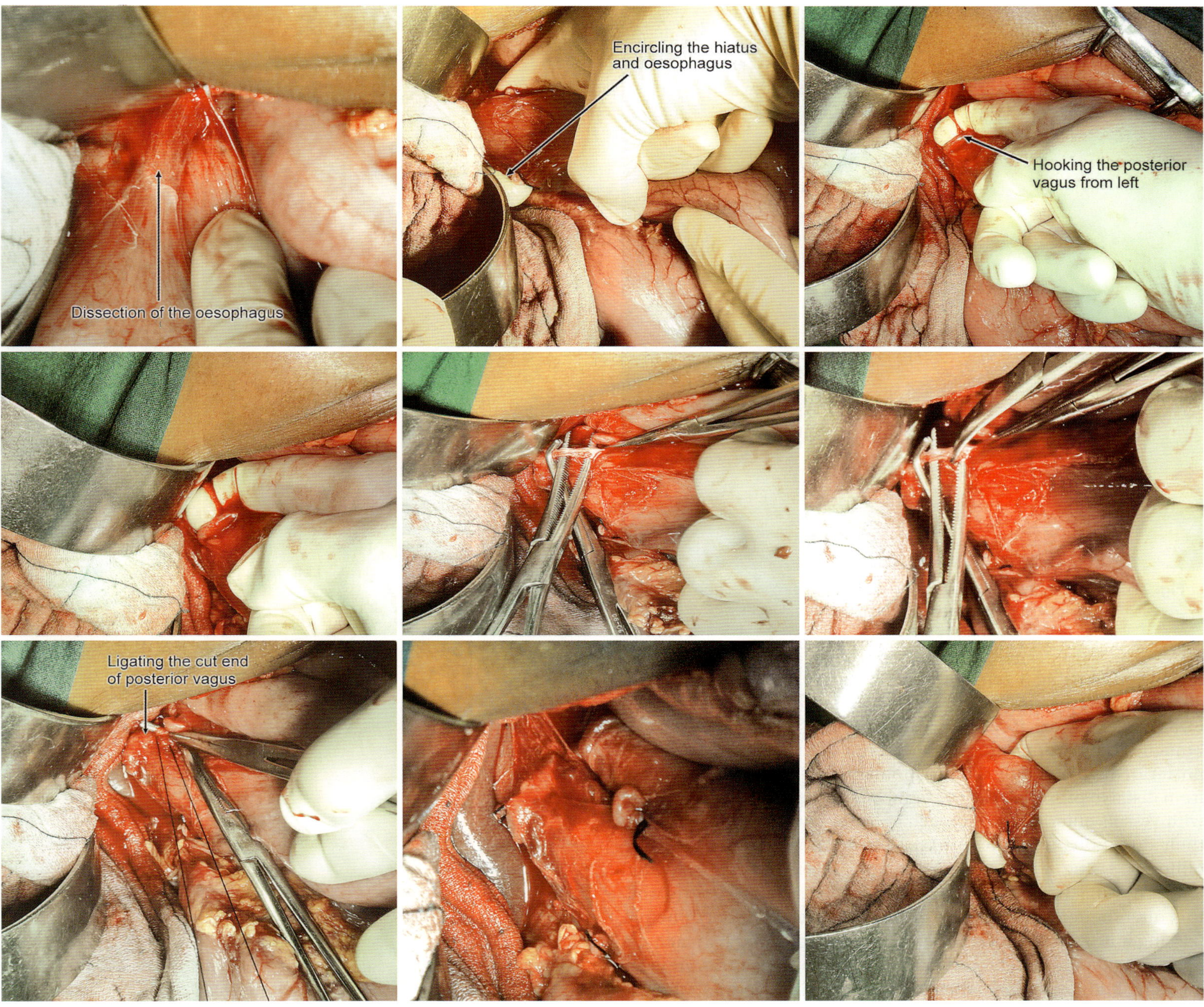

Figs. 21-33(2)

Figs. 21-33(1 and 2): Technique of open truncal vagotomy.

Advantages

It is safer with less than 0.3% mortality. Dumping syndrome or diarrhoea is not known. Antral pump is retained and so drainage procedure is not needed. Basal acid secretion reduces to 80%; maximum acid response to stimuli (pentagastrin) is reduced to 60%. Developing anaemia, tuberculosis, osteoporosis, and carcinoma are not present.

Disadvantages

Lesser curve necrosis even though is rare but is a definitive complication. Ulcer recurrence rate is higher which is 10–15%. Dissection on the proximal part along the OG junction, angle of His and distal 7–8 cm of oesophagus is most crucial to prevent recurrence or to avoid failure due to incomplete vagotomy.

Technique

Preparation, position, incision are same as truncal vagotomy. Many surgeons suggest that hiatus should be dissected early with identification and dissection of vagal trunks first. It is probably not necessary or may be an option for individual surgeon. Oesophageal hiatus is mobilised using index finger and encircled with a Penrose or infant feeding tube. Anterior vagal trunk is carefully felt and identified; it is dissected gently and slinged using silk suture material or vascular slings. Similarly posterior vagus is dissected on the right side of the hiatus, and slinged. Greater curvature is mobilised; posterior surface of the stomach is also mobilised. Anterior PGV is done first. Crow's foot is identified. PGV begins from uppermost branch of the crow's foot; if crow's foot is not obvious then at a point of 6 cm from the prepyloric vein of Mayo (pylorus) dissection begins.

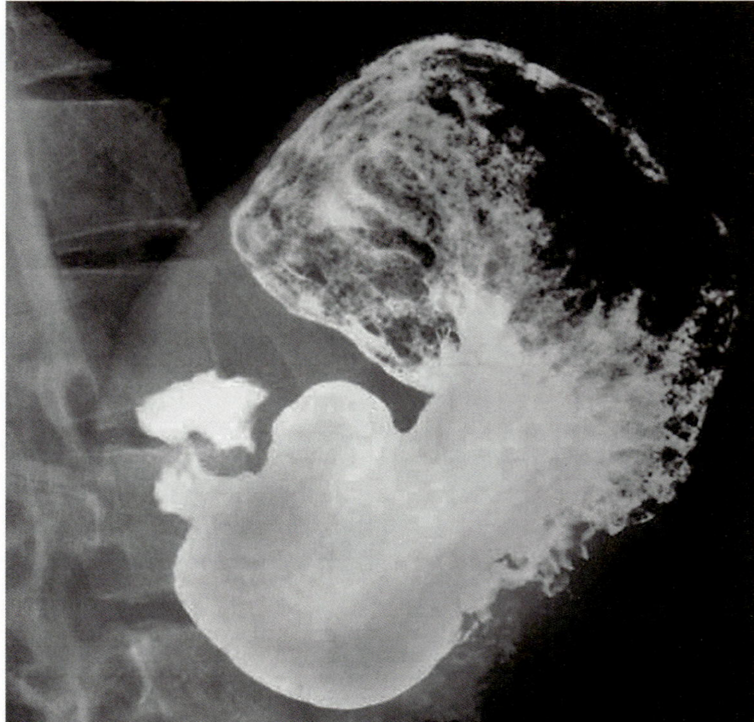

Fig. 21-34: Barium meal X-ray showing gastric outlet obstruction due to pyloric stenosis due to chronic duodenal ulcer.

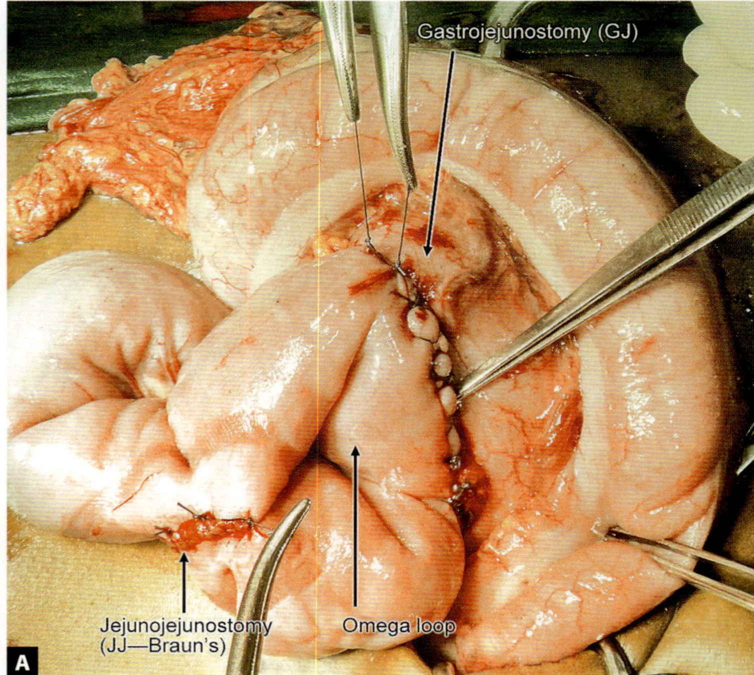

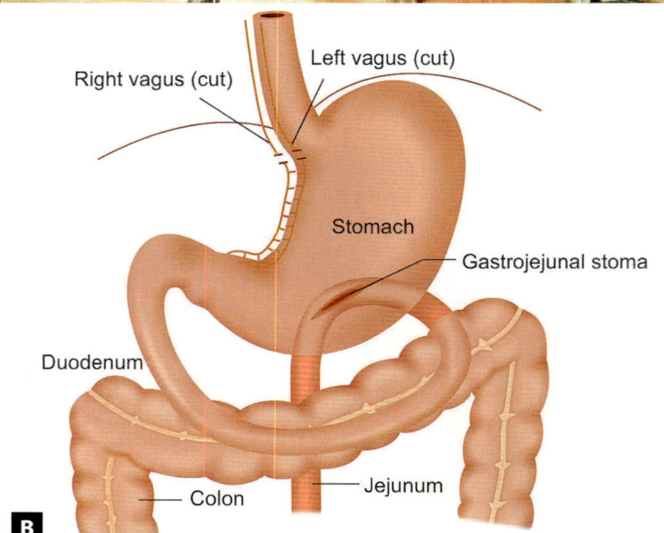

Figs. 21-35A and B: Posterior, vertical, short loop, retrocolic gastrojejunostomy of Mayo. Vagotomy should be combined with gastrojejunostomy.

A stay suture using 3-zero silk is placed at this point on the lesser curvature. Lesser omentum where it joins the lesser curve shows three distinct layers, if carefully dissected; first anterior layer gastric branches of anterior vagus; 3rd posterior layer gastric branches of posterior vagus; middle a loose areolar tissue. PGV begins always from distal to proximal. Gastric branches are very closely associated with vessels entering the stomach at lesser curvature, even though their directions are different (vessels are transverse; nerves are oblique). Using a fine haemostat, vessels are clamped, divided and tied using 3-zero silk individually very close to the gastric wall. It is often better to dissect the vessels for adequate length before passing a ligature towards lesser curve side followed by placing a haemostat on the lesser curve side to cut in between. This prevents bleeding and haematoma formation. It is continued up to the OG junction and later extended in front of the oesophagus towards left beyond the angle of His. Haemoclips and cautery should not be used. Haemoclip may slip causing bleeding and preventing further dissection properly. Cautery may transmit the energy along the nerve of Latarjet. Once anterior leaf is dissected and denerved properly, posterior vagotomy begins. Crow's foot in posterior vagus is not identified. Dissection begins 6–7 cm from the pylorus towards proximally along the posterior leaf of the lesser omentum very close to the lesser curvature of the stomach. Devascularisation with denervation is done similarly from below upwards towards OG junction; near OG junction criminal nerve of Grassi is identified which crosses behind the oesophagus. Often stomach is rotated to dissect the posterior part properly; but it is not necessary. One has to remember that stomach wall should not be included in ligatures.

Distal 8 cm oesophagus should be denerved properly and completely. Anterior vagus is gently retracted towards right and all nerve fibres are felt and divided carefully. Often fibres embedded in the oesophageal muscle are also divided; fibres along the angle of His are also divided. Posterior vagus is retracted towards right and OG junction towards left; distal 8 cm of posterior oesophagus is again cleared of all nerve fibres.

Entire length of both vagi are completely dissected and both nerves of Latarjet are visualised. Slings and Penrose rain are removed. Lesser curvature of the stomach is imbricated with 3-zero silk suture to prevent the devascularisation, perforation or lesser curve necrosis; it also prevents the nerve regeneration.

Gastroepiploic nerve along with the right gastric and epiploic artery when present should be divided. It is divided at the junction of the right and left gastroepiploic artery. Adding this, is called as extended proximal gastric vagotomy.

Ontable tests (intraoperative) are often used to confirm the completion of vagotomy. *Burge test*; ontable oesophagus and pylorus is closed to convert into a closed system; vagus nerve is electrically stimulated; intragastric pressure is recorded using a manometer; pressure rises in incomplete vagotomy. *Grassi test*; pentagastrin is injected intravenously during intraoperative period; gastrotomy is done; pH of the gastric mucosa is assessed before and after vagotomy; pH is less than 2.5 before, but more than 5.5 after vagotomy.

Complications of Vagotomy

Intraoperative

When left triangular ligament is mobilised more than usual, it may cause injury to the hepatic and phrenic veins causing bleeding.

Splenic injury even though rare can occur while retracting spleen towards left. It is more often seen in enlarged spleen. It can occur also during traction over the greater curvature of the stomach and whenever there are fibrous adhesions between spleen and greater curvature of the stomach.

Oesophageal laceration can occur when hiatus is mobilised from left side with index finger. Laceration usually occurs on the right posterolateral oesophageal wall. Tear should be exposed by rotating the oesophageal wall and is sutured with interrupted silk sutures. Often Nissen's fundoplication wrap may be useful. Nasogastric tube should be kept in situ for 7–10 days postoperatively. Injury is more while doing revagotomy or in patients with any previous upper abdominal surgery.

Other rare but known complications are—pneumothorax; oesophagogastric disruption; distal pancreatic injury; thoracic duct injury.

Early Complications

Gastric atony can occur due to altered gastric pacesetter potential, and normal propagation of peristalsis is altered. Ectopic pacemaker may appear which reduces the normal fundal pacemaker function leading into gastric atony. Atony leads into delayed emptying. Contrast (water soluble) study will show emptying of the gastric content but slowly. Endoscopy reveals widely opened stoma.

Transient dysphagia is seen in 10% of patients. It is due to temporary operative trauma; less commonly due to vagotomy.

Lesser curve necrosis (0.3%) occurs in 72 hours. They present with toxicity and features of perforation. It is initially thought due to devascularisation; but probably, it is due to gastric distension which causes compression on vascular network in already ligated vascular area. It requires reexploration, excision of the necrosed area, until it bleeds and resuturing. Jejunostomy may be required. Gastrectomy may also be needed.

Subphrenic abscess formation due to sepsis can occur. Occasionally infection may spread above to cause dreaded mediastinitis.

Long-term Complications

Twenty percent of truncal, 3% of selective, 1% of proximal gastric vagotomy will develop bowel disturbances like diarrhoea. It is episodic, with urgency of passage of mucus, flatus and stool. Truncal vagotomy can cause severe disabling diarrhoea in 1% of patients. Stasis, hypoacidity with bacterial overgrowth, changes in intestinal villi, altered biliary and pancreatic exocrine function, dysmotility of small bowel are the probable causes. It usually gets controlled with passage of time. Restriction of fluid, carbohydrate and milk products, neomycin, loperamide, codeine, cholestyramine are the treatments for vagotomy diarrhoea. Severe disabling persistent incapacitating diarrhoea (20 times a day stool with incontinence) needs surgical correction. Reverse jejunal interposition is the treatment.

Disruption of crural fibres due to dissection may cause reflux oesophagitis and later stricture formation.

Truncal vagotomy increases the incidence of gallstone formation. Because of hepatic divisions, gallbladder becomes hypotonic; decreased release of cholecystokinin from the duodenum is also the cause for gallstone formation.

PYLOROPLASTY

It is done in case of bleeding duodenal ulcer. Though this bleeding is controlled by various methods. It is also done as part of the procedure in creation of gastric reservoir for oesophageal substitution or bypass, if pyloromyotomy is not undertaken or not possible **(Fig. 21-36)**.

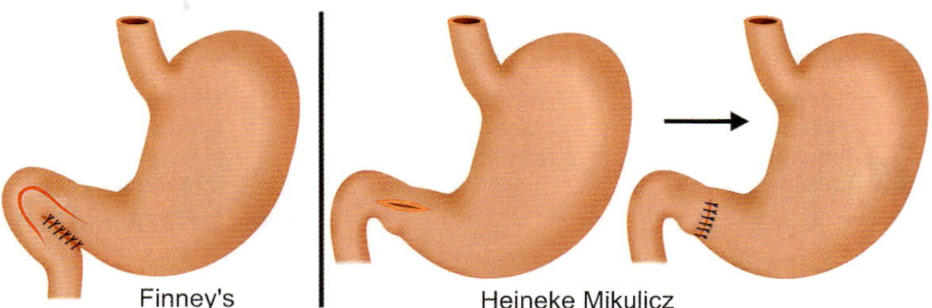

Fig. 21-36: Types of pyloroplasty.

Types of Pyloroplasty

Heineke–Mikulicz Pyloroplasty

Upper midline incision is used for laparotomy. Duodenum is mobilised by Kocherisation. Peritoneum is held on the lateral part of the 2nd part of duodenum and is incised along the margin of the duodenum. Finger dissection further facilitates the mobilisation. Avascular lateral duodenal ligament that runs between duodenum and retroperitoneum is also divided. Curved scissor and cautery can be used for the same. About 5–6 cm incision is made along the lower antrum, pylorus and 1st part of the duodenum longitudinally to its entire thickness. Bleeding points are cauterised using bipolar cautery. Opened pyloroduodenotomy wound is closed transversely as full thickness interrupted 3-zero vicryl or silk sutures **(Figs. 21-37A and B)**.

First midpoint suture is placed; then sutures are placed on either side. Once midpoint suture is placed and is held long with a haemostat, remaining sutures are placed from one corner towards middle on either side. Second seromuscular suture is also placed often but it is difficult as it often tears. If no tear occurs interrupted, seromuscular sutures can be placed, but it is not mandatory. Omentum is wrapped around it to secure. Stapling closure also can be done easily using 55–4.8 mm linear stapler.

Emergency Surgical Management of Bleeding Duodenal Ulcer

Bleeding from duodenal ulcer is either from the small vessels in the wall of ulcer crater or due to erosion into the gastroduodenal artery.

Precipitating causes are—alcohol, NSAIDs, steroids, excessive fibrosis and atherosclerotic disease.

Forrest classification of bleeding or bled ulcer

- Ia Spurting and bleeding
- Ib Non-spurting but active bleeding
- IIa Visible vessel with red or blue protrusion or pulsatile pseudoaneurysm
- IIb Non-bleeding ulcer with clot overlying
- IIc Ulcer with haematin base
- III Clean ulcer—no clot, no vessel

Usually posterior duodenal ulcer bleeds; bleeding from small vessels in the wall of ulcer is due to sloughing of the ulcer. It is less severe,

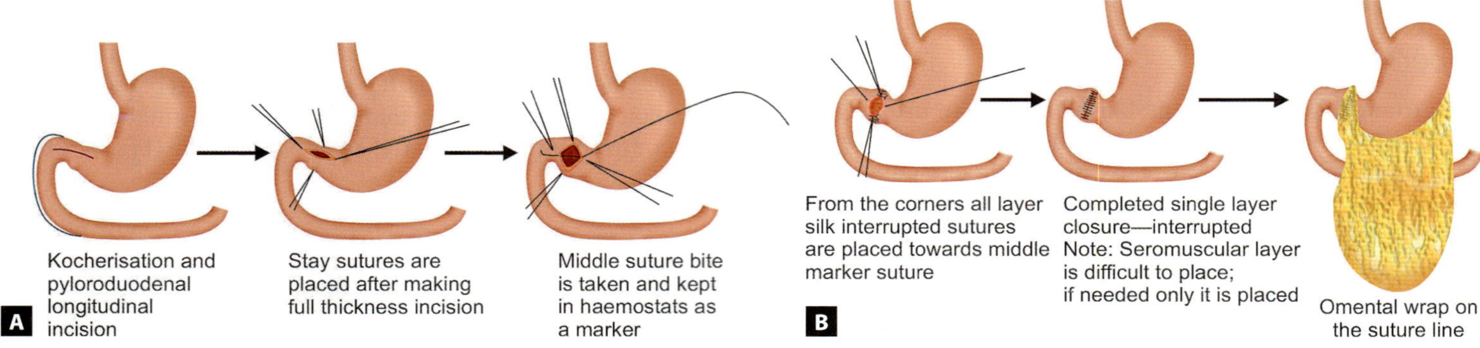

Figs. 21-37A and B: Heineke–Mikulicz pyloroplasty.

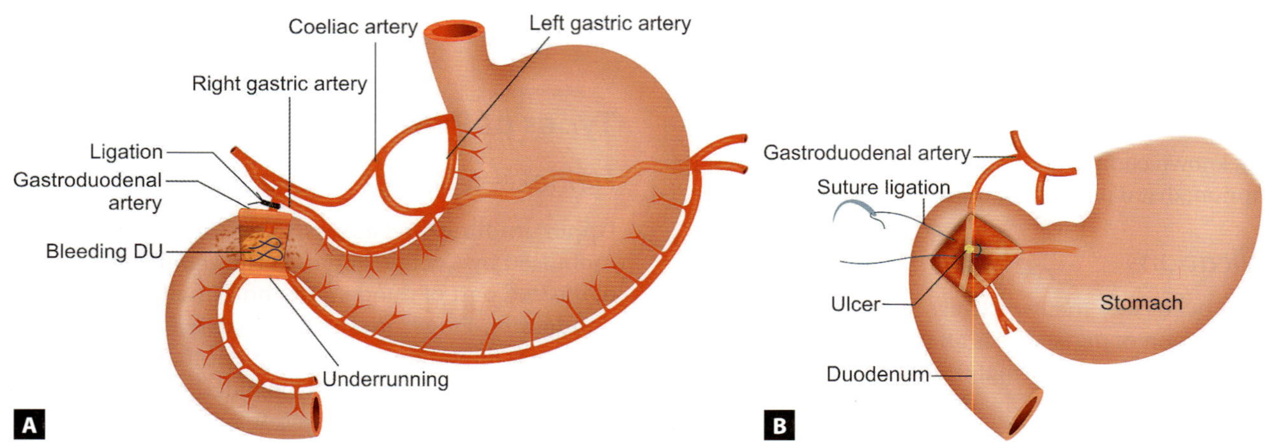

Figs. 21-38A and B: Bleeding duodenal ulcer (DU) is treated by underrunning the ulcer bed or ligating the gastroduodenal artery in two places.

gradual and often well-controlled by conservative treatment. Bleeding from erosion of gastroduodenal artery is severe, torrential and almost always needs early surgical intervention **(Figs. 21-38A and B)**.

Indications for surgical treatment: In spite of conservative treatment, condition of patient deteriorates; bleeding from gastroduodenal artery; recurrent bleeding; elderly patient; if more than 4 units of blood required immediately.

Technique

After laparotomy, adequate Kocherisation is done. Pyloric channel and first part of the duodenum (gastroduodenum) are opened longitudinally, bleeder is identified. Underrunning of the bleeding area with 2-zero silk or vicryl is done. Proximal and distal bleeding points are transfixed using 2-zero silk sutures. Deep transverse pancreatic artery which is a deep posterior branch of gastroduodenal artery should be occluded by placing a deep middle transfixing suture in the ulcer bed. If the bleed is from gastroduodenal artery, then it has to be ligated to stop the bleeding. It is done by dissecting above the duodenum where it originates from the common hepatic artery. Aneurysm needle may be used to pass a secure ligature around. Gastroduodenal artery also often needs to be ligated inferiorly to prevent backflow of blood; it is ligated below after defining and dissecting just above the origin of the right gastroepiploic artery. Keeping 5 mm distance from the origin, it is securely ligated with transfixation sutures using 2-zero silk. Opened gastroduodenum is closed by ***Finney's pyloroplasty.*** Truncal vagotomy may be done together, if only the general condition of the patient is good.

Finney's Pyloroplasty (1922)

It is done in bleeding duodenal ulcer and when wide pyloroplasty is needed.

Upper midline incision is used. Kocherisation is done adequately. Junction of the pylorus and first part of the duodenum is held at its upper margin with a Babcock's forceps or stay suture. Distal part of the greater curvature is brought closer to the pancreatic side of the 2nd part of the duodenum. Seromuscular sutures (3-zero silk) are placed between distal part of the greater curvature of the stomach and proximal inner part of the duodenum which are tied either after placing all sutures or individually after placing sutures one by one. A 'U'-shaped incision is made from greater curvature towards proximal duodenum which is deepened to have a full thickness gastroduodenotomy. Inner all layer suturing is done using 3-zero silk or vicryl from upper most apex part of the posterior layer towards downwards direction. Once lowermost part is reached, it is continued in front as anterior all layer continuous Connell sutures from below upwards. Anterior seromuscular interrupted 3-zero silk sutures are placed at the end. It is supported with omental patch. Truncal vagotomy may be added **(Figs. 21-39A to D)**.

Complications

Bile leak due to anastomotic dehiscence is possible, especially when pyloroplasty is done in a scarred duodenum. Infection, subphrenic abscess formation, delayed gastric emptying are other complications.

Note:

Kennedy duodenoplasty is similar to pyloroplasty but distal to the pylorus on the proximal part of the first part of the duodenum;

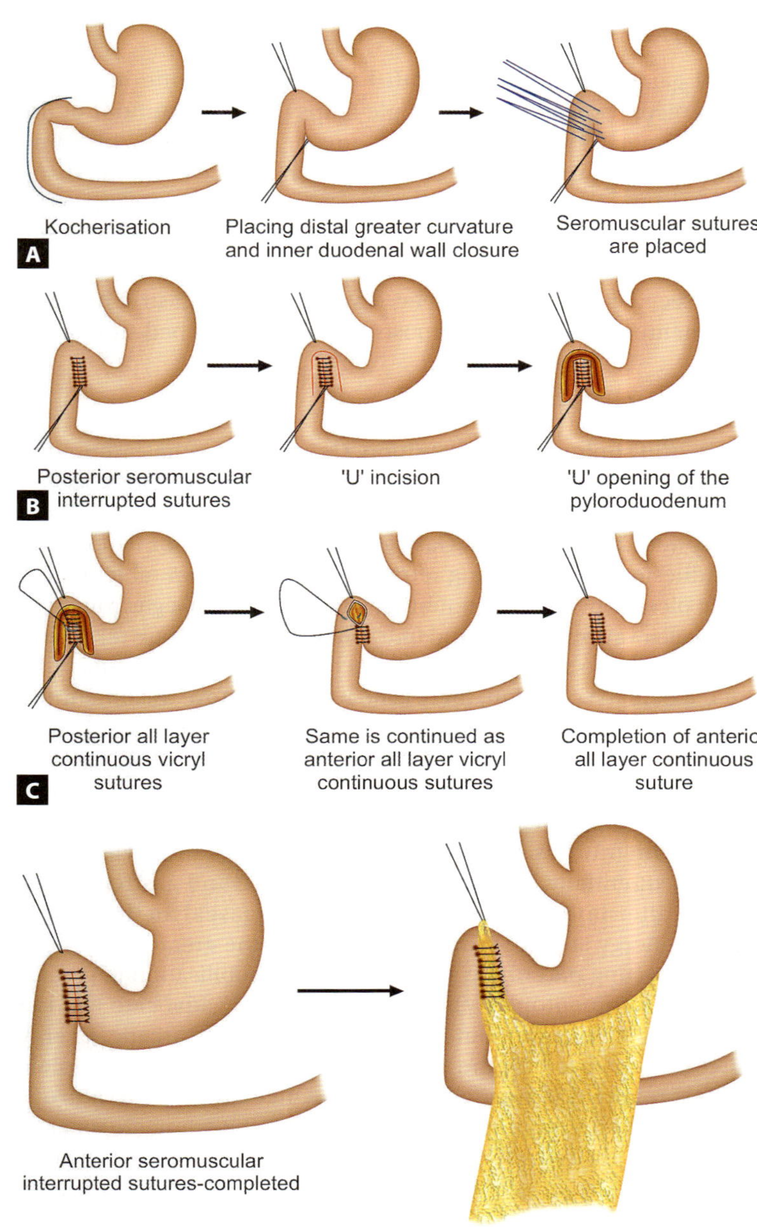

Figs. 21-39A to D: Finney's pyloroplasty.

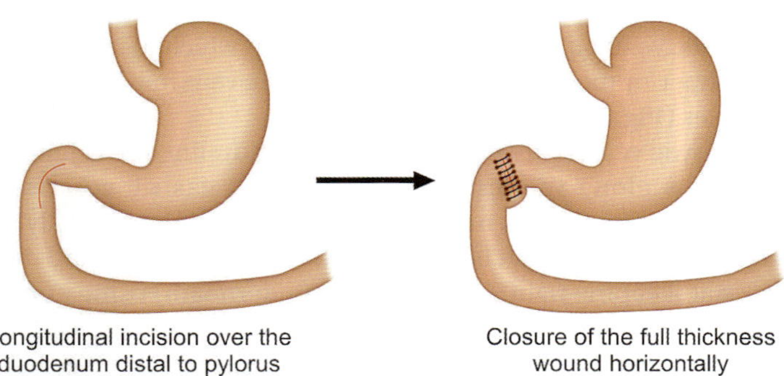

Fig. 21-40: Duodenoplasty is done distal to pylorus (Kennedy).

longitudinal full thickness incision is closed transversely **(Fig. 21-40)**.

Dudd pylorectomy: Here ulcer crater is excised by a diamond-shaped incision along with pyloroplasty.

Antrectomy (hemigastrectomy): Here ulcer bearing area in the stomach is removed and pyloric antrum with either gastroduodenal or gastrojejunal anastomosis is done. It is done in case of recurrent ulcers or in Zollinger Ellison syndrome. It removes the gastrin secreting area (G cells). Antrectomy as a primary procedure is not routinely done for duodenal ulcer.

Gastric mucosal resection (Kirk, 1972): It is done in recurrent ulcers. Here antral mucosa is dissected and removed without ligating vessels externally. It is done after vagotomy. Anterior gastrotomy is done from pylorus 8 cm proximally and 3 cm distally to open entire distal stomach and duodenum. Using pH probe, proximal acid secreting mucosa and distal alkali secreting mucosa is marked at junction. Around 300–500 mL of 1 in 2,00,000 saline with adrenaline is injected into the submucosa. It distends and separates the mucosa and also prevents bleeding. Onto this mucosa, only circumferential incision is made at the pylorus junction and mucosa proximal is dissected off from the submucosa like tube for 8 cm. Proximal part is also transected circumferentially. Small bleeders are fulgurated using bipolar cautery. Mucosal edges proximal and distal are brought together using 3-zero vicryl sutures continuously taking bites deeply up to muscular layer.

GASTRECTOMY

Removal of the part or entire stomach surgically is called as gastrectomy. It can be antrectomy (hemigastrectomy), partial (65%), subtotal (80%), total or radical (nodal clearance) gastrectomy.

Gastrectomy reconstruction can be Billroth I or Billroth II type. Billroth I is gastroduodenostomy; Billroth II is gastrojejunostomy.

Professor Hans Theodor Billroth did first gastrectomy with gastroduodenostomy in 1881 **(Figs. 21-41 to 21-43)**.

Gastrectomy with Billroth I Methods of Anastomosis

Classical Billroth I operation is partial gastrectomy with gastroduodenostomy with closure of lesser curve and anastomosis at greater curvature side. Horsley, von Haberer–Finney, von Haberer, Schoemaker, Kocher are different Billroth I modifications.

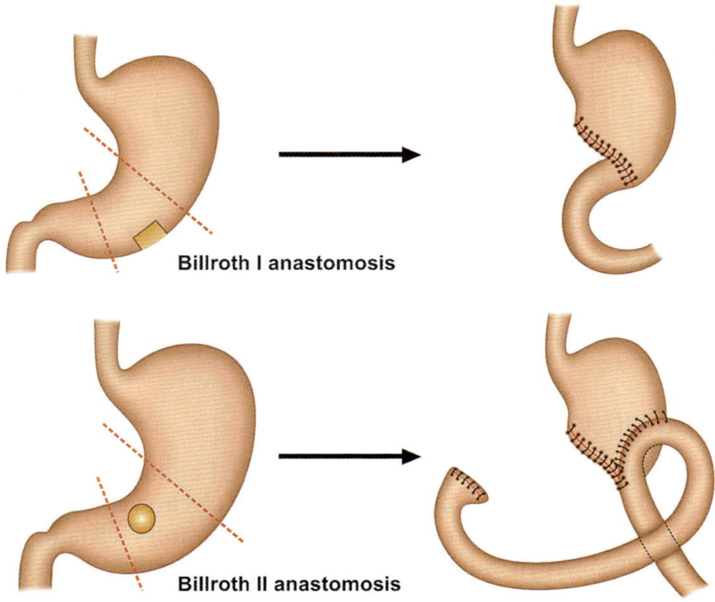

Fig. 21-41: Billroth I and II anastomosis after gastrectomy.

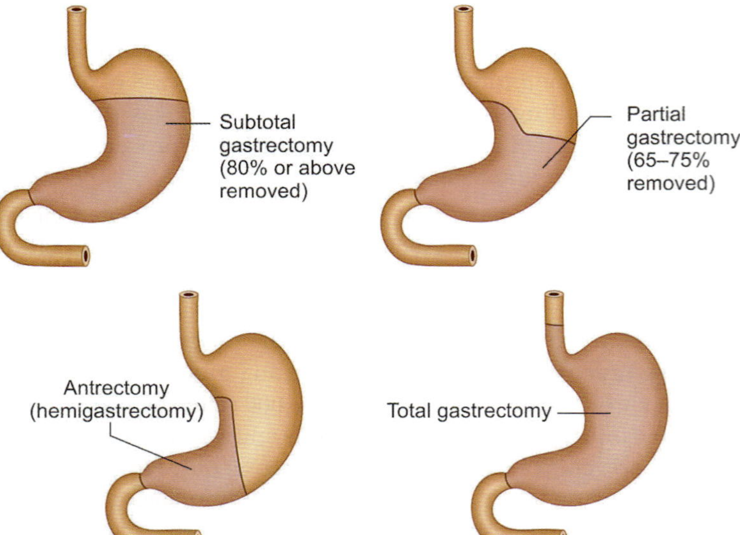

Fig. 21-42: Anatomical meanings of hemigastrectomy, partial, subtotal and total gastrectomies.

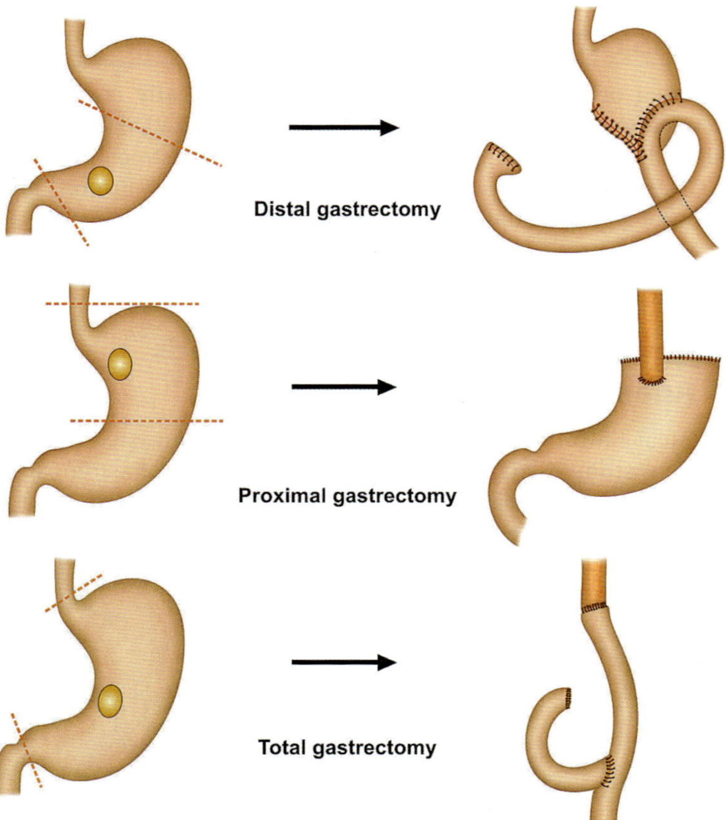

Fig. 21-43: Technical meanings of distal, proximal and total gastrectomies. Proximal gastrectomy is done rarely now; probably done in OG junction growths only; even there, total gastrectomy is preferred by many.

Preparation

Gastroscopy and adequate biopsy are must; CT abdomen to detect any additional pathology; adequate hydration; electrolyte imbalance management; evaluation of cardiac and respiratory systems are needed. Nasogastric tube and urinary catheter should be passed. Preoperative/perioperative antibiotics are a must as once stomach is opened, field gets contaminated.

Indications

Partial gastrectomy with Billroth I procedure is done in benign gastric ulcer (proved by endoscopic biopsy), benign tumour of the distal stomach, trauma to distal stomach, recurrent or bleeding duodenal ulcer, if pyloroplasty is not feasible. In carcinoma distal stomach, Billroth I anastomosis is usually not done as recurrence in bed when it occurs will cause obstruction due to encasement of the relapsed (local) tumour; whereas in Billroth II gastrojejunostomy, stoma recedes upwards and leaves away from the gastric bed and also omentum; and colon interposes between gastric bed and stoma.

Technique

Patient is in supine head up position. General anaesthesia/epidural are given. Abdomen is approached through upper midline incision extending down towards left of the umbilicus. Abdomen is explored for any additional findings. Gastric ulcer area is felt for its location and adhesion. Self-retaining retractor is placed. If on table benign gastric ulcer appears to be doubtfully malignant then a gastrotomy is done well away proximally and four quadrant biopsies are taken and sent for frozen section biopsy and proceeded further accordingly.

For a benign condition, there is no need to remove the omentum. Kocherisation is done adequately. Gastrohepatic ligament (lesser omentum) is opened using index finger and gently posterior wall of the stomach is separated using finger dissection; adhesions if present, are released after release of greater omentum under direct vision. Greater omentum is clamped with two haemostats, divided and ligated sequentially between greater curvature and gastroepiploic arcade; alternatively bipolar cautery or ligaseal or harmonic scalpel (energy sources) can be used to free the greater omentum on the resecting part of the stomach (like in mobilisation of greater omentum in omentoplasty); alternatively, many advocate ligation of the greater omentum outer to the gastroepiploic arcade. Energy sources can be used for the same (harmonic). Right gastroepiploic artery is retained if arcade is retained. Once greater curvature is freed off the omentum, posterior surface of the stomach is easily seen by everting it; if any adhesions present, they should be divided either with sharp dissection using scissor or cautery or harmonic scalpel. These adhesions if forced with finger for release will cause troublesome bleeding. Dissection close to the origin of the right gastroepiploic vessels should be done with care as small multiple veins may get torn causing bleeding. Middle colic vessels are very close and care should be taken not to injure them; especially middle colic artery if injured will cause transverse colon ischaemia. Middle colic vein joins right gastroepiploic vein which joins the portal vein or superior mesenteric vein. Middle colic vein may be ligated if need arises **(Fig. 21-44)**.

Left gastric vessels are ligated usually at midpoint of OG junction and pylorus along the lesser curvature. Left gastric vessels are clamped together; two haemostats (medium or large) proximally and one distally are applied; it is divided in between proximal and distal haemostat (keeping right angled forceps underneath) using number 15 blade or fine scissor. Proximal part is transfixed once with silk and another ligated. Distal part is also ligated using silk. One should confirm that there is no bleeding or loosening of the ligature. Often alternatively, left gastric vessels are dissected using right angle forceps for 1.5 cm and ligature is passed and ligated both proximally (2 or 3) and distally (one) and divided in between; lengthy ligature ends are held with traction during division. But now it is practiced that left gastric artery and vein are individually dissected, isolated and ligated separately, however it is technically difficult. Left gastric vein

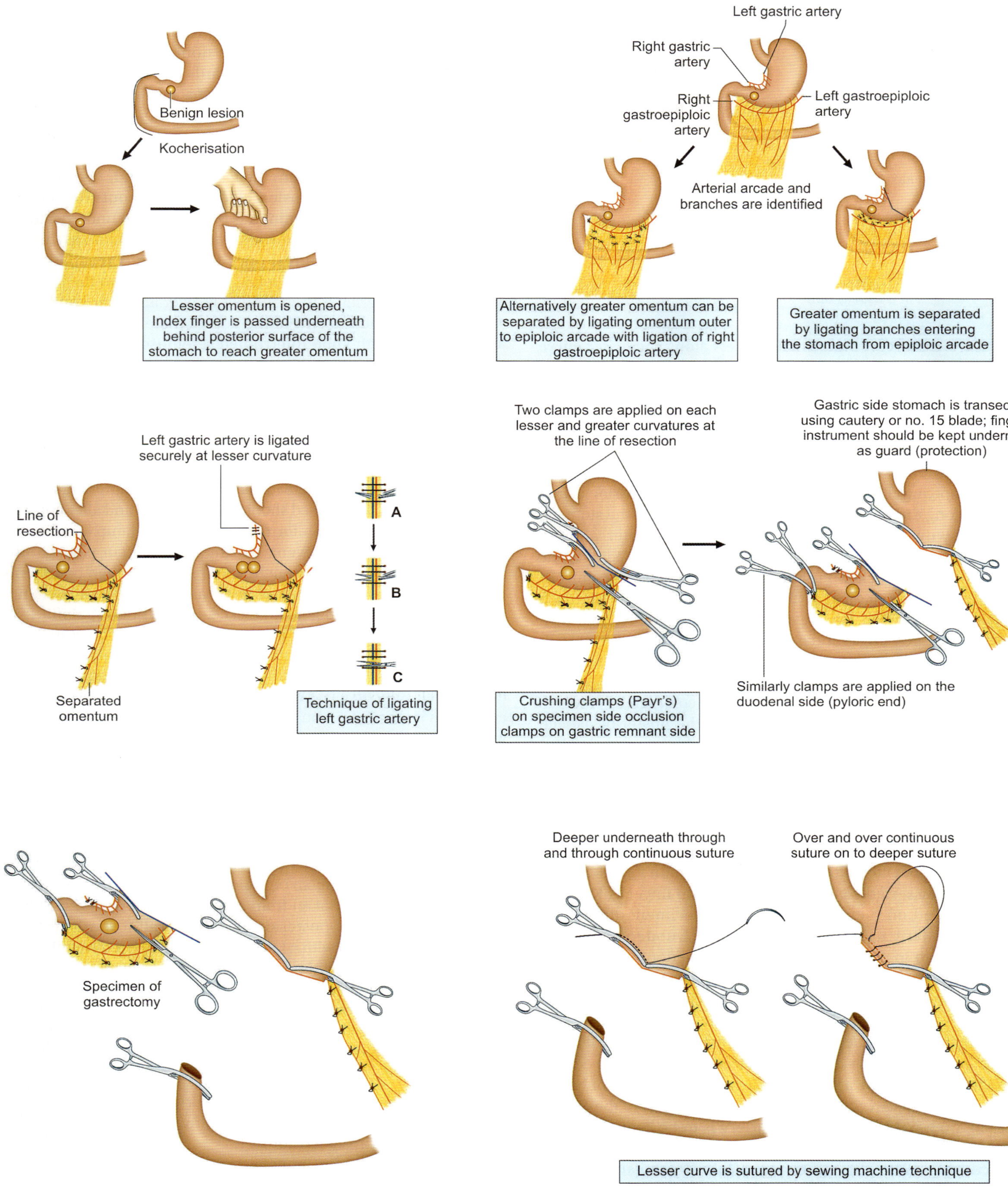

Benign lesion
Kocherisation
Lesser omentum is opened, Index finger is passed underneath behind posterior surface of the stomach to reach greater omentum
Left gastric artery
Right gastric artery
Right gastroepiploic artery
Left gastroepiploic artery
Arterial arcade and branches are identified
Alternatively greater omentum can be separated by ligating omentum outer to epiploic arcade with ligation of right gastroepiploic artery
Greater omentum is separated by ligating branches entering the stomach from epiploic arcade
Left gastric artery is ligated securely at lesser curvature
Line of resection
Separated omentum
A
B
C
Technique of ligating left gastric artery
Two clamps are applied on each lesser and greater curvatures at the line of resection
Crushing clamps (Payr's) on specimen side occlusion clamps on gastric remnant side
Gastric side stomach is transected using cautery or no. 15 blade; finger or instrument should be kept underneath as guard (protection)
Similarly clamps are applied on the duodenal side (pyloric end)
Specimen of gastrectomy
Deeper underneath through and through continuous suture
Over and over continuous suture on to deeper suture
Lesser curve is sutured by sewing machine technique

Figs. 21-44(1)

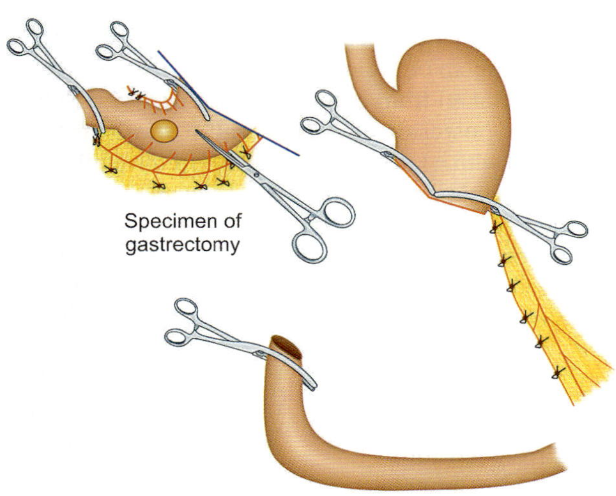

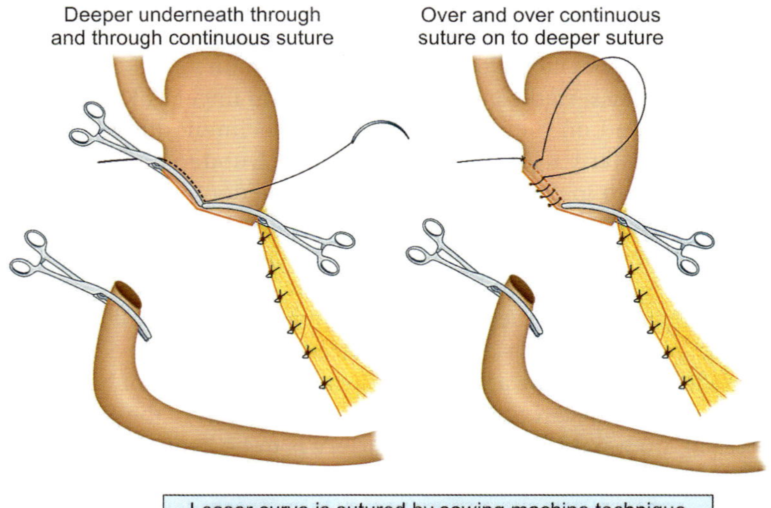

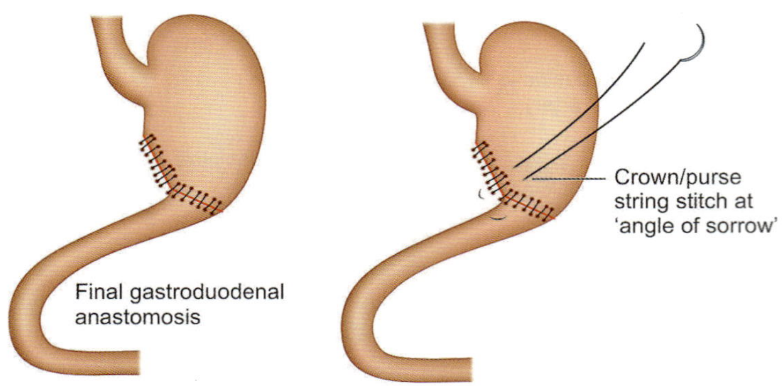

Figs. 21-44(2)

Figs. 21-44(1 and 2): Gastrectomy with Billroth I anastomosis—technique. It is usually done for benign lesions.

is caudal to artery. Few more small vessels along the lesser curve at this point are also ligated and divided. Remaining gastric stump is supplied by the ascending branch of left gastric artery, left gastro-epiploic and short gastric arteries. Similarly left gastroepiploic vessels (commonly two veins will be present at this level) are ligated along the greater curvature side at the point of resection of the stomach.

Nasogastric tube is palpated and pulled out proximally away from the line of applying clamps and line of division. One occlusion clamp is applied along the lesser curvature towards middle of the stomach directed downwards from lesser curve side; another applied horizontally from greater curvature side towards middle of the stomach. Large Payr's clamp is applied or (two Kocher's clamps or Parker Kerr crushing clamps) on the specimen side below. Stomach is transected in between, leaving clear margin on the proximal side; transection is done using number 15 blade from lesser curve towards greater curve with keeping finger or flat instrument behind as a guard to prevent inadvertent injury to deeper structures. Cautery can be used for the division. Antral mucosa should be completely removed.

Distal part is lifted upwards to visualise the posterior aspect. Small vessels between pancreas and stomach are cauterised or ligated and divided. Right gastric artery on the upper margin of the pylorus is dissected, ligated and divided. Other vessels in the lesser curve are also ligated and divided. Often instead of single right gastric artery, there will be leash of right gastric vessels which are ligated and divided. An occlusion clamp is applied on the 1st part of the duodenum after mobilising duodenum for 1.5–2.0 cm. Duodenum is dissected gently using bipolar and finger. A Kocher's clamp is applied on the distal part of the specimen; duodenum is divided similarly using number 15 blade. Duodenal clamp is removed once to inspect its mucosa for completion of removal of entire antral mucosa; finger is passed inside to feel for orifice of duct of Santorini and ampulla of Vater (which is 7 cm from the pylorus). Care should be taken not to injure the bile duct. If duodenal division is done within gastroduodenal artery level (not beyond) then it is less likely that pancreatic ducts are injured. Bleeding from the cut edge of the duodenum should be adequate. If greater omentum is mobilised outer to the epiploic arcade by dividing fat and vessels of the greater omentum, then right gastroepiploic artery is to be ligated close to pancreas and where it enters the lower margin of duodenum and greater curvature. There is a rare chance of loss of omental viability by ligating both right and left gastroepiploic arteries; in such situation, omental excision can be added. Right gastroepiploic vessels can be ligated and divided as a bulk (mass tie) between proximal two and distal one ligatures; but present practice is identifying vessels individually and dissecting and ligating.

Alternatively duodenal part of the dissection and ligating of right gastric artery and separation from the pancreas, clamping and dividing the duodenum can be done first, later lifting the specimen upwards, forwards and towards left. Left gastric and left gastroepiploic vessels are addressed. Stomach is similarly transected between clamps.

Lesser curve oblique clamp is held upwards; using 2 or 3 zero silk or vicryl, this part of the lesser curve is closed using sewing machine suturing technique. Here from the lesser curve end, needle bite is taken underneath the occlusion clamp and tied outside; tail end is held with a haemostat; continuous bites are taken underneath the clamp from lesser curve side towards the tip of the clamp as through and through running sutures; once this suture is reached up to the tip of the clamp, clamp is released; knot is tied to the last loop of the suture material; it is continued as over and over continuous suture towards the tail end of the suture material at lesser curve where it is tied with knot. Interrupted seromuscular layer suturing (Lembert) is also done on this layer.

During mobilisation and dissection of stomach, care should be taken to protect spleen, pancreas, duct of Santorini, common bile duct, middle colic artery. Duodenal mobilisation should not go beyond the gastroduodenal artery. Adhesion between pancreas and stomach distally is most crucial; care should be taken not to pull the stomach and do blunt dissection; instead sharp or bipolar cautery dissection should be done. Clamps used should be ellipsoidal and after applying compression should be uniform on the bowel. Clamp steadies the gut, prevents spillage, prevents oozing from the cut edges of the stomach and duodenum. Straight clamps even though commonly used are more damaging than ellipsoidal. These occlusion clamps when applied on your finger and locked, should not be painful.

Billroth I gastroduodenal anastomosis is done. Posterior interrupted silk stay sutures are placed; later tied after taking all bites. Posterior all layer through and through vicryl continuous suture is done from lesser curve end towards greater curve end; bites are taken at 3–5 mm interval, 3–5 mm from the cut edges; locking is done once in 3 or 4 bites to prevent purse string and for haemostasis. Same is continued as anterior all layer through and through sutures towards lesser from greater curve. Connell sutures can be placed to invert the mucosa. In lesser curve, it is sutured to the tail end of the suture material. Anterior seromuscular interrupted silk sutures are placed afterwards. *Angle of sorrow* (***Jammerecke***) is angle where lesser curve end meets the sutured upper duodenal end. It should be reinforced with *crown stitch/purse string stitch/triple seromuscular stitch.* Bite (seromuscular) is taken from anterior gastric wall to posterior gastric wall and from posterior duodenal wall towards anterior duodenal end and tied with a knot. Often this stitch alternatively can be taken prior to completion of the suturing of the angle of sorrow which is kept untied and tied only at the end. Patency of lumen is confirmed by admitting the tip of the thumb. Usually nasogastric tube is negotiated across gastroduodenal stoma. Tube drain may be kept and is removed after 5–7 days.

Note:

Stapler can be used for closure of lesser curvature.

Present concept is gastroduodenostomy should be performed without clamps to avoid tension.

In olden days for suturing inner layer, *Moynihan atraumatic straight intestinal needle* were used (not now). They were used with hand for suturing.

Tanner's method: Twin gastroenterostomy clamps (Lane's) can be used for anastomosis by applying their blades on both duodenal and gastric sides.

Pauchet's operation/maneuver is used in high gastric ulcer with distal stomach lifted upwards to visualise the ulcer bearing area on the lesser curvature and tongue-like piece of lesser curve containing ulcer is excised and immediately sutured.

In a high lesser curve ulcer where access is difficult especially in obese individual, lesser curve can be created without application of the clamp. Here suturing begins from lower part of the proposed lesser curve, continuous sutures are applied upwards as '*open climbing*' technique until lesser curve end is reached. It is often guided by nasogastric or orogastric tube.

In von Haberer method, reefing and purse string is done to lower greater curvature part of the cut end of the stomach so that it is buried to avoid angle of sorrow.

In Schoemaker modification, entire lesser curve and antrum are removed; new lesser curve is created by hand suturing or stapling device.

In Horsley's modification, duodenum is anastomosed to lesser curve end of the stomach.

In von Haberer Finney's modification, opened entire cut end of the stomach is sutured to the side of the mobilised 2nd part of the duodenum with closure of the duodenal stump.

In Maingot's modification of von Haberer Finney's technique, duodenal stump is not closed; but its end is given a cut on its inner part (like a Cheatle's cut in small intestine) to widen the duodenal stoma which is anastomosed to the lower cut end of the stomach towards greater curvature after suturing lesser curvature.

Pylorus preserving Billroth I procedure and vagus preserving Billroth I procedures are advocated in Japan for early gastric cancers **(Figs. 21-45 to 21-51)**.

Postoperative care

Nasogastric aspiration is done for 5 days. Then oral sips are started. Respiratory exercise, early mobilisation and deep vein thrombosis (DVT) prophylaxis should be given. Antibiotic coverage, fluid and electrolyte management, observations are mandatory. Drain is removed in 5–7 days.

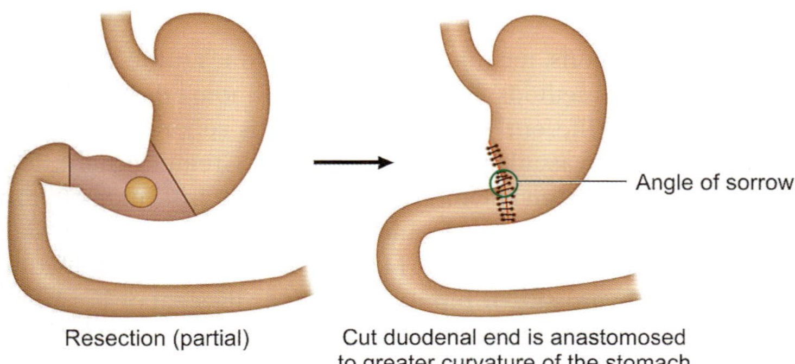

Fig. 21-45: Gastrectomy with Billroth I anastomosis.

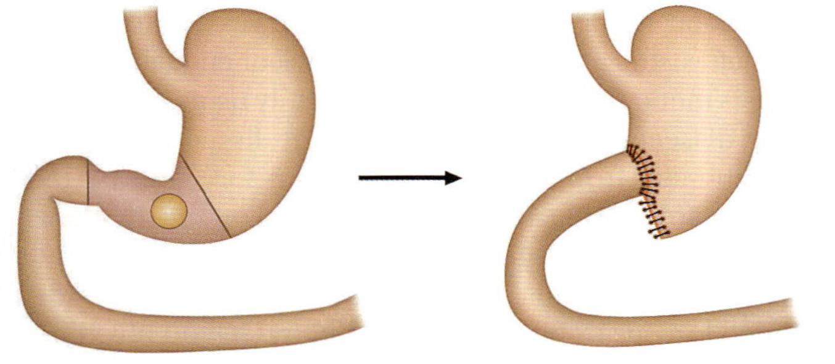

Fig. 21-46: Gastrectomy with Horsley's modification of Billroth I anastomosis.

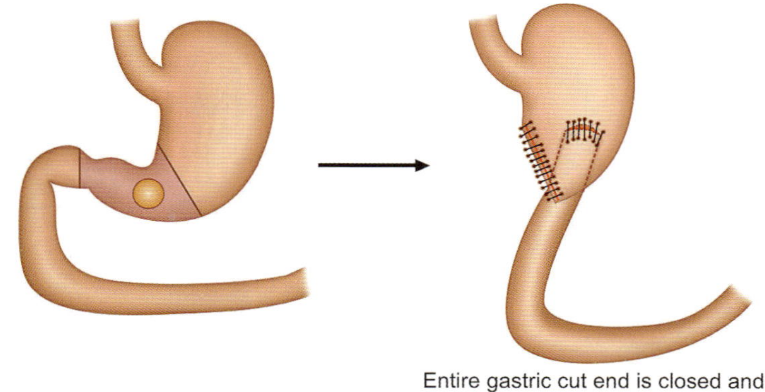

Fig. 21-47: Gastrectomy with Kocher's modification of Billroth I anastomosis.

Complications

Stomal oedema, gastric paresis, stomal obstruction, anastomotic dehiscence and bile leak, sepsis, subphrenic abscess formations are known complications.

Gastrectomy with Billroth II Methods of Anastomosis

It is partial/subtotal gastrectomy with closure of the duodenal stump and achieving the continuity by doing gastrojejunostomy. Billroth first did this procedure on 1885 January 15. It was anterior antecolic gastrojejunostomy. So many modifications were done at a later period on this. Kronlein (1887); Von Eiselsberg (1889), Braun (1892); Roux (1893); Reichel (1908; Polya (1911); Hofmeister-Finsterer (1914); Balfour (1917); Moynihan (1923) are different modifications.

Indications

Gastric ulcer where Billroth I is not possible; carcinoma pylorus and antrum as a radical or palliative procedure; recurrent ulcers; trauma to distal stomach and duodenum are different indications.

Preparation

Gastroscopy and biopsy are a must; CT abdomen to stage the tumour; adequate hydration; electrolyte management; evaluation of cardiac and respiratory systems are needed. Nasogastric tube and urinary catheter should be passed. Preoperative/perioperative antibiotics are a must as once stomach is opened, field gets contaminated.

Technique

After doing laparotomy through midline incision, thorough exploration of the abdomen is done to look for secondaries in liver, assess the omentum, transverse colon, mesocolon, pancreas, primary tumour fixity, resectability, operability, nodal status, etc. Operability means amenable for radical cure. Resectability means even though advanced, primary tumour which is not fixed posteriorly can be removed. Resection of growth (partial gastrectomy) is the best palliation even though it is advanced. In a fixed non-resectable tumour, palliative anterior gastrojejunostomy or Devine's exclusion procedure can be done to relieve vomiting due to gastric outlet obstruction by the tumour **(Fig. 21-52)**.

Kocherisation is usually not necessary for Billroth II anastomosis; if at all needed, only limited Kocherisation should suffice.

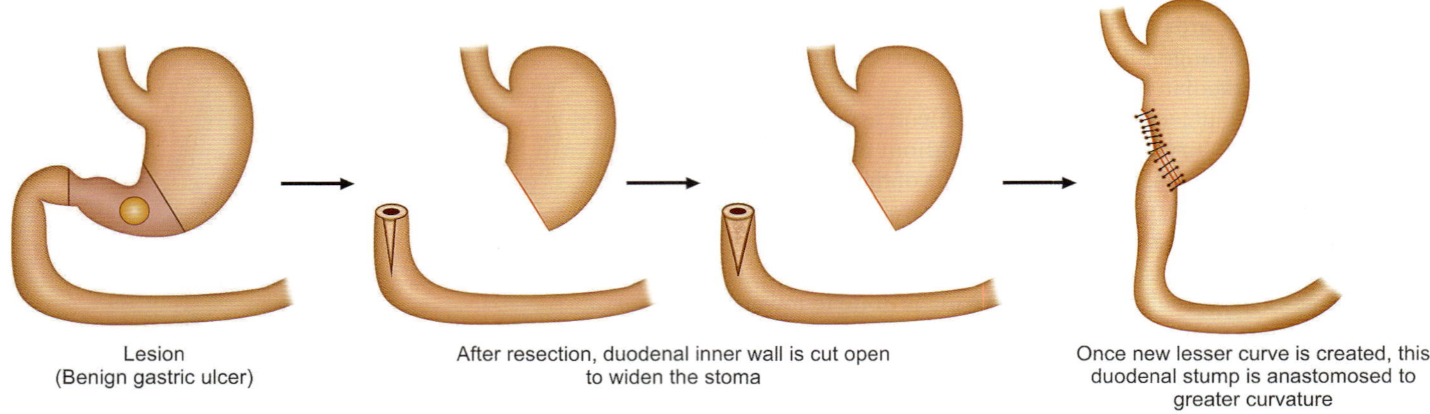

Fig. 21-48: Gastrectomy with Maingot's modification of Billroth I anastomosis.

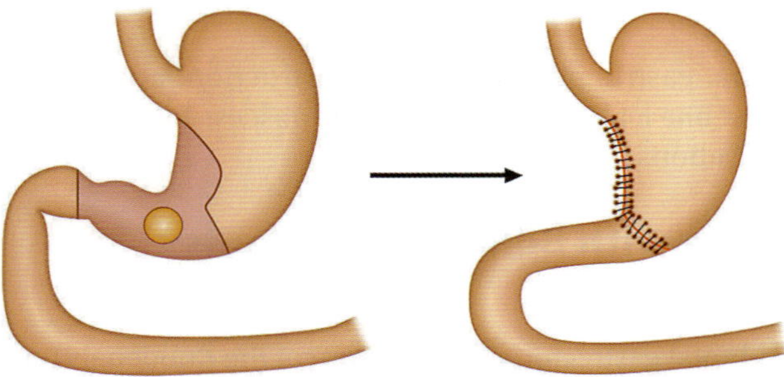

Fig. 21-49: Gastrectomy with Schoemaker's modification of Billroth I anastomosis.

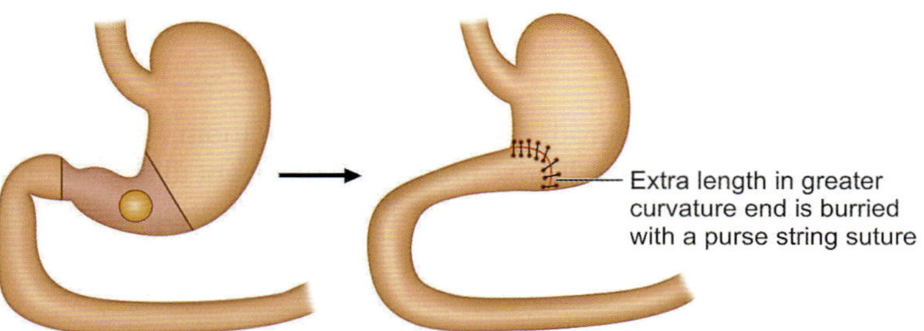

Fig. 21-50: Gastrectomy with von Haberer modification of Billroth I anastomosis.

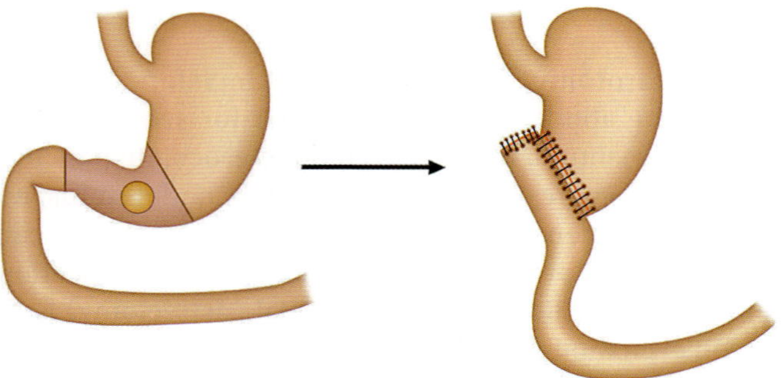

Fig. 21-51: Gastrectomy with von Haberer Finney's modification of Billroth I anastomosis.

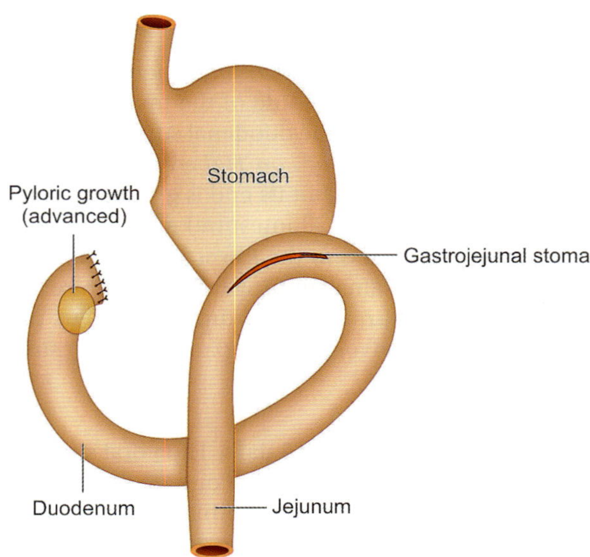

Fig. 21-52: Devine's exclusion procedure.

For benign lesions, technique of mobilisation is same as detailed above in Billroth methods. For confirmed carcinoma distal stomach, mobilisation is different. Greater omentum is separated from the colon along the avascular plane completely. Greater omentum is included in the specimen. Omental bursa is carefully separated from the transverse mesocolon and pancreatic bed. Care should be taken not to injure middle colic artery. Ligation and division of individual vessels using 3 zero silk or bipolar cautery or ligaseal or harmonic scalpel may be used as techniques to achieve this.

Right gastroepiploic vessels, right gastric artery, descending branch of left gastric artery (left gastric vascular pedicle) and left gastroepiploic vessels are doubly ligated and divided. Gastric remnant attains its blood supply through short gastric vessels and ascending branch of left gastric artery—which are sufficient enough. Retrogastric dissection is meticulously carried out carefully using bipolar cautery and sharp dissection is better (never blunt dissection). Duodenal part is mobilised from the pancreatic bed for 2 cm by rotating stomach upwards. Occlusion clamp is applied on the duodenal side at 1st part of the duodenum. Payr's crushing clamp is applied on the gastric side; duodenum is cut in between using no. 15 blade with right angled forceps or flat instrument behind. Good bleeding from the cut edge should be ensured from the duodenal stump, otherwise duodenal leak may occur at later period. If tissue is not healthy, edge is trimmed until it bleeds properly.

Duodenal stump closure

Duodenal stump closure is an important step. It is done by different methods.

Using 2-zero or 3-zero vicryl or silk from superior to inferior part *sewing machine technique* closure is done; here continuous bites alternatively from right and left sides are taken underneath the occlusion clamp close to it to reach the inferior margin; then clamp is gently released, suture is looped and tightened; same suture material is again passed as over and over suture on the previous suture to reach the superior part and is tied to the tail end with secure knot. If needed, few additional interrupted sutures are placed. There is usually space, and length of the stump is not present to place interrupted Lembert sutures to bury/invert the duodenal stump. Often anterior part of the stump is buried on the prepancreatic fascia with interrupted vicryl sutures to secure the stump further **(Fig. 21-53)**.

Alternatively, clamp placed on the duodenal stump is gently lifted; loose over and over vicryl suture loops are placed from superior margin of the stump towards inferior margin under and over the clamp which is held loosely; clamp is loosened and gently removed by sliding and traction off the duodenal stump; suture is pulled tight. Then purse string thin small seromuscular suture is placed around the stump to invert it. A third layer purse string is placed to invaginate the stump completely (*Tanner's method*). Or Lembert seromuscular suture can also be placed using silk **(Fig. 21-54)**.

Open closure of the duodenal stump without applying the clamp using Connell suture is also practiced. Second layer of mattress silk suture is also required **(Figs. 21-55A and B)**.

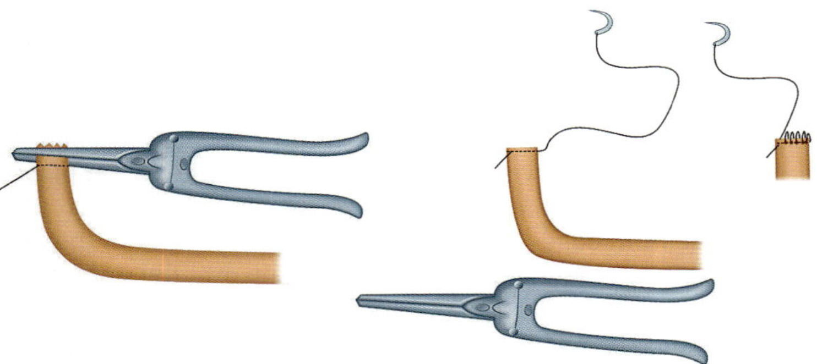

Fig. 21-53: Closure of duodenal stump using sewing machine technique.

Both inner and outer layers are closed using interrupted 3-zero or 2-zero silk sutures and is considered safer.

Stapler closure of duodenal stump is safer and saves time with a good apposition. Usually, there is no need to invaginate stapler line **(Fig. 21-56)**.

Catheter duodenostomy: It prevents build up of intraduodenal pressure and sutured stump will not distend. It is done in difficult duodenal stump and when there is doubt about the integrity of the stump. Usually lateral duodenostomy is done. Prior to closure of the duodenal stump, right angle clamp is passed into the lumen and 3 mm incision is made at lateral wall in 2nd part of duodenum on its tip; 14 Foley's catheter is passed into the duodenum. Duodenotomy around the catheter is closed by purse string vicryl/silk suture; and is also fixed to abdominal wall and brought out of abdominal wall through a stab incision and fixed to skin. It is usually kept for 10 days. Catheter is irrigated with 5–10 mL of warm normal saline. On 10th day catheter is partly withdrawn to the adjacent of the duodenum; if drainage after low suction becomes less than 100 mL it is gradually removed step by step in 2 days. In case if duodenal stump is impossible to close then catheter duodenostomy is done directly across the stump and is closed around it **(Fig. 21-57)**.

Nissen-Cooper technique: When there is fibrotic ulcer crater (benign) which could not be mobilised and removed, it is left in place on the surface of the pancreas and duodenum, if could not get adequate length, stump should be sutured to the ulcer crater itself in three layers. First layer is from anterior and anterolateral duodenal margin to the distal end of the fibrotic edge of the ulcer crater; 2nd layer is interrupted silk sutures between seromuscular duodenal wall to the proximal edge/lip of the ulcer crater; 3rd layer often is used to appose onto the thickened peripancreatic tissue. It is not done nowadays.

Bancroft Plenk operation: It is done when there is scarred duodenum which cannot be dissected or mobilised; 7.5 cm proximal to pyloric sphincter, circular seromuscular incision is made in the antrum. Muscular tube is dissected off from the mucosa circumferentially up to the pyloric sphincter; entire mucosa is made like tube; seromuscular purse string is placed at the pyloric sphincter excluding antral mucosal tube. Antral mucosal tube is cut and included in the gastrectomy specimen. Duodenal stump is further invaginated over seromuscular purse string suture. It is not done nowadays.

Lahey's method: Here in difficult distal stump, common bile duct is opened; Bake's dilator is passed to identify the duct during duodenal stump mobilisation and closure. Bile duct is closed with T tube.

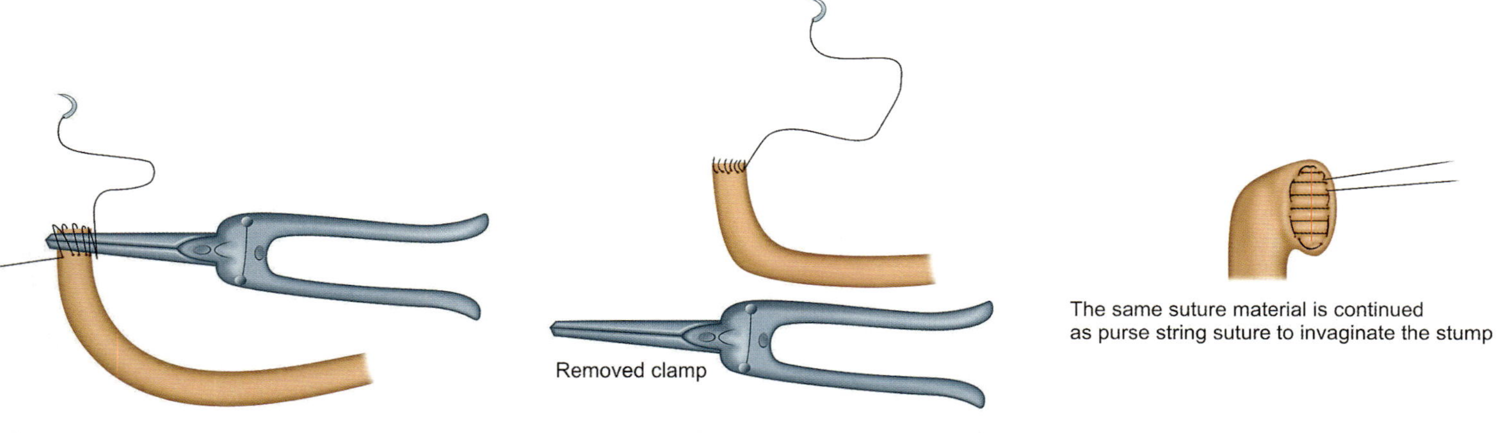

Fig. 21-54: Duodenal closure by Tanner's method.

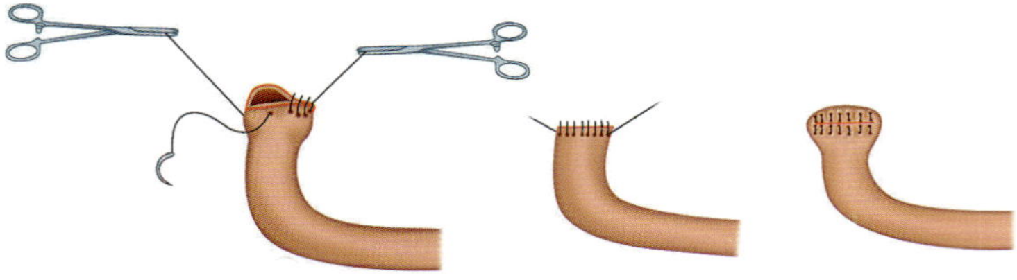

Clamp is not applied to duodenal stump; stump corners are held with stay sutures; continuous or interrupted silk or vicryl sutures are placed. Final 2nd layer interrupted silk sutures are placed as seromuscular.

A

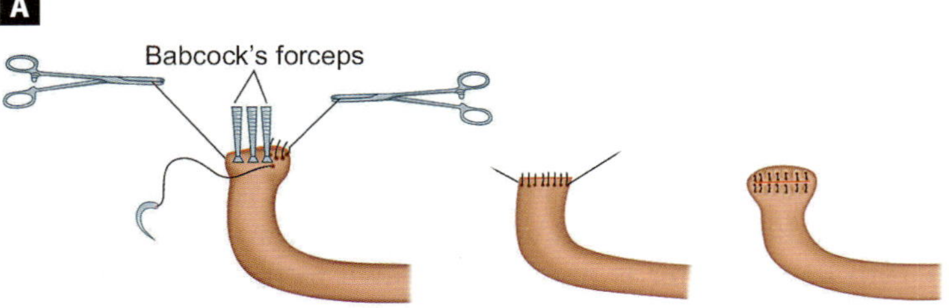

Clamp is not applied to duodenal stump; Babcock's forceps are applied to both edges of the stump together; stump corners are held with stay sutures; continuous or interrupted silk or vicryl sutures are placed; while sutures are on place adjacent Babcock's forceps are removed. Final 2nd layer interrupted silk sutures are placed as seromuscular.

B

Figs. 21-55A and B: Technique of stump closure of duodenal stump without using occlusion/crushing (Payr's clamp).

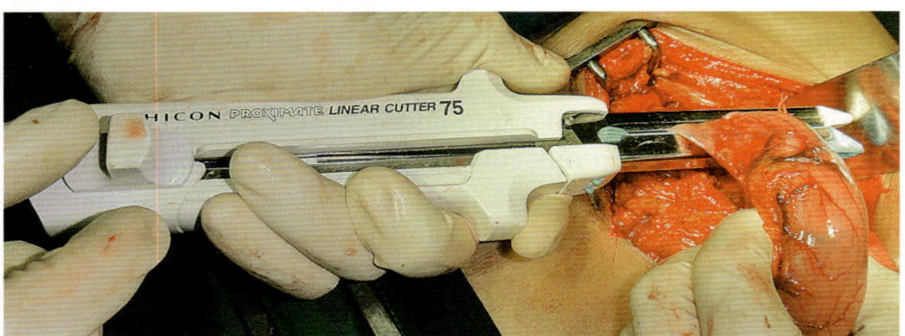

Fig. 21-56: Stapler duodenal closure.

Completion of gastrectomy and Billroth II anastomosis

Distal end of the specimen (duodenal side) is held upwards and towards left to visualise anatomy posteriorly. Descending branch/ left gastric artery is identified and ligated after proximal two secure ligatures. Left gastroepiploic vessels are ligated. Gastric remnant derives its blood supply from the oesophageal branches of inferior phrenic artery, short gastric arteries, proximal gastric branches of the left gastric artery (in 65% partial gastrectomy left gastric artery is ligated distally unlike in subtotal (75–80%/4/5th) gastrectomy wherein left gastric artery is ligated at its origin).

Stomach is fully drawn upwards on to the abdominal wound. Duodenojejunal junction is identified in similar way through ligament of Treitz and inferior mesenteric vein. First loop of the jejunum is taken making afferent loop of about 15–20 cm. Lengthy afferent or efferent loop may stand behind gastric remnant causing obstruction. Antecolic or retrocolic approach may be used; antecolic is preferred than retrocolic, because if stomal ulcer develops chances of penetration or formation of the gastrojejunocolic fistula is higher in retrocolic. However different surgeons prefer different approaches. If retrocolic then loop is brought through the transverse mesocolon left of the middle colic artery. Occlusion clamps applied on the lesser curve, on the greater curve and on the jejunal loop. Alternatively twin clamp can be applied. Posterior seromuscular sutures are placed using continuous or interrupted (seromuscular) silk sutures. This suture line runs through the entire length of the stomach curvature and selected loop of the jejunum from greater curvature towards lesser curve. Alternatively only greater curvature side of the stomach is sutured at the stomal length of around 4–5 cm. Crushing Payr's clamp is placed on the specimen side of the stomach. Specimen is cut between occlusion clamps and crushing clamp. Anterior flap of the gastric edge is kept longer than posterior flap. Lesser curve is closed using continuous 2- or 3-zero vicryl sutures as standard sewing machine technique or over and over two layer closure. Earlier placed continuous seromuscular silk suture is continued on the created lesser curve from edge of the lesser curve towards apex of the new lesser curve kept carefully for later continuation over the stoma. One should confirm that jejunum is correctly placed with antimesenteric margin properly aligned otherwise oblique anastomosis can cause stomal obstruction at afferent or efferent level. Around 4 cm length of the jejunum is opened on the greater curvature (left) side.

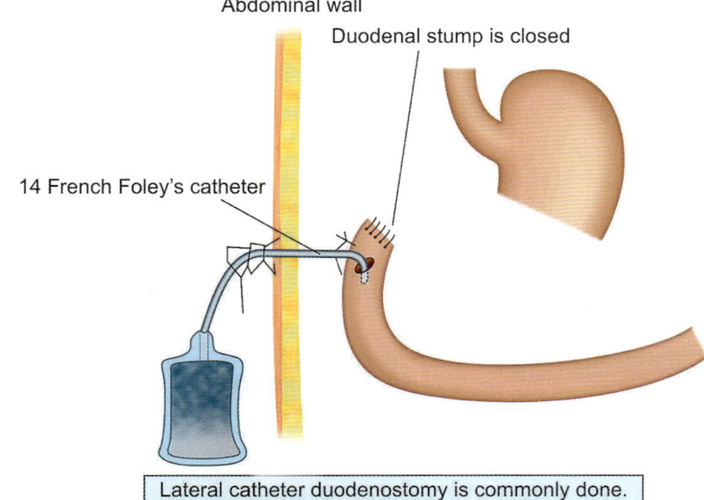

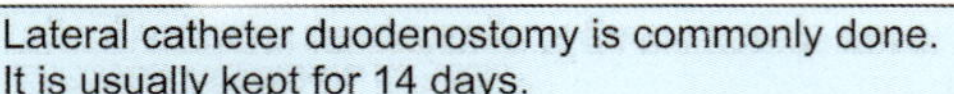

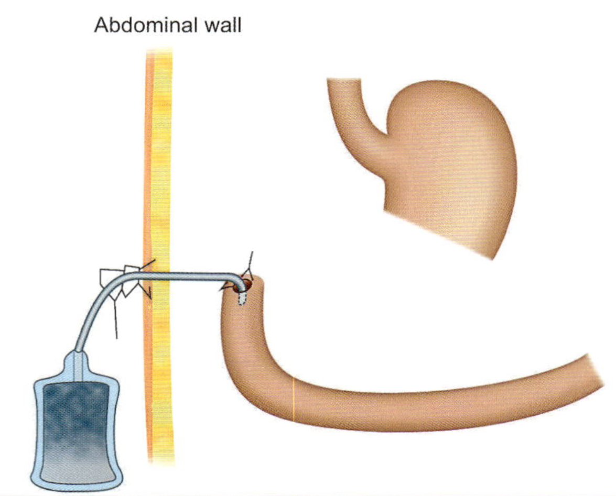

End duodenostomy is done on to the duodenal stump.
It is done only if duodenal stump can not be closed due to fibrosis.

Fig. 21-57: Catheter duodenostomy used to decompress the duodenal stump.

Posterior all layer through and through continuous sutures are placed using vicryl from greater curvature side towards lesser curve angle; it is continued as anterior layer all layer suture (using Connell suture) to reach greater curvature again and tied with a knot. Anterior seromuscular continuous suture is placed as a continuation of the already placed seromuscular suture on the new lesser curve, thus completing the anastomosis. Clamps are removed. Nasogastric tube should be passed across the stoma along the efferent limb. Any bleeders if present are secured with transfixation. Adequacy of the stoma is checked.

In order to prevent enterogastric bile reflux, jejunojejunostomy is done between afferent and efferent limbs—*Braun's enteroenterostomy*. This prevents bile reflux but diverts bile only partially unlike in *Roux-en-Y anastomosis which is more ulcerogenic.*

Ligatures at all four main vessel sites are observed for its security. Subphrenic spaces are sucked out and cleaned. Duodenal stump closure is observed. Abdomen is closed in layers after placing a tube drain.

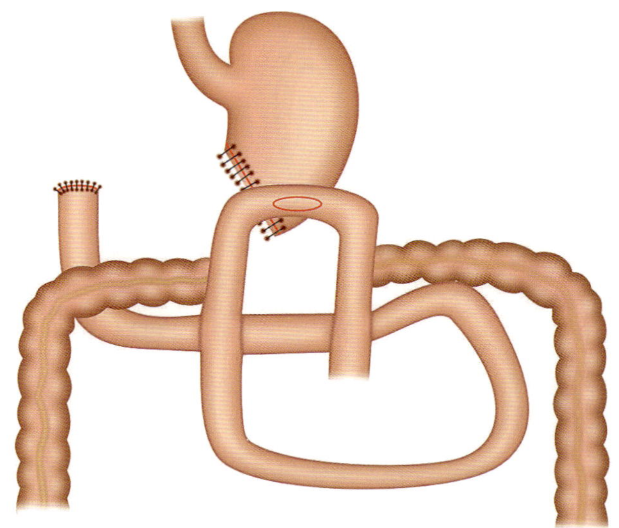

Fig. 21-59: Gastrectomy with classical Billroth II anastomosis.

Postoperative Care

Nasogastric tube aspiration; observation of vitals, drain site and urinary catheter; respiratory monitoring.

Nasogastric tube is removed in 5 days; oral sips started; drain removed in 7 days.

Note:

Antecolic is said to be better than retrocolic after gastrectomy and Billroth II anastomosis. However both are used all over equally.

Valve is found to be not helpful during anastomosis **(Fig. 21-58)**.

Single layer closure is universally accepted now as far as Billroth II anastomosis.

When placing afferent loop towards greater or lesser curve, it will not make much difference as far functioning of the stoma is considered. Moynihan's placing afferent loop towards greater curvature has gained popularity. Different modifications are shown in figures **(Figs. 21-59 to 21-68)**.

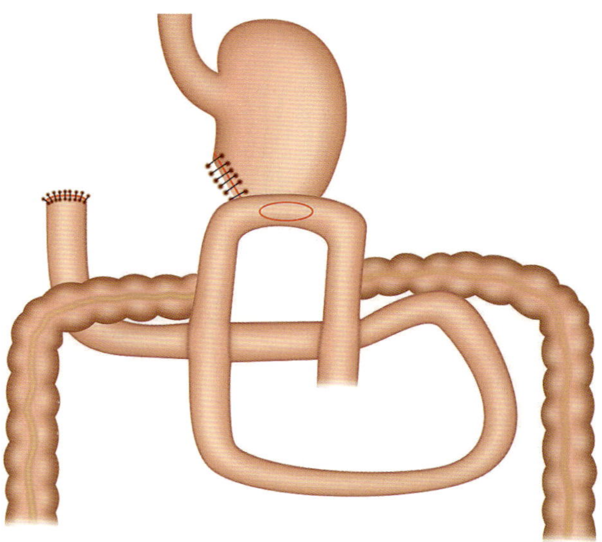

Fig. 21-60: Gastrectomy Von Eiselsberg's modification of Billroth II anastomosis.

Distal Gastrectomy with Roux-en-Y Anastomosis

Cesar Roux, Swiss surgeon from Lausanne described Roux-en-Y anastomosis in 1897. Jejunum is transected 20 cm from duodenojejunal junction; distal cut part of the jejunum is brought upwards towards gastric remnant and anastomosed; proximal cut end is anastomosed to distal cut part of the jejunum 45 cm from its cut margin to maintain the continuity.

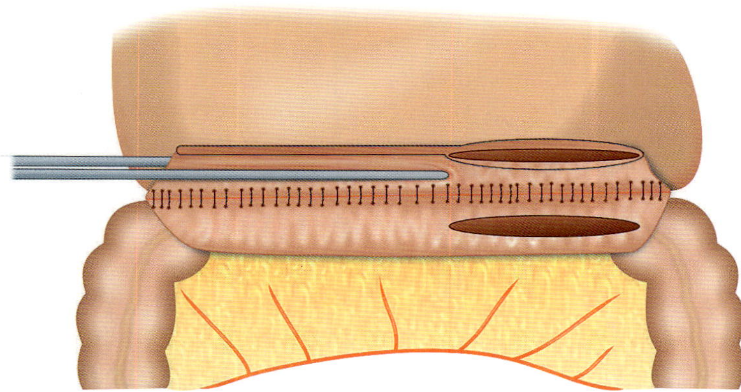

Fig. 21-58: Valved gastrojejunostomy.

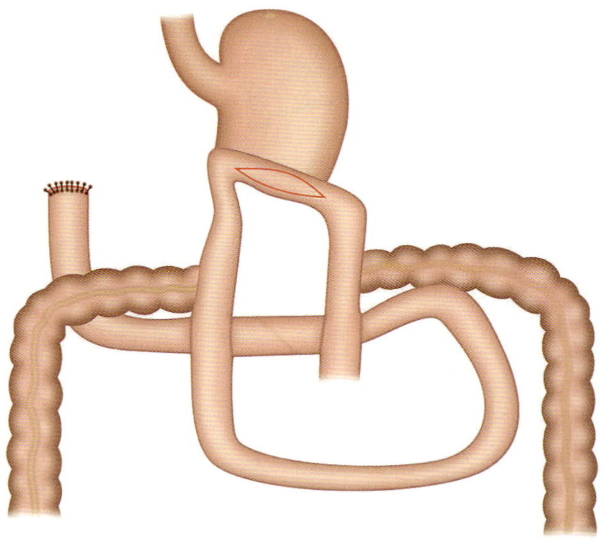

Fig. 21-61: Gastrectomy Kronlein modification of Billroth II anastomosis.

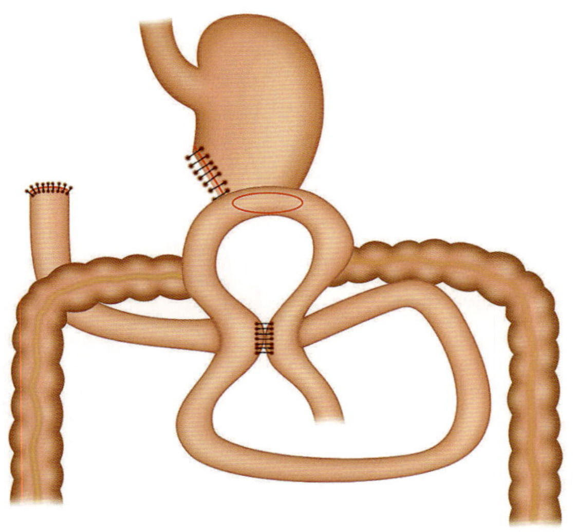

Fig. 21-62: Gastrectomy Braun modification of Billroth II anastomosis.

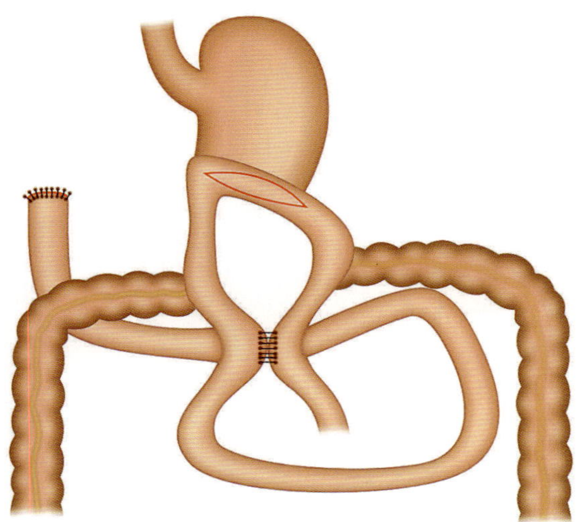

Fig. 21-63: Gastrectomy Balfour modification of Billroth II anastomosis.

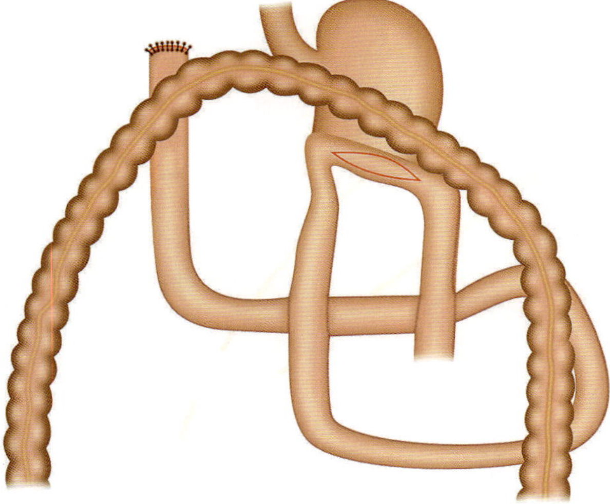

Fig. 21-64: Gastrectomy Reichel and Polya modification of Billroth II anastomosis.

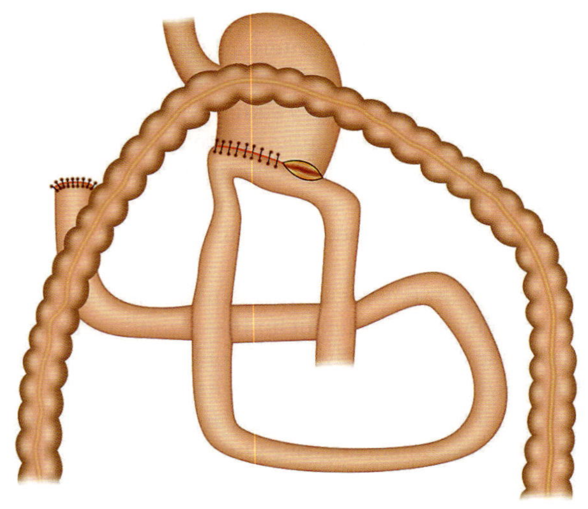

Fig. 21-65: Gastrectomy Finsterer Hofmeister modification of Billroth II anastomosis.

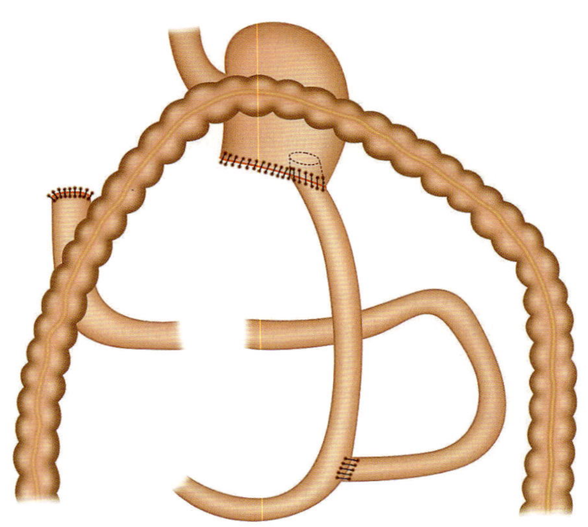

Fig. 21-66: Gastrectomy Roux modification of Billroth II anastomosis.

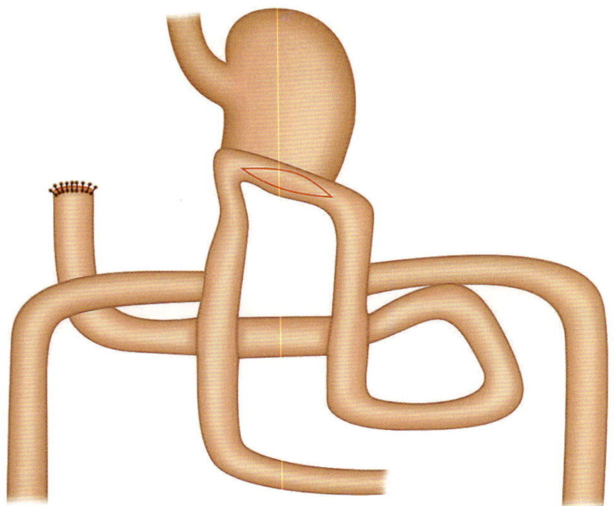

Fig. 21-67: Gastrectomy Moynihan modification of Billroth II anastomosis.

Csendes procedure

Type IV gastric ulcer within 2 cm of oesophagogastric (OG) junction. Gastrectomy is done with removal of entire lesser curve up to OG junction. Much of the greater curve is preserved; antecolic Roux-en-Y gastrojejunostomy is done to entire cut end of the stomach from OG junction to greater curve.

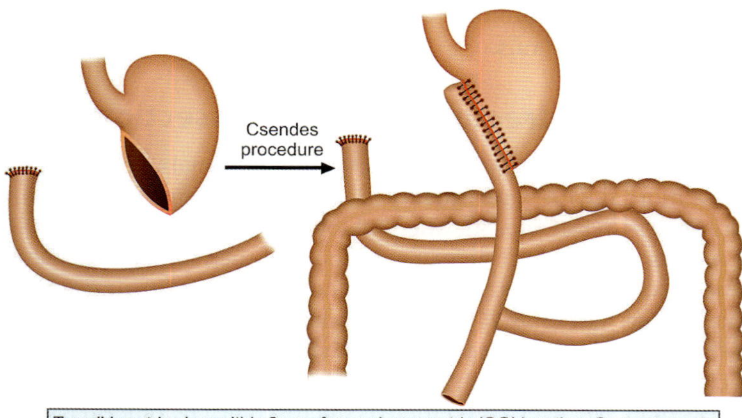

Fig. 21-68: Csendes procedure—with gastrectomy, Roux-en-Y antecolic gastrojejunostomy to entire cut end of stomach.

Indications

Early gastric cancer is a good option but with lymph node dissection. Gastrointestinal stromal tumour (GIST) and leiomyoma are other indications. It has been opined by many that Roux-n-Y anastomosis should be reserved to only subtotal gastrectomy with less gastric remnant. But presently proved that Roux-n-Y anastomosis is better; but Roux syndrome and gastric stasis are the major drawbacks.

Advantages

It shows very less enterogastric reflux and lower incidence of *H. pylori* infection. Gastritis and dumping is less in Roux-en-Y.

Disadvantages

Development of stomal ulcers; gallstone formation; technically additional anastomosis; endoscopic access to ampulla of Vater is lost or difficult; Roux stasis syndrome (25%, inadequate jejunal limb peristalsis).

Technique (Fig. 21-69)

Under general anaesthesia with head up position laparotomy is done with upper midline incision. Thorough exploration of the peritoneal cavity is done. Greater omentum is separated from the transverse colon through avascular plane using scissor or cautery.

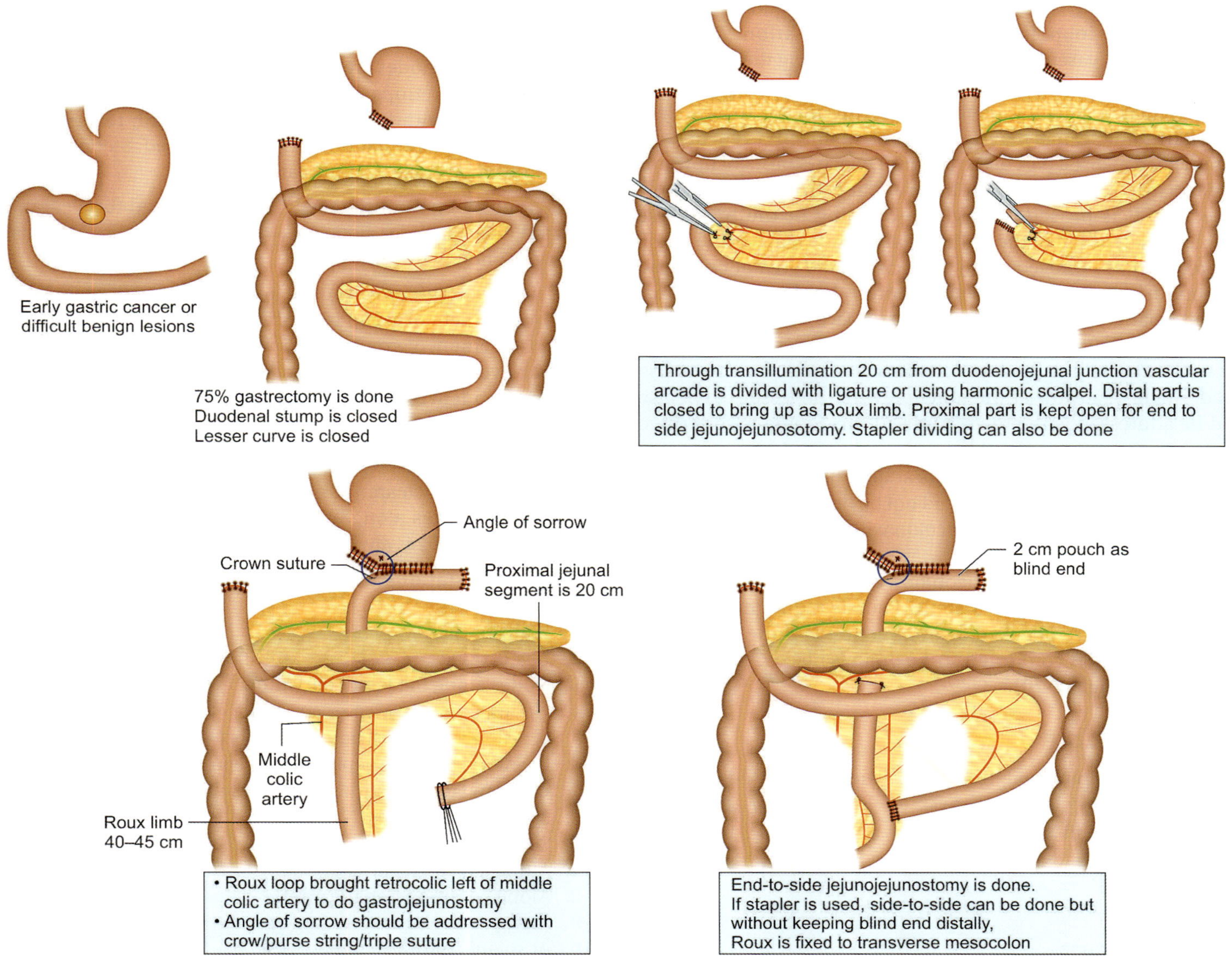

Early gastric cancer or difficult benign lesions
75% gastrectomy is done
Duodenal stump is closed
Lesser curve is closed
Through transillumination 20 cm from duodenojejunal junction vascular arcade is divided with ligature or using harmonic scalpel. Distal part is closed to bring up as Roux limb. Proximal part is kept open for end to side jejunojejunosotomy. Stapler dividing can also be done
Angle of sorrow
Crown suture
Proximal jejunal segment is 20 cm
Middle colic artery
Roux limb 40–45 cm
• Roux loop brought retrocolic left of middle colic artery to do gastrojejunostomy
• Angle of sorrow should be addressed with crow/purse string/triple suture
2 cm pouch as blind end
End-to-side jejunojejunostomy is done.
If stapler is used, side-to-side can be done but without keeping blind end distally,
Roux is fixed to transverse mesocolon

Fig. 21-69: Roux-en-Y anastomosis after subtotal gastrectomy.

Middle colic artery should be taken care of. While using cautery, care should be taken not to transmit heat to adjacent colon which may be dangerous. Lesser omentum is divided. Omental bursectomy is done by peeling off the omental layer from the superior part of the transverse mesocolon and in front of the pancreas. Line of proximal resection is marked; descending branch of left gastric artery and vein are ligated securely and divided; branch of left gastroepiploic artery along the arcade is ligated and divided. Stomach is transected using linear stapler device at two levels to create lesser curve and to achieve Roux-en-Y gastrojejunostomy. This can be done by applying pairs of clamps on each part and dividing in between using number 15 blade or cautery. Clamp distal to the resected line with the distal stomach is lifted upwards and towards right to expose posterior aspect of the stomach and duodenum in front of the pancreas. All adhesions between distal stomach and pancreas are divided with cautery or harmonic scalpel. Right gastroepiploic and right gastric arteries are ligated and divided. Right gastric artery may be like leashes of vessels often. Duodenum is mobilised up to the gastroduodenal artery level, not beyond. Small vessels entering the proximal duodenum should be tackled using bipolar cautery. Duodenum is transected using stapler. It can also be transected between two clamps and can be closed by hand suturing. Specimen is removed. Lymph node dissection is also carried out along with gastric mobilisation in case of distal gastric cancer.

Ligament of Treitz is identified; 20 cm from the duodenojejunal junction jejunal loop is selected for mobilisation. Through transillumination, vascular arcades are ligated along the mesentery to get adequate length of the distal jejunum. Jejunum is divided after ligating vascular arcade. It is better to ligate this arcade using 3-zero silk; but harmonic scalpel may be sufficient. About 40–45 cm of Roux limb is selected at distal part of the jejunum which is brought upwards towards gastric remnant. It can be brought retrocolic commonly or antecolic. It is passed through an opening in the transverse mesocolon towards left of the middle colic artery. Stapler line in the gastric remnant is removed partly for 4 cm on the greater curvature side; jejunum is opened on the antimesenteric border 2 cm proximal to the terminal end for 4 cm using cautery. Two layer anastomosis using outer continuous or interrupted silk and inner all layer vicryl sutures. Alternatively single layer continuous vicryl or silk can also be used. Angle of sorrow at the junction with the lesser curve also should be addressed with crown/triple suture. Stoma is confirmed using fingers. Continuity of gut below is maintained by end-to-side jejunojejunostomy after removing the stapler line (side-to-side also can be done wherein stapler line need not be removed). Roux jejunal loop is fixed to the transverse mesocolon with interrupted sutures to prevent herniation.

Nasogastric tube is gently negotiated across gastrojejunostomy stoma distally which acts as a stent. Pedicles, duodenal stump, anastomotic lines are checked again. Suction is done in surgical field. Mop counting is confirmed. Tube drain is placed. Abdomen is closed in layers **(Fig. 21-70)**.

Postoperative Care

Nasogastric tube is removed in 72 hours. Oral sips started and later solid food.

Drain is removed in 5 days.

Complications

- Gastroparesis.
- Dumping syndrome.
- Roux stasis syndrome.
- Afferent loop syndrome.
- Other complications.

Subtotal Gastrectomy with D2 Dissection

Subtotal gastrectomy is still an acceptable reasonable option as it is less morbid with better quality of life than total gastrectomy with equivalent survival rate. But when subtotal gastrectomy is not possible or microscopic margin clearance is doubtful then total gastrectomy is better option, especially when tumour is large occupying almost entire lesser curve or 75% of the stomach or tumour of the body of the stomach. Microscopic margin clearance is most important deciding factor, along with lymph node involvement which should be less than five. Even when there is microscopic clearance if lymph nodes are positive in more than 5 nodes, then there is no benefit as far as prognosis is considered.

D2 gastrectomy includes—removal of stomach with growth, omental bursa, greater and lesser omentum, anterior layer of mesocolon, anterior pancreatic capsule, D2 lymphadenectomy. D2 dissection is better than D1 dissection of lymph nodes.

Presently newer staging for dissection is practiced in Japan—D1, D2, D3, D4, depending on levels of lymph nodes cleared ('D' for dissection). D1 or D2 dissections are commonly done.

D1 is done when nodes are N0. It is removal of nodes along the lesser and greater curves and pylorus (Group I: Stations 3–6).

D2 is done when nodes are N1. Here nodes like left gastric/common hepatic/splenic/retropancreatic are removed. Splenic nodes can be cleared with or without splenectomy along with removal of tail of pancreas. Here node stations 1–11 are removed. Stations 12–18 are not removed. Average 27 nodes are removed.

D3 is done when nodes are N2. Nodes removed for clearance are hepatoduodenal, nodes along mesentery, middle colic (1–16 stations). Average 43 nodes are removed.

D4 is *not commonly advocated*. It is removal of stations 1–18.
D1—involvement of group I lymph nodes.
D2—involvement of group I and II lymph nodes.
D3—involvement of group I, II and III lymph nodes.
D4—involvement of group I, II, III and para-aortic nodes.

Note:
All lymph nodes are numbered differently as 'stations' or 'echelons'.

D1 gastrectomy is clearance of perigastric nodes; *D2 gastrectomy* is clearance of nodes along major vessel trunks—along coeliac and splenic arteries. D2 is always better than D1.

Lymph node stations in gastric carcinoma (Japan)—18 stations are there:

1. Right cardiac
2. Left cardiac
3. Nodes along the lesser curvature
4. Nodes along the greater curvature
   a. Along short gastric vessels—4sa
   b. Along left gastroepiploic vessels—4sb
   c. Along right gastroepiploic vessels—4sc
5. Suprapyloric nodes
6. Subpyloric nodes
7. Along left gastric artery
8. Along common hepatic artery
9. Along coeliac axis
10. At splenic hilum
11. Along splenic artery

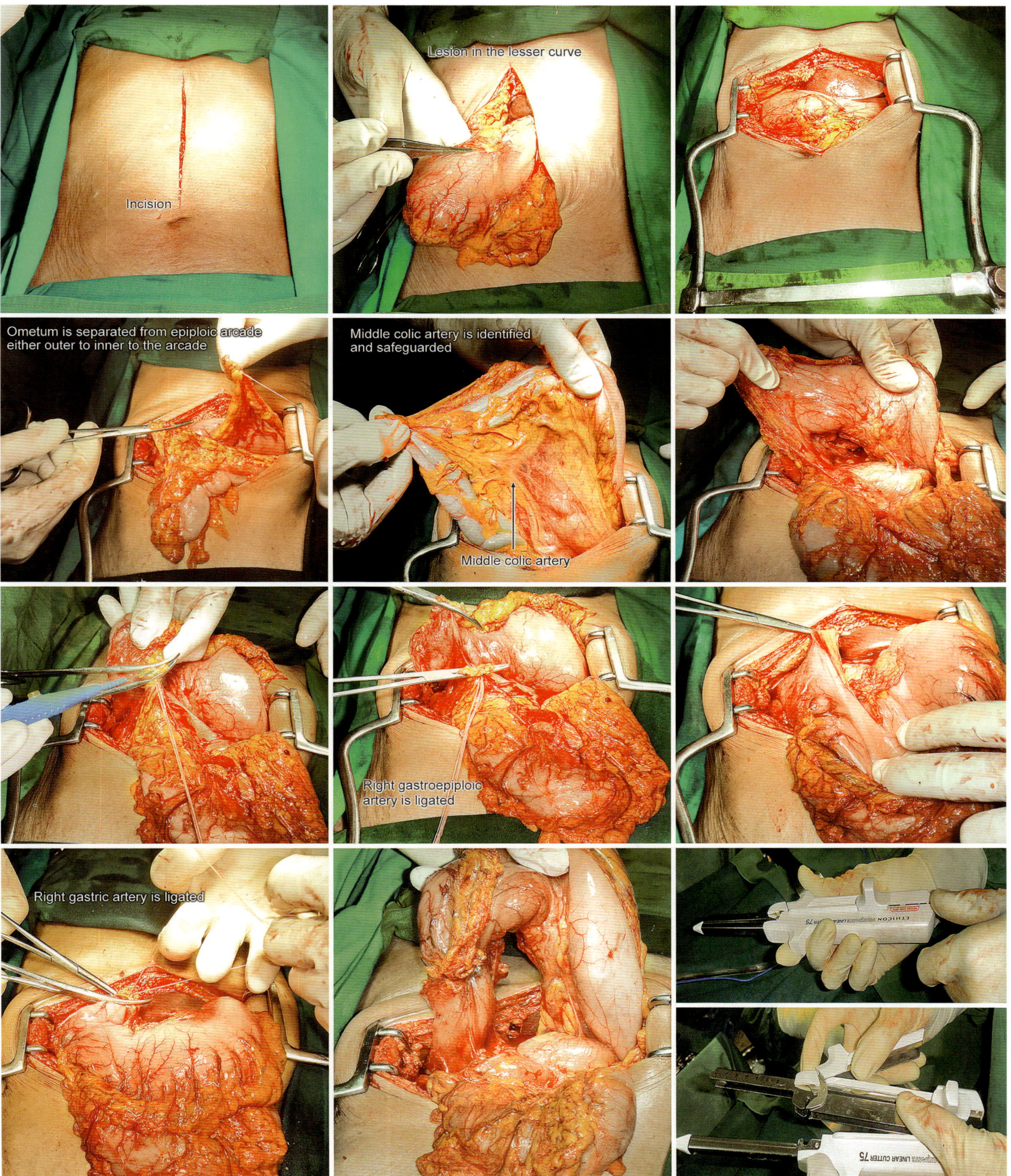
Incision
Lesion in the lesser curve
Ometum is separated from epiploic arcade either outer to inner to the arcade
Middle colic artery is identified and safeguarded
Middle colic artery
Right gastroepiploic artery is ligated
Right gastric artery is ligated
ETHICON
LINEAR CUTTER 75

Figs. 21-70(1)

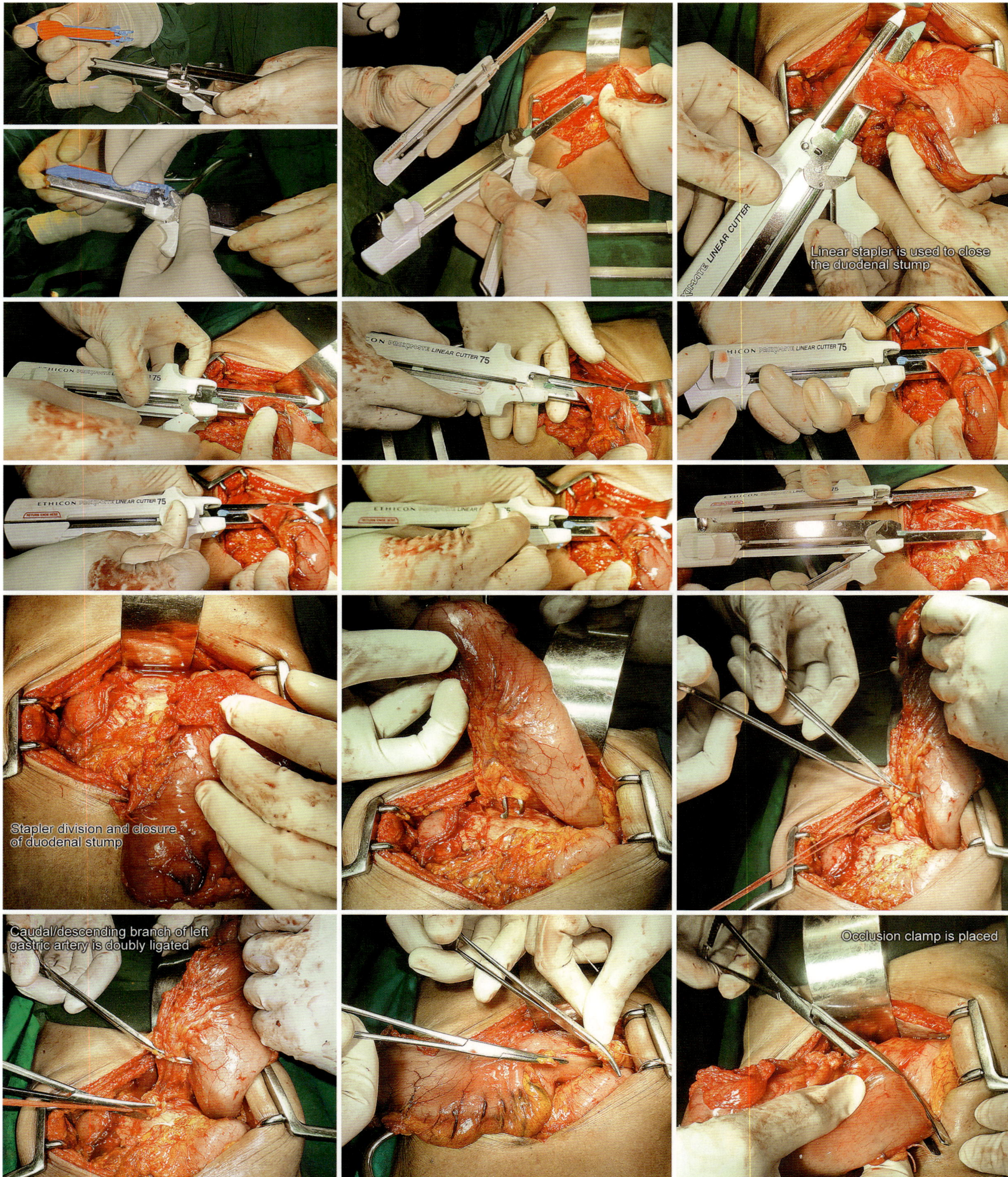
Linear stapler is used to close the duodenal stump
Stapler division and closure of duodenal stump
Caudal/descending branch of left gastric artery is doubly ligated
Occlusion clamp is placed

Figs. 21-70(2)

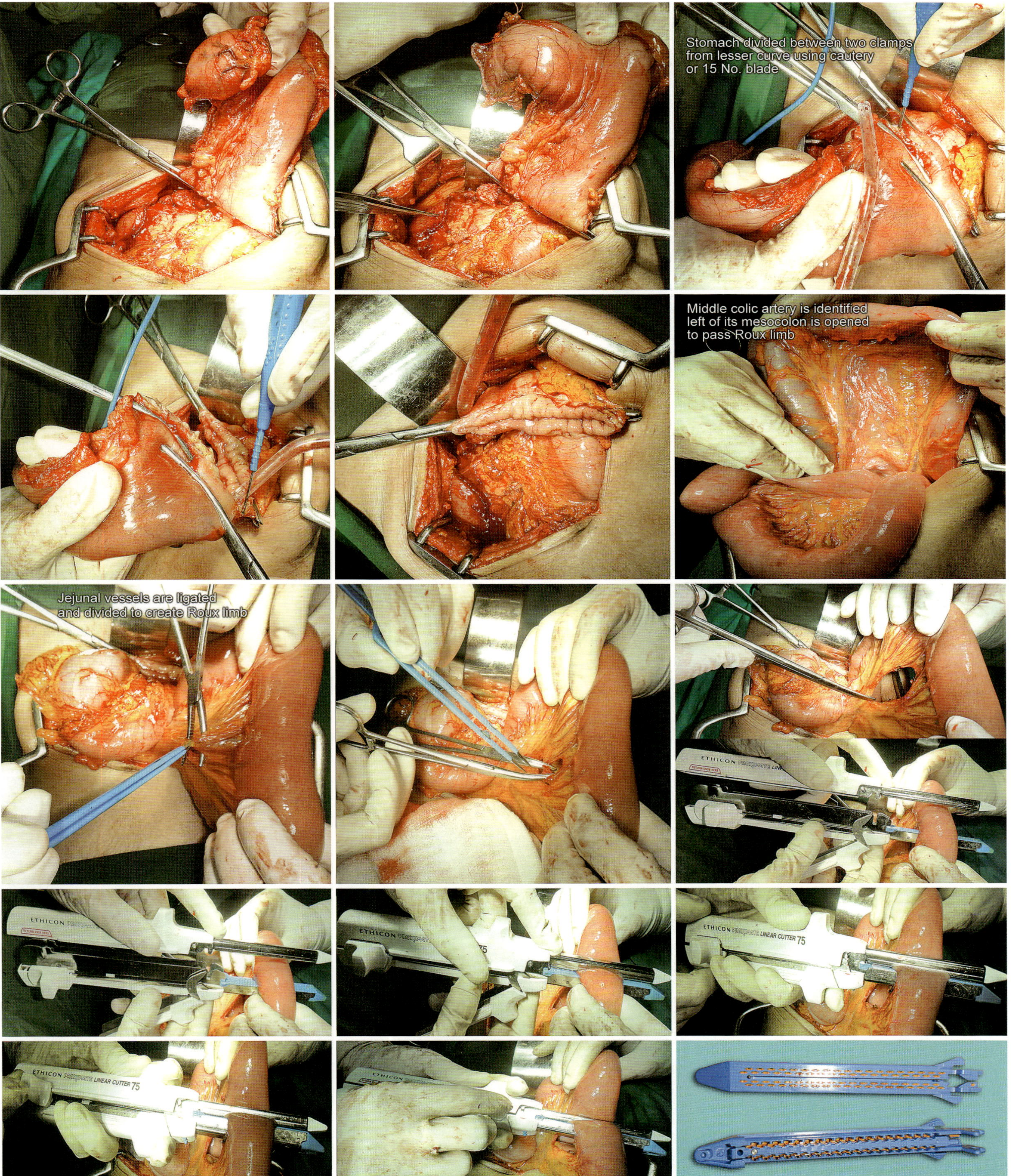
Stomach divided between two clamps from lesser curve using cautery or 15 No. blade
Middle colic artery is identified left of its mesocolon is opened to pass Roux limb
Jejunal vessels are ligated and divided to create Roux limb
ETHICON
ETHICON LINEAR CUTTER 75

Figs. 21-70(3)

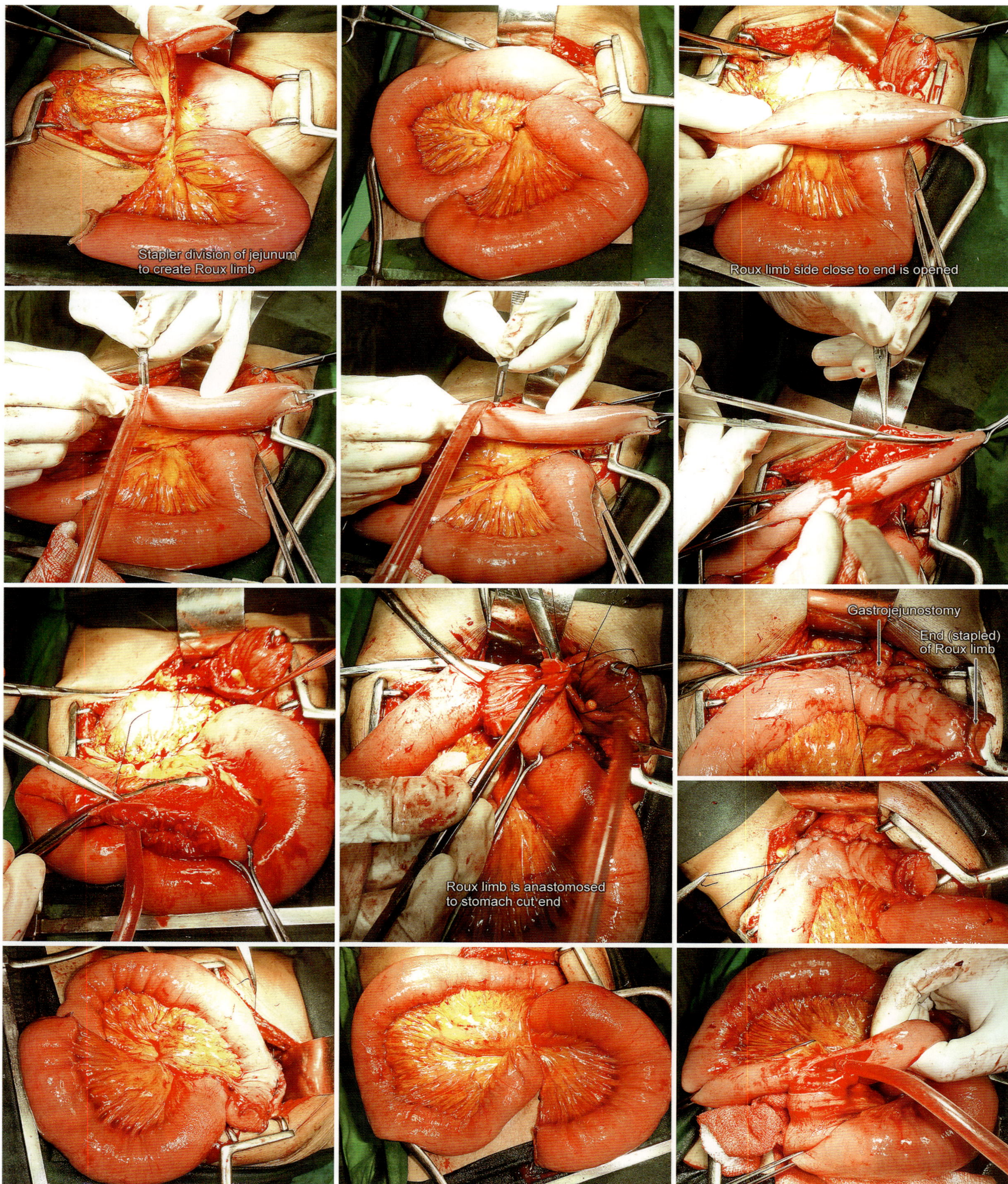
Stapler division of jejunum
to create Roux limb
Roux limb side close to end is opened
Gastrojejunostomy
End (stapled)
of Roux limb
Roux limb is anastomosed
to stomach cut end

Figs. 21-70(4)

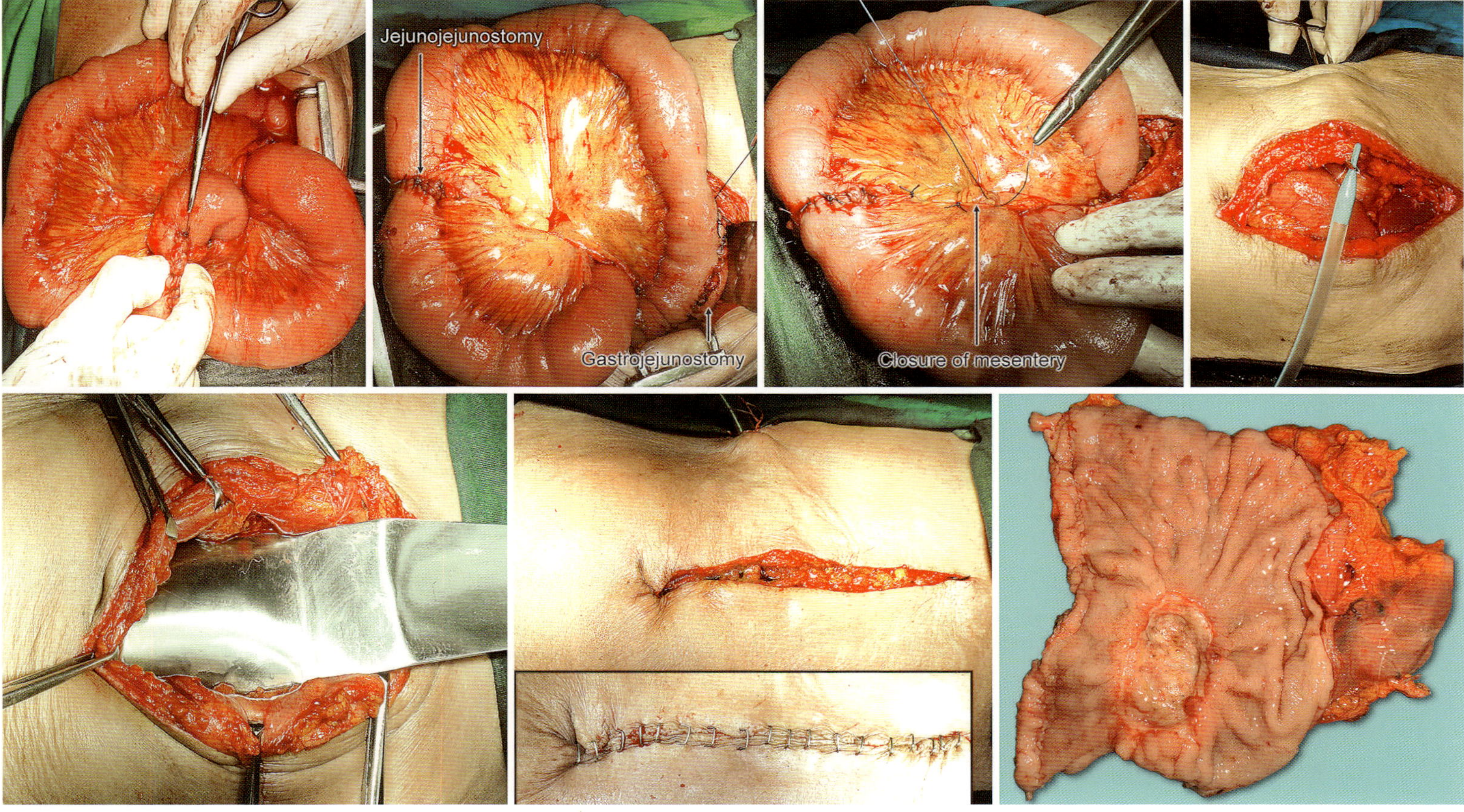

Figs. 21-70(5)

Figs. 21-70(1 to 5): Gastrectomy with Roux-en-Y gastrojejunostomy.

12. At hepatoduodenal ligament
13. Retroduodenal lymph nodes
14. At root of mesentery
15. Around middle colic artery
16. Para-aortic nodes
17. Around lower oesophagus
18. Supradiaphragmatic

TNM staging—7th edition, 2010

Tumour – T
- Tx – tumour cannot be assessed
- T0 – no evidence of tumour
- Tis – carcinoma in situ, intraepithelial tumour without invasion
- T1a – invades lamina propria or muscularis mucosa
- T1b – invades submucosal
- T2 – invades muscularis propria
- T3 – invades subserosal connective tissue without invasion of visceral peritoneum or adjacent structures
- T4a – invades serosa/visceral peritoneum
- T4b – invades adjacent structures

Nodes – N
- Nx – cannot be assessed
- N0 – no nodal spread
- N1 – 1–2 regional nodes
- N2 – 3–6 regional nodes
- N3a – 7–15 regional nodes
- N3b – 16 or more nodes

Metastases – M
- M0 – no distant spread
- M1 – distant spread present

Contd…

First tier nodes: Nodes within 3 cm from primary tumour (stations 1-6)—N1 (old TNM).

Second tier nodes: Nodes in main and intermediate arterial trunk (stations 7-11)—N2 (old TNM).

Contd…

Staging
- 0 – Tis N0 M0
- IA – T1 N0 M0;
- IB – T1 N1 M0/T2 N0 M0
- IIA – T1 N2 M0; T2 N1 M0; T3 N0 M0
- IIB – T1 N3 M0; T2 N2 M0; T3 N1 M0; T4a N0 M0
- IIIA - T2 N3 M0; T3 N2 M0; T4a N1 M0
- IIIB - T3 N3 M0; T4a N2 M0; T4b N0-1 M0
- IIIC – T4a N3 M0; T4b N2-3 M0
- IV: Any T Any N M1
- Stage I, II, II: Locoregional disease
- Stage IV: Systemic disease

Japanese Classification of Gastric Carcinoma (JCGC)

It includes following principles:
- Basic rules for clinical, surgical, pathological, and final features
- Specific rules for histology
- Gastric biopsy specimen group classification
- Chemo RT response

Nodal spread as per JCGC:
- Nx – Nodes unknown/cannot be assessed
- N0 – No nodal spreads
- N1 – Group I nodes only involved
- N2 – Group II nodes are involved but not group III
- N3 – Group III nodes are involved

Lymph node stations in relation to gastric carcinoma

Station	*Lymph nodes*
1	Right paracardial nodes
2	Left paracardial nodes
3	Nodes along the lesser curvature
4	Nodes along the greater curvature
	4sa: Along short gastrics
	4sb: Left greater curvature lymph nodes along the left gastro-epiploic artery
	4d: Right greater curvature lymph nodes
5	Suprapyloric lymph nodes
6	Infrapyloric lymph nodes
7	Nodes along the left gastric artery
8	Nodes along the common hepatic artery
9	Nodes around the celiac axis
10	Splenic hilar nodes
11	Nodes along the splenic artery
12	Nodes in the hepatoduodenal ligament, in the caudal half between the confluence of the right and left hepatic ducts and the upper border of the pancreas
	12a: Nodes along the proper hepatic artery
	12b: Nodes along the bile duct
	12p: Nodes along the portal vein
13	Lymph nodes at the posterior aspect of the pancreatic head
14	Lymph nodes at the root of the mesentery
	14v: Nodes along superior mesenteric vein
	14a: Nodes along superior mesenteric artery
15	Lymph nodes in the mesocolon of the colon transversum
16	Para-aortic lymph nodes
17	Lymph nodes on the anterior surface of the pancreatic head
18	Lymph nodes along the inferior border of the pancreatic body
19	Infradiaphragmatic lymph nodes predominantly along the subphrenic artery
20	Hiatal paraesophageal lymph nodes
110	Paraesophageal lymph nodes in the lower mediastinum
111	Supradiaphragmatic lymph nodes distant from the oesophagus
112	Posterior mediastinal lymph nodes distant from the oesophagus and the hiatus

Source: Adapted from Japanese Gastric Cancer Association. Japanese Classification of Gastric Carcinoma, 3rd English edition. Gastric Cancer. 2011;14: 101-12.

Concept of D (dissection) in gastrectomy for gastric cancers

Type of gastrectomy	*Extend of lymphadenectomy*	*Lymph node stations*
Total gastrectomy	D1	No. 1–7
	D1+	D1 + No. 8a, 9, 11p + No. 110 for tumours invading the oesophagus
	D2	D1 + No. 8a, 9, 11p, 11d, 12a + No. 19, 20, 110, 111 for tumours invading the oesophagus
Distal gastrectomy	D1	No. 1, 3, 4sb, 4d, 5, 6, 7
	D1+	D1 + No. 8a, 9
	D2	D1 + No. 8a, 9, 11p, 12a
Pylorus-preserving gastrectomy	D1	No. 1, 3, 4sb, 4d, 6, 7
	D1+	D1 + No. 8a, 9
Proximal gastrectomy	D1	No. 1, 2, 3a, 4sa, 4sb, 7
	D1+	D1 + No. 8a, 9, 11p + No. 110 for tumours invading the oesophagus

Source: Adapted from Japanese Gastric Cancer Association. Japanese Classification of Gastric Carcinoma, 3rd English edition. Gastric Cancer. 2011;14: 101-12.

Birmingham staging

1 – Confined to mucosa/muscularis propria
2 – Muscularis/serosal involvement
3 – Nodal spread
4a – Residual disease; 4b – Metastatic disease

Third tier nodes: Nodes at stations 12–18 (para-aortic and above)—N3 (old TNM).

Note: 15 lymph nodes must be removed for adequate staging of nodes.

Technique

Preparation is same as other gastrectomy. But CT scan and other modalities of evaluation in relation to secondaries and lymph node status should be done thoroughly.

Under general anaesthesia, laparotomy is done through lengthy upper midline incision which is extended below across the umbilicus. Head up position is preferred (reverse Trendelenburg).

Greater omentum is mobilised from the transverse colon through avascular plane. Anterior leaf of the peritoneum of the transverse mesocolon and peritoneum over the anterior surface of the pancreas is removed (omental bursectomy). Need for omental bursectomy is controversial. Omentum is dissected from splenic flexure of colon and inferior pole of the spleen to expose the tail and body of the pancreas. Left gastroepiploic vessels are divided at their origin from splenic vessels. Short gastric vessels are also ligated and divided. Energy sources like harmonic scalpel are of great use in such situation.

Right gastroepiploic vein is carefully dissected; bleeding is common here as many fragile tributaries are present. Right gastroepiploic vein after being joined by the middle colic vein forms gastrocolic vein which is short and joins the superior mesenteric vein. Right gastro-epiploic vein is ligated at this junction where it joins middle colic vein. If tear and bleeding occur, gastrocolic trunk vein or middle colic vein can be ligated (middle colic artery should be safeguarded). Superior mesenteric vein is dissected on its front, medial and lateral aspects to clear lymph node stations. Right gastroepiploic artery is dissected at its origin from the gastroduodenal artery. Tissues with lymph nodes in front of the head of pancreas and behind the pylorus are cleared.

Gastrohepatic ligament is dissected. Aberrant hepatic artery if present should be preserved. Hepatoduodenal ligament is opened. Common hepatic artery, proper hepatic artery, right gastric artery, gastroduodenal arteries are identified and dissected to remove fat lymph nodes adjacent to it. Right gastric artery is ligated and divided at its origin. It usually arises from proper hepatic artery; but as variation, it can arise from gastroduodenal artery. Small vessels are common in this area which cause troublesome bleeding; so bipolar cautery or harmonic scalpel are better to be used. Kocherisation is needed for proper nodal clearance in relation to duodenum.

Duodenum is transected using stapler in similar way as mentioned earlier. Stapler is ideal; otherwise duodenum is cut between clamps and duodenal stump is closed by one of the suitable methods discussed earlier.

D2 lymphadenectomy is done. It begins by removing fat and lymph nodes lateral to the proper hepatic artery; tissues in front of the portal vein, superior border of the pancreas, in front and behind the common hepatic artery; left gastric vein (coronary vein) is ligated where it joins the portal vein which courses behind the lesser curvature; tissues along and above the splenic artery are also cleared. Coeliac axis is identified; nodes in front of it are cleared; left gastric artery is dissected, doubly ligated and divided and nodes along its origin are cleared. Lymph nodes along the right side of the OG junction along the crura of diaphragm and anterior surface of the abdominal oesophagus (lower 3 cm of abdominal oesophagus) should be cleared. Dissection continues along the splenic artery and posterior surface of the stomach. Dissection is continued towards splenic hilum, if nodes are suspiciously involved. Splenectomy is not necessary **(Fig. 21-71)**.

Gastric division is done as *subtotal gastrectomy* (75–80%) by dividing the stomach 2 cm distal to OG junction along lesser curve and 5 cm distal along the greater curvature. Straight occlusion clamp is placed along the greater curvature towards remnant side and along lesser curve obliquely to create lesser curve. Crushing (Payr's) or Kocher's clamps are placed towards specimen side. Stomach is cut using no. 15 blade. Specimen is placed in orientation grid. Intraoperative frozen section biopsy is done to confirm the clearance at margins. Stapler device can be used to divide the stomach at two places. Usually lesser curvature part is transected with stapler. Stomal part is cut with knife between clamps.

Reconstruction is done by omega loop gastrojejunostomy with Braun jejunojejunostomy (ideally antecolic but retrocolic can be used)

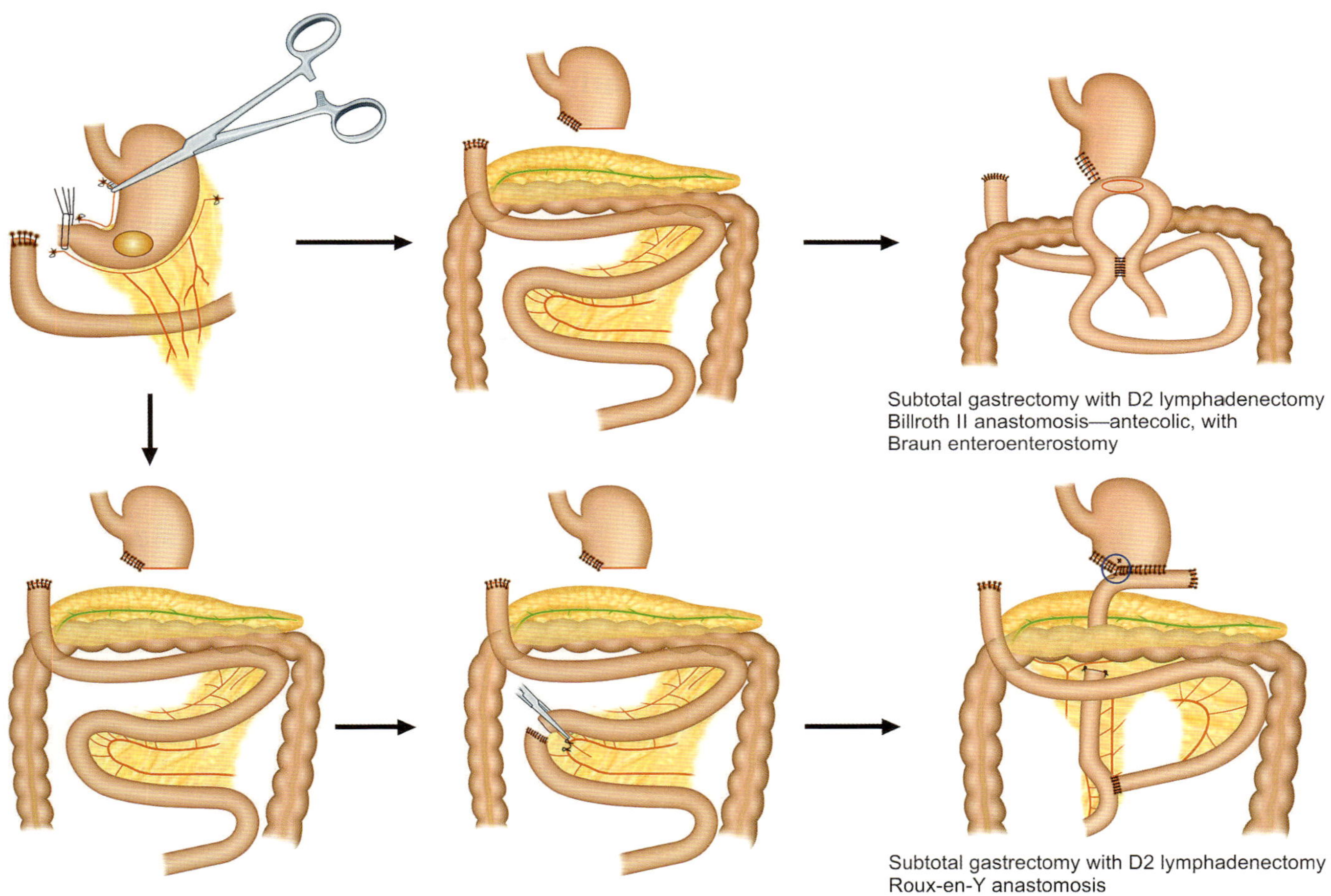

1. Mobilisation of greater omentum
2. Infrapyloric dissection with ligation of right gastroepiploic vein where it forms gastrocolic trunk; ligation of right gastroepiploic artery at its origin from gastroduodenal artery
3. Suprapyloric dissection with ligation of right gastric artery at its origin from proper hepatic artery; ligation of right and left gastric vein where they join the portal vein
4. Duodenal stump is closed—stapler or hand sewn
5. D2 lymphadenectomy clearing all nodes at proper hepatic artery level towards left at superior part of pancreas along splenic artery, along left gastric artery, along right side of cardia mainly; coeliac lymph node; nodes which originate along the splenic artery—may be removed, if possible
6. Occlusion clamp applying 2 cm distal to OG junction at lesser curve and 5 cm at greater curve
7. Completion of subtotal gastrectomy with D2 lymphadenectomy

Fig. 21-71: D2 lymphadenectomy with subtotal gastrectomy.

or Roux-en-Y gastrojejunostomy. Angle of sorrow/angle of death is addressed with crown/purse string/triple suture to stabilise the angle. Nasogastric tube is negotiated into efferent or Roux limb. Feeding jejunostomy may be required. Tube drain is placed. Even though gastric remnant is small, it maintains the function of OG junction function and remnant acts as small but significant reservoir.

TOTAL GASTRECTOMY

Removal of entire stomach (with cardia, distal oesophageal tube and cuff of duodenum) with nodal clearance may be the oncologically right surgery for carcinoma stomach. Palliative total gastrectomy, even though is done, often is doubtful about its advantages.

Connor did first total gastrectomy in 1884. Brigham, Richardson, Moynihan, Ravitch, etc. started doing total gastrectomy.

Indications

Carcinoma involving most of the lesser curvature, carcinoma of body or proximal part of the stomach are probably the indications.

Preoperative preparations are same as subtotal gastrectomy.

Technique

Under general anaesthesia with double lumen, endotracheal tube is used. Patient is positioned supine with left chest upwards in case if extension is needed at a later period. Entire chest and abdomen are cleaned and draped. Upper midline incision with provision for extension into the thorax or bilateral subcostal incision or left upper oblique incision towards left chest wall or left thoracoabdominal incision is used. Lengthy incision is preferred to achieve good exposure **(Fig. 21-72)**.

Procedure is almost same as for subtotal gastrectomy. Mobilisation of the greater omentum from the transverse colon, infrapyloric dissection with ligation of right gastroepiploic vein and artery; suprapyloric dissection with ligation of right gastric artery at its origin and removing fat and lymph nodes along these vessels; duodenal transection; dissection along the cardia and lower oesophagus with clearance of all lymph nodes; ligation of left gastric artery at its origin; left gastric vein is ligated at its joining with the portal vein. Nodes along the splenic artery up to the hilum are cleared. Splenectomy is usually not indicated; but if inevitable it should be done. Lymph nodes along the crus of the diaphragm and coeliac artery are removed. Vascular clamp is applied at the line of resection of the lower oesophagus 3 cm proximal to the OG junction. With crushing clamp on specimen side, specimen is removed.

Reconstruction is done by Roux-en-Y oesophagojejunostomy. Roux limb should be 40–45 cm. Oesophagojejunostomy should be end-to-side. Nasogastric tube should be passed across the oesophageal stoma. Distal jejunojejunostomy is done at 20 cm from the duodenojejunal junction. End-to-side anastomosis is done. If stapler resection of the loop was done earlier then side-to-side anastomosis is done.

COMPLICATIONS OF GASTRIC SURGERIES

Early Complications

Intragastric haemorrhage occurs usually from anastomotic site. It is identified by blood in the nasogastric tube. If it is mild, it can be left alone as it will subside in a day or two. If it is severe then patient develops shock with tachycardia and hypotension. Blood transfusion is required. If persists such patient needs relaparotomy, identification of bleeding point from the anastomotic site and secure suturing of

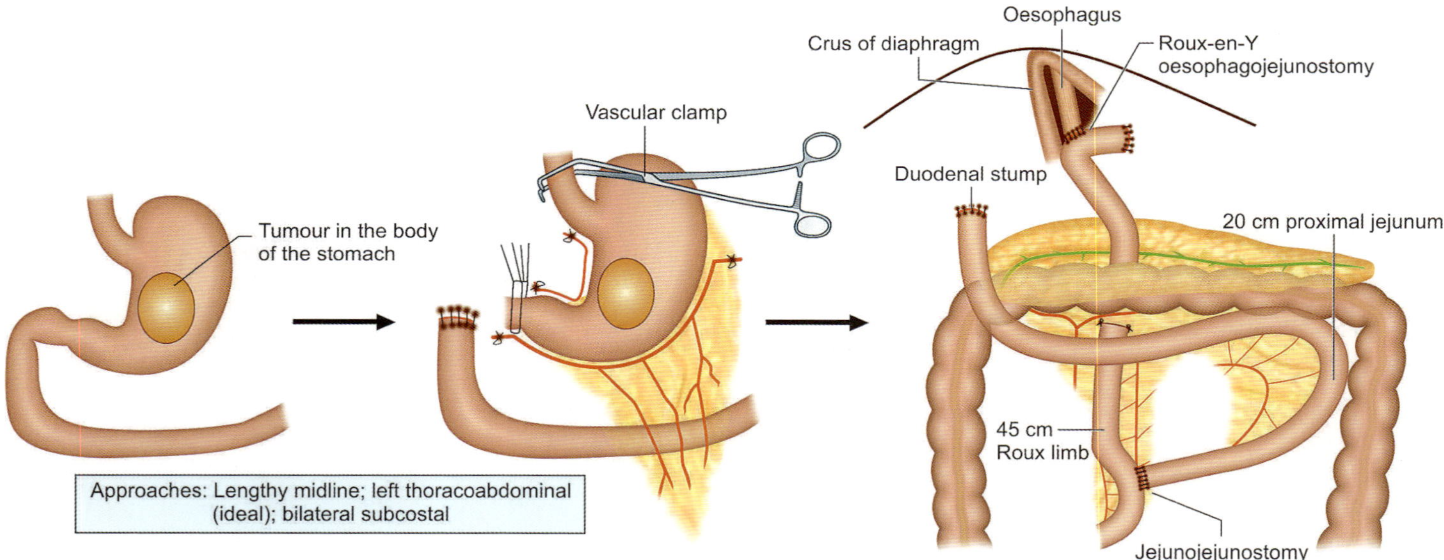

1. Mobilisation of greater omentum
2. Infrapyloric dissection with ligation of right gastroepiploic vein where it forms gastrocolic trunk; ligation of right gastroepiploic artery at its origin from gastroduodenal artery
3. Suprapyloric dissection with ligation of right gastric artery at its origin from proper hepatic artery; ligation of right and left gastric vein where they join the portal vein
4. Duodenal stump is closed—stapler or hand sewn
5. D2 lymphadenectomy clearing all nodes at proper hepatic artery level towards left at superior part of pancreas along splenic artery, along gastric artery, along both sides or cardia mainly right side; coeliac lymph nodes; ligation of left gastric artery at its origin; ligation of the left gastroepiploic artery and posteror gastric artery which originates from splenic artery
6. Vascular clamp applying 3 cm proximal to OG junction to the oesophagus
7. Completion of total gastrectomy

Fig. 21-72: Total gastrectomy with oesophagojejunostomy—Roux-en-Y anastomosis.

the area using silk or vicryl. Occasionally bleeding can occur from the existing ulcer (duodenal ulcer) which usually subsides once acid level comes down and ulcer starts healing.

Extragastric haemorrhage occurs either from slipping of ligatures of left gastric/right gastric or epiploic arteries. Bleeding can occur from pancreatic bed, omental site or organs like spleen or liver. Nasogastric tube will not show the blood. Signs like shock, palor and low haemoglobin confirms the diagnosis, blood transfusion, relaparotomy and addressing the bleeding area accordingly is needed.

Duodenal blow out/duodenal stump leakage occurs in Billroth II anastomosis. It occurs in 5th–7th postoperative period commonly. Incidence is 3–5%. It is due to duodenal fibrosis, poor blood supply of the stump, pancreatitis, infection, raised intraduodenal pressure. It can also occur if there is obstruction at afferent limb of the loop Billroth II anastomosis without Braun enteroenterostomy. Leak causes sudden pain, tachycardia and initial sepsis; but gradually gets localised. Conservative treatment usually is sufficient. Additional feeding jejunostomy, creation of jejunojejunostomy between afferent and efferent loops usually is sufficient **(Fig. 21-73)**.

Leak from the Billroth I anastomosis is due to partial disruption of the anastomosis, probably few sutures have disrupted. Usually subsides gradually on its own. If it causes leak, it is problematic. Gastrografin study provides a clue for leak. In such situation, relaparotomy is needed. Omental patch over the suture site with a drain placement is often sufficient. Occasionally needs conversion of Billroth I to Billroth II anastomosis. Feeding jejunostomy is needed.

Disruption of gastrojejunostomy is usually seen after Billroth II anastomosis; occasionally occurs after simple gastrojejunostomy also. It needs CT study/gastrografin study, reopening and omental patch if it is small. Often needs conversion to Roux-en-Y anastomosis. Disruption of pyloroplasty needs gastric resection.

Stomal obstruction: Stomal obstruction is due to stomal oedema; afferent loop obstruction; herniation of afferent or efferent limbs; kinking and adhesions at efferent loop level; afferent or efferent loop interposition behind the gastric remnant (herniation into lesser sac). Gastroduodenostomy obstruction if persists (Billroth I) for more than 10 days then it needs intervention by relaparotomy. It is not possible to dismantle the gastroduodenostomy stoma as it will cause leak. It is better to leave it like that and do a gastrojejunostomy as antecolic in the gastric remnant. Stomal oedema usually subsides over the period of time. Thirty percent of stomal obstruction when persists need relaparotomy. Release of kinking and adhesions, correction of internal herniations of afferent or efferent or both limbs; conversion into alternate procedures like Billroth II or Roux-en-Y or adding one more gastrojejunostomy to gastric remnant are alternatives used.

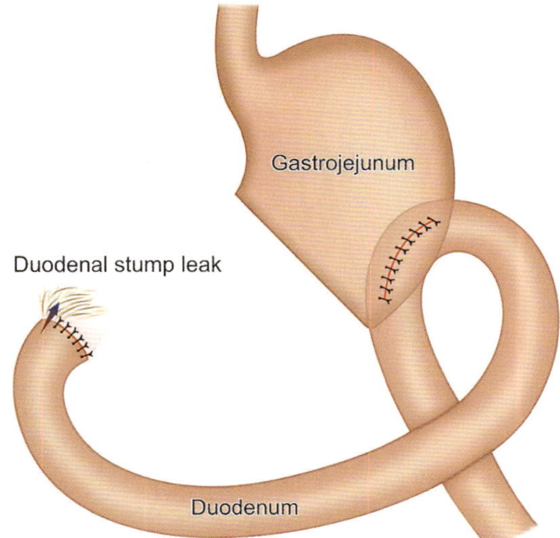

Fig. 21-73: Duodenal blow out after gastrectomy with Billroth II anastomosis.

Afferent loop obstruction: It is due to long afferent loop. Afferent loop is usually taken as 8–10 cm for posterior and 15 cm for anterior gastrojejunostomy. Roux-en-Y anastomosis eliminates afferent loop. Long afferent loop causes kinking of the loop at its junction with anastomosis which leads into duodenal obstruction. This leads into duodenal blow out in case of Billroth II anastomosis. Long afferent loop also can lead into twist, internal herniation, jejunogastric intussusception. All these lead into closed loop obstruction proximally in the duodenum raising intraduodenal pressure exceeding pancreatic duct pressure, abdominal pain, vague tender mass in the abdomen, raised total count and serum amylase mimicking acute pancreatitis. But in reality, there is enormous dilatation of the loop and duodenum which needs immediate laparotomy and surgical decompression or diversion. *Afferent loop obstruction cannot be diagnosed by endoscopy. Surgical treatment:* If loop is viable on laparotomy then creation of jejunojejunostomy between dilated afferent and normal efferent limb is suffice. Otherwise resection, dismantling the gastrojejunostomy and creation of Roux-en-Y anastomosis is needed **(Fig. 21-74)**.

Jejunal loop herniation after Billroth II anastomosis can occur as early complication or as late complication also. Herniation occurs in either afferent or efferent loop or both. If afferent loop is short, efferent loop will herniate; if afferent loop is long then afferent loop will herniate behind the gastrojejunostomy or efferent loop. Both loops if fixed to posterior parietal structures, it can be prevented. Relaparotomy is needed; hernia is reduced; mesentery is closed; if needed, afferent, loop is shortened and Roux-en-Y anastomosis is done.

Gastric remnant necrosis occurs in gastrectomies in which left gastric artery is ligated at its origin or splenectomy is also undertaken which compromises the blood supply of the gastric remnant. Gastric remnant after ligation of the left gastric artery maintains the viability through branch from left inferior phrenic artery. As a known variation, if inferior phrenic artery arises from left gastric artery which is already been ligated at its origin, gastric remnant necrosis is most likely to occur. Entire or part of the gastric remnant goes for necrosis leading to acute peritonitis with features of coffee ground vomitus which needs immediate surgical intervention. Condition is diagnosed by MDCT abdomen. If part of the gastric remnant is necrosed then resection of that part and creating Roux-en-Y gastrojejunostomy is done; viability of remaining stomach should be adequate. If entire gastric remnant is involved which often may extend to distal oesophagus, then gangrenous part is resected with dismantling of the anastomosis; lower oesophagus is formed into a tube ostomy; cervical oesophagostomy is also done.

Intra-abdominal abscess is not uncommon. It can be subphrenic abscess, pelvic abscess, interloop abscess; it can be single or multi-loculated. CT abdomen is diagnostic. Higher generation antibiotics, percutaneous drainage or open surgical drainage is needed **(Fig. 21-75)**.

Postoperative pancreatitis can occur (2–5%). It is usually not due to trauma but due to close proximity. But can occur while dissecting the pancreas in front, while removing the pancreatic capsule. It is treated conservatively. Postoperative jaundice is known to occur after gastric surgeries. It may be due to pancreatitis, anastomotic leak (bile gets absorbed from peritoneal cavity); haemolysis, sepsis, injury to bile duct, cholangitis, anaesthesia toxicity.

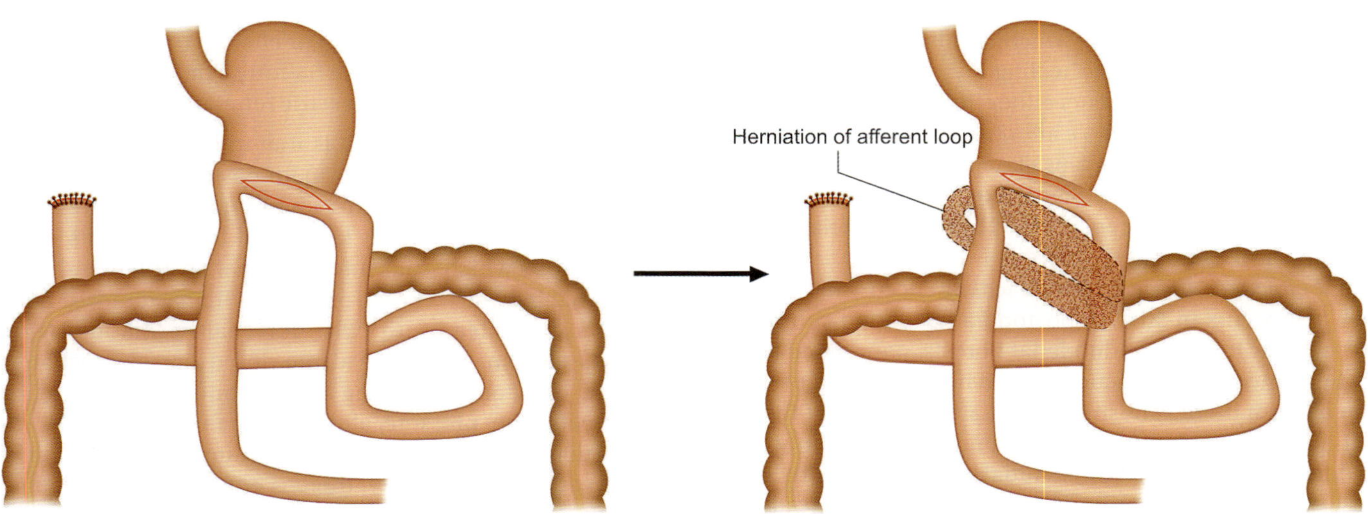

Fig. 21-74: Afferent loop obstruction occurs due to long afferent loop which may herniate or twist or kink.

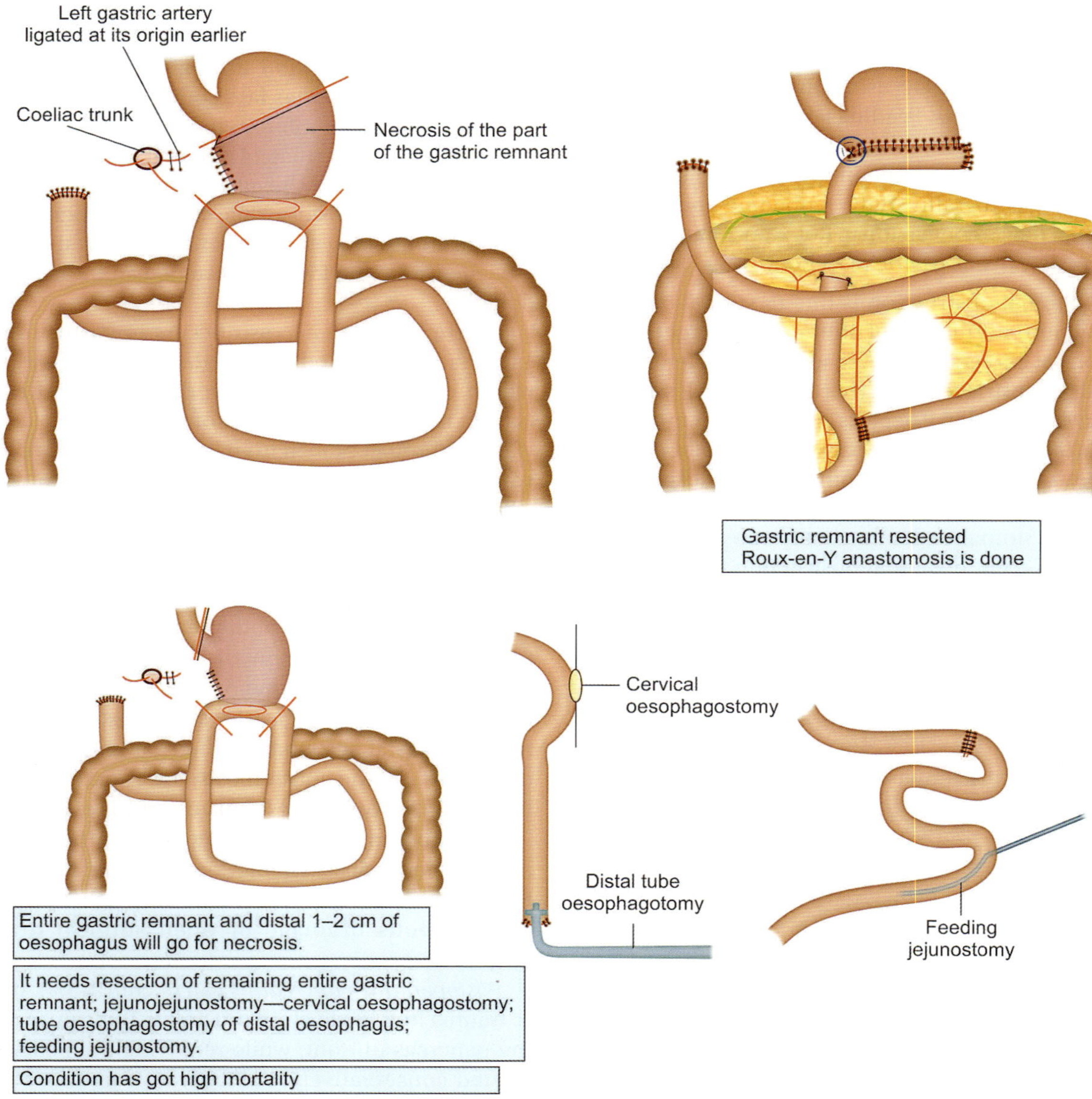

Left gastric artery ligated at its origin earlier

Coeliac trunk

Necrosis of the part of the gastric remnant

Gastric remnant resected
Roux-en-Y anastomosis is done

Cervical oesophagostomy

Distal tube oesophagotomy

Feeding jejunostomy

Entire gastric remnant and distal 1–2 cm of oesophagus will go for necrosis.

It needs resection of remaining entire gastric remnant; jejunojejunostomy—cervical oesophagostomy; tube oesophagostomy of distal oesophagus; feeding jejunostomy.

Condition has got high mortality

Fig. 21-75: Gastric remnant necrosis. It is managed by resection of necrosis non-viable part and remaining part is anastomosed with jejunum as Roux-en-Y with feeding jejunostomy. If entire gastric remnant is disrupted then it is managed by cervical oesophagostomy, distal tube oesophagostomy and feeding jejunostomy. Later once patient recovers from shock and sepsis, after 3 months, colonic bypass is required.

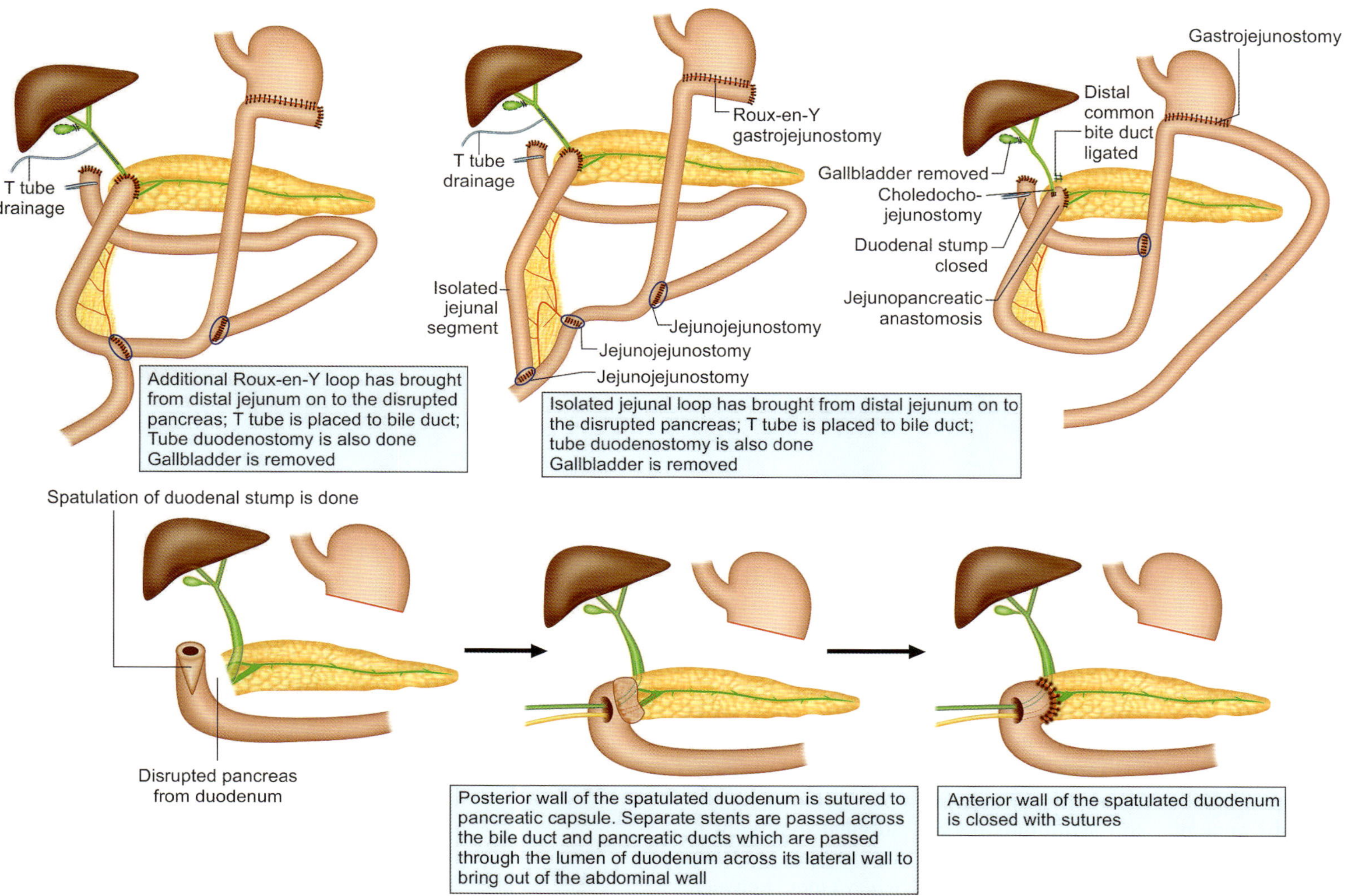

Fig. 21-76: Different procedures used for duodenopancreatic disconnection.

Common bile duct injury and injury at ampulla of Vater is uncommon but can occur. It is difficult to manage. Duodenum is opened; common bile duct is exposed; opened duodenum is sutured to head of the pancreas over the disrupted part as a coverage ostomy. T-tube drainage and stenting of ducts on table are other options. Isolated jejunal loop harvested from distal to existing anastomosis can be sutured to the head of the pancreas on to disrupted area. Second Roux loop can be taken to suture to the area **(Fig. 21-76)**.

Omental infarction, stress ulceration, inadvertent gastroileostomy are rare complications.

Late Complications

Alkaline reflux gastritis is commonest postgastrectomy late problem. Bile, pancreatic and duodenal juice is injurious to gastric mucosa. Reflux gastritis can occur in Billroth II (commonly), Billroth I, gastrojejunostomy alone when done and, pyloroplasty. Burning epigastric pain, bilious vomiting, anaemia, bleeding from the stomach are the features. Endoscopy with biopsy is diagnostic which shows oedema and friability of gastric mucosa. There will be acute and chronic inflammation with decrease in parietal cell mass but increase in mucus secreting cells. Prokinetic drugs may help. Measurement of bile acid in fasting gastric aspirate is useful. Surgical treatment is conversion to Roux-en-Y anastomosis; if patient has had pyloroplasty or gastrojejunostomy (after vagotomy) alone, then antrectomy and Roux-en-Y anastomosis to be done as Roux-en-Y perse is ulcerogenic. Many patients may have additionally reflux oesophagitis. Antireflux surgery may be needed in these patients.

Delayed gastric emptying can occur in any type of gastric bypass. It is probably alteration in the gastric pacemaker activity. In these patients, endoscopy shows normal stoma **(Fig. 21-77)**.

Dumping syndrome can be early or late.

Early dumping syndrome is due to loss of pyloric sphincter mechanism allowing rapid passage of food across the duodenum or proximal jejunum causing vasomotor and gastrointestinal disturbances. It causes palpitation, sweating, increased bowel movements and borborygmi, colicky pain, tachycardia, hypotension, hypovolaemia, vomiting and diarrhoea. There is rapid passage of food. It is common (10%) and more severe type. It occurs in 30–60 minutes of food intake. It is a primary disorder of carbohydrate metabolism. Initial transient hyperglycaemia prevents further absorption of glucose, which in turn draws fluid from the bowel wall by high osmolarity resulting in increased intestinal activity, diarrhoea, and fall in blood pressure. Radionuclide studies show rapid emptying from the stomach; if patient is asked to drink 100 mL of 50% glucose in water, it will show the early symptoms. In late dumping syndrome, 3 hours after intake of 50% glucose in 100 mL of water will show drop in blood sugar below 50 mg% with concomitant raise in plasma insulin level.

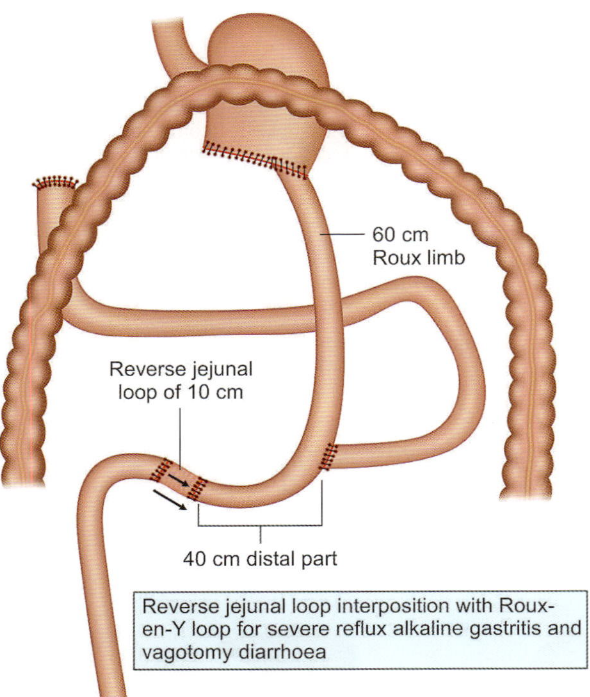

Fig. 21-77: Reverse jejunal loop interposition with Roux-en-Y loop is done for severe alkaline gastritis and vagotomy diarrhoea.

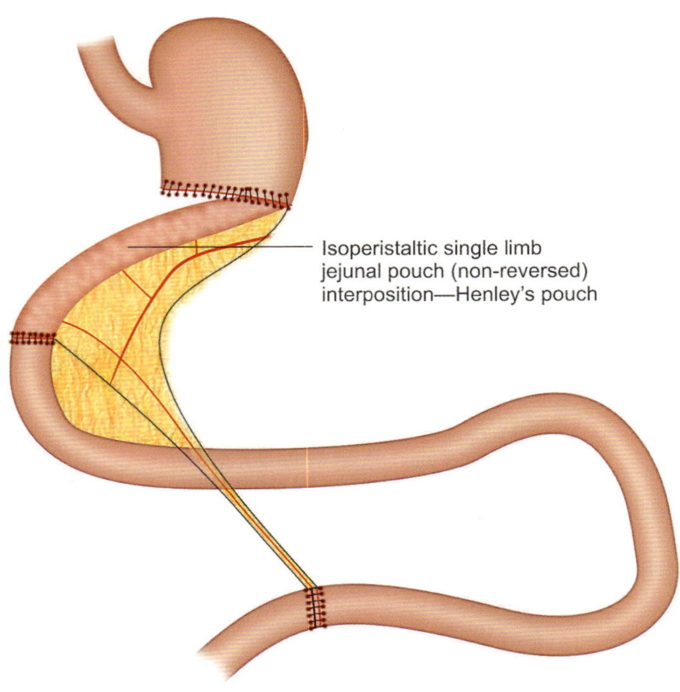

Fig. 21-78: Henley's isoperistaltic jejunal loop interposition (non-reversed). It does not give good results compared to reversed jejunal loop interposition.

Treatment is small, frequent diet that includes dry food, carbohydrate diet avoided, octreotide 100 microgram taken before food subcutaneously; surgical treatment may be required if patient looses weight, develops anaemia, and symptoms persist. Surgical treatment is conversion into Roux-en-Y anastomosis or interposition of 25 cm of proximal jejunal segment as isoperistaltic (*Henley's loop*) between stomach and duodenum or jejunum itself. Vagotomy should be completed in these patients. Poth's double limb pouch is better and satisfactory than Henley's loop. Ulcer formation in the pouch/loop, stasis, obstruction are the problems. Triple limb pouches have also been tried. All these pouches have been tried along with Roux-en-Y anastomosis. Antrectomy is a must if Roux limb is planned. Ligidakis modification of Hunt Lawrence pouch has also been tried. It is similar to Henley's loop interposition but loop is reversed during interposition giving better result. Ligidakis pouch is said to provide normal pouch motility, required delayed gastric emptying, without any pouch dilatation and stasis **(Figs. 21-78 and 21-79)**.

Late dumping syndrome is of less severe type (5%). It is due to initial hyperglycaemia-induced insulin release which in turn causes hypoglycaemia 2–3 hours after meals. Diarrhoea and boborygmi are not present. Features of hypoglycaemia occur 2 hours after the food intake with tremor, fatigue, nausea, sweating, and drowsiness. It is a reactive hypoglycaemia. Symptoms are relieved by glucose but aggravated by exercise. Treatment is reduced carbohydrate meal; increased protein diet; small intake of glucose between meals. Usually, surgical correction is not needed for late dumping syndrome.

Dumping syndrome may be associated with postvagotomy diarrhoea. It is corrected by Roux-en-Y anastomosis and creating short jejunal reversal loop 100 cm distal to the ligament of Treitz. Dumping syndrome may be associated with reflux gastritis. It is treated with Roux-en-Y anastomosis. Occasionally dumping syndrome, reflux gastritis and vagotomy diarrhoea may be associated together.

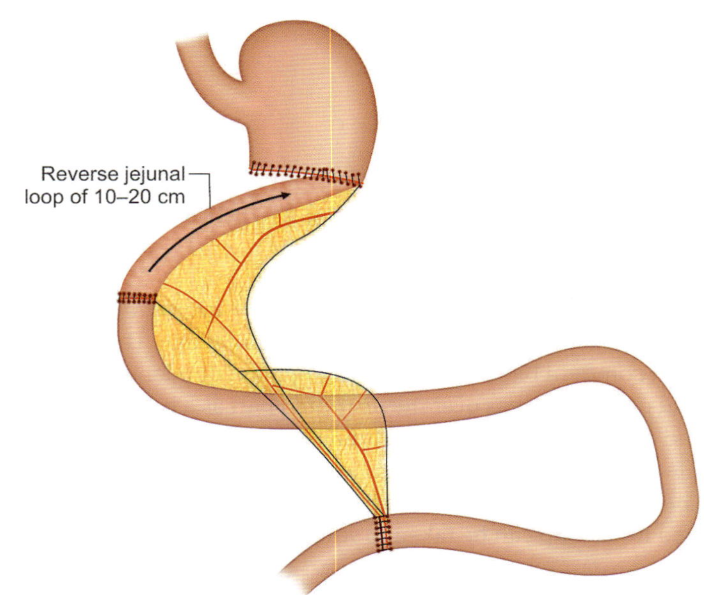

Fig. 21-79: Reverse jejunal interposition is better than isoperistaltic.

It is treated by Roux-en-Y anastomosis, creation of short reversed jejunal segment distal to the 40 cm end-to-side anastomosis.

Recurrent ulcer: Recurrent ulcer after vagotomy with drainage procedure is treated with antral resection and completion vagotomy. Recurrent ulcers due to Zollinger Ellison syndrome is treated with total gastrectomy with Roux-en-Y anastomosis.

Small gastric remnant syndrome: It is due to reduced gastric reservoir. Patient develops abdominal discomfort after taking food and so restricts caloric diet. Gastric reservoir function is increased by doing different pouches using jejunum. Hunt Lawrence or Tanner Roux 19 pouches are often used **(Figs. 21-80 to 21-85)**.

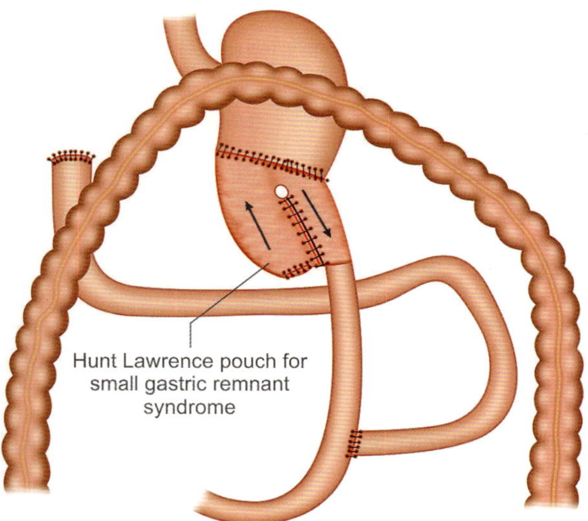

Fig. 21-80: Hunt Lawrence pouch as a reservoir for small gastric remnant.

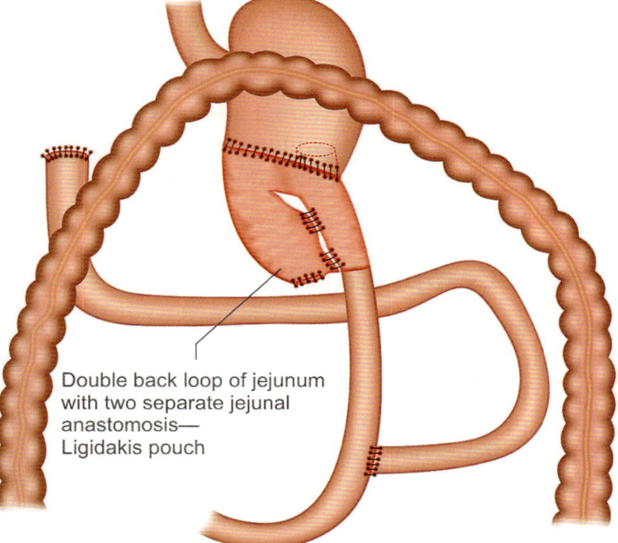

Fig. 21-81: Ligidakis pouch. Ligidakis modification of Hunt Lawrence pouch is said to provide normal pouch motility, required delayed gastric emptying, without any pouch dilatation and stasis.

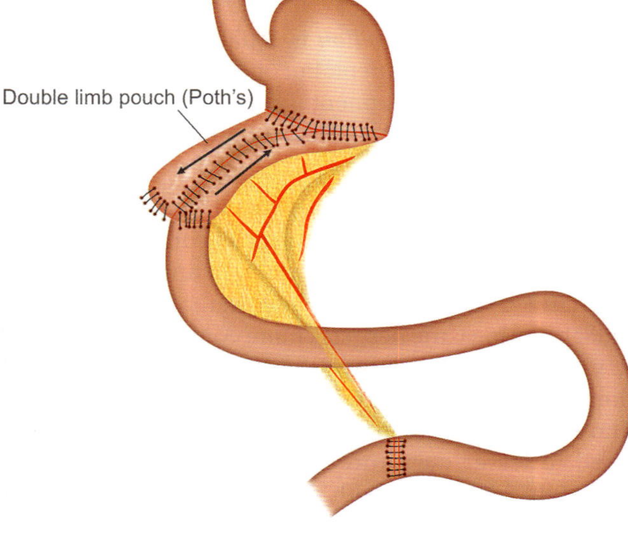

Fig. 21-82: Double limb jejunal pouch—Poth's.

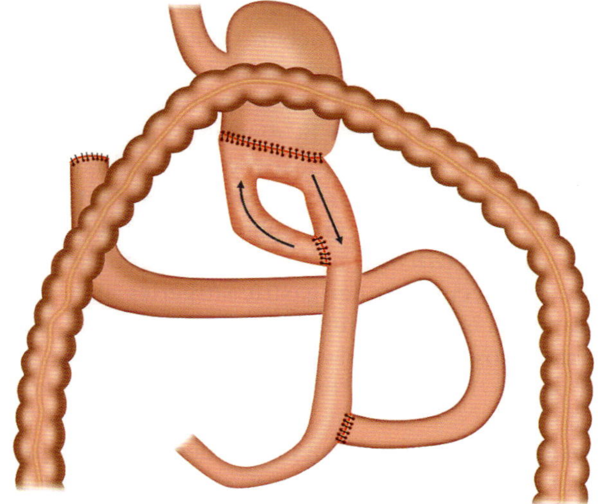

Fig. 21-83: Tanner Roux 9 technique for small gastric remnant.

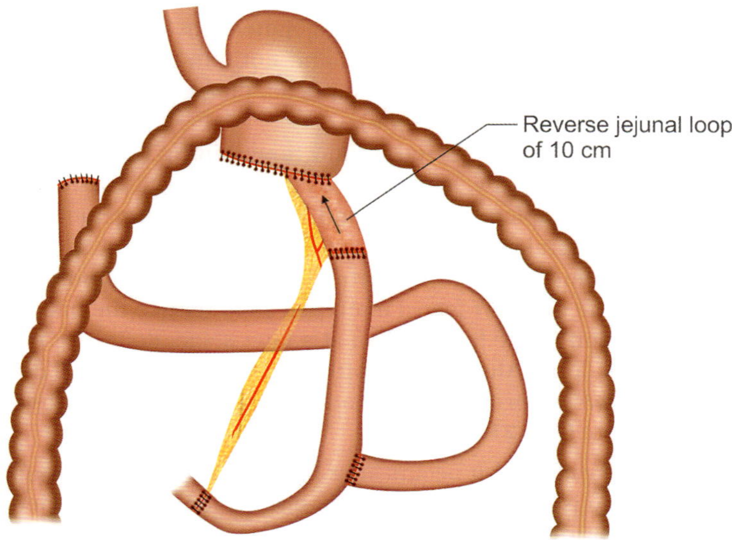

Fig. 21-84: Terrence Kennedy reverse jejunum technique. Reverse jejunal loop is interposed in the Roux limb at gastrojejunostomy level.

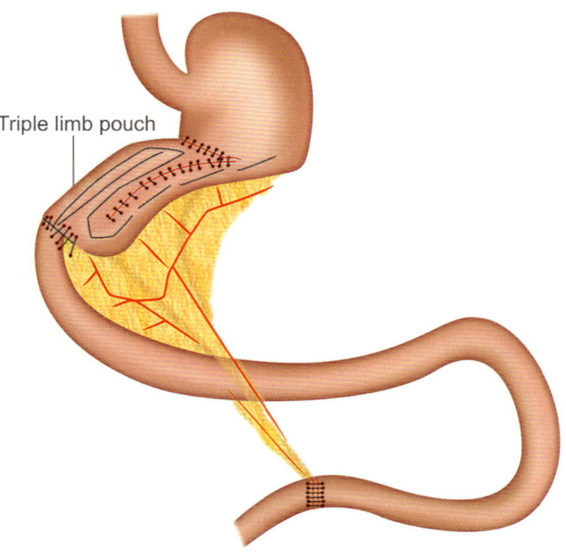

Fig. 21-85: Triple limb pouch across the Roux limb.

Malabsorption, gastric remnant bezoar formation, motility problems are also known to occur. Gastric remnant bezoar is common in Billroth I anastomosis and pyloroplasty. It is commonly phytobezoars (vegetable matter). Bezoar causes bleeding, perforation and malnutrition. It is treated by digestive agents like enterases, papase and other enzymes. Endoscopy removal may be required. Low fibre diet is required to prevent recurrence. Motility disorders can be treated by prokinetics, urecholine, coherin peptide, etc.

Gastric remnant carcinoma: It is more common after Billroth I operation, can occur in other gastric surgeries also. Reflux with deconjugation of bile acids with hypoacidity; bacterial reduction of nitrates into nitrosamines, and vagotomy—are the causes. Incidence is 5%. It occurs 10 years after the gastrectomy. It carries poor prognosis.

Gastrojejunocolic fistula occurs in retrocolic gastrojejunostomy. It can occur after Billroth II anastomosis or simple gastrojejunostomy (retrocolic) also. Incidence is 5%. Initially marginal ulcer occurs on the anterior wall/rim of the stoma which gradually deepens/penetrates to erode into the anteriorly located colon to create gastrojejunocolic fistula. As marginal ulcer occurs on the anterior aspect of the stoma in antecolic gastrojejunostomy this ulcer erodes anteriorly into the abdominal wall and not into the colon. Faecal belching, vomiting, emaciation, anorexia, diarrhoea, gross weight loss—are the features **(Fig. 21-86)**.

Treatment is triple resection and maintaining the continuity with gastrojejunostomy, jejunojejunostomy, colocolic anastomosis. It is better to complete vagotomy and Roux-en-Y gastrojejunostomy if patient's general condition permits. In severely ill patient, initial ascending colostomy (*Phiffer*) proximal to colonic component of fistula is done to divert faecal matter so as to reduce the bacterial contamination in the fistula, then at a later stage, definitive triple resection is done. Alternatively often ileosigmoidostomy (*Lahey*) is done between terminal ileum and sigmoid colon to divert the faecal content **(Fig. 21-87)**.

Roux stasis syndrome: It occurs after Roux-en-Y gastrojejunostomy. Its incidence is 10–30%. When Roux limb is longer, its incidence increases. Intolerance for solids is typical. Distressing bilious vomiting, loss of weight and recurrent pain are common. Gastroscopy shows patent stoma. Contrast study shows normal flow of dye. Radionuclide study reveals severe impairment of the gastric emptying. Roux limb in these patients acts as a barrier for gastric emptying. It shows severe gastric atony. It is common in females. Ectopic pacemaker in the Roux limb gets activated and delays the gastric emptying. There is uncoordinated peristalsis of Roux limb preventing progressive peristalsis. Uncoupled myoelectric complex, increased non-peristaltic and retrograde waves cause dysmotility of Roux limb. Prokinetic drugs will not benefit. Erythromycin may be beneficial. Treatment is conversion into Billroth I or II loop gastrojejunostomy.

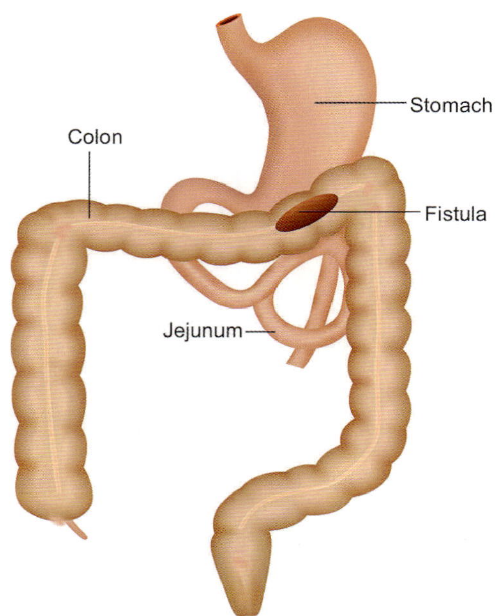

Fig. 21-86: Gastrojejunocolic fistula.

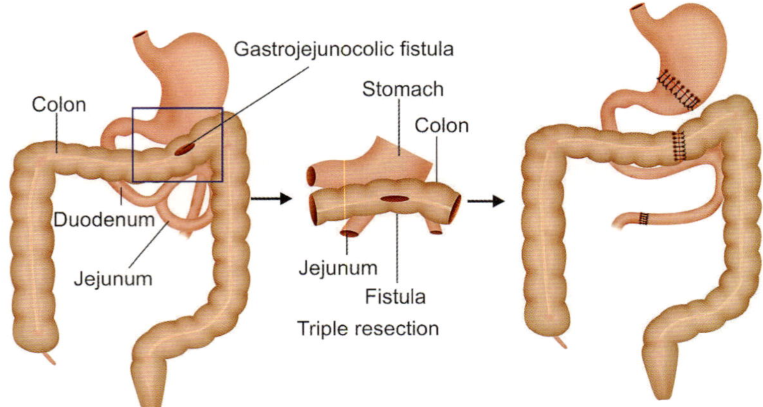

Fig. 21-87: Triple resection for gastrojejunocolic fistula. Condition has got high mortality.

Long-term Complications

Chronic afferent loop obstruction: It is due to long afferent loop design in Billroth II reconstruction. It causes recurrent twist or kink at gastrojejunostomy site. Internal herniation of afferent under efferent, stenosis of afferent at junction with stomach, volvulus of the redundant afferent loop, adhesions of afferent loop are common causes. It is recurrent repetitive obstruction. There is projectile vomiting; and vomitus contains bile. Upper abdominal pain develops after meals. Pain is relieved by vomiting. (In reflux gastritis, pain is constant; pain is not relieved by vomiting. Anaemia and bleeding are not uncommon in reflux gastritis). Treatments modalities of chronic afferent loop obstruction are jejunojejunostomy, suspension of afferent loop, resection and shortening of the afferent loop, conversion into Roux-en-Y (ideal) or Billroth I anastomosis.

Chronic efferent loop obstruction is usually due to adhesions and kinking. It is usually intermittent; but often, it may be severe causing efferent loop gangrene. Treatment is surgical. Release of adhesions, conversion into Roux-en-Y anastomosis; require resection if there is gangrene.

Internal hernias after gastric surgery: It can occur as afferent or efferent loop hernias. It is seen in Billroth II anastomosis or simple gastrojejunostomy. It is common in antecolic anastomosis. Here afferent loop is taken larger and there is large space behind the stomach. Retrogastric hernia is more common in such situation. Ideally in antecolic anastomosis, jejunal loops should be fixed to abdominal wall parietes (*Gry and Morton method*) to prevent herniation. But it is not commonly practiced. When afferent loop is sutured to lesser curvature then hernia chances are higher. When anastomosis is done with afferent from greater curvature to lesser curvature side (left to right), herniation of afferent loop is less likely. It is treated by surgical correction.

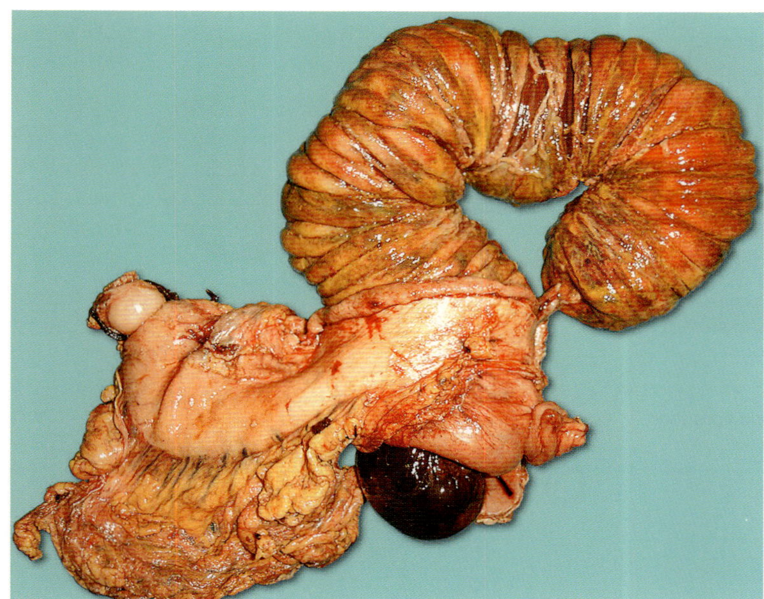

Fig. 21-88: Retrograde jejunogastric intussusception.
Courtesy: Dr Arunkumar, MCh, Gastrointestinal surgeon.

Jejunogastric intussusception: It is the retrograde intussusception of efferent jejunal loop into the stomach or gastric remnant. It occurs only in loop gastrojejunostomy. It is rare but severe. In 80% cases, efferent limb is involved. Rarely afferent limb or both can be involved. Palpable tender mass on left of the umbilicus, haematemesis, pain on left side of umbilicus radiating towards back are typical. Contrast study shows coiled spring appearance. Laparotomy should be done. Intussusception is reduced; if it is viable, it is fixed to abdominal parietes. If it is gangrenous, resection is done; with Roux-en-Y anastomosis **(Fig. 21-88)**.

RAMSTEDT'S PYLOROMYOTOMY FOR CONGENITAL HYPERTROPHIED PYLORIC STENOSIS

It is the manifestation of progressive hypertrophy of muscular wall of the pyloric sphincter muscle. Clinically non-bilious vomiting, palpable olive shaped pyloric mass in upper abdomen in a male infant of 3–4 weeks age; visible gastric peristalsis, with hypokalaemia and metabolic alkalosis sonologically pyloric channel >3 mm thickness and pyloric length >2 cm is 100% diagnostic. *In 1912, Ramstedt* did pyloromyotomy but could not suture transversely as infant was severely ill; but surprisingly infant recovered well, without a need for any further surgery.

Preparation

Initial electrolyte and fluid management is needed.

Technique

General anaesthesia is used. Infant is in supine position. Nasogastric tube (narrow/fine tube) is passed. Right upper quadrant transverse incision is used. External and internal oblique muscles are cut; transverse abdominis muscle is split. All layers muscle splitting incision also can be used. Peritoneum is opened. Body of the stomach is identified and held out of the wound. Pyloric hypertrophied mass should not be held as it will cause serosal tear and bleeding. If stomach is not clearly identifiable, then 30 mL of air is insufflated into the stomach to make it distend and visible. Greater curvature of the stomach is held and drawn towards left with traction. Mass extends distally up to the pyloric vein of Mayo. Middle of pylorus and mass on the anterior aspect is relatively avascular and is incised longitudinally along its entire length and thickness. Often muscle may invaginate into the duodenal bulb distally. Care should be taken not to injure the mucosa. If mucosal perforation occurs, mucosa is closed using 3- or 4-zero vicryl and omental patch is placed over it. Small venous ooze can occur due to venous congestion. Monopolar cautery should not be used; if needed, only bipolar cautery should be used. Benson pyloric spreader instrument is very useful to do proper pyloromyotomy. When superior and inferior margins of the cut pylorus move independently then pyloromyotomy is said to be complete.

If mucosal injury prevents further continuation of myotomy procedure, Graham patch of omentum is placed over it and sutured. Myotomy is done by rotating the pylorus to 180° **(Figs. 21-89A and B)**.

Problems

Mucosal perforation, incomplete myotomy, postoperative vomiting and electrolyte imbalance, infection, pneumonia—are ontable and postoperative problems.

Postoperative Care

Feeding is started in 12 hours with graded protocol. Pyloric muscle regresses to its normal thickness in 12 weeks. Final result and cure rate is excellent.

Laparoscopic pyloromyotomy is equally good and technique is similar but through laparoscopic instruments. Umbilical port is placed for camera. Two 5 mm working ports are placed. Arthroscopy knife is used to make incision over the pylorus. Laparoscopic spreader similar to Benson spreader is available to spread the incised pyloric muscle completely to allow protrusion of the mucosa outwards. One should avoid perforation. Two edges are held apart to confirm the completion of myotomy. Stomach is insufflated with air using orogastric or nasogastric tube to confirm no leak through laparoscopic vision **(Fig. 21-90)**.

DUODENUM

Duodenum is derived from Latin-Greek word *dudekadaktulos* that means 12 fingers. It lies at the level of 1st, 2nd and 3rd lumbar vertebrae and at and above the level of the umbilicus in front. It is C-shaped with head of pancreas attached to its inner part. It is widest (2.5 cm), shortest, most fixed part of small intestine. The *duodenum* is 20–30 cm in length. It extends from pyloric sphincter to *ligament of Treitz*. It is divided into four parts. Ninety percent of duodenal ulcer occurs in the 1st part of duodenum (duodenal bulb/cap). CBD and pancreatic duct merges to form *ampulla of Vater* and enter the 2nd part of duodenum. The 3rd part of duodenum is wedged between aorta and superior mesenteric artery.

Proximal part (2.5 cm) of the 1st part of the duodenum is intraabdominal and is mobile; its distal part (2.5 cm) is retroperitoneal. First part is related to the common bile duct, portal vein, gastroduodenal artery and inferior vena cava on its posterior aspect. In front, it is related to caudate lobe of liver and gallbladder; above to the epiploic foramen and below to head and neck of the pancreas.

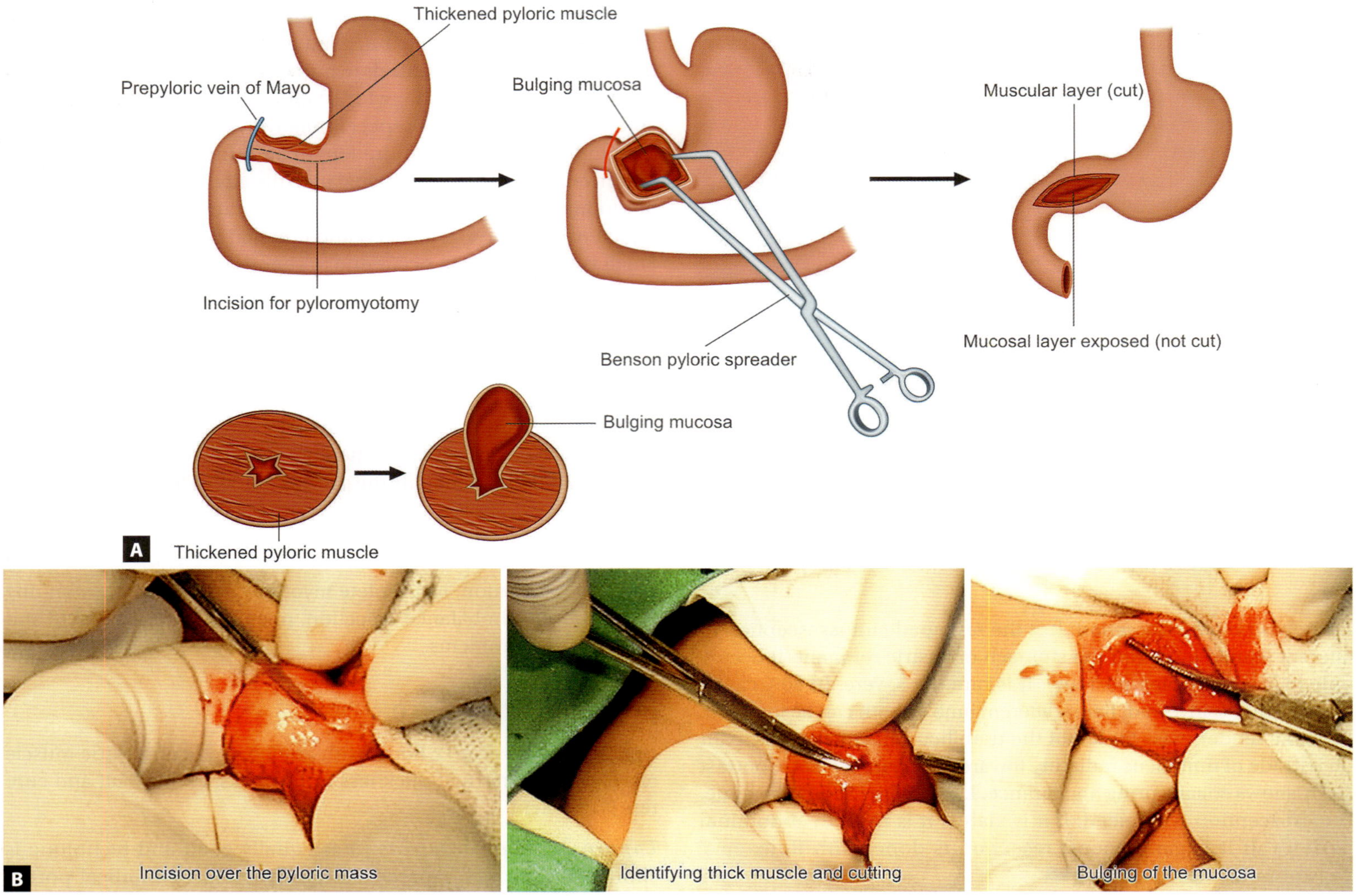

Figs. 21-89A and B: Ramstedt's pyloromyotomy technique.

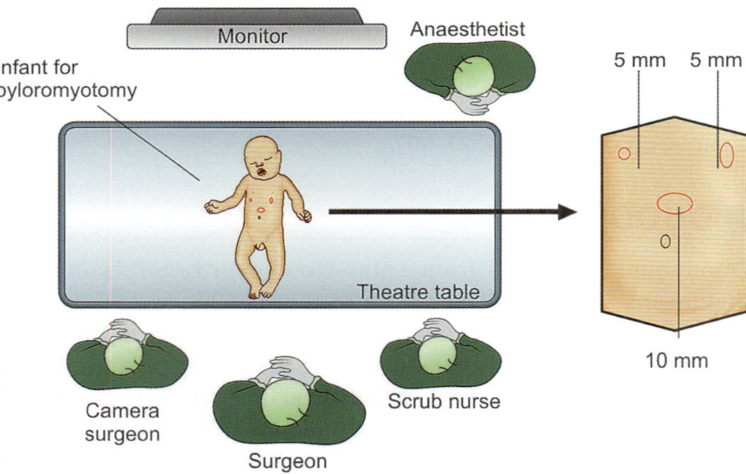

Fig. 21-90: Laparoscopic cardiomyotomy.

At gastroduodenal junction, submucosal glands of Brunner appear which are not present in gastric mucosa. First part is 5 cm long. At superior duodenal flexure, it continues as 2nd part.

Second part is 7.5 cm long that begins at superior duodenal flexure runs downward; at the level of 3rd lumbar vertebra and at inferior duodenal flexure, it turns towards left to continue as 3rd part. Anteriorly, it is covered with peritoneum except in the middle where it is directly related to transverse colon. Other anterior relations are right lobe of the liver; transverse colon, root of transverse mesocolon, and small bowel. Posteriorly, it is related to right kidney, right renal vessels, inferior vena cava, right gonadal vein (joins the inferior vena cava behind 2nd part of the duodenum) and right psoas major. Medially, it is related to head of pancreas and bile duct. Major duodenal papilla is located 10 cm distal to pylorus as an elevation. Accessory pancreatic duct opens at minor duodenal papilla, 6 cm from distal to pylorus.

Third part is 10 cm long that begins at inferior duodenal flexure at the level of the right margin of the lower border of the 3rd lumbar vertebra. It runs horizontally and upwards to continue as 4th part. In front, it is related to superior mesenteric vessels and root of mesentery (vein is medial to artery); behind right ureter, right psoas major, right testicular or ovarian vessels; inferior vena cava; abdominal aorta with inferior mesenteric artery; above to head of pancreas and uncinate process; below to coils of jejunum.

Fourth part is 2.5 cm long; travels upwards left of the aorta up to superior margin of 2nd lumbar vertebra. Here it curves to form jejunum. Its terminal part is mobile. In front, it is related to transverse colon, transverse mesocolon, lesser sac and stomach; behind to left sympathetic chain, left psoas major, left renal vessels, left testicular vessels and inferior mesenteric vein; to the right upper part of the mesentery; to the left kidney (left) and ureter; above is body of the pancreas.

Suspensory ligament of Treitz is a fibromuscular band which arises from right crus of the diaphragm, passes downward behind the pancreas and splenic vein in front of the left renal vein. It is attached to the upper posterior surface of the duodenojejunal flexure and 3rd and 4th part of the duodenum. It may insert only to duodenojejunal flexure or 3rd or 4th parts only or may have multiple attachments. Its proximal part is skeletal muscle; distal part is smooth muscle and in between elastic fibres **(Fig. 21-91)**.

Arterial supply of duodenum: Foregut part of the duodenum is supplied by superior pancreaticoduodenal artery (anterior and posterior), a branch of gastroduodenal artery; hindgut part is by inferior pancreaticoduodenal artery (anterior and posterior), a branch superior mesenteric artery. Other branches are supraduodenal artery of Wilkie, a branch of proper hepatic artery; retroduodenal artery of Edwards Michel, a branch of common hepatic artery. Inferior pancreaticoduodenal artery may arise from 1st jejunal branch of superior mesenteric artery or as a common trunk with 1st jejunal branch **(Fig. 21-92)**.

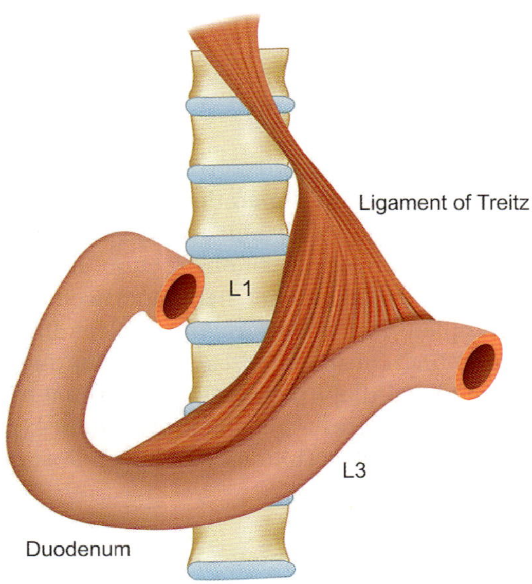

Fig. 21-91: Suspensory ligament of Treitz.

Venous drainage is mainly portal, superior mesenteric and splenic veins. Venous arcade is superficial to arterial arcade **(Fig. 21-93)**.

Lymphatic drainage is to pancreaticoduodenal nodes; to hepatic nodes; coeliac nodes; often to pyloric and aortic nodes.

Surgical Significance

Kocherisation is needed in many oesophageal, gastroduodenal and pancreatic surgeries to mobilise the duodenum. It is done by incising the right peritoneal reflection of the 2nd part of the duodenum and mobilising it towards left in front of inferior vena cava and right renal vein and aorta. It is mobilised along the head of the pancreas. Even though plane is avascular, care should be taken not to injure the vena cava and right gonadal vein.

Mobilisation of the hepatic flexure and transverse colon from the 2nd and 3rd parts of the duodenum to expose duodenum proximal to superior mesenteric vein is necessary in colectomy and pancreatic surgeries—*Cattell manoeuvre.*

Only 2 cm of 1st part of the duodenum can be skeletonised so as to retain the blood supply of the stomach.

Suspensory ligament of Treitz can be divided without any problem.

Duct of Santorini is close to gastroduodenal artery and may get injured in gastrectomy while mobilising the duodenum. Accessory pancreatic duct passes under the gastroduodenal artery (*water under the bridge*); while ligating the gastroduodenal artery (bleeding ulcer), one should avoid anterior medial duodenal wall to avoid injury to gastroduodenal artery. Duodenum should not be mobilised beyond the gastroduodenal artery.

One of the pancreaticoduodenal arteries should be retained ideally to keep head of pancreas viable, otherwise head may go for necrosis.

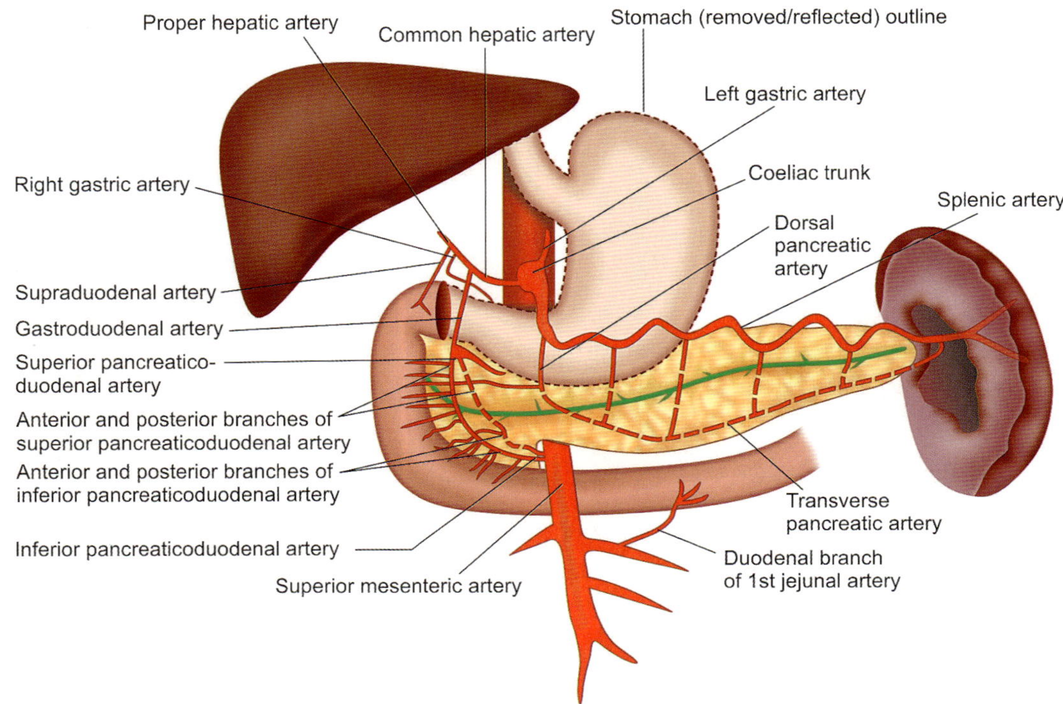

Fig. 21-92: Arterial supply of duodenum.

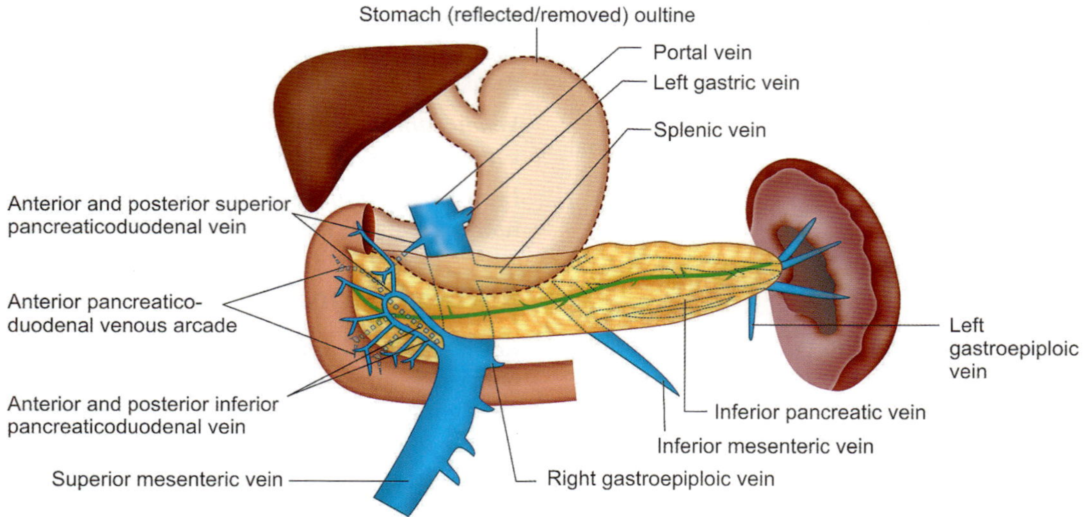

Fig. 21-93: Venous drainage of the duodenum.

SURGICAL TREATMENT OF SUPERIOR MESENTERIC ARTERY SYNDROME (WILKIE'S/VASCULAR COMPRESSION OF THE DUODENUM)

It is the compression of the 3rd part of the duodenum between aorta and emerging of superior mesenteric artery which is in front of the duodenum. It is due to acute angulation between SMA and Aorta leading into compression. Bilious vomiting, distension, electrolyte imbalance are the features. Contrast imaging is diagnostic.

Treatment is release of suspensory ligament of Treitz and duodenojejunostomy between proximal dilated 2nd part of the duodenum and jejunum 10–15 cm from the duodenojejunal flexure. Side-to-side anastomosis is done. Gastrojejunostomy should not be done **(Figs. 21-94A and B)**.

DUODENAL ATRESIA

It is the commonest site of intestinal atresia. It is usually a complete stenosis of the second part of duodenum at the level of ampulla of Vater. It is defective fusion of foregut and midgut with failure of recanalisation. Incidence is one in 10,000 live births.

Types (Figs. 21-95A to D)

Type 1: Complete duodenal atresia: It is the commonest type (50%). It is usually complete separation with intact wall. In 25% cases, complete separation with wall also occurs. Type 2: Fibrous cord. Type 3: Incomplete or partial obstruction. It can be stenosis or web with an aperture. Duodenal diaphragm/web can present as complete; incomplete with a fenestra; incomplete diaphragm with central aperture which causes '*windsock' deformity* due to proximal dilatation. Here actual diaphragm will be proximal to the site of obstruction. Duodenal atresia may be *preampullary* (non-bilious vomiting) or *postampullary* (bilious vomiting). Postampullary is common (80–90%).

Associations

Duodenal stenosis is often associated with annular pancreas. It can be isolated with duodenal atresia or in association with Down's syndrome (30%)/incomplete rotation of gut (20%)/congenital heart diseases (30%)/trisomy (30%)/anorectal malformations (10%), etc. It is commonly associated with maternal polyhydramnios (50%). Antenatal ultrasonography can confirm it. Fifty percent infants are premature.

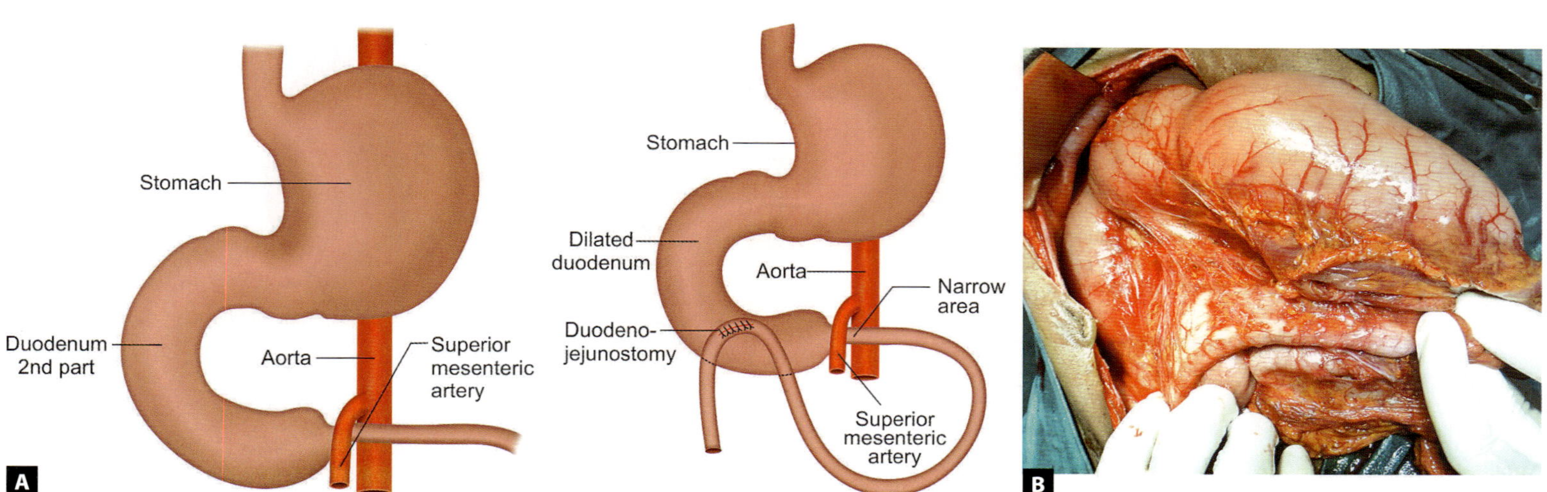

Figs. 21-94A and B: Vascular compression of the duodenum—Wilkie's syndrome.

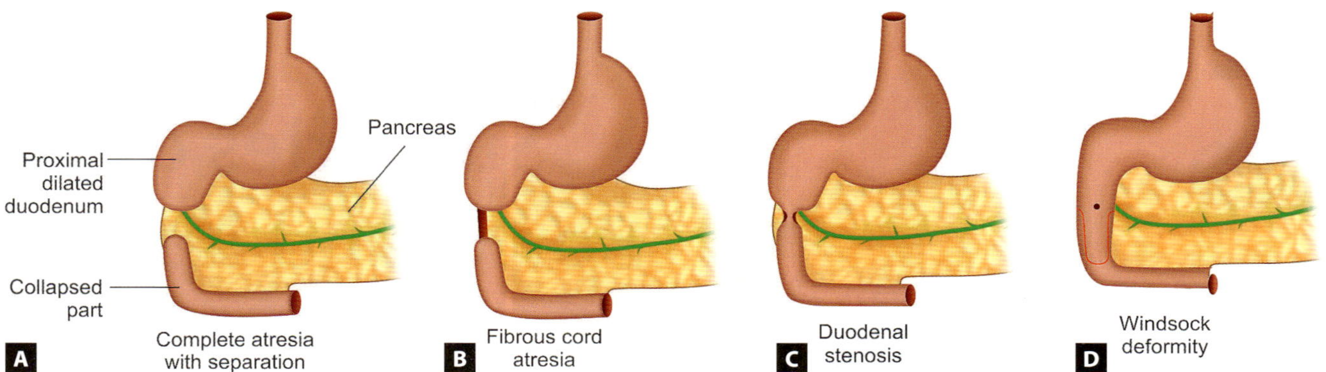

Figs. 21-95 to D: Types of duodenal atresia—(A) Complete; (B) Fibrous cord; (C) Duodenal stenosis; (D) Windsock deformity.

Features

Jaundice, bilious/non-bilious vomiting immediately after birth, features of gastric outlet obstruction, dehydration, electrolyte changes are common, growth retardation of newborn due to deprived nutrition (by swallowed amniotic fluid in foetus).

Investigations

Plain X-ray shows classic *double-bubble sign with absence of air in the distal part*. In partial obstruction, air may be present in distal loop and so contrast study has to be done. Risk of aspiration in newborn infant should be remembered. Ultrasonography will show distended stomach and proximal duodenum, *rail road track* duodenum and features of associated anomalies. Maternal and foetal ultrasound in pregnancy may identify the pathology and also maternal polyhydramnios.

Treatment

Proper preoperative preparations like correction of fluid and electrolytes; gastric decompression; TPN; injection vitamin K; evaluation for associated anomalies.

Duodenoduodenostomy is done. Associated malrotation should be corrected in these patients (Ladd's operation).

Side-to-side duodenoduodenostomy may cause dilated duodenum (megaduodenum—30%); anastomotic dysfunction; and delayed transit of the content. *Kimura's diamond-shaped anastomosis* between transversely opened proximal pouch and longitudinally opened distal pouch reduces the problems of anastomosis. Presence of bile in the duodenum and proximal and distal patency should be confirmed by saline irrigation. Horizontal incision on the proximal dilated part; vertical incision in the lower collapsed part to create diamond-shaped gap which is sutured above with middle of the lower diamond-shaped edge will appose to corner of the proximal upper wound to create duodenoduodenostomy. Interrupted 4-zero or 5-zero vicryl or PDS is used for suturing. Transanastomotic nasojejunal or gastrostomy tube for feeding purpose is needed as prolonged postoperative ileus is the usual problem. *Tapering duodenoplasty* may be required if there is persistent duodenal dysmotility with a megaduodenum **(Fig. 21-96)**.

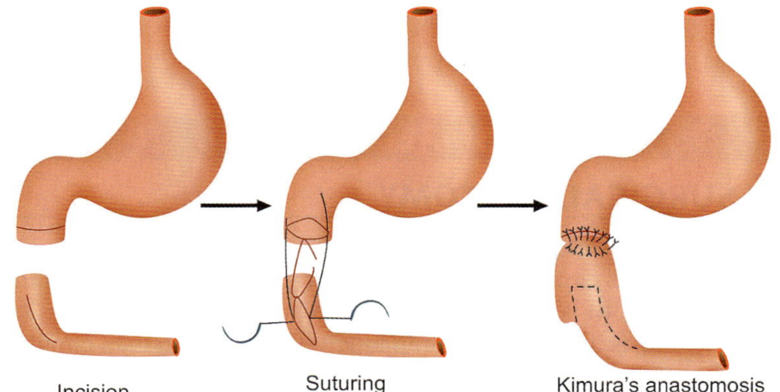

Fig. 21-96: Duodenal atresia is treated by duodenoduodenostomy ideally. Kimura's duodenoduodenostomy gives good results.

Duodenojejunostomy may cause blind loop problems. When gap and defect are long, retrocolic loop jejunojejunostomy is done. Gastrojejunostomy should not be done due to high incidence of marginal ulceration and bleeding.

22

CHAPTER

Surgeries of Small Bowel and Appendix

A. SMALL BOWEL

SURGICAL ANATOMY

The small intestine is 6 m in length. This includes upper fixed part (duodenum, 25 cm) and lower mobile part (proximal 2/5th is jejunum and distal 3/5th is ileum). Soon after death intestine elongates as muscle tone is lost much faster in longitudinal muscle than circular muscle. Through small bowel is 6 meters in length, its mesentery is only 15–25 cm in length at its *root*. Mesentery attaches the small intestine to the posterior abdominal wall, contains blood vessels, lymphatics and fat. Line of attachment of the mesentery is an oblique line starting from a point 2.5 cm left of the midline and 1.0 cm below the transpyloric line extending downwards to the right iliac fossa. It extends from ligament of Treitz at the level of L2/L3 vertebra to right sacroiliac joint **(Fig. 22-1)**.

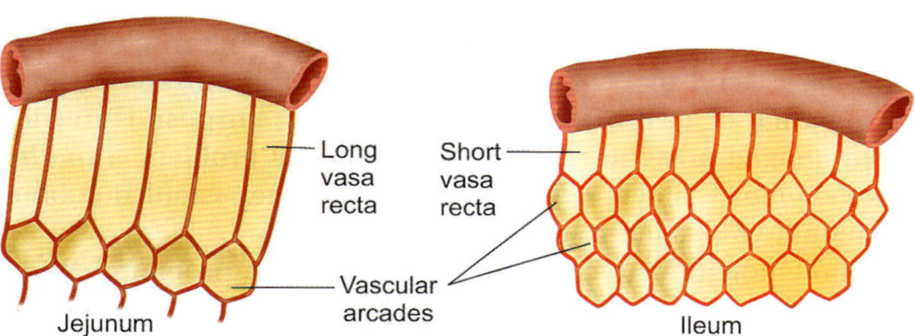

Fig. 22-1: Surgical anatomy of small bowel.

Differences Between the Features of Jejunum and Ileum

Jejunum	*Ileum*
1. Long and few vasa rectae	Short and numerous vasa rectae
2. Long plicae	Small plicae
3. Thick wall	Thin wall
4. Mesentery transparent	Mesentery contains fat
5. Peyer's patches are scanty	Peyer's patches are abundant, located in the antimesenteric border
6. Villi, leaf like and more abundant	Villi, finger like and less abundant
7. Proximal 40% of small bowel	Distal 60%

Small bowel wall contains serosa, longitudinal and circular muscles, submucosa, mucosa with muscularis mucosa. Submucosa should be included to achieve optimum integrity in anastomosis **(Figs. 22-2 and 22-3)**.

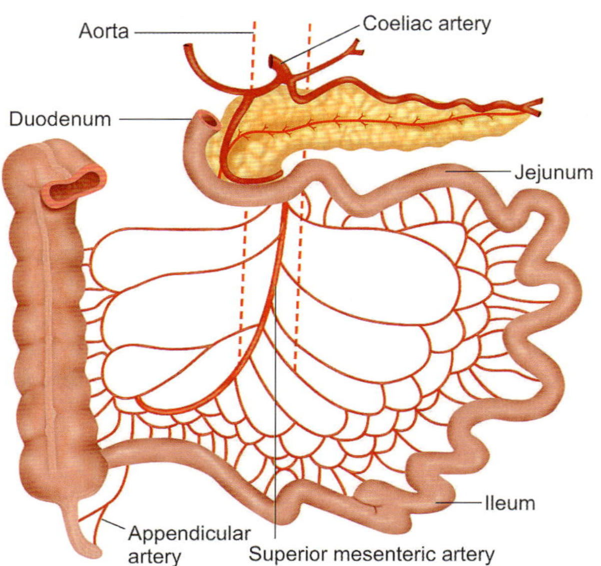

Fig. 22-2: Arterial supply of the small bowel.

Nerve Supply

Sympathetic supply is from T9-T11 and parasympathetic supply is from vagus. Both pass through coeliac and superior mesenteric plexus. Bowel wall contains the myenteric plexus of Auerbach which lies between the circular and longitudinal muscle coats; and submucous plexus of Meissner. Sympathetic nerves are motor to sphincter, inhibitory to peristalsis; parasympathetic nerves are inhibitory to sphincter and stimulates peristalsis.

Normal gastrointestinal tract (GIT) secretions

Saliva: 1000 mL
Gastric: 1500 mL
Intestinal: 4000 mL
Bile: 1000 mL
Pancreas: 1500 mL

Cell type function

Goblet cells: Mucous
Paneth cells: Lysozyme, tumour necrosis factor, cryptidins
Enterocytes: Absorption
Enteroendocrine cells: Different hormones

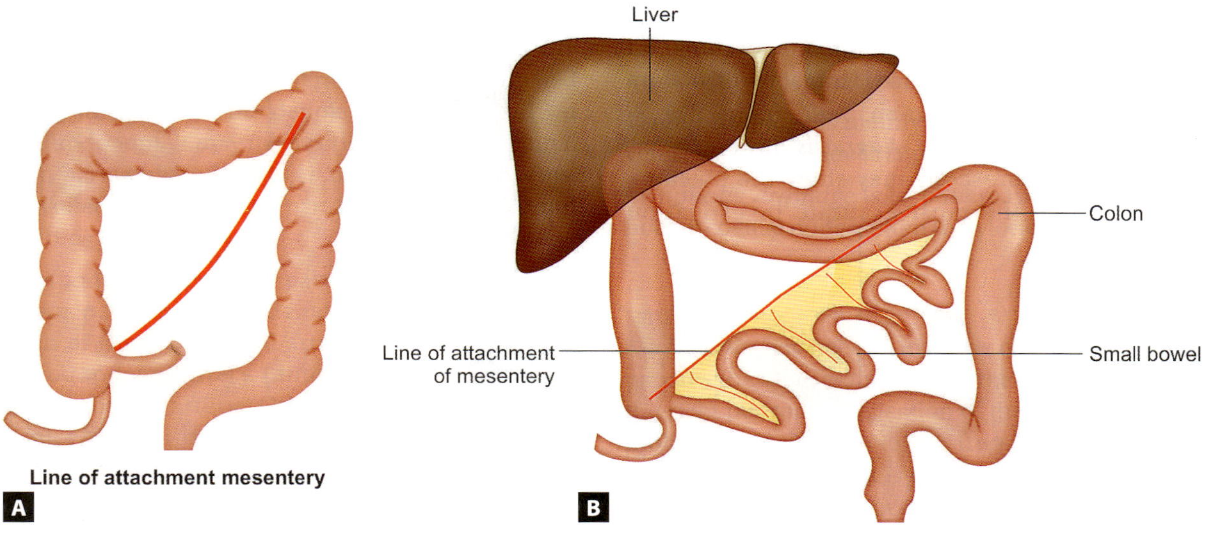

Figs. 22-3A and B: Attachment of the mesentery (small bowel).

SURGICAL TREATMENT OF MECKEL'S DIVERTICULUM

It is a congenital diverticulum arising from the terminal ileum and is part of the unobliterated proximal portion of the vitellointestinal duct **(Fig. 22-4)**.

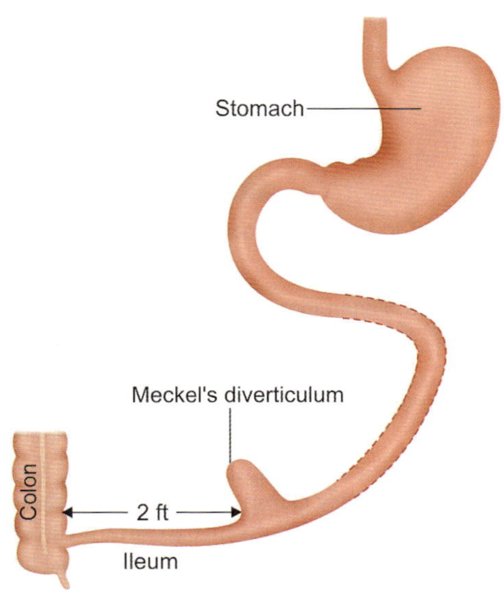

Fig. 22-4: Anatomy of Meckel's diverticulum.

It is 2% common; 2 feet from the ileocaecal valve; 2 inch in length; 2% of Meckel's diverticulum only will be symptomatic; 50% of symptomatic are below 2 years of age; 2:1 female preponderance is seen. It is congenital, results from incomplete closure of vitellointestinal duct. It is the most common congenital anomaly of small intestine. It arises from the antimesenteric border of the ileum, containing all three layers of the bowel with independent blood supply. In 20% of cases mucosa contains heterotopic epithelium like gastric (commonest—50%), colonic and pancreatic tissues (5%). It may be connected to or communicates with the umbilicus through a band or fistula. It may be associated with oesophageal atresia, exomphalos, and anorectal malformations **(Fig. 22-5)**.

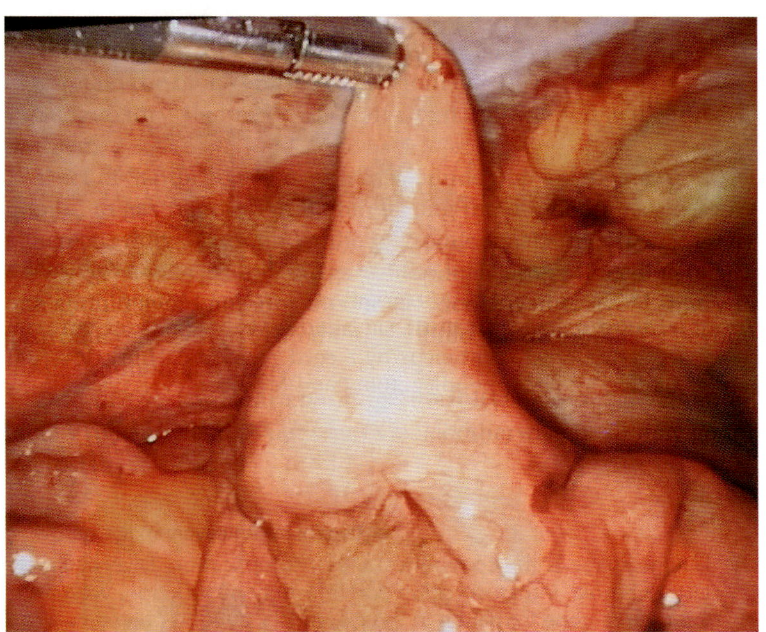

Fig. 22-5: Meckel's diverticulum—laparoscopic view.

Presentations in Meckel's Diverticulum

It is asymptomatic in majority of the cases. Severe haemorrhage is most common, presentation seen in children aged 2 years or younger *(Maroon coloured blood)*. It can cause intestinal obstruction due to bands/adhesions/intussusception, perforation, volvulus of small bowel, peptic ulceration, diverticulitis (20%)—features mimic acute appendicitis. *Littre's hernia*—it is the presence of Meckel's diverticulum in hernial sac as content. It is observed in inguinal/femoral hernia. Silent Meckel's diverticulum may be found during laparotomy or laparoscopy or by radioisotope study. Carcinoid or gastrointestinal stromal tumour (GIST) can occur in Meckel's diverticulum.

It is diagnosed by Technetium (Tc99) radioisotope scan which is very useful (90–95% accuracy). About 90% of heterotrophic gastric mucosa can be identified in Meckel's diverticulum by radioisotope study. It can detect Meckel's diverticulum with minimal bleeding also (0.1 mL/minute). So it is very useful investigation in children presenting with bleeding. X-ray abdomen is taken to see complications like obstruction, perforation. *Laparoscopy is very useful way to confirm the diagnosis.* Enteroclysis/small bowel enema under fluoroscopy may show the Meckel's diverticulum. It is probably the most accurate investigation **(Fig. 22-6)**.

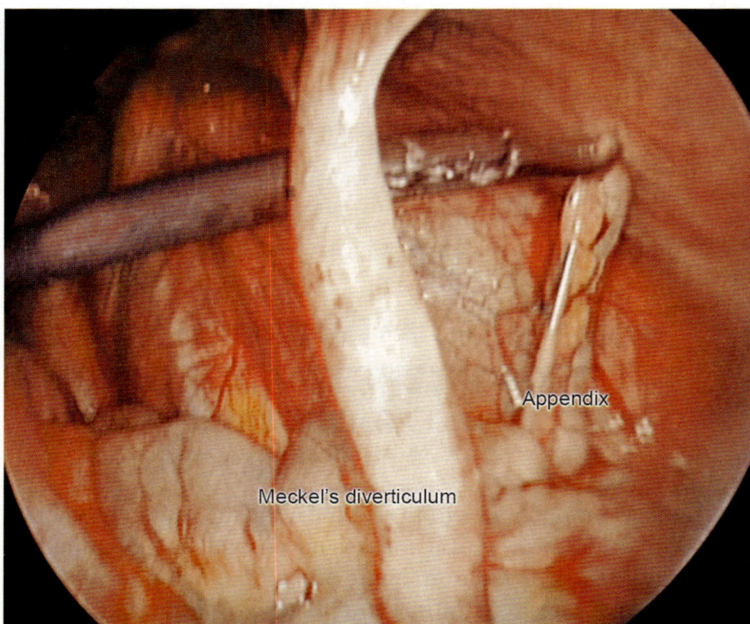

Fig. 22-6: Laparoscopic view of Meckel's diverticulum. Patient presented with features of acute appendicitis. On laparoscopy, Meckel's diverticulum which was adherent to umbilicus by a cord was found. Appendix was identified separately. Appendicectomy and Mecklian diverticulectomy was done.

Complications

Haemorrhage is the commonest (30%) complication. Diverticulitis, Littre's hernia, intussusception and intestinal obstruction, volvulus, adhesions, stone formation in the diverticula, daughter diverticula in the Meckel's, vesicodiverticular fistula formation, ulceration, perforation, neoplasm (carcinoid—45%) formation, presence of ectopic tissues [gastric (50%) and pancreatic] in the diverticula, phytobezoar formation in the diverticula—are other complications.

Treatment

Asymptomatic Meckel's diverticulum can be left alone when identified during laparotomy.

Surgical treatment

Surgery is done whenever the base is narrow, in lengthy diverticulum, in presence of adhesions or band which may precipitate obstruction, intussusception or volvulus in symptomatic patients or presence of complications, when found in children below 2 years.

Resection of a short segment of ileum containing Meckel's diverticulum and end-to-end anastomosis is done.

Meckelian diverticulectomy with closure of enterotomy also can be done, but chances of retaining heterotopic tissues and stenosis are higher **(Figs. 22-7 and 22-8)**.

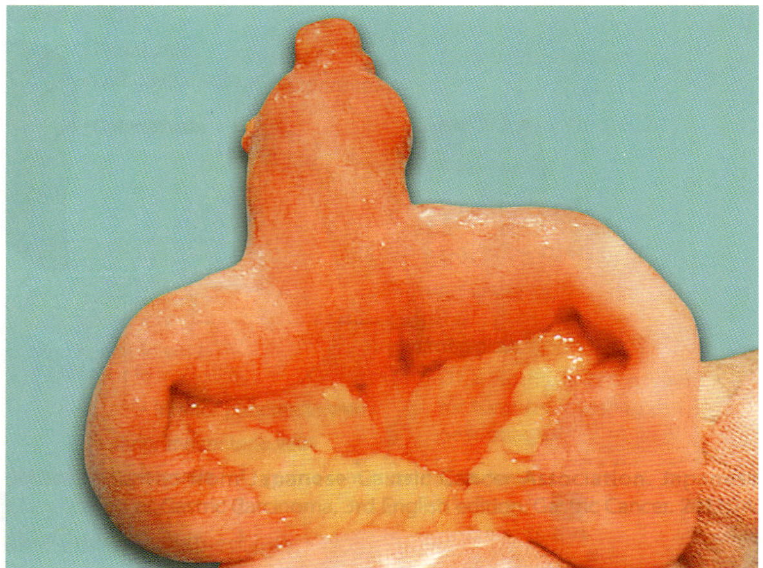

Fig. 22-7: Meckel's diverticulum on table look. Patient underwent resection and anastomosis.

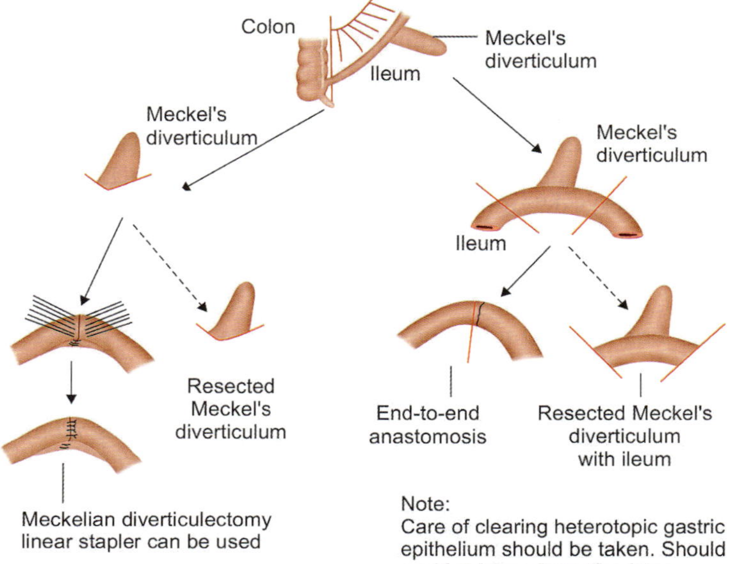

Fig. 22-8: Meckel's diverticulum—surgical treatment. Meckelian diverticulectomy is done by obliquely clamping beyond the base of the Meckel's diverticulum. Care should be taken not to retain heterotopic gastric (or other) epithelium which can be felt like indurated area. Enough precaution should be taken so that stricture will not form later. When heterotopic tissues extend beyond the Meckel's diverticulum into the ileum, then resection of ileum with Meckel's and anastomosis is done. Clamping distal to the base of the Meckel's diverticulum like appendicectomy should not be done. It will cause stricture, leak or retaining heterotopic tissues in the part.

SMALL BOWEL RESECTION

It is one of the common surgeries done in the abdomen. It may be in an emergency situation or an elective one.

Indications: Small bowel tumour, multiple perforation, trauma, bowel ischaemia, strangulation, Crohn's disease, intussusception **(Figs. 22-9 and 22-10)**.

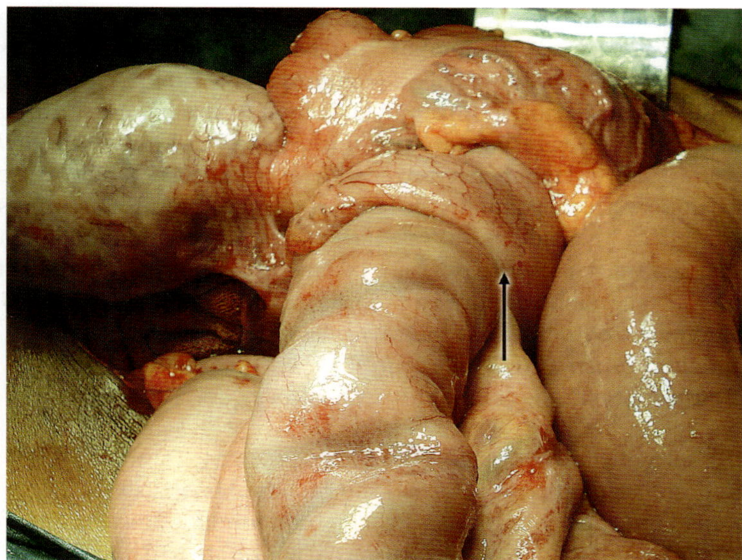

Fig. 22-9: Intussusception.

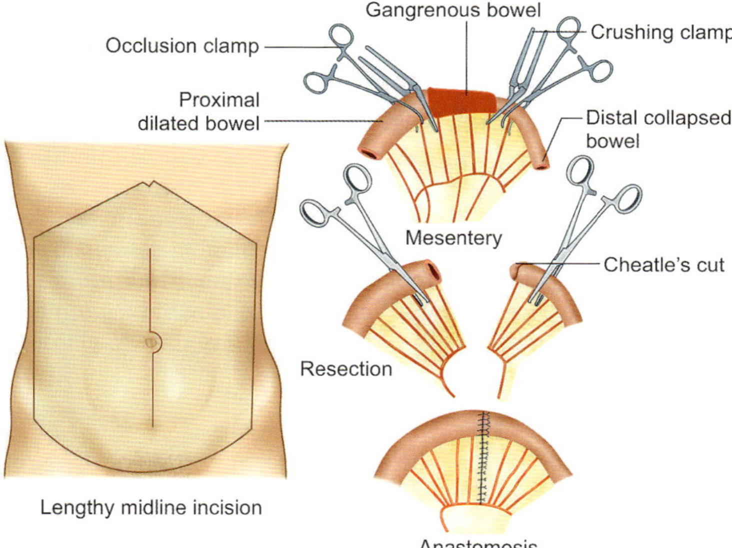

Fig. 22-10: Bowel resection and anastomosis for gangrene in case of intestinal obstruction. Cheatle's cut on the antimesenteric margin of the collapsed distal segment is often needed to avoid discrepancy in luminal width. Single layer interrupted (silk/vicryl) or two layered continuous sutures can be used. Single layer is better in acute conditions.

Principles in Bowel Surgery

Antimesenteric border has least blood supply and is so critical point in bowel anastomosis. So antimesenteric border should be cut obliquely while doing bowel anastomosis. Mesenteric arterial pulsation should be checked. Cut edge bleeding is very important. If surgeon is not satisfied about cut edge bleeding then one should trim the edge adequately. Blood supply is absolute deciding factor in bowel anastomosis.

Colour, peristalsis, pulsation in the arcade, bleeding suggests adequate blood supply. This is often confirmed by asking anaesthetist to give 100% oxygen for few minutes or by placing warm mop over the bowel or by on table Doppler study.

Serosal area should be *cleared off from fat* for 1 cm margin before doing bowel anastomosis. Fat will interfere with proper apposition of the cut edges. It also reduces the blood supply.

Luminal size of the anastomotic segments should be near equal to have proper serosal apposition. If it is not then narrower segment should be widened by incising antimesenteric border obliquely to widen the lumen (*Cheatle's cut*). Usually distal collapsed part will be narrower compared to proximal dilated segment; so commonly distal part needs Cheatle's cut.

Anastomotic edges should have free mobility; once anastomosis is done, stoma should not be under any tension. Release of adhesions, adequate mobilisation by incising the peritoneal layer of the mesentery may be occasionally needed.

Knot should be tied with only optimum force. Excessive force will strangulate the cut edges. Loose knot will leave a gap causing inadequate apposition.

While suturing anterior layer one should be careful in avoiding inadvertent bites of the posterior layer which will block the lumen partially causing stricture and obstruction. Bites should be taken at 5 mm gap with 5 mm thickness of tissue from the cut edge.

Handling: Bowel should be handled carefully using non-toothed dissecting forceps or finger; one should not use toothed dissecting forceps or Allis forceps.

Clamps over the bowel should be placed at 30 degrees at antimesenteric border. Clamps should not extend far into the mesentery. Occlusion clamps are applied at viable part to prevent spillage of contents into peritoneal cavity, to prevent oozing from cut edges of the bowel and to stabilise the gut. Crushing clamps are placed after ligation of mesentery just prior to cutting the bowel; it is applied on the specimen side. One should take care about avoiding twisting of mesentery prior to anastomosis after resection.

Corners of the cut edge of the bowel should be held with seromuscular sutures or Babcock's forceps to allow posterior layer to drop behind and to facilitate proper bite taking of the cut edges.

Anastomosis can be done as continuous layer or interrupted sutures. In acute conditions as there is oedema interrupted one is better. Single layer interrupted sutures are safer and equally good. If two layer anastomosis is done outer interrupted silk sutures are used; inner continuous absorbable sutures like vicryl or polydioxanone suture (PDS) are used.

Posterior layer knots are placed inside the lumen; anterior layer knots are placed outside. Posterior layer knots can be placed outside also but it is technically tedious and it does not make any difference in outcome. In interrupted sutures bites should be taken as all layers through and through and kept long untied; once all bites are taken along one (posterior) layer, they are tied together. In the same way anterior layer is sutured. But it needs more suture material and becomes costly. It is possible to place suture and knot immediately and consecutively to complete the anastomosis of one layer in elective cases. Probably in acute conditions where there is oedema and inflammation in the cut edge of the bowel all layer tying together should be done.

In two layer anastomosis first posterior seromuscular interrupted sutures are taken which should include submucosa (which is strongest); then posterior 2nd layer of all layer through and through continuous sutures are taken at 5 mm gap with 5 mm tissue thickness bites. It is locked in between to prevent purse string effect on the stoma (*posterior continuous locking sutures*). Usually this suture begins at mesenteric end, runs towards antimesenteric end where it can be adjusted for size discrepancy; same suture material is continued as anterior layer towards again mesenteric end from antimesenteric end; anterior layer is sutured as outside in and inside out each from opposite side as inverting suture (anterior inverting sutures) or as outside in and inside out each from side looping over the cut edge towards opposite (*Connell suture*). Anterior layer is sutured afterwards as interrupted seromuscular silk sutures **(Figs. 22-11 and 22-12)**.

Suture materials usually used are silk or polyglactic acid (vicryl) or PDS. Usually 3-zero suture materials are used. In difficult situations

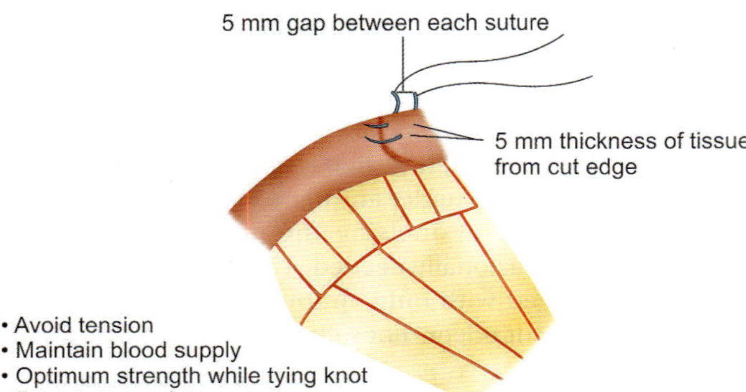

- Avoid tension
- Maintain blood supply
- Optimum strength while tying knot
- Do not strangulate
- Handle bowel carefully with non-toothed dissecting forceps or finger
- Do not use Allis forceps or toothed dissecting forceps
- Hold the corners with stay sutures on each side or Babcock's forceps
- Both two layers or single layer anastomosis are acceptable
- Continuous or interrupted sutures; interrupted sutures are preferred
- In acute condition like in gangrene interrupted single layer is ideal as due to oedema seromuscular layer suturing is difficult
- Knots in posterior layer can be inside the lumen in bowel; knot in anterior layer is placed outside; however, posterior layer outside knot placing can be done but it is technically tedious and there is no difference between two in relation to outcome

Fig. 22-11: Principles in taking bites in cut edges.

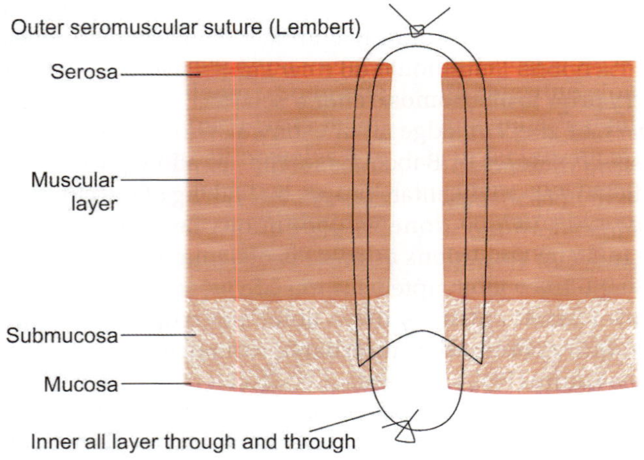

Fig. 22-12: Two layer suturing of the bowel wall.

2-zero may be needed. In children 4-zero is used. Curved round body needle is used.

After completion of the anastomosis, additional sutures at corners may be added to prevent possible leak.

Mesenteric defect should be closed using interrupted or continuous sutures.

In emergency conditions tube drain may be required.

To check for viability of bowel, look for:
- Peristalsis
- Pulsations
- Bleeding in mesentery and bowel wall
- Friability—friable, flabby muscle is seen in ischaemia
- Colour (black/pink)
- Dull, lusterless, without shining serosa is seen in ischaemia

Different suturing used in bowel are:

Single layer seromucosal suture of bowel: It is now well practiced method of suturing of the bowel. Interrupted seromucosal sutures using 3-zero/2-zero vicryl or PDS takes up well. Non-absorbable silk or linen can also be used. *These non-absorbable sutures are good old suture materials which are even now accepted well.* Only drawback presumed is formation of suture granuloma at the anastomotic site **(Fig. 22-13)**.

Gambee single layer full thickness (all layers) sutures using vicryl are also used in bowel anastomosis. It can also be used as continuous sutures especially during gastrojejunostomy. *Continuous suturing* is quicker; alternate bites should be locked to prevent purse string effect; anterior layer is closed with inverting sutures. *Interrupted suture* is more stable and stronger with less chances of anastomotic disruption. It also maintains the blood supply better than continuous sutures. Width of suture bite taken should be less over mucosal part than seromuscular part. Bites are taken 3 mm from the cut edge of the serosa; each bite is taken in a 5 mm gap **(Figs. 22-14A to D)**.

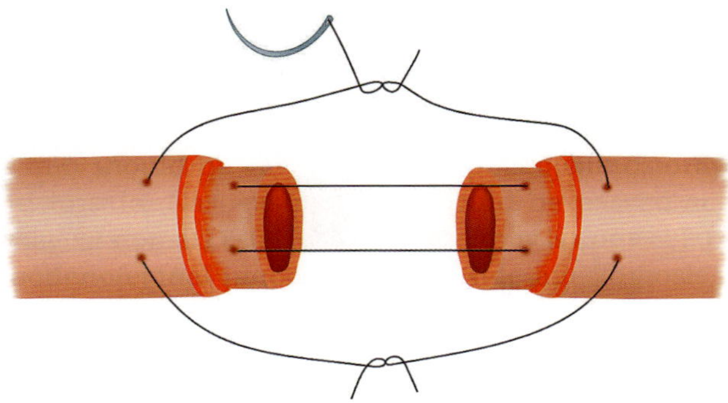

Fig. 22-13: Single layer seromucosal suturing of the bowel.

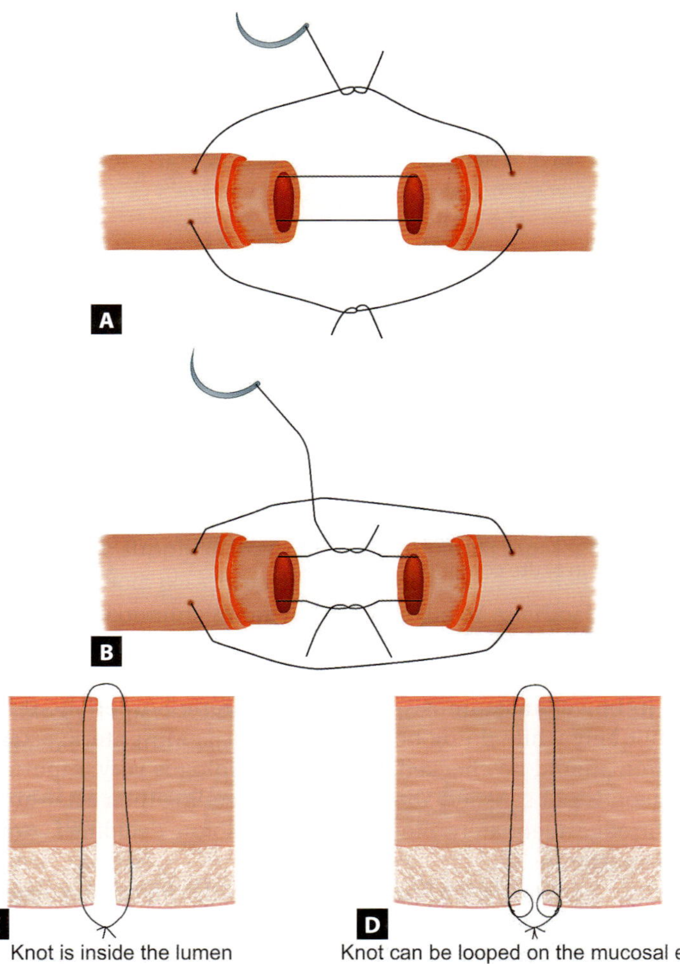

Gambee stitch is placed as all layers interrupted sutures.
It may be placed as **(A)** All layers interrupted suture from outer serosal through inner mucosa and from inner mucosa towards outer serosa with knot placing outside; ***OR*** as **(B and C)** All layer interrupted sutures from inner mucosal to outer serosa and from outer serosal to inner mucosa with knot placing inside the lumen; **(D)** Often here a knot can be looped inside the mucosa also.

Figs. 22-14A to D: Gambee suture.

Lembert suture: It is the commonly used seromuscular suture. Silk 3-zero or vicryl 3-zero is used. Deep seromuscular suture including submucosal layer is taken at a point 5 mm from the cut edge of the serosa; this bite emerges at same line (2 mm) from the cut closer edge of serosa; bite is taken on the opposite part of the bowel at 2 mm from the serosal cut edge as seromuscular which emerges at 5 mm point away in the same longitudinal line and knot is placed. It can be used as continuous suture also **(Fig. 22-15)**.

Cushing suture: It is similar to Lembert suture wherein seromuscular bites are taken parallel to the cut edge of the serosa (at 2 mm from the cut edge). Thickness of tissue taken is 5 mm. Both interrupted and continuous sutures can be taken **(Fig. 22-16)**.

Halsted suture: It is actually seromuscular horizontal mattress suture. Care must be taken to avoid excessive tension over the suture line as this may lead to ischaemia of the anastomotic site **(Fig. 22-17)**.

Connell suture: Here suture material passes through all the layers of the intestine from serosa to mucosa; again brought out through all layers of the intestine on the same side from mucosa to serosa; passed over opposite segment of the bowel; passing from serosa to lumen/mucosa and from mucosa to outside towards serosa; again coming towards same side to repeat the technique. It is very good technique to invert the mucosal part of the anterior layer. It is commonly used in double layer anastomosis but can be used in single layer anastomosis. Connell suture apposes well; achieves good mucosal inversion. But it is *not adequately haemostatic* and so bleeders on the cut edge of the bowel should be ligated or cauterised individually **(Fig. 22-18)**.

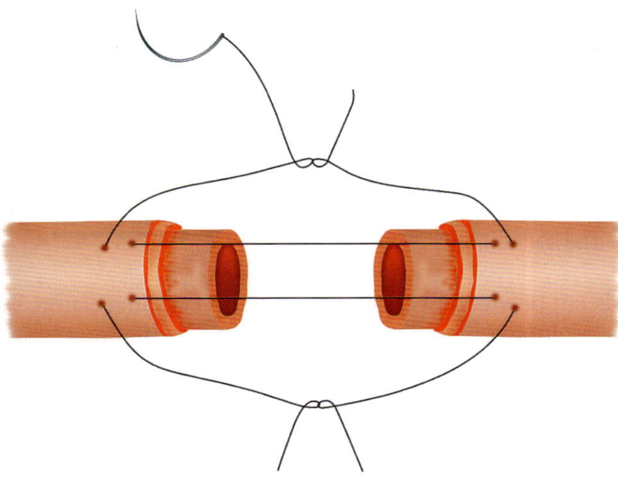

Fig. 22-15: Lembert suture.

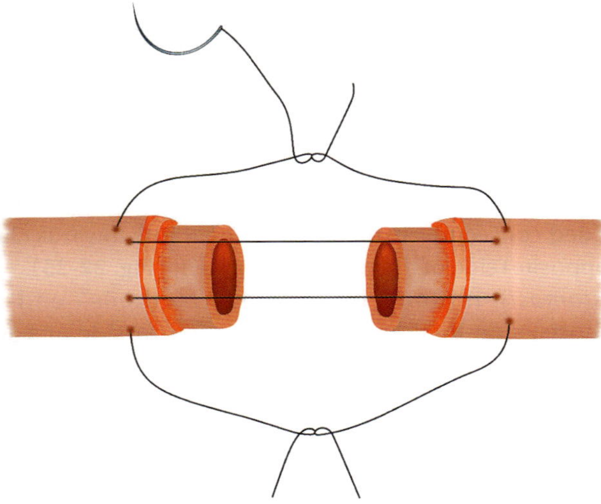

Fig. 22-16: Cushing suture.

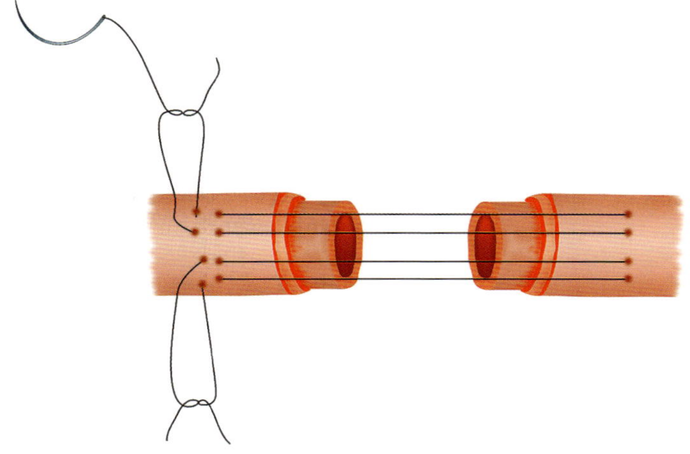

Fig. 22-17: Halsted suture.

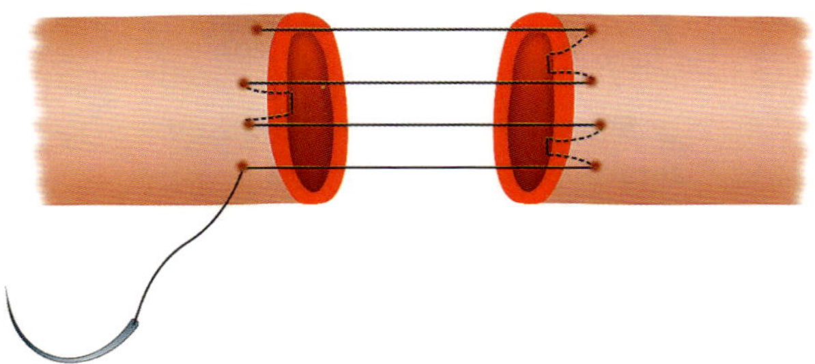

Fig. 22-18: Connell suture for bowel anastomosis.

Resection for gangrenous bowel should be done with division of mesentery very close to the bowel wall. In *small bowel tumour* mesentery is divided away at main branch vessel level with adjacent mesenteric lymph node clearance **(Figs. 22-19 to 22-21)**.

Any serosal tear during small bowel surgery should be invaginated transversely using interrupted silk sutures. It prevents adhesion formation and possible chance of postoperative perforation from serosal tear site.

Technique

Nasogastric tube and urinary catheter is passed. Under general anaesthesia with patient in supine position, upper midline incision or middle midline incision running over left side of the umbilicus is made **(Fig. 22-22)**.

After laparotomy abdomen is explored routinely. In obstruction, junction of the proximal dilated segment and distal collapsed segment is identified. In tumour, site of tumour is recognised. Entire small and large bowel should be inspected and palpated for additional pathology. Mesenteric lymph nodes should be looked for. Bowel to be resected is clamped using occlusion clamps on either side at the line of resection. Clamps should not extend far into the mesentery. These clamps should be placed obliquely. Mesenteric vasculature is studied using transillumination. Once vascularity is identified, small windows are made in avascular area using artery forceps and is clamped with artery forceps, divided and ligated. If mesentery is bulky it is better to place two clamps proximally and two ligatures; often it is also necessary to transfix proximal sides of the windows with transfixation sutures to avoid slippage of ligature and bleeding. In resection of tumour, main branch vessel close to that particular loop is clamped, ligated and divided to achieve nodal clearance.

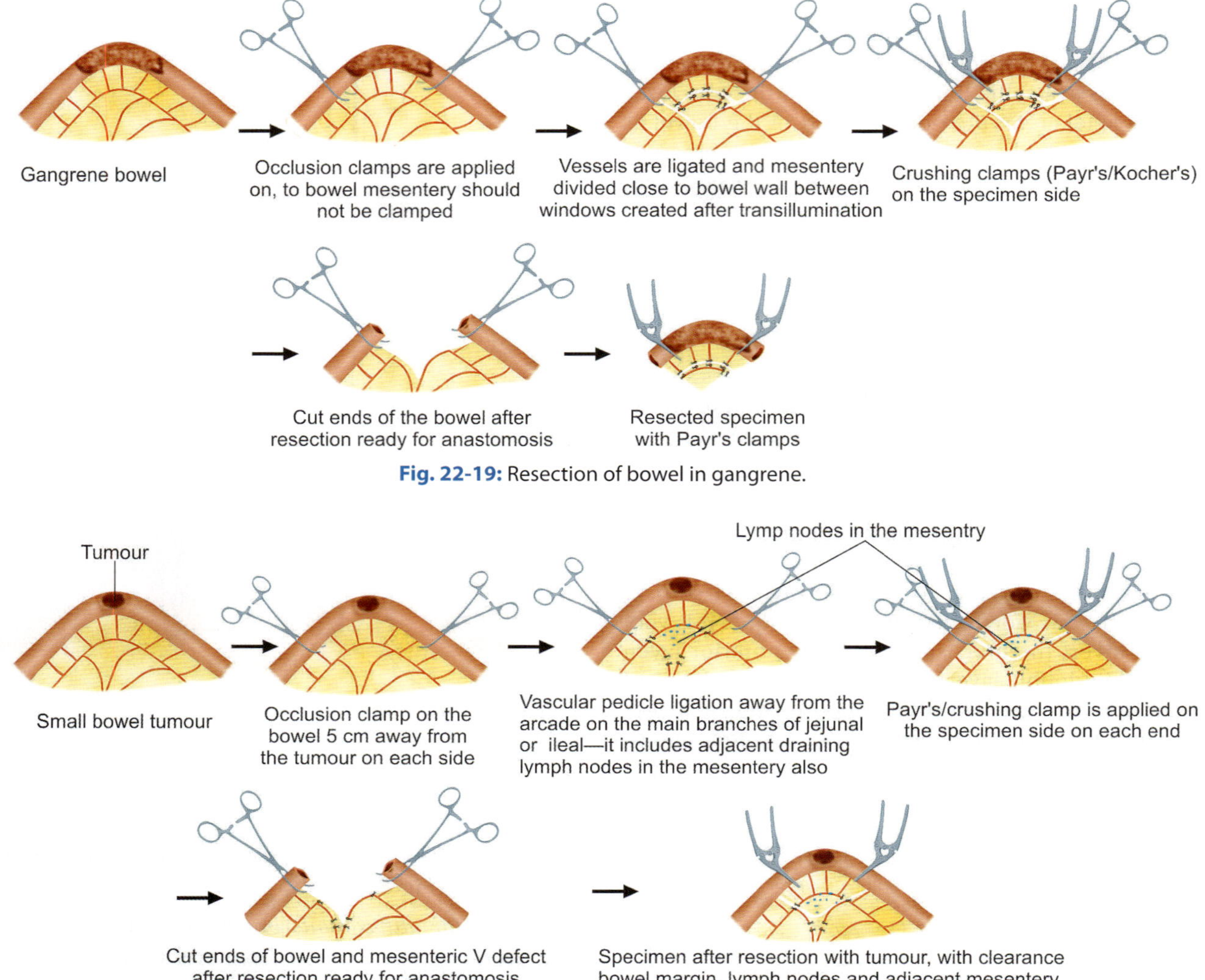

Fig. 22-19: Resection of bowel in gangrene.

Fig. 22-20: Resection of bowel in small bowel tumour.

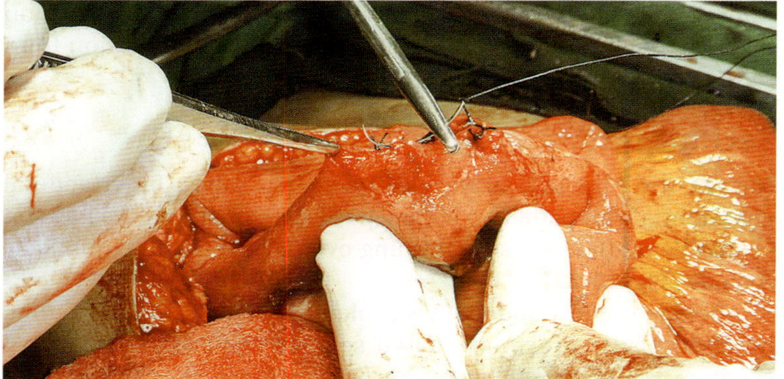

Fig. 22-21: Serosal tear suturing should be done as interrupted seromuscular suture using silk—3-zero.

Alternatively after creating two consecutive windows silk ligatures are passed and tied, two proximally and one distally and divided between proximal two ligatures and distal one; these tied ligatures should be cut only after dividing the pedicle/vessel. Instead of distal ligatures, artery forceps can be kept and left like that as it will come out with the specimen at the end which will avoid additional ligature passage but it is cumbersome because of so many instruments in the surgical field. In gangrene arcades are ligated close to bowel wall. All vessels entering the bowel are ligated and divided between two clamps. *Payr's* crushing clamp is applied on the specimen side; bowel is cut between occlusion clamp and crushing clamp. Division of bowel is done using no. 15 blade or cautery from mesenteric side to antimesenteric side; it is advisable to keep mop or flat instrument underneath to prevent injuring the deeper structures. Clamps should be at 30° angle to the antimesenteric part of the bowel and specimen is removed with the crushing clamp. In tumour, mesentery is ligated proximal to the arcade level away from mesenteric margin of the bowel at main vessels (jejunal or ileal branches) to include adjacent lymph nodes in the specimen; bowel should be divided 5 cm away from the outer margin of the tumour on both sides. Superior mesenteric vessels will be much closer to dissecting area in such situation and so should be careful while applying clamps in such situation. Bulk clamping should be avoided. Large area of mesenteric clamping also can lead to mesenteric tear and cause difficulty in placing ligatures. Small mesenteric segments are clamped, ligated and divided consecutively till one reaches across towards clamp on other (opposite) side of the resecting segment **(Fig. 22-23)**.

Anastomosis is done by different methods—end-to-end anastomosis; side-to-side anastomosis; end-to-side anastomosis **(Fig. 22-24)**.

Commonly *end-to-end anastomosis* is used. First step is to place a seromuscular Lembert suture at mesenteric side 1 cm from the mucosal cut edge; often this stitch is taken as a through and through all layer single suture which also acts as stay suture and is held with a small haemostat. If there is discrepancy in size between two ends

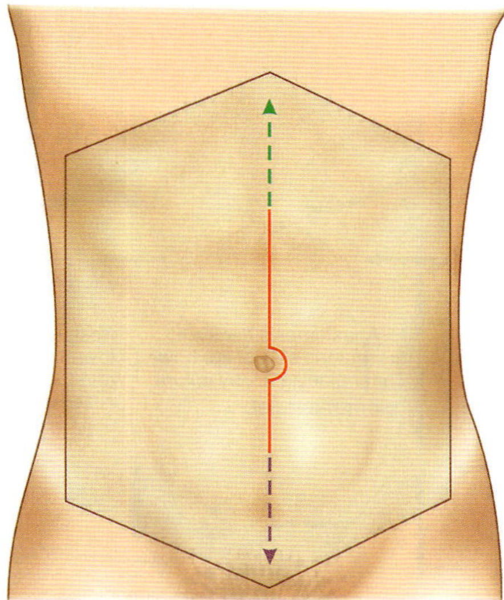

Fig. 22-22: Incision for bowel resection.

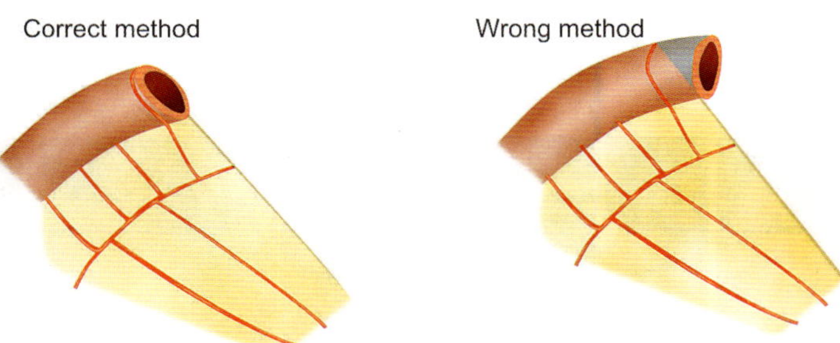

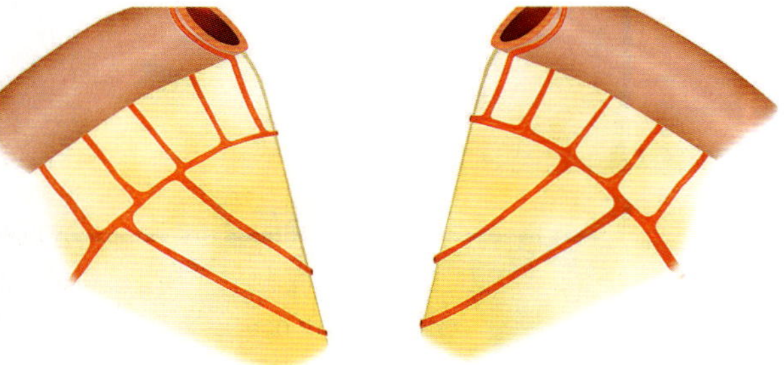

Fig. 22-23: Correct and wrong methods of dividing bowel margin.

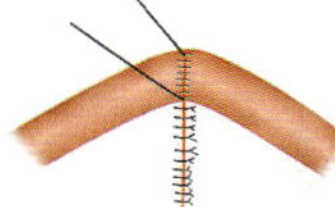

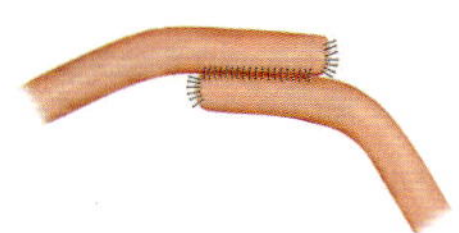

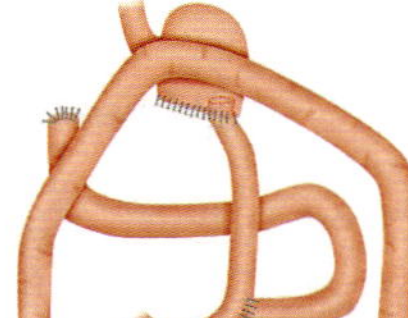

Fig. 22-24: Different types of bowel anastomosis.

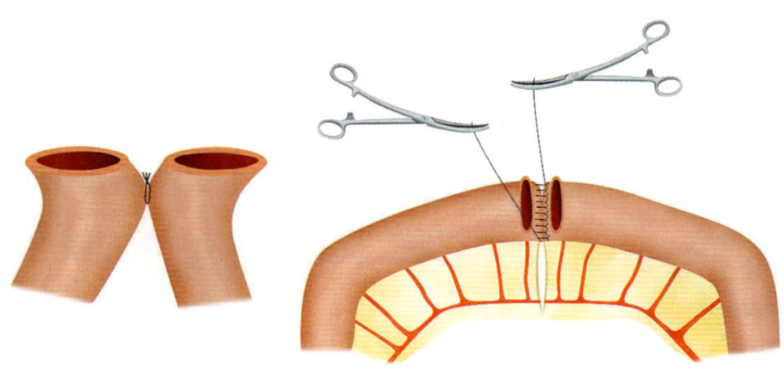

Fig. 22-25: Interrupted posterior outer seromuscular layer suture.

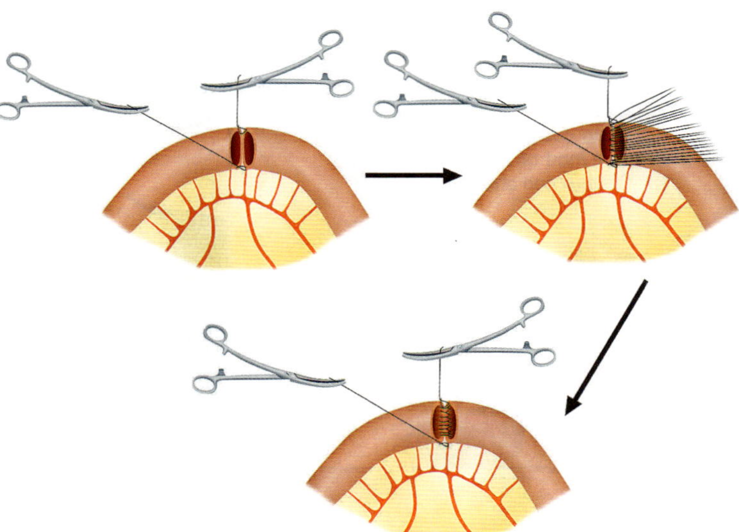

Fig. 22-26: Posterior all layer suturing is done as either interrupted full thicknes sutures (silk—3-zero); or continuous locking sutures using vicryl.

then *Cheatle's cut* is given to distal collapsed smaller sized bowel. Either single layer interrupted full thickness all layer sutures with 3-zero silk are placed or outer interrupted silk sutures with inner continuous vicryl sutures as two layers is used. After completion of the anastomosis stoma should be checked for patency and adequacy by placing fingers (two fingers); it is important to look whether sutured part is pink and healthy or dusky and unhealthy. If it is dusky then anastomosis is disconnected and edges are trimmed until it bleeds and anastomosis is redone. Supportive *crown stitch* is placed on the mesenteric side of the anastomotic site to avoid any possible leak. Tube drain is placed in difficult cases **(Figs. 22-25 to 22-31)**.

In single layered interrupted anastomosis, *Gambee stitch* is used as all layers through and through interrupted sutures which are placed in one of the two ways—(1) As bite is taken from outside serosa into the mucosa, then mucosa and serosa of opposite edge to get knot outside. (2) Another way is by taking bite from mucosa inside through the bowel wall towards serosa then through serosa and mucosa of opposite edge to place the knot inside the bowel lumen; here again before placing the knot additional loop can be taken at the mucosal edge as a loop to achieve better mucosal inversion. In single layer anastomosis often four quadrant (two on each side) seromuscular sutures are placed to relieve tension on inner layer.

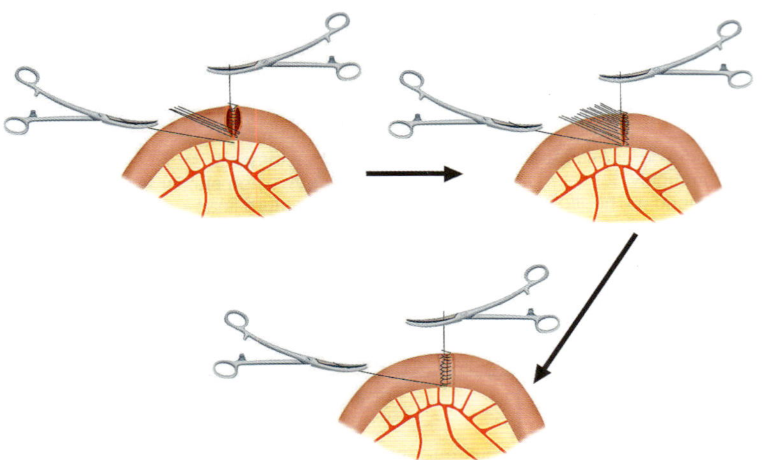

Fig. 22-27: Anterior layer interrupted suture in bowel anastomosis.

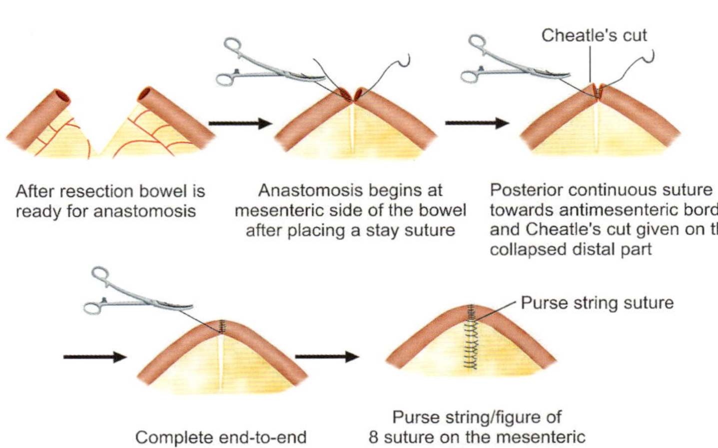

Fig. 22-28: Technique of end-to-end anastomosis.

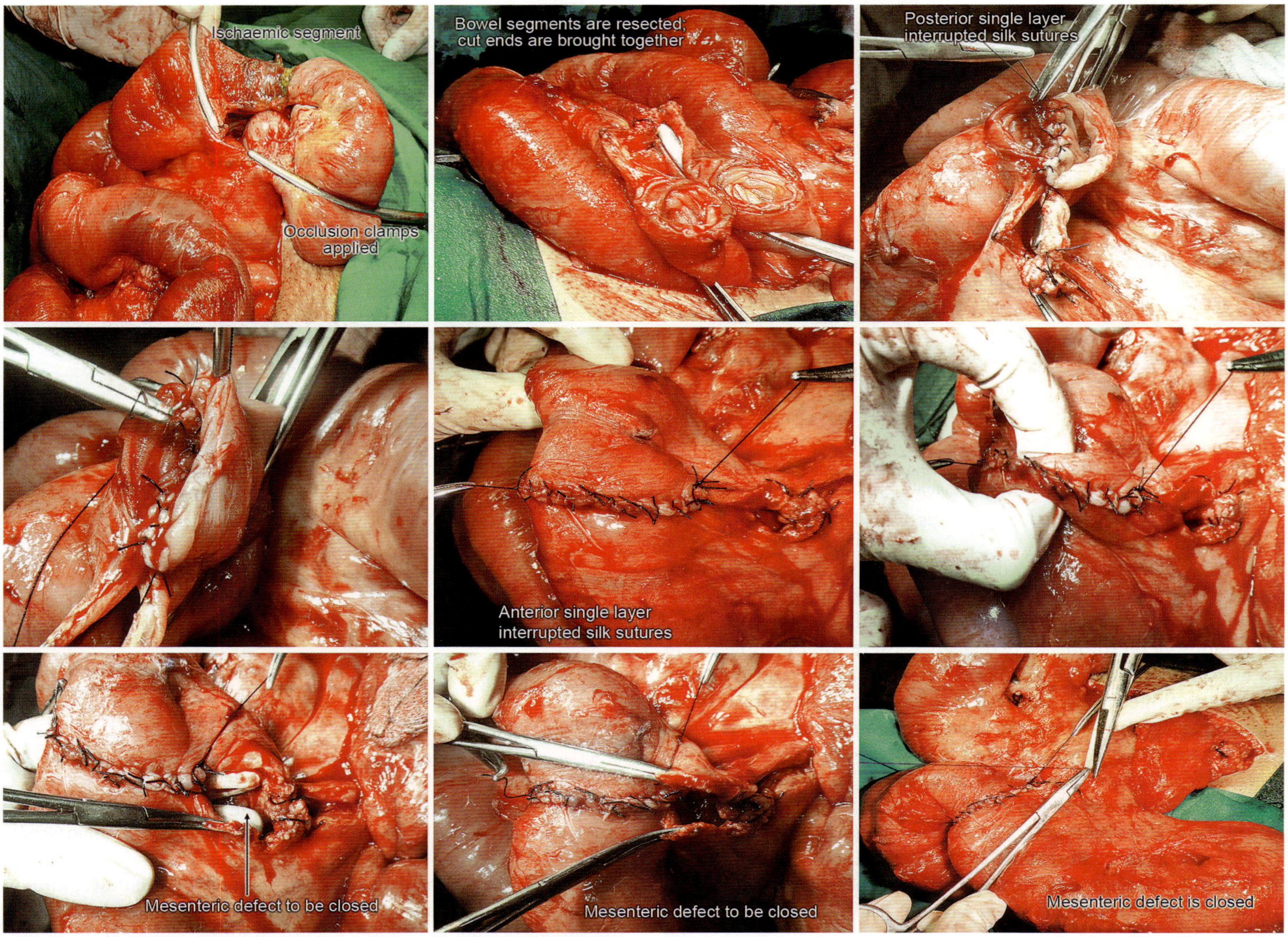

Fig. 22-29: Technique of resection and anastomosis.

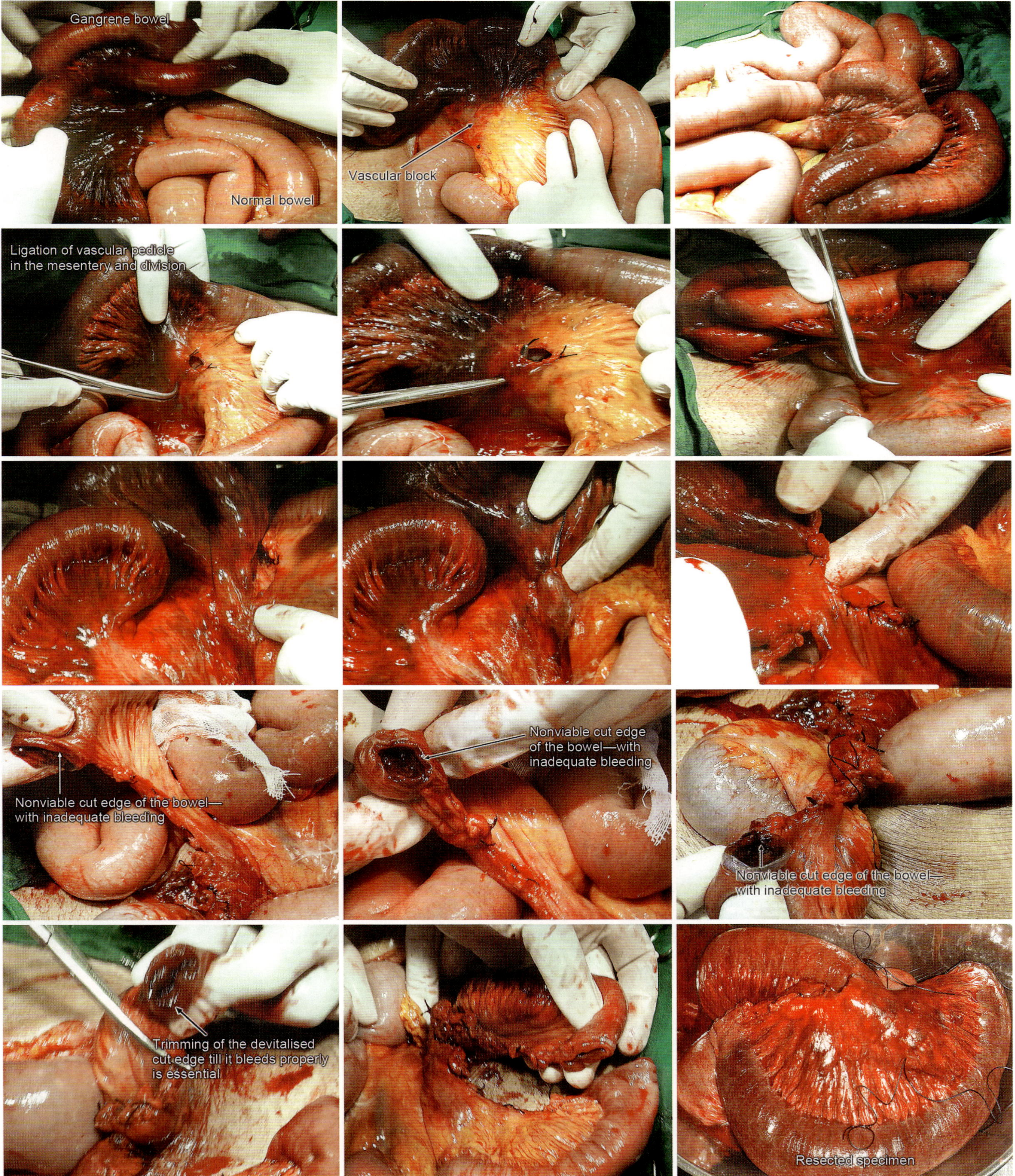

Gangrene bowel
Normal bowel
Vascular block
Ligation of vascular pedicle in the mesentery and division
Nonviable cut edge of the bowel—with inadequate bleeding
Nonviable cut edge of the bowel—with inadequate bleeding
Nonviable cut edge of the bowel—with inadequate bleeding
Trimming of the devitalised cut edge till it bleeds properly is essential
Resected specimen

Figs. 22-30(1)

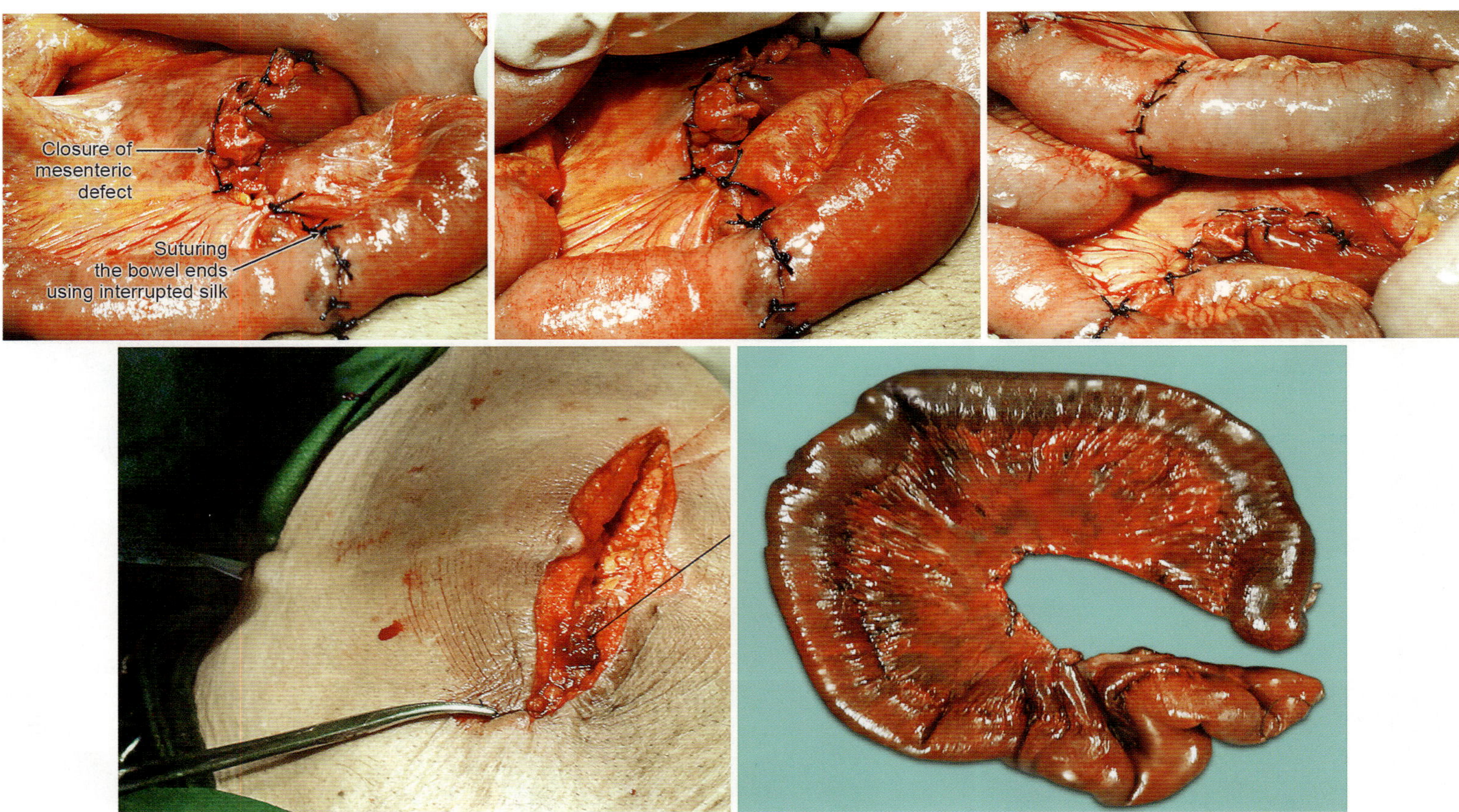

Figs. 22-30(2)

Figs. 22-30(1 and 2): Resection of bowel in (massive resection) extensive gangrene due to mesenteric artery thrombosis.

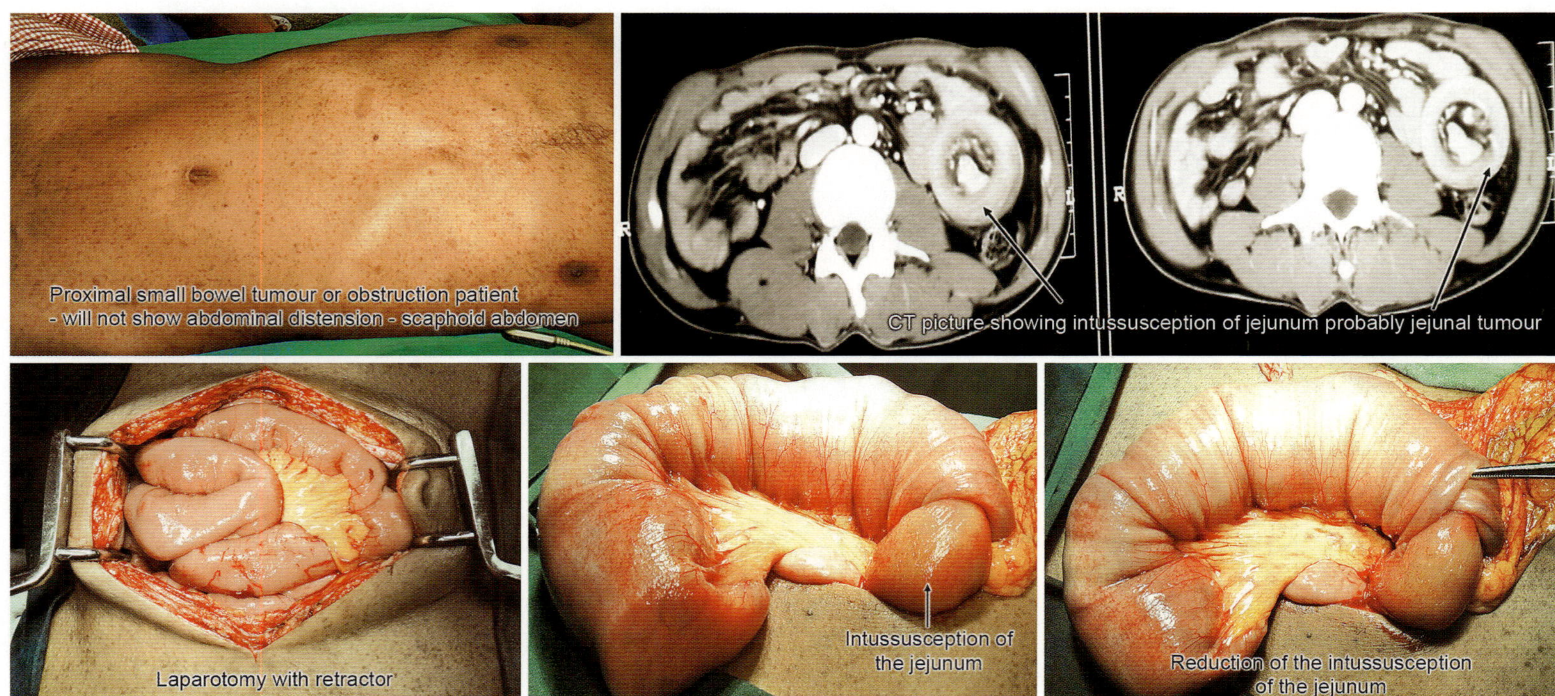

Figs. 22-31(1)

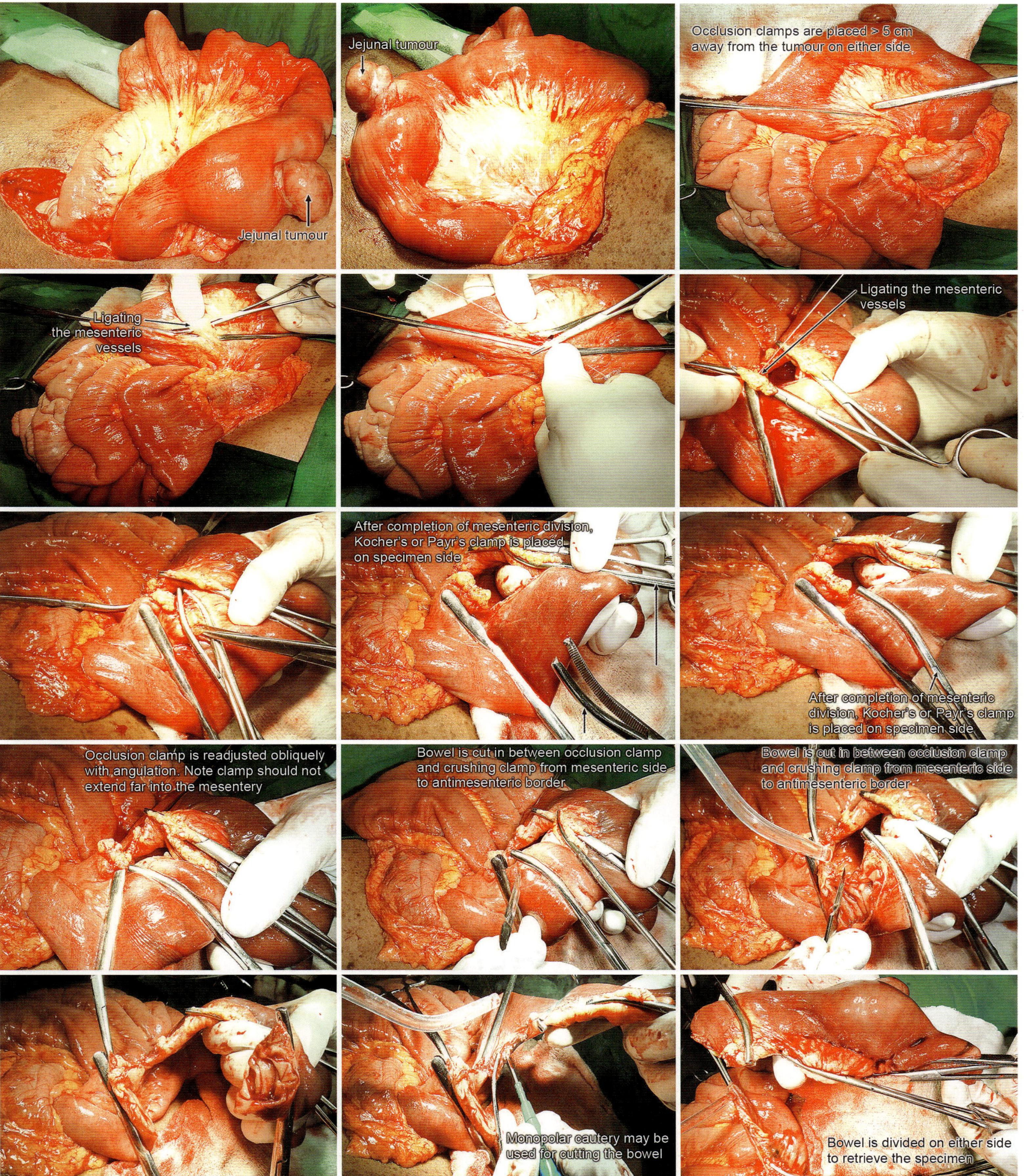
Jejunal tumour
Jejunal tumour
Occlusion clamps are placed > 5 cm away from the tumour on either side
Ligating the mesenteric vessels
Ligating the mesenteric vessels
After completion of mesenteric division, Kocher's or Payr's clamp is placed on specimen side
After completion of mesenteric division, Kocher's or Payr's clamp is placed on specimen side
Occlusion clamp is readjusted obliquely with angulation. Note clamp should not extend far into the mesentery
Bowel is cut in between occlusion clamp and crushing clamp from mesenteric side to antimesenteric border
Bowel is cut in between occlusion clamp and crushing clamp from mesenteric side to antimesenteric border
Monopolar cautery may be used for cutting the bowel
Bowel is divided on either side to retrieve the specimen

Figs. 22-31(2)

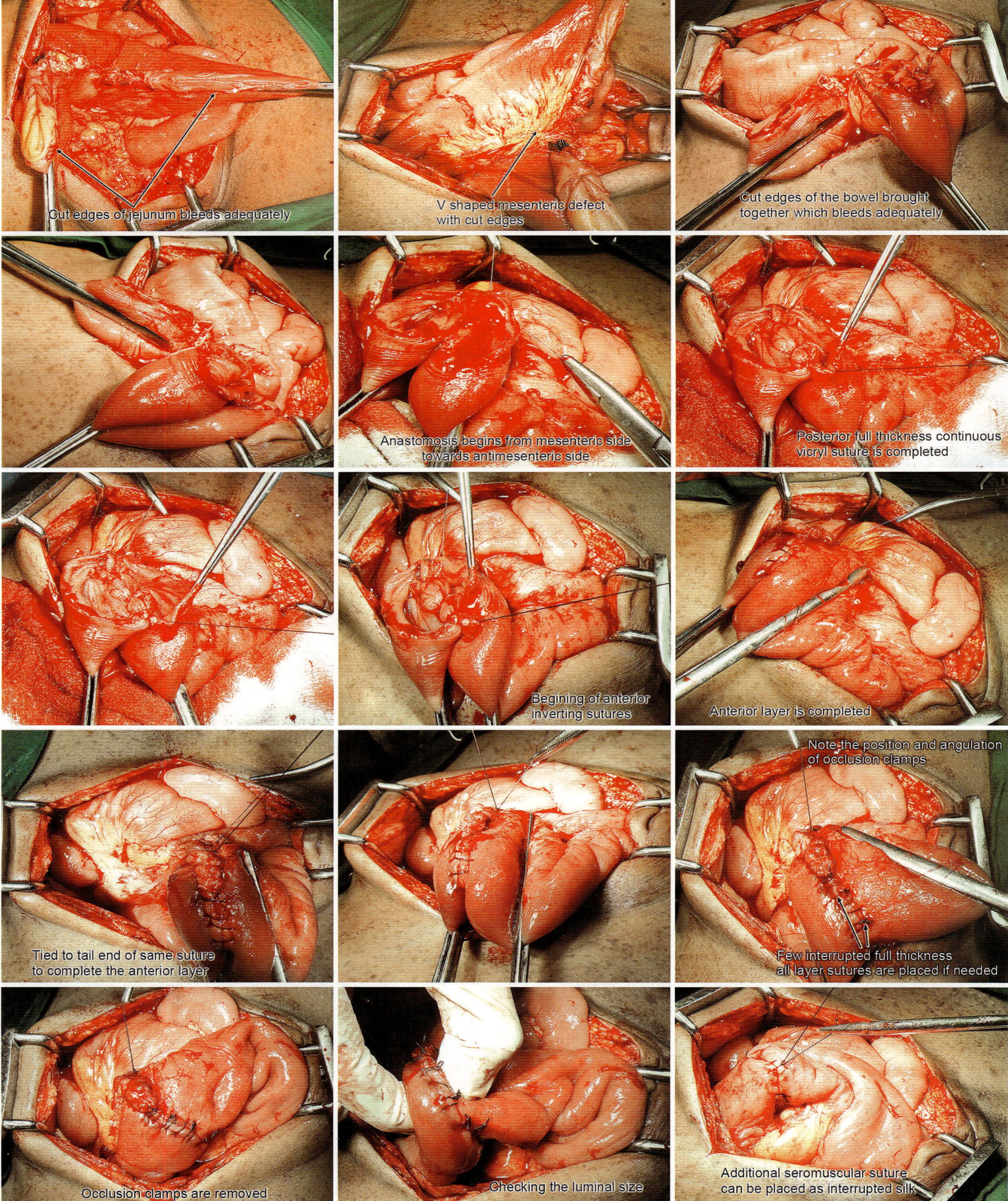
Cut edges of jejunum bleeds adequately
V shaped mesenteric defect
with cut edges
Cut edges of the bowel brought
together which bleeds adequately
Anastomosis begins from mesenteric side
towards antimesenteric side
Posterior full thickness continuous
vicryl suture is completed
Begining of anterior
inverting sutures
Anterior layer is completed
Tied to tail end of same suture
to complete the anterior layer
Note the position and angulation
of occlusion clamps
Few interrupted full thickness
all layer sutures are placed if needed
Occlusion clamps are removed
Checking the luminal size
Additional seromuscular suture
can be placed as interrupted silk

Figs. 22-31(3)

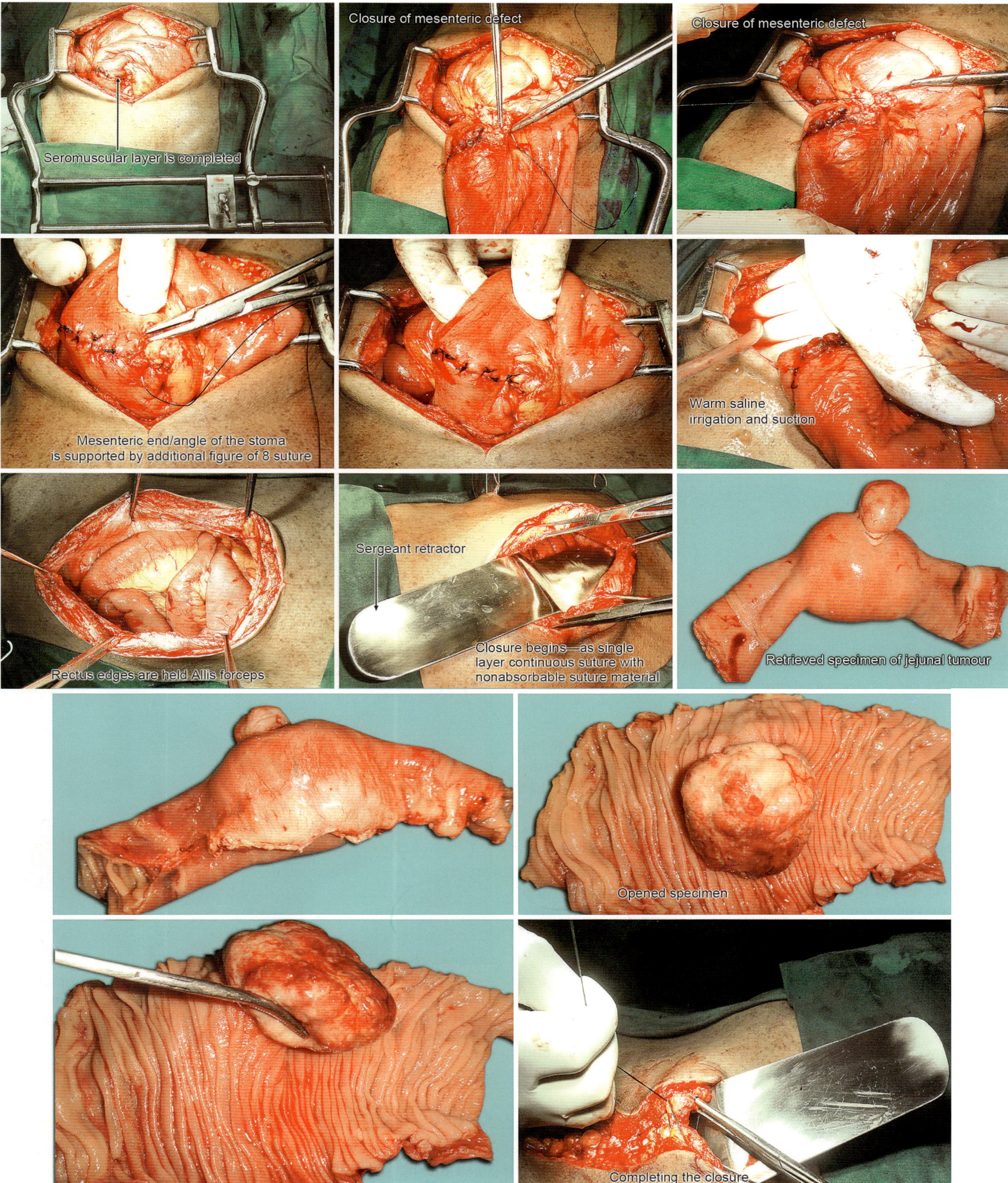

Figs. 22-31(4)

Figs. 22-31(1 to 4): Resection of jejunal tumour and end-to-end anastomosis.

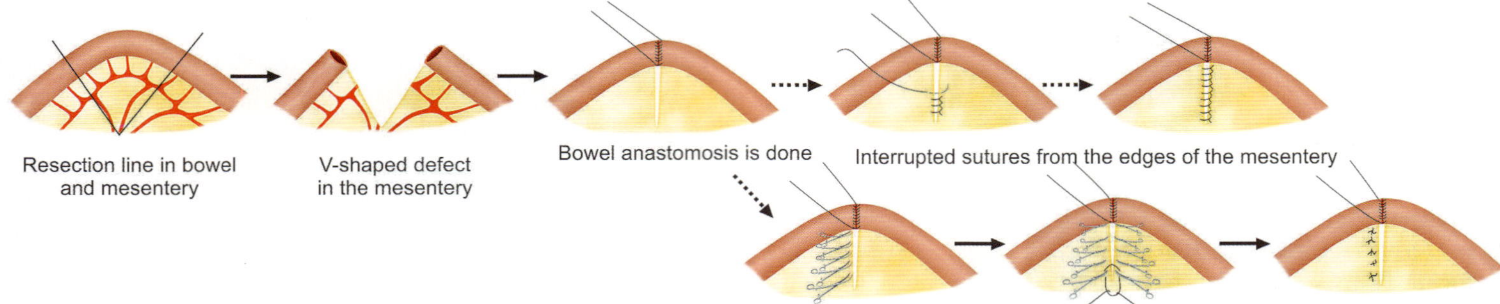

Fig. 22-32: Closure of mesenteric defect using interrupted sutures.

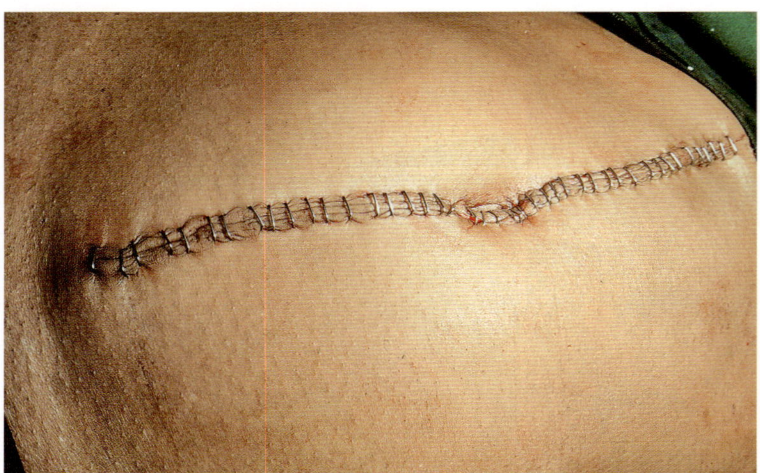

Fig. 22-33: Laparotomy wound closed after resection and anastomosis.

Parker Kerr basting stitch previously was in use; after applying Parker Kerr clamps, basting Cushing's continuous suture bites are taken on the seromuscular layer over the clamp on each side circumferentially and then clamps are released.

V-shaped mesenteric defect is closed with interrupted silk sutures (ideal); often corresponding parts of the edges are held together with haemostats and ligature is tied around each pair to close the mesenteric defect (as here needle bite is not taken needle bite bleeding and haematoma of the mesentery will not occur—Devine's technique of closing the mesenteric defect). Continuous suturing even though mesenteric practiced causes troublesome tear at mesenteric edge and bleeding **(Figs. 22-32 and 22-33)**.

Problems and Complications

Friable bowel wall with poor blood supply can lead into leak and enterocutaneous fistula. Ileostomy may be better in such situation rather than doing anastomosis.

Sepsis, subphrenic abscess and pelvic abscess can occur.

ENTEROLYSIS/ADHESIOLYSIS

Adhesions and bands are the most common causes of intestinal obstruction in Western countries. In India, hernia and then adhesions are the two common causes of intestinal obstruction **(Fig. 22-34)**.

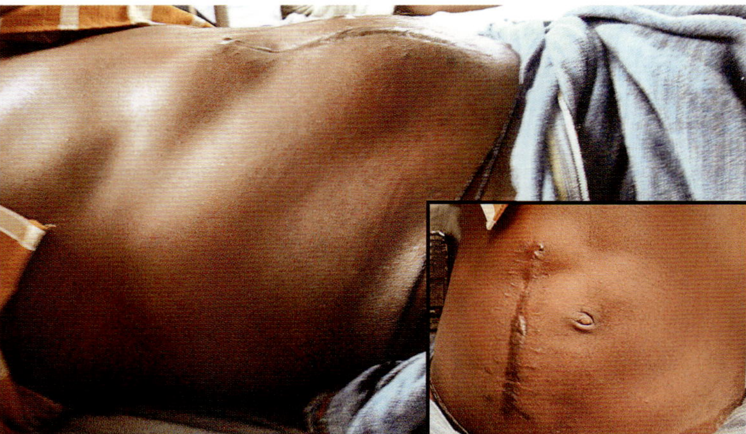

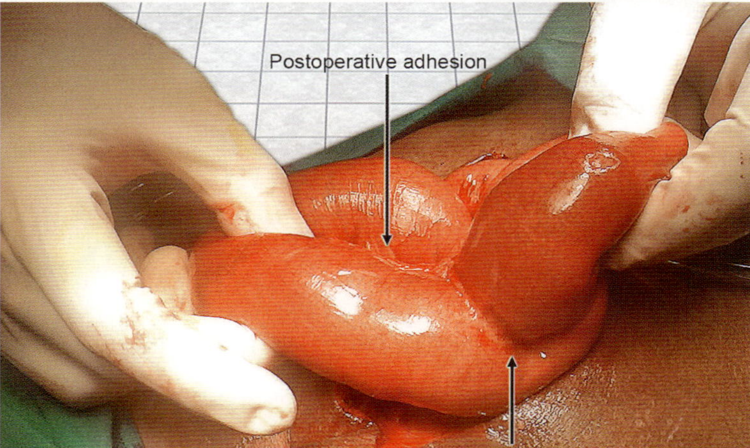

Fig. 22-34: Step ladder peristalsis in intestinal obstruction. Postoperative adhesions have become commonest cause of intestinal obstruction. Note the abdominal distension in a previous laparotomy patient and on table adhesions.

Causes

Infection due to peritonitis; appendicitis; postlaparotomy; materials used during surgery can cause dense inflammatory reactions—suture materials like silk, thread, and foreign body, mop, and gauze, talc powder; drugs like sulphonamides and penicillins; ischaemia of bowel due to poor blood supply; gynaecological conditions;

bowel injury; radiation-induced enteritis, Crohn's disease and other inflammatory bowel diseases; specific conditions like tuberculosis, malignancy **(Figs. 22-35 and 22-36)**.

Note:

- It is often called as *adhesive small bowel obstruction* (ASBO). 80% cases showed earlier laparotomies; 35% multiple laparotomies. In such patients 75% of surgeries are emergency ones.
- *Causes may be classified as: Congenital* adhesions; *Ischaemic*—reduced blood supply of the bowel, *Traumatic*—patients have undergone laparotomies for intra-abdominal injuries; *Irritants*—talc powder used for gloves, starch, antibiotics, non-absorbable suture materials, gauze and cotton filaments, barium; *Inflammatory*—appendicitis, cholecystitis, pelvic infection, Crohn's disease, tuberculosis; *Others*—serosal denudation during surgery precipitates adhesions.
- Initial cause ischaemia/injury → inflammatory exudates → fibrinous adhesions → fibrous adhesion → fibrinolysis. Fibrinous adhesion is avascular. Often thick vascular adhesions develop. Adhesions can be localised or extensive.

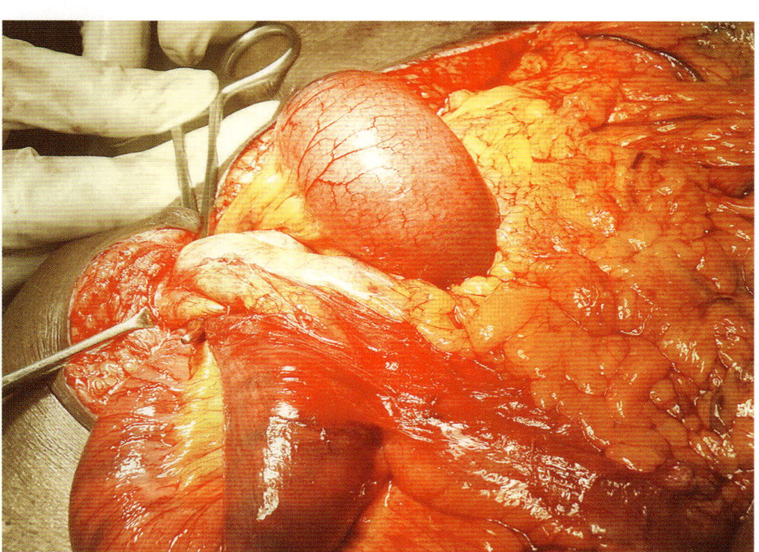

Fig. 22-35: Band with adhesions causing intestinal obstruction.

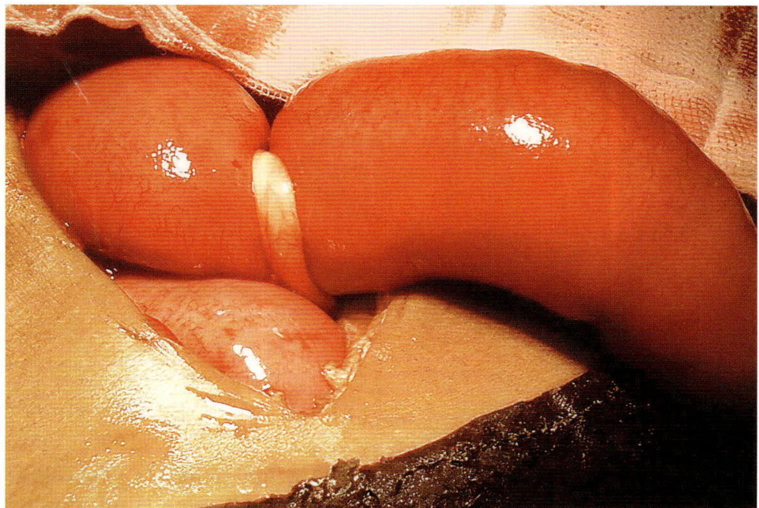

Fig. 22-36: A band causing stricture of small bowel.

Types

Type I: Fibrinous adhesions occur during 5th to 10th postsurgical period. It usually gets resolved completely. It is avascular and flimsy.

Type II: Fibrous adhesions. Due to lack/poor blood supply, bowel gets attached to part of the peritoneum or omentum or other parts of the bowel with dense vascular adhesions to maintain blood supply. It will persist and precipitate intestinal obstruction, often subacute and recurrent type.

Adhesions due to tuberculosis are severe, dense and difficult to separate.

Obstruction due to Bands

These are *dense fibrous strings* attached from one portion of the abdomen to another area or bowel causing entrapment of intestines leading into obstruction and often dangerous *strangulation*. Common causes are vitellointestinal duct, Ladd's band, omental band, postsurgical fibrous band, tuberculous band.

Clinical features are like that of intestinal obstruction. Management is release of the band either through laparoscopy or through laparotomy.

Features

Pain abdomen—colicky type and recurrent and episodic; distension, vomiting, constipation; reduced bowel sounds on auscultation; previous surgical scars commonly observed; dehydration, tachycardia, hypotension.

Commonest symptom in adhesions is ***pain*** which is sharp, sudden, recurrent, episodic and colicky. Colicky pain is more common in midlevel obstruction. *Gilroy Bevan triad* of adhesive pain is: (1) Pain may get aggravated or relieved on change of posture. (2) Pain in the region of old abdominal scar. (3) Tenderness is elicited by pressure over the scar.

Lower adhesions will have more distension compared to proximal adhesion.

Often it presents with features of obstruction initially, later features of strangulation (toxicity, fever, tachycardia, guarding, rigidity, rebound tenderness). Adhesions may be asymptomatic for many years but later become symptomatic.

Plain X-ray abdomen shows dilated bowel loops; oral contrast with CT scan is very useful; only in partial obstruction enteroclysis with water-soluble iodine dyes can be done.

Level of obstruction should be assessed probably by X-ray and CT scan; CT may show radiological features of strangulation—intramesenteric fluid; mesenteric oedema, congestion, bowel wall thickening more than 2 mm, reduced mural enhancement in strangulated bowel compared to adjacent bowel. Small bowel loop may go for volvulus showing *Whirl sign* in CT scan which is due to whirlpool mesentery of that part of the bowel. Electrolyte estimation, total count, serum creatinine, blood grouping—are needed **(Figs. 22-37 and 22-38)**.

Treatment

Initial Treatment

Intravenous fluids, nasogastric aspiration, antibiotics, often per anal flatus tube insertion, commonly patient responds in 4–5 days of therapy.

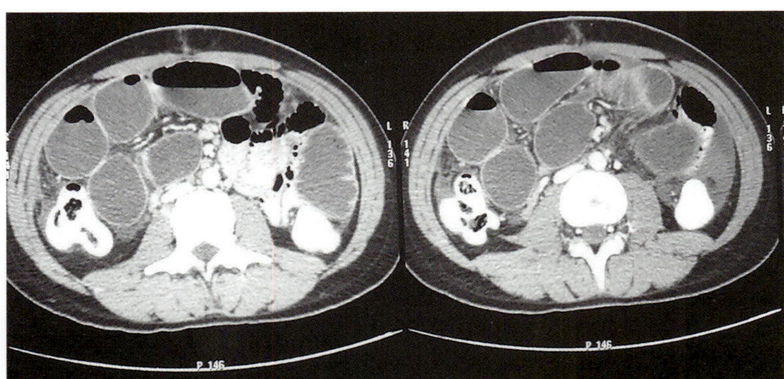

Fig. 22-37: CT is ideal and diagnostic for intestinal obstruction.

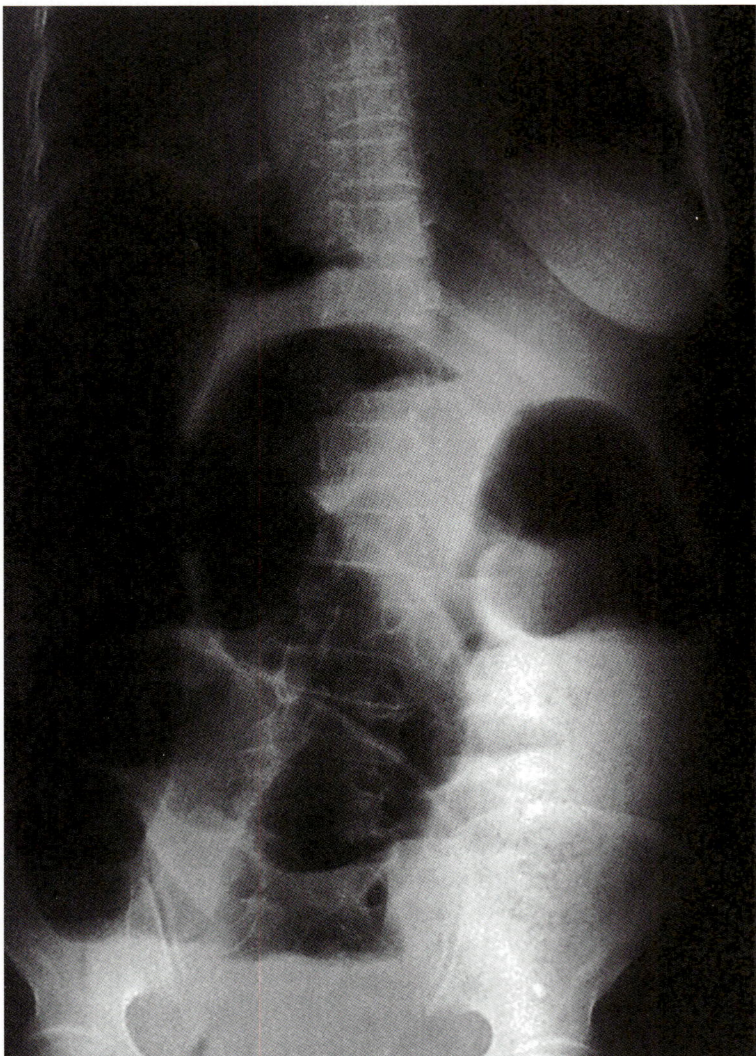

Fig. 22-38: X-ray showing small bowel obstruction with multiple air fluid levels.

Later Treatment

Open surgical adhesiolysis using fingers gently.

Laparoscopic adhesiolysis is becoming popular, safer, and ideal with less recurrent adhesion rate and good results **(Fig. 22-39)**.

Noble's plication of intestines—wherein adjacent coils of small bowel are sutured to prevent going in for further recurrent adhesions.

Childs-Phillips mesenteric plication is a similar way of plication of intestinal mesentery, which will prevent crumpling of bowel and adhesion formation.

Passing long stiff tube from exterior through an opening in the proximal bowel up to the entry into the large bowel, which acts as intraluminal splinting **(Figs. 22-40 and 22-41)**.

Intestinal intubation is technically difficult with chances of perforation and fistula formation. *Baker's tube* insertion through *jejunostomy* site; *Stewardson insertion of Baker tube* through nasogastric route; In *Nelson and Nyhus* method, 2nd balloon to Baker tube 25 cm proximal to the first to facilitate easier insertion of the tube—are different tubes and techniques used **(Figs. 22-42 and 22-43)**.

Expandable polytetrafluoroethylene (PTFE) membrane barriers or hyaluronic acid and carboxymethyl cellulose membrane barriers are also used.

Surgical Treatment for Adhesions—Enterolysis

Adhesions are common causes of intestinal obstruction. Usual treatment is adhesion release either through open or laparoscopic approach. Laparoscopic approach has become standard now. However principles of adhesiolysis are similar in both approaches.

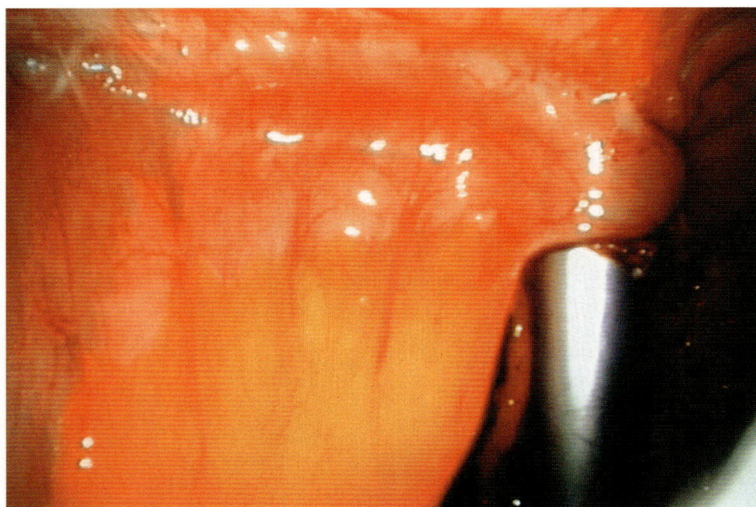

Fig. 22-39: Laparoscopic view of dense adhesions—postoperative cause.

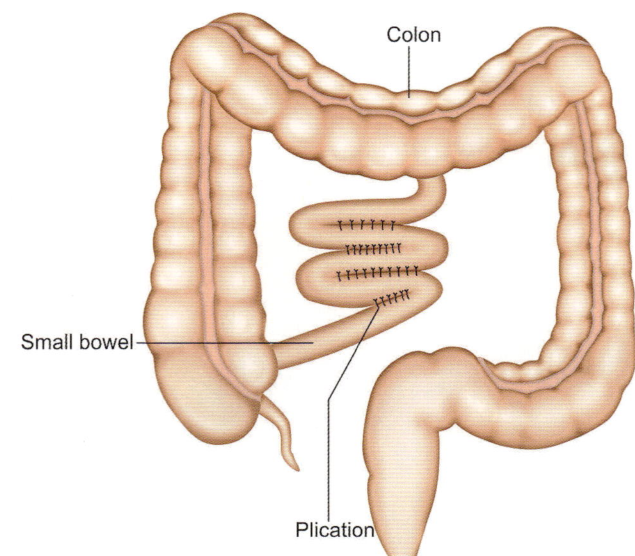

Fig. 22-40: Methods used to prevent recurrent adhesions and so to reduce the chances of intestinal obstruction. Noble's plication is plication of intestines.

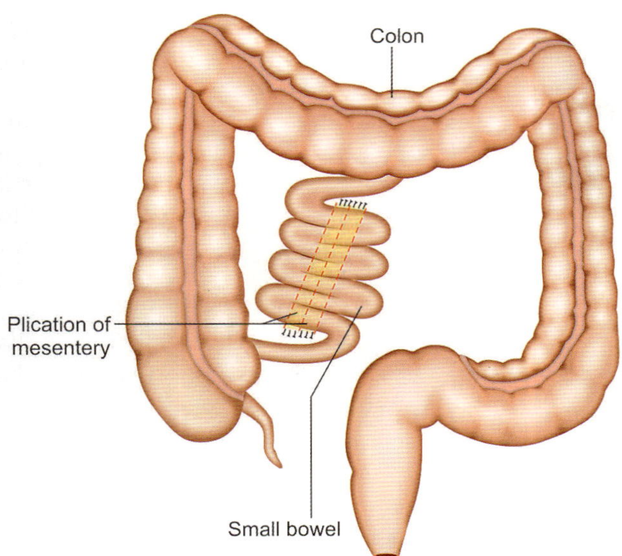

Fig. 22-41: Childs-Phillips operation done to prevent adhesive obstruction by plicating mesentery.

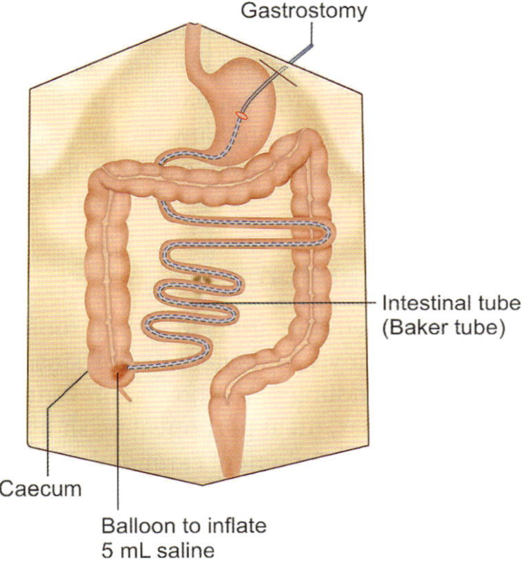

Fig. 22-42: Intestinal intubation via a gastrostomy tube used for adhesions.

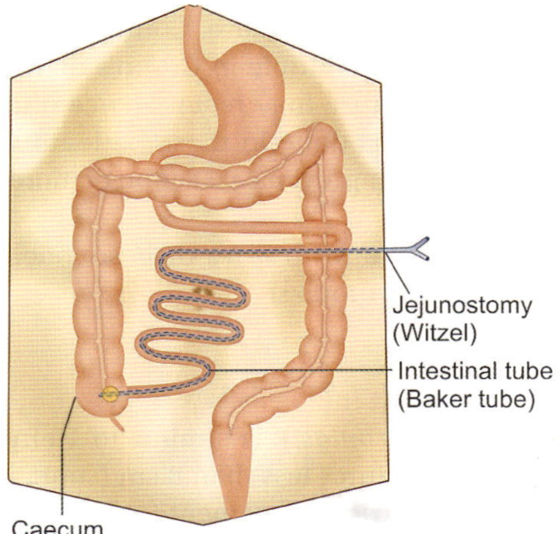

Fig. 22-43: Intestinal intubation via a jejunostomy tube used for adhesions.

Open Method

Usually, it is diagnosed by recurrent pain, distension, vomiting. CT scan confirms the diagnosis. Approach is through same previous scar with extension on either ends. But peritoneum should be opened through normal part of the incision not through the old scar area. Once peritoneum is opened remaining part of the wound is opened under vision with release of any adherent omentum or bowel.

Sharp dissection is better if adhesions are fibrous and thick. In bowel adhesions to abdominal wall, dissection should be carried out very close to the abdominal wall; it is better to incise the abdominal wall peritoneum rather than creating a non-existing plane between adherent bowel and abdominal wall; if it is tried it will surely create a rent in the bowel. While cutting adhesion finger is used underneath for guidance.

Flimsy thin fibrinous adhesions are dissected using index finger. *Gentle finger dissection* is carried out with care to avoid serosal or deeper tears in the bowel wall. *Oozing* while releasing adhesions usually subside after keeping a mop on the site.

Vascular adhesions need *bipolar cautery* to prevent bleeding. *Harmonic scalpel* can be used to release vascular adhesions. Monopolar cautery *should be avoided* as much as possible as bowel injury is likely to occur.

Release of omentum often needs ligature and division or harmonic scalpel. Adherent omentum pulls transverse colon along with it; colon will be often very close to crumpled adherent omentum; during dissection care should be taken not to injure colon inadvertently.

Adhesions very close to mesenteric vessels often will be thick and release should be careful to avoid injury to vessels.

Adhesions especially after hysterectomy and pelvic surgery will be mainly in the pelvis; such adhesions commonly involve terminal ileum and omentum. These adhesions are often stiff and difficult to release as they are deep in pelvis. Finger dissection may be helpful but has to be done with care. Undue traction to the bowel causes tear in the bowel.

Always adhesion release should begin from *easier area to difficult area*. Once all easier area is released, difficult area becomes easier to release.

Mesenteric peritoneal tear often occurs while releasing the bowel; placing a mop on the mesentery usually controls any ooze if occurs; definitive bleeding needs bipolar cautery fulguration or transfixation stitch using 3-zero silk or vicryl.

Entire small bowel from suspensory ligament of Treitz (duodenojejunal junction) to ileocaecal junction should be released.

Any small *serosal tear* is sutured using vicryl or silk seromuscular Lembert suture to invaginate the raw area. Lengthier tear should be sutured transversely using Lembert suture. Perforated bowel segment should be closed using interrupted 2-zero silk sutures. If certain part of the released bowel wall looks non-viable and dusky it should be resected and anastomosed without any doubt or debate. If bowel wall is oedematous and friable and difficult to undertake the resection and anastomosis then loop or end ileostomy is done; closure of ileostomy is done at a later stage after 3–6 months.

On table *Doppler evaluation* should be done if there is doubt about the viability of the bowel.

Some adhesive parts if it looks like to form adhesions again, such part can be *diverted* by doing enteroenterostomy or ileotransverse anastomosis. But it creates a blind pouch and may cause blind loop syndrome.

On table intestinal decompression is often needed if bowel is distended enormously. *Baker intestinal tube* (270 cm long with a 5 mL balloon) is passed by nasogastric route by anaesthetist or by operating surgeon through a gastrostomy incision creating a Stamm gastrostomy. Tube is gently negotiated across the pylorus into the duodenum gently and balloon is inflated partially to negotiate it into the entire length of small intestine by slow milking into the caecum

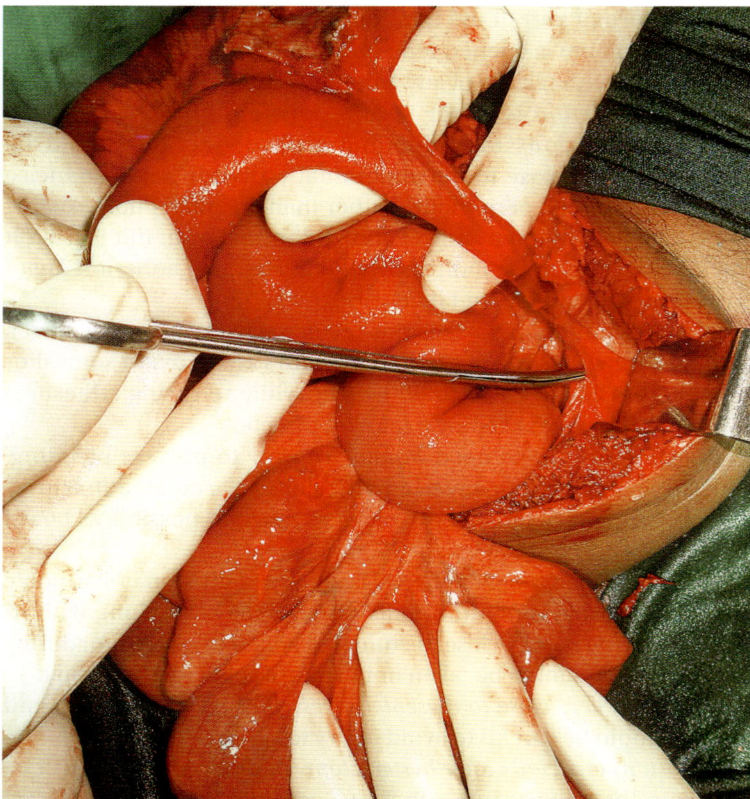

Fig. 22-44: Releasing adhesions through open method.

across the ileocaecal valve. Balloon is fully inflated with 5 mL of saline. Suctioning of the tube should be done while negotiating it through the small bowel to decompress it. It can be kept for 3 weeks to create a *stitchless plication* of the small bowel. Tube is adjusted to make bowel as multiple 'S'. Tube is removed after 3 weeks. While removing it should be deflated completely otherwise it will create reverse intussusception of the small bowel **(Fig. 22-44)**.

Laparoscopic Method

Laparoscopy is better than open method. However, if bowel resection is needed open method is preferred or conversion has to be done. Camera port is placed away from previous scar. Usually it is placed in *left Palmar point* (left subcostal point) or right upper abdomen. Open method is ideal for placing first port. Visiport can be used safely. Stomach should be decompressed. Nasogastric tube and urinary catheter should be passed. Once main port is passed remaining ports (5 mm) are placed depending on the location of adhesions. One on each side and additional 5 mm on left side may be needed. First abdominal wall adhesions are released using scissor and bipolar cautery keeping scissor very close to abdominal wall. 30° telescope is ideal for this purpose. After releasing all abdominal wall adhesions bowel loop adhesions which are bands are released. Initially easier part is released with sharp scissor dissection. Later dense and difficult adhesions are released slowly, carefully and gently with patience. Entire small bowel is dissected off to complete the adhesiolysis. Serosal tear is sutured with intracorporeal Lembert suture using 3-zero vicryl. If perforation occurs it is better to convert into open method; however, if the surgeon is experienced and confident the perforation can be sutured laparoscopically using silk or vicryl by intracorporeal suture. But proper closure should be ensured otherwise peritonitis due to leak will occur **(Fig. 22-45)**.

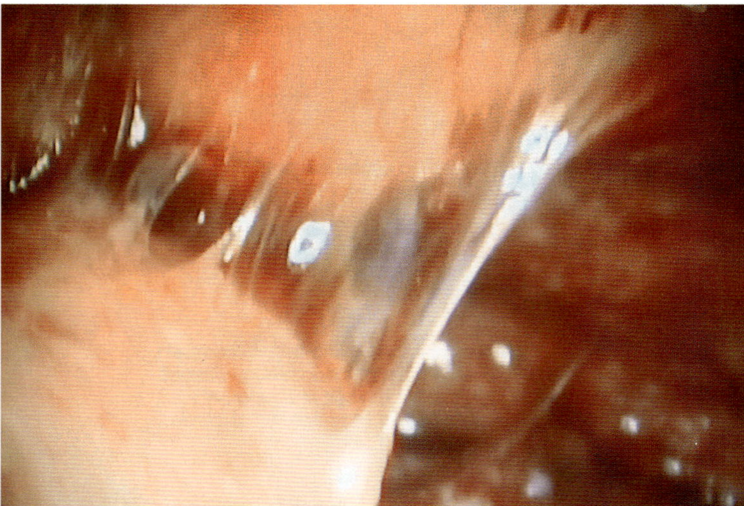

Fig. 22-45: Adhesion seen through laparoscopy.

Problems and Complications

Serosal tear may be missed or overlooked and may leak at a later period causing peritonitis. Recurrent obstruction after adhesiolysis is 15%. Many patients undergo repeated laparoscopic or open surgeries to relieve the obstruction. Slow recovery, prolonged ileus requiring many days nasogastric tube placement, long time intravenous fluids and lengthy hospitalisation are the problems.

Prevention of Adhesions

Prevention is done by instilling drugs like hyaluronidase, steroids, dextrans, dextrins, polyvinyls, silicone, fibrinolysins, chondroitins, streptomycins; gentle handling of the bowel; prevention of spillage of contents like bile, faeces; ideal peritoneal wash using 8–10 litres of saline before closing the abdomen; careful placing of the drains; *Laparoscopic procedures has got lesser chance of adhesions than open method.*

STRICTUROPLASTY

It is commonly done for ileal stricture. Common cause is Crohn's disease. Strictures may be multiple in Crohn's disease. Even after resection disease or stricture may recur. Hence often, instead of resection stricturoplasty is done in these patients. It is useful in recurrence of stricture after previous resection of more than 100 cm; short fibrotic stricture.

Perforation, fistula due to Crohn's disease, haemorrhage are contraindications for stricturoplasty.

Types

Heineke Mikulicz stricturoplasty is similar to Heineke Mikulicz pyloroplasty, used in strictures less than 8 cm (short segment). It is longitudinal incision of stricture segment for its full thickness and transverse closure as a single layer with interrupted silk suture. Stricture is incised longitudinally 2 cm beyond the stricture on to the normal bowel on either side.

Finney's stricturoplasty is done for longer segment stricture. It is similar to Finney's pyloroplasty. Adjacent strictured bowel loops are brought together; U incision is made on the antimesenteric border of the bowel segments; anastomosis is done as in pyloroplasty

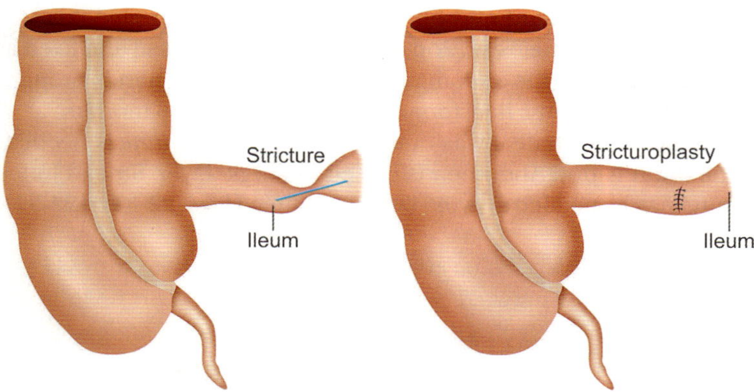

Fig. 22-46: Heineke Mikulicz stricturoplasty.

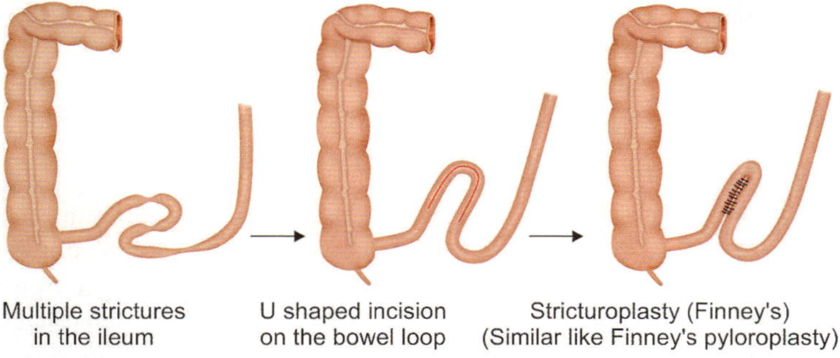

Fig. 22-47: Finney's stricturoplasty.

with posterior seromuscular interrupted silk sutures, posterior all layer continuous or interrupted vicryl sutures, anterior all layer continuous or interrupted sutures and anterior seromuscular interrupted silk sutures **(Figs. 22-46 and 22-47)**.

Problems and Complications

Recurrence, failure, re-obstruction at same segment, leak and peritonitis due to anastomotic dehiscence as anastomosis is on a scarred segment.

JEJUNOSTOMY

Jejunostomy for enteral nutrition is becoming more popular because of its comfort, easy to do, can be kept for long time, lesser complication than gastrostomy. *Indications* are same as gastrostomy.

Types

Witzel jejunostomy: Site of placing jejunostomy is 20 cm from duodenojejunal junction. It is usually done after major abdominal surgeries. After finishing procedures like pancreatic surgery, a stab incision is made on the left side of the abdomen at the level or above the umbilicus. Catheter tip is passed from outside across the abdominal stab wound using a long artery forceps. Loop of jejunum 20–30 cm from the duodenojejunal junction is selected and held with Babcock's forceps. A small incision is made on the antimesenteric border of the selected jejunum of 5 mm in size; entire thickness of the bowel is opened using cautery; jejunostomy catheter (Foley's catheter 16 F or 18 F or feeding tube or nasogastric tube) is passed into the jejunum for adequate length beyond next loop. A purse string seromuscular suture using vicryl is placed around it and tightened securely around the catheter. A seromuscular tunnel of 5 cm length is created around the tube using 3-zero silk interrupted sutures. Serosa at proximal part of the tunnel may be fixed to parietal peritoneum at the abdominal wall. Tube outside is fixed to the skin **(Fig. 22-48)**.

Problems are: tube dislodgement, jejunal obstruction, intestinal juice leak, torsion of the bowel loop, catheter block, leak into the peritoneal cavity, diarrhoea, abdominal discomfort, abscess formation, metabolic problems. Problems may be mechanical, metabolic, gastrointestinal and infectious.

Jejunostomy can be done using gastroduodenoscopy (gastroscopy) similar like percutaneous endoscopic gastrostomy (PEG). Gastroscopy is passed across the duodenum to jejunum; under visualisation and guidance percutaneous needle is punctured into the jejunum and fine catheter through the needle is passed which is held using endoscopic snare and pulled out; jejunostomy catheter is tied.

Laparoscopic jejunostomy is done similar to needle jejunostomy under laparoscopic vision.

Needle catheter jejunostomy using catheter of small gauge can be done. Here percutaneous needle is passed across the abdominal wall into the abdominal cavity which is then inserted into the jejunum 20 cm from duodenojejunal junction. Fine catheter is passed through it; needle is removed. Purse string suture is placed. Jejunum is fixed to abdominal wall to prevent torsion. Tube is fixed to skin **(Fig. 22-49)**.

SMALL BOWEL PERFORATION

Perforation of small bowel can occur by various causes like trauma, typhoid ulcer, enteritis, roundworm infestation, bands causing initial obstruction and later perforation. Patients present with features of peritonitis. Typhoid perforation which occurs on 3rd day after

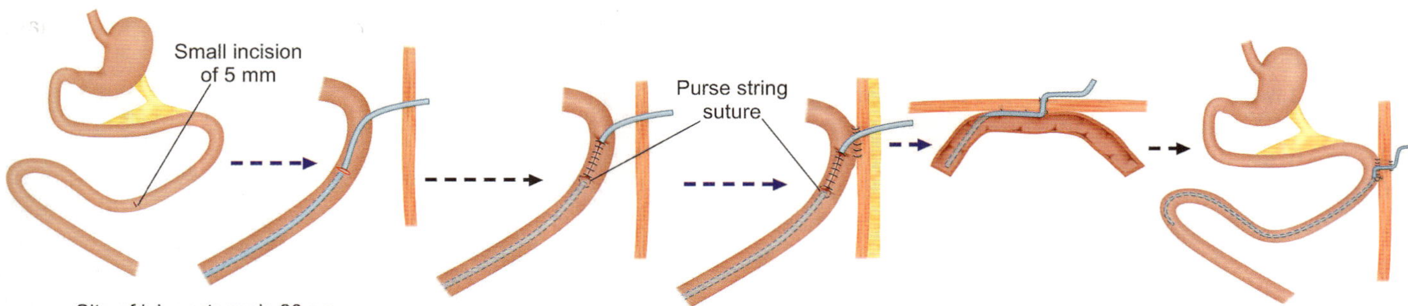

Fig. 22-48: Witzel jejunostomy.

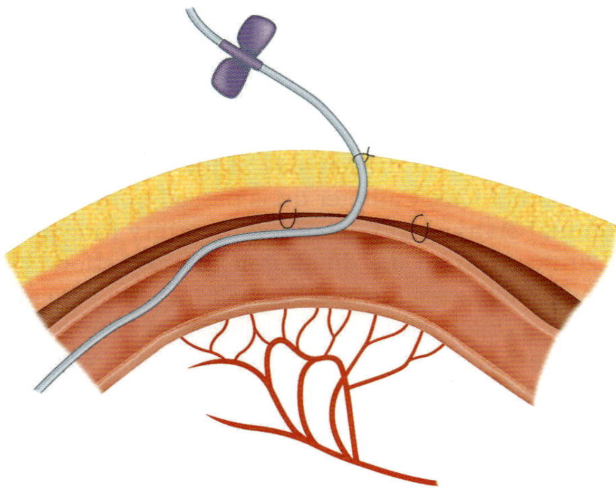

Fig. 22-49: Needle catheter jejunostomy.

the infection, are usually multiple, along the antimesenteric border on the Peyer's patch. Guarding, rigidity which are definitive features of perforation may not be present in typhoid perforation. Traumatic perforation may be due to stab injury or blunt injury. Blunt injury causes traction at duodenojejunal junction leading to disruption of the bowel on the first loop of the jejunum; often it may be in ileocaecal region also for the same reason. Occasionally specific diseases like Crohn's or tuberculosis or malignancy or lymphoma of bowel can cause perforation **(Fig. 22-50)**.

Perforations should be treated surgically. After laparotomy entire small bowel should be inspected. Peritoneal cavity contains pus and intestinal juice. Pus should be collected for culture and sensitivity. Site should be held with Babcock's forceps. Peritoneal infected fluid is sucked out. Perforation edge is trimmed off. Perforation is closed transversely using interrupted 2- or 3-zero silk sutures. Often biopsy from the edge of the perforation should be taken especially when perforation is at ileal site. Seromuscular Lembert interrupted suture may be placed; but it is often difficult in a friable oedematous bowel. Any mesenteric tear if present should be sutured. In multiple perforations resection of the ileum is necessary. If patient's general condition is not good and bowel is friable then loop ileostomy is preferred. Often after resection distal end may be closed and fixed at definitive point in the abdominal wall; and proximal part is brought out as end ileostomy. Ileostomy closure is done in 3–6 months.

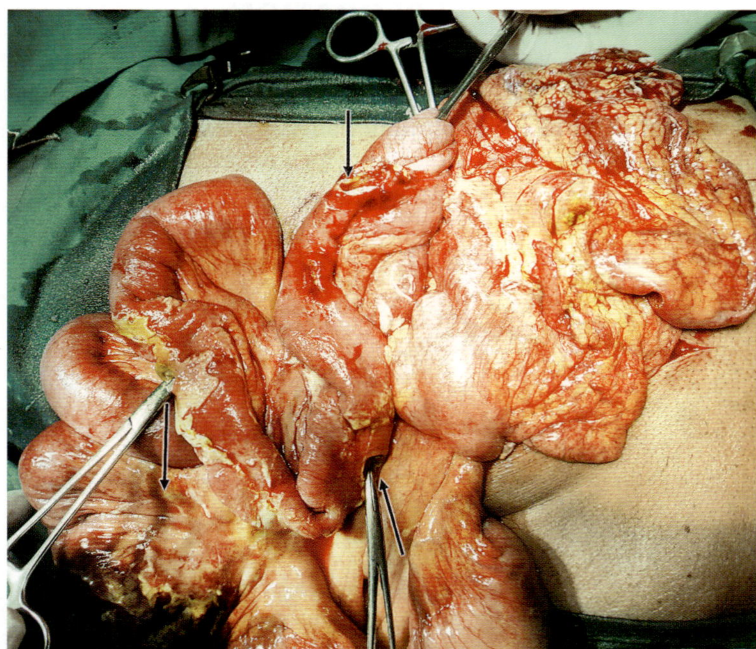

Fig. 22-50: Multiple perforations in the ileum; could be due to typhoid.

Adequate peritoneal wash using *warm normal saline* is needed. Tube drain is put. Abdomen is closed as single layer. Smead Jones suture may be needed to avoid burst abdomen **(Figs. 22-51 to 22-54)**.

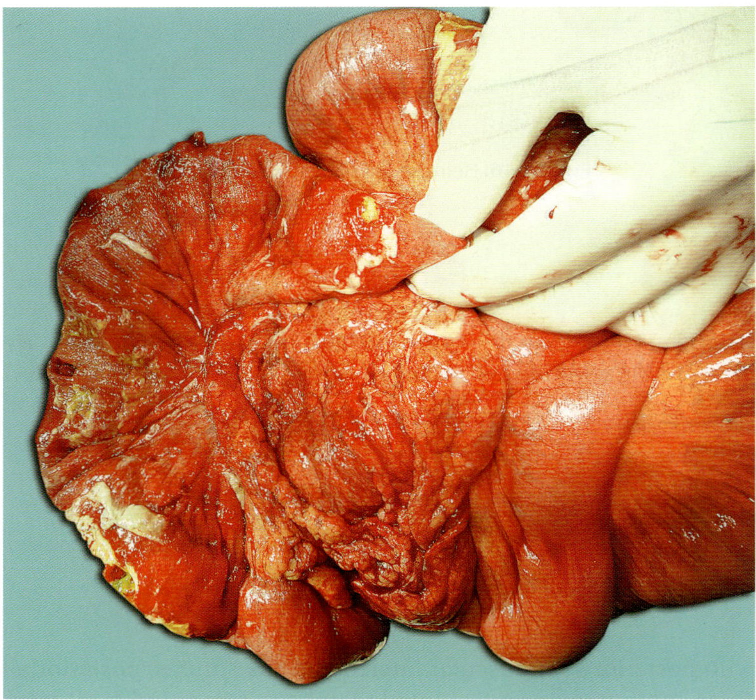

Fig. 22-51: When bowel is viable in multiple perforations, it is nor resected but individual perforations are closed.

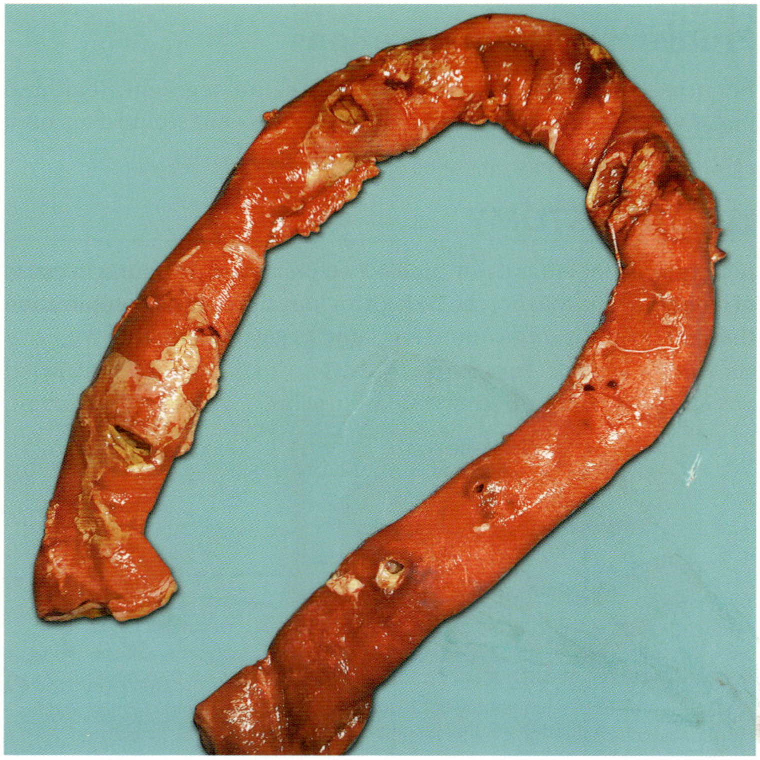

Fig. 22-52: When multiple perforations are present and bowel is ischaemic and non-viable, resection is done. Either primary anastomosis is done; or ileostomy is done (better when there is severe sepsis); or primary anastomosis with proximal diversion ileostomy may be done.

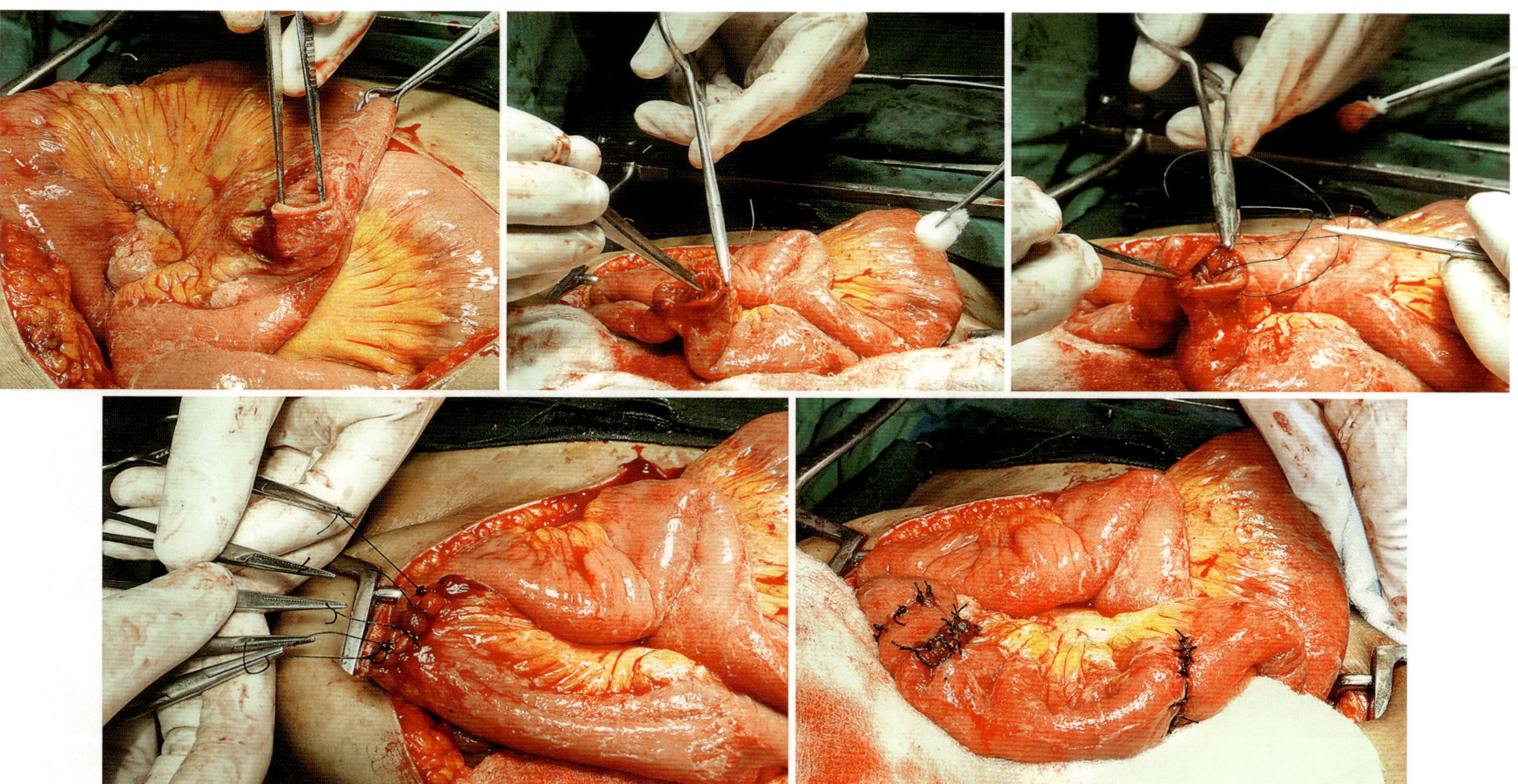

Fig. 22-53: Closure of ileal perforation.

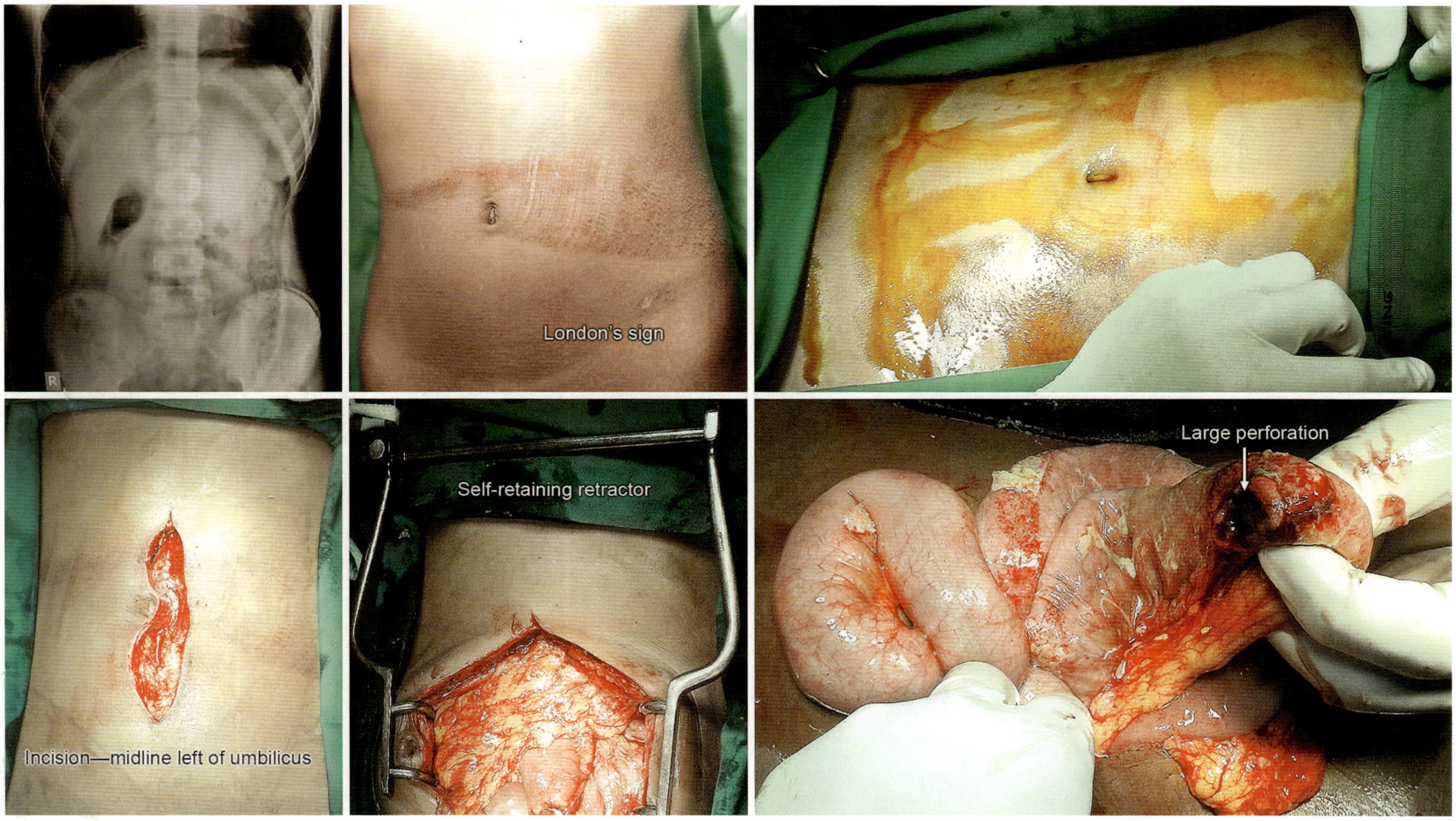

Figs. 22-54(1)

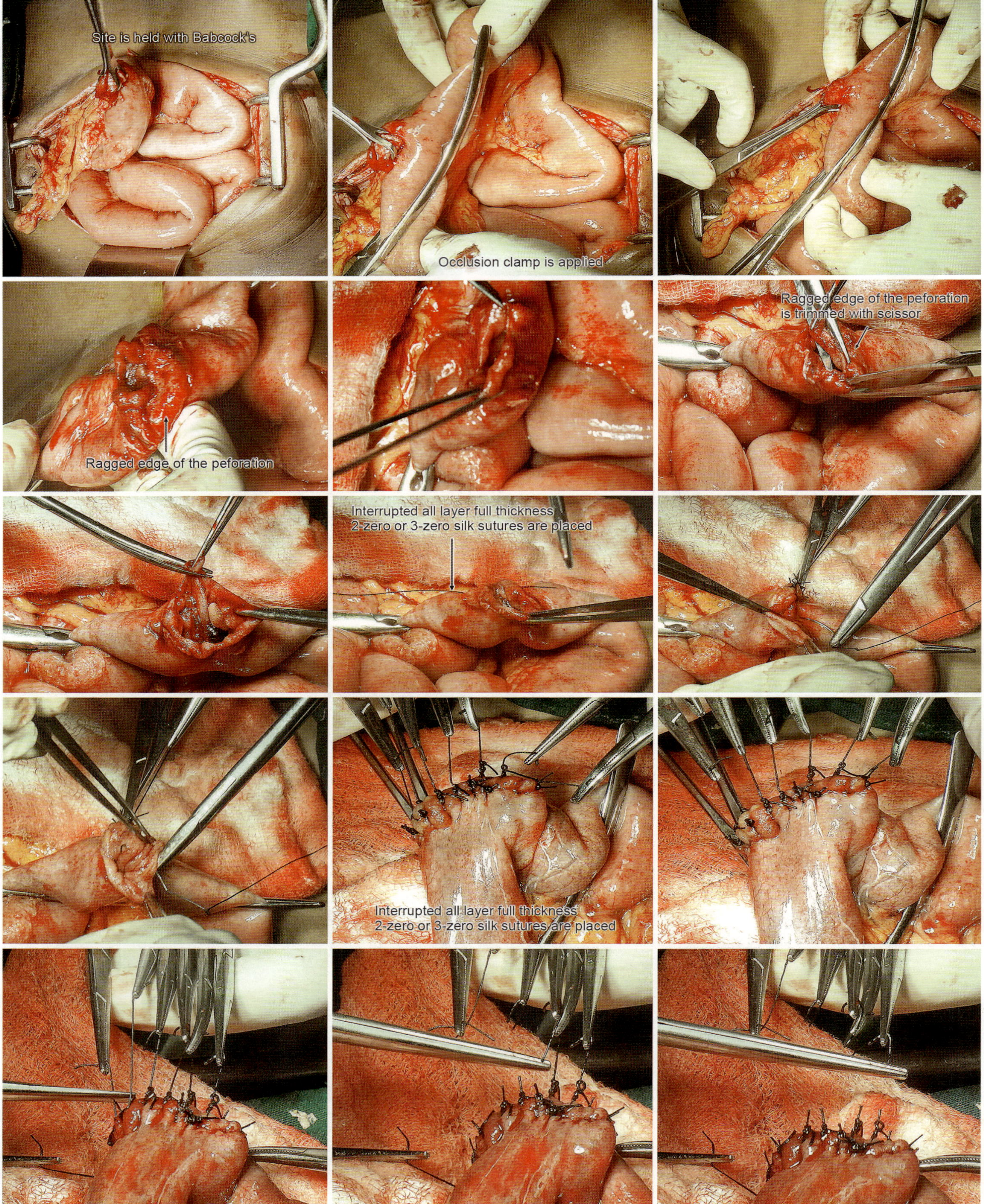
Site is held with Babcock's
Occlusion clamp is applied
Ragged edge of the peforation
Ragged edge of the peforation
is trimmed with scissor
Interrupted all layer full thickness
2-zero or 3-zero silk sutures are placed
Interrupted all layer full thickness
2-zero or 3-zero silk sutures are placed

Figs. 22-54(2)

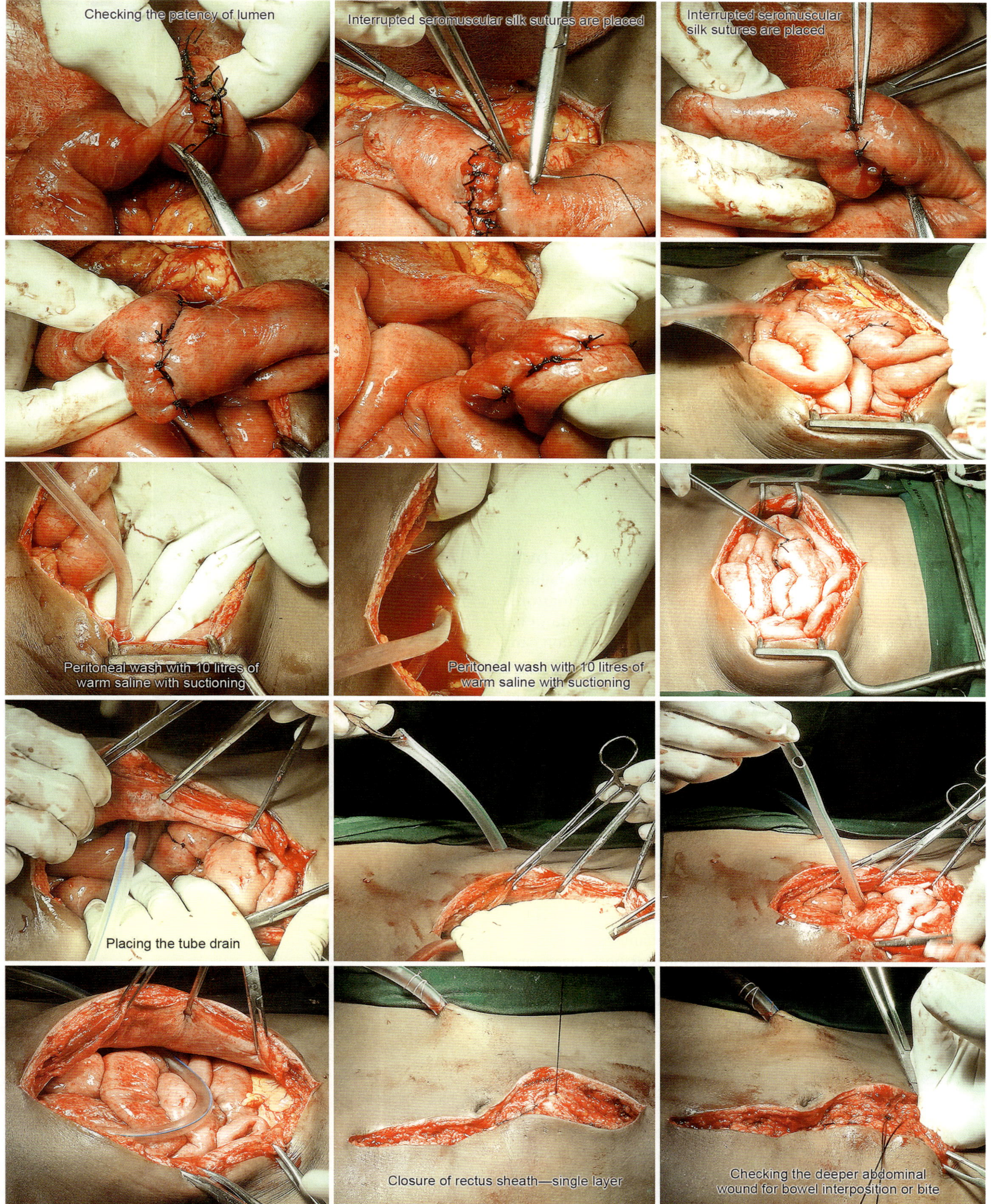
Checking the patency of lumen
Interrupted seromuscular silk sutures are placed
Interrupted seromuscular silk sutures are placed
Peritoneal wash with 10 litres of warm saline with suctioning
Peritoneal wash with 10 litres of warm saline with suctioning
Placing the tube drain
Closure of rectus sheath—single layer
Checking the deeper abdominal wound for bowel interposition or bite

Figs. 22-54(3)

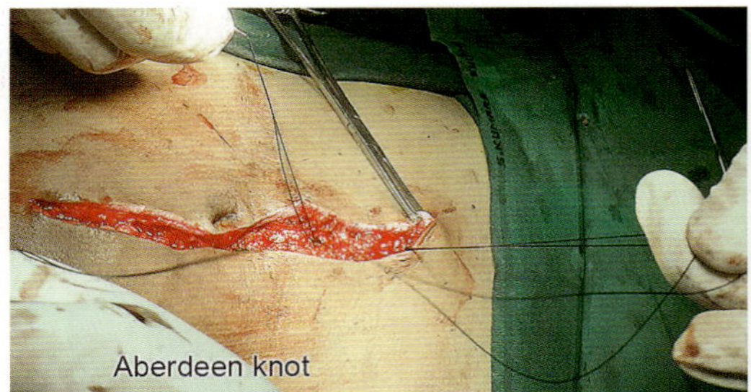

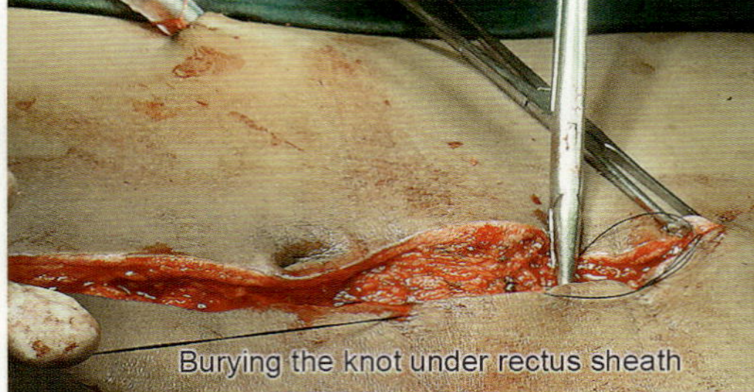

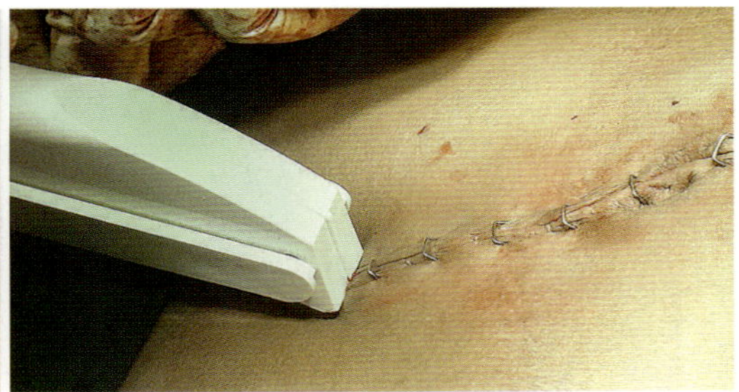

Figs. 22-54(4)

Figs. 22-54(1 to 4): Traumatic perforation of the small bowel due to blunt injury abdomen; London's sign with ecchymotic patch in the abdomen; X-ray showing gas under diaphragm; closure of perforation as shown.

Postoperative Care

Antibiotics, intravenous fluids, total parenteral nutrition (TPN), central line—central venous pressure (CVP), urinary output measurement, monitoring and ICU care is needed. Nasogastric tube is kept in place. Prevention of deep vein thrombosis (DVT) using low molecular heparin is better. Drain is removed in 5 days as well as nasogastric tube once bowel sounds appear. Observation for complications is very important.

Problems and Complications

Septicaemia, acute respiratory distress syndrome (ARDS), DVT, disseminated intravascular coagulation (DIC), acute renal failure, subphrenic abscess, pelvic or interloop abscess formation. Reperforation and peritonitis is a real threat. Burst abdomen, enterocutaneous fistula, are again a problem. Wound infection can occur.

INTESTINAL BYPASS PROCEDURE

Diverting a loop which is non-functioning or creating problem may be required as a surgical technique so as to relieve the obstruction or complication like leak. It is done in severe localised adhesions, malignancy, trauma, tuberculosis or Crohn's disease. However, formation of blind loop and its consequences like malabsorption, recurrent infection in blind loop are the problems and setback to this procedure. Small bowel bypass, ileotransverse anastomosis, ileosigmoid anastomosis are few bypass procedures usually advocated in selected patients. All these procedures are done as side-to-side anastomosis. It can be done as two layer anastomosis hand sewn or through stapler. In two layer anastomosis both layers are done as interrupted sutures using silk or inner vicryl and outer silk. While doing ileotransverse anastomosis transverse colon is opened longitudinally along its taenia **(Figs. 22-55 and 22-56)**.

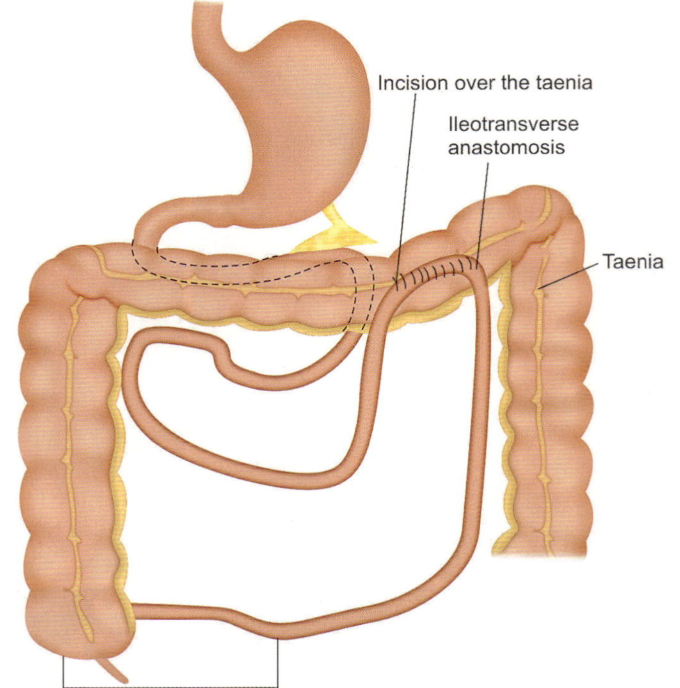

Fig. 22-55: Ileotransverse anastomosis.

ILEOSTOMY

There two types of ileostomy—end and loop. Usually end ileostomy is done as a permanent one after total proctocolectomy if ileal pouch to anal canal is not contemplated. Occasionally temporary end ileostomy is done; in such situation distal segment is closed and kept in right iliac fossa with a fixation stitch to abdominal wall. Temporary end ileostomy may be indicated in Crohn's disease, complex fistulas, ileocaecal trauma. While creating urinary diversion as ileal conduit ileostomy is needed.

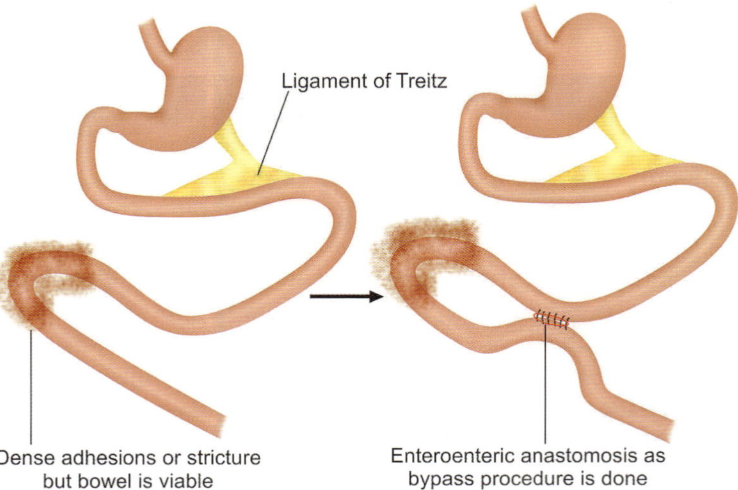

Fig. 22-56: Small bowel bypass.

Loop ileostomy is always temporary for diversion of small bowel content in any terminal ileal disease or proximal colonic disease.

Principles in Ileostomy

Stoma site should be marked in individual patient prior to surgery. It should be clearly discussed with patient. Stoma therapist should do rehabilitation and counselling.

Stoma site is right iliac fossa with infraumbilical mould of fat as summit. Incision should be marked at the surface on the rectus abdominis muscle. Stoma site should be away from scars, umbilicus, bony points, burn injury, etc.

Stoma is marked as round line using a faceplate placed in proposed site.

Muscle should only be split not cut.

Creation of *spout* is important.

Types (Fig. 22-57)

- End ileostomy
- Loop ileostomy
- Loop end ileostomy

End Ileostomy

It is usually done after total proctocolectomy in ulcerative colitis, familial adenomatous polyp (here ileal pouch is contraindicated), multiple synchronous carcinomas, occasionally as temporary end ileostomy in Crohn's disease, ileocaecal trauma, right colonic obstruction.

Terminal ileum is brought out as ileostomy. Terminal ileum is mobilised from its mesentery keeping its arcade and blood supply intact. Terminal ileum is very important for absorption and so one should avoid unnecessary excision of terminal ileum.

Stoma site is in the right iliac fossa over the outer half of the right rectus extending downwards for 2 cm. *Skin is excised* for about a 2 cm circle. Subcutaneous fat is not excised **(Fig. 22-58)**.

Vertical (3–3.5 cm) or cruciate incision is made in the rectus sheath. Only vertical incision on the rectus sheath is sufficient; it is not mandatory to place the cruciate incision. With haemostat and finger dissection peritoneum is reached which is opened to enter the peritoneal cavity. Muscle should be *only split*, never cut. Through laparotomy wound a mop is firmly kept and pressed over the rectus muscle to prevent muscle getting slipped while splitting the rectus muscle. Vertical incision is made in the posterior rectus sheath and peritoneum. Peritoneal opening should be of *two finger size (index and middle)* snugly fitting; it should not be more as it will cause parastomal hernia. As laparotomy wound already exists access can be made easily through it. Injury to inferior epigastric vessels should be avoided. Terminal ileum is transected 2 cm from the ileocaecal valve in case if ileal pouch is being planned later; maximum up to 10 cm of terminal ileum can be removed but not beyond that in any type of ileostomy. *Stapler division* of the ileum is done to prevent the contamination. Stoma is fashioned by retaining the arcade; proximal to arcade few vessels are ligated. Incised rectus sheath is retracted. Babcock's forceps is passed across the ileostomy wound into the peritoneal cavity and cut end of the ileum is held and gently pulled out through the wound *for 6 cm* **(Fig. 22-59)**.

Mesentery may be fixed to the lateral abdominal wall using interrupted 2-zero vicryl sutures. *Seromuscular interrupted stitches* are placed between the ileum and peritoneum as stabilisation stitch. It is not done in case of Crohn's disease as fistula may form. This suture is placed through laparotomy wound from inside by everting the cut edge of laparotomy wound. Laparotomy wound is closed. Stapler line is excised from the terminal end. Often another seromuscular bite is taken from ileum 1 cm from the ileal cut end and superficial fat layer (Camper); it prevents formation of the *parastomal gully*.

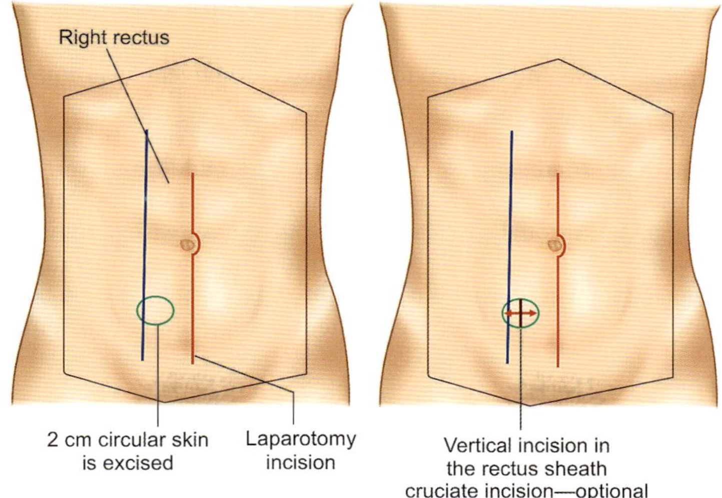

Fig. 22-58: Incision site for ileostomy.

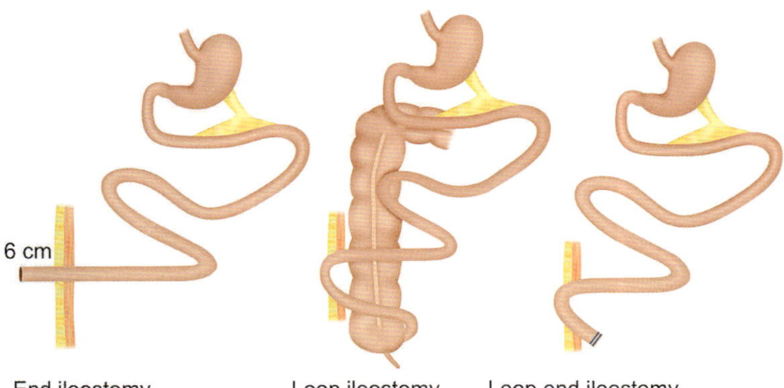

Fig. 22-57: Ileostomy types—end, loop, loop end.

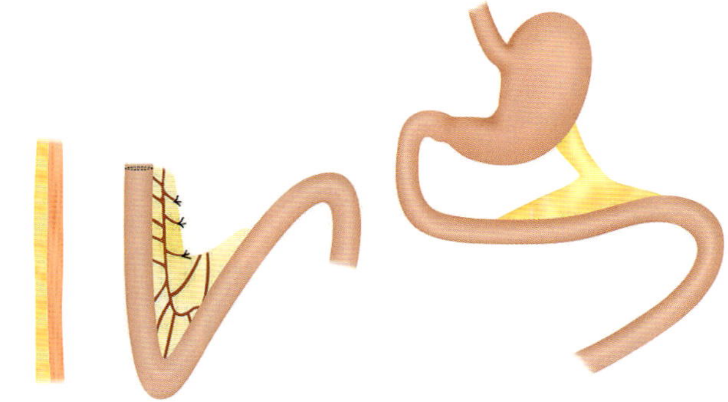

After total protocolectomy during retrieval of specimen terminal ileum at 2–10 cm from ileocaecal valve is transected using stapler.
Stoma is fashioned by retaining the closure arcade to the stapled end.
Ensure that blood supply at the end is optimum.

After circular skin excision of 2 cm at stoma site vertical incision is made in the rectus sheath; muscle is only split; peritoneum with posterior rectus sheath is opened.
By passing Babcock's forceps stapled ileal end is brought out through ileostomy wound.

Fig. 22-59: Ileostomy stoma fashioning.

Cut edge of the ileum (full thickness all layer interrupted) is apposed to subcuticular part of the skin (not full thickness skin) with initial four points then additional four sutures in between (*maturation*) **(Fig. 22-60)**.

After placing all sutures, knots are tied one by one. In a different method, alternate sutures are placed with an additional seromuscular stitch prior to passing through the skin subcuticular part. Through and through skin is better avoided otherwise there will be chances of mucosal island implantation and early separation of stoma appliances. Placement of two myotomies of the stoma before suturing to skin will also prevent the recession of the ileostomy to create needed *spouting*. While taking seromuscular suture, care should be taken not to enter mucosa to avoid stoma fistulas at the edge.

Often *spout is created* in such a way that stoma is made *to face downwards* which is ideal. It is done while placing seromuscular—outer fat suturing where in the proximal part is taken shorter while in the caudal part it is longer and it is in between at sides. It can also be achieved while taking final bite between subcuticular and cut edge of ileum, additional seromuscular bites are taken at different levels **(Fig. 22-61)**.

• Staple line is divided using scissor-maturation
• 1 cm from cut end of ileum seromuscular bite is taken to again pass into the outer fat layer to prevent parastomal gully formation

• Mesentery is sutured to abdominal wall
• Stabillisation stich is placed from seromuscular suture of ileal wall to peritoneum; placed through the laparotomy wound
• Laparotomy is closed

8 interrupted sutures at 8 corners from full thickness ileal cut end to subcuticular part of the skin (not through the entire skin)

Fig. 22-60: Maturation of ileostomy.

Midline laparotomy → definitive procedure (proctocolectomy) → *marking the stoma site* on the right lower rectus → 2.5 cm *circular skin is excised* → fat is *not* removed → *vertical* 3.5 cm or cruciate incision in the *rectus sheath* → rectus muscle is *split* → mop with finger support through the laparotomy wound to prevent slipping of the rectus → posterior rectus sheath and peritoneum is incised vertically for *two finger breadth only* → *stapler transection* of the terminal ileum at 2–10 cm from ileocaecal valve → *stoma fashioning* is done with retaining the arcade → *Babcock's forceps* is passed from outside into the peritoneal cavity across the ileostomy wound → stapled ileum is held → brought out gently for *6 cm exteriorisation* → mesentery may be obliterated by suturing it to abdominal wall → through laparotomy wound *stabilisation interrupted stitches* are placed between seromuscular ileum and peritoneum all round → laparotomy wound is closed → ileostomy maturation is done by cutting stapled area → seromuscular stitch 1 cm away from the cut end of ileum is sutured to outer fatty layer to avoid parastomal gully by creating concertina effect → full thickness cut edge of the ileum is sutured to subcuticular part of the skin with interrupted sutures (8 sutures).

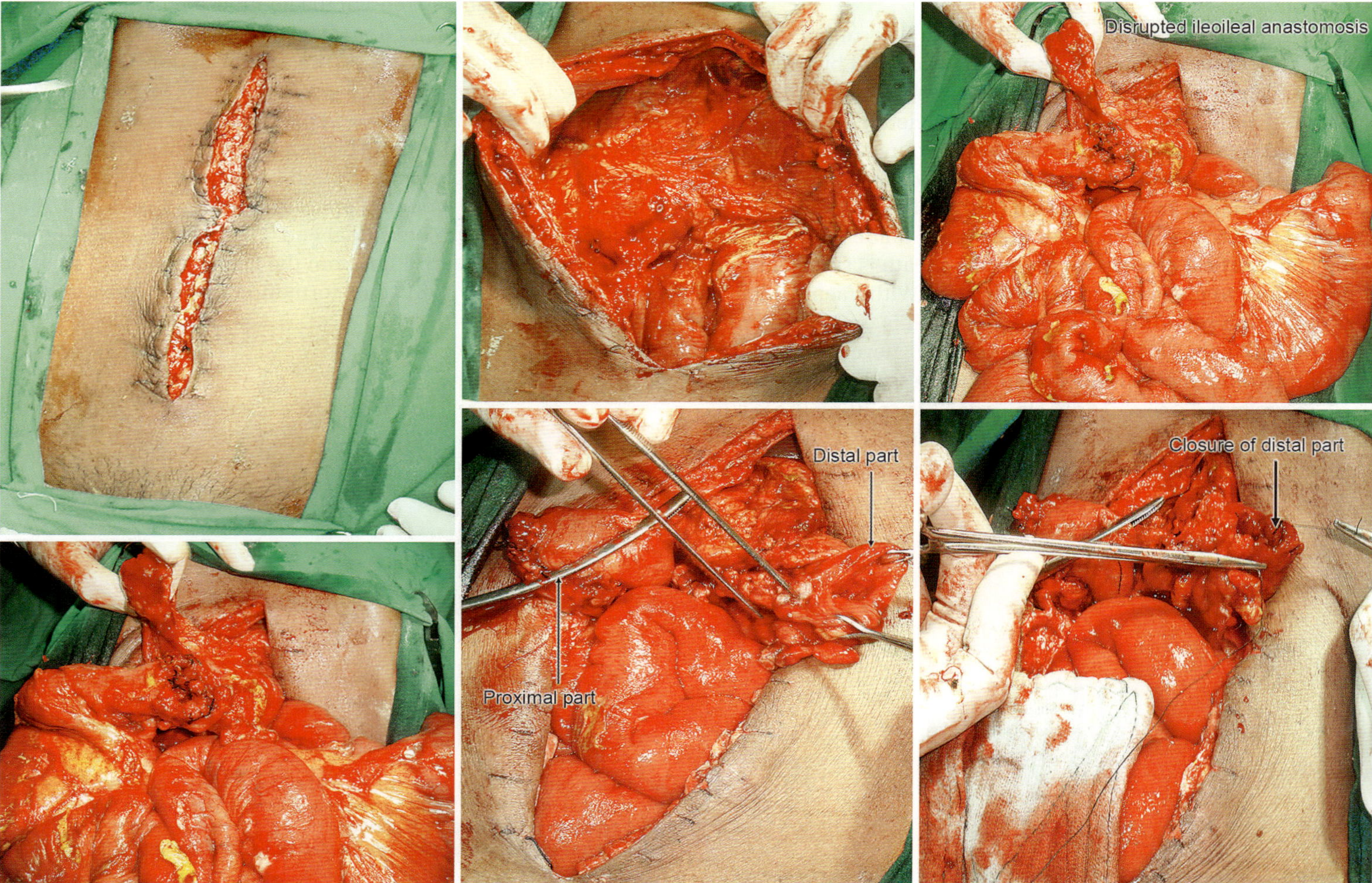

Figs. 22-61(1)

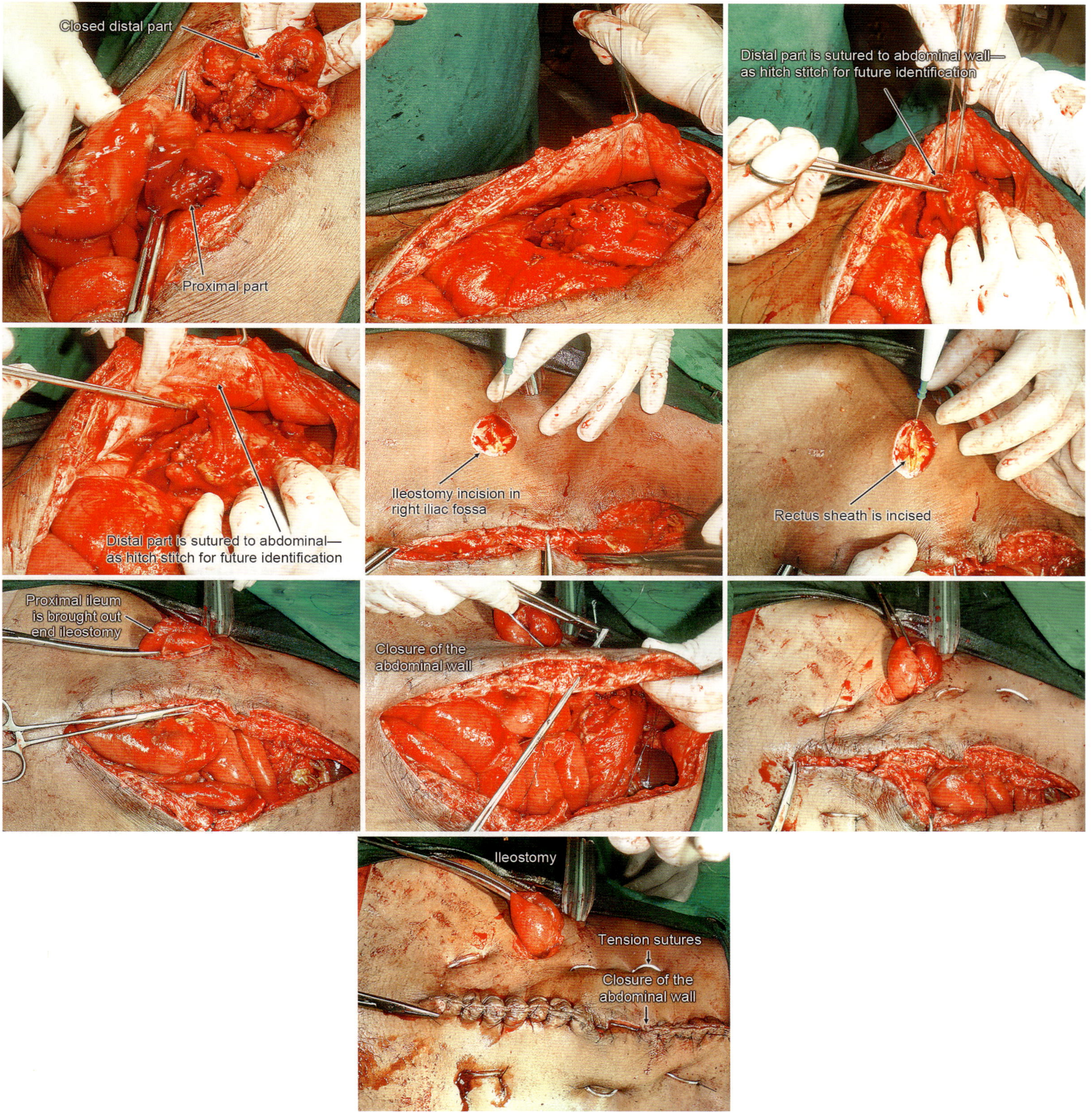

Figs. 22-61(2)

Figs. 22-61(1 and 2): End ileostomy done for critically disrupted earlier closed ileal perforation.

Loop Ileostomy

It is done to create diversion as temporary method. After ileal pouch with pouch anal canal anastomosis, covering diversion loop ileostomy is placed for 3–6 months. It is used in enterocutaneous fistula, ascending colon or caecal sepsis or gangrene, in radiation related severe pelvic problems. In multiple perforations of terminal ileum where severe sepsis prevents from doing primary anastomosis, diversion ileostomy is always better. Mesenteric vessels are not divided here. Loop ileostomy is done 15–20 cm proximally as ileum is not resected and later repositioned once its purpose is served **(Fig. 22-62)**.

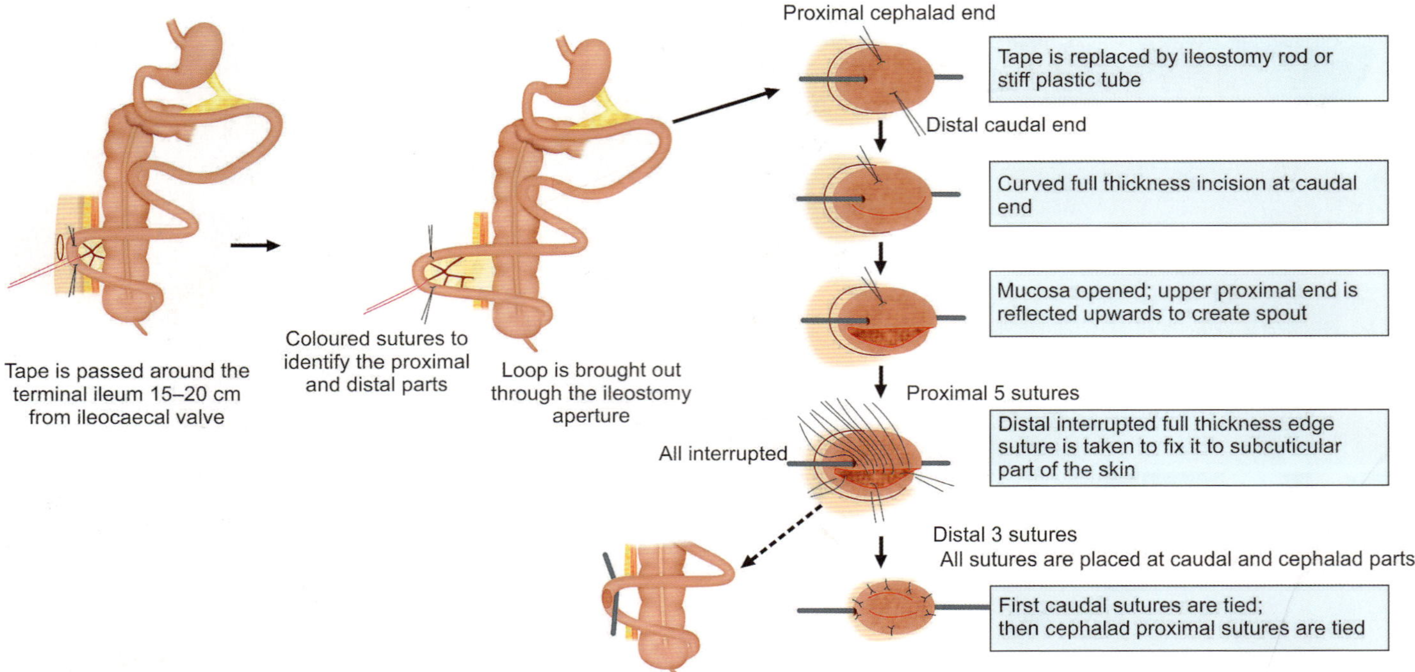

Fig. 22-62: Technique of doing loop ileostomy.

Midline laparotomy is done for definitive condition. Once loop ileostomy is planned; stoma site is marked alike in end ileostomy on the right iliac fossa at lower rectus muscle area. Site in the ileum is identified and antimesenteric part is held with a Babcock's forceps. A small window is made in the small bowel mesentery and a tape is passed around it. Proximal and distal parts are tagged with stay stitches of different colours for identification purpose when it is brought out of the ileostomy aperture. Loop is brought out of the ileostomy wound. Rotation or twist or tear in the mesentery should not occur while pulling out. Proximal end is identified and oriented at cephalad direction; distal end at caudal end. Tape is replaced with ileostomy rod; or stiff plastic tube can also be placed. Laparotomy wound is closed. After proper identification of loops coloured stiches can be removed. Incision is made on the distal caudal end transversely using no. 15 blade or cautery 0.5 cm from the distal skin margin. Incision extends 5 mm in front of the mesenteric attachment. Scissor is often better to the needed enterotomy. 3-zero vicryl interrupted sutures are placed from full thickness cut edges to the subcuticular part of the skin; caudally 3 sutures are needed; cephalad 5 sutures are needed. Sutures are kept long untied. Once all sutures are placed first caudal sutures are tied; then cephalad sutures are tied. Only proximal functioning part of the loop is everted, not distal non-functioning part. *Spouting* is thus created to place a proper stoma appliance.

Complications

Mucosal sloughing, pseudo-obstruction, later cutaneous stenosis (Bishop's collar deformity), high output, electrolyte imbalance, parastomal infection by bacteria, *candida*, ileostomy fistula, paraileostomy ulceration, ileostomy obstruction, ileostomy recession, ileostomy prolapse and hernia. Many of these complications need revision ileostomy.

CLOSURE OF ILEOSTOMY

Closure of ileostomy is done after 3 months not prior to that. In closure of loop ileostomy distal part of the bowel should be assessed by doing colonoscopy and contrast X-ray. Bowel preparation may be needed with clear liquids for 24 hours prior to surgery. Nasogastric tube and urinary catheter is passed.

Under general anaesthesia in supine position after cleaning and draping, a circumferential incision is made close to mucocutaneous junction leaving 2 mm skin margin. Transverse or vertical extension if needed should be done. These extensions will help in proper adequate mobilisation of bowel proximally and distally. Bowel wall is held with Allis forceps and traction is given to facilitate the dissection between bowel margin and abdominal wall to enter the peritoneal cavity. Usually sharp dissection using no 15 blade or scissor is used to cut through the planes. Cautery usage should be carefully done only to avoid the bowel injury. Counter traction on skin margin is achieved using retractor. Traction on the bowel edge with countertraction on the abdominal wall is essential to open the planes by sharp dissection. Once abdominal cavity is reached, adhesions are released by finger dissection with index finger being kept close to the abdominal wall and with sweeping action. Once mobilised loop is brought out of the wound, proximally on both sides adequate mobilisation should be done to avoid tension on the ileostomy closure. Adhesions on the part of the mesentery of that particular loop are also freed carefully without tearing the mesentery. This prevents kinking, angulation and tension on the bowel wall. Mucosal eversion is reversed. Cut edge of the bowel is trimmed to remove attachments of the skin and fat on to it. Adequate bleeding from the trimmed cut edge of the bowel is essential. Bowel wall serosa is also carefully dissected off from fat and adherent tissue. This facilitates the closure of anastomosis. Any tear in the bowel wall should be checked which might have occurred during dissection. It may be confirmed by infusing the normal saline into the lumen. Edge of the ileum should be cut properly using fine scissor. Defect in the bowel wall is closed transversely using 3-zero vicryl as interrupted sutures. Initially corner stitches are placed which are held up as stay stitches. Next middle stitch is placed to appose the defect. Further stitches are placed at 3–5 mm gap. Usually full thickness suturing is done; but it is often advisable to place seromuscular sutures including proper bites on submucosa but mucosa is spared. This ensures accurate approximation. Often outer interrupted silk sutures are placed as additional seromuscular but it is not necessary **(Figs. 22-63 and 22-64)**.

Bowel kept outside the wound is gently pushed inside without disruption. Drain (peritoneal) is usually not kept; but often is kept in practice by many. Rectus sheath is closed as interrupted single layer. Full thickness bites using non-absorbable suture material (1-zero) is used. Skin is often kept open instead of primary suturing. Secondary suturing is done once wound granulates well after 3 weeks. Often wound heals by scarring without secondary suturing. Whenever primary skin closure is done using 1-zero polypropylene interrupted sutures, subcutaneous drain should be placed.

In difficult situation, abdominal wound is extended adequately transversely or vertically. Complete mobilisation of the ileum and ascending colon is done. Resection and anastomosis is done. Anastomosis is either ileoileal or ileocolic type depending on bowel retained **(Figs. 22-65 and 22-66)**.

Stapler closure of the loop ileostomy can be done. It is usually done as side to side.

Postoperative Care

Oral liquid is started after 48 hours. Low residue diet is used for 8 weeks. Antibiotics, heparin, urinary catheter is kept in place. Nasogastric tube is removed in 48 hours.

Complications

Anastomotic disruption and faecal fistula through the wound is the complication. Usually it settles down with conservative therapy. Occasionally, it needs ileostomy again and later period resection and anastomosis.

Wound infection is common which settles with regular dressing and antibiotics.

SEROSAL PATCH TECHNIQUE

It is used in enterocutaneous fistula and intestinal perforations. In 1959 to 1963 Austin Jones and Kobald and Thal started this technique. This is useful in difficult cases. Serosa has got high ability to seal the perforations of any nature-recent, chronic or with severe sepsis. But it is not routinely used; it is reserved for cases where nothing else is possible.

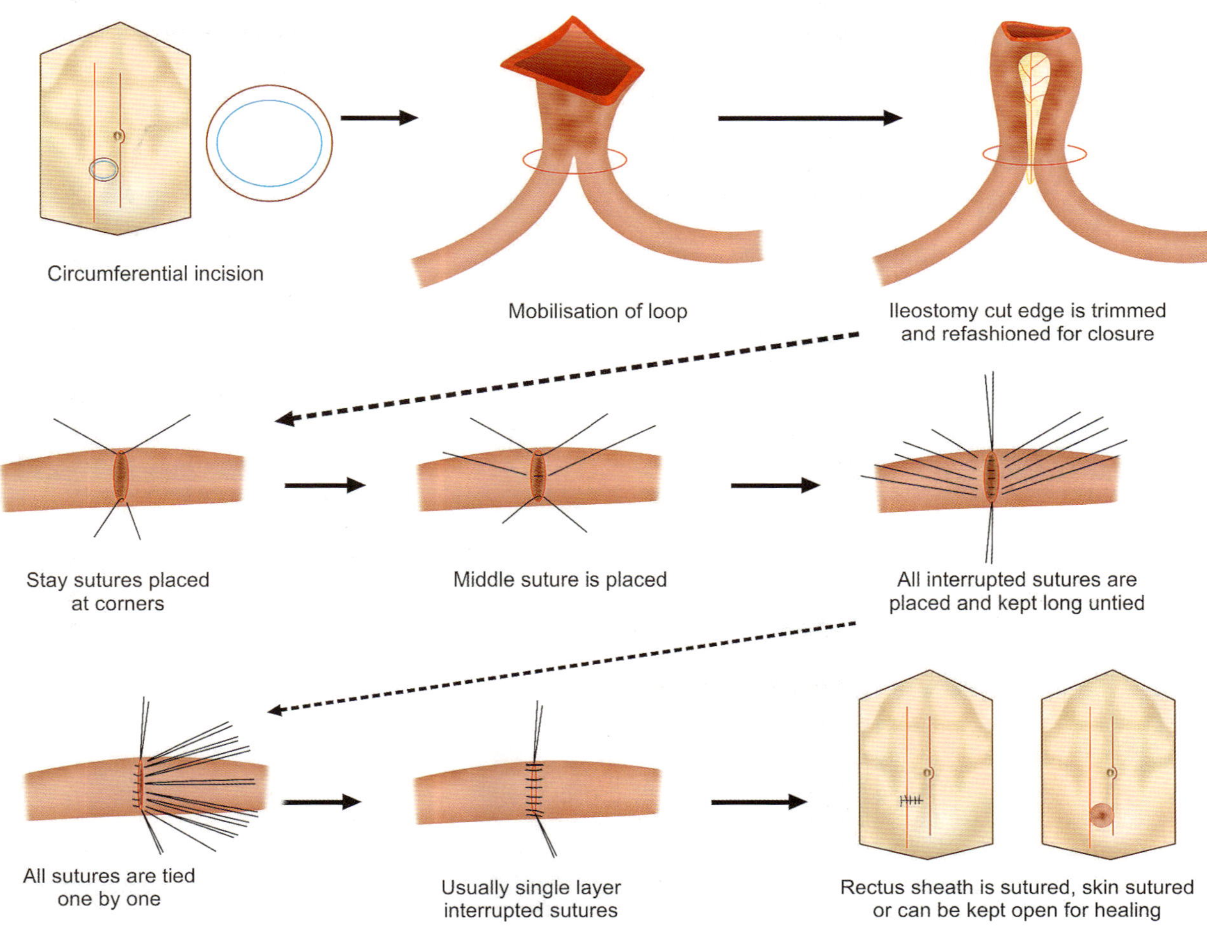

Fig. 22-63: Technique of ileostomy closure—loop type.

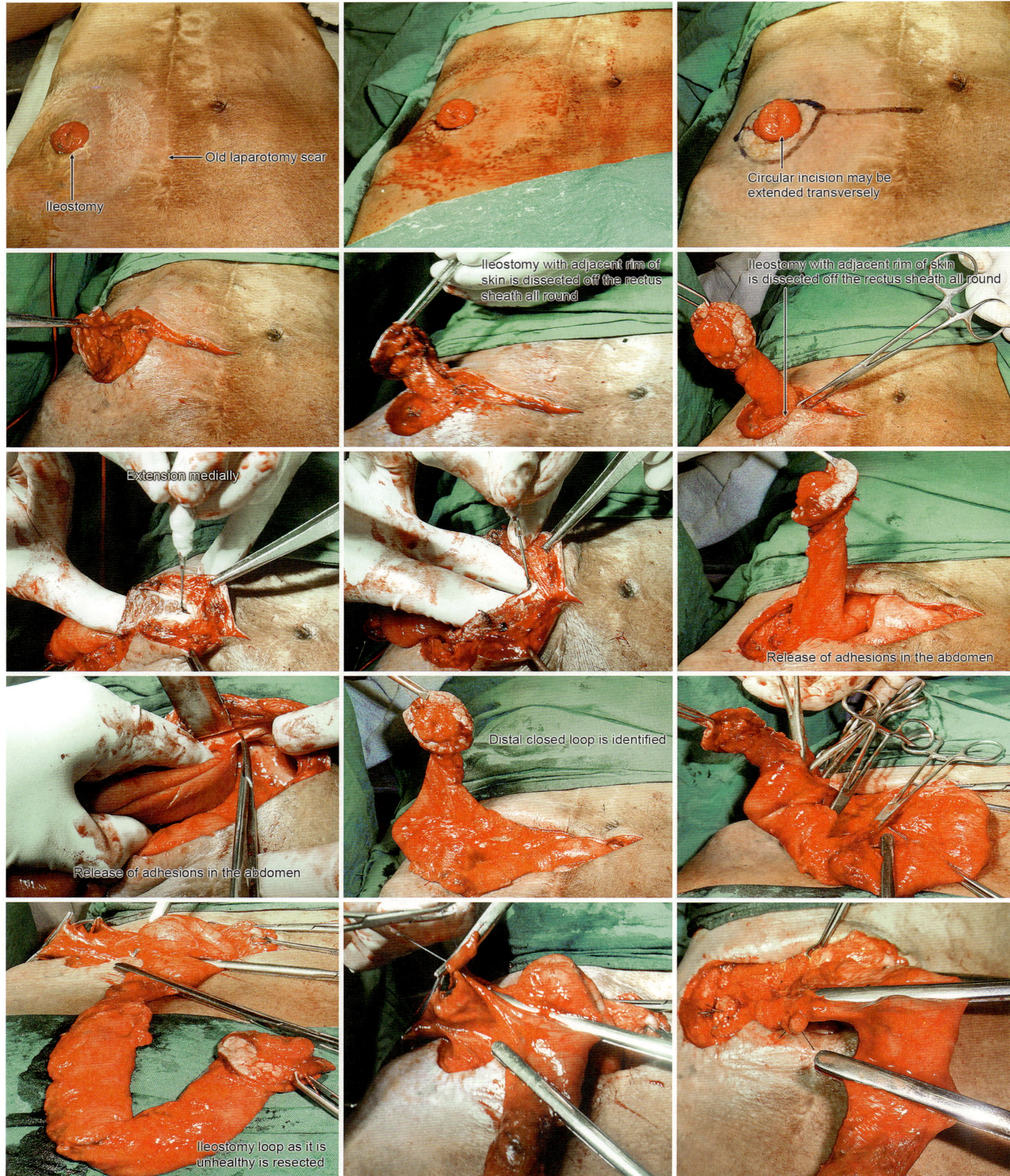
Old laparotomy scar
Ileostomy
Circular incision may be extended transversely
Ileostomy with adjacent rim of skin is dissected off the rectus sheath all round
Ileostomy with adjacent rim of skin is dissected off the rectus sheath all round
Extension medially
Release of adhesions in the abdomen
Release of adhesions in the abdomen
Distal closed loop is identified
Ileostomy loop as it is unhealthy is resected

Figs. 22-64(1)

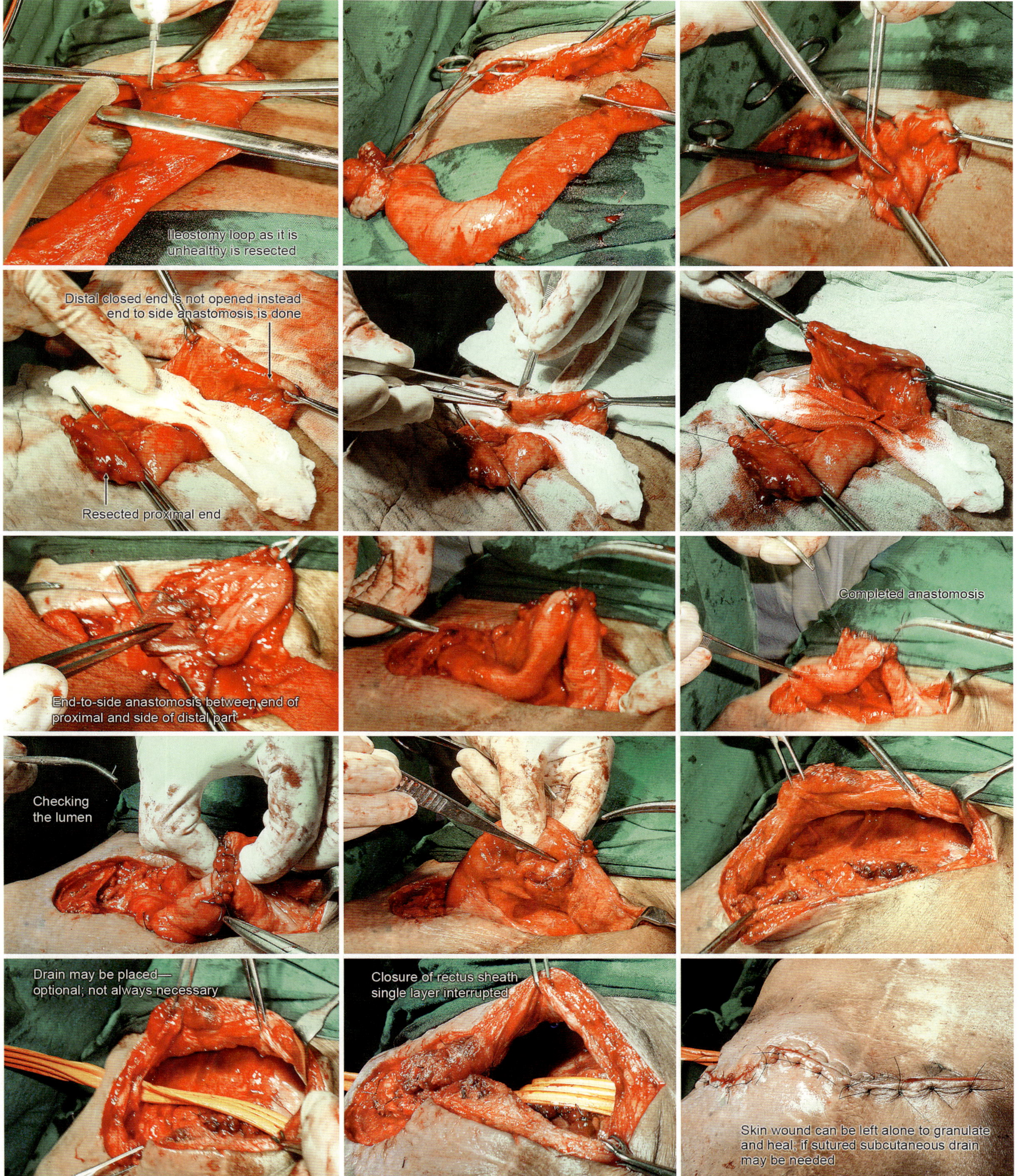

Figs. 22-64(2)

Figs. 22-64(1 and 2): Closure of the ileostomy.

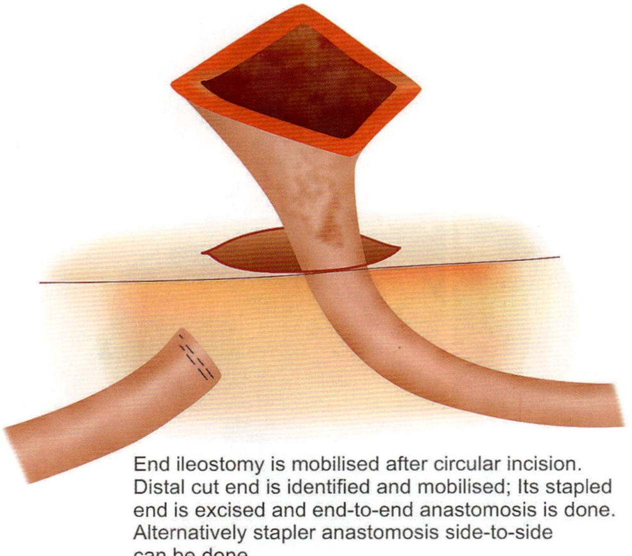

Fig. 22-65: Ileostomy closure—in loop end type.

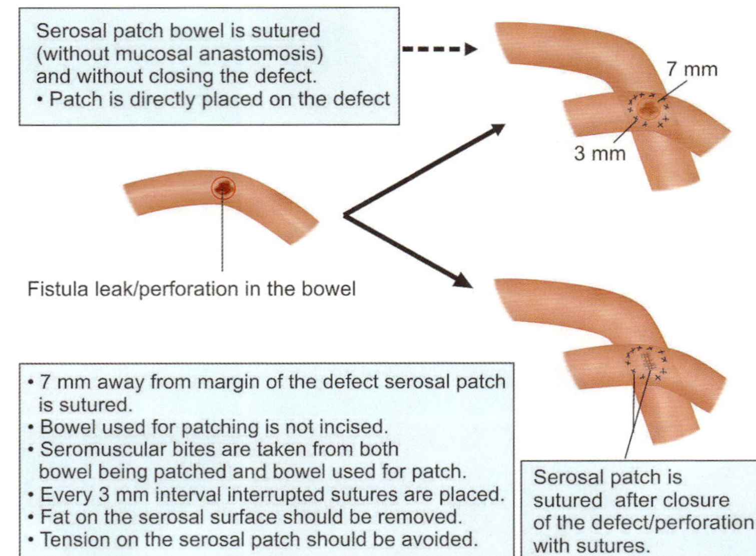

Fig. 22-67: Serosal patch technique.

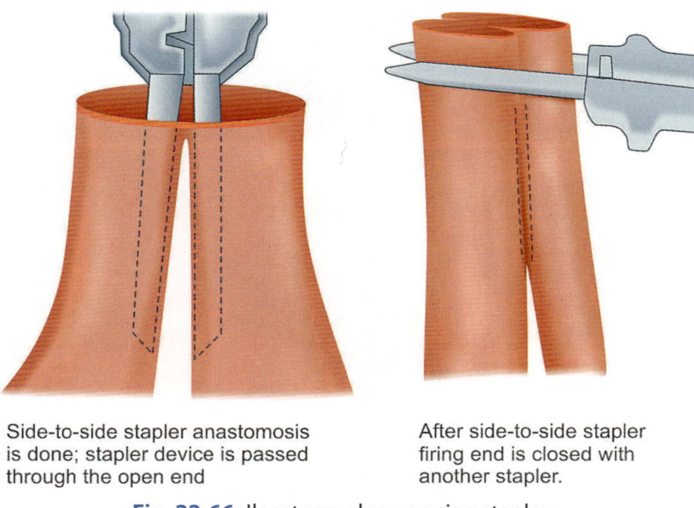

Fig. 22-66: Ileostomy closure using stapler.

It is used when there is difficulty in closing duodenal stump, large perforations; enterocutaneous fistulas where in spite of proper conservative therapy patient is not responding.

It is used in leaking or difficult duodenal stump after Billroth II anastomosis; in duodenal perforation if closure is not possible or pyloroplasty is not possible; in already done pyloroplasty that has disrupted in enterocutaneous fistula.

Procedure

Serosa of the small bowel (usually jejunum) is used. Loop (omega) or Roux loop is used. Serosal surface of the bowel is cleared of all fat by gentle dissection. Perforated site is debrided and edge is trimmed. If possible, if there is no tension perforated edge can be sutured; otherwise site is directly kept ready for serosal patch. Serosal patch is sutured 7 mm away from the edge of the defect/perforation. Interrupted seromuscular bites are taken both from the perforated bowel and the intestine which is being used for patching. 3-zero silk is used for suturing. Sutures are placed at 3 mm interval **(Figs. 22-67 to 22-69)**.

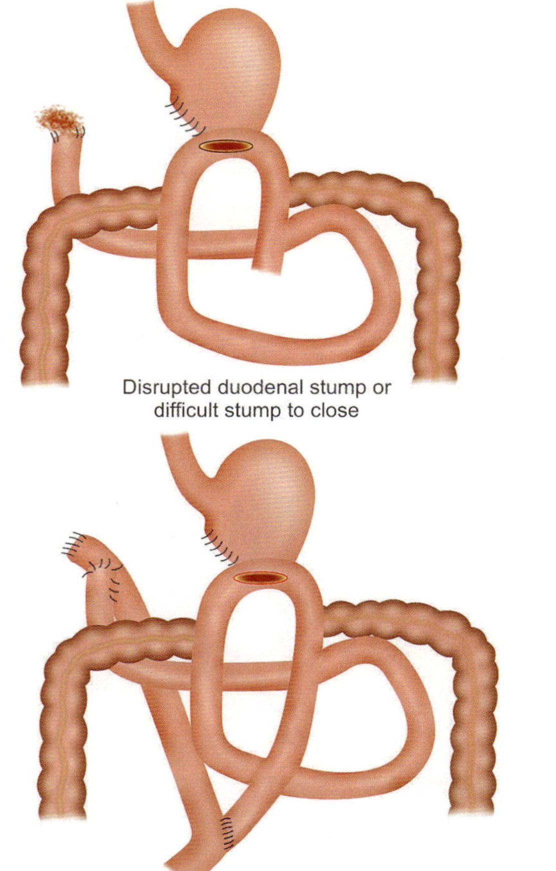

Fig. 22-68: Serosal patch technique for duodenal stump problems after Billroth II anastomosis.

Problems

It is technically demanding. Recurrence of fistula and disruption may occur.

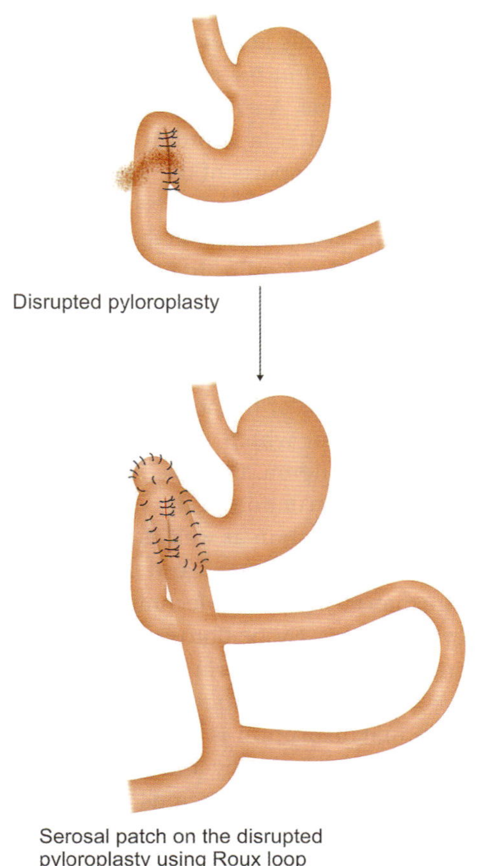

Fig. 22-69: Serosal patch technique for disrupted Finney's pyloroplasty.

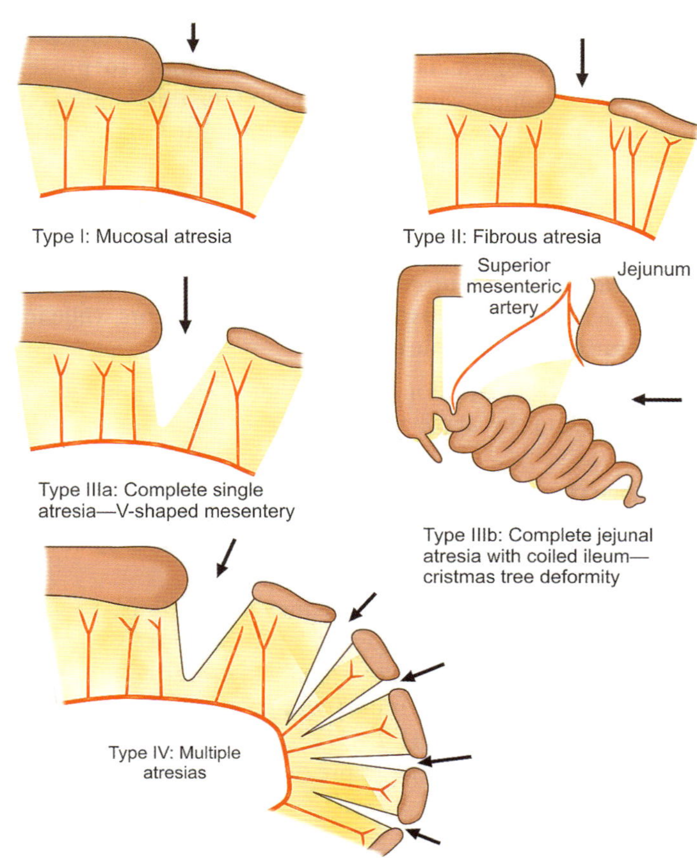

Fig. 22-70: Intestinal atresia.

SMALL INTESTINE ATRESIA (INTESTINAL ATRESIA)

It is jejunoileal atresia. It is due to intrauterine mesenteric vascular accidents (occlusion) of the segments affected. V-shaped mesentery; presence of bile pigments in the distal segments suggesting earlier period of patency—are supportive for the above theory. It is often associated with malrotation, gastroschisis, volvulus—20%. Common site is proximal jejunum; next common is distal ileum. Maternal polyhydramnios occurs in 35% of jejunal atresia. Proximal bowel wall is dilated with hypertrophy but villi are normal. Distal bowel is collapsed but with hypertrophied villi. Narrow collapsed large intestine (microcolon) is seen in proximal atresia.

Griesfield Modification of Martin's Classification of Intestinal Atresia (Fig. 22-70)

- Type I: Membranous/mucosal with normal mesentery—20%.
- Type II: The lumen is atretic—fibrous cord between proximal and distal parts of the segment involved (only one atretic segment) but mesentery is normal—40%.
- Type III (a): Atresia with complete separation of proximal and distal ends and V-shaped defect of mesentery—35%.
- Type III (b): Atresia with Christmas tree-shaped defect in mesentery with distal bowel being supplied by single artery—right colic/ileocolic/superior mesenteric—*apple peel atresia.*
- Type IV: Multiple atresias—5%.

Treatment

Resection and anastomosis is the choice of therapy. Treatment of associated anomalies; tapering proximal jejunoplasty is done if extensive length of jejunum is involved. Prognosis depends on length of atretic bowel; multiple atresias; associated anomalies.

MALROTATION

It is interference in the process of normal rotation of midgut in foetus and its mesenteric fixation.

Stages of Normal Rotation of Midgut

Stage 1: In 4th–8th week of intrauterine period, midgut supplied by superior mesenteric artery (SMA) grows rapidly. As coelomic cavity cannot accommodate growing midgut during that period, it protrudes into the umbilical cord as *physiological hernia.*

Stage 2: In 10th–12th week, midgut migrates into coelomic cavity. First, small bowel returns towards the left side of the abdomen. Then caecocolic loop returns to left lower abdomen. It rapidly rotates 270° counterclockwise to reach right iliac fossa. Then duodenojejunal segment rotates 270° counterclockwise to reach left of SMA and behind the colon.

Stage 3: Fusion of different parts of mesentery and posterior peritoneum.

Different Errors of Rotation

Stage 1: Exomphalos major/minor or gastroschisis.

Stage 2: Errors of rotation in this stage is important and is usually considered under malrotation.

Non-rotation: Causing small bowel in right side; colon in left side; caecum in midline as suspension.

Incomplete rotation: It is the *most common type* of malrotation. Caecum is subhepatic located in right hypochondrium. *Ladd's peritoneal band* connects from caecocolic loop to posterior abdominal wall compressing the 2nd part of the duodenum. Entire midgut is hanging down along with SMA with a narrow based mesentery causing midgut volvulus.

Reverse rotation: Final 180° rotation occurs clockwise bringing colon posterior to duodenum and SMA.

Hyperrotation: Rotation up to 360° or 450° causing caecum on left side of the abdomen. Encapsulated small bowel occurs while foetal midgut returns into coelomic cavity.

Stage 3: Final defect in fixation causes mobile caecum and ascending colon leading into caecal volvulus **(Fig. 22-71)**.

Treatment

Resuscitation, antibiotics, replacement of fluid and electrolytes, blood transfusion as initial therapy **(Fig. 22-72)**.

Laparotomy through horizontal incision is done. Clockwise rotated midgut which is congested and cyanotic is identified. Untwisting of the midgut in counterclockwise direction is done. Viability of bowel is confirmed (colour, vessels in mesentery, peristalsis, on table Doppler). *Ladd's band* is divided, *large bowel is repositioned on left side.* The entire duodenum is *Kocherised* and the ligament of Treitz is divided so that *duodenum becomes straight towards right* iliac fossa. This achieves *wide root of the mesentery* and places the *small bowel in the right* side of the abdomen thus preventing further volvulus. A *complementary appendicectomy* is done—*Ladd's operation.* After laparotomy, if bowel is gangrenous, it is resected and remaining parts of the bowel are exteriorised as enterostomies. A second look operation is done to look for viability of remaining bowel and also to maintain the continuity. Often it will be extensive bowel resection leading to poor prognosis.

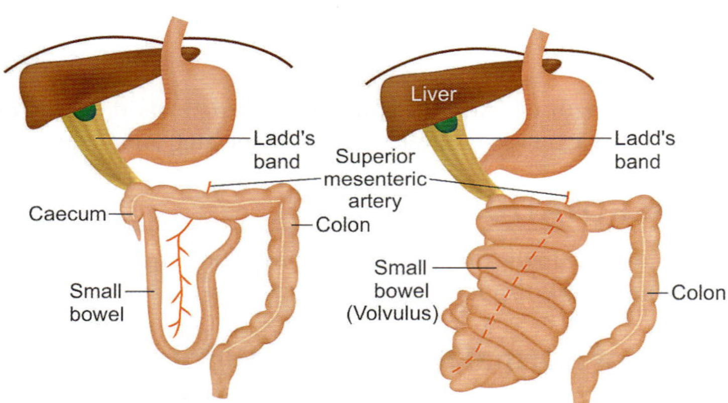

Fig. 22-71: Diagram showing incomplete gut rotation and small bowel volvulus.

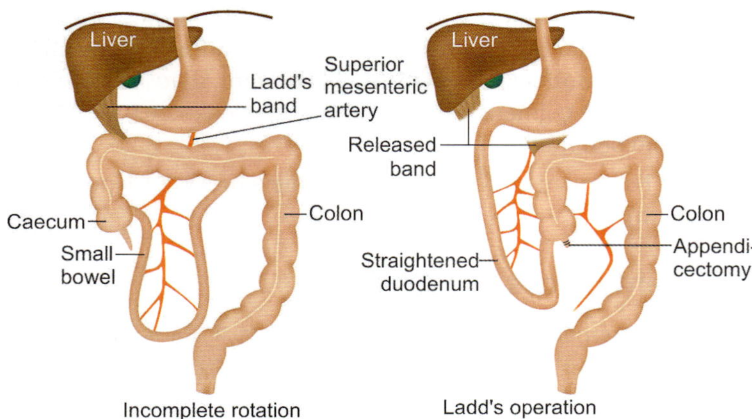

Fig. 22-72: Ladd's operation for incomplete gut rotation. Ladd's band is released. Duodenum is straightened. Appendicectomy is done.

MECONIUM ILEUS

It is neonatal manifestation of fibrocystic disease of the pancreas wherein thick meconium, which is viscid and paste like, gets collected in the terminal ileum. Because of inspissation it forms a firm bolus leading to obstruction of the ileum. Neonates present with features of ileal obstruction as well as respiratory dysfunction, exocrine pancreatic insufficiency, and high salt in the sweat (Na^+ and Cl^- more than 90 mmol/L). Meconium ileus occurs in 15% of patients with cystic fibrosis. Cystic fibrosis is an autosomal recessive disease involving bronchioles, exocrine pancreas and sweat glands.

Condition is common in Caucasians. Exocrine pancreatic insufficiency and malabsorption is seen in 90% of patients with cystic fibrosis. There is hypertrophy and dilatation of the proximal ileum containing thick, viscid, tenacious dark green meconium. Distal ileum and colon are narrow and contracted having greyish meconium pellets. Meconium gets calcified very rapidly. Gangrene, perforation, volvulus can occur in 50% of cases. Intra-uterine perforation causes foetal meconium peritonitis which leads to dense adhesions and calcification in peritoneum. Foetal meconium peritonitis is sterile. Plain X-ray shows calcified meconium pellets with multiple air fluid levels which appear as 'soap-bubbles' (*Neuhauser sign*). Vomitus of the patient which does not contain trypsin, when poured on the exposed X-ray film will not digest the gelatin of the film whereas the vomitus of individual with normal pancreas will digest the gelatin of X-ray film—*very useful test.* Pilocarpine, a cholinergic drug is injected into skin to stimulate the sweating and collected sweat (100 μg sweat) is analysed for sodium and chloride. Elevated albumin level in meconium, sodium level assay in nail clipping, serum immune active trypsin assay are other investigations **(Fig. 22-73)**.

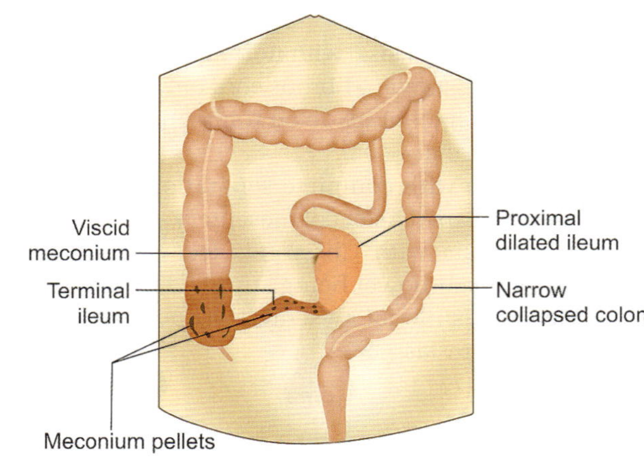

Fig. 22-73: Pathology of meconium ileus. Note the meconium pellets in the distal ileum and colon; thick viscid meconium in proximal ileum.

Treatment

Non-operative Measures

Dissolution through enema can be tried using *gastrografin* which is hyperosmolar and contains Tween 80 as dissolving agent. *Gastrografin* is diatrizoate meglamine with Tween 80 (polysorbate 80) as dissolving agent.

Acetylcholine (2–4%) also can be used for irrigation per-anally. Acetylcholine wash through nasogastric tube also can be used—5–10 mL 6th hourly. Treatment for cystic fibrosis is needed.

Operative Measures

When patient's condition is critical with obstruction, *Bishop-Koop operation* is done. Proximal dilated segment is resected and resected end is anastomosed to side of the distal collapsed ileum. End of the distal ileum is brought out as ileostomy. Through the ileostomy gastrografin or acetylcysteine wash is given regularly to dissolve meconium pellets. This ileostomy can be kept for long time. Continuity is maintained at later period **(Fig. 22-74)**.

Santulli operation is done where proximal ileum is brought as ileostomy for irrigation using a fine tube and distal ileum is sutured to proximal ileum as end-to-side anastomosis **(Fig. 22-75)**.

Resection and anastomosis is ideal if patient is fit and if proximal bowel is suitable for anastomosis.

SHORT BOWEL SYNDROME (SHORT GUT SYNDROME)

It is the symptom complex after massive small bowel resection, i.e. *resection more than 70% of the bowel.* Minimum bowel required is 1.2 meters. Proximal jejunal resection is better tolerated than distal ileal resection. Ileum is more adaptive and has got capacity to increase the absorption capacity more efficiently. So in massive resections, patients with retained ileum will do better. Adaptation is better if ileum and caecum is preserved.

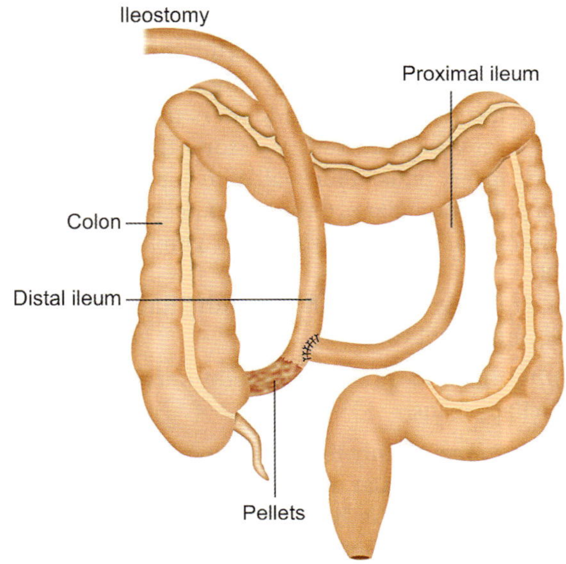

Fig. 22-74: Bishop-Koop operation. Here distal ileum is brought as ileostomy and proximal part sutured to distal bowel.

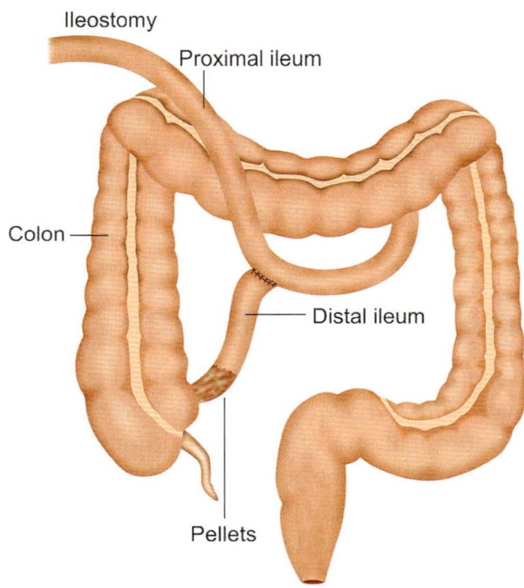

Fig. 22-75: Santulli operation done for meconium ileus wherein proximal ileum is brought out as ileostomy. Distal ileum is sutured to proximal.

Causes

Massive small bowel resection as in superior mesenteric artery ischaemia; multiple sequential resections; recurrent Crohn's disease—common cause, necrotising enterocolitis in neonates and children, intestinal atresia, midgut volvulus, radiation enteritis.

Adaptive Changes in the Retained Small Bowel

Villous hypertrophy and hyperplasia, increased absorptive surface, increased capacity of small bowel, lower transit time of bowel content are different changes.

Factors Deciding the Outcome in Short Gut Syndrome

Age: Infants tolerate massive resection better. Retaining ileocaecal valve shows better outcome as ileocaecal resection interrupts the enterohepatic circulation of bile salts which in colon gets metabolised to secondary bile salts. Secondary bile salts block the absorption of water and electrolytes. Delayed clearance of gastrin causes hyperacidity and peptic ulcer. Adaptability of the small bowel—adaptation is better if ileum and caecum are preserved. Additional colectomy increases the morbidity. In such occasion retained jejunum will function as either of two ways.

'Net absorbers' have adequate absorption of water and sodium and usually will have more than 100 cm of jejunum retained. *'Net secretors'* have less than 100 cm of jejunum retained and lot of sodium and water are secreted into the lumen from plasma. These patients should avoid hypotonic solutions like water/tea; instead should take hypertonic saline with glucose containing 90 mmol sodium/L. WHO cholera fluid is ideal (contains 90 mmol sodium/L).

Clinical features: Diarrhoea, fluid and electrolyte deficiency, severe malnutrition, recurrent bacterial enteritis.

Outcome of Short Bowel Syndrome

Severe malabsorption, severe dehydration, gallstone formation due to altered bile metabolism, urinary calculi due to increased oxalate level, water and electrolyte imbalance, diarrhoea is common, recurrent bacterial enteritis, fulminant hepatic failure often can occur, osteomalacia, tetany, hypomagnesaemia, bleeding diathesis, peripheral neuropathy.

MASSIVE BOWEL RESECTION

Resection of *more than 200 cm* of small bowel is called as massive resection. *Metabolic sequelae* in massive resection depends on—extent and anatomical site of resection, functional capacity and adaptation of the small or large bowel, cause for the resection. It causes gastrin hypersecretion, increased parietal cell mass in stomach, peptic ulceration; increased endocrine pancreatic secretion; hypoalbuminaemia, oedema. *Resection of more than 100 cm of distal ileum* causes diarrhoea and steatorrhoea (steatorrhoea is faecal fat >6 g/day), increases bile lithogenicity, causes deficiency of vitamins A, D, E, K; colonic bacteria converts unabsorbed fatty acids and conjugated bile salts into hydroxy fatty acids and deconjugated bile salts. *Ileum* maintains enterohepatic circulation of bile salts, absorption of vitamin B12 and vitamin D. Resection of middle part of small bowel is better tolerated. *Removal of ileocaecal valve* reduces the intestinal transit time; reduces absorption of vitamin B12, calcium, magnesium, zinc; increases diarrhoea and contamination of shortened small bowel by bacteria. In massive resection, *colonic bacteria* degrade fatty acids into lactate and short chain fatty acids; lactate reduces colonic pH which inhibits bacteroides; due to this acid resistant anaerobes will increase in colon which produces large amount of D lactate which is absorbed causing *D lactic acidosis* presenting with confusion, ataxia and nystagmus. *TPN* was introduced by Dudrick. It is very useful in short gut syndrome.

Treatment

Early Phase

Total parenteral nutrition.

Fat and fibre free but protein rich liquid diet with essential fatty acids; diarrhoea is controlled by loperamide/codeine phosphate; oral cholestyramine to bind bile salts is needed in massive resection which includes ileum; parenteral vitamin B12 injection regularly; H2 antagonists/PPIs/somatostatin (to reduce secretions from stomach, liver and pancreas); octreotide reduces the secretion and reduces GI motility; fluid and electrolyte management; control of diarrhoea.

Late Phase

Enteral nutrition is used to stimulate intestinal adaptation; TPN supplement—often permanently required; *home parenteral nutrition* is universally used method in western countries. But in Asian countries it is not yet practicable. Hormones and glutamine administration are under trial.

Surgical techniques to delay the intestinal transit time or small bowel transplantation are under trial but with less success. *Reversal of 10 cm intestinal segment* to delay transit time can be useful. *Intestinal lengthening* to delay transit time and increase the absorption surface is done. *Small bowel transplantation*, ideal but graft rejection and failure is the problem. Antiperistaltic colonic interposition into the small bowel segment also tried. Regeneration of intestinal mucosa over denuded serosa is a new method. Longitudinal splitting of the intestine and closing of these as separate tubes which are anastomosed to each other to achieve lengthening—*Binachi's surgery*; Mucosal *stem cell transplantation using enterocytes* without lymphoid tissue; Seeded mucosal autografts in prosthetic tubes are other newer methods on trial.

B. APPENDIX

SURGICAL ANATOMY OF APPENDIX

It is a worm-like diverticulum, located at the terminal end of the caecum where three taeniae join, about 2 cm below the ileocaecal orifice. Usually, it is around 2–20 cm in size but can be variable (9/10 cm average). Size of its lumen is that of matchstick. Diameter of appendix is 3–8 mm; diameter of lumen is 1–3 mm (matchstick). It is longer in children. *Base of the appendix is located 2 cm below the junction of the transtubercular and right lateral planes. McBurney's point is only site of maximum tenderness in appendicitis* **(Figs. 22-76 and 22-77)**.

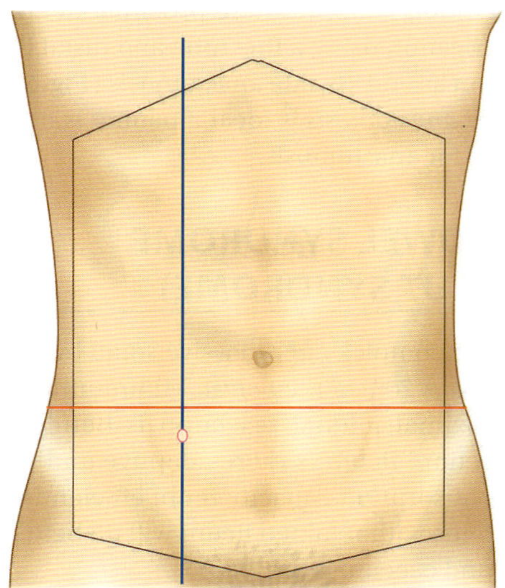

Fig. 22-76: Base of the appendix is located 2 cm below the junction of the transtubercular and right lateral planes.

Mesoappendix is extension of the mesentery containing appendicular artery, a branch of ileocolic artery. Artery runs behind the terminal part of the ileum and enters the mesoappendix near base where it gives a recurrent anastomotic branch to posterior caecal artery. Artery ends in the wall of the appendix near tip. Often an accessory appendicular artery (*of Seshachalam*) may be present. Thrombosis of these vessels leads to gangrenous appendicitis **(Fig. 22-78)**.

Venous drainage is through appendicular, ileocolic, superior mesenteric and portal vein.

Nerve supply: T9 and T10 sympathetic nerves supply appendix through coeliac plexus.

Lymphatic drainage: Mainly to ileocolic nodes. Often drainage may occur through appendicular nodes.

Mucosa of appendix is lined by columnar cells with crypts. Submucosa contains numerous lymphatic aggregations (follicles) *('Abdominal Tonsil')*. Opening of the appendix into caecum is guarded by *'valve of Geralch'* **(Fig. 22-79)**.

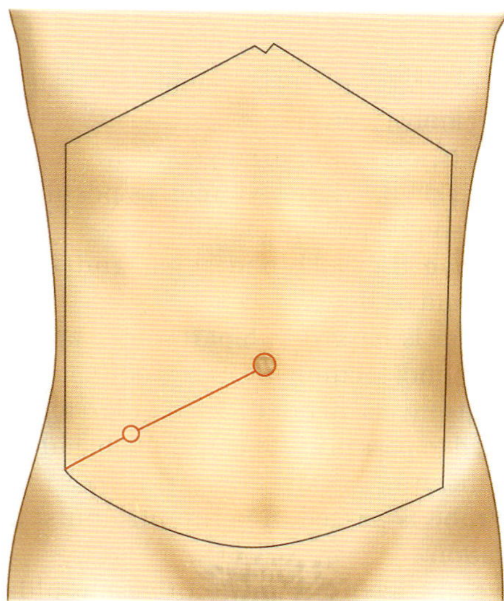

Fig. 22-77: McBurney's point is only site of maximum tenderness in appendicitis. It is at the junction of lateral 1/3rd and medial 2/3rd of right spinoumbilical line.

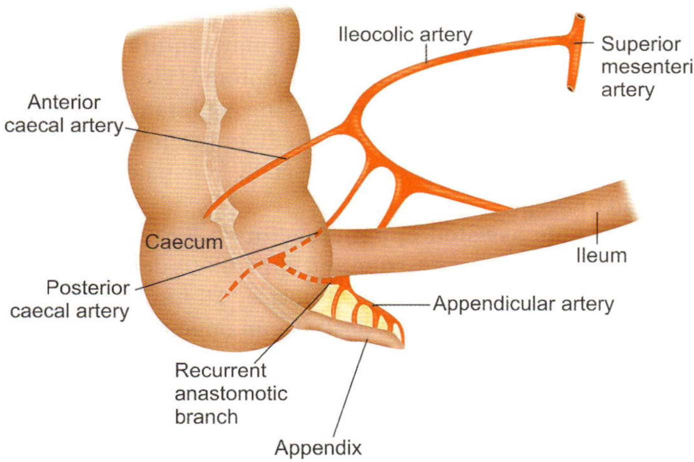

Fig. 22-78: Appendicular artery.

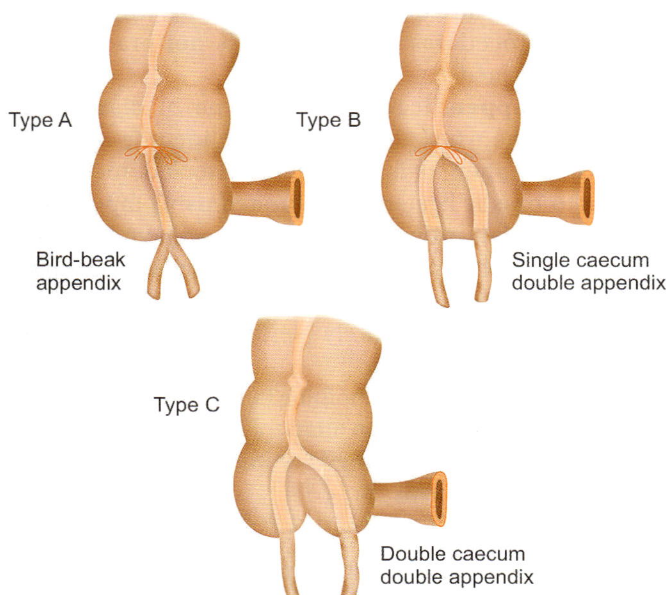

Fig. 22-79: Wallbridge classification of duplication of appendix.

Duplication of appendix (Wallbridge classification)
- Type A: Partial duplication in a single caecum.
- Type B: Two separate appendices in a single caecum.
- Type C: Double caecum with each one having one appendix.

Different Positions are

Most common position *is retrocaecal (65–75%). Next common is pelvic (21–31%). Other sites are:* Preileal (anterior)—rare (1%); postileal (splenic)—rarest (0.4%); paracaecal; subcaecal (2.2%); subhepatic.

Often it may be in subserosal plane leading to difficult dissection during appendicectomy. In situs inversus appendix is on *the left side* **(Fig. 22-80)**.

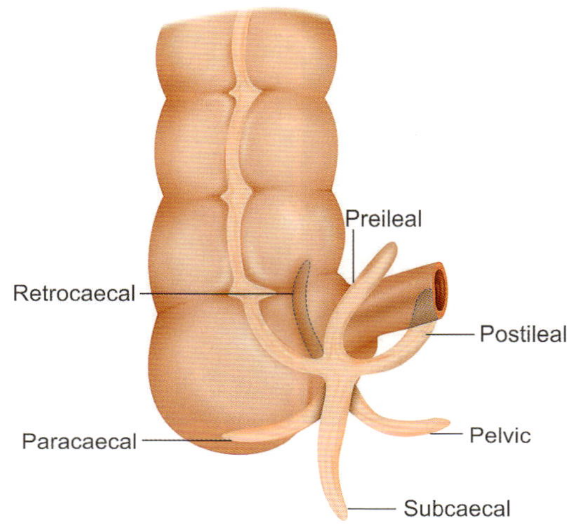

Fig. 22-80: Different positions of the appendix.

APPENDICECTOMY

Reginald Fitz from Boston coined the term appendectomy in 1886. Chester McBurney started early surgery for acute appendicitis with muscle splitting incision (1884-1889).

Indications

- Acute appendicitis.
- Recurrent appendicitis.
- Appendicitis in pregnancy—done in 2nd trimester ideally.
- Appendicectomy as a part to give colonic lavage (Doodley's lavage). Appendicectomy along with other procedures—in correcting the malrotation of the gut (Ladd's procedure).
- Appendicectomy in carcinoid tumour involving the tip of appendix and tumour size less than 2 cm.
- Appendicectomy is done in *Munchausen syndrome*—a psychological condition.

Contraindications for Appendicectomy

- Appendicectomy is contraindicated in appendicular mass when formed after an attack of appendicitis. Here appendicectomy is done after 6 weeks as interval appendicectomy.
- Appendicectomy is not done in acute phase of Crohn's disease; however, it should be done if appendix and caecum is diseased.

Investigations

- Total leucocyte count is increased.
- Ultrasound is done to rule out other conditions like ureteric stone, pancreatitis, ovarian cyst, ectopic pregnancy and also to confirm appendicular mass or abscess **(Fig. 22-81)**.

Sonographic criterias for appendicitis (85% specificity)

- Non-compressible appendix of size >6 mm AP diameter,
- hyperechoic thickened appendix wall >2 mm—target sign.
- Appendicolith.
- Interruption of submucosal continuity.
- Periappendicular fluid.

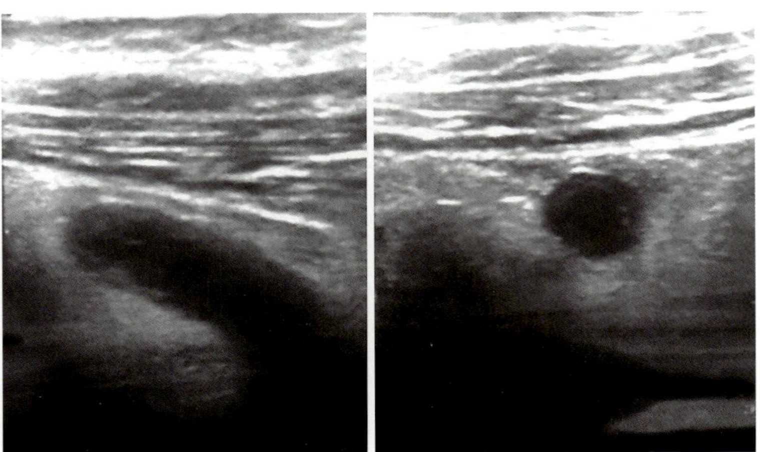

Fig. 22-81: Ultrasound showing dilated non-compressible appendix.

- Contrast CT scan is very much useful when diagnosis is difficult especially in old people. Dilated appendix; dilated lumen; thickened wall; non-filling of the lumen by contrast or air; periappendicular fluid collection; presence of mass/abscess/ associated pathology like carcinoma can be identified. It has 95% sensitivity and specificity with 95% accuracy. *Dirty fat thickened mesoappendix*, appendicular *phlegmon*, appendicular *faecolith* and thickened caecum funnelling contrast into the orifice of the appendix as *arrowhead sign*—are all relevant features in CT scan.
- MRI is very useful in diagnosing appendicitis in *pregnancy*.
- *C-reactive protein*, even though non-specific increases in acute phase. *99mTc HMPAO labelled leucocyte* imaging may give guidance in deciding the management.
- Laparoscopy is the most useful method **(Fig. 22-82)**.

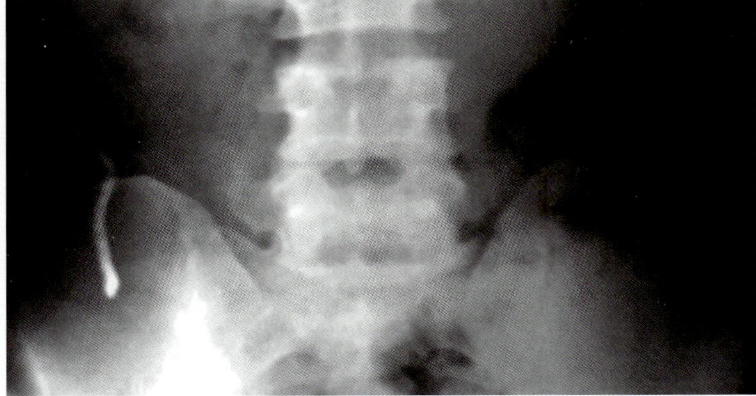

Fig. 22-82: Calcified appendix/faecolith in plain X-ray.

Preparation

- Preoperative diagnosis by US abdomen; CT scan; total leucocyte count and by clinical features.
- Nil per oral for 6 hours prior to surgery.
- Preparation of skin of entire abdomen as possibility of extension of the incision should be kept in mind.
- Fitness for anaesthesia; blood sugar and serum creatinine estimation should be done.
- Urinary catheter is passed in laparoscopic appendicectomy or in difficult appendicectomy or in appendicitis with peritonitis where laparotomy is needed. In regular appendicectomies patient is asked to pass urine to empty the bladder before coming to operation theatre.
- Nasogastric tube is passed in peritonitis, burst appendicitis or with suppuration.
- Preoperative intravenous antibiotics should be started—amoxycillin, metronidazole or higher antibiotics depending on the need of individual case basis.

Types of Appendicectomy

- **Open appendicectomy:** Good old method. Here entire peritoneal cavity cannot be visualised. Often it may require extension of incision or converting into formal laparotomy **(Fig. 22-83)**.
- **Laparoscopic appendicectomy:** It is the gold standard approach for appendicectomy. Incision is small; entire peritoneal cavity can be seen which is important especially in females. Recovery is faster in this type.
- **Laparoscopic assisted appendicectomy:** Peritoneal cavity is visualised through laparoscope and appendix is delivered outside under vision through umbilical port or 10 mm working port. Mesoappendix and stump is dealt like in open appendicectomy. It is faster and meantime diagnosis is also confirmed. But it is often difficult to bring out the appendix with mesoappendix outside as mesoappendix may get torn.
- Appendicectomy can be done through **single incision laparoscopic surgery (SILS)**.
- **Interval appendicectomy** is done after initial conservative treatment for appendicitis or appendicular mass.
- **Incidental appendicectomy** is done along with some other abdominal procedures. Nowadays it is not practiced unless genuinely indicated.
- **Retrograde appendicectomy** is a type of dissection (not approach) done when tip is difficult to identify or to dissect. Here base of appendix is identified, dissected, mesoappendix adjacent to base is ligated or fulgurated using bipolar cautery. Base is crushed; transfixed using 2-zero vicryl and dissection is proceeded towards tip by repeated clamping and ligating tissue close to the appendix and ligating repeatedly until tip is dissected and appendix is freed entirely (serial clamping, division and ligation).
- **Elective appendicectomy** is nothing but interval appendicectomy done after recovering from an attack of acute appendicitis.
- **Emergency appendicectomy** is doing appendicectomy at the time of acute appendicitis.

Note:

- There is no role for prophylactic appendicectomy.
- But removal of normal appendix in an exploration for presumed appendicitis is accepted based on following reasons:

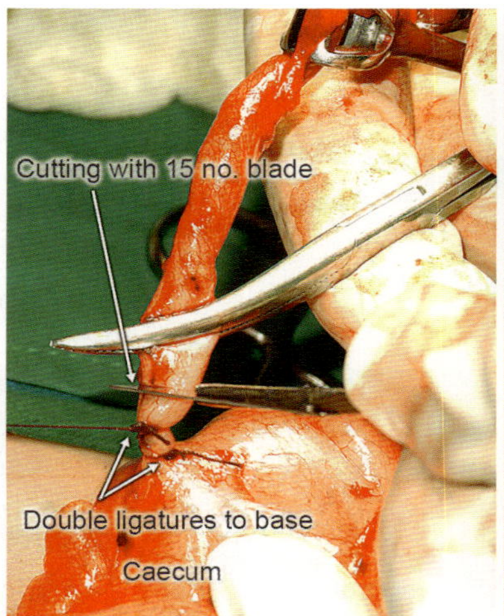

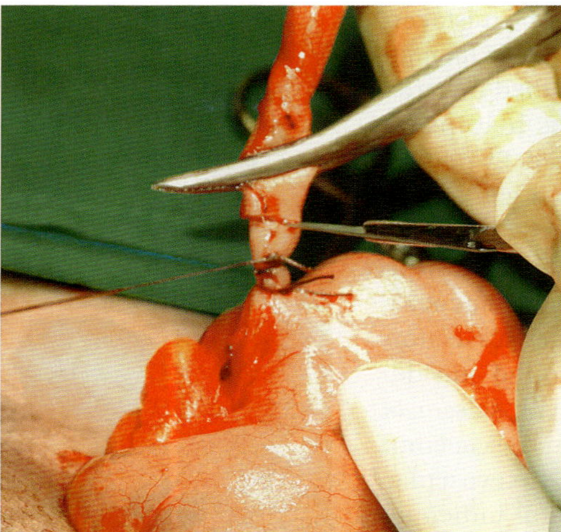
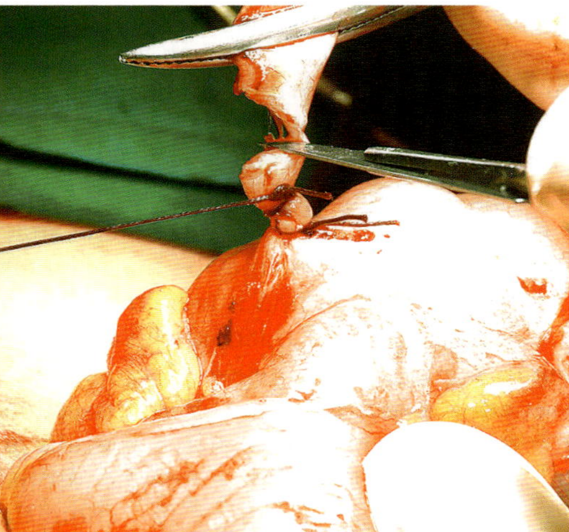

Fig. 22-83: Open appendicectomy.

- Early acute appendicitis (catarrhal/mucosal) on gross inspection is difficult to determine accurately; so grossly normal looking appendix still can have early appendicitis.
- It avoids future diagnostic dilemma in chronic pain in right iliac fossa. Pain may be due to inflammatory bowel disease or gynaecologic conditions.
- A scar in right iliac fossa in any patient is assumed by surgeon that appendicectomy is done.
- Long kinked appendix or presence of faecolith may justify appendicectomy.

OPEN APPENDICECTOMY

Anaesthesia: However, even spinal anaesthesia is satisfactory general anaesthesia is ideal.

Incision

- *McBurney's incision* is used (McArthur; Gridiron). McBurney's point is at junction of lateral 1/3rd and medial 2/3rd of right spinoumbilical line. At this point, incision of 5 cm in length is made perpendicular to this line 2.5 cm on each side. It is muscle splitting incision. Gridiron is a frame of cross beams to support a ship during repairs.
- *Lanz crease incision* is curved horizontal incision of 5 cm in length. Deeper dissection is same as McBurney's incision. It is cosmetically better as it is in the crease line.
- *Rutherford Morrison's muscle cutting incision:* It is usually modification done in an originally placed McBurney's incision as an extension to have better approach. Here internal oblique and transverse abdominis muscle are cut laterally. It is often done in higher or difficult or subhepatic appendix.
- *Fowler-Weir (Fowler-Davis; Rockey-Davis) approach:* Here extension of the original McBurney's incision is done medially and below by cutting lateral part of the rectus sheath. It is used in pelvic appendix or to feel the right ovary properly.
- *Right paramedian or lower midline incision:* It is used in case of peritonitis due to burst appendicitis **(Fig. 22-84)**.

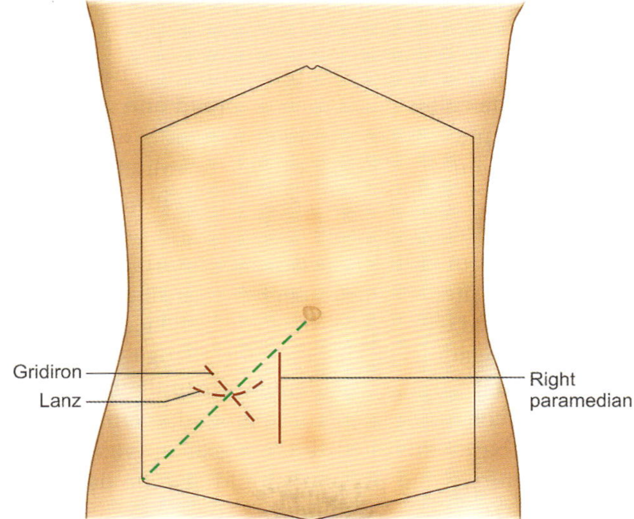

Fig. 22-84: Different approaches for open appendicectomy.

Procedure

Skin is incised. Outer Camper fascia with subcutaneous fat is incised. Inner membranous scarpa's layer is also incised. Often superficial epigastric and superficial circumflex veins may require to be ligated. External oblique aponeurosis is visualised. It is incised laterally using blade. Medially it is cut along the line of incision using scissor or cautery. Cut edges are held using haemostats. Two Langebeck retractors are placed deep to the aponeurosis to visualise internal oblique muscle. Internal oblique muscle is split in the line of fibers using curved haemostat (curved medium sized artery forceps). Direction of the tip of the instrument should be laterally to prevent inadvertent opening of the rectus sheath and muscle and also to avoid injuring the inferior epigastric vessels. Similarly transversus abdominis muscle is split to reach the peritoneum. Often two fingers are passed deep into the wound and stretched away from the wound line to increase the space underneath. Often extraperitoneal fat may be present which needs careful blunt dissection with finger. Small vessel bleeding can occur which should be controlled using cautery. It is confirmed that the bowel is not close under the peritoneum by feeling peritoneum with two fingers. Peritoneum is opened by an oblique incision using blade or scissor; fluid if exudes out should be collected for culture. Omentum at the site under the peritoneum suggests that appendix is inflamed. Peritoneum incision is extended along the line of skin incision (wound) to enter the peritoneal cavity.

Caecum is located in the right iliac fossa which is identified by the presence of 3 taeniae. Often summit of the sigmoid colon when it is redundant will be towards the right iliac fossa and may be mistaken for caecum and leads into futile search for appendix. Once taeniae of caecum is identified; caecum is held and gently pulled towards the wound without causing serosal tear. Caecum is held using Babcock's forceps. Base of the appendix will be identified. By putting the index finger inside the peritoneal cavity one can gently feel tubular structure which has got blind end and attached to caecum. But fallopian tube in females may be mistaken for that. Once the base of appendix is identified it is held with another Babcock's forceps. Gentle continuous traction with careful finger dissection makes entire appendix to be delivered through the wound outside. Whenever adhesions are present sharp dissection with scissor is better to prevent tear in the base of the appendix or in the caecum. Adhesions anywhere other than mesoappendix part are avascular and will not bleed much by sharp dissection. Careful judicious cautery dissection is allowed but one should not cause cautery injury to caecum or base which may lead to late necrosis, perforation and peritonitis which is life-threatening. During dissection, bowel should be held using non-toothed forceps.

In females by passing right index finger, right ovary and fallopian tube should be palpated to confirm that they are normal. If there is fluid it should be collected. If there is blood one should suspect ectopic gestation and in such situation appendix will look grossly normal. It is also important to pull out terminal ileum for the presence of Meckel's diverticulum; and also to inspect and palpate ileal mesentery for enlarged lymph nodes.

Mesoappendix is often thick, oedematous and friable. Appendicular artery can be often seen through light transillumination which is dissected, clamped with haemostats, cut and ligated using 2-zero silk or vicryl (first ligation can be done by passing two ligatures and then can be cut). If it is difficult to identify appendicular artery which is a branch of ileocolic artery then mesoappendix clamped at several places up to the base and transfixed using silk or vicryl. Accessory appendicular artery when present should also be dealt similarly **(Figs. 22-85A to D)**.

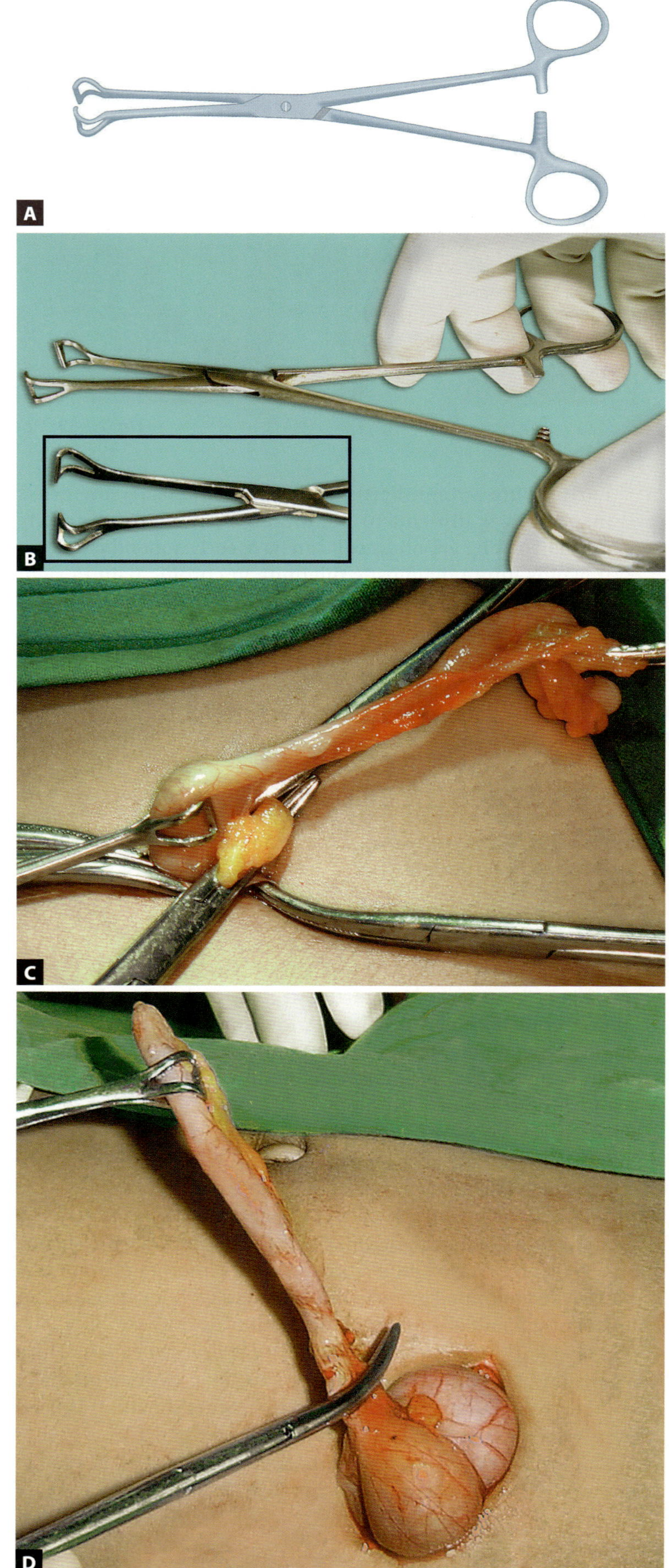

Figs. 22-85A to D: Babcock's instrument is used to hold appendix and caecum during appendicectomy. Caecum should be held at taenia.

Appendix is held with Babcock's with proper visualisation of the base of the appendix with adequate caecal wall. Base, 3–5 mm from the caecal junction is crushed using curved artery forceps (haemostat) and released and applied again 1 cm distally. Crushed part of the base of appendix is transfixed using figure of eight suture by 2-zero vicryl suture. Crushing the base was good old practice, which is done to appose the mucosal surface firmly. But now it is argued that crushing is not necessary and transfixation is done without crushing the base. Additional simple (not transfixation) ligature using vicryl or silk is done 2 mm proximal to this to have double ligation of the base. Appendix is cut between distally applied artery forceps and transfixation ligature using no 15 blade. Stump is cleaned with normal saline or povidone iodine solution. Two ligatures are safer to prevent giving way and it is practiced commonly; evidence suggests one strong proper ligature at the base is sufficient enough to hold **(Fig. 22-86)**.

Base of the appendix can be ligated with two firm ligatures using silk or vicryl without any transfixation also, like what is practiced in laparoscopic appendicectomy **(Figs. 22-87A and B)**.

Invagination or Burial of the Appendix Stump

Burial of the stump can be done by various methods. Need for invagination or burial and its advantages are controversial. It was earlier thought that burial prevents the exposure of the stump to free peritoneal cavity which may lead into adhesion/band or sepsis.

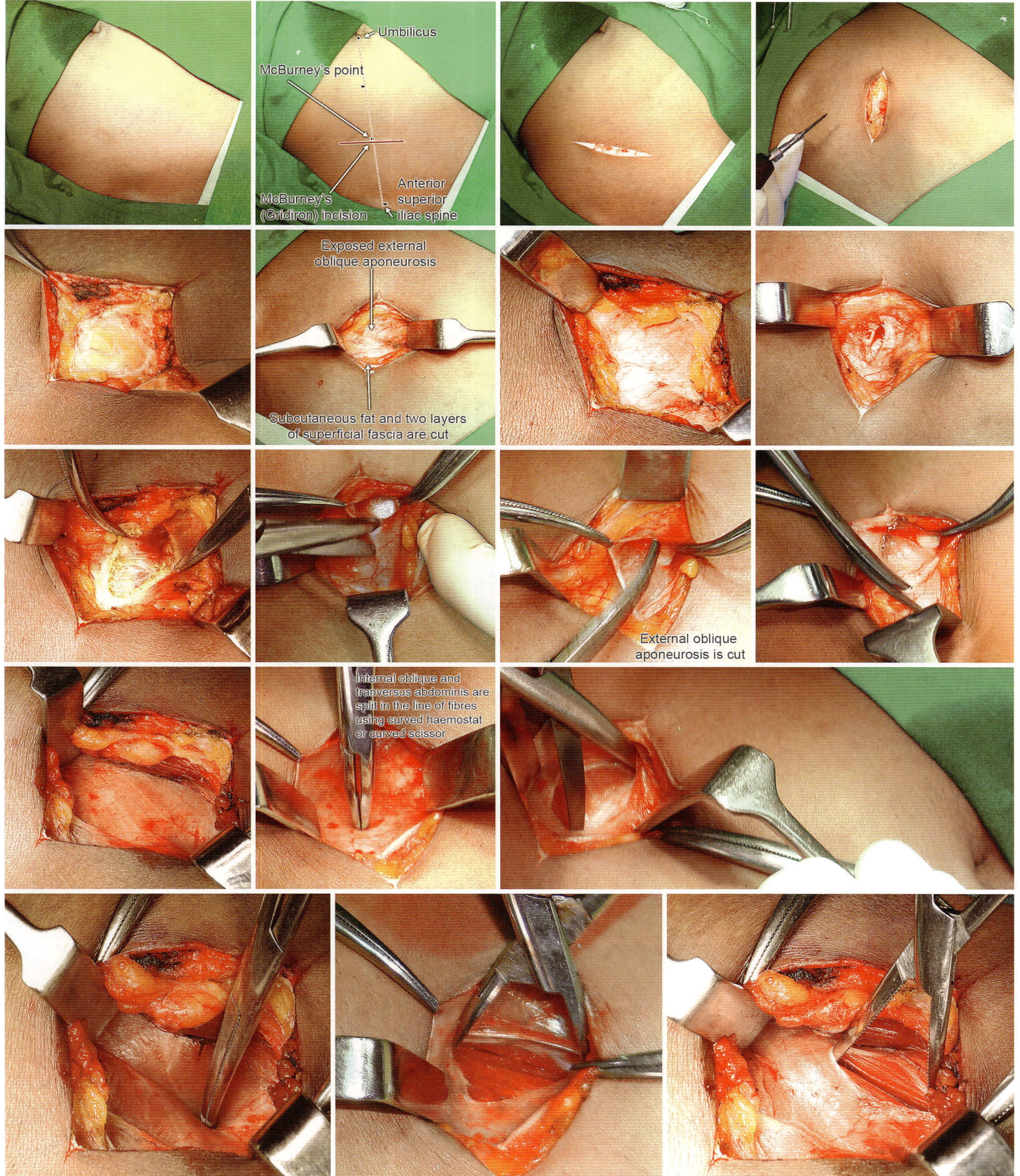
Umbilicus
McBurney's point
McBurney's (Gridiron) incision
Anterior superior iliac spine
Exposed external oblique aponeurosis
Subcutaneous fat and two layers of superficial fascia are cut
External oblique aponeurosis is cut
Internal oblique and tranversus abdominis are split in the line of fibres using curved haemostat or curved scissor

Figs. 22-86(1)

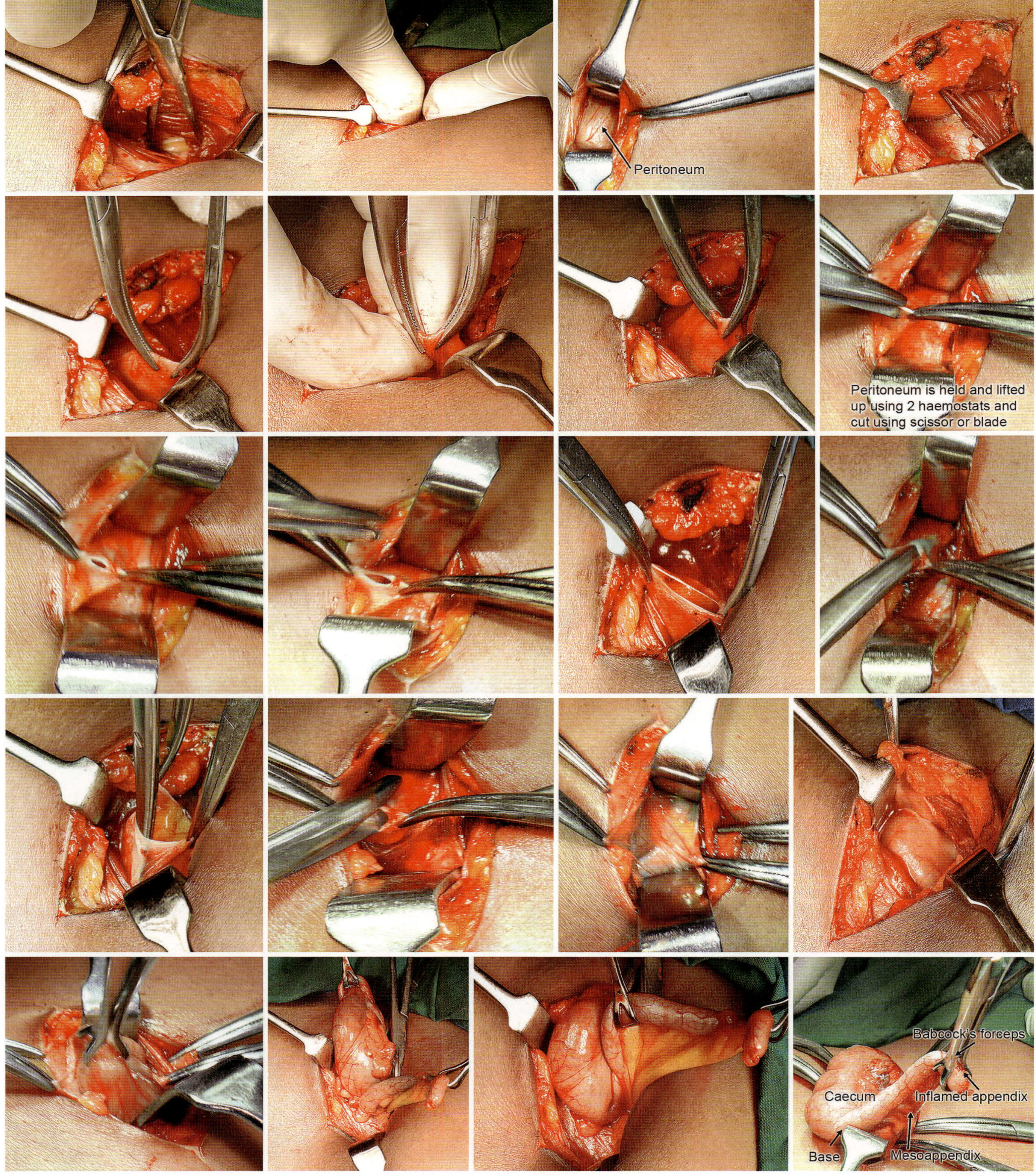
Peritoneum
Peritoneum is held and lifted up using 2 haemostats and cut using scissor or blade
Babcock's forceps
Caecum
Inflamed appendix
Base
Mesoappendix

Figs. 22-86(2)

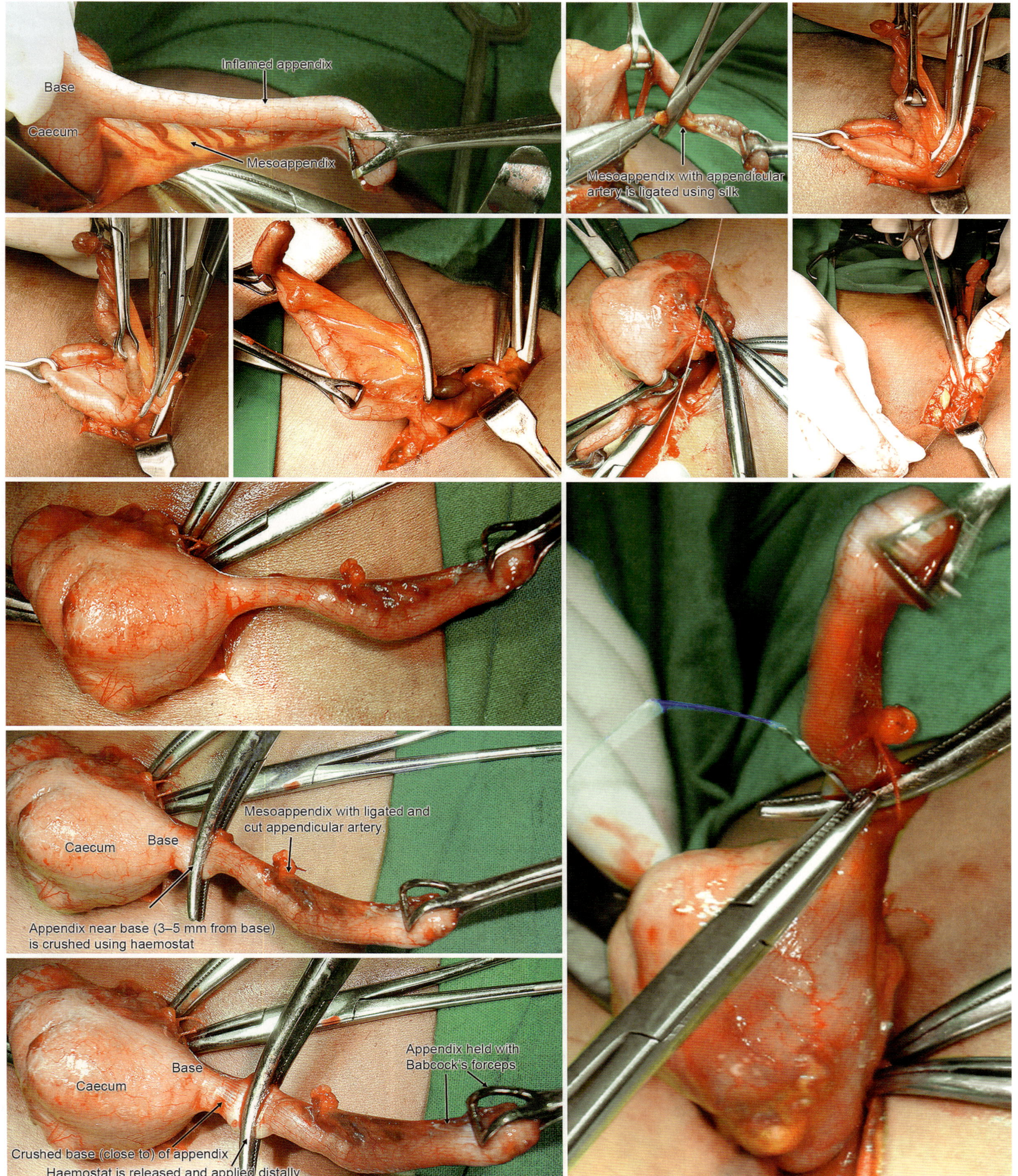
Inflamed appendix
Base
Caecum
Mesoappendix
Mesoappendix with appendicular artery is ligated using silk
Mesoappendix with ligated and cut appendicular artery
Caecum
Base
Appendix near base (3–5 mm from base) is crushed using haemostat
Appendix held with Babcock's forceps
Base
Caecum
Crushed base (close to) of appendix
Haemostat is released and applied distally

Figs. 22-86(3)

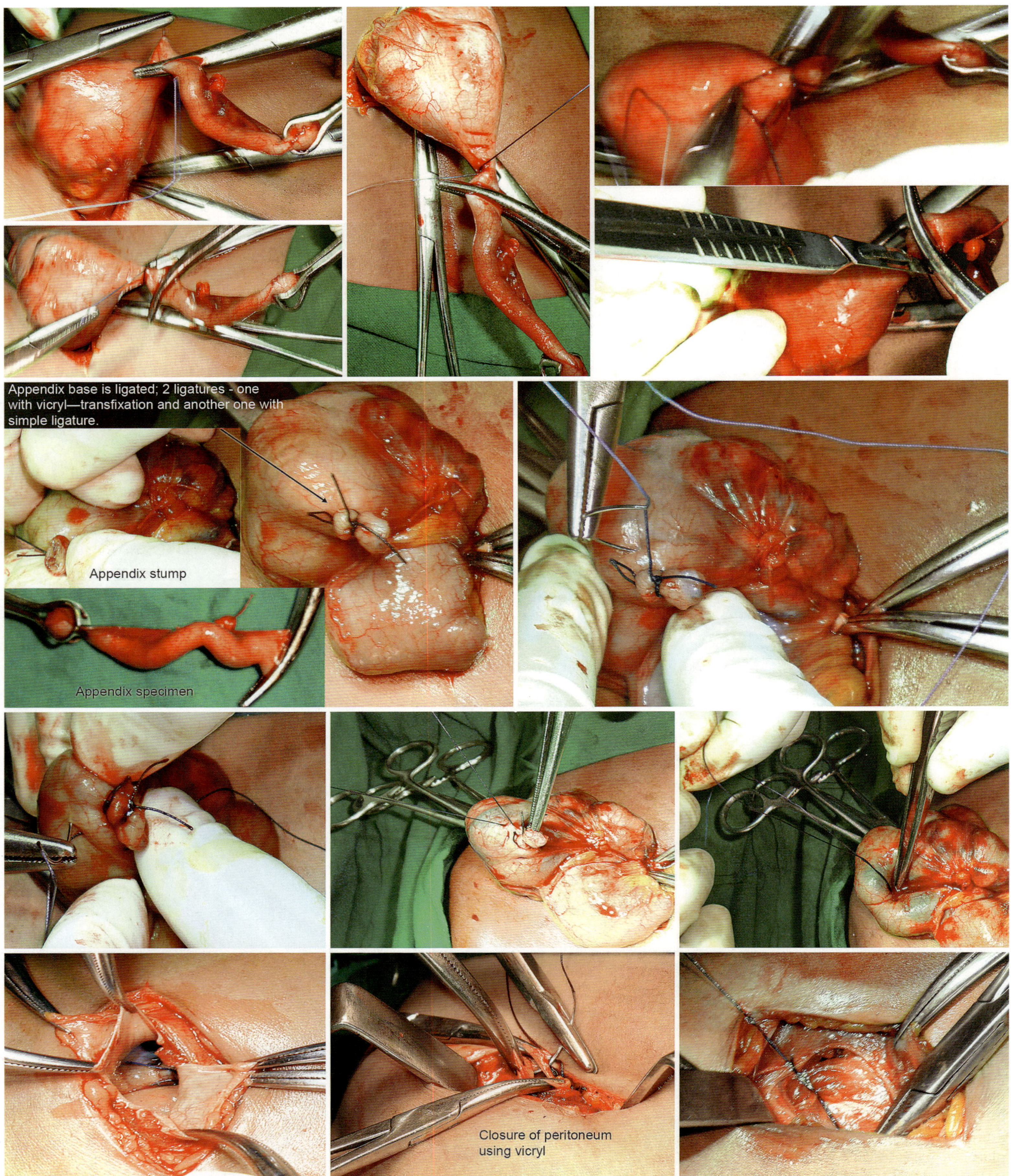
Appendix base is ligated; 2 ligatures - one with vicryl—transfixation and another one with simple ligature.
Appendix stump
Appendix specimen
Closure of peritoneum using vicryl

Figs. 22-86(4)

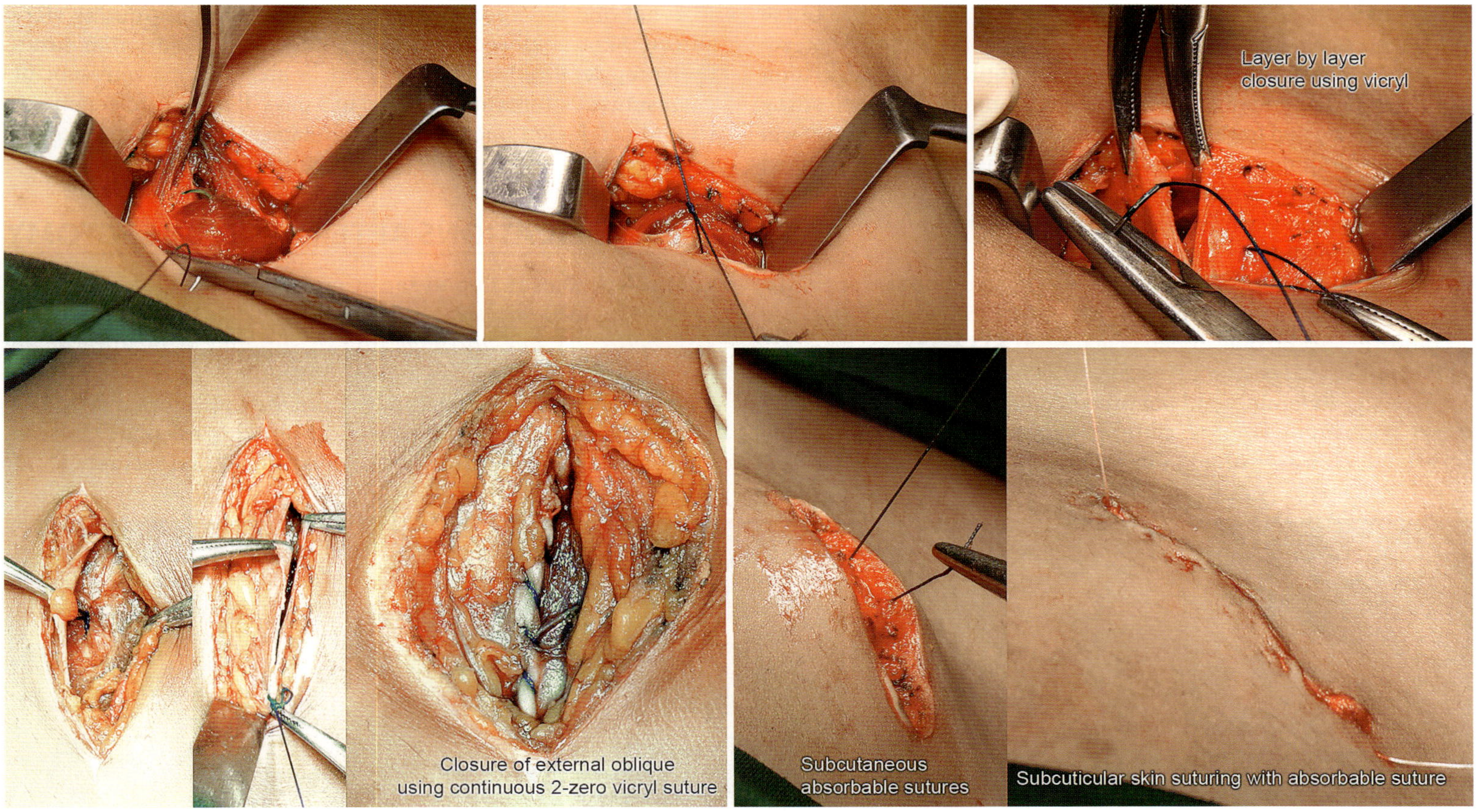

Layer by layer closure using vicryl

Closure of external oblique using continuous 2-zero vicryl suture

Subcutaneous absorbable sutures

Subcuticular skin suturing with absorbable suture

Figs. 22-86(5)

Figs. 22-86(1 to 5): Technique of open appendicectomy.

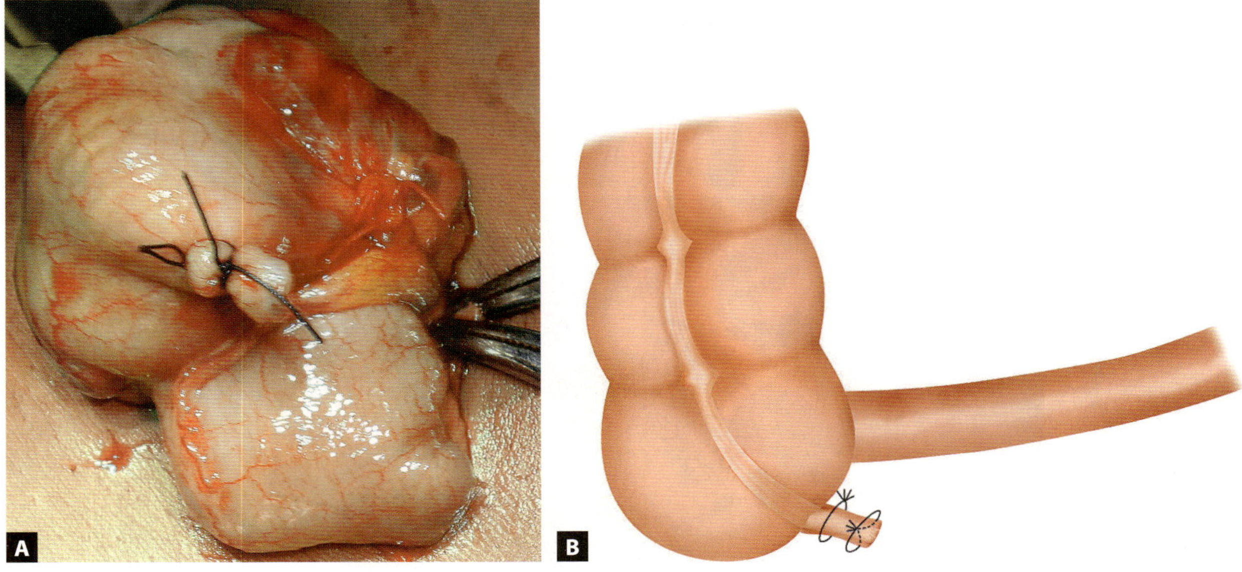

Figs. 22-87A and B: Ligation of the stump of the appendix.

But present antisepsis, antibiotics use proved it is not so and there is no need to invaginate the stump. There is a debate that burial itself may precipitate abscess formation by creating closed cavity within the stump—serosa area. But again it is also controversial; however, present accepted trend/method is not to use invagination/burial; but place two ligatures with one of them may or may not be transfixation.

Burial when used is done by various methods—Simple 2–3 seromuscular Lembert interrupted sutures or purse string sutures. Purse string suture is taken using 2-zero silk or vicryl. Bites are taken circumferentially around the base starting from one point 5–10 mm away from the base on the caecal wall beginning from a taenia and ending (last bite) again at same taenia usually last bite passes beyond the first seromuscular caecal bite. Ends of the suture material are kept long with small haemostats. It is usual practice to take seromuscular invagination purse string circumferential sutures before transfixing the appendix but after freeing the appendix from mesoappendix.

Many surgeons also practice taking seromuscular caecal purse string sutures after transfixation and cutting the appendix. Whatever the way it does not make much difference until burial/invagination is proper and adequate. Once appendix stump is cut purse string suture is gently tied towards the base; in the meantime, assistant will push the stump deep to serosa using a haemostat or non-toothed forceps. Burial knot is placed.

Normal saline wash is given to the cavity and suction is done **(Figs. 22-88 to 22-90)**.

If appendix is perforated and there is pus around the appendix drain (tube/corrugated) is placed in the right iliac fossa. But its use is controversial and questioned **(Figs. 22-91 to 22-93)**.

Wound is closed in layers: Peritoneum with continuous 2-zero vicryl. Transversus abdominis and internal oblique with 2 or 3 interrupted vicryl apposition sutures. Sutures should be loose and fascia covering the muscle should be included (not just muscle bundle). External oblique aponeurosis is closed using continuous vicryl suture. Skin is closed with interrupted non-absorbable suture (polypropylene/polyethylene) suture or absorbable 3-zero subcuticular suture. Sutures are removed in 7 days. If there is infection skin wound can be left open until it granulates. When infection comes under control it is closed by secondary suturing.

COMPLICATIONS AFTER APPENDICECTOMY

- *Paralytic ileus* is due to sepsis and bowel handling. It usually subsides in 2–3 days.
- *Reactionary haemorrhage* due to slipping of ligature of the appendicular artery can be life-threatening. Tachycardia, palor, dropping haemoglobin and PCV are the indicators. Emergency re-exploration with transfusion of blood is needed. Clots are removed. Bleeding artery is identified and ligated securely.

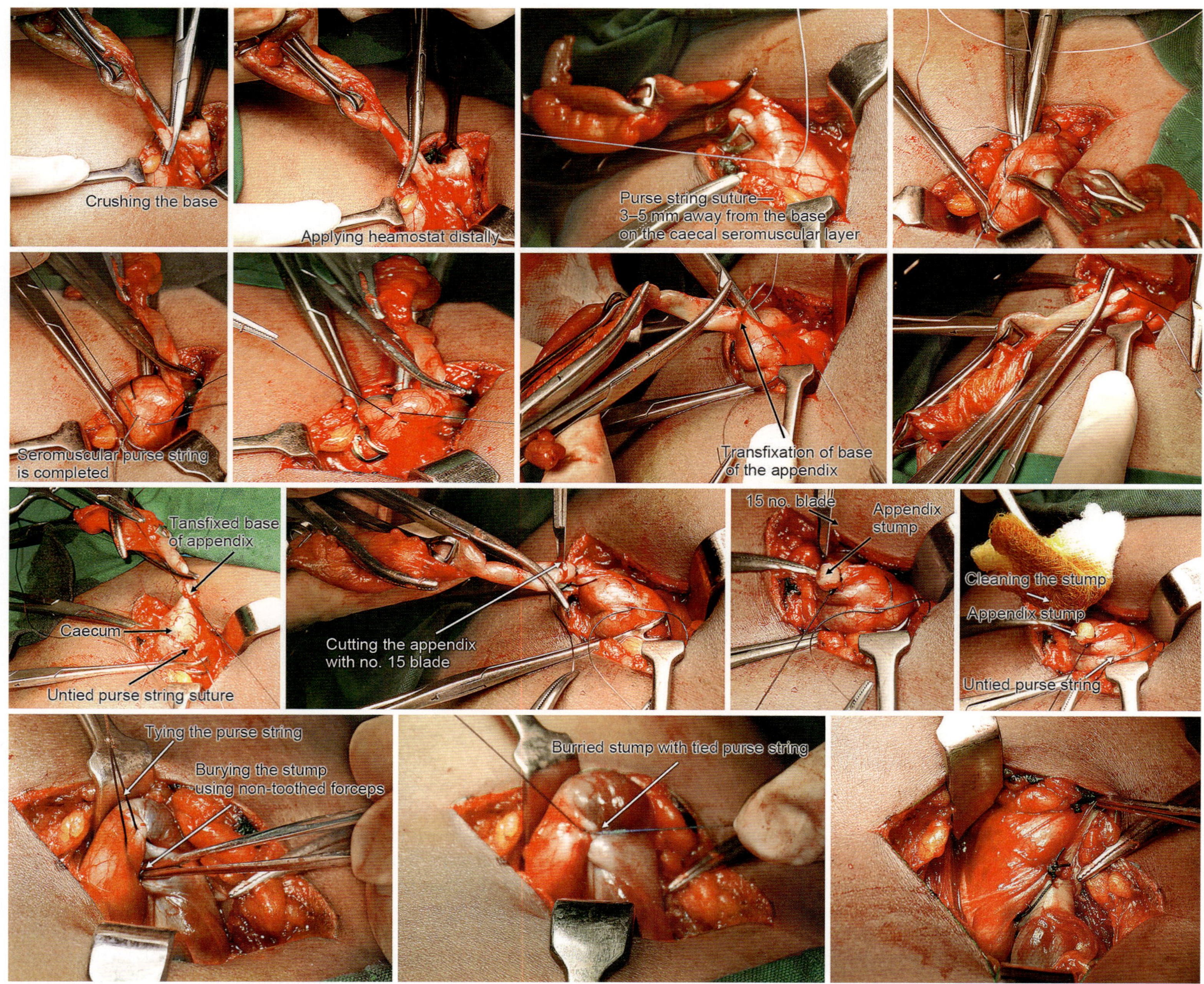

Fig. 22-88: Invagination of appendicular stump using purse string suture.

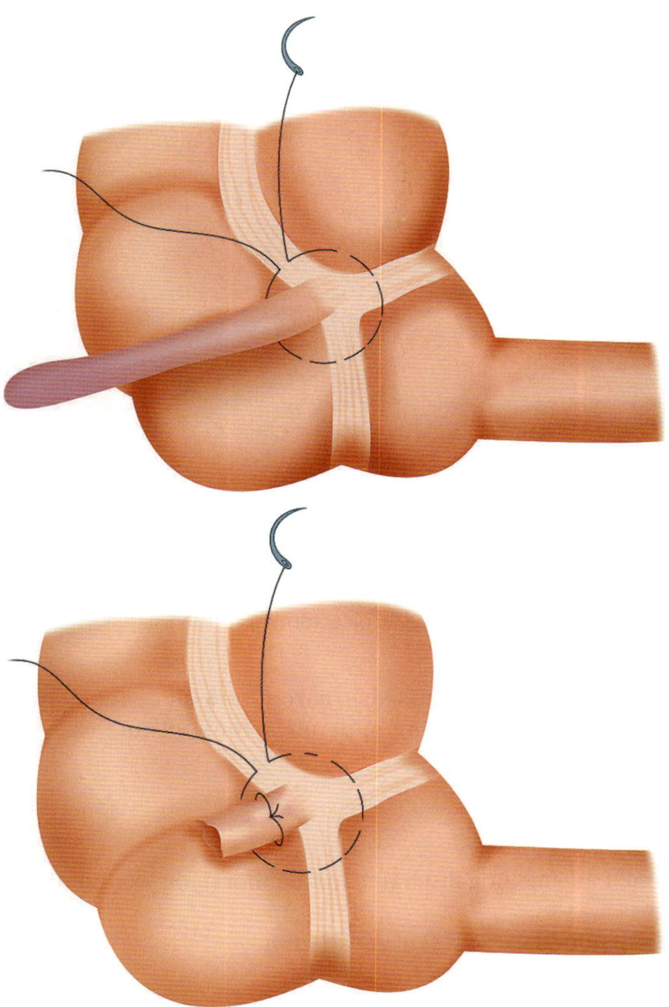

Fig. 22-89: Purse string suture is passed using vicryl or silk by taking bite from taenia then seromuscular bites 5 mm away from the base of appendix circumferentially to reach same taenia again; appendicectomy is done then purse string suture is tied to invaginate the stump of appendix.

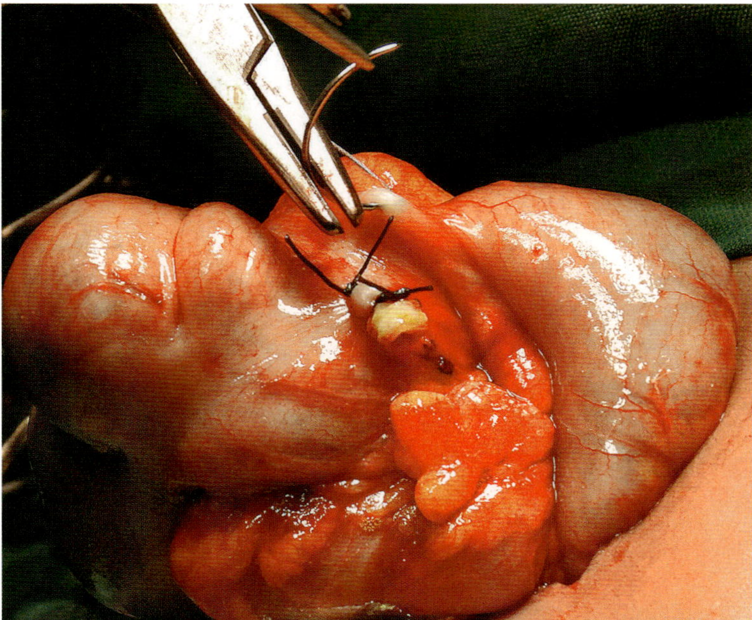

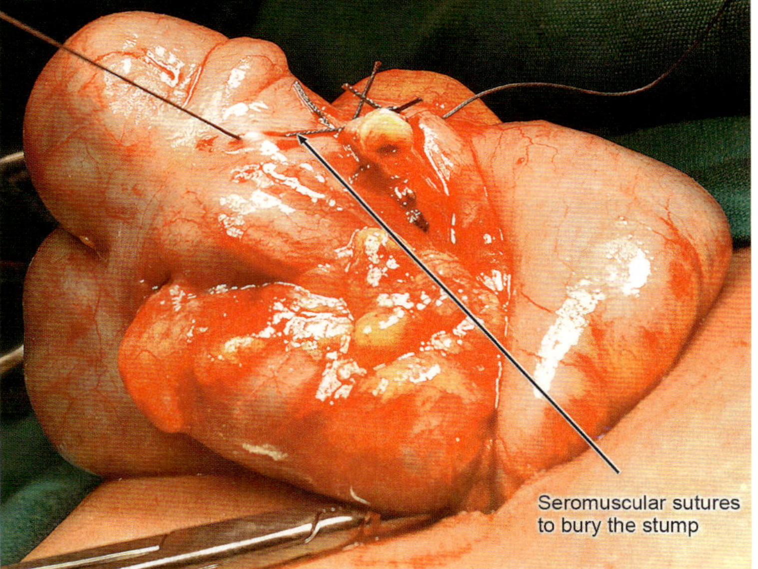

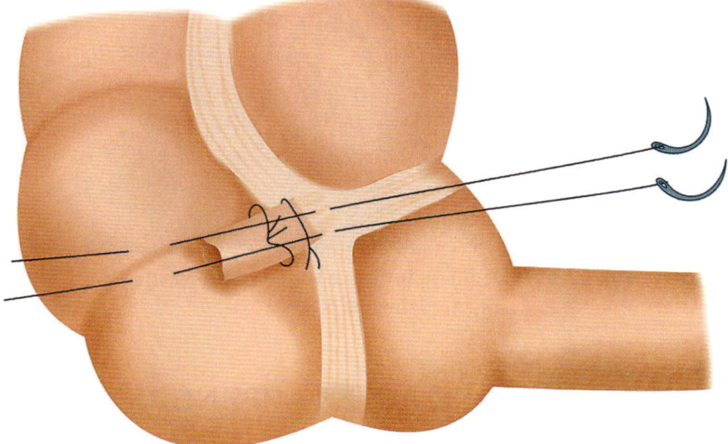

Fig. 22-90: Invagination of stump of appendix using seromuscular Lembert suture.

- *Residual abscess* (pelvic, paracolic, local, subdiaphragmatic) can occur. Its severity depends on the virulence and load of the bacteria. It is initially treated with antibiotics. If it persists or progresses, CT scan is done to confirm it and later appropriately drainage is done depending on the location of the abscess.
- *Pylephlebitis (Portal pyaemia)* is nowadays rare due to availability of proper antibiotics. However, it can occur if there is immunosuppression. It presents with fever, chills, jaundice and tender, smooth, soft palpable liver. It is treated with adequate antibiotics.
- *Adhesions, kinking* and intestinal obstruction can cause recurrent spasmodic/colicky pain with vomiting. It is initially treated conservatively; but may require laparoscopic adhesiolysis later.
- *Right inguinal hernia (direct)*—due to injury to ilioinguinal nerve can occur.
- *Wound sepsis* 10%, faecal fistula can occur. Wound is laid open and later secondary suturing is done in case of wound sepsis. Faecal fistula usually subsides in few weeks. If there is distal obstruction or specific causes like tuberculosis or malignancy fistula will persist which should be dealt appropriately **(Fig. 22-94)**.
- *Respiratory problems*, DVT can occur.

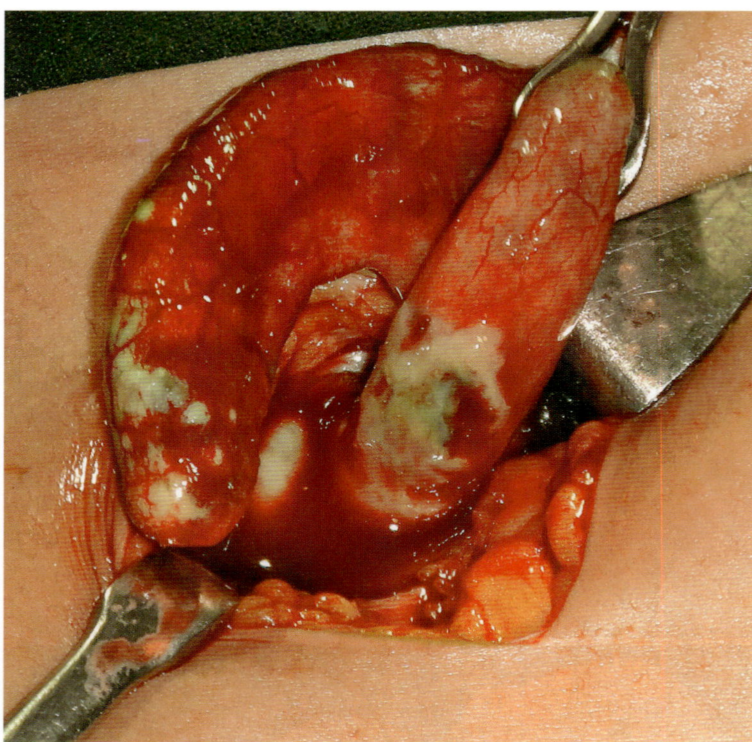

Fig. 22-91: Suppurative appendicitis.

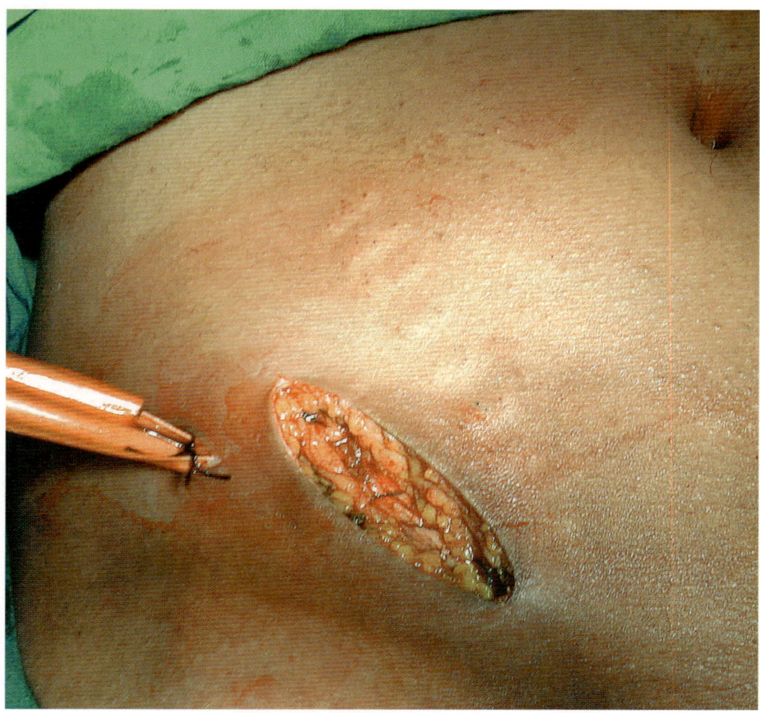

Fig. 22-92: Placing drain after appendicectomy. Ideally tube drain is placed.

FAECAL FISTULA AFTER APPENDICECTOMY

Causes

It can occur when appendicectomy is done in gangrenous/perforated/friable base appendix. It can occur after drainage of appendicular abscess. It can occur if appendicectomy is done/attempted in appendicular mass. If there is underlying additional pathology like Crohn's disease/carcinoma/ileocaecal tuberculosis/actinomycosis during appendicectomy, fistula can occur **(Fig. 22-95)**.

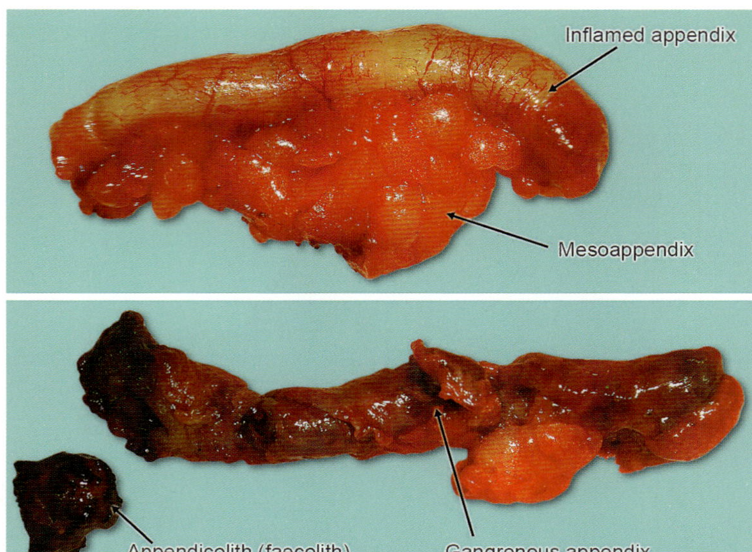

Fig. 22-93: Appendicectomy specimen.

Features

Faeculent, foul smelling discharge from either main wound or drain site.
Features of infection, with skin excoriation.
Features suggestive of cause.

Investigations

CT fistulogram to delineate the track.
CT scan abdomen to find out the other pathology.
Other relevant investigations, Hb%, albumin level, etc.

Treatment

Initially conservative—antibiotics, IV fluids, dressing, zinc oxide cream over the skin, observation.

Most of the time fistula subsides, provided there is no distal obstruction by adhesions or kinking or specific causes like carcinoma or tuberculosis. If persists even after 6 weeks, resection of ileocaecal segment and anastomosis is done.

TROUBLES IN APPENDICECTOMY

During surgery if appendix is found normal, other cause for symptoms should always be looked for like Meckel's diverticulum, Crohn's disease, ovarian/pelvic causes in females, malignancy, etc.

Appendicular tumour may be found. If it is in the tip, appendicectomy is sufficient. It could be carcinoid tumour. If it is in the base right hemicolectomy is done.

Absence of appendix—a rare occasion can occur. Caecum and taeniae should be traced properly before finalising it.

Appendicular abscess/pelvic abscess formation may create difficulty in managing the situation.

Malignancy in the caecum if identified on table—right hemicolectomy should be done.

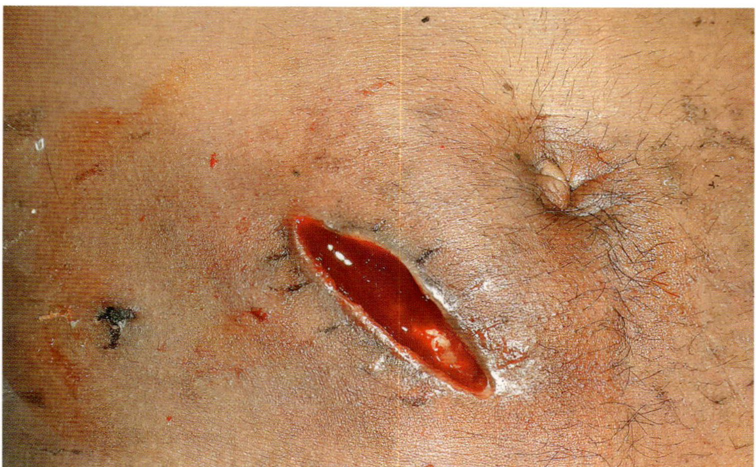

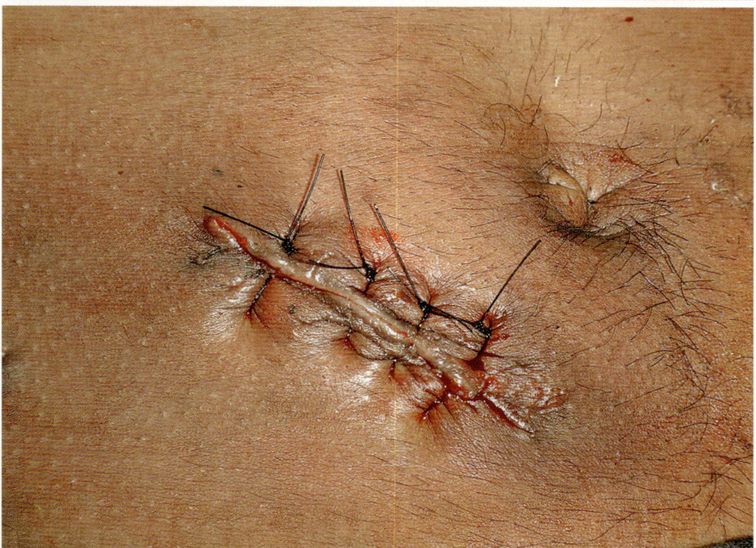

Fig. 22-94: Wound infection after appendicectomy; secondary suturing is done at a later period.

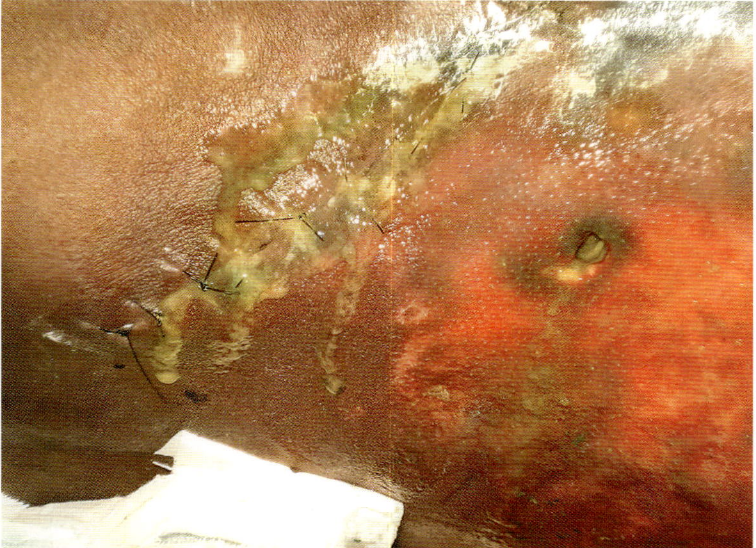

Fig. 22-95: Faecal fistula after appendicectomy.

If Crohn's disease is identified during surgery, appendicectomy can be done with care, if base of the appendix is normal. But in rare occasion where appendix is involved by Crohn's disease, appendicectomy should not be done but treated only with antibiotics and steroids, otherwise fistula can develop.

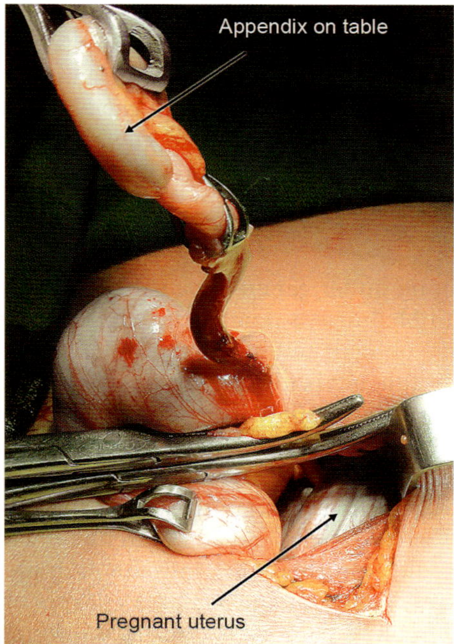

Fig. 22-96: Appendicectomy in pregnancy—it is usually done through laparotomy.

Mortality rate of appendicectomy is less than 1%. Morbidity and complications are more after surgery for perforated appendicitis.

Surgical site infection is 5% in uncomplicated appendicitis; 20% in perforated appendix after surgery.

Small bowel obstruction postoperatively is 1% with simple appendicitis; 3–5% in perforated appendicitis after surgery.

More than 50% of obstruction occurs in first year of postoperative period. In children with appendicitis, there is poor localisation and so peritonitis is common. So conservative therapy should be avoided. Surgery is the only choice of treatment otherwise early peritonitis is the danger. Appendicular mass is initially treated with *Ochsner Sherren* regime. After 6 weeks, *interval appendicectomy* is done.

Children, old age, faecolith, laxative abuse, diabetes mellitus, immunosuppression and pelvic appendix are high-risk factors for perforation in appendicitis. In pelvic and retrocaecal appendicitis, adjacent ureteral inflammation can occur in which urine on analysis shows blood cells and pus cells. Incidence of removal of normal appendix is 30%. *Stump appendicitis* is inflammation and infection in the remaining portion of the appendix stump after appendicectomy. It is a rare entity. If on table normal appendix is found during surgery, it is called as '*Lily white appendix*'. Then other pathology like Meckel's diverticulum, ileal/mesenteric lymph node/ ovarian disease should to be looked for.

Appendicitis is the commonest acute abdominal condition found in pregnancy, their site of pain and features vary. They need appendicectomy by laparotomy. Laparoscopic appendicectomy is under trial in pregnancy. It is more common in 1st and 2nd trimester. Guarding and rebound tenderness will be absent. Risk of premature labour is 15%. Foetal death is 5%; but if appendix bursts it raises to 29%. Maternal mortality raises to 10 times after 6 months **(Fig. 22-96)**.

SMALL INCISION OPEN APPENDICECTOMY

Often many surgeons do open appendicectomy using a very small incision of 1.5 to 2.0 cm in length. Even though cosmetically it is good, due to availability of laparoscopic appendicectomy this procedure should be avoided. And also it is a blind forcible procedure which is against surgical principle as appendix is pulled out through the wound forcibly and mesoappendix also tied forcibly with traction. There are chances of tearing of the mesoappendix, and serosa of the caecum. Moreover, once mesoappendix and stump of the appendix are tied and pushed into the peritoneal cavity, it is impossible to visualise the stump for its security and integrity making the entire procedure as presumption and blind **(Fig. 22-97)**.

Procedure

Procedure is done under general anaesthesia; a small incision of 2 cm is made in McBurney's point. Skin, superficial fascia, external oblique, internal oblique and transversus abdominis are separated accordingly. Peritoneum is identified and is held using haemostat. Once peritoneum is opened its edges are held securely with 4–6 artery forceps (haemostats). These arteries should never be removed until appendicectomy is complete and peritoneum is closed. Using Babcock's appendix is gently pulled out into the wound with traction. Caecum is also pulled out to identify the base of the appendix. Caecum is pushed back into the peritoneal cavity with base being held using Babcock's forceps. Mesoappendix is clamped and ligated up to the base. Base is transfixed using vicryl. Another simple ligature is also placed to the base. After cutting the appendix stump is pushed back into the peritoneal cavity. Peritoneum is closed using purse string vicryl suture. Muscles apposed using one or two vicryl sutures. External oblique is closed. Skin apposed using absorbable subcuticular suture.

LAPAROSCOPIC APPENDICECTOMY

History

In 1983, Semm from Germany did first incidental laparoscopic appendicectomy. In 1987 Schrieber reported laparoscopic appendicectomies in women in acute appendicitis.

Principles and Indications

Laparoscopic appendicectomy is a relatively controversial topic as most of the surgeons including those in the West still favour open appendicectomy in all cases. The main point of concern especially for cases that present late or those with burst appendix is the failure to give adequate peritoneal toileting and the formation of abscesses in the peritoneum. This fear can be alleviated by the use of thorough irrigation with antiseptic solution and insertion of drain through lateral port for evacuation of debris. It is still recommended that the beginner have a low threshold for conversion if he finds that the appendix is not visualised, is very friable, is perforated or the peritoneum is severely contaminated. Even though most experienced surgeons are capable of taking out the appendix via a very small incision there are situations where laparoscopic appendicectomy scores over open procedure. These are:

- Vague chronic abdominal pain where diagnostic laparoscopy culminates in an appendicectomy.

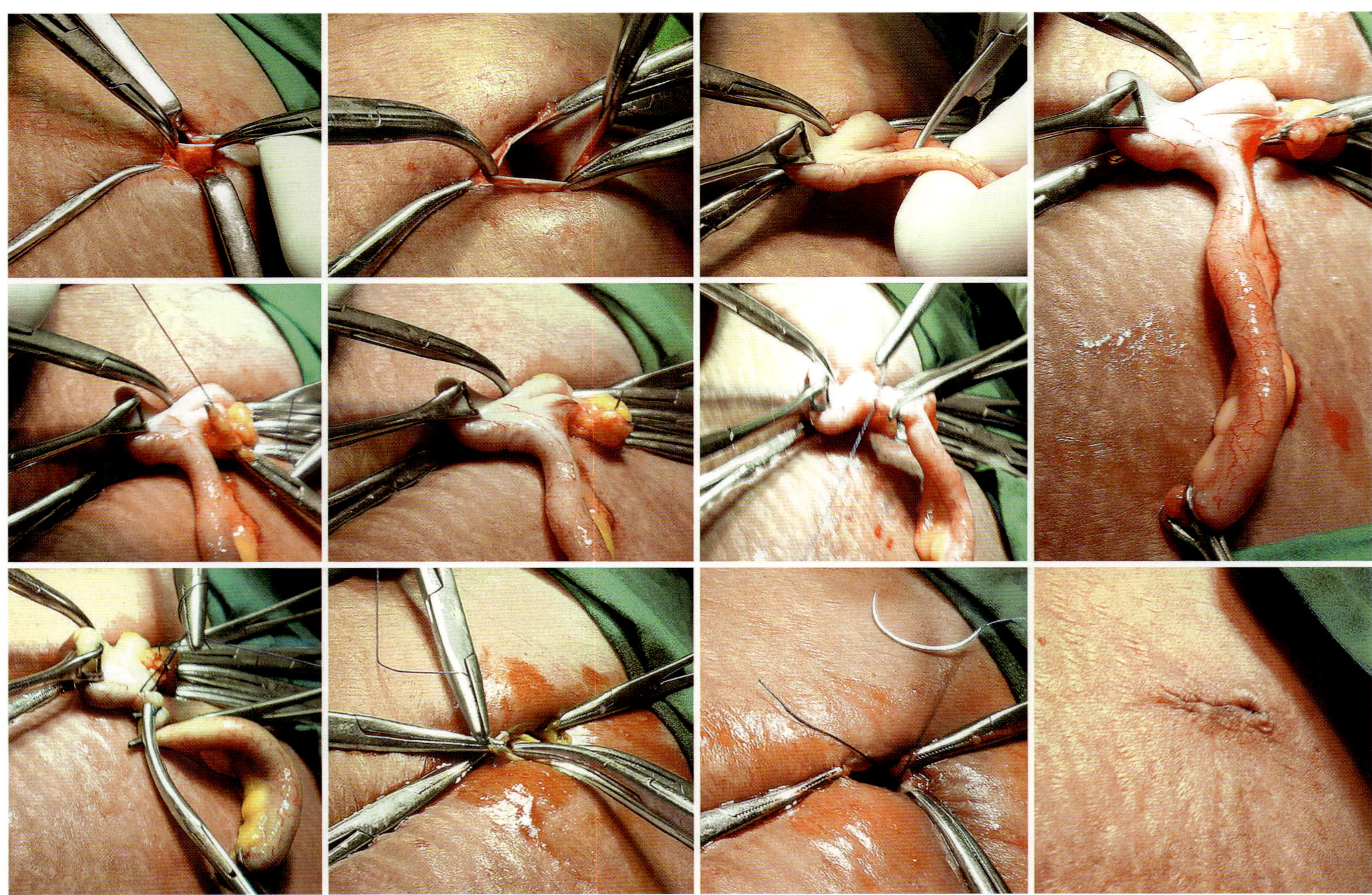

Fig. 22-97: Small incision open appendicectomy technique.

- Right iliac fossa pain in young women where the cause is of doubtful appendicular or ovarian/fallopian tube origin.
- Patients with atypical pain where there is chance of abnormal position of appendix such as subhepatic or in situs inversus.
- Obese individuals where a large incision may be required to access the abdomen.
- Diabetics where there is a chance of wound infection.
- Interval appendicectomy where recovery and discharge is faster in laparoscopic appendicectomy.

Note:
In spite of all these debate laparoscopic appendicectomy has become gold standard due to its added advantages compared to disadvantages.

Cases which should be taken up with caution (preferably by an experienced laparoscopic surgeon) are:

- Patients who are poor risk for general anaesthesia.
- Patients whose abdominal scan shows formation of abdominal mass.
- Patients with previous lower abdominal surgery.
- Patients with stump appendicitis or burst appendix.

Ideal case for a beginner would be a young adult with pain of less than 48 hours of duration when you will find a turgid appendix which is still mobile in the peritoneal cavity without much of omental adhesion and pus formation. The routine work up of the patients is done as for open surgery. Consent is taken for laparoscopic surgery as well as for conversion in each case irrespective of the nature of the case. A nasogastric tube is not routinely placed if open access technique is used but it is used if surgeon uses Veress needle to create pneumoperitoneum. Catheterisation is done to evacuate the bladder. It may be discontinued for routine cases when the surgeon has got enough experience to cut down the operating time. In these cases, the patient is asked to void just before the procedure to keep the bladder empty.

Advantages of Laparoscopic Appendicectomy

- It allows thorough exploration of the contents of the peritoneal cavity especially in females. It also facilitates treatment for additional pathology identified like ovarian cyst in same sitting.
- It allows easier approach in subhepatic appendix and appendix in situs inversus.
- It allows lesser hospital stay (24 hours); can be done as day care surgery in uncomplicated cases.
- Pain in postoperative period is less with faster recovery period and also early return to work. Trauma of access is less.
- It reduces/prevents the incidence of wound complications.
- It is cosmetically better and avoids unnecessary laparotomy.

Disadvantages of Laparoscopic Appendicectomy

Technical difficulties in mobilising the appendix; clearing the adhesions; cauterising the mesoappendix; placing ligatures around appendix; extraction of the appendix.

One should always take prior consent for conversion into open appendicectomy.

Contraindications

It is relatively contraindicated in previous lower abdominal surgery, pregnancy with appendicitis, malignancy, palpable appendicular mass, immunosuppressed individual, comorbid status.

Instruments

1. Veress needle.
2. 10 mm port—2 in no.
3. 5 mm port—1 in no.
4. 30° camera; xenon light source; 3 chip camera; monitor; CO_2 cylinder; CO_2 insufflator.
5. Maryland dissector.
6. Babcock dissector.
7. Bipolar forceps.
8. Scissors.
9. Suction irrigation.
10. Endoloops.
11. Endo bag.

Position of the Patient and Operating Room Setting

The patient is in supine position with Trendelenburg position to start with. Once the ports are in place and surgeon is ready to proceed with actual procedure the patient's right side is tilted up so as to clear right iliac fossa of small bowel. This can be done by tilting the table or placing a sand bag under the patient.

Monitor is kept on foot end towards right. Surgeon stands on left side facing downwards. Camera surgeon will stand on right side of the surgeon or diagonally opposite side (right side) depending on the convenience. Scrub nurse will stand on right side at distal end. Additional monitor may be placed on the left side, left of the surgeon to facilitate the proper view of the video images to people standing on the right side.

Laparoscopic appendicectomy is done under general anaesthesia **(Fig. 22-98)**.

Procedure

The first trocar (10 mm or 5 mm depending on the telescope being used) is inserted via a periumbilical incision. Access to the peritoneum can be gained by either insertion of Veress needle followed by trocar or direct insertion of trocar by open Hasson's method. After insertion of the first port, the telescope is inserted and entire abdominal cavity is inspected. 10 mm 30° camera is always better; but 0° is sufficient to do usual appendicectomies. After this the attention is directed towards the right iliac fossa. Adequate tilt is required to clear the small bowel from the field. The secondary ports are inserted under direct vision so as to prevent injury to underlying bowel. The positions of the working trocars vary widely from person to person and from case to case. It is better for the surgeon to place the trocars according to the findings inside the abdomen. The position of the appendix can vary widely and also the amount of adhesions depends on factors such as number of previous attacks and duration of present attack.

The first port is inserted via an 11 mm infraumbilical incision either by open or closed technique. Subsequent two 5 mm ports are placed under vision. One port is commonly in the midline between umbilicus and pubic symphysis. The other is variable. Some surgeons prefer another port at the level of the umbilicus in the right almost in the anterior axillary line while others place it in right iliac fossa. Many other surgeons also in West prefer the working port to be placed in left iliac fossa. The point for consideration here is that the basic triangulation which is preferred in performing laparoscopy should be maintained. Any of the above mentioned port placement is correct as long as the surgeon is comfortable and performs a safe surgery.

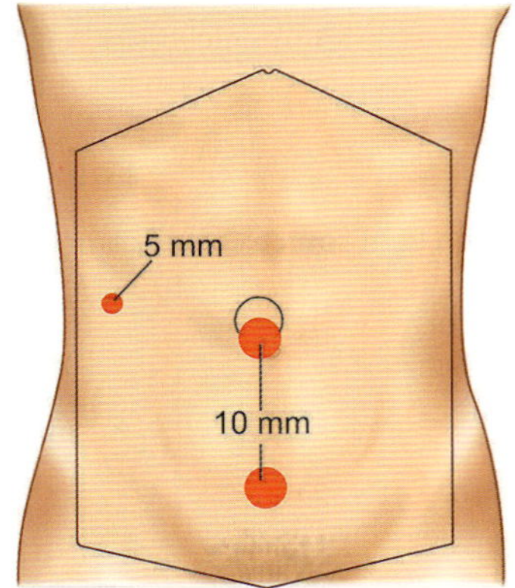

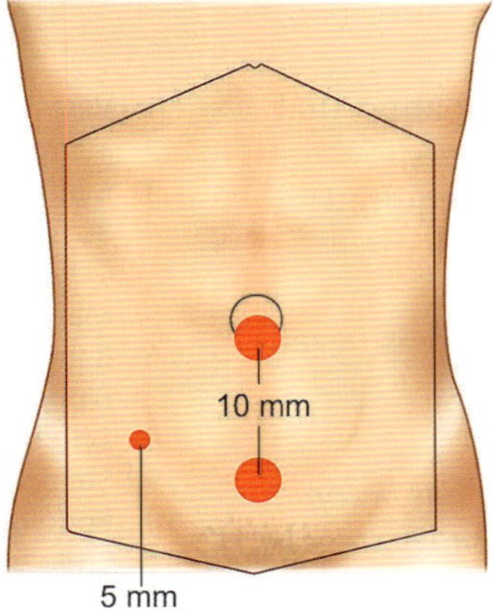

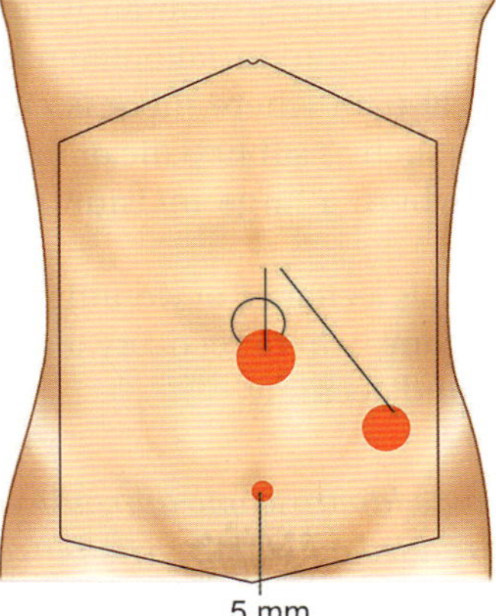

Fig. 22-98: Approaches for laparoscopic appendicectomy.

One should not go in with a fixed idea for the ports as very often the surgical field demands alteration in the port placement. If endoloops are used as ligatures, left-sided two additional working ports suffice (10 mm and 5 mm); if intracorporeal ligatures or transfixation are used then one port on midline below the umbilicus or in left iliac fossa and other on the right iliac fossa is a need to facilitate taking needle bites and putting ligature. Working ports are inserted always under vision. Additional 4th 5 mm working port can be used in difficult appendicectomies which will facilitate retraction of bowel or holding the appendix.

The left hand Babcock's forceps is used to hold the appendix and right hand Maryland dissector is used to trace the entire length of the appendix and reach the base of the appendix. Different energy source can be used to coagulate and divide the mesoappendix. For the basic set up and also most often bipolar coagulation forceps is adequate for the process.

Bipolar forceps is applied to the free edge of the mesoappendix and curved scissors is used to divide the same. This dissection is continued up to the base of the appendix. Harmonic scalpel may ease and quickens the job.

Use knot pusher to place three ties around the base of appendix. Grasping the appendix through the loop is an easy method to do this. Preformed endoloops can also be used. Many surgeons place intracorporeal ligatures using vicryl often with transfixation. Stump should have two ligatures in situ after appendicectomy. If faecolith is present it should be milked distally towards body using Maryland forceps **(Fig. 22-99)**.

After this the base of the appendix is secured with preformed endo loop or suture passed via the knot pusher. Three ties are placed. Between proximal most ligature and 2nd ligature gap should be less than 5 mm. The appendix is divided using curved sharp scissor between 2nd and 3rd ligatures. Intestinal stapling device can be used to cut and close the stump with two rows of staples. But stapling is not very popular and not cost effective. Specimen is removed through 10 mm working port using an extraction bag or finger of no 7.5 or 8 sterile gloves or using sterile condom **(Fig. 22-100)**.

If the appendix is friable or is badly infected then specimen retrieval bag should be used to prevent infection at port site. A thorough wash is given to the area using normal saline. A good look at the pelvis should be done before finishing the procedure. Choice of leaving a drain is dictated on case to case basis. It is recommended to close all fascial defects made by 10 mm ports as lot of subsequent hernias are been reported. Difficulty arises whenever there is a phlegmon or abscess or perforation. Subserosal appendix should be identified by incising the serosa carefully. Postileal, subhepatic and situs inversus appendix should be remembered **(Fig. 22-101)**.

A rapid recovery from ileus is noted in almost all patients when compared to open appendicectomy and early commencement of oral intake is not associated with higher complications. The patient is usually discharged within 48 hours of surgery.

After putting telescope through umbilical port, if appendix mobilisation looks easier and not a very turgid appendix, then both working ports can be 5 mm. In such occasions after cutting, appendix is extracted through the umbilical 10 mm port. 5 mm telescope is attached to the camera and can be used to visualise extraction procedure.

Key steps

1. Camera port at umbilicus.
2. Two working ports one in midline and one in right flank.
3. Divide the mesoappendix after cauterising with bipolar forceps.
4. Secure the appendix with endoloop.
5. Divide and retrieve appendix. Use endobag, if needed.
6. Wash the area.
7. Keep drain if needed.

Complications

- Injury to bowel, vessels while passing the ports.
- Complications of pneumoperitoneum.
- Accidental cautery injury to bowel, vessels and other vital structures.
- Bleeding, bowel perforation, peritonitis.
- Slipping of ligature, leak, peritonitis, fistula formation.

All complications need re-evaluation with US/CT abdomen; total count; liver function tests; platelet count. Higher generation antibiotics may be needed and one should not be hesitant to use it to control/prevent distressing septicaemia. Reopening if needed should be done at the earliest. Re laparoscopy can be ideal to observe what went wrong and amount of collection in the peritoneal cavity. Laparotomy with adequate midline incision should be done. Any pus collection should be drained. Perforation should be identified, is usually located in the caecum or ileum; it is closed using interrupted silk sutures. Adhesions, bands should be released. Thorough normal saline wash is given. Resection of the ileocaecal segment may be needed occasionally. Occasionally ileotransverse colon bypass anastomosis may be considered if caecal and appendicular stump

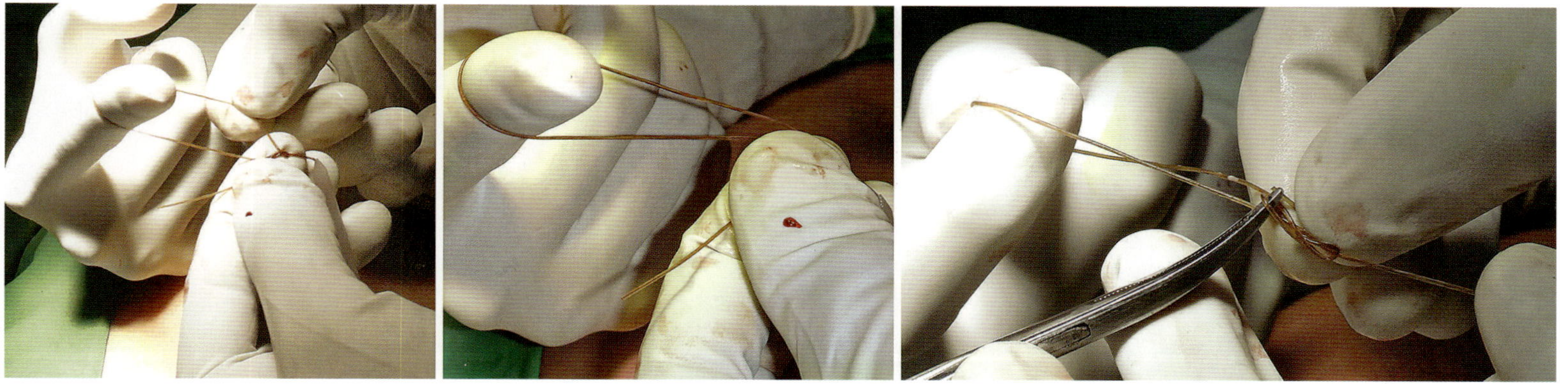

Fig. 22-99: Creating the Roeder's knot.

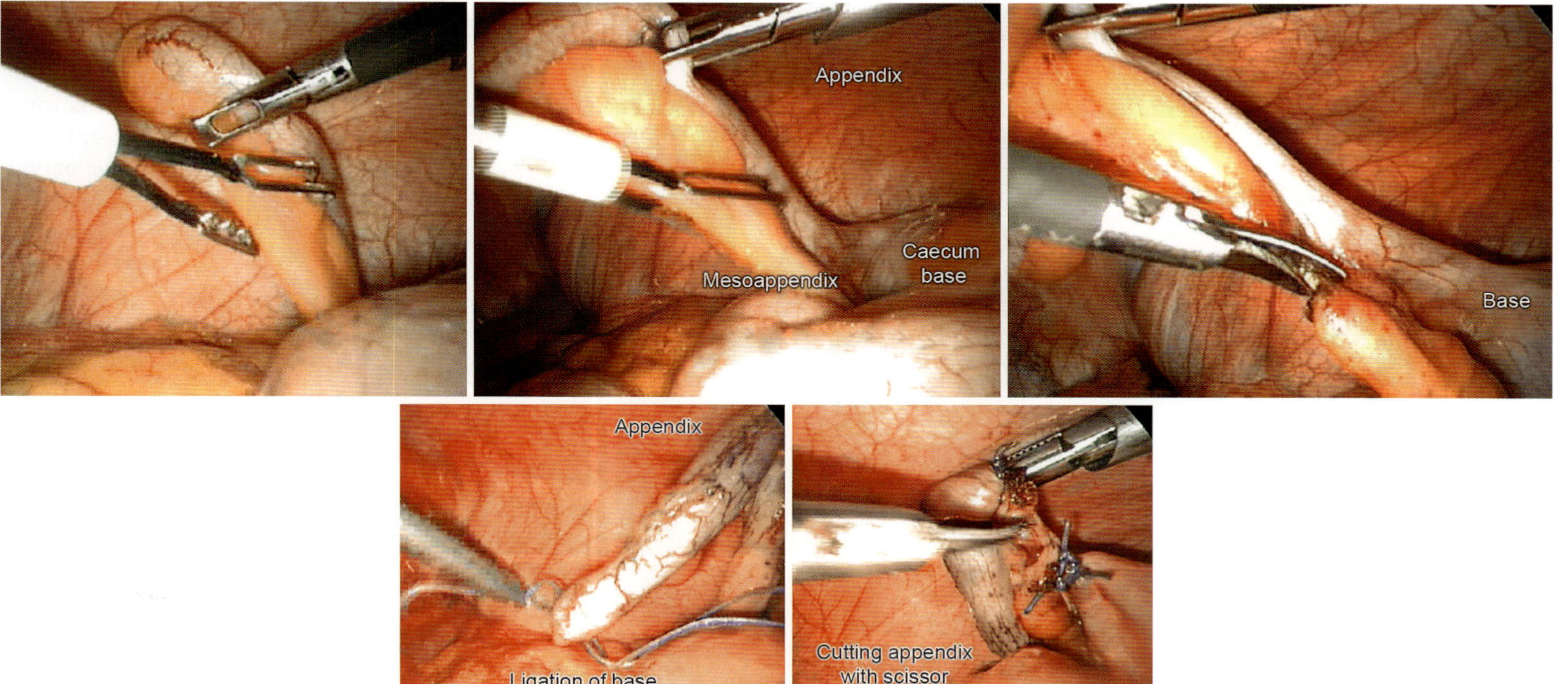

Fig. 22-100: Suturing of base in laparoscopic appendicectomy.

area looks unhealthy. Proper assessment of the problem and proper decision on table should be taken to achieve an optimum recovery as 3rd reopening after 2nd will be more troublesome and often may be disastrous. So all possible options should be kept in mind to achieve complete control of the problem.

Note:

It is ideally always better to use bipolar cautery while dissecting the mesoappendix. Additional precaution should be taken while cauterising close to the caecum adjacent to base of the appendix.

When uncomfortable, conversion to open procedure should be done without hesitation; otherwise one should call and request another laparoscopic surgeon for help.

LAPAROSCOPY ASSISTED APPENDICECTOMY

This technique combines the advantage of visualisation of internal anatomy and confirmation of appendicitis and also fast completion of the procedure by open method. The inflamed appendix is brought out to the exterior via a 10 mm trocar and the procedure of appendicectomy is carried out as in open surgery. The first trocar is placed around the umbilicus **(Fig. 22-102)**.

After inspection of the abdomen the nature of the appendix is assessed. Appendix which is around 6–8 mm, turgid, freely mobile in the peritoneal cavity and with minimal non-purulent fluid collection in RIF are easily and ideally removed via this approach **(Fig. 22-103)**.

In these cases, it is easy to apply some amount of traction on the appendix to deliver out through the trocar wounds. It is important to assess how much traction the appendix can take (as a friable appendix can get cut when traction is applied). Such appendix which is very turgid and friable should be removed by dividing inside the peritoneal cavity as already described. The appendix is delivered through the umbilical port after mobilisation or is brought out through a port placed in right iliac fossa. The position of the second trocar in right iliac fossa is variable and is dictated by the position of the base of the appendix which is seen on the inside. The tip of the appendix is grasped with a Babcock forceps on a reducer and delivered out of the wound. The gas flow to the abdomen is stopped

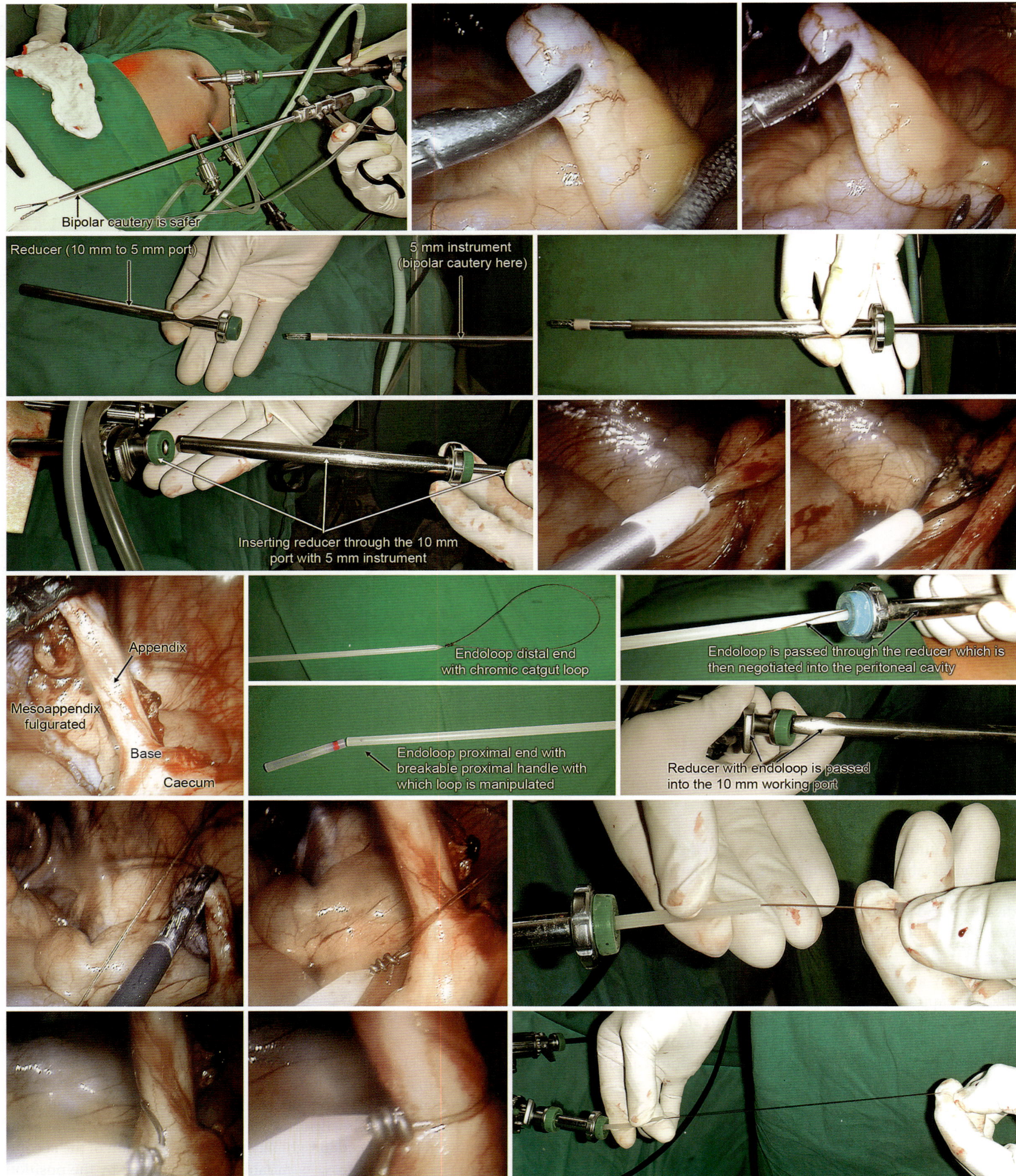
Bipolar cautery is safer
Reducer (10 mm to 5 mm port)
5 mm instrument
(bipolar cautery here)
Inserting reducer through the 10 mm
port with 5 mm instrument
Appendix
Mesoappendix
fulgurated
Base
Caecum
Endoloop distal end
with chromic catgut loop
Endoloop is passed through the reducer which is
then negotiated into the peritoneal cavity
Endoloop proximal end with
breakable proximal handle with
which loop is manipulated
Reducer with endoloop is passed
into the 10 mm working port

Figs. 22-101(1)

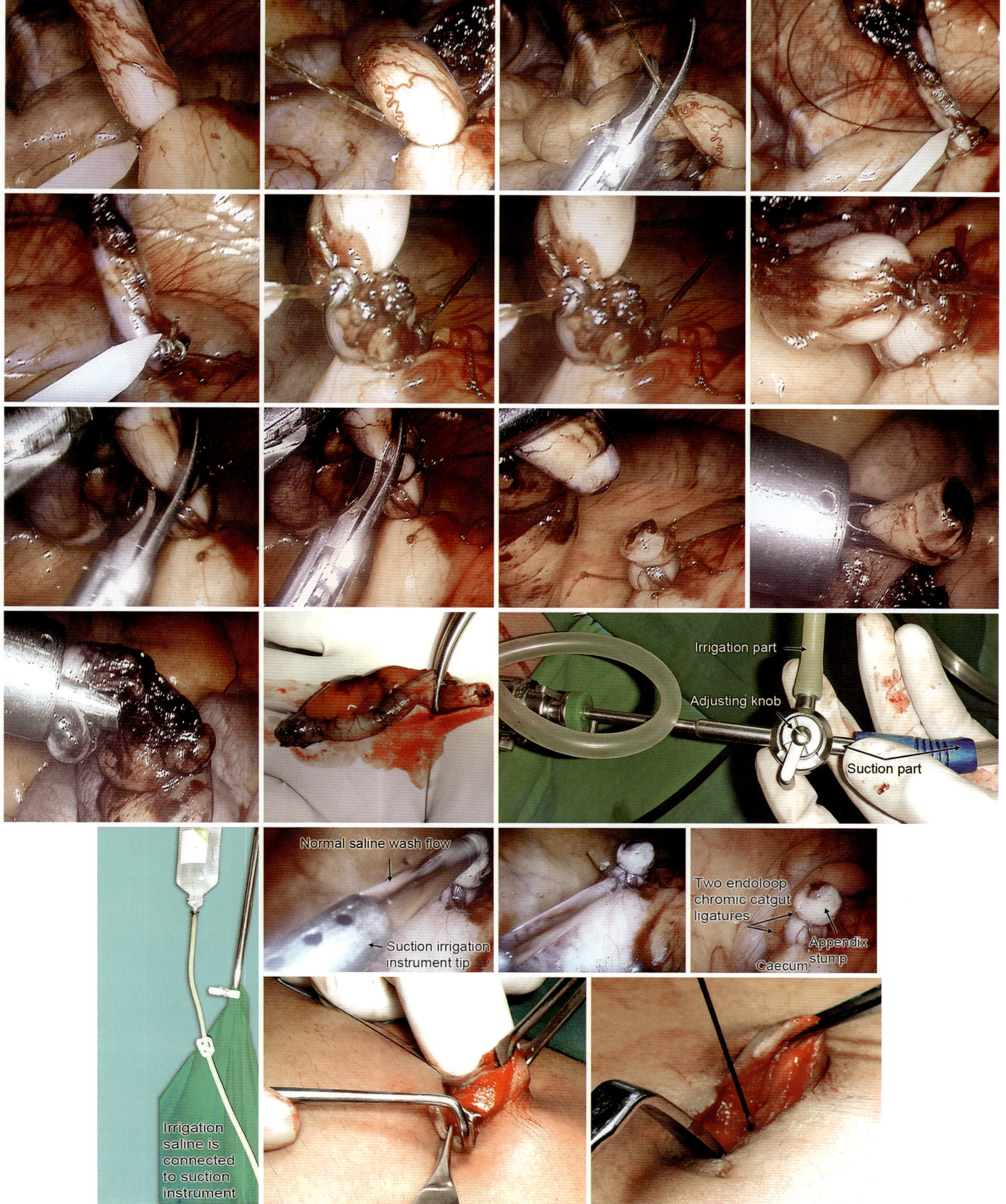

Figs. 22-101(2)

Figs. 22-101(1 and 2): Laparoscopic appendicectomy.

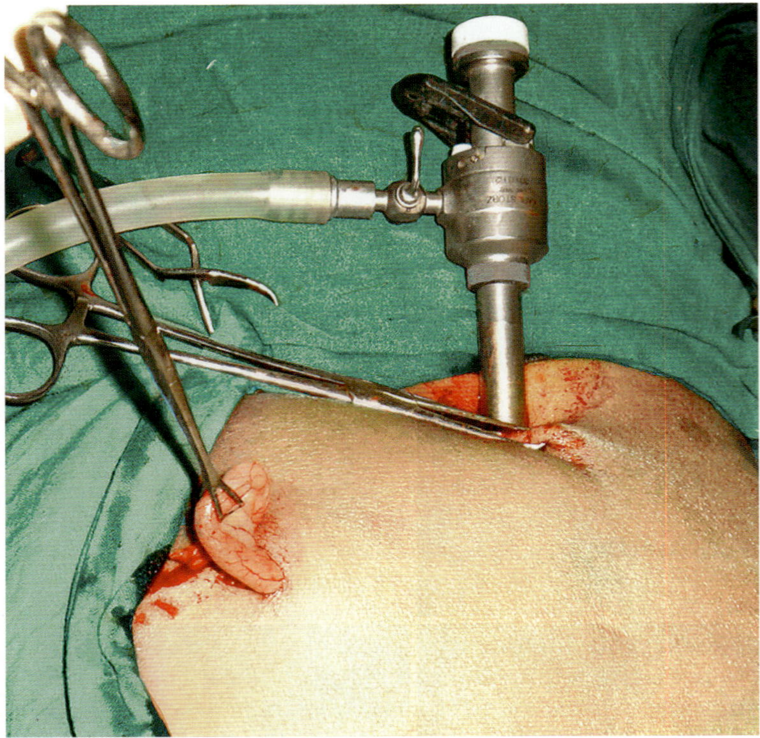

Fig. 22-102: Laparoscopic-assisted appendicectomy.

and the pneumoperitoneum is evacuated. This step is important to facilitate the delivery of the appendix through the wound. After this the procedure is same as for open appendicectomy. The mesoappendix is ligated and divided up to the base of the appendix and then appendicectomy is carried out. The stump is inspected for bleeding and caecum is pushed back into the abdomen. Pneumoperitoneum is recreated and the appendicular stump is again inspected to make sure that there is no bleeding. The pelvis can be washed with normal saline if any collection is seen. The right paracolic gutter is also inspected for any purulent collection and wash is given to the area. Keeping a drain is not a routine practice but the operating surgeon is the best judge to assess the same. Keeping a drain through the trocar site is simple and this can be removed after 24 hours. This is reassuring for surgeons performing initial few cases of laparoscopic appendicectomy.

Key steps

1. Camera port at umbilicus.
2. Second port over the base of the appendix.
3. Grasp the tip of the appendix with Babcock.
4. Evacuate pneumoperitoneum.
5. Deliver the appendix out via the working port.
6. Proceed with a routine appendicectomy.
7. Check the abdomen after procedure.

SUBMUCOSAL APPENDICECTOMY

In difficult appendicectomy wherein if there is dense adhesions and plane is impossible to create to go ahead with formal appendicectomy either by open or through laparoscopic approach, submucosal appendicectomy is performed as an alternative but definitive surgical procedure.

Here an incision is made on the antimesenteric wall of the appendix and the mucosal sleeve was pulled out, leaving the muscular wall. The base is then ligated flush with the caecum and divided distally, leaving the muscular tube. Drain may be placed, depends on the surgeon's discretion and situation. It avoids injury to adjacent structures like ileum and major vessels; it also prevents injuring the unidentified (due to inability to identify) appendicular artery. Inner mucosal tube is sleeve resected as distally as possible; distal part should not be closed to avoid creating blind tube. With laparoscopic approach it may avoid conversion into open technique.

APPENDICULAR ABSCESS

It occurs due to suppuration in an acute appendicitis or suppuration in an already formed appendicular mass. Abscess commonly

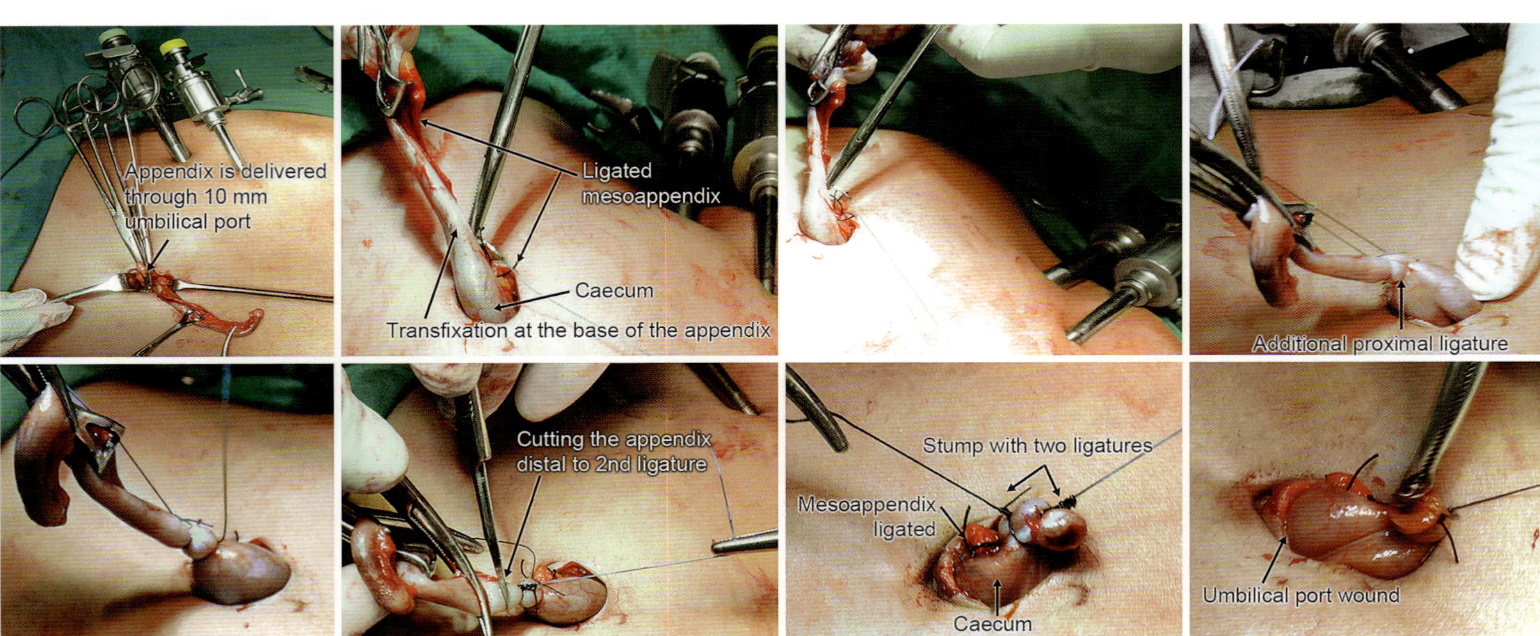

Fig. 22-103: Laparoscopic-assisted appendicectomy—technique.

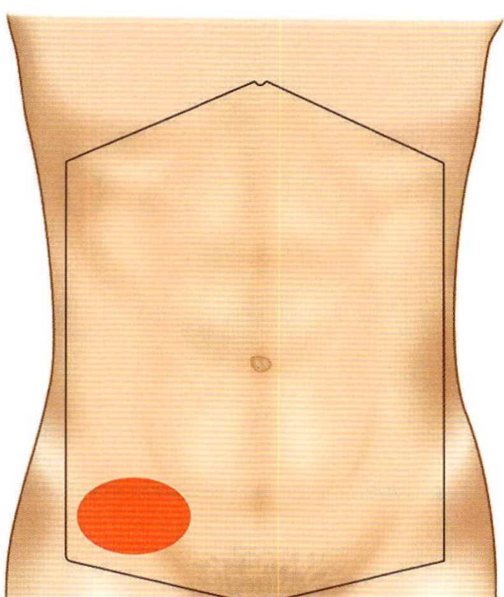

Fig. 22-104: Appendicular abscess.

occurs in retrocaecal region but often can occur in subcaecal, preileal lumbar or postileal regions. *Pelvic abscess is also common after an attack of acute appendicitis* **(Fig. 22-104)**.

Features

High fever, features of toxicity with a soft, tender, swelling which is dull to percuss in right iliac fossa lying towards right lateral and lower side with clear upper margin but indistinct lower margin. Ultrasound confirms the diagnosis.

Treatment

Antibiotics are started. US or CT guided catheter drainage initially followed by interval appendicectomy in 12 weeks is quiet useful.

If patient is not responding then under general anaesthesia, incision is made in the lower lateral aspect of the swelling above the inguinal ligament. Skin, external oblique muscle is cut. Abscess cavity is opened and pus is drained *extraperitoneally*, which is sent for culture and sensitivity. Wound is closed. A drain is placed through a separate incision. Antibiotics are continued. *Interval appendicectomy is done after 3 months.*

Recent study has confirmed that immediate appendicectomy in appendicular abscess showed higher rates of complication and hospital stay compared to initial percutaneous/open drainage followed by interval appendicectomy at 12 weeks.

23

CHAPTER

Surgeries of Liver and Biliary System

A. LIVER

- Surgical anatomy
- Liver resection
  - Principles and indications
  - Left hepatectomy
  - Right hepatectomy
  - Extended hepatectomy
  - Segmetectomies and non-anatomical resections
- Liver transplantation
- Surgical treatment of portal hypertension
- Surgical treatment of hydatid cyst

SURGICAL ANATOMY

The liver has always been noted to have the power of regeneration even from the time of Greek mythology where Prometheus was chained to a rock and an eagle would feast on his liver and it would regenerate each night in time for the eagle's return. It is a unique organ which can regenerate as well as be replaced with transplantation. Surgery of the liver is both easy and tough at the same time.

Grossly liver can be divided into right, left, quadrate and caudate lobes. It weighs around 1500 g. It is the largest organ of the body. It extends downwards from 5th intercostal space mainly on the right side partly on the left side. It is wedge-shaped like a pyramid of 4 sides. The falciform ligament divides the liver into right and left lobe on the diaphragmatic surface and ligamentum teres divides the same on the inferior surface. The quadrate lobe is situated between the gallbladder fossa and the porta hepatis. And the caudate lobe is situated between the inferior vena cava, the porta and fissure carrying ligamentum venosus. This division, however, does not represent the functional anatomy of the liver **(Figs. 23-1A and B)**.

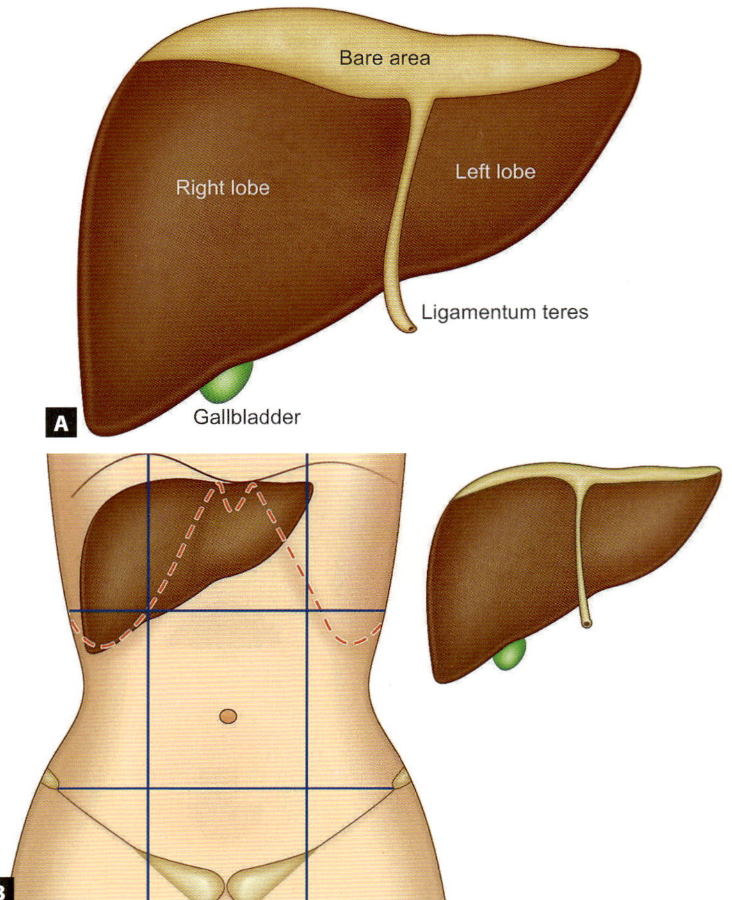

Figs. 23-1A and B: Anatomy of liver—surface and gross.

Different peritoneal attachments of the liver are called as ligaments of the liver which are important in initial mobilisation of the liver. Anterior and posterior reflections of the liver are called as anterior and posterior coronary ligaments. Between these two lies the 'bare area' without peritoneal coverage and is directly related to the diaphragm. On right and left side two reflections join and form right and left triangular ligaments. Anteriorly it reflects on the superior surface of the liver and abdominal wall and forms falciform ligament; in between folds of falciform ligament, embryonic left umbilical vein forms round ligament/ligamentum teres; it also forms a fissure in the liver to separate liver into apparent right and left lobes **(Fig. 23-2)**.

On the visceral surface, it extends as fissure for the ligamentum venosum. Between ligamentum venosum and gallbladder lies the quadrate lobe; between it and porta hepatis posteriorly lies the caudate lobe. At porta hepatis peritoneum extends as lesser omentum extending into the stomach and duodenum as hepato-gastric and hepatoduodenal ligaments. Free right margin of the lesser omentum contains common bile duct, hepatic artery and portal vein with foramen Winslow communicating lesser sac into free peritoneal cavity **(Figs. 23-3 and 23-4)**.

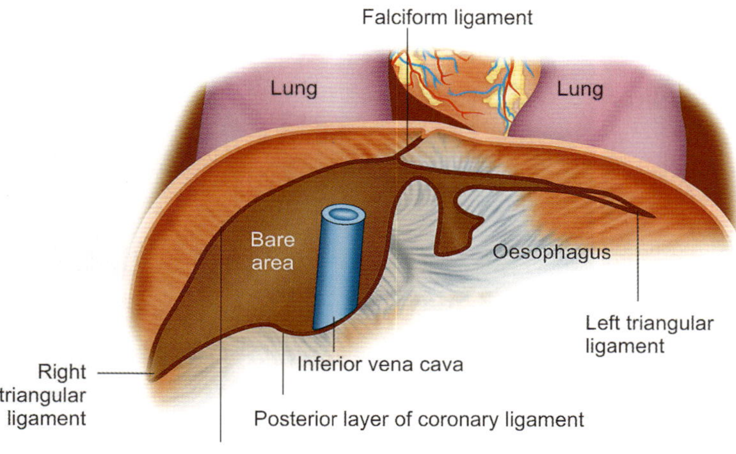

Fig. 23-2: Inferior surface of the diaphragm showing bare area; IVC position; coronary ligament; right and left triangular ligaments.

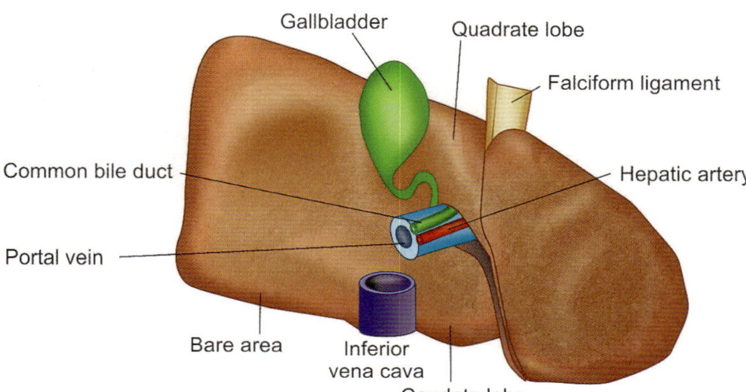

Fig. 23-3: Visceral surface of the liver.

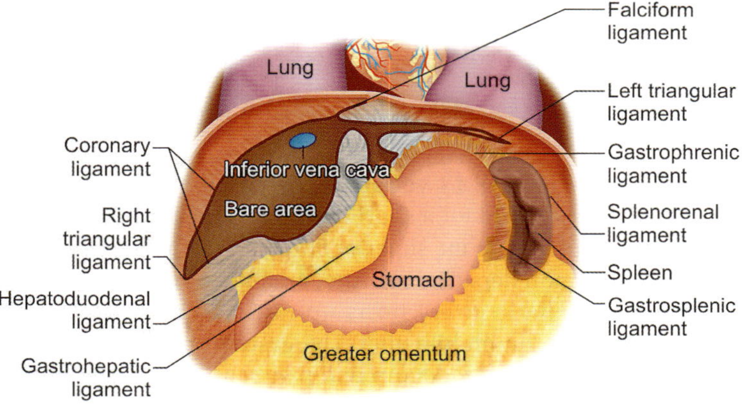

Fig. 23-4: Peritoneal reflections and ligaments of the liver.

True left lobe contains left lateral and medial segments; each is divided into superior and inferior subsegments. Right lobe is divided into anterior and posterior segments by invisible imaginary intersegmental fissure; each again is divided into superior and inferior subsegments **(Fig. 23-5)**.

Caudate lobe is in direct contact with inferior vena cava (IVC) on its left side; it is often divided into right and left parts and caudate process. Caudate lobe derives its connections from bile duct, hepatic artery and portal veins of both right and left lobes. Caudate lobe is a separate region as such. It is segment 1, and is anatomically and functionally separate from right and left lobe. It is behind the liver hilum and in front of retrohepatic IVC. Caudate lobe proper is

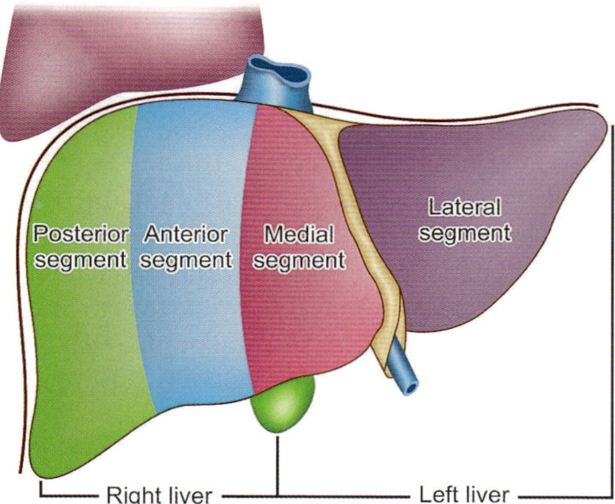

Fig. 23-5: Right lobe of liver (right liver) contains anterior and posterior segments; left lobe (left liver) contains medial and lateral segments.

called as *spigelian lobe*. In front, it is fused to segment 4; right side to segments 6 and 7. It is not draining into the hepatic veins; but drains directly into the retrohepatic IVC at its left front aspect. It derives its portal blood supply from three branches from main, right and left portal veins. Three branches arise from right and or left hepatic arteries. Ducts from caudate lobe run in front of the portal branch vein to drain into right or left hepatic duct or both.

Left lobe may be diminished in size as anomaly. Usually right lobe is 2/3rd of total liver mass. *Riedel's lobe* is an elongated tongue of liver extending from the right lobe to or below the umbilicus. It presents as an asymptomatic right upper abdomen unexplained mass in a middle-aged lady **(Fig. 23-6)**.

Grossly liver has got diaphragmatic and visceral surfaces. Diaphragmatic surface has got anterior, superior, posterior and right parts. Anterior part is related to diaphragm, costal margins, xiphoid process, and anterior abdominal wall; its inferior margin has got a deep notch for ligamentum teres and a wider notch for gallbladder. Superior part is related to diaphragm and is separated from right pleura and lung, pericardium, left pleura and lung. Posterior part is related to diaphragm and ribs; bare area and sulcus for IVC is located here. Right part is related to diaphragm, right pleura and lung, 7th to 11th ribs. Visceral surface is related to hepatic flexure and transverse colon in front; hepatorenal pouch (Morrison's) right kidney and right adrenal behind; gallbladder in gallbladder fossa of liver; 1st and 2nd part of the duodenum; oesophagus and stomach.

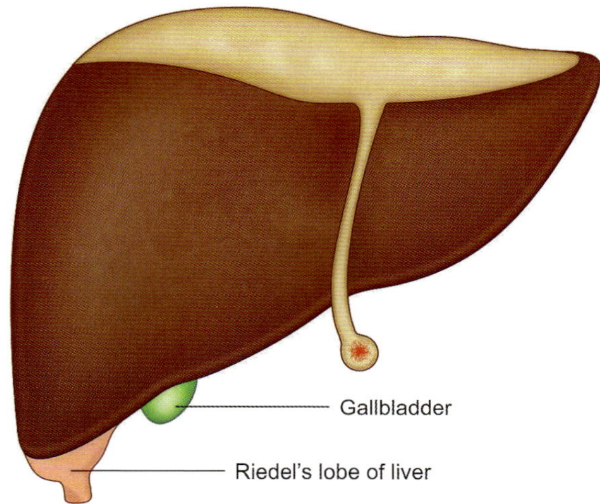

Fig. 23-6: Riedel's lobe of liver. It is common in females; presents as unexplained mass.

All the surgical techniques are based on the functional anatomy of the liver. The foundation of which was laid by J Cantlie in 1898 when he described *Cantlie's line* which passes to the left of the gallbladder fossa to the left of inferior vena cava. *Claude Couinaud* then divided into 8 functional units based on separate vascular and biliary pedicle (in clockwise direction). This has laid the foundation to all anatomical resection of liver. At the hilum, the right portal vein pursues a very short course (1–1.5 cm) before entering the liver. Once entering the hepatic parenchyma, the portal vein divides into a right anterior sectoral branch that arches vertical in the frontal plane of the liver, and a posterior sectoral branch that follows a more posterolateral course. The right portal vein supplies the anterior (or anteromedial) and posterior (or posterolateral) sectors of the right lobe. The branching pattern of these sectoral portal veins subdivides the right liver into 4 segments—segments V (anterior and inferior) and VIII (anterior and superior) form the anterior sector, and segments VI (posterior and inferior) and VII (posterior and superior) form the posterior sector. In contrast to the right portal vein, the left portal vein has a long extrahepatic length (3–4 cm) coursing beneath the inferior portion of the quadrate lobe (segment 4B) enveloped in a peritoneal sheath (the hilar plate). Upon reaching the umbilical fissure, the left portal vein runs anteriorly and superiorly within the liver substances, and gives off horizontal branches to the quadrate lobe medially segments IV A (superior) and B (inferior) and to the left lateral segment segments III (inferior) and II (superior). The caudate lobe (segment I) is neither part of the left nor right lobes, though it lies mostly on the left side. To avoid confusion and bring uniformity in nomenclature of hepatic surgeries, the International Hepato-Pancreato-Biliary Association (IHPBA) which promotes understanding of causes, investigation and treatment of liver, pancreas and biliary tree disorders in 2000, during the recent World Congress of IHPBA in Brisbane presented their recommendations (for example, right hemiliver = right hepatectomy, right anterior section = right anterior sectionectomy, segments = segmentectomy) **(Figs. 23-7 to 23-10)**.

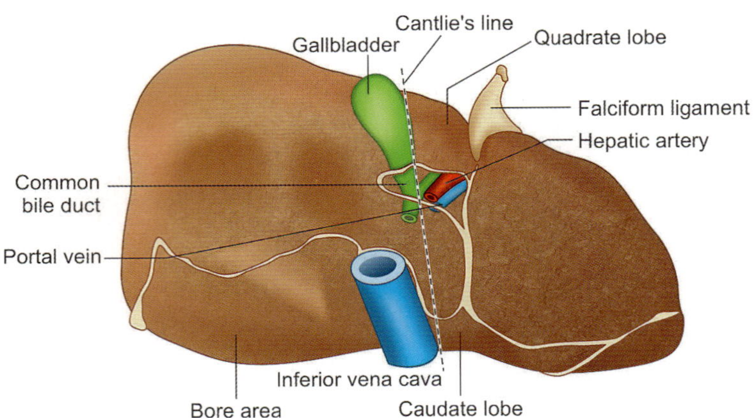

Fig. 23-8: Cantlie's line. It passes from left of the gallbladder to left of the inferior vena cava.

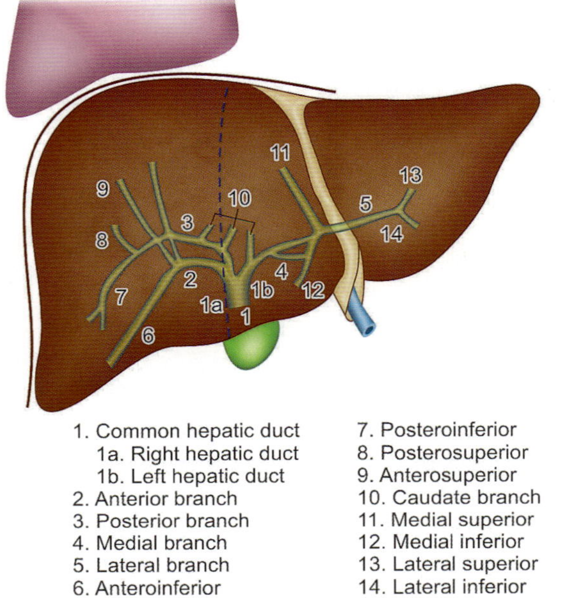

Fig. 23-9: Distribution of biliary tree intrahepatically and portal plate.

Blood Supply

Hepatic Artery

Hepatic artery supplies around 20% of total inflow to the liver. The anatomy of hepatic vasculature is standard only in about 60% of the patients. Several anomalous vessels supply segments of liver where they are termed as replaced hepatic arteries. The hepatic artery is one of the three branches of coeliac trunk arising from the aorta at the level of L1 vertebra. The common hepatic artery typically passes forward for a short distance in the retroperitoneum where it then emerges at the superior border of the pancreas and left side of the common hepatic duct. After arising from the coeliac axis, the common hepatic artery turns upward and runs lateral and adjacent to the common bile duct. The gastroduodenal artery that supplies the proximal duodenum and pancreas is typically the first branch of the common hepatic artery. The right gastric artery takes off shortly thereafter and continues within the lesser omentum along the lesser curve of the stomach. At this point, the common hepatic artery is referred to as the proper hepatic artery. The proper hepatic artery courses towards the hilum, and soon divides into the right and left hepatic arteries. Prior to the bifurcation, a small cystic artery branches off to provide blood supply to the gallbladder **(Fig. 23-11)**.

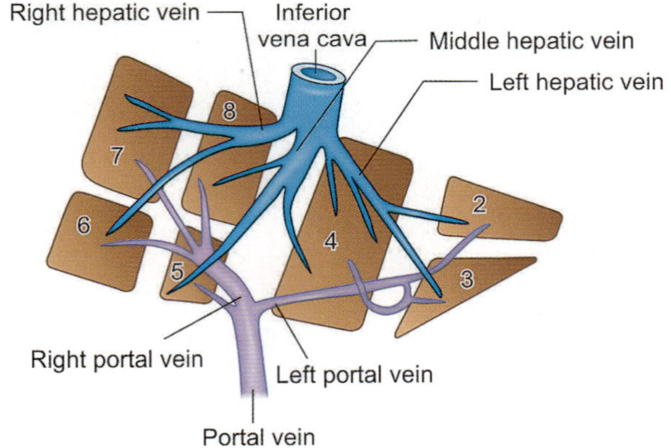

Fig. 23-7: Cantlie's line and Couinaud's segments in liver. Caudate lobe is segment 1.

The proper hepatic artery bifurcates earlier than the common bile duct and portal vein. In 80% of cases, the right hepatic artery courses posterior to the common hepatic duct before entering the hepatic parenchyma. In 20% of cases, the right hepatic artery may lie anterior to the common hepatic duct. Upon reaching the hepatic parenchyma, the right hepatic artery branches into right anterior (segments V and VIII), and right posterior sectoral branches (segments VI and VII). The posterior sectoral branch initially runs horizontally through

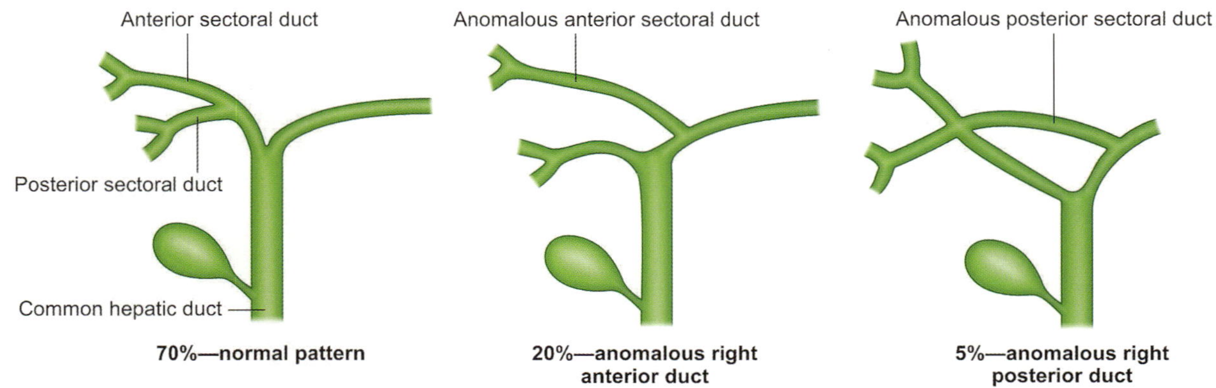

Fig. 23-10: Usual pattern and anomalies which can occur in sectoral ducts in the liver.

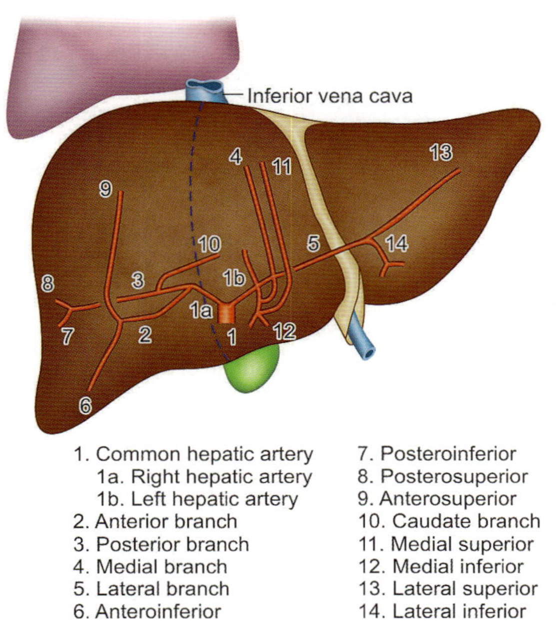

Fig. 23-11: Arterial supply of the liver—distribution of hepatic artery.

the hilar transverse fissure (of Gunz), normally present at the base of segment V and adjacent to the caudate process. The left hepatic artery runs vertically towards the umbilical fissure where it gives off a small branch (often called the middle hepatic artery, also often it arises from right hepatic artery) to segment IV, before continuing on to supply segments II and III. Additional small branches of the left hepatic artery supply the caudate lobe (segment I), although caudate arterial branches may also arise from the right hepatic artery. The most common hepatic arterial anomaly involving a replaced vessel is a replaced right hepatic artery (25%). In this situation, the replaced right hepatic artery usually arises from the superior mesenteric artery and runs lateral and posterior to the portal vein within the hepatoduodenal ligament. In rare instances, the entire common hepatic artery, or its individual branches may arise directly off the coeliac trunk or aorta.

Middle hepatic artery is an extrahepatic arterial branch originates at liver hilum from *right hepatic artery (45%) or left hepatic artery (25%)* or when there is anomaly of either of right or left hepatic arteries then it arises from normal of the two branches. It is present in 70% of individuals and supply segment 4.

Hepatic arteries are not end arteries; translobar and subcapsular collateral circulation can exist. Right gastric and gastroduodenal may maintain hepatic blood flow. *Hepatic artery ligation needs cholecystectomy.*

Portal Venous System

The portal vein contributes about 80% of total inflow to the liver. The portal vein is formed by a union of the superior mesenteric vein (SMV) and splenic vein behind the neck and body of the pancreas. In up to one third of all individuals, the inferior mesenteric vein may also join this confluence. Venous tributaries from the pancreas may also drain directly into the portal vein, and generally correspond to the arterial supply. More precisely, there are anterior, posterior, superior and inferior pancreatic vessels. Access to the portal vein is typically obtained by identifying the superior mesenteric vein on the inferior surface of the pancreas. In some circumstances, it is necessary to first locate the middle colic vein within the transverse mesocolon and follow it inferiorly to the SMV **(Figs. 23-12 and 23-13)**.

Right portal vein lies in front of the caudate lobe entering the right liver across the hilar plate divides into right anterior and posterior branches, right anterior branch runs vertically, divides into descending branch to segment 5 and ascending branch to segment 8. Right posterior branch runs horizontally and posterolaterally to supply segment 6 and 7. Right portal vein gives a branch to right side of caudate lobe. Left portal vein runs in portal plate for 3 cm and turns towards front and left in the umbilical fissure to join the round ligament anteriorly. It supplies segment 4 from its right side and segment 2 and 3 from its left side. Anatomical variations are common especially in right portal vein. Left portal vein is commonly extraparenchymal. Portal vein and hepatic artery branches to segment 4 can be isolated

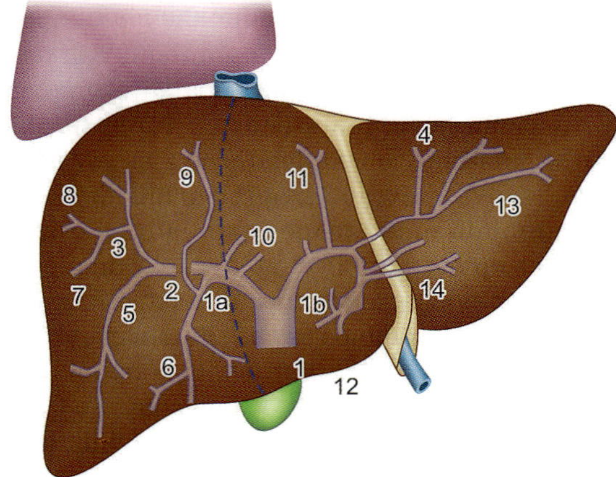

1. Portal vein	7. Posteroinferior
1a. Right portal vein	8. Posterosuperior
1b. Left portal vein branch	9. Anterosuperior
2. Anterior branch	10. Caudate branch
3. Posterior branch	11. Medial superior
4. Medial branch	12. Medial inferior
5. Lateral branch	13. Lateral superior
6. Anteroinferior	14. Lateral inferior

Fig. 23-12: Portal venous system—intrahepatic course.

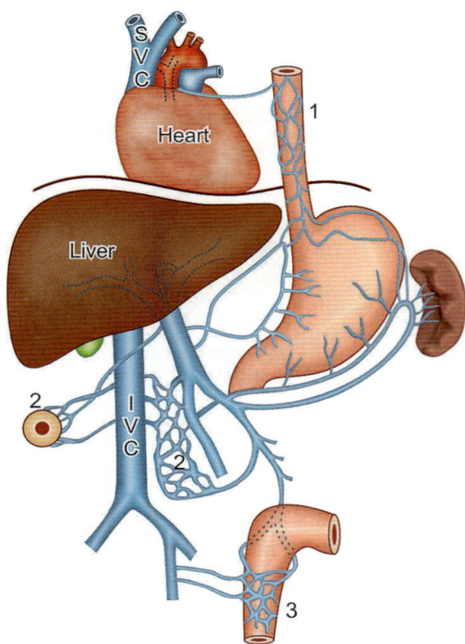

Fig. 23-13: Anatomical sites of porta systemic collaterals: 1. Lower end of oesophagus; 2. Around umbilicus; 3. Around anorectum.

in the umbilical fissure outside the liver capsule. The left portal vein is narrower and longer compared to right portal vein. It divides into medial and lateral branches, each divides into superior, inferior branches; left portal vein gives a branch to left side of caudate lobe.

Reduction in portal blood flow increases the hepatic arterial flow but reduction in hepatic arterial flow will not increase the portal flow. Portal vein ligation can cause atrophy of liver.

Hepatic Veins (Outflow)

The three major hepatic veins (right, middle and left) comprise the main outflow tract for the liver, although additional veins (5–20) of varying size are always present as direct communications between the vena cava and the posterior surface of the right lobe. Uniquely, the caudate lobe (segment I) drains principally through direct communications with the retrohepatic vena cava. The right hepatic vein lies within the *right scissura* (or right segmental fissure) and divides the right lobe into a posterior (segments VI and VII) and anterior (segments V and VIII) sector. The middle hepatic vein lies within the *main hepatic scissura* separating the right anterior sector from the quadrate lobe. The middle hepatic vein occupies the plane separating true right and left lobes and does not follow the branches of the biliary tree. The middle hepatic vein drains from segments 5 and 6 (right anterior) and segment 4 (left medial section). The left hepatic vein lies within the *left scissura* in line with or just to the right of the falciform ligament. Left hepatic vein is formed by veins from segment 2 (transverse branch) and segment 3 (sagittal branch) **(Figs. 23-14A and B)**.

The right hepatic vein drains directly into the suprahepatic vena cava, while the middle and left hepatic veins join to form a short common trunk of 1 cm in length prior to entry. Venous branches from segment 4 drains into middle hepatic vein but can drain left hepatic vein as a variation. Segment 4 vein is often called as umbilical vein but is misnomer. The umbilical vein represents an additional alternative site of venous efflux. It is located beneath the falciform ligament and eventually terminates in the left hepatic vein, or less commonly in the confluence of the middle and left hepatic veins. Large accessory right hepatic vein can often be present which drains to the vena cava directly. The caudate lobe has independent venous outflow directly draining into IVC. All three major hepatic veins (right, middle, left) drain into

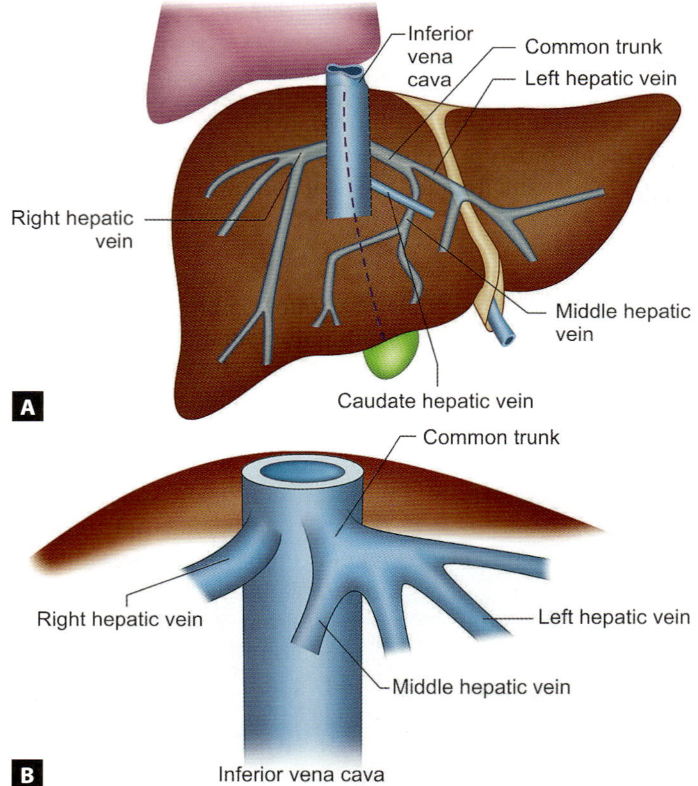

Figs. 23-14A and B: Distribution of hepatic veins—outflow/venous drainage of liver.

suprahepatic part of IVC. Suprahepatic IVC with junction of the three major hepatic and phrenic veins joining the IVC is enclosed with thick fibrous sheath extending from diaphragm. Division of this sheath is necessary to expose the major hepatic veins. In right hepatectomy, after mobilisation of the liver, this sheath has to be identified and divided before parenchymal transection. There is also a fibrous band extending from the posterior part of retrohepatic IVC at the level of junction with right hepatic vein called as *Makuuchi IVC ligament* which courses from dorsal edge of left side of the caudate lobe and right liver. Left and middle hepatic veins in left hepatectomy are usually approached after parenchymal dissection. Ligation of one hepatic vein is not necessarily to proceed with hepatic resection.

Hepatic Plate

It is fibrous sheath continuing from the Glisson's capsule, covering hepatic artery, portal vein and bile duct. Portal pedicle contains these three structures with lymphatics. Bile duct and hepatic artery are closely bounded together. Portal vein is separated from these two by a separate loose areolar fascial sheath. Hilar plate is bounded above by segment 4 and right by cystic plate and left it continuous as umbilical plate. Umbilical plate contains left hepatic duct left hepatic artery and left sided portal vein. Middle hepatic artery is also located in umbilical plate.

Anatomical speciality

- Arterial anomalies occur up to 60% of times mostly with right hepatic artery but replaced left hepatic artery in lesser omentum (from left gastric) must also be looked for.
- Each segment is supplied by portal triad and drained by hepatic vein based on which segmentectomy can be performed.
- Glisson's capsule invests within hepatic parenchyma along with separate portal triad leading to glissonian approach to resection.
- Vascular control is fundamental to safe liver resection.

Lymphatic Drainage of Liver

Superficial lymphatics lie on the surface of the liver deep to peritoneal coverings. Deep lymphatics drain into the right middle phrenic nodes; nodes of porta hepatis; these portal hepatis nodes in the transverse fissure are closer to portal vein and hepatic artery than bile duct.

LIVER RESECTION

In 1888, Langenbuch successfully removed solid left lobe tumour. Tiffany from America in 1890 removed a left lobe mass lesion. Keen removed a cystic lesion, angioma and a primary carcinoma of liver. In 1952, Lortat-Jacob and Robert designed thoracoabdominal approach and extrahepatic ligation of vascular pedicle to control bleeding prior to parenchymal dissection. In 1953, Quattelbaum described breaking of the liver tissue by finger fracture/digitoclasia. Finger or handle of knife is used for liver transection. In 1956, Finberg and associates started parenchymal dissection using back of scalpel. In 1958, Tien Yu Lin et al. started the technique of dividing the tissue between thumb and fingers; once resistant structures are felt (either vessel or ducts), they are ligated on both sides and divided.

Indications

Benign Neoplasms

- Hemangiomas
- Adenomas
- Focal nodular hyperplasia
- Cystadenoma

Malignant Tumours

- Primary
  - Hepatocellular carcinoma
  - Cholangiocarcinoma
- Metastatic tumours from
  - Colorectal cancers
  - Non-colorectal and neuroendocrine tumours
- Tumours directly invading liver
  - Adrenal, renal, gastric, colonic, retroperitoneal and IVC sarcoma
- Gallbladder carcinoma
- Hilar cholangiocarcinoma

Benign Conditions

- Intrahepatic biliary stricture/fistulae
- Intrahepatic biliary stones
- Recurrent pyogenic cholangitis
- Caroli disease
- Liver cysts/polycystic liver disease
- Parasitic cysts

Trauma

Liver Resection in Living Donors for Transplantation (Fig. 23-15)

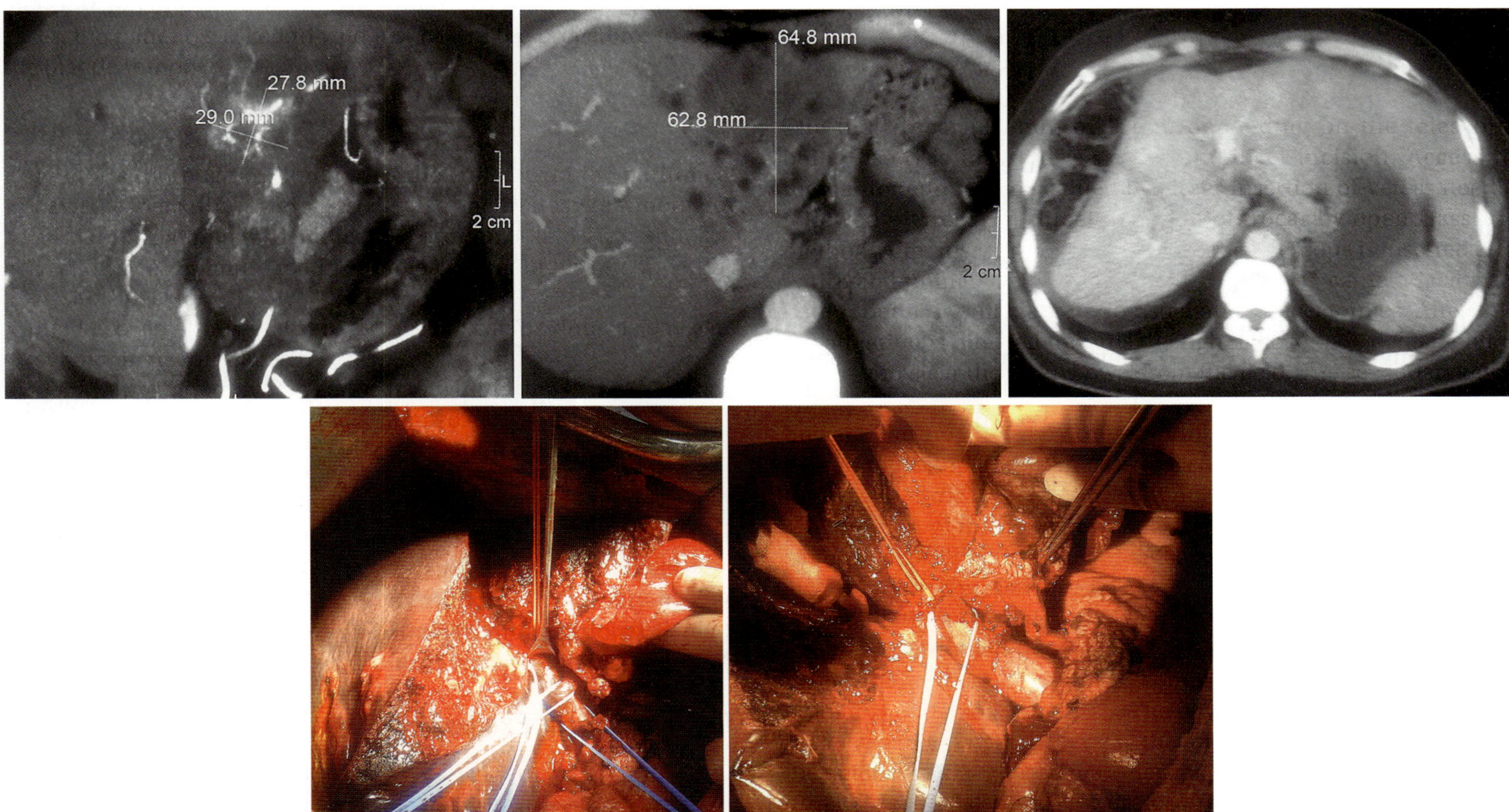

Fig. 23-15: CT and operative pictures of cholangiocarcinoma undergoing resection.
Courtesy: Dr Arunkumar, MCh, Gastro, Kochi.

General Considerations in Liver Resection

Case selection and perioperative management of patients with liver disease is as important as performing a safe surgery of liver. With advances in critical care management and surgical advances, it is now, however, possible to subject patients to liver resection in conditions like liver cirrhosis. Preoperative assessment of patients must include good preoperative imaging and volumetry (in case of major resection). High resolution triphasic CT scan should be obtained to delineate the portal anatomy, biliary anatomy and hepatic venous anatomy. Detailed discussion on hepatic imaging is beyond the scope of this book and only surgical aspect of liver resection is discussed. Major liver resection can be done only in patients who fall under CTP (Child-Turcotte-Pugh)—A class. Patients who are CTP B should be assessed carefully and additional ICG clearance may be needed to decide upon surgery. A minimum clearance of 10% is required for patients undergoing major resection. Patients who are CTP C class are generally not fit for any type of liver resection. A minimum of 30% of functional liver must be left behind (FLR—future liver remnant) for adequate recovery of the patient. This value can be higher than 40% in case of cirrhotics in whom the volume of liver does not correlate with functional liver. In cirrhotic patients, preoperative portal vein embolisation (2 weeks prior) is a good strategy to induce compensatory hypertrophy of remnant liver in order to increase the FLR.

Liver resection is classified as *anatomical and non-anatomical.* Anatomical is along the functional segmental anatomy of parenchyma with defined boundaries. When resection is done without taking into consideration of the segments is called as non-anatomical. Anatomical resections are termed as sectionectomy/segmentectomy; hepatectomy/hemihepatectomy. Hepatectomies are right and left. Sectionectomies are left lateral; left medial; right anterior; right posterior. Resection of three consecutive sections is called as trisectionectomy. Extended right hemihepatectomy includes middle hepatic vein with the part of segment 4. Extended left hemihepatectomy included middle hepatic vein with part segments 5 and 8.

Resection of three or more liver segments is called as *major* hepatic resection. Middle hepatic vein is the landmark between right and left liver. It begins in gallbladder fossa and ends in IVC either after joining left hepatic vein as common trunk or independently. It receives hepatic veins from segments 5 and 8 on right side and segment 4a and 4b from left side. Major resection is done when tumour is more than 5 cm or when tumour is close to liver hilum involving the portal pedicles. Major hepatic resection is often done in selected patients with en bloc removal of part of IVC or right adrenal gland or diaphragm or right kidney or duodenum.

In right hepatectomy when remnant liver in left lobe is inadequate then preoperative right portal vein embolisation is done to induce the hypertrophy of left liver which is future remnant liver.

Evaluation in Liver Resection

Multidetector CT scan is ideal imaging method in terms of assessing the resectability and CT volumetry of the remnant liver. *Urata formula* is used to estimate the liver volume. It is important in cirrhotics. If liver volume is less than 40% in cirrhotics then major resection becomes high risk. Hepatic angiogram is not necessary unless MDCT shows vascular anomalies.

Assessment of liver and kidney function (LFT/RFT) is important. *Child-Pugh grading* is done to decide the selection of the patient for resection.

Indocyanine green (ICG) clearance test is more valuable than Child's grading or prothrombin time or platelet count. But high ICG retention rate can occur if there is partial compression of portal vein or bile duct.

Screening preoperatively for other comorbid diseases is also essential.

Vascular Control

The crux of good liver surgery lies in haemostasis. Liver vascular control has two components—*inflow control and outflow control.*

Pringle Manoeuvre

The inflow to the liver can be controlled using the *Pringle manoeuvre.* As described in anatomy, the whole hepatic pedicle including the artery lies in the free border of hepatoduodenal ligament. Here it can be encircled using an umbilical tape or vascular tape by making a window in the lesser omentum. The tape is threaded over a red rubber catheter and clamped. Tightening the clamp allows to stop inflow to the liver [Pringle's manoeuvre (PM)]. The PM has relatively little general haemodynamic effect and no specific anaesthetic management is required. However, bleeding can still occur from the backflow from the hepatic veins and from the liver transection plane during unclamping. The other concern is the ischaemic-reperfusion injury to the liver parenchyma, especially in patients with underlying liver diseases. The Pringle's manoeuvre can be applied either continuously or intermittently. Continuous occlusion is safely applied for up to 60 minutes in healthy liver and for up to 30 minutes in diseased liver (fatty liver/cirrhosis). In intermittent Pringle's manoeuvre, the inflow is occluded for 15 minutes followed by 5 minutes of reperfusion. There is no difference in blood loss during surgery in both the manoeuvres; however, there is more ischaemic injury to the liver in patients with pre-existing liver disease.

Hemihepatic clamping (half-Pringle manoeuvre) interrupts the arterial and portal inflow selectively to the right or left liver lobe that is to be resected. It can be performed with or without prior hilar dissection. It can also be combined with simultaneous occlusion of the ipsilateral major hepatic vein. The advantage of this technique is that it avoids ischaemia in the remnant liver, avoids visceral congestion and allows clear demarcation of the resection margin. The disadvantage is that bleeding from the parenchymal cut surface can occur from the non-occluded liver lobe. Segmental vascular clamping entails the occlusion of the ipsilateral hepatic artery branch and balloon occlusion of the portal branch of a particular segment.

It is often claimed that Pringle manoeuvre prepares the liver for eventual ischaemia—ischaemic preconditioning. Now newer gadgets like ultrasonic dissector allows liver transection without Pringle manoeuvre.

Total Vascular Exclusion

Total vascular exclusion (TVE) combines total inflow and outflow vascular occlusion of the liver, isolating it completely from the systemic circulation. It is done with complete mobilisation of the liver, encircling of the suprahepatic and infrahepatic IVC, application of the Pringle manoeuvre, and then clamping the infrahepatic IVC followed by clamping of the suprahepatic IVC.

Occlusion of the IVC leads to marked reduction of venous return and cardiac output, with a compensatory 80% increase in systemic vascular resistance and 50% increase in heart rate and thus, not every patient can tolerate it. TVE can be applied to a normal liver for up to 60 minutes and for 30 minutes in a diseased liver. Lumbar veins will not be present in retrohepatic IVC. Right adrenal vein needs ligation.

Retrocaval ligament bridging the segments 6 and 7 should be completely divided to expose right hepatic vein. Hepatic veins should be exposed only after proper inflow control.

Parenchymal Transection

Maximum blood loss during liver surgery occurs during parenchymal transection. The toughest structure in the liver is the Glisson's capsule. The rest of the liver does not have much connective tissue and parenchyma is packed within lattice of biliary radicles and vascular structures. Even though the segments have independent vascular supply, there is still bleeding from adjacent side when inflow occlusion is not applied. Portal veins are less fragile than hepatic veins. The advance in surgical instrumentation has definitely made parenchymal transection easy. Though the simplest of techniques is sufficient energy sources may be needed in certain cases. The choice of device, however, remains personal and also depends on availability as many of these devices are expensive to procure and maintain **(Fig. 23-16)**.

The main modality of parenchymal transection are:
1. Kelly clamp and bipolar forceps.
2. Water jet dissection—contact method.
3. Cavitron ultrasonic surgical aspirator (CUSA)—contact method.
4. Ultrasonic dissection.
5. Bipolar vessel sealer.
6. Staplers.
7. Finger fracture—compression method.
8. Electrocautery and laser—thermal method.
9. Suture ligation.

Before starting parenchymal dissection, stay sutures are taken on either side of line of parenchymal transection. This aids greatly in applying traction especially in the initial dissection. Capsule of the liver is marked/scored along the line of planned resection with cautery. Parenchymal transection is better begun at relatively thin liver free edge.

Kelly Clamp and Bipolar Forceps

A small clamp (Kelly) is used to crush parenchyma between its blades in order to isolate vessels and bile ducts. Fine branches of Glisson's tree or tiny tributaries of hepatic veins (<3 mm) are coagulated using a bipolar forceps and are cut by scissors. Bipolar forceps cautery is equipped with a channel for water dripping, which prevents adhesion of debris to the cautery blades. Bigger identified vessels or bile ducts (>3 mm) are ligated or clipped on the remnant liver slice before cutting.

Water Jet Dissection

A jet of water (saline) is used for dissection of liver parenchyma. The saline is delivered on parenchyma at 30–50 atmospheric pressure which washes off soft tissue leaving behind more resilient biliary radicles and vessels. The device tip also hosts a suction device which clears the field for further dissection. The biliary radicles and vessels are either cauterised or ligated depending on their size as mentioned earlier. The device is held near but not in contact with liver parenchyma and dissection is done using gentle paintbrush-like strokes.

Cavitron Ultrasonic Surgical Aspirator

Cavitron ultrasonic surgical aspirator (CUSA) is a multifunctional instrument that is used to perform ultrasonic cavitation, stanching, debridement and liposuction. The CUSA absorbs cells with high water content such as adipose tissue and protects tissues with a high collagen content that has got good elasticity. So damage to healthy surrounding tissues is reduced. CUSA is currently used for liver and spleen resection, transplantation, and neurological surgery. It is found to be useful in nerve sparing radical hysterectomy.

The device delivers ultrasonic shock to the tissue in contact with the vibrating tip and the tissue is then suctioned off the field by an inbuilt suction at the tip of the device. The ultrasonic probe divides parenchymal cells (because of their high water content) by the cavitational effect with less injury to structures with a high content of fibrous tissue, e.g. bile ducts and blood vessels. These structures are taken down using clips or suture ligation in the usual way. CUSA is more precise but slow. It acts as a mechanical disrupter and suction; it is useful in hilar area dissection. Ultrasonic dissector may damage hepatic veins when power is kept very high; so power should be set between 40–60% with short range amplitude **(Fig. 23-17)**.

Ultrasonic Cutting Devices

These devices have two blades at the tip of which one moves at high frequency (55 kHz) against the other producing sealing and cutting effect due to protein denaturation. Many companies now make these devices each one similar to the other. In practice, the device works partly like the Kelly crushing technique. When the Jaws of the device are approximated, they crush the parenchyma and then the small biliary radicles and vessels are sealed. Additional ties or bipolar may be required if the parenchyma is divided in fast cutting mode.

Bipolar Vessel Sealer

Bipolar vessel sealing device is also an excellent tool for parenchymal transection. The jaws initially act as a Kelly clamp in crushing liver tissue and then the biliary and small vascular channels are coagulated. The larger (10 mm) instrument has got an inbuilt blade which can then be used to divide the sealed tissue. The smaller (5 mm) jaw blade does not have an inbuilt blade, and hence, tissue is divided by sharp dissection using scissors or electrocautery.

Stapling Devices

Vascular load of stapler (same as those used in gastrointestinal surgery) can also be used for liver transection. These, however, are used mainly towards the posterior part of dissection where one encounters the hepatic veins. This helps to take the hepatic veins within the liver parenchyma which reduces the risk of vascular complications when compared to extrahepatic take of the hepatic veins. The jaws are approximated and stapler is fired across the tissue after making sure the field is clear and no inadvertent tissue is caught in the stapler.

Finger Fracture

It is pinching and compressing about 1 cm of parenchyma between thumb and forefinger. It disrupts the normal liver with preserving the

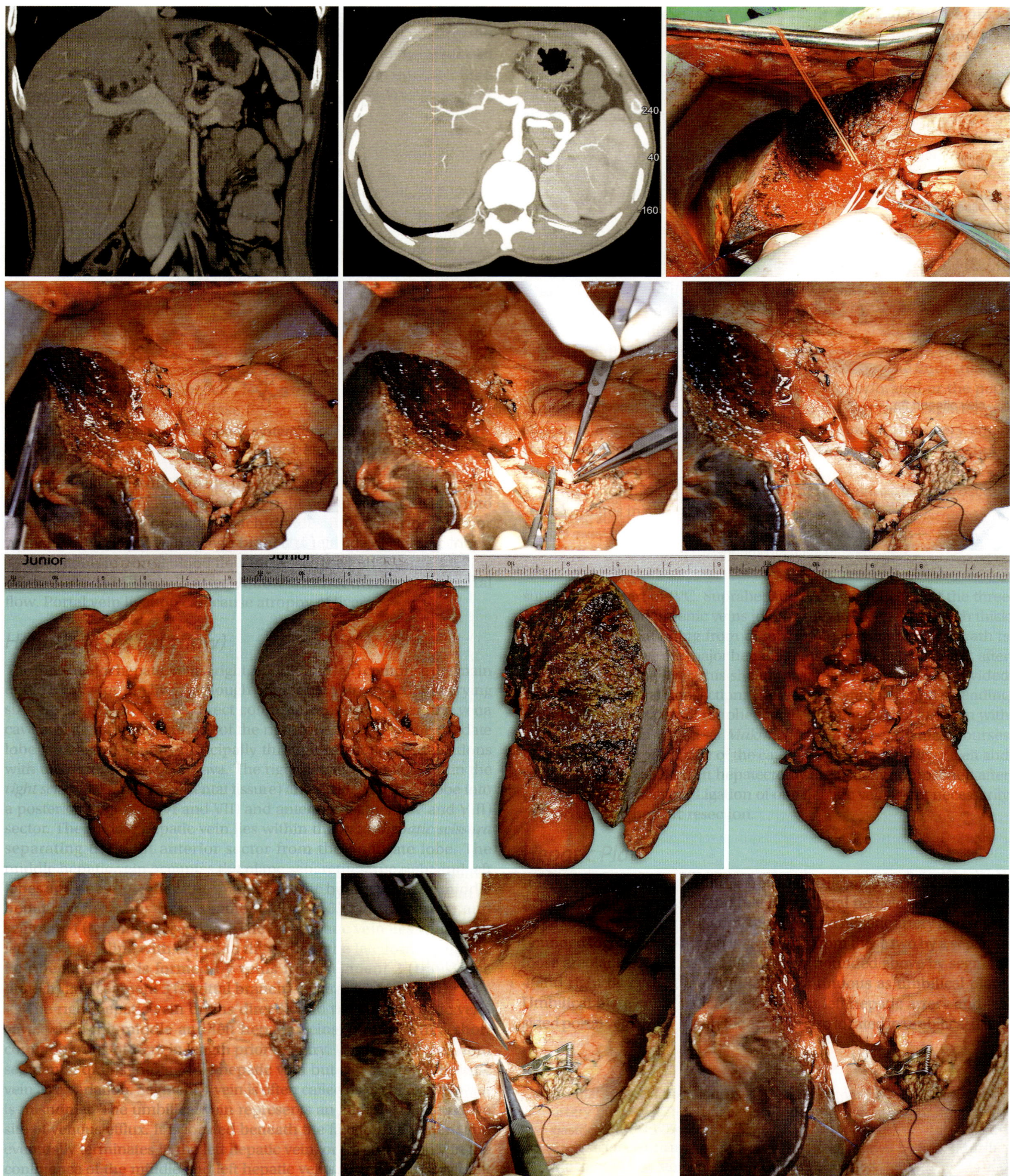

Figs. 23-16(1)

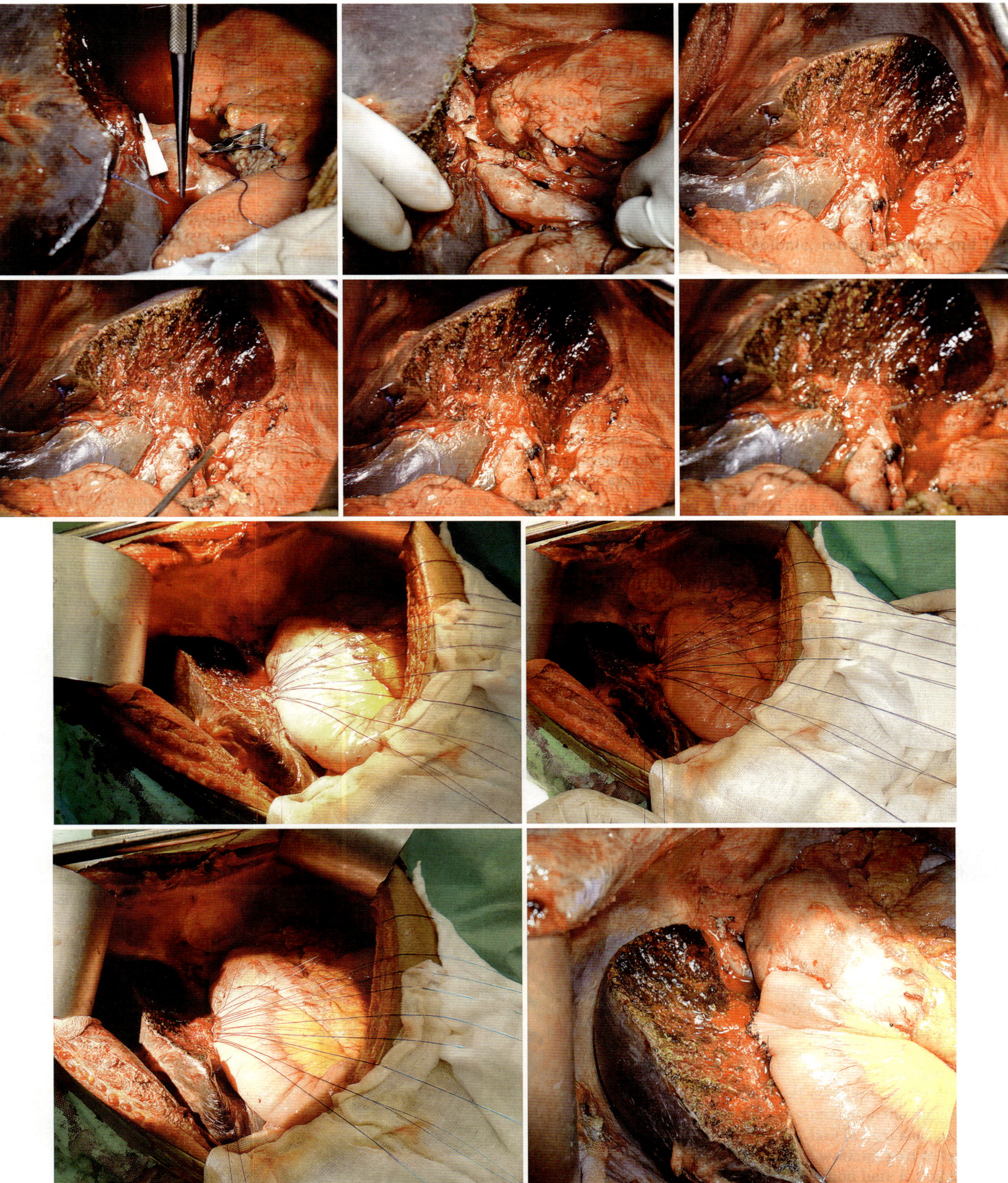

Figs. 23-16(2)

Figs. 23-16(1 and 2): Cholangiocarcinoma—arterial resection.
Courtesy: Dr Arunkumar, MCh, Gastro, Kochi.

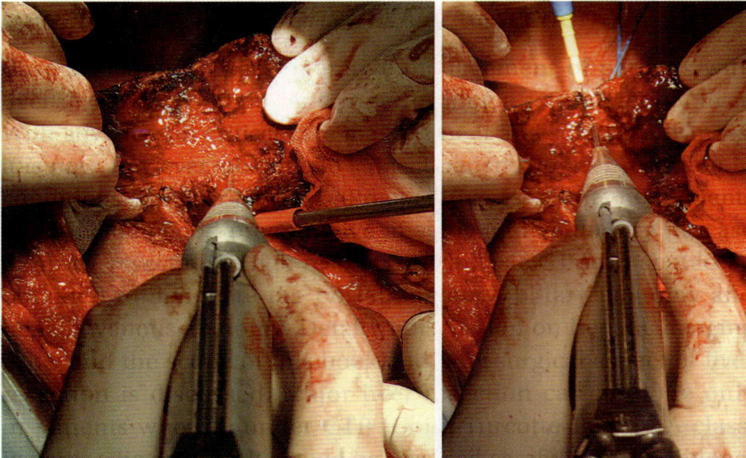

Fig. 23-17: Cavitron ultrasonic surgical aspirator (CUSA).

vascular and ductal structures. Both surgeon and assistant do finger fracture together.

Suture Ligation

Any structure more than 2 mm in liver needs suture ligation or clipping. Circumferential and adequate length exposure is essential prior ligation. Fine silk, vicryl or metal clips can be used. All small portal and hepatic branches should be ligated on either side and divided in between. Avulsion of small hepatic veins can bleed significantly. Avulsed hepatic vein opening should be identified using suction and carefully sutured using 5-zero polypropylene suture material.

Argon Beam Coagulator

Argon beam coagulator can be used to control small bleeds on the surface. It is also used to stop bleeders on the surface of middle hepatic vein through tiny holes.

Preservation of Hepatic Ducts

It is very important to preserve the hepatic duct of the remnant; for that entire biliary tree until entering the liver parenchyma should be dissected especially in liver parenchyma. Branches are isolated; but ligation is done only after major part of parenchymal transection. Parenchyma around major duct is dissected using CUSA device. Choledochotomy and cannulation may safely identify the ductal anatomy.

Incisions Used for Liver Resection

Patient is in supine position with both upper limbs on the side of the table or at least right side should be on the side of the table. Warming devices should be placed on the body. Perioperative antibiotics are given. Bilateral subcostal incision with an upper midline extension; thoracoabdominal incision; extension as sternotomy are different incisions used.

Mercedes Benz incision, Makuuchi J incision and bilateral roof top bucket handle incision—are different incisions used to expose field adequately **(Fig. 23-18)**.

Upper hand or Thomson retractor is used to elevate the rib cage; additional retractors are used in abdominal cavity. All perihepatic attachments are released—both triangular ligaments and falciform ligament. Mops are placed between diaphragm and liver to displace the liver downwards **(Figs. 23-19 to 23-22)**.

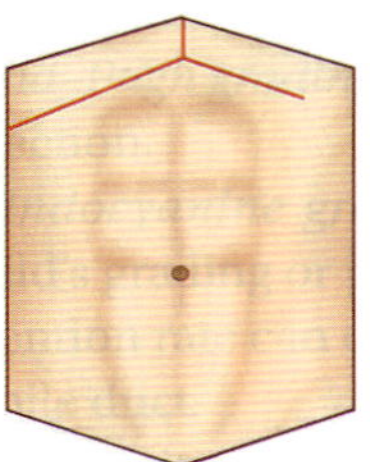

Roof top incision with extension upwards (Mercedes Benz)

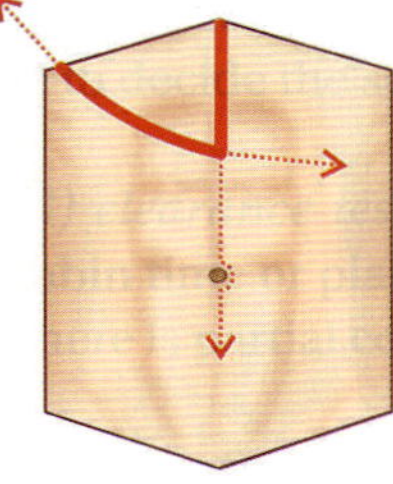

Makuuchi J incision—can extend towards left or downwards

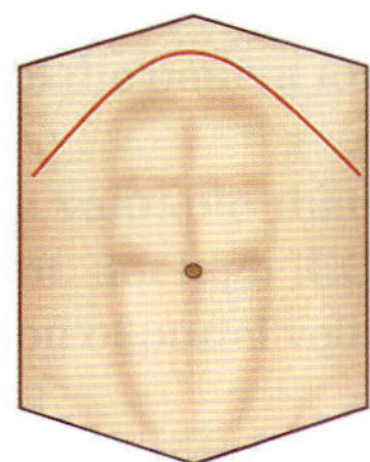

Roof top bucket handle incision

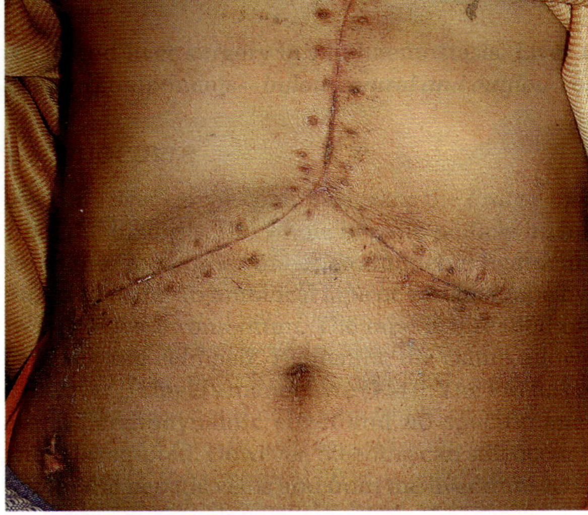

Fig. 23-18: Incisions used to approach liver for resection and other procedures.

Nomenclature for liver resection

Segments	*Brisbane—2000*	*Couinaud—1957*	*Goldsmith and Woodburne—1957*
V-VIII	Right hemihepatectomy	Right hepatectomy	Right hepatic lobectomy
IV-VIII	Right trisectiontectomy	Right lobectomy	Extended right hepatic lobectomy
II-IV	Left hemihepatectomy	Left hepatectomy	Left hepatic lobectomy
II, III	Left lateral sectionectomy	Left lobectomy	Left lateral segmentectomy
II, III, IV, V, VIII	Left trisegmentectomy	Extended left hepatectomy	Extended left lobectomy

Starlz nomenclature: Entire right liver with complete resection of segment 4 is right trisegmentectomy; entire left liver with complete resection of segments 5 and 8 is left trisegmentectomy.

Indications	*Contraindications*
• Primary/secondary malignancy from gallbladder or colorectum or carcinoids • Benign tumours of liver • Parasitic/non-parasitic cysts—hydatid cysts/simple liver cysts • Refractory abscess/Caroli disease/recurrent pyogenic cholangitis (RPC) • Living donor liver transplantation (LDLT) • Klatskin's tumour • Trauma to liver	• Acute hepatitis—viral/alcoholic • Severe chronic hepatitis • Poor liver reserve • Severe portal hypertension • Severe coagulopathy • Severe thrombocytopenia—platelet count less than 30,000/-

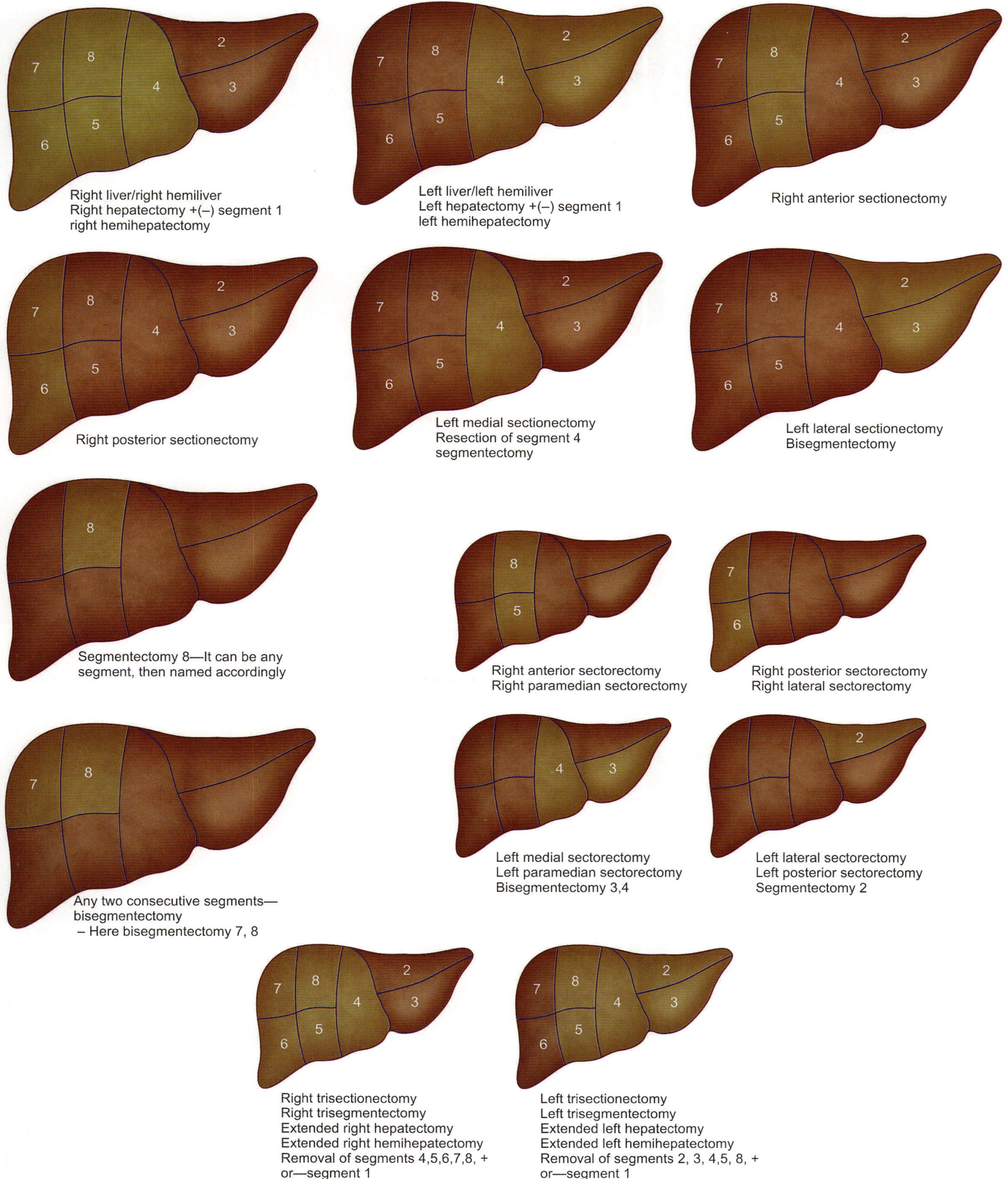

Fig. 23-19: Different types of hepatic resections.

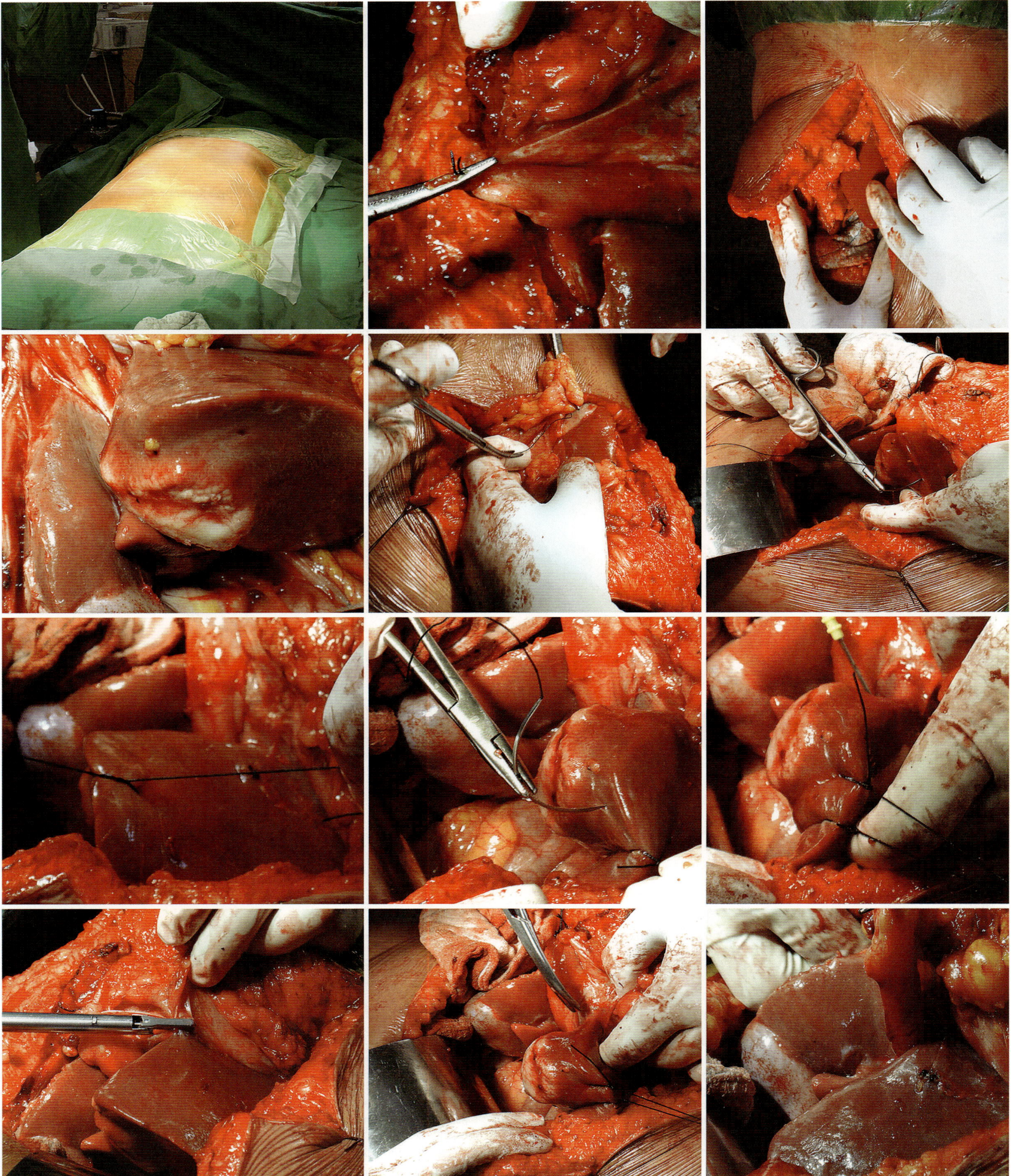

Figs. 23-20(1)

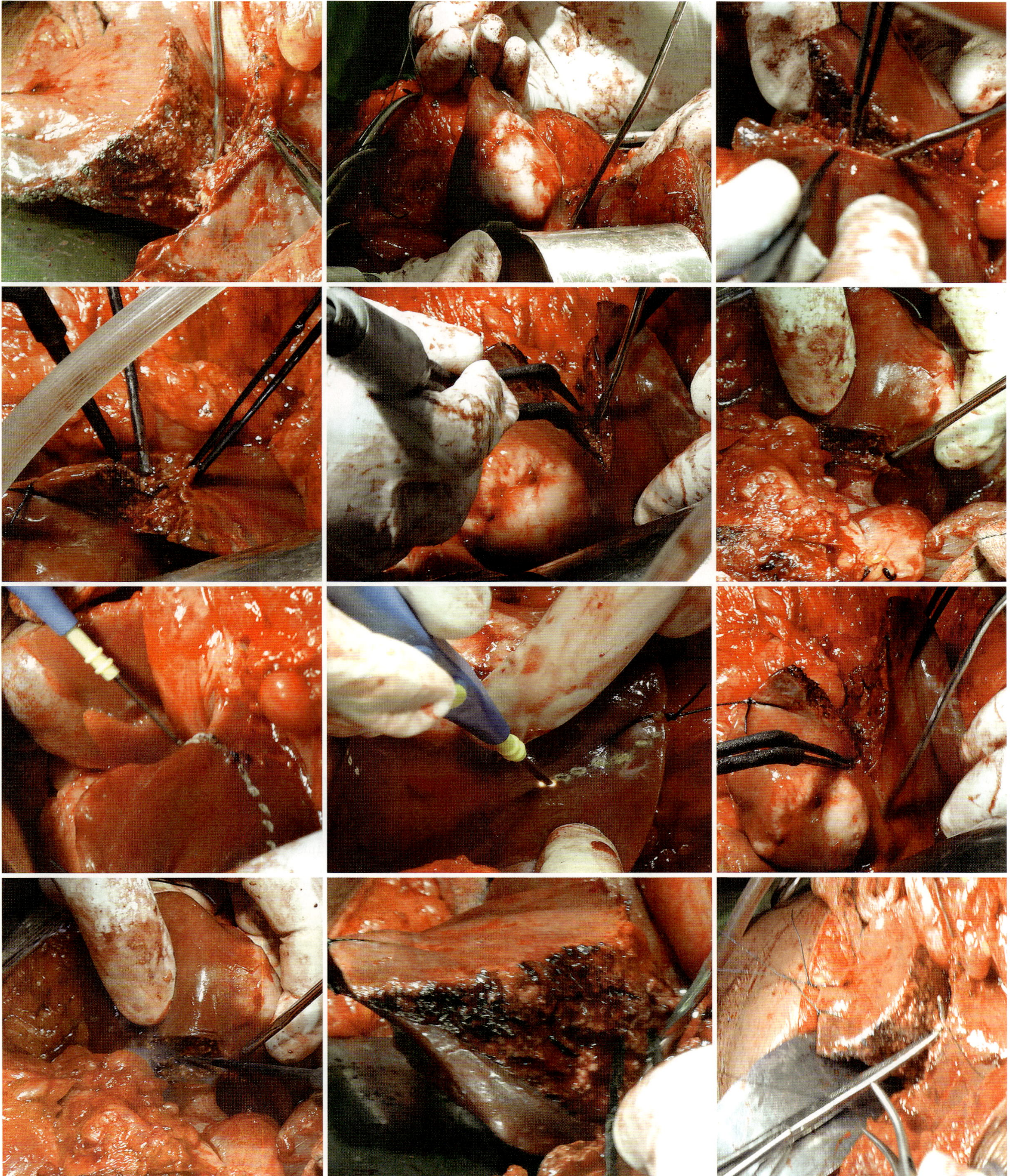

Figs. 23-20(2)

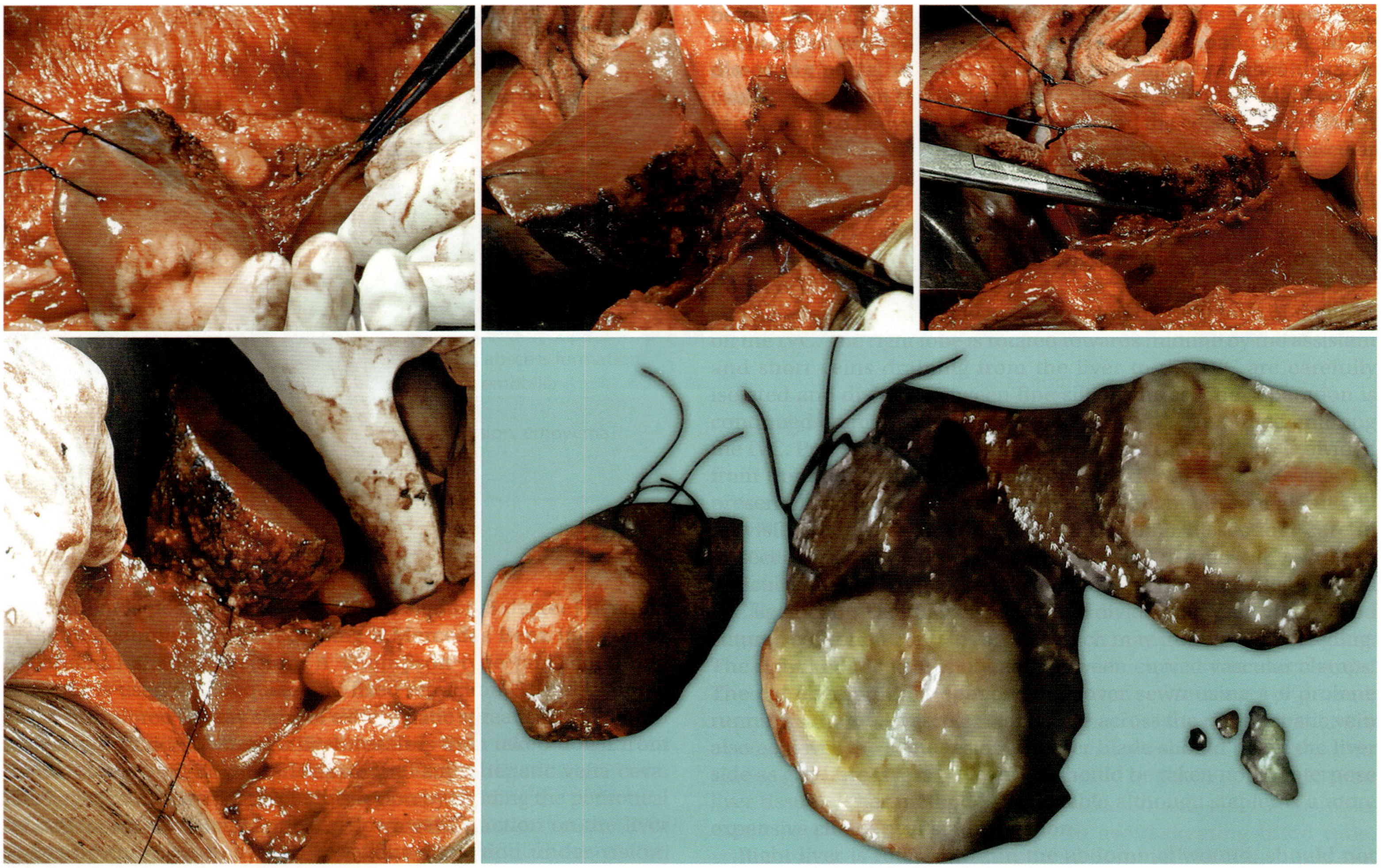

Figs. 23-20(3)

Figs. 23-20(1 to 3): Segmental liver resection—for secondaries (single) in liver from carcinoma of colon.

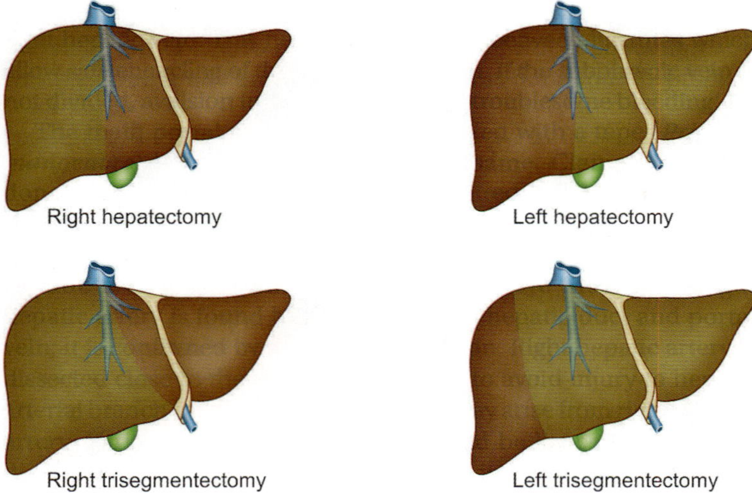

Fig. 23-21: Major hepatic resections.

Types of hepatectomy techniques

- Preliminary vascular section (Lortat-Jacob).
- Primary parenchymal transection (Ton That Tung in 1965).
- Selective clamping.
- Total vascular exclusion.
- Pedicular clamping (Pringles).
- Suprahilar clamping (Glissonian approach).
- Intrahepatic portal control.

Technical principles

Inflow (portal vein, hepatic artery) control; outflow (hepatic veins) control; parenchymal transection; preservation of adequate sized liver remnant with intact inflow, biliary drainage and venous outflow; mobilisation of left and right triangular ligament; ligation of branches of portal vein and hepatic artery and resection of hepatic duct branch of the side; ligation of hepatic vein at a later period; proper haemostasis and ligation of individual biliary ductules. Retrohepatic caval dissection includes—dissection of right adrenal vein, inferior hepatic veins and IVC ligament. Preservation of the bile duct to the remnant liver is also equally important.

Vascular control

↓

Parenchymal dissection

↓

Precise anatomical identification

↓

Division of biliary tree (ducts/branches) with preservation of bile drainage of remnant liver

Resection along the main portal fissure (Cantlie's line) and removal on right side is *right hemihepatectomy* and removal on left side is *left hemihepatectomy*. Resection on right of the ligamentum teres is called as *right trisegmentectomy* (older—right lobectomy); and left of the ligamentum teres is called as *left lateral segmentectomy* segment II and III (older left lobectomy). Removal of single segment is called as *unisegmentectomy. Plurisegmentectomy* is removal of two or more segments. Segments IV and V are removed in carcinoma of gallbladder. Removal of small portion of liver either within the segment or traversing segments is called as *wedge resection* of the liver.

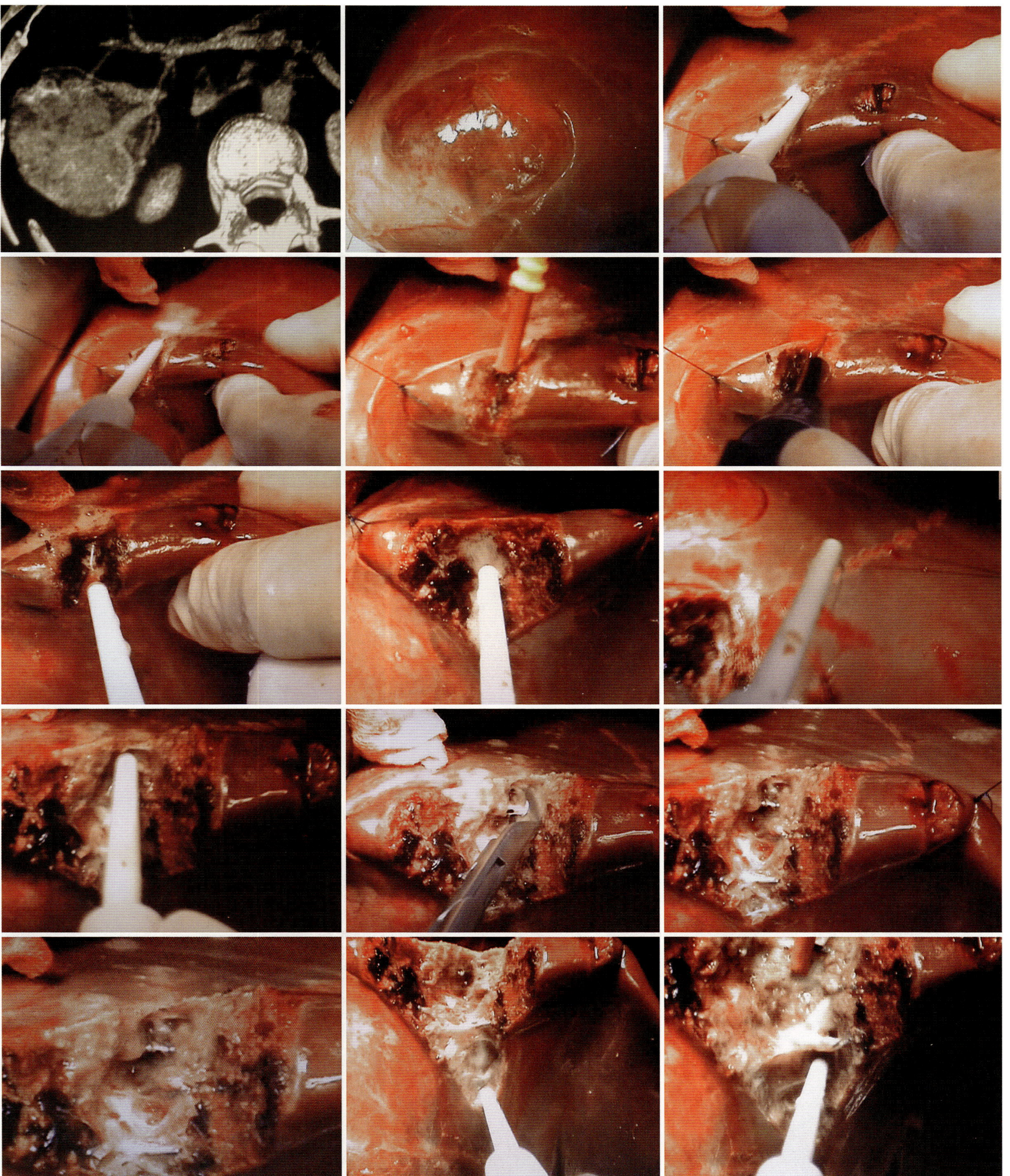

Figs. 23-22(1)

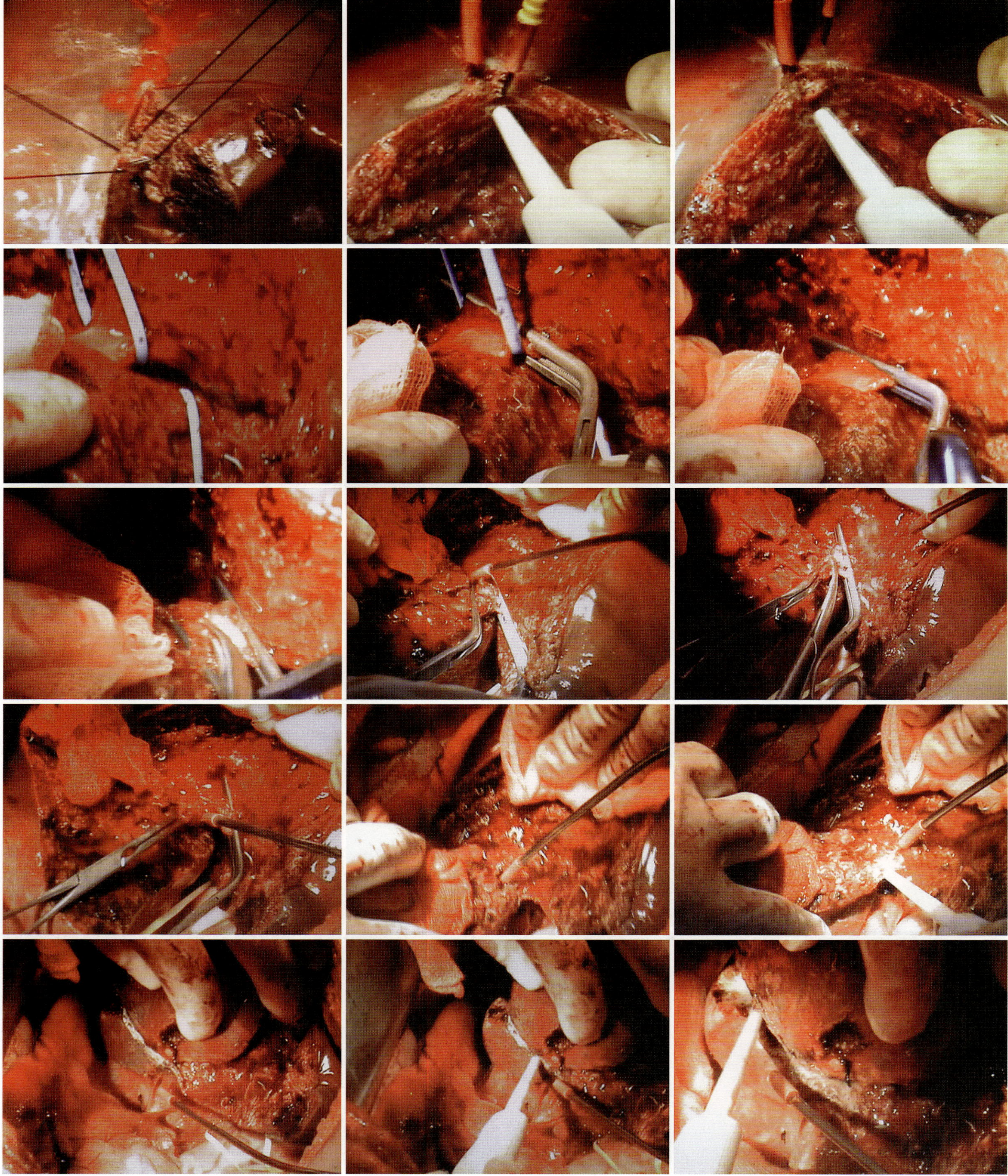

Figs. 23-22(2)

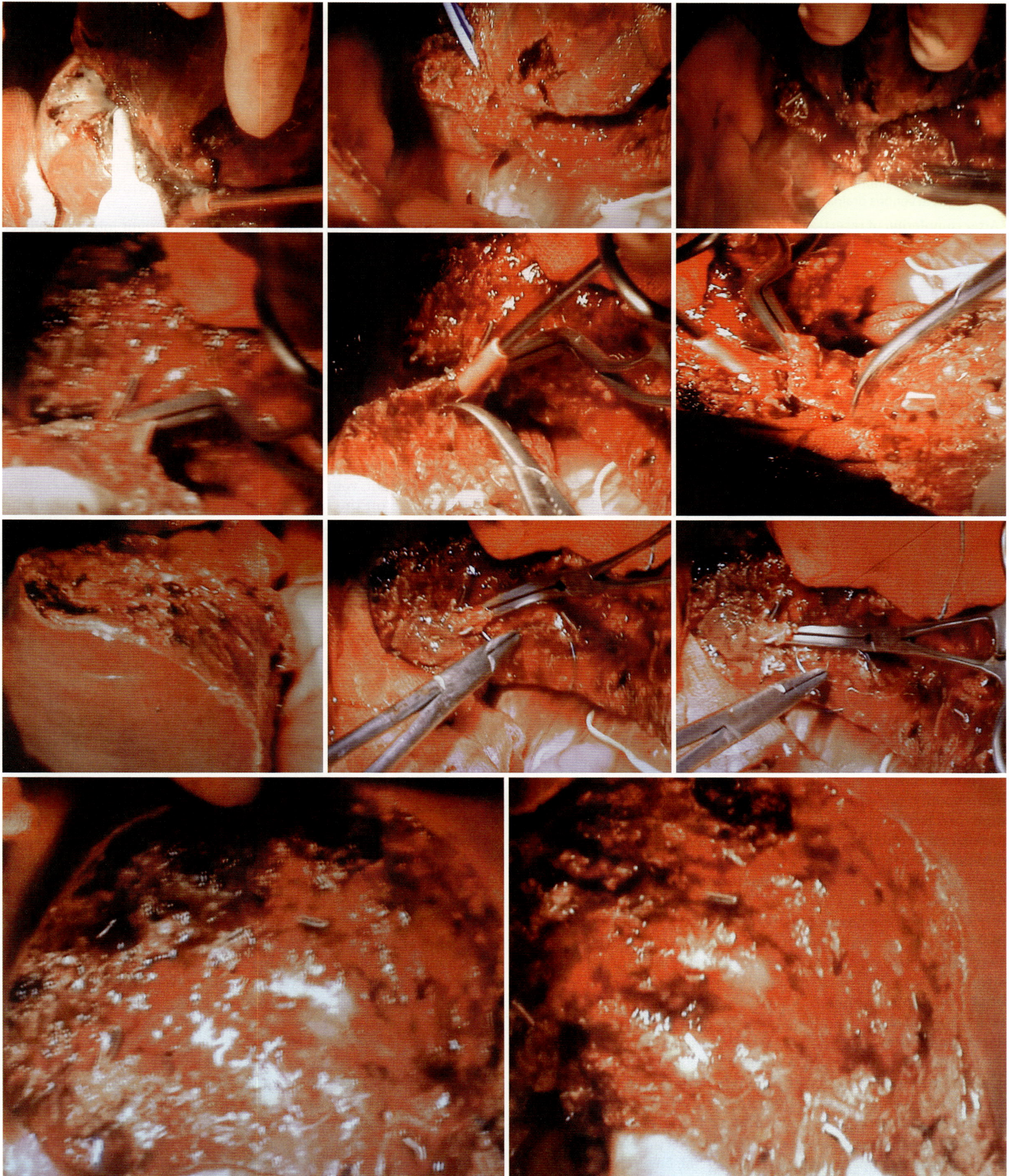

Figs. 23-22(3)

Figs. 23-22(1 to 3): Technique of liver resection—note the usage of waterjet for parenchymal transection.
Courtesy: Dr Ravishankar, MCh, Gastro, Bengaluru.

Techniques of parenchyma dissection	Intraoperative ultrasound
♦ Kelly clamp and bipolar forceps ♦ Water jet dissection ♦ Ultrasonic dissection ♦ Ultrasound cutting ♦ Dissecting sealer **How much to cut** ♦ Remnant liver— ≥30% of the original liver volume with complete venous drainage is safe	♦ Identifying tumour ♦ Recognising the anatomy ♦ Unexpected contralateral tumour ♦ Intrahepatic selective vascular control using a balloon catheter ♦ Guided biopsy
After completion of resection	**Complications**
♦ Check for bile leak by injecting dye through cystic duct ♦ Check for absolute haemostasis ♦ Cholangiogram to confirm contralateral biliary patency ♦ Fix the left lobe through falciform ligament	♦ Bleeding, infection, septicaemia ♦ Subphrenic abscess formation ♦ Bile leak, haemobilia ♦ Liver failure ♦ Pleural effusion, empyema

Right Hepatectomy

The patient is positioned supine with a slight (15 degree) head up tilt. The abdomen is opened using a Mercedes Benz incision or Makuuchi J shaped incision. A Thompson type table mounted retractor is used for adequate and fixed retraction. The abdominal cavity is explored for any signs of extrahepatic spread. The falciform ligament is divided between ligatures. It is then taken down from the diaphragm till its posterior extent of suprahepatic vena cava. The hepatic veins are defined in this region by dividing the peritoneal reflection under vision. Applying downward traction on the liver opens up this space so as to carry out dissection under vision. The right triangular ligament is then divided which allows us to rotate the liver towards the left to expose the posterolateral side of the right liver. The right hepatic vein can be seen entering the IVC at the apex. The right subphrenic vein enters the IVC just above the insertion of the right hepatic vein. This needs to be divided between ligatures which allow safe encircling of the right hepatic vein. If the subphrenic vein is not divided, avulsion injury to it can cause troublesome bleeding.

The main portal pedicle is now encircled with a tape (*Pringle's manoeuvre*) but without clamping the same. Clamping can be done any time during the surgery if required. Cholecystectomy is performed and the cystic duct is cannulated with an infant feeding tube and secured. The portal plate is now lowered and the right hepatic artery and common hepatic duct are identified. Right hepatic artery is found between common hepatic duct and portal vein; it is confirmed by feeling the pulsation. Right hepatic artery is dissected close to the hilum of right liver to avoid injury to hepatic arterial branch to segment 4 which often may arise from right hepatic artery. Variations can occur which should be kept in mind while dissecting it. Right branch of portal vein is situated behind these structures and is also identified and looped. Arterial supply of hepatic duct is preserved while dissecting by staying away from it. A temporary vascular occlusion of right hepatic artery confirms the vascular anatomy in the patient. Initially bulldog clamp is applied to right hepatic artery; left hepatic artery pulsation should be checked now to confirm that inadvertent clamping of proper hepatic artery has not occurred. On table, Doppler study may be helpful for this purpose. The line of demarcation will appear along the Cantlie's line on arterial occlusion.

The right liver is now rotated to the left by the assistant so as to expose the retrohepatic IVC. The right hepatic artery is then divided between ligatures; two ligatures on either side should be placed before dividing. The right portal vein is now exposed. Atraumatic retractor is gently used to retract common hepatic duct while dissecting portal vein and its divisions. Small branches towards caudate lobe from right portal veins should be divided. Right portal vein is divided between vascular clamps and the edge over sewn with 6-0 polypropylene sutures. Alternately it can be divided with vascular stapler; or two ligatures are placed with more than 1 cm gap and two transfixation sutures are placed between two ligatures and divided in between. The right hepatic duct is not divided extrahepatically (at this juncture). It is divided during parenchymal division away from the hilar plate **(Fig. 23-23)**.

The attention is now given to separate the right lobe of the liver off the IVC. The right lobe is rotated towards midline by the assistant and short veins draining from the liver to the IVC are carefully isolated and divided between fine silk ligatures. The separation is continued cranially till the right hepatic vein is identified entering the IVC. Process and paracaval portion of the caudate lobe is divided from front and right side of the IVC. Inferior hepatic vein may be present if so should be carefully divided. Right adrenal gland will be visible and may interfere with the proper dissection; careful dissection is done between liver adrenal gland to expose the IVC; in a difficult situation, right adrenal gland may be removed. Right side of IVC ligament is carefully dissected and divided between clamps and sutured as it often contains a vein which may trouble with bleeding. The right hepatic vein is divided between curved vascular clamps. The cut edge on the hepatic vein is over sewn using 4-0 prolene running sutures. A vascular stapler fire across the right hepatic vein also achieves the same result. Thinner blade should be on the liver side as gap here is less but caution should be taken not to interpose liver tissue. Either method is acceptable although stapler is a more expensive choice over suture ligation.

Right liver is rotated within the abdominal wound; should not be brought out of the wound to prevent ischaemia of left liver. After devascularising the right lobe, clear line of demarcation is seen on the liver surface which is scored using electrocautery. If demarcation is not there then right anterior hepatic artery or portal vein may be present. The parenchymal dissection is now carried out under low CVP (<5 mm Hg). Dissection is done along the middle hepatic vein plane rather than towards left. Transection plane is not vertical in relation to IVC but oblique in right hepatectomy. The choice of method for liver transection depends on the preference of surgeons and the available gadgets at his disposal. In fibrotic cirrhotic liver, dissection along the middle hepatic vein is difficult and troublesome. The small biliary radicles and vascular branches are secured within liver parenchyma by bipolar coagulation or fine silk sutures if more than 3 mm in diameter. After parenchymal transection careful inspection of the cut surface is done to look for any bile leaks. It is usual to place a fresh piece of gauze on the cut surface and look for any biliary stains on the same after few minutes. Such points are then suture ligated using 4-0 vicryl sutures. At this point a saline leak test can be done using the already cannulated cystic duct stump. Saline is pushed from the cystic duct and any leak from the cut surface of the liver is looked for. Dilute methylene blue injection also can be used. Right hepatic duct is now dissected from the surrounding hilar plate and is divided with scissor and sutured with vicryl. It is usual to apply a pair of vascular clamps across the right hepatic duct and divide it; but care should be taken not to clamp part of the confluence; so after clamping, dye is injected into the cystic duct cannula to delineate the left hepatic duct properly under C arm image intensifier. Once again after inspecting the cut surface of the remnant liver dye is injected through cystic duct across the left hepatic duct to rule out bile leak. Any significant bile leak is suture

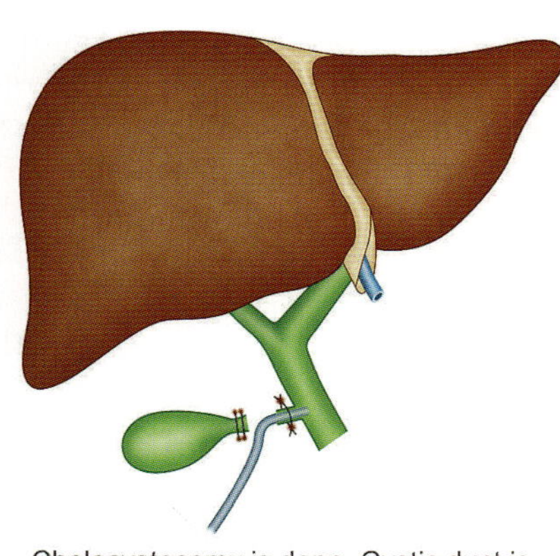

Cholecystecomy is done. Cystic duct is cannulated with fine tube for eventual cholangiogram to delineate biliary system

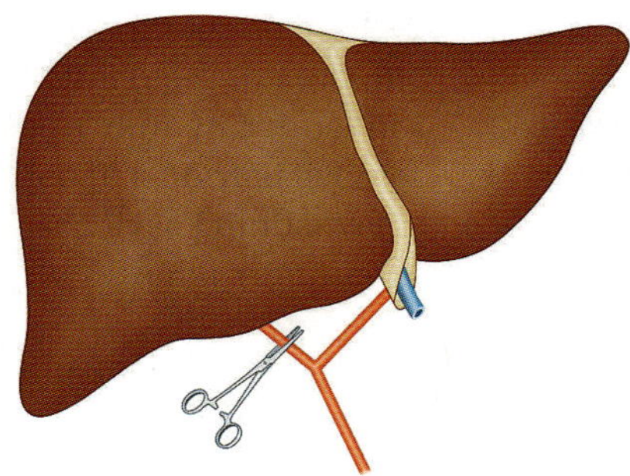

Right hepatic artery is dissected after retracting the right hepatic duct. Soft vascular clamp or bulldog clamp is applied to right hepatic artery Presence of left hepatic artery pulsation should be confirmed Doppler on table will help to identify this and anomalies and also segments — 2,3,4 hepatic arterial branch and flow

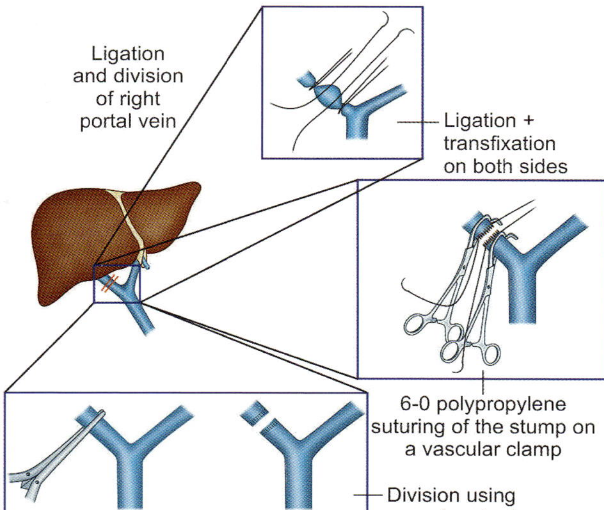

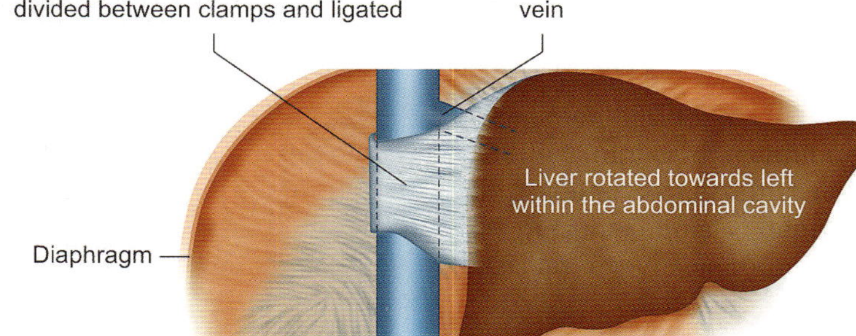

Right hepatic vein should be transected ideally with stapler or using sutures When stapler is used, thinner blade should pass between liver and right hepatic vein

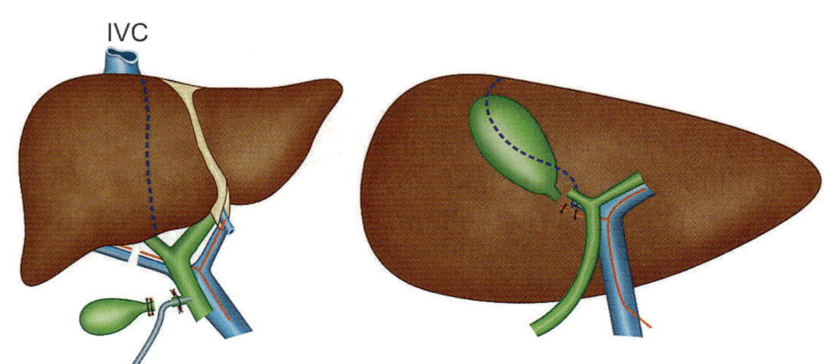

Scoring is done the superior and inferior surface along the Cantlie's line—while doing parenchymal dissection in this plane, middle hepatic vein terminal branches are identified and ligated, divided

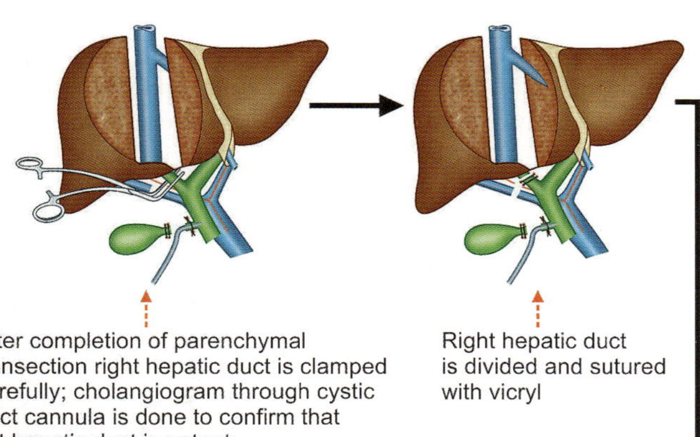

After completion of parenchymal transection right hepatic duct is clamped carefully; cholangiogram through cystic duct cannula is done to confirm that left hepatic duct is patent

Right hepatic duct is divided and sutured with vicryl

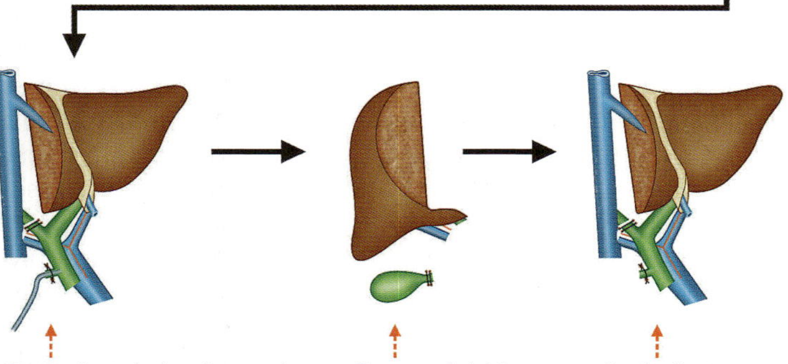

Cystic duct cholangiogram is repeated or dilute methylene blue or saline is injected to identify possible bile leak from the surface of remnant liver; if present site is ligated with fine suture

Removed right hepatectomy specimen with gallbladder

Cystic duct cannula is removed and ligated securely

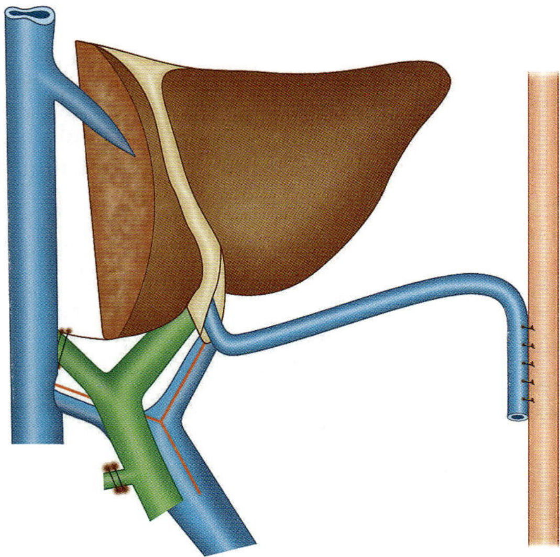

Falciform ligament should be fixed to the anterior abdominal wall to avoid falling of left lobe towards right and so torsion of remnant liver

Fig. 23-23: Technique of right hepatectomy.

ligated using fine polypropylene or vicryl. Argon beam coagulation is used to control fine bleeders on the surface.

Cystic duct cannula is removed and stump is ligated securely. The falciform ligament is now sutured back to the underside of the diaphragm. This is an important step to make sure that the remaining left liver does not rotate to the right thus causing torsion. The cut surface of liver is then covered by a single sheet of surgicel. A drain is placed in the subhepatic space and the abdomen is closed.

Anterior Approach Hepatectomy (Right or Left)

It is done in large tumour of right liver where it may be adherent to diaphragm, adrenal or mobilisation becomes tougher.

To begin with prior standard liver mobilisation is not done. First hilar dissection is done. Cholecystectomy is done by ligating cystic artery and cystic duct; cystic duct is cannulated temporarily till the end of the procedure to identify left hepatic duct and bile leaks after resection in the remnant liver. Right hepatic artery, right portal vein and right hepatic duct is ligated after proper dissection. Liver is transected from anterior surface towards the liver hilum; initially scoring on both superior and inferior surface is done. Caudate lobe may be retained or excised depending on the need. Parenchymal dissection is done with ligation of segment 8 hepatic vein on the right side of middle hepatic vein. IVC is exposed in front on its entire length. Hepatic veins of segment 6 (inferior right) and 7 (middle right) and right hepatic vein is exposed. All three veins are dissected carefully, ligated and divided from front. IVC ligament is identified, ligated and divided. Right triangular ligament and right adrenal gland is dissected from the liver.

Problem with anterior approach is bleeding during parenchymal transection **(Figs. 23-24 and 23-25)**.

Belghiti et al. Liver Hanging Manoeuvre

Belghiti et al. liver hanging manoeuvre when done very carefully will have control on bleeding during parenchymal dissection. Curved forceps is passed gently between liver tissue and anterior surface of liver to allow passage of a tape between suprahepatic IVC and infrahepatic IVC. It creates compression, guides the transection of liver and safeguards the IVC to some extent. But initial passage of forceps may injure the veins on the anterior surface of the IVC causing torrential haemorrhage.

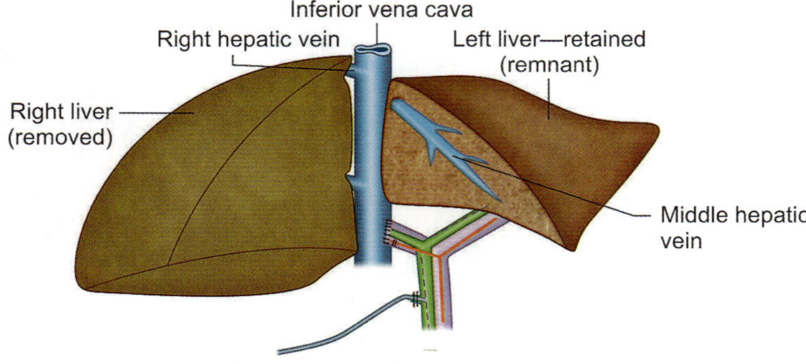

Fig. 23-24: Right hepatectomy—anterior approach.

Right hepatectomy—technique

- Incision is subcostal—Mercedez Benz.
- Retract costal cartilage, lower abdomen properly.
- Assess the abdomen.
- Free the liver from all ligaments coronary, triangular of both lobes using harmonic.
- Small veins should be ligated or fulgurated.
- Dissect the gastrohepatic ligament and free the foramen Winslow for inflow control.
- Do cholecystectomy. If needed cannulate the cystic duct.
- Dissect the portal plate and cystic plate to reach the hilum.
- Identify right hepatic duct, right hepatic artery, right portal vein. Dissect carefully, isolate and sling them.
- Score the liver surface for parenchymal dissection.
- Do parenchymal dissection; do inflow control for 15 minutes and release for 10 minutes; can be done for three sessions. Finger, haemostat or ligasure, harmonic, etc. can be used.
- Ligate branches of the middle hepatic veins; save middle hepatic vein main trunk.
- Reach IVC anterior surface slowly and carefully.
- Ligate the right portal vein, right hepatic artery, right hepatic duct.
- At the end ligate the right hepatic vein and small branches.
- Make sure perfusion and biliary system of the left lobe.
- Keep a drain and close.
- Check for leak from the left lobe surface.

Left Hepatectomy

The abdomen is opened by either a Mercedes Benz incision or J (Makuuchi) incision and preliminary exploration is done to make sure the lesion is operable. Any evidence of peritoneal involvement precludes resection. A table mounted abdominal retractor system is essential to relieve the assistants hands from retraction in a long procedure and it gives better and sustained exposure of the operative field especially at the hiatus and the suprahepatic IVC area. The falciform ligament is ligated and divided up to the suprahepatic IVC. Care must be taken during the posterior dissection near IVC. Then the left lobe of the liver is mobilised by dividing the left triangular ligament using scissors or electrocautery. A mop placed behind the left lobe prevents inadvertent injury to the stomach or spleen. Attention is now given to taking down the hilar plate (dividing the peritoneum along the inferior surface of the liver at the hilum) which exposes the hilar structures.

The left pedicle is easy to identify and control as it runs a long and more horizontal extrahepatic course. The hepatic artery is temporarily clamped to confirm the anatomy and to look for any aberrant left hepatic artery (if present from the left gastric artery,

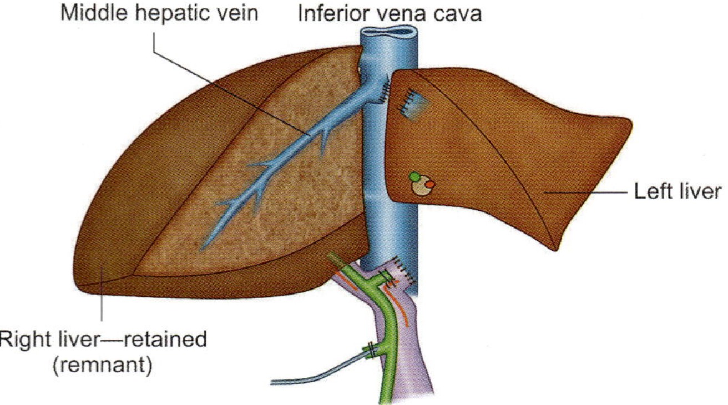

Fig. 23-25: Left hepatectomy—anterior approach.

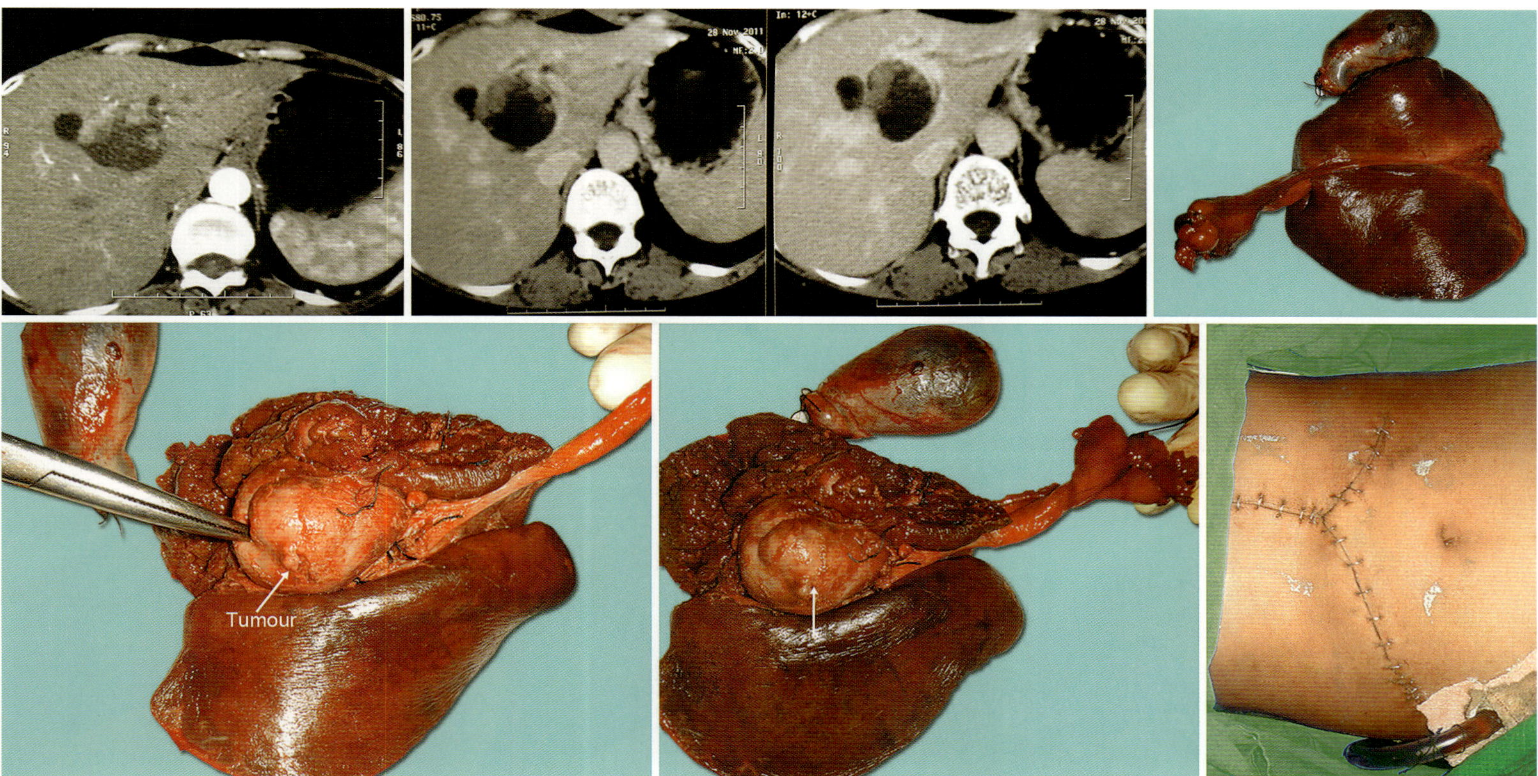

Fig. 23-26: CT scan picture of left lobe HCC with resected left hepatectomy specimen and sutured incision.

the liver parenchyma will appear perfused despite clamping of the normal left hepatic artery) and after confirming anatomy divided between double ligature of 1-0 silk. The left hepatic vein is then identified behind the artery and isolated. Tributaries draining the caudate lobe may drain close to the bifurcation and they can be preserved or divided between fine ligatures. The left portal vein is taken down around 5 mm distal to the bifurcation to avoid any stenosis of the right portal branch. The vein can be suture ligated with 1-0 silk or divided with vascular staplers or closed with running 5-0 prolene suture **(Fig. 23-26)**.

Cholecystectomy is performed and cystic duct can be cannulated and kept for performing a leak test at the end of the parenchymal transection. The biliary duct is often taken down higher up in the liver parenchyma during dissection to avoid any damage to the right bile duct. Bile duct is extremely prone to ischaemic injury and every precaution is taken to avoid it. Hence the ducts are always taken inside liver be it right or left hepatectomy. The left hepatic vein also runs a horizontal course and joins the middle hepatic vein within the liver on most of the occasions. The vein is usually divided at the end of parenchymal transection. Once the left hepatic artery is divided, the plane of parenchymal transection is obvious on the surface of the liver. This is a good time for requesting a low central venous pressure from your anaesthetist colleague. CVP lower than 5 mm Hg decreases blood loss during parenchymal transection. The line of transection is scored using monopolar cautery. Stay sutures are taken on either side of line of demarcation which helps in applying traction during parenchymal dissection. The liver capsule is the toughest structure during transection and it needs to be divided using electrocautery. Further parenchymal transection is carried out in one of the methods as described above. Our preferred method of transection still remains Kelly clamp method as it is economical and fast. In cirrhotic patients, however, CUSA or water jet dissection is preferred. As the parenchymal transection is towards completion, Satinsky vascular clamp is applied to include the left hepatic vein. The left hepatic vein is then closed with running sutures using 5-0 prolene. Alternately, the left hepatic vein can be divided using a vascular stapler load. Meticulous haemostasis is achieved with bipolar coagulation. In some situations, a figure of eight suture using 4-0 prolene may be required to achieve haemostasis **(Fig. 23-27)**.

The cut surface of liver is observed carefully for any biliary leaks. A fresh piece of gauze is placed over the cut surface. Any yellowish discouloration should be looked into very carefully and identified biliary radicles should be ligated. A simple saline leak test can be performed at this stage as well. Saline is injected via the cannulated cystic duct and cut surface of liver is observed for any leaks. Various methods of managing the cut surface of liver have been described such as using argon beam coagulation, use of surface cauterisation using ball cautery and use of tissue glue on cut surface but none have been proved superior to one another. We cover the raw surface with single sheet of surgicel (oxidised cellulose). A single drain is placed in the subhepatic space and brought out via a separate stab incision in the right subcostal region. Abdomen is closed routinely after haemostasis. Patient is extubated as early as possible as this decreases the overall ICU stay of the patients and helps in early recovery of the patient. The patient is shifted out of high dependency unit by postoperative day 2 when his drain output has decreased and bowel sounds return. The drain is removed by postoperative day 5 or when the drain output is less than 50 mL over 24 hours. Patients liver function test, prothrombin time and INR are monitored and fresh frozen plasma is given for correcting any abnormality. Albumin infusion is given only if the plasma albumin falls below 3 g/dL **(Fig. 23-28)**.

Postoperative Complications

Biliary leaks: Incidence of bile leak and biliary duct injury is more in left hepatectomy as confluence is towards left side; and right anterior and posterior hepatic duct may join left hepatic duct.

Liver failure: It is the failure of remnant liver may be due to less volume or sepsis or ischaemia. Renal failure develops as a after effect of the liver failure or sepsis.

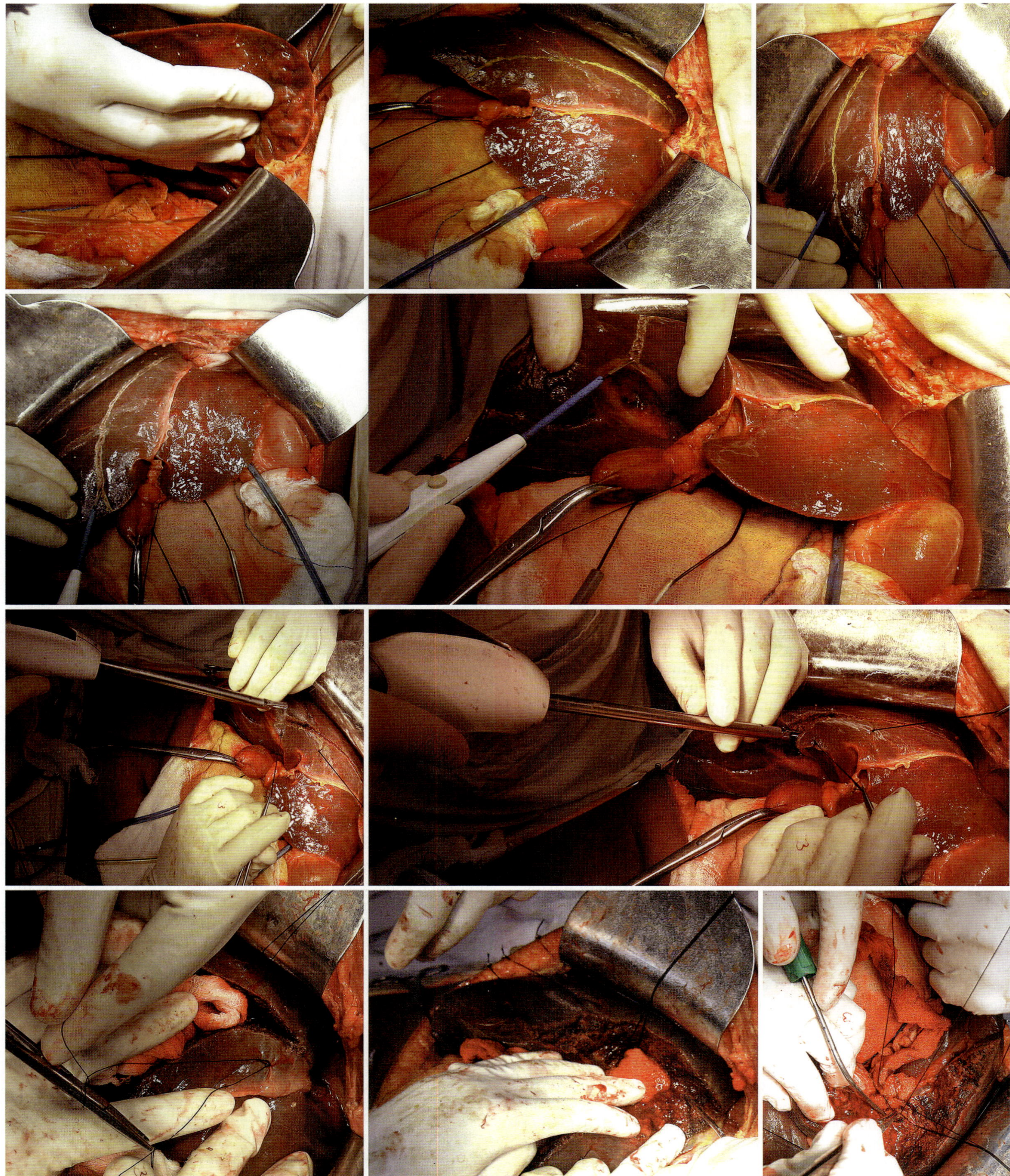

Figs. 23-27(1)

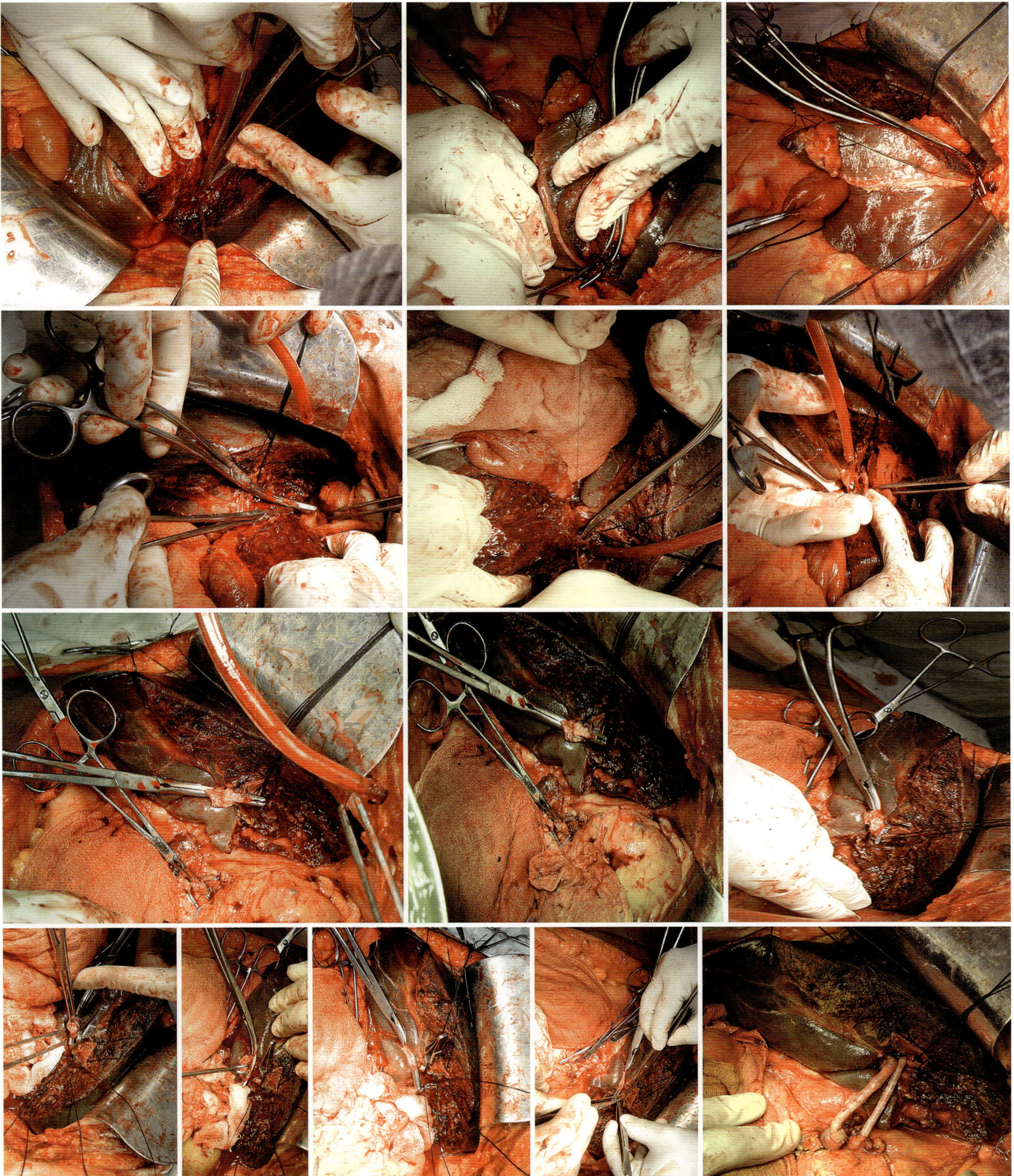

Figs. 23-27(2)

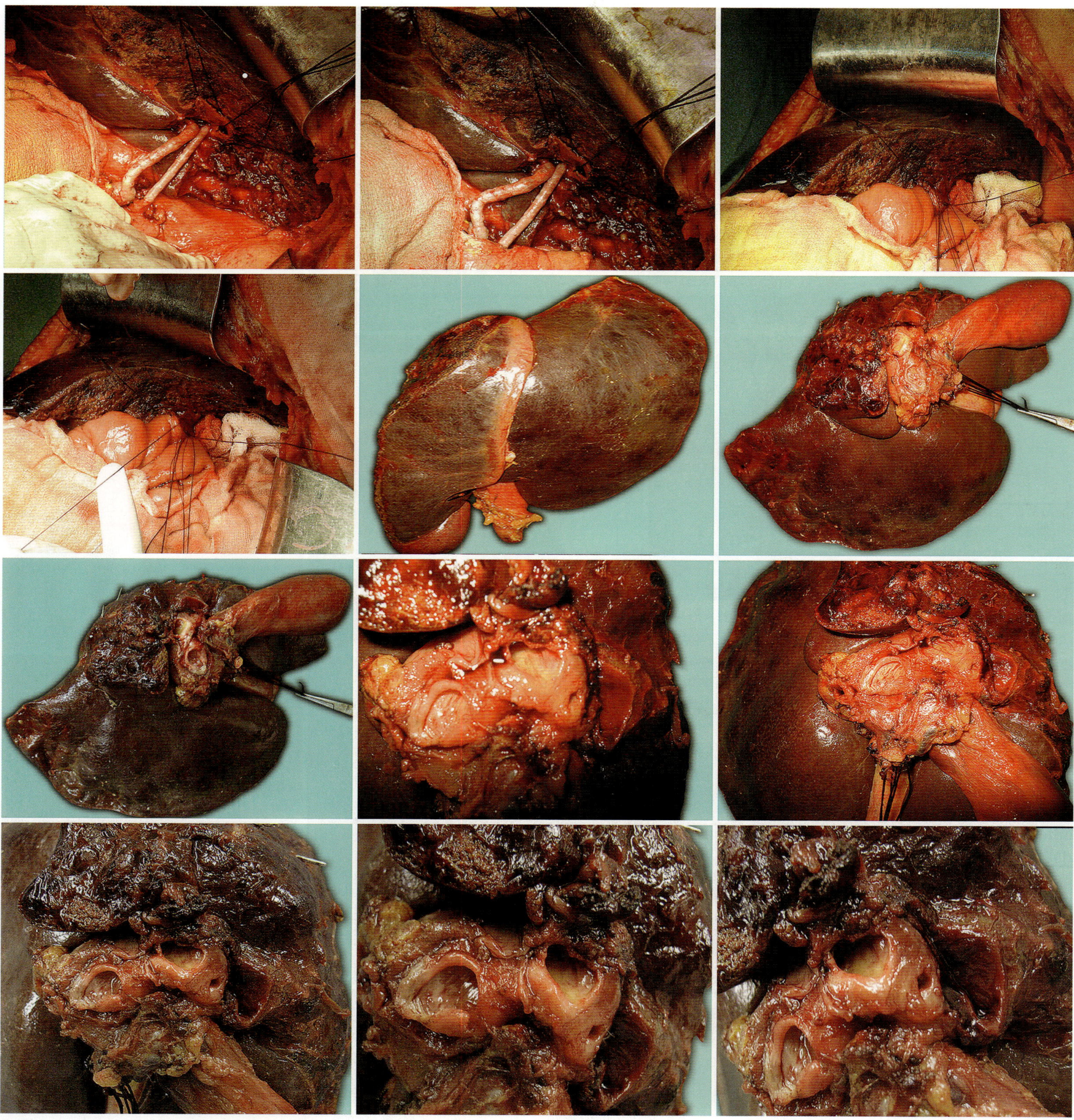

Figs. 23-27(3)

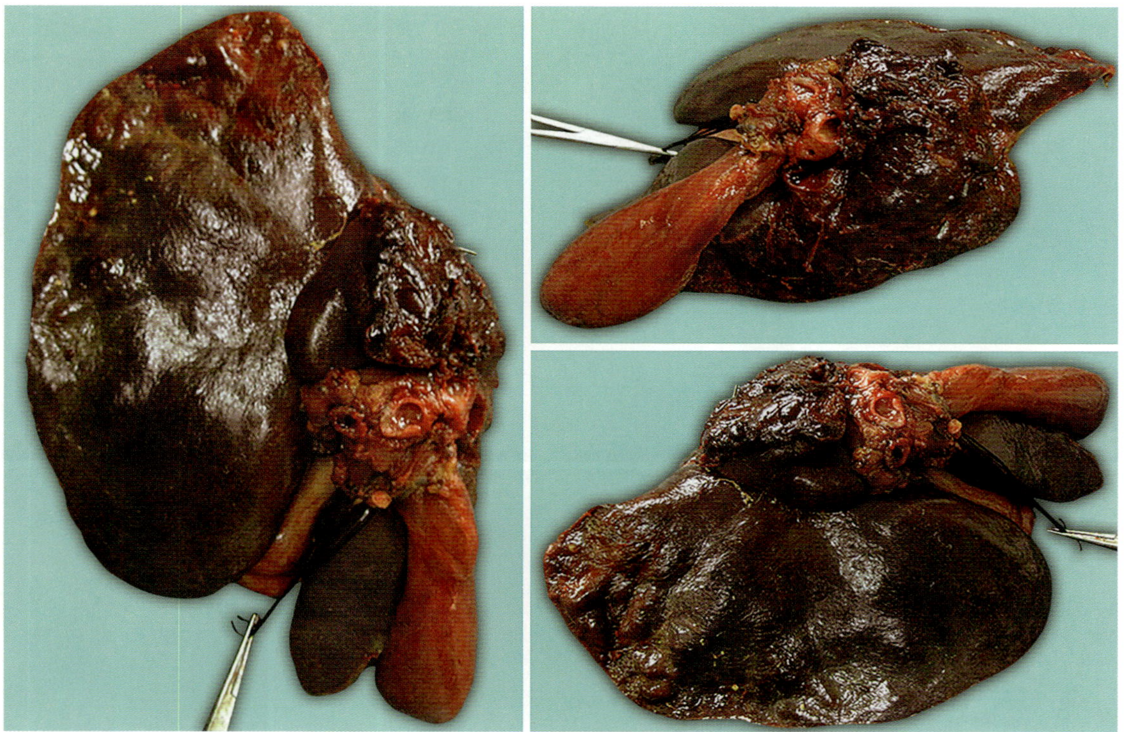

Figs. 23-27(4)

Figs. 23-27(1 to 4): Klatskin tumour—underwent left hepatectomy with resection of hepatic artery and portal vein with saphenous vein grafts to both.
Courtesy: Dr Arunkumar, MCh Gastro, Kochi.

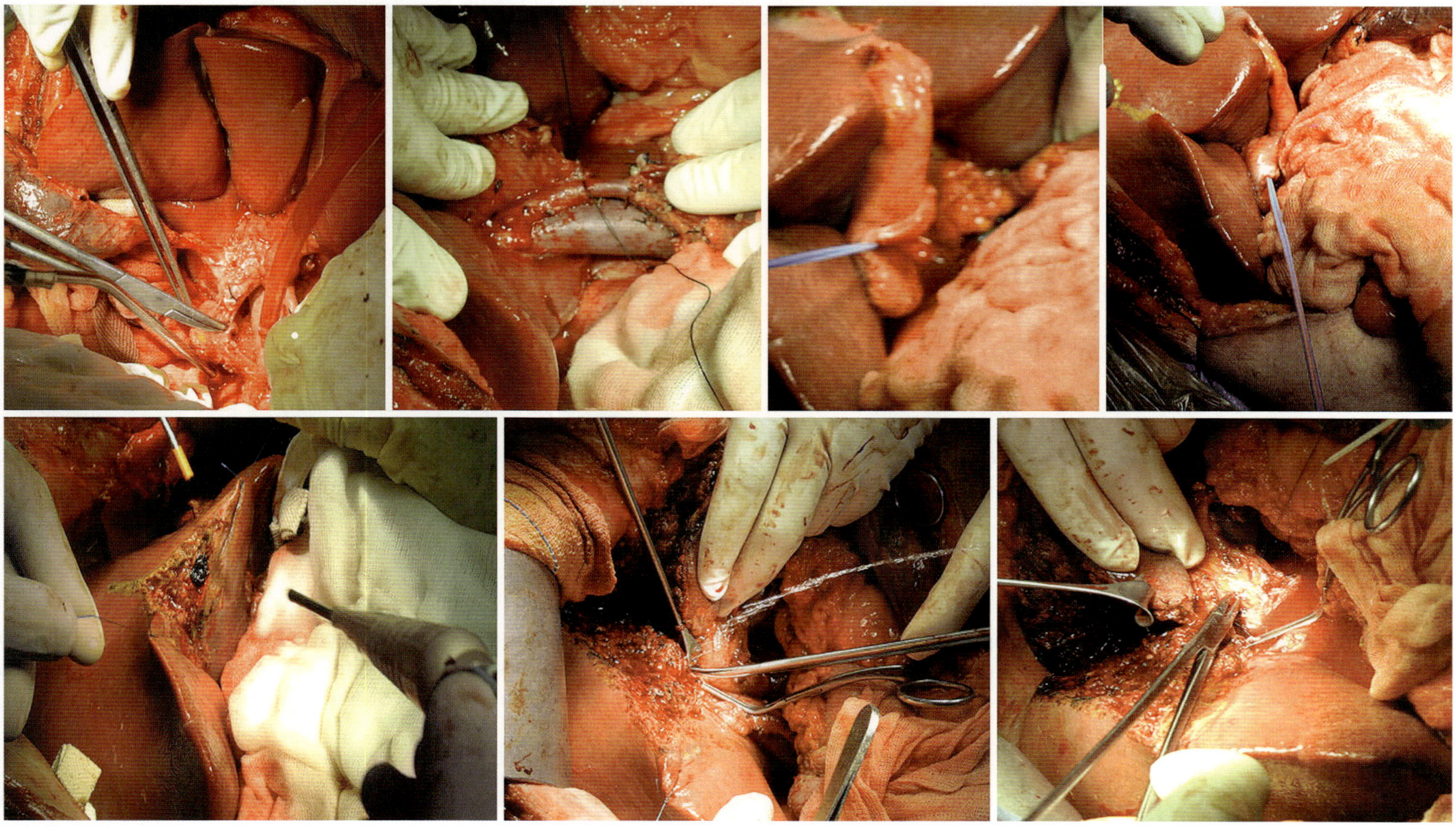

Figs. 23-28(1)

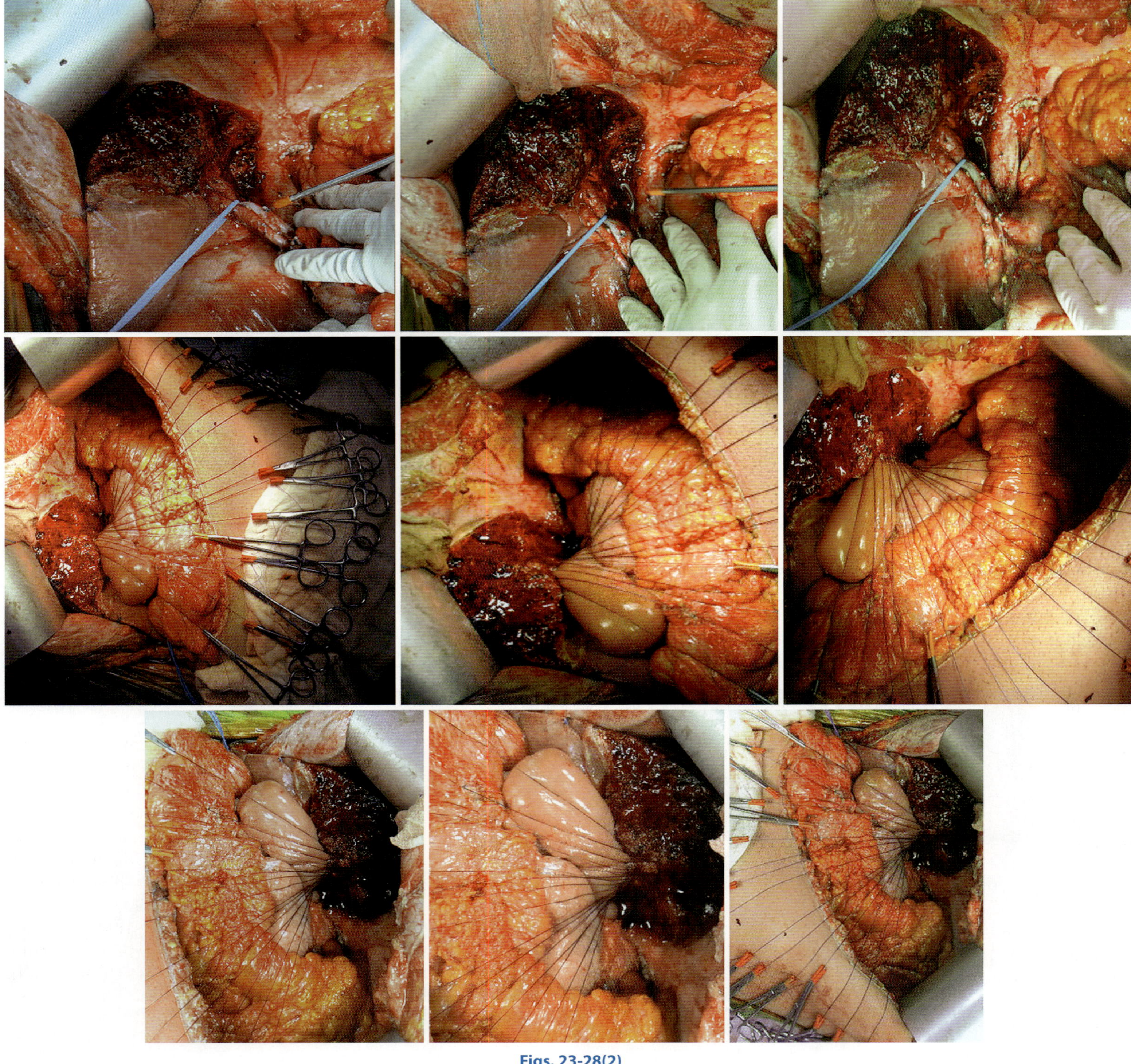

Figs. 23-28(2)

Figs. 23-28(1 and 2): Hilar cholangiocarcinoma—left hepatectomy.
Courtesy: Dr Arunkumar, MCh Gastro, Kochi.

Intra-abdominal bleeding: Usual bleeding is 500 mL to 800 mL in hepatectomies; but torrential bleeding can occur at any stage of the surgical dissection.

Delayed gastric emptying and intolerance to oral feeding is common after liver resection.

Ascites; portal vein thrombosis; other pulmonary complications; bililary strictures; biliomas are other complications which are addressed and evaluated accordingly.

Infection and intra-abdominal abscess formation: Sepsis is due to liver failure or sepsis may precipitate liver failure. Bronchopneumonia is also common other than intra-abdominal sepsis.

Postoperative Care

Postoperatively patient is kept in critical care unit for 48 hours with monitoring urine output, liver function, hydration, blood pressure, body temperature, etc. High ammonia level, metabolic acidosis, respiratory distress, hypoglycaemia are indicators of inadequate remnant liver cell function. Dopamine or noradrenaline should be used to maintain blood pressure. Meantime fluid overload is also should be avoided. Parenteral nutrition with branched chain amino acids, phosphate and medium chained triglyceride emulsions and vitamin infusion is better. Phosphate is essential for liver regeneration and energy release. Intravenous potassium phosphate or oral sodium phosphate is given. Early enteral feeding promotes liver regeneration but tolerance for food especially medium chained triglycerides which is essential in postoperative period otherwise parenteral nutrition to be continued.

Extended Hemihepatectomy

Extended Right Hepatectomy

The extended right hepatectomy or right trisectionectomy includes liver segments 4 to 8 (segment 4 with right liver). It is usually done for resection of hilar cholangiocarcinomas or resection for carcinoma of gallbladder. Any extended hemihepatectomy is carried out after confirming that the remnant liver will be able to withstand the demand. In the classical approach, the segment 4b pedicle is secured before the parenchymal transection. The right pedicles are isolated and divided as for right hepatectomy (described earlier). The right hepatic vein is also taken down after mobilising the liver from the IVC posteriorly. For isolating the segment 4 pedicle, after lowering the hilar plate dissection is carried out to the right of portal pedicle going cranially. The pedicle is identified in the liver substance, isolated and divided between ligatures. The plane of parenchymal dissection is to the right of falciform ligament and is now identified by the ischaemic line. Parenchymal dissection is done in the usual fashion. As the right hepatic vein is already divided, the middle hepatic vein is the one major vessel to be encountered. It joins the left hepatic vein most of the times within the liver substance and hence, taking it needs careful attention. Care should be taken not to damage the left hepatic vein which joins it just within the liver. The falciform ligament is now sutured back to the underside of the liver. Drain is placed in the cavity. Rest of the procedure and postoperative care is the same as in major hepatic resection.

Extended Left Hepatectomy

This involves removal of liver segments 2, 3, 4, 5 and 8 (segment 5 and 8 with left liver). The residual liver 6 and 7 segment volume must be adequate to warrant a safe resection. In this case, the right hepatic vein needs to be preserved to provide drainage to the remnant segments. Portal vein embolisation with delayed hepatectomy (about 4 weeks) should be considered prior to resection, if the remnant liver is judged too small. The left portal pedicle is identified and tackled similar to left hepatectomy. The right anterior segmental pedicle is identified as it runs a horizontal course to the right after bifurcating from the posterior sectoral duct which runs deep into the liver cranially. After ligation of the pedicle, the transection line is demarcated on the liver surface and the parenchymal dissection is carried out in the usual fashion. The location of the right hepatic vein should be known at all the times and dissection should be to the left of the vein. At the end of parenchymal transection, the middle and the left hepatic vein are divided using a vascular stapler or suture ligated with continuous 4-0 prolene suture. Attention should be given to identify and points of biliary leaks from the cut surface of the liver. The abdominal cavity is drained and the postoperative monitoring done in routine fashion.

Right Anterior Sectionectomy

This is the resection of segments V and VIII which is supplied by anterior segment of the right portal pedicle. After performing cholecystectomy, the right main portal pedicle is identified and isolated. The anterior segmental pedicle is identified as going to the right and horizontally compared to the posterior pedicle which enters liver parenchyma cranially and posteriorly. The pedicle is isolated and clamped to produce the line of ischaemia which is seen on the liver surface. The parenchymal dissection is started and the anterior pedicle is ligated. The branches draining to the right hepatic vein are ligated intraparenchymally and at the end of parenchymal transection, the middle and the right hepatic vein are seen exposed in the field.

Left Lateral Sectionectomy

This procedure includes the removal of segments II and III of the left lobe of liver. These segments are situated to the left of the falciform ligament. The procedure is started with the mobilisation of the left liver by releasing the left triangular ligament and dividing the falciparum ligament. By pulling up the left liver via the round ligament, hepatic parenchymal transection is done along the left edge of the falciform ligament. The portal pedicle of the segment 3 is situated within 2 cm of liver transection and it is taken down intraparenchymally. The segment 2 pedicle is reached during more cranial dissection and it is usually thicker than the segment 3 pedicle. After dividing it, the left hepatic vein is reached. It is divided by using a vascular stapler or with help of a Satinsky clamp and cut edge is over sewn using 4-0 prolene.

Non-anatomical Wedge Resection

This is usually indicated in patients who have peripherally situated tumours which are easy to access on the surface. In patients who are not candidates for anatomical resections and in cirrhotic patients as well, these wedge resections are helpful. A resection margin of 1 cm is adequate in such situations. The line of resection is marked around the tumour and the depth is confirmed by an on table ultrasound. Parenchymal transection is begun without any vascular clamping whenever the lesion is large or significant bleeding is anticipated, the portal inflow can be taped (not clamped) and prepared should any inflow occlusion be needed. The biliary radicles and vessels are secured and divided as and when they cross the operative field **(Fig. 23-29)**.

Laparoscopic Liver Resection

There are three types of laparoscopic liver resections—pure laparoscopic (75%); hand-assisted laparoscopic resections; hybrid method.

Usually done procedures are—segmentectomy, left lateral sectionectomy, right and left hepatectomies, metastasectomy in colorectal malignancies.

It should have similar ***indications***, technical principles are same as of open procedure. Safety and outcome should be considered. Patient selection, size of tumour (<5 cm), location (in segments 2, 4, 5, 6), number of lesions, status of the liver, condition of patient, facilities available and skilled expertise are important.

Contraindications: Central tumours; right posterior lobe tumours; tumours at hilum/close to major vessels; not fit for laparoscopic procedures.

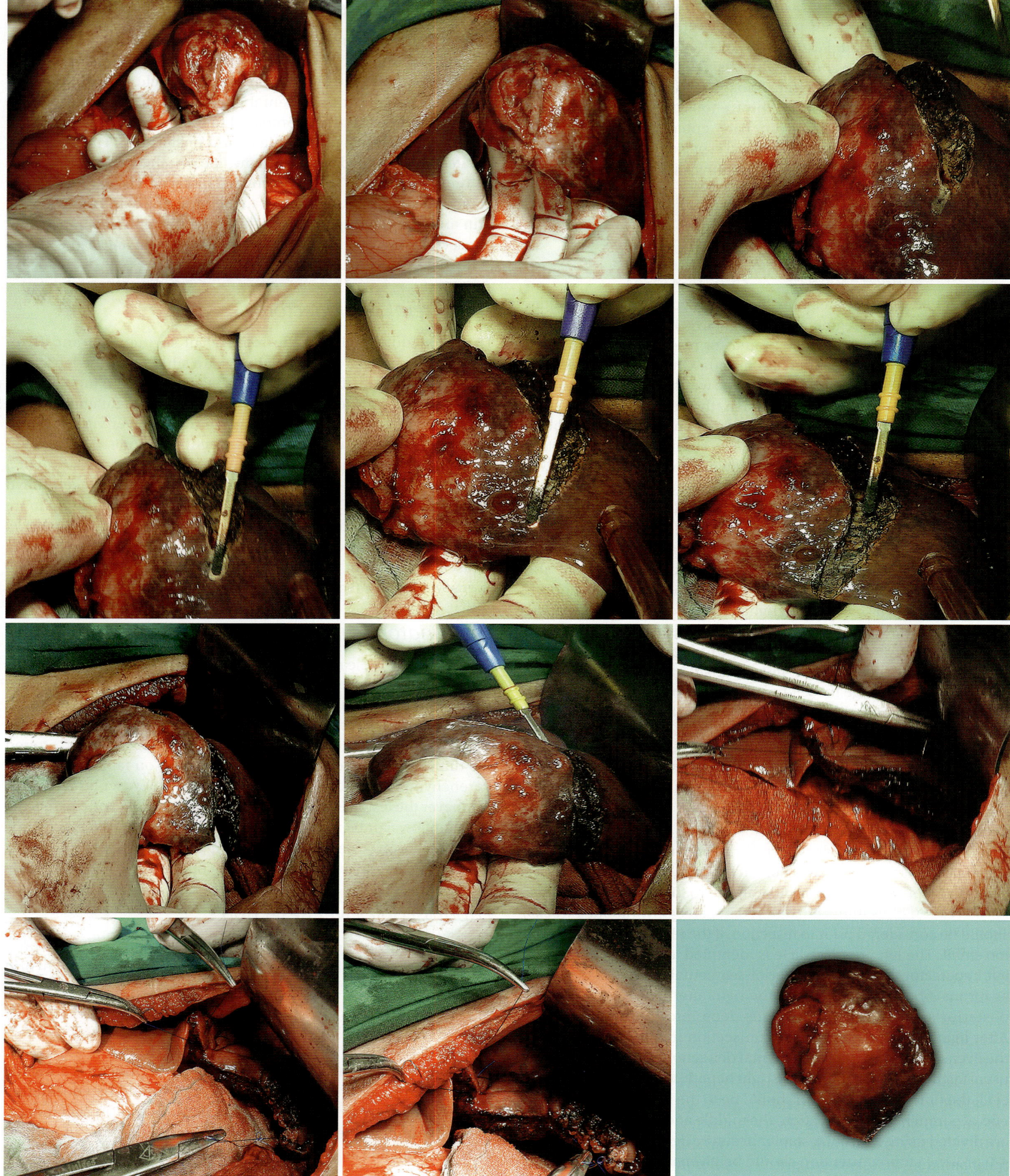

Fig. 23-29: Non-anatomical resection for secondaries in liver; primary is in colon.

Technique: Right side of the patient is elevated with surgeon standing on the left side and first assistant on the right side. Surgeon can also stand between legs of the patient.

A 12 mm port is introduced just above the umbilicus by open method. After laparoscopic exploration, additional 12 mm ports are placed in the right subcostal region. Laparoscopic ultrasound is essential. 5 mm ports are not used usually; but it is individual surgeon's choice. Parenchymal transection is done using ligaseal, harmonic or ultrasonic dissector or endovascular stapler. Cholecystectomy is done with fundus first method to reach Calot's. Blood vessels and bile duct branches are managed with endoclips or endostaplers. Raised pneumoperitoneum controls the oozing from the parenchymal surface. Portal inflow occlusion is usually not necessary. Hepatic veins are divided with cutting endovascular stapler. Intraoperative cholangiogram is done to identify biliary leak. Liver surface of the remnant liver may be covered with fibrin glue. Specimen is removed using a retrieval bag which is removed through a lengthened port incision. Drain is placed through the laparoscopic port. All other technical steps and principles are same as open procedure but through laparoscopy. Here tissue feel is not present; only magnified vision is present.

Conversion when needed—undue bleeding; difficulty in proceeding with dissection should be done without hesitation.

Complications are—pulmonary embolism; bleeding; biliary injuries; respiratory infections; bowel, diaphragm, pericardium, pleural injuries; air embolism and CO_2 embolism can occur. Air embolism is more risky.

Postoperative care—ICU management; electrolyte management; sepsis control; monitoring liver and renal functions; nutrition support; analgesia, prevention of DVT; daily biochemical assessment; when needed imaging evaluation.

LIVER TRANSPLANTATION

Introduction

Liver transplantation is the choice for end stage liver disease. Liver transplant is an accepted and effective treatment. Many tumours can be treated by transplantation. Cirrhosis, hepatitis, sclerosing cholangitis, biliary atresia, tumours are indications. In Budd-Chiari syndrome, if portacaval shunt has failed with progressive liver damage liver transplantation is indicated.

CTP (Child-Turcotte-Pugh) scoring system (ascites, encephalopathy, bilirubin, albumin, PT-INR), model for end stage liver disease (MELD score) consists of total bilirubin, INR, creatinine, paediatric end stage liver disease scoring (PELD) are different scorings used to assess the patients.

MELD Score = $0.957 \times \text{Log}_e(\text{creatinine mg/dL}) + 0.378 \times \text{Log}_e(\text{bilirubin mg/dL}) + 1.120 \times \text{Log}_e(\text{INR}) + 0.643$

Transplantation of the liver is among the most technically demanding surgical procedures. TE Starzl performed the first human liver transplantation in 1963. Since then continuous improvements in surgical techniques, immunosuppressant's, prolongation of ischaemic tolerance and experience with indications/timing, liver transplantation has become a standard modality of treatment for chronic and acute end stage liver disease. The majority of liver transplantation is performed orthotopically. The shortage of organs has led to development of reduced size, split liver and living related (donor) liver transplantation techniques. Given the overall broad nature of the topic, the focus will be on deceased donor liver transplantation procedure along with a brief description of other techniques. For further reading, readers should refer to references at the end of the chapter.

Contraindications for Liver Transplantation

Active sepsis, SBP and HIV; extrahepatic malignancy; large hepatocellular carcinoma and cholangiocarcinoma; unfit for surgery—severely advanced cardiopulmonary disease, active alcohol or substance abuse, inability to comply with immunosuppression protocols because of psychosocial situations—are the contraindications.

Donor Criteria

They are related to donor liver function, hepatitis screening, history of consumption of alcohol and toxic substances. Marginal donor and expanded donor criteria are in use in places due to very high demand for donor for transplantation. ABO compatibility is important. HLA matching is not necessary unlike in renal transplantation.

Deceased donor liver transplantation donor (DDLT)	*Living donor liver transplantation donor (LDLT)*
♦ 50 years or younger ♦ No hepatobiliary disease ♦ Haemodynamic and respiratory stability (systolic blood pressure >100 mm Hg, and central venous pressure >5 cm/H_2O); an acceptable PaO_2 and haemoglobin level ♦ No severe abdominal trauma, systemic infection, or cancer ♦ Normal kidneys—diuresis greater than 50 mL/h and normal creatinine; and finally, a dopamine requirement less than 10 µg/kg/min ♦ Simple technically ♦ Recipient complication is low (of bile duct) ♦ Graft quality is average ♦ Donor's complication—nil	♦ Young ♦ Non-obese, tall ♦ No infection and malignancy ♦ No fatty liver ♦ Enough liver to donate ♦ Enough residual liver ♦ Suitable anatomy ♦ Technically complex procedure ♦ Recipient complication is higher ♦ Graft quality is good ♦ Donor's complication—25% morbidity; 0.4% mortality

Back—Table Preparation of Liver Graft—Donor Operation

It is by a midline incision from suprasternal notch to pubic symphysis. Initially, dissection is done with a beating heart; but later with a cold preservation into aorta and portal vein and local ice application. UW solution extends cold ischaemic time for 24 hours but usually within 10 hours transplantation is done. IVC segment is removed with hepatic veins. Portal vein is transected. Coeliac artery with branches along through hepatic artery is dissected and transected at coeliac artery origin. Bile duct is transected.

Note:

Remnant liver—≥30% of the original liver volume with complete venous drainage is safe for donor survival.

The donor liver is prepared on the back table for implantation. Bench preparation includes resection of the donor diaphragm and adrenal gland off of the bare area of the liver and vena cava. Meticulous ligation of tributaries from the vena cava (adrenal vein, phrenic vein, and lumbar branches) is performed. The artery is dissected free from the Carrel patch of the aorta up to the gastroduodenal artery. Dissection near the right or left hepatic arteries is avoided to prevent unnecessary injury. The portal vein is circumferentially dissected free.

The gallbladder may be removed at this stage or following reperfusion. Tissues surrounding the common bile duct are left intact to avoid injury of the blood supply.

Recipient Operation

Bowel preparation, prophylactic antibiotics, administrative immunosuppressive agents are needed before surgery. Bilateral subcostal incision is used with midline upward extension. Falciform ligament, left lateral ligaments, hepatogastric and hepatoduodenal ligaments are divided. Right and left branches of hepatic arteries are ligated. CBD and cystic ducts are divided with ligatures. Portal vein is dissected. Infra and suprahepatic vena cava are exposed. Portal vein and suprahepatic vena cava are clamped. Venovenous bypass between portal and femoral veins and internal jugular vein is created with a flow of blood through it more than 2.5 mL/minute. Warming circuits and ultrafiltration is needed. Suprahepatic vena caval cuff is created at the opening of the right, middle and left hepatic veins. Donor IVC is sutured to recipient IVC first above and then below as end to end. Recipient IVC can be preserved entirely and donor IVC is sutured to recipient IVC as end to side. Preservation solution is passed. Portal vein is sutured. Reperfusion injury can occur at this stage with hyperkalaemia and acidosis. Arterial reconstruction is done between donor coeliac artery to recipient gastroduodenal artery. Bile ducts are sutured as end to end with or without T tube. Often choledochojejunostomy is also done.

Graft should be:

- 40% of the estimated standard liver volume.
- 0.8% to 1% of the body weight of the recipient is necessary for the recipient recovery.

Details of the Technique

The recipient's abdomen and bilateral groins are prepped and draped in a standard fashion. The most commonly used incisions are bilateral subcostal incision with a midline extension to the xiphoid process and reverse 'L'. The ligamentum teres is carefully divided between clamps and ligated because a large recannulised umbilical vein is often present in patients with severe portal hypertension. After dividing the falciform ligament with cautery, a mechanical retractor (Thompson) is used to retract the bilateral costal margins anteriorly and superiorly for excellent exposure of the upper abdomen. The abdominal cavity and liver are then inspected for any abnormalities including unsuspected malignancy. Following this, liver transplantation occurs in three stages:

a. Recipient hepatectomy.
b. Anhepatic phase and implantation of donor liver.
c. Post-revascularisation phase.

Recipient Hepatectomy

The liver is mobilised from its ligamentous attachments and the portahepatis is skeletonised. The peritoneum overlying the portal triad is divided with electrocautery near the liver edge. The right and left hepatic arteries are dissected free, ligated, and divided, leaving adequate length to form a branch patch for the arterial anastomosis. The proper hepatic artery is also dissected free to the level of the gastroduodenal artery allowing enough length for clamping during the anastomosis. A replaced or accessory right hepatic artery, which arises as a branch off the superior mesenteric artery travels in a posterior position to the common bile duct and lateral to the portal vein, can usually be palpated if present and can be ligated and divided. When the replaced right hepatic artery is relatively large and the proper hepatic artery is diminutive in size, the replaced right hepatic artery can be left long and used for arterial inflow for the donor liver.

The common bile duct and common hepatic duct should be dissected free with as much length as possible and without injuring the blood supply to the bile duct. Leaving the recipient bile duct as long as possible allows the length of the donor bile duct, which may have a tenuous blood supply, to be shorter and still avoids tension at the time of anastomosis. This is accomplished by first ligating and dividing the cystic duct. The common bile duct and common hepatic duct are then circumferentially dissected free, leaving the surrounding tissue to preserve the bile duct blood supply. The common hepatic duct is then ligated as close to the native liver as possible.

Once the bile duct and the hepatic artery are freed from surrounding tissues, the portal vein can be easily approached from its anterior, medial, and lateral aspects. In general, the portal vein is freed circumferentially from the edge of the duodenum up to its bifurcation of the right and left portal veins. Small branches may arise near the pancreas and excessive bleeding may arise if these are inadvertently injured. In situations where there is small bowel oedema, the portal vein should be left in continuity for as long as possible, particularly when the use of venovenous bypass is not intended.

The ligamentous attachments of the liver are then divided using electrocautery. Care must be taken to avoid injury to the phrenic or hepatic veins when freeing the suprahepatic inferior vena cava where it traverses the diaphragm. The liver is then dissected off of the anterior aspect of the inferior vena cava. Small venous branches from the inferior vena cava to the caudate lobe are ligated and divided. Division of the portal vein facilitates exposure for this dissection but is not required. The liver may be gradually retracted and dissected from either the right or left aspects until the right, middle, and left hepatic veins are reached. If a venacaval resection technique will be used, the vena cava can be circumferentially mobilised near the diaphragm above the hepatic veins as well as in an infrahepatic position. However, if a piggyback or cavocavostomy (side-to-side caval anastomosis) technique is intended, the dissection of the posterior aspect of the vena cava should be avoided to prevent bleeding from collaterals or lumbar vessels.

Anhepatic Phase and Implantation of the Donor Liver

At this point, the liver has been completely mobilised except for its attachments of the hepatic veins to the inferior vena cava and, in some cases, the portal vein. The decision should now be made whether to use venovenous bypass. Most patients will tolerate clamping of both the portal vein and the inferior vena cava without difficulty. At this point, communication with the anaesthesiologist is essential and the vena cava should be test clamped before division to make sure that adequate cardiac filling and blood pressure can be maintained. If the patient becomes hypotensive during test clamping, the clamp should be removed and additional volume or pressor support can be administered. Occasionally, patients will require venovenous bypass, but its use is no longer routine at most centres.

If necessary, venovenous bypass can be accomplished from both the portal vein and inferior vena cava simultaneously, or a single cannula in either the portal vein or the inferior vena cava may be used. Inferior vena caval and mesenteric blood is delivered to the superior vena cava by a centrifugal pump. Flow rates of 1 to 2 L/min are usual.

Once venovenous bypass has been established or the decision to forego bypass has been made, the recipient hepatectomy is completed. If still intact, the portal vein is divided as high in the hilum as possible. Three methods are commonly used for orthotopic liver transplantation: (1) the segmental IVC resection (bicaval) technique, (2) the piggyback technique, and (3) cavocavostomy (side-to-side caval anastomosis) technique.

1. For the segmental IVC resection technique, the recipient liver is excised en bloc with the retrohepatic inferior vena cava after caval clamps have been placed in a suprahepatic and infrahepatic position. The hepatic veins are divided within the substance of the liver to allow the creation of a large suprahepatic cuff compromising the left, middle, and right hepatic veins. This technique has the disadvantages of (a) totally obstructing inferior vena cava flow, resulting in renal ischaemia and decreased cardiac filling with associated hypotension, possibly leading to the requirement of venovenous bypass; (b) requiring two vena caval anastomoses, prolonging the warm ischaemic time; and (c) requiring dissection posterior to the vena cava, possibly leading to bleeding. However, complete dissection of the caudate lobe off of the vena cava is not necessary, making the recipient hepatectomy phase somewhat easier and faster.
2. For the piggyback technique, a clamp is placed transversely, partially occluding the vena cava at the level of the hepatic veins. The vena cava is left in continuity and the hepatic veins are divided within the substance of the liver, allowing the creation of a common patch of the right, middle, and left hepatic veins for a wide anastomosis. This technique does have the advantage of only requiring a single vena caval anastomosis, helping to limit warm ischaemic time.
3. For the cavocavostomy technique, clamps can be placed on the right hepatic vein as well as the junction of the left and middle hepatic veins. The liver is excised and these venous branches are oversewn and the clamps are removed. Alternatively, the hepatic veins can be divided using an Endo GIA stapler. Advantages of the cavocavostomy anastomosis include (a) minimalisation of the time that the vena cava is clamped; (b) the vena caval clamp is placed longitudinally, only occluding the anterior third of the vena cava, leading to minimal or no changes in the recipient's hemodynamics; (c) a cavoplasty with long anastomosis over 6 cm is performed, limiting the likelihood of caval stenosis and minimising the risk for hepatic vein outflow complications; and (e) exposure during suturing of the anastomosis is considerably improved compared to the piggyback or bicaval technique.

After removal of the recipient liver, the right upper quadrant is carefully inspected and haemostasis is obtained. Complete haemostasis in the bare area is essential at this time because this region is easily visualised when the liver is absent but may be relatively inaccessible once the donor liver is implanted, especially if the donor liver is relatively large or the recipient is obese.

The donor liver is then brought onto the operative field. The vascular anastomoses are performed using a running monofilament polypropylene suture. If an IVC resection technique is planned, two caval anastomoses are required. For the piggyback technique, the donor infrahepatic vena cava is either oversewn or stapled and donor suprahepatic vena cava is then sewn in to the recipient hepatic vein cuff. For the side-to-side caval technique, a clamp is placed longitudinally on the anterior third of the recipient vena cava. A longitudinal venotomy is made on the anterior surface of the recipient vena cava. The donor suprahepatic and infrahepatic vena cava are either oversewn or stapled closed. A longitudinal posterior venotomy is then made matching the length of the recipient venotomy. The liver is then placed in the right upper quadrant and the left lateral segment is elevated. The two vena cava are then sutured in a side-to-side fashion.

During the caval anastomosis, the donor liver may be perfused with cold fluid via a cannula placed within the donor portal vein to wash out the preservation solution and helps to maintain the cold temperature of the liver. This step is not required but may be considered if the liver was preserved with a solution containing a high concentration of potassium or if a prolonged warm ischaemic time is anticipated.

Once the caval anastomosis or anastomoses are completed, the portal anastomosis, arterial anastomosis, or both can be performed prior to reperfusion. In theory, reperfusion with arterial blood would limit the extent of warm ischaemia to the biliary tree, which, unlike the remainder of the liver, receives its blood supply exclusively from the arterial blood and not along with portal venous blood. However, neither sequence has been clearly shown to be an advantage over the other, so the choice is made based on the surgeon's preference and the patient's anatomy. Most commonly, the portal venous anastomosis is completed and the liver is reperfused. The portal anastomosis is usually performed in an end-to-end fashion using a running technique. To avoid narrowing, an air knot (growth factor) is used when the suture is tied. For those patients with portal vein thrombosis, portal venous flow can be restored in most cases. Often, the thrombus can be evacuated with the use of forceps or by placing a Yankauer suction tip within the lumen of the portal vein. If the thrombus is more mature, an eversion endovenectomy may be necessary. If these manoeuvres are unsuccessful, the junction of the splenic vein and superior mesenteric vein may be patent. Dissection of the portal vein behind the pancreas to this junction can then be performed to allow for future anastomosis. In rare cases, all of these manoeuvres may be unsuccessful and a venous bypass graft using donor iliac vein from the superior mesenteric vein may be necessary. If the superior mesenteric vein is also occluded, either inferior vena cava (cavoportal hemitransposition) or left renal vein can be used for portal inflow.

At the time of revascularisation, flow is restored to the liver through the portal vein and/or the hepatic artery. Alternatively, the caval clamp can be "flashed" and the anastomosis inspected for bleeding and repaired if present. Portal blood should be restored gradually to minimise cardiac irritability, bradycardia, and hypotension. Close coordination between the surgeon and anaesthesiologist is necessary during this phase as hypotension and bradycardia are routinely encountered and cardiac arrest may rarely occur. If venovenous bypass has been used during the anhepatic phase, it can now be discontinued.

Once haemostasis is obtained and the patient has stabilised, attention can now be turned toward the arterial anastomosis if it has not already been performed. Hepatic artery (HA) anastomoses can be performed in variety of different ways due to variations in recipient and donor vascular anatomy, the need to optimise arterial inflow and surgeon's preference. At the end of HA reconstruction, one needs to avoid excessive looping, redundancy or twisting, especially so after release of retractors. For a donor HA with a standard anatomy either coeliac axis with or without aortic carrel patch or shortened coeliac artery near splenic artery origin with subsequent joining of coeliac and splenic arterial orifice to form a patch, can be used. On recipient side, a patch created between the orifice of right and left hepatic arteries or between that of common hepatic and gastroduodenal arteries is used. Anastomosis is usually performed using a fine, non-absorbable, monofilament, running suture. Variations in donor arterial anatomy require back-table reconstruction. If the recipient arterial inflow is inadequate, an aortic conduit may be constructed. This is often performed using a graft consisting of the donor common and external (or internal) iliac artery. A partially occluding aortic clamp can either be placed in a supracoeliac or infrarenal position and the common iliac artery is sutured in an end-to-side fashion to the recipient aorta. The donor Carrel patch can then be sutured in an end-to-end fashion to the external iliac artery of the conduit.

Post-revascularisation Phase

Following revascularisation, the liver should assume a normal colour and consistency within several minutes. Bile production should be seen while in the operating room and is among the first evidence for liver function. Inspection for surgical bleeding should be performed. If bleeding continues after all surgical bleeding has been resolved, attention should be directed toward correction of coagulopathy as described earlier.

Because of the relatively high complication rate associated with biliary reconstruction, it has been referred to as the "Achilles heel" of liver transplantation. There are several options for biliary reconstruction. The simplest and most common technique is currently an end-to-end choledochocholedochostomy from the donor to the recipient bile duct. If a size discrepancy exists, the narrower duct can be spatulated. Absorbable monofilament suture is most commonly used to avoid a nidus for future stone formation within the bile duct. While T-tubes were commonly used in the past to stent the anastomosis, evidence now suggests that more leaks or strictures develop as a result of the T-tube than are prevented. Alternative biliary reconstruction methods may be necessary for those with a bile duct of inadequate quality or size or in those whose primary disease is biliary pathology such as primary sclerosing cholangitis or biliary atresia. The most common option employed in these situations includes a standard Roux-en-Y choledochojejunostomy. Placement of drains is optional. Abdominal wall and skin closure is then performed in the standard fashion.

Reduced Size and Split Liver Transplantation

In the 1980s, the waiting list mortality for small, paediatric liver candidates was relatively high because the number of suitably sized small liver donors was inadequate. As a result, techniques to reduce the size of an adult liver, based on Couinaud's segmental anatomy were developed so that the left lobe, left lateral segment could be used for a recipient smaller by weight than the donor. During the early experience, the donor hepatectomy was performed in a standard fashion and the liver was brought back to the recipient hospital. The needed segments of the liver were cut down on the back table with the organ on ice, the vessels were left intact to the future transplant graft, and the remainder of the liver was discarded. Techniques have now developed so that both sides of the liver can be transplanted into two recipients, either a child and an adult or two adults. In addition, the liver may be split in situ at the donor hospital, allowing coagulation of the cut edge of the liver so that bleeding is minimised following reperfusion. Perfusion to both sides of the liver can be inspected prior to flushing, ensuring that blood flow to all segments of each future graft has been preserved. Split liver transplantation has been associated with a decreased survival rate and the potential for increased risk of complications, including primary non-function, hepatic artery thrombosis, and biliary complications. Because of this split, liver transplantation only accounts for a small proportion of transplants performed. In addition, only grafts from "ideal donors" are thought to be suitable for this form of transplantation. Current criteria for splitting include that the donor should be less than 40 years of age, to be on a single pressor or no pressors, have transaminases no greater than three times normal, and have a body mass index of 28 or less.

Segmental/Lobar/Split/Living Donor Liver Transplantation

Experience with deceased donor split liver transplantation as well as the success with living donor kidney transplantation led to the adoption of the techniques for split liver transplantation to living donor liver transplantation. The first living donor liver transplantation allowed an adult volunteer to donate the left lateral segment of the liver to a child. Based on the success of living donation in the paediatric population as well as the increased waiting list mortality rate for adults, these techniques have also been applied to adult recipients receiving either the right or left lobe from an adult volunteer. Living donor liver transplantation now accounts for approximately 5% of all liver transplants performed in the United States. In south East Asian countries including India, where deceased donor transplantation has developed more slowly because of cultural difficulties living donor transplant is the rule rather than the exception.

It is newer beginning but becoming preferred one. It is based on segmental anatomy and liver regeneration capacity. Minimum liver mass required is more than 1% of graft to body weight ratio. Right lobe is better. It is basically used in children; but useful in adults also. MELD score in donor should be less than 20 for living donor transplantation. Regeneration occurs very significantly in recipients in first 2 weeks reaching standard in 1 month. Regeneration is slow in living donor liver in 1 year. Graft to standard liver ratio should be more than 40%. Function of liver in living donor should be optimum. Proper imaging of the donor for entire anatomy including vasculature is important. Individual branches of portal vein, hepatic artery and bile duct are dissected and isolated. Liver is carefully separated from IVC; small branches of hepatic vein are ligated. Main hepatic vein is isolated; liver parenchyma is dissected with finger/Kelly fracture technique. After completion of parenchymal division, vessels are transected; dissected liver is perfused with cold preservation. Diseased liver of the recipient is removed completely. Graft is anastomosed in usual manner hepatic vein, portal vein, hepatic artery, bile duct. Living donor transplantation has got higher chances of morbidity, complications compared to cadaveric transplantation.

In many respects, transplantation of a graft from a living donor is similar to transplantation of a whole liver from a deceased donor. However, an IVC segmental resection technique is not possible given that the donor vena cava is not available for replacement of the recipient's retrohepatic inferior vena cava. Therefore, the recipient vena cava must be left intact. A direct hepatic vein to vena caval anastomosis is used. Establishing adequate outflow of hepatic venous blood is necessary to prevent oedema of inadequately drained segments of the liver possibly leading to small-for-size syndrome. Therefore, any accessory veins greater than 5 mm in diameter should be reconstructed either by direct anastomosis to the vena cava or by using an interposition graft. In addition, the lengths of the portal vein, hepatic artery, and bile duct on the donor graft are considerably shorter than those available from a deceased donor. Therefore, during the recipient hepatectomy, considerable care should be given to preserving the length of the recipient bile duct as well as the right and/or left hepatic artery and portal vein that are intended for future anastomosis.

Auxiliary/Heterotopic/Ectopic Liver Transplantation

Under selected circumstances, there is a good rationale for placing the donor allograft in heterotopic rather than orthotopic position, leaving the native liver in place. This procedure is known as auxiliary liver transplantation. Auxiliary liver transplantation has occasionally been used for cases in which liver transplantation is indicated for enzymatic deficiency but the native liver is otherwise normal in all other respects. It has also been used in cases of fulminant hepatic failure where the liver candidate is expected to die in the near future without transplant but if adequate time was allowed, the native liver may recover and return to normal. In this situation, immunosuppression can slowly be weaned, the transplanted liver will atrophy, and the recipient can be taken off of all immunosuppression. Another option, auxiliary partial orthotopic liver transplantation (APOLT), has been developed. For this technique, part of the native liver is resected, often the right trisegment, leaving only the left lateral segment intact. The donor liver is then transplanted in an orthotopic position. If the native left lateral segment recovers, immunosuppression can be weaned, leading to hypertrophy of the left lateral segment and involution of the allograft.

Postoperative Management

Antirejection drugs are given. Liver shows low immunogenicity and high regeneration capacity causing long-term outcome. Initially cyclosporine or tacrolimus with mycophenolate mofetil (MMF) or azathioprine with prednisolone is given. ICU care is needed.

Electrolyte and fluid management, sepsis management, prevention of encephalopathy, observation for complications are important.

Complications and Problems of Liver Transplantation

- Bleeding on table and postoperatively can occur especially when recipient liver is cirrhotic. FFP, platelet and blood are needed. Re-exploration is needed if bleeding persists postoperatively.
- Hepatic artery thrombosis is the common vascular complication leading into graft failure, common bile duct (CBD) necrosis and anastomotic dehiscence.
- Immediate graft failure as primary non-functional graft can occur (5% liver grafts).
- Bile leak due to CBD ischaemia which can be identified by hepatobiliary iminodiacetic acid (HIDA) scan, endoscopic retrograde cholangiopancreatography (ERCP), revision anastomosis is needed.
- Infection is common especially enterococci, staphylococci, gram-negative organisms, *Candida*, *Aspergillus*, etc. Antibiotic and antifungal therapy is needed.
- Acute rejection (30%) of T cell-mediated is seen within 10 days commonly but can occur up to 6 months. Liver biopsy confirms the rejection. Higher steroid therapy, polyclonal anti T cell antibodies are used.
- Chronic rejection is seen after 6 months; appears gradually with liver cell dysfunction and hyperbilirubinaemia. Liver biopsy shows less numbered biliary radicles—vanishing bile duct syndrome. It is due to humoral immunity. It is difficult to control; eventually needs retransplantation.
- Recurrent of the earlier disease to the transplanted liver like hepatitis, biliary sclerosis, sclerosing cholangitis. Hepatitis can be controlled by lamivudine (antiviral DNA polymerase for HBV), interferon α, ribavirin for HCV.
- Complications of immunosuppressive drugs like hypertension, hyperglycaemia, hyperlipidaemia, osteoporosis, malignancy, infection, bone marrow suppression, are often difficult to manage.

Survival

5 year survival is 70% in adults and 80% in children. It depends on age, general condition, earlier disease, associated problems, MELD scoring. The risk of rejection is highest (40%) during the first 3–6 months after transplantation and decreases significantly thereafter.

SURGICAL TREATMENT FOR PORTAL HYPERTENSION

Liver Transplant (Orthotopic)

Liver transplant is becoming popular for cirrhosis with varices. It is ideal, final and best. But donor availability and cost is the problem. If patient is for orthotopic liver transplantation (OLT), open shunt surgeries should not be done as liver hilum should be kept virgin for effective transplantation. TIPSS can be done as a bridge in such patients.

Shunt Surgery

Prophylactic shunt surgery should not be done. Shunt surgeries should not be done if the varices have not bled before.

Indications

Child's Grades A and B status with portal hypertension which has bled earlier at least once. Budd-Chiari syndrome with ascites is an indication. Familial heterozygous hypercholesterolaemia and glycogen storage disorders in olden days were indications for portacaval shunting (Child's grading is used for selecting patients for surgery and predicting prognosis).

Surgery is contraindicated in Child C.

Non-selective Shunt Surgeries

Portacaval shunt (end-side, side-to-side); mesentericocaval shunt with or without graft; mesentericorenal shunt.

Proximal splenorenal shunt—Linton's shunt.

Non-selective shunts control and prevent further bleeding as well as reduce the ascites. But since it diverts the blood from liver, *there is high incidence of encephalopathy.*

Note:
End-to-side portacaval shunt is called as Eck fistula (Eck, 1877).

Non-selective shunt surgeries are done in supine position with right side slightly elevated. Right subcostal incision extending on to left side is commonly used. Thoracoabdominal incision is used in patient with significant hepatomegaly or in obese patients. Liver is retracted upwards; duodenum is mobilised by Kocherisation; hepatoduodenal ligament is dissected.

Common bile duct is dissected and isolated. Kocherisation should be done. Posterior part of the portal vein is dissected first as front aspect is having mainly collateral which may cause torrential haemorrhage (it is often found that collaterals are so tortuous and friable and creates difficulty on dissecting the portal vein); these collaterals are more on the anterior aspect. Once portal vein is dissected all around an umbilical tape is passed around it. Adequate posterior dissection is essential to prevent angulation during anastomosis with IVC. Portal pressure should be measured through an omental vein.

Retroperitoneum is incised; IVC in front, lateral and medial aspect is dissected from a point where right renal vein joins the IVC to a point where IVC becomes retrohepatic. Vascular clamps are applied to portal vein proximally just above the pancreas and distally prior to bifurcation. ***In end-to-side portacaval shunt*** distally portal vein is divided and distal end is sutured using continuous 5-0 polypropylene suture. Two stay sutures are placed to proximal cut end of portal vein. Satinsky vascular clamp is applied to the anterior aspect of the IVC. IVC is incised. Often an ellipse of the wall in front of IVC may be excised. Incision in IVC should be at least *1½ times the size of the portal vein. Posterior part of the portal vein is sutured to the medial part of the IVC using 5-0 continuous polypropylene sutures.* It is easier if many sutures are taken and then tightened to slide the portal vein into IVC. Anterior suturing is done between anterior aspect of the portal vein to lateral part of the IVC incision. This should be done always from upper part towards lower part. Continuous or interrupted sutures are used. End-to-side will decompress the splanchnic pressure but keeps sinusoids under high pressure; it will control the variceal bleeding; but will not relieve ascites. End-to-side is not done now. It is a total shunt. Hypertrophied caudate lobe creates problem in side-to-side anastomosis. Future liver transplantation may become difficult **(Fig. 23-30)**.

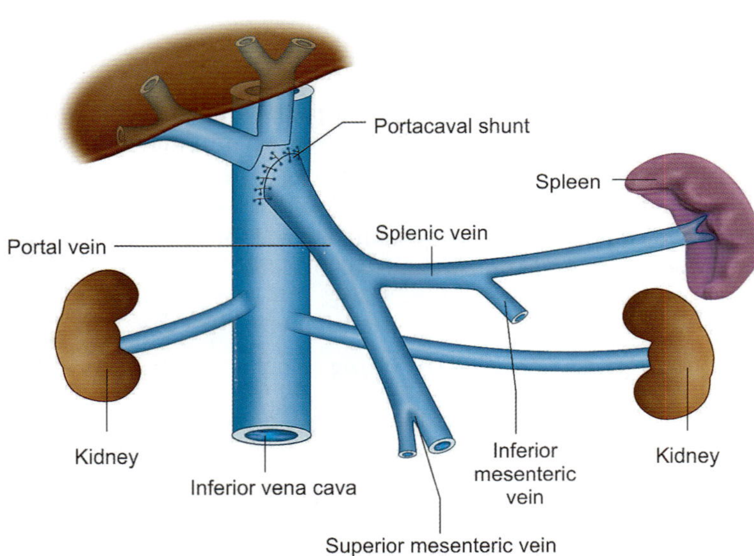

Fig. 23-30: End-to-side portacaval shunt.

Side-to-side shunt is also done similarly without transecting the portal vein. Longitudinal incisions in both portal vein and IVC are done. IVC incision should be 1½ times more than that of portal vein. Posterior continuous and anterior continuous or interrupted sutures are placed from above downwards. Shunt size should be minimum 10 mm. This shunt reduces the obstruction of sinusoids and so relieves ascites also along with control of variceal bleeding. It is a total shunt. *Total shunt* should have a shunt diameter not less than 10 mm.

Side-to-side shunt with an interposition graft (PTFE 8 mm size graft, 3 cm long) diverts blood causing reduction in portal pressure. Since its size of shunt is less than 10 mm, it controls the variceal bleeding well and also maintains the portal perfusion significantly reducing the incidence of the hepatic encephalopathy. It is a partial shunt. *Partial shunt* should have a shunt diameter not more than 8 mm; usually 8 mm **(Fig. 23-31)**.

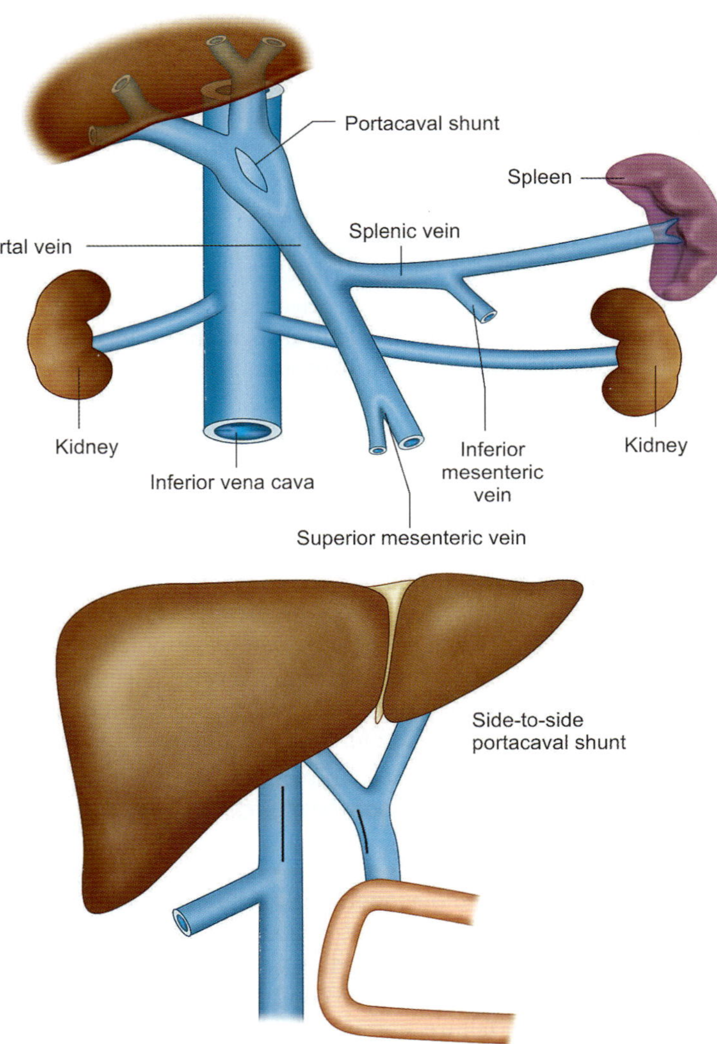

Fig. 23-31: Side-to-side portacaval shunt surgery.

Mesocaval shunt can be side-to-end or side-to-side with a graft. In portal cavernoma in children side-to-side mesentericocaval shunt is used. In adult side to side with a graft is used. Midline laparotomy incision is used. When transverse colon is held and stretched upwards superior mesenteric vein can be seen; it is dissected and isolated. Ligament of Treitz is divided to mobilise small bowel forward and right **(Fig. 23-32)**.

Duodenum should be mobilised by Kocherisation. A 2 cm long superior mesenteric vein (SMV) unobstructed segment is needed; large tributary vein on the left side of SMV should not be present; artery should not cross or override the SMV. Peritoneum in the right paracolic gutter is incised; entire ascending colon and proximal transverse colon is mobilised medially to identify IVC. IVC is dissected from iliac vein confluence to right renal vein level.

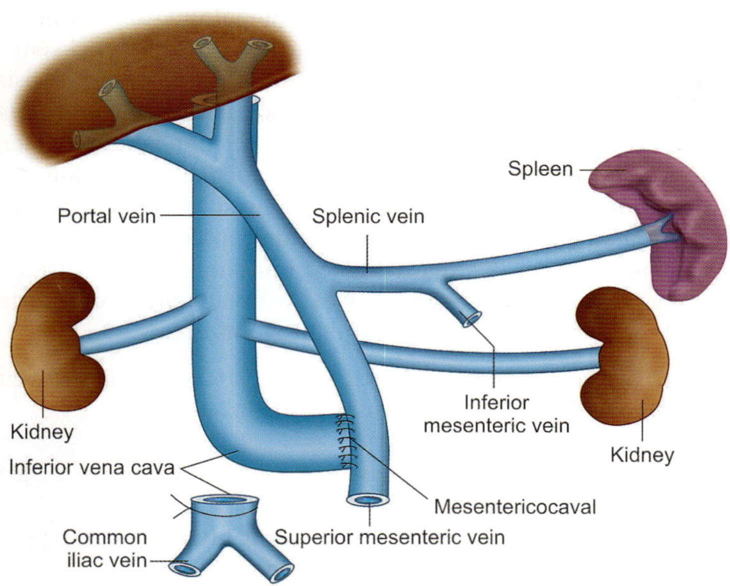

Fig. 23-32: Side-to-end mesentericocaval shunt.

Vascular clamps are applied across the IVC one at close to its iliac confluence, another just below the renal vein level. IVC is transected just above the lower clamp; it is passed through the small mesentery through a created window between distal ileal vessel and ileocolic vessel. SMV is incised after applying a vascular clamp; incision is made on posterolateral part of it longitudinally proximal to right colic vein level. Anastomosis is done using 5-zero polypropylene continuous sutures.

Mesentericocaval shunt with an *interposition graft* is side to side. Graft used is woven Dacron or PTFE. IVC is similarly dissected; side of IVC is incised after applying Satinsky clamp; IVC is anastomosed to graft as side to end with continuous 5-0 polypropylene suture. Other end of the graft is passed through the mesentery and is anastomosed to the side of mobilised SMV. Mesocaval shunt is preferred for isolated hepatic vein obstruction; technically easier; hilar dissection is not present **(Fig. 23-33)**.

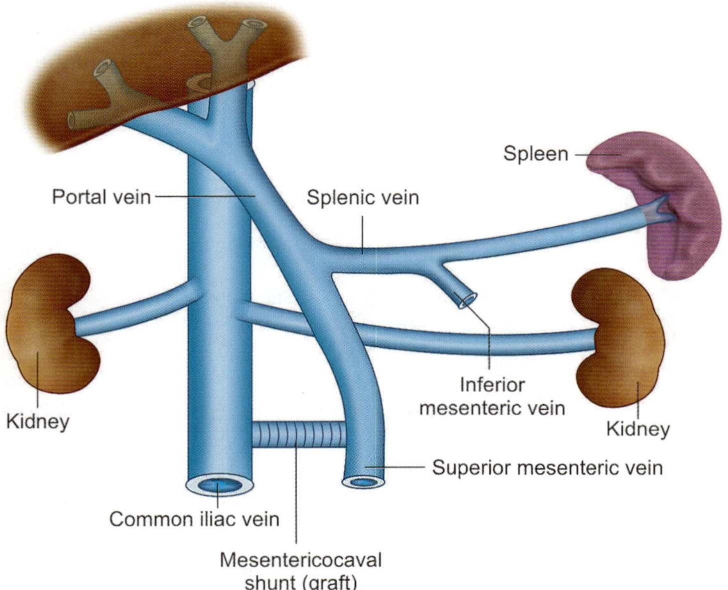

Fig. 23-33: Side-to-side mesenteric caval interposition graft to create a shunt.

Proximal (central) splenorenal shunt: Here blood flows from high pressure portal system towards the low pressure systemic venous system through renal vein. It is presumed that it allows part of blood to course through the liver to reduce effects of the encephalopathy. Patient under general anaesthesia with left side up or oblique; left lengthy subcostal or left thoracoabdominal incision is made. Splenic flexure and transverse colon is mobilised to retract them downwards. Short gastric vessels are ligated and divided; splenophrenic and splenorenal ligaments are divided to reach the splenic hilum to identify splenic vessels. Splenic artery is ligated. Splenic vein is dissected proximally by ligating and dividing all branches entering into it so as to free it until it joins the superior mesenteric vein. Inferior mesenteric vein entering the splenic vein can be ligated and divided safely if needed. Vascular clamp is applied to the splenic vein; spleen is removed **(Fig. 23-34)**.

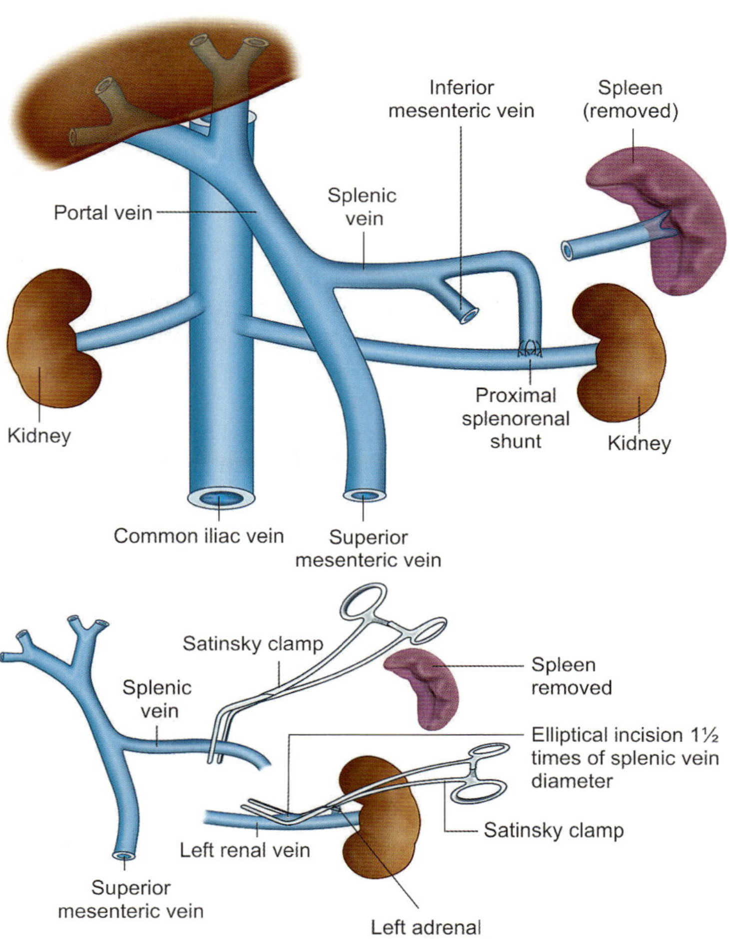

Fig. 23-34: Proximal splenorenal shunt surgery. It is a non-selective shunt (Linton's).

The retroperitoneum is incised to identify the left renal vein just at lower margin of the pancreas. Left renal artery and renal vein is isolated with vascular tapes. Left adrenal vein often needs ligation and division for proper mobilisation of the left renal vein. Left renal vein is mobilised adequately. Left renal artery is often occluded with vascular bulldog clamp to reduce renal vein flow temporarily. A Satinsky clamp is placed obliquely across the renal vein; incision is made on the anterosuperior aspect of the left renal vein often to remove elliptical piece of it; incision should be 1½ times the diameter of the splenic vein end. End of splenic vein is anastomosed to the left renal vein using continuous 5-0 polypropylene sutures posteriorly and interrupted sutures anteriorly to complete the proximal/central splenorenal shunt. Tapes and clamps are removed from the left renal artery, renal vein and splenic vein.

Portacaval Shunt with Arterialisation

This is done in end-to-side portacaval shunt as there is abrupt stop of hepatic blood flow. So hepatic blood flow is maintained by interposition of the saphenous vein graft or synthetic PTFE graft between infrarenal aorta and hepatic stump of portal vein in end-side shunt. Arterialisation also can be achieved by turning end of splenic artery to the portal vein to create end-to-end anastomosis. As end-to-side portacaval shunt is not done now, arterialisation procedure has also no role at present **(Fig. 23-35)**.

Selective Shunts

Distal splenorenal shunt (DSRS)—Warren's shunt *(Warren, 1967)*. Size of the splenic vein should be 10 mm or more to do distal splenorenal shunt; if less, then shunt may develop thrombosis and shunt failure can occur. End of splenic vein is shunted to the side of the left renal vein. Splenic vein should be more than 10 mm in size (diameter). It selectively decompresses the portal bed near oesophagogastric area (so that it prevents bleeding). Liver is also perfused adequately and so possibility of encephalopathy is less. But it may augment incidence of ascites. Left subcostal or chevron incision is used with left side up position. Incision extends from left anterior axillary line extending across the right rectus up to the right margin of the right rectus muscle. Through gastrocolic ligament lesser sac is entered. Gastroepiploic arcade is divided to prevent later formation of collaterals (arcade is divided towards gastric side). Short gastric vessels should be retained (should never be interrupted; it is through this, variceal bed is decompressed into splenic vein). Plane is created between 3rd part of the duodenum and pancreas by dividing peritoneum over it. When gland is reflected upwards, splenic vein is identified which is dissected carefully by ligating all branching vessels individually and divided. A venous catheter is passed into the splenic vein to measure the splenic vein pressure. Inferior mesenteric vein is identified and, dissected, doubly ligated and divided. Splenic vein is mobilised up to its entry into the superior mesenteric vein. Vascular clamp is applied to the splenic vein. Splenic vein is divided at its junction with SMV. Small pancreatic branches entering the splenic vein are ligated and divided **(Fig. 23-36)**.

Left renal vein is dissected similarly; left adrenal vein is ligated but left gonadal vein is retained. Average length of the renal vein is 8 cm; 5 cm of it should be mobilised for proper shunt anastomosis. Portal side of the cut end is sutured with continuous polypropylene sutures. Left gastric (coronary) vein at its junction where it enters the portal or splenic vein is ligated and divided; all veins along the retroperitoneum above the pancreas, along splenocolic ligament, along greater and lesser omentum are interrupted effectively; right gastroepiploic vein is already ligated but should be confirmed. Efficacy in control of bleeding is 94%; with 90% preserved portal blood flow. Incidence of encephalopathy is 15% or less.

Inokuchi shunt is a selective shunt between IVC and left gastric vein (using a graft).

Unconventional shunts:

Modified Rex shunt: It is done between left portal vein and SMV using autologous IJV graft.

Alternative splanchnic drainage is done using inferior mesenteric or gastroepiploic veins; coronary vein to left portal vein.

Alternative systemic route: Mesogonadal or lienoadrenal shunts.

Unconventional shunts cause partial non-selective decompression; yield effective shunting; does not preclude liver transplantation. But need is vein of good quality adequate length and caliber (>5 mm).

Splenectomy

Left sided portal hypertension also called as *segmental portal hypertension* (sinistral portal hypertension) is due to splenic vein thrombosis (If partial channels are present within it, it is called as *splenic vein cavernoma*). Here liver is normal and *splenectomy* alone will correct the condition. Banti in 1894 originally suggested splenectomy for portal hypertension.

Transjugular Intrahepatic Portosystemic Stenting/Shunt (TIPSS)

Size of stent must be 10 mm. It is a non-surgical, interventional radiological method, wherein, a stent is placed in the liver between hepatic venule and portal through a guidewire following dilatation. It is a simple and easier method to reduce portal pressure. It can cause hepatic encephalopathy, bleeding, bile leak and infection.

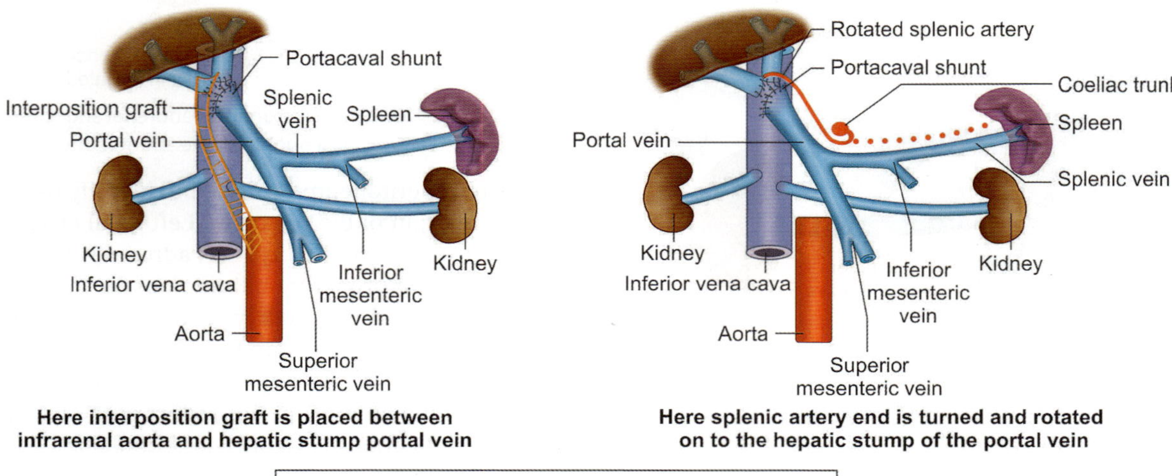

Fig. 23-35: Portacaval shunt with arterialisation being done.

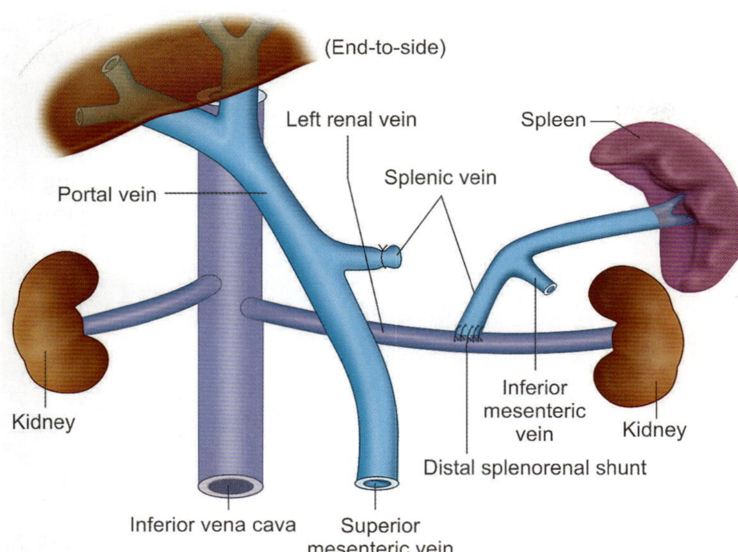

Fig. 23-36: Distal splenorenal shunt (DSRS)—Warren's shunt.

It is contraindicated in encephalopathy, tumours and liver cysts. It is quite useful as a temporary measure to reduce portal bed pressure, before doing orthotopic liver transplantation in cirrhotic patients.

Problems with TIPSS

Post-stent encephalopathy—40%; stenosis (50%) and recurrent varices; bleeding; bile leak; sepsis **(Fig. 23-37)**.

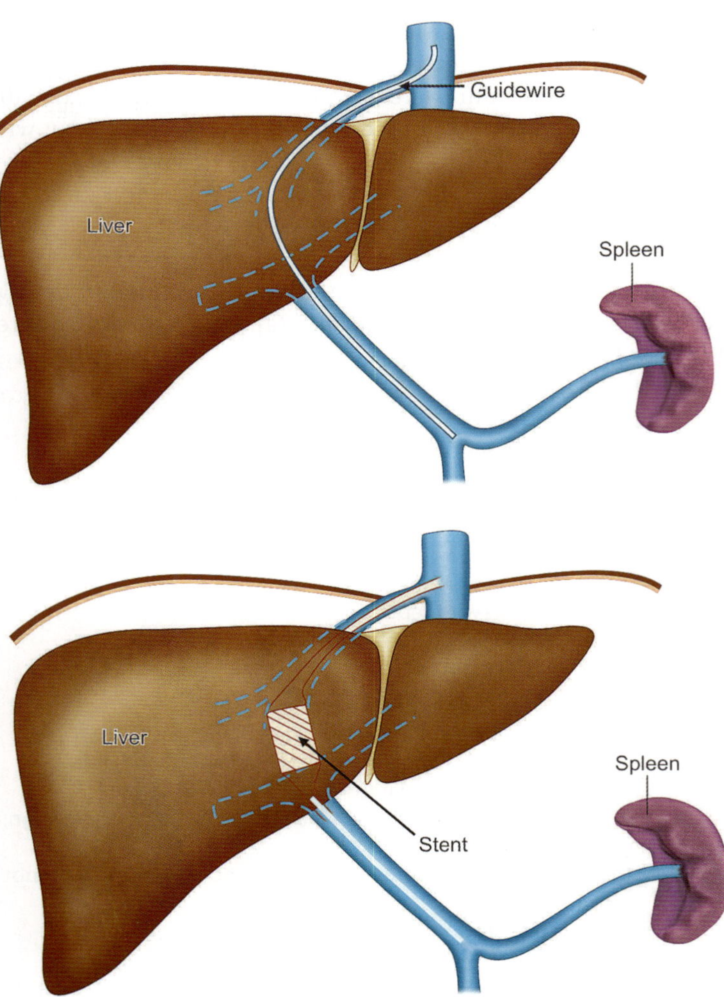

Fig. 23-37: Transjugular intrahepatic portosystemic stenting/shunt (TIPSS).

Mesoatrial Shunt

When hepatic vein and IVC block are present, mesoatrial shunt or caval stenting and portacaval shunt or cavoatrial shunt with portacaval shunt is needed. Mesocaval shunt is indicated when there is IVC block that is not amenable for stenting; prerequisite is a pressure gradient of 15 mm Hg or more between IVC and right atrium. Shunt placement in low pressure system may precipitate shunt thrombosis.

TABLE 23-1: Child's grading of severity of liver disease

Clinical and biochemical measurement	*Points scored*		
	1	2	3
Serum bilirubin (mg/dL)	<2.0	2.0–3.0	>3.0
Serum albumin (g/dL)	>3.5	3.0–3.5	<3.0
Ascites	None	Controlled	Uncontrolled
Mental status	Normal	Disoriented	Coma
Nutrition	Very good	Good	Poor
Total score	<6 Child's A	7–9 Child's B	10–19 Child's C
Pugh's modification			
Prothrombin time prolonged in seconds	Increased up to 3	Between 3–6	>6

Surgeries for portal hypertension
- Orthotopic liver transplant (OLT)
- Devascularisation surgeries
- Decompression surgeries

Surgeries for oesophageal varices and portal hypertension

Decompression procedures
- Non-selective shunts
  - End-to-side portacaval shunt (Eck fistula)
  - Side-to-side portacaval shunt
  - Mesentericocaval shunt
  - Mesentericocaval shunt with graft
  - Proximal splenorenal shunt—Linton's shunt
  - TIPSS

Selective shunts
- Distal splenorenal shunt—Warren's shunt
- Inokuchi shunt between left gastric vein and IVC through a graft

Devascularisation procedures
- Oesophageal stapler transection; Boerema Crile operation; Tanner's oesophageal gastric transection; Milnes Walker transection; Sugiura Futagawa/Hassab/Orozco and colleagues operations

Porta-azygos Disconnection/ Devascularising Procedures

They are inflow control that act effectively by devascularising the portal bed. It is useful in extensive portal and splenic vein thrombosis. Incidence of encephalopathy is very low here.

Oesophageal stapler transection of Johnston: Through an anterior gastrotomy incision end-to-end stapler is passed across the oesophagogastric (OG) junction into the oesophagus and stapler is fired to transect, interrupt all varices, disconnect azygos and portal connection at oesophageal level and reanastomose automatically through the stapler. It is simple to do **(Fig. 23-38)**.

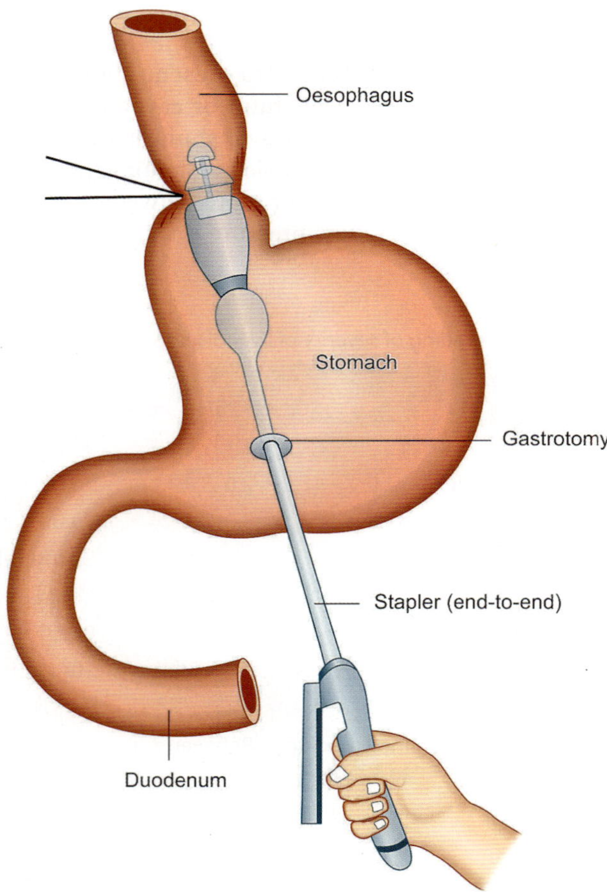

Fig. 23-38: Stapler transection—devascularisation procedure.

Boerema-Crile operation: It is a thoracic approach. With patient in right lateral position, thoracotomy is done through 8th rib; oesophagus is dissected and isolated; clamp is applied at cardia; oesophagus is opened longitudinally to hold edges with stay sutures. Varices columns are underrun using continuous vicryl sutures. Incised muscle layer of oesophagus is resutured again. Usually hiatus is not opened across the diaphragm to abdominal cavity as if ascites is present, it may communicate into the pleural cavity.

Milnes-Walker thoracic oesophageal transection: It is done through left sided thoracic approach; vagi are safeguarded. Oesophageal muscle is incised longitudinally; mucosa and submucosa are dissected and isolated as like longitudinal tube which is resected to interrupt the mucosal and submucosal varices. This tubular structure is resutured and muscle incised is sutured back again. Below this, transection done at the level of hiatus and resutured again.

Tanner's abdominal oesophagogastric transection: It is done through abdominal approach. All communications between the portal system and azygos systemic veins are interrupted after transection the stomach 5 cm below the OG junction. After proper interruption reanastomosis is done between the cut ends of stomach.

***Sugiura-Futagawa operation* (1977, Japan):** Vagotomy, pyloroplasty, devascularisation, splenectomy. Laparotomy is done; can also use thoracoabdominal incision. Spleen is removed; devascularisation begins at lesser curvature of stomach; left gastric artery and vein (coronary vein) are ligated; greater curvature, posterior part of the stomach are devascularised. Paraoesophageal devascularisation is done by disconnecting all vessels passing between hemiazygos and azygos veins up to inferior pulmonary vein (in original Sugiura method, devascularisation was done up to arch of aorta) for at least 7 cm of lower oesophagus. Highly selective vagotomy is done (in original Sugiura truncal vagotomy and pyloroplasty is done). Oesophagus is transected using EEA stapler; anastomosis is covered with Nissen's fundoplication. Hassab from Egypt did similar devacularising procedure. Orozco and colleague from Mexico did similar devascularisation procedure without splenectomy with good results.

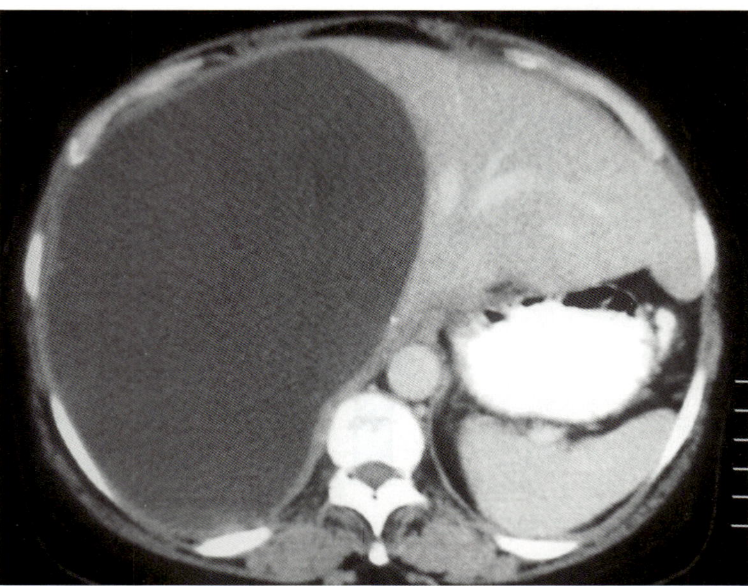

Fig. 23-39: Hydatid cyst CT scan—large cyst in liver.

SURGERIES FOR HYDATID CYST

Hydatid cyst is managed by chemotherapy; minimally invasive techniques (PAIR); open surgeries; laparoscopic procedures **(Figs. 23-39 to 23-43)**.

Classifications

Hassen Gharbi's ultrasound-based classification of liver hydatid cysts (1981)

Type 1 – Pure fluid collection
Type 2 – Fluid collection with split wall
Type 3 – Fluid collection with septa
Type 4 – Heterogeneous appearance
Type 5 – Reflecting thick walls

WHO classification of liver hydatid cyst

Type – CL – Active; unilocular; no cyst wall; early stage; not fertile
Type – CE 1 – Active; cyst wall present; hydatid sand present; fertile
Type – CE 2 – Active; multivesicular rosette-like cyst wall; fertile
Type – CE 3 – Transitional; detaching laminated membrane; *water-lily* sign; beginning of degeneration
Type – CE 4 – Inactive; degenerative contents; no daughter cysts; not fertile
Type – CE 5 – Inactive; thick calcified wall; not fertile

Cyst is common in right lobe (65%); left lobe is (18%); both (16%). Segment 8 is commonly involved (30%); then segment 5 (22%).

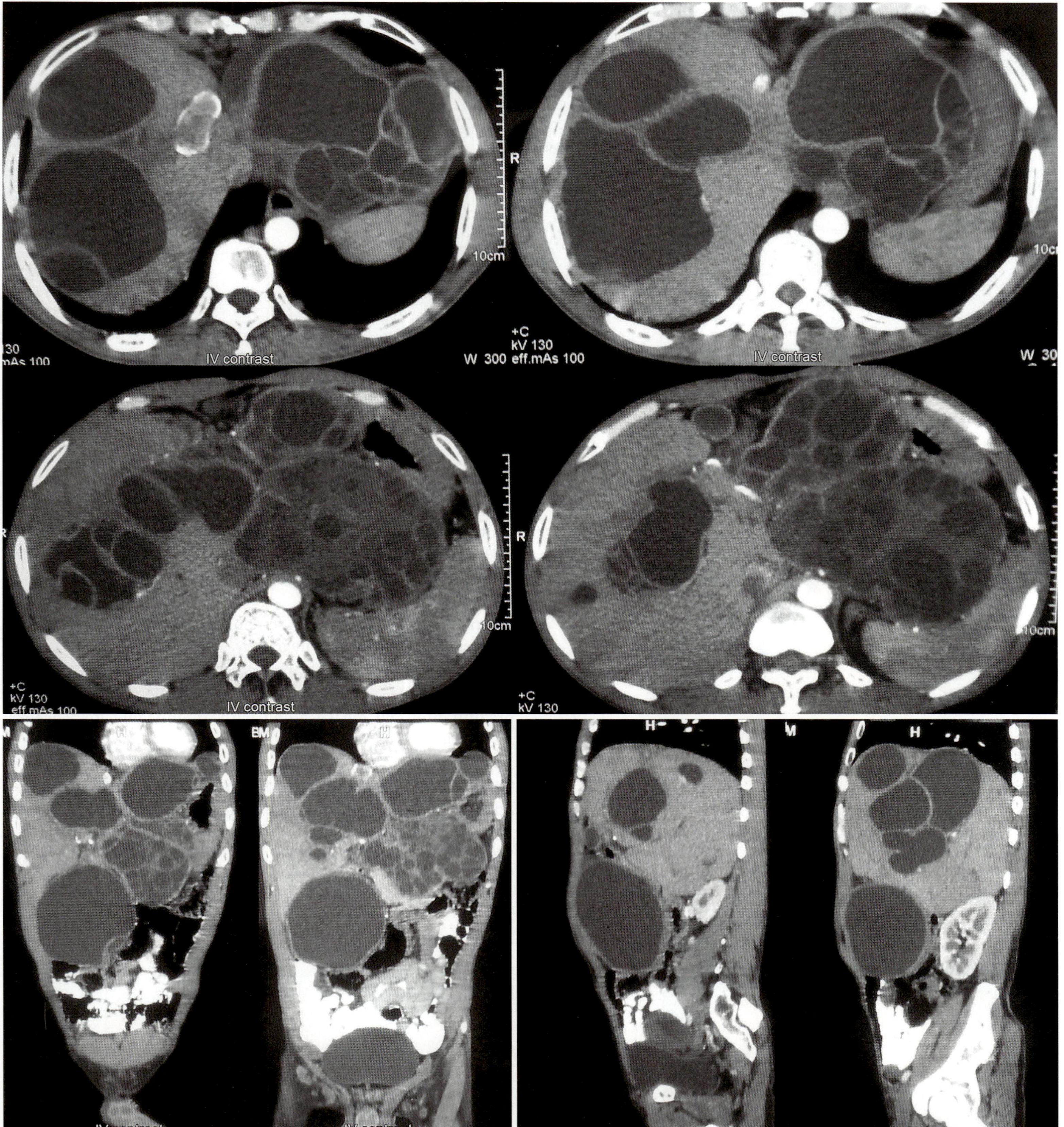

Fig. 23-40: Hydatid cyst—multiple in liver and extrahepatic region.

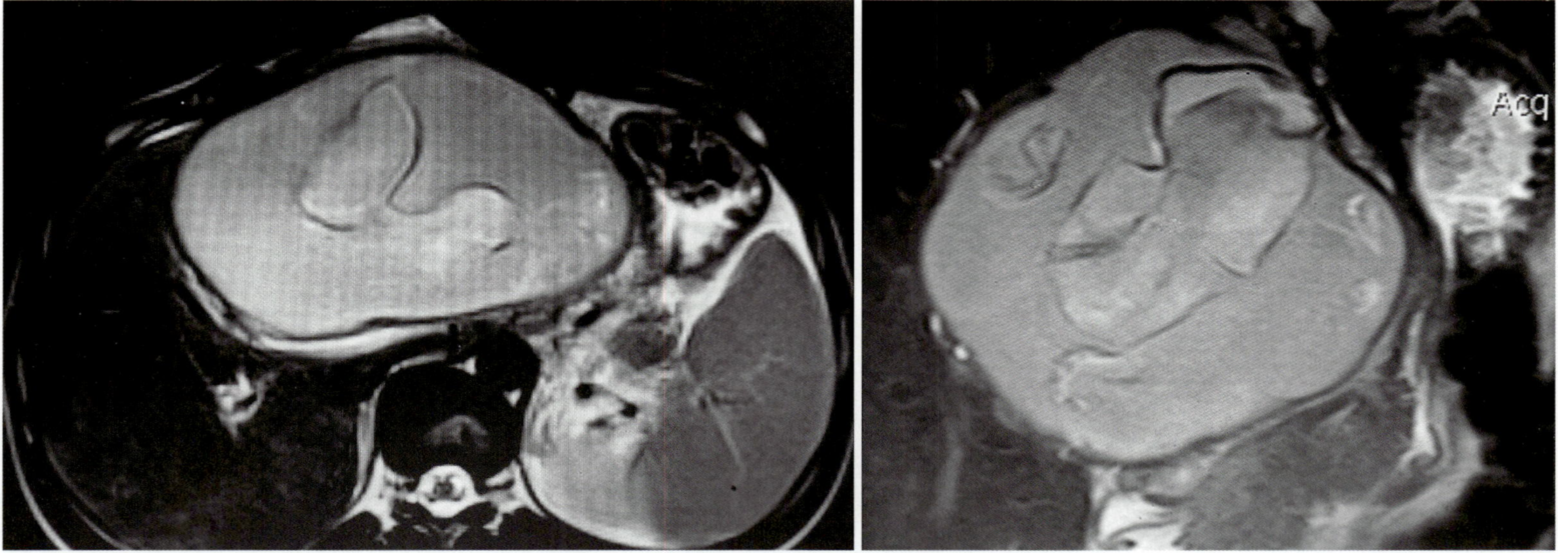

Fig. 23-41: Hydatid cyst—MRI is ideal and better than CT scan.

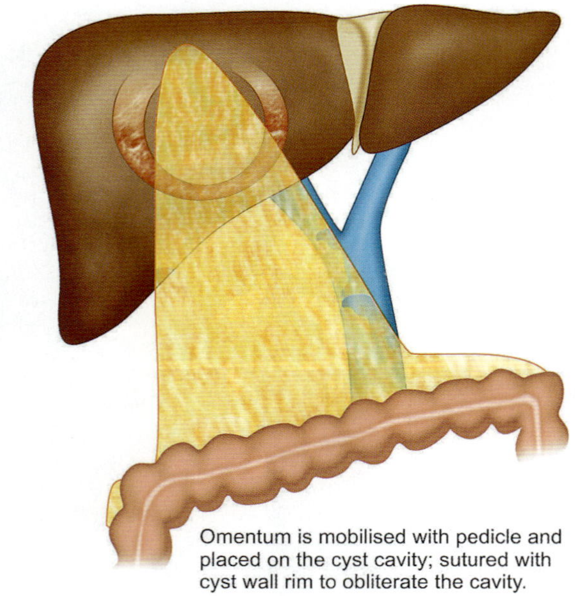

Fig. 23-42: Hydatid cyst—cavity obliteration by omentoplasty.

Drugs

Indications for drug therapy: 4 days prior to intervention and continue it for 1 month (albendazole) to 3 months (mebendazole) after the intervention; inoperable cysts; multiple or multiorgan cysts; recurrent hydatids; surgically unfit patients; cysts in lungs, bone, brain and eyes.

Contraindications: Large cysts; honeycomb cysts (with septae); infected or calcified cysts; pregnancy.

Drugs used are: Albendazole 4 weeks cycles with 2 weeks drug free interval. It is ovicidal/larvicidal/vermicidal. Commonly used; praziquantel—60 mg/kg along with albendazole for 2 weeks; mebendazole—600 mg daily for 4 weeks.

Puncture–Aspiration–Injection–Reaspiration (PAIR)—Percutaneously Done (1980)

Aspiration of the cyst should not be done due to risk of anaphylaxis but presently Puncture-aspiration-injection-reaspiration (PAIR) is done effectively.

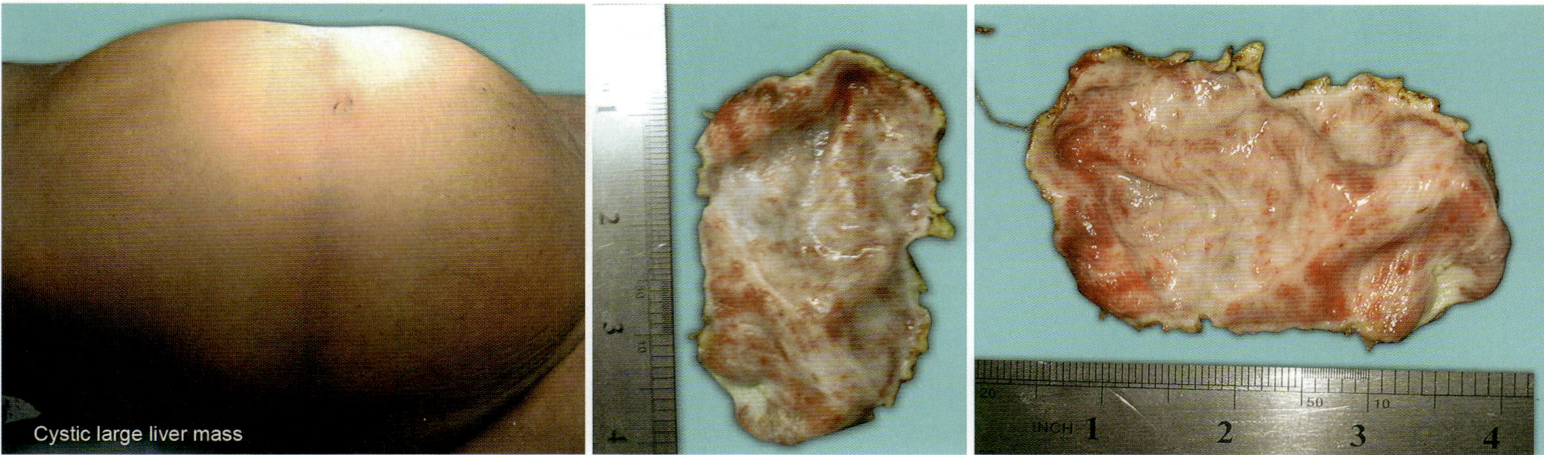

Fig. 23-43: Simple cyst of liver; it is removed through laparoscopy easily. It is a differential diagnosis for hydatid cyst of liver.

Indications for PAIR	Results and problems of PAIR
♦ Inoperable patients ♦ Patients who refuse surgery ♦ CL, CE 1, CE 2 and CE 3 types/ Gharbi type 1 and 2 ♦ Relapse cysts ♦ Infected cysts ♦ In pregnant women; children less than 3 years ♦ Cysts more than 5 cm in different liver segments	♦ Complication rate—10–40% ♦ Mortality rate—0.9–2.5% ♦ Fever—35%, disappears in 72 hours ♦ Anaphylaxis—0.1–0.2%, same as open surgery, but drugs should be kept ready for ♦ Anaphylaxis ♦ Infection—10% well-controlled by antibiotics ♦ Local recurrences—4%, repeat PAIR can be done

Contraindications for PAIR
- Inaccessible cysts
- Cysts with multiple septae—honeycomb cysts
- Hyperechogenic cysts
- Communicating cysts to bile duct
- Calcified cysts
- Cysts in the lung

Technique of PAIR

It is done under US/CT guidance; under local anaesthesia, cyst is punctured using a cholangiography 22-gauge needle through thickest route/part of cyst wall; cyst is entered through non-dependent wall and 50% of fluid is aspirated. All multiple/daughter cysts are aspirated. Radiopaque dye is injected to see if any communications are present. Scolicidal agents—15-20% hypertonic saline is injected into the cyst. After 20 minutes reaspiration is done. A sclerosant—alcohol is injected. If cyst is 6 cm or more, a drainage catheter is placed for 24 hours for complete drainage and later alcohol sclerosant is injected. Double-puncture aspiration and injection (D-PAI) or modified PAIR/PEVAC (Percutaneous EVAcuation of Cyst) are other procedures done. PAIR has gained wide acceptance as it is safe, less invasive, and easier to do, with low morbidity and mortality. Complications and results are same as open surgery.

SURGERY

Surgery is the best treatment for hydatid disease as it removes the parasite, cystobiliary communications are addressed, less morbidity and mortality and low recurrence rate.

Procedures are conservative and radical.

- Surgery is still the choice and gold standard therapy for hydatid disease. The abdomen is opened, and the peritoneal cavity is packed with mops (black or colored mops are used to identify white scolices clearly so as to pick up all and prevent any spillage). Fluid from the cyst is aspirated and scolicidal agents (cetrimide, chlorohexidine, alcohol, hypertonic saline (15–20%), 10% povidone iodine or H_2O_2) are injected into the cyst cavity (formalin should not be used). Hypertonic saline should be left within the cavity for 15–20 minutes to have effective scolicidal effect.
- Detection of cystobiliary communications is very crucial as it may cause caustic sclerosing cholangitis when scolicidal agent like formalin is used. Communicating openings may be single or multiple. Cyst more than 10 cm is likely to have cystobiliary communications. Often clinically features of communications may not be present. Preoperatively there may be recurrent cholangitis; dilated bile duct. Factors important are—its size, number, site, involvement of hepatic/bile ducts and liver dysfunction.

Contd...

Contd...

Bile stained cyst on table during aspiration is highly suggestive of communication. White mops soaked with hypertonic saline are kept in the cyst cavity and gallbladder is gently squeezed to see for the bile staining of the mop in the cavity which confirms communication.
- Pericystectomy is ideal, but technically demanding.
- Laparoscopic pericystectomy is becoming more popular. Contraindications are deeply situated cyst, densely adherent cyst, and inaccessible cysts; more than 3 cysts; calcified cysts and cysts in other organs. Main problems with laparoscopic pericystectomy is spillage and difficulty in preventing it.
- Liver resection—only occasionally segmental or hemihepatectomy is done.

Scolicidal agents

- Cetrimide—can cause acidosis
- Alcohol 80%—can cause cholangitis
- Hypertonic saline—hypernatraemia
- Sodium hypochlorite—hypernatraemia
- Hydrogen peroxide

In cases with biliary communication, only hypertonic saline (15–20%) is used (not other agents)

Features of formed abscess are

Procedures used to correct the cystobiliary communications and to obliterate the cavity are:
- Suturing of the communication—simple suture using vicryl/PDS suture with T tube drain of bile duct.
- Pericystectomy (Pericystectomy is done by peeling off the cyst wall and abdomen is closed with or without a drain), marsupialisation.
- Tube drainage of the cavity; capitonnage—spiral suturing of the bottom of the cavity upward from base of cavity to the edge of the cyst wall; introflexion—inverting the rim of the cyst edge without apposition; omentoplasty.
- Internal drainage procedures like choledochojejunostomy; transduodenal sphincteroplasty; Roux-en-Y cysto/intracystic hepatico jejunostomy; Roux-en-Y hepaticojejunostomy.
- In cystobiliary communication (fistula), cystobiliary disconnection is achieved anatomically between cyst and fistula and a multiperforated transparenchymal drain is placed into the fistula through the cyst and another multiperforated drain is placed into the cyst cavity. A T tube drain is placed into the bile duct (perdomo procedure) to achieve complete external drainage with facilitation of closure of the communication.
- Bipolar drainage: A drain is placed to cyst cavity and a T tube is placed into common bile duct.
- Reconstructive procedure like pericystojejunostomy; bile duct repair.
- ERCP sphincterotomy.

Conservative Surgical Approach

It is technically easier; hepatic specialised surgeons are not necessary; safer; liver parenchyma is not entered; multiple bilateral cysts can be approached; cost-effective; tissue sparing; acceptable in relation to recurrence, morbidity and mortality.

Cyst should be exposed completely; cyst should be sterilised properly (scolicidal); should be evacuated completely; cystobiliary communications and cyst cavities are to be managed effectively.

Right subcostal with often extension towards left side is needed for adequate exposure. Liver should be released of all adhesions and made mobile.

Entire field surrounding the liver should be packed with hypertonic saline (20%) soaked black/blue/green drapes/mops (to identify white scolices). Cyst wall is punctured carefully; often specialised cones are used for this purpose (Saidi Nazarian cryogenic cone (1971); Aaron's cone by Aaron's and Kune, Australia). Aaron's suction cone is better, safer and effective. But it is not necessary to use these devices. Stay sutures are placed on the cyst wall; cyst wall incised for 5 cm. Large sump suction is used to suck all fluid in the cavity. All laminated membranes are removed using forceps or hand or spoon.

Cyst roof which is redundant is excised. Cut edge of the cyst should be underrun with sutures (oversewing) to block small vessels and ducts in the cyst wall. Inside cyst cavity wall is gently scraped using hypertonic saline soaked gauze. All daughter cysts should be removed by this method with care, gentleness and patience. Cavity is washed with hypertonic saline repeatedly. Saline soaked packs are kept in the cavity for 10 minutes.

Different scolicidal agents are used. Different types have got different efficacy and exposure time. 30% hypertonic saline is safer with 10 minutes exposure time; lesser concentration needs more exposure time. Cetavlon has got shortest exposure time—5 minutes. Other scolicidal agents used are—povidone-iodine, hydrogen peroxide, formalin (not used) with different exposure timings. Scolicidal agents can cause severe sclerosing cholangitis, methhaelmoglobinaemia, acute toxicity, hypernatraemia, air embolism, anaphylaxis, metabolic acidosis, and may cause death rarely. Hypertonic saline is ideal. Partial pericystectomy is done usually in many situations; subtotal pericystecomy is also done occasionally. Pericyst adherent to biliary and vascular structures are left behind.

Cystobiliary communications (CBC) should be identified and managed properly. It may be single or multiple. Its management depends on the number, type, depth, site, size (minute or wider orifice), duct involved, and status of liver. On table, bile-stained cyst suggests communication. In such situation, with careful repeated saline wash staining site of bile can be identified. It is better to pass a needle into the CBD and inject saline or saline and air or dilute methylene blue to the bile duct to identify the site. Intraoperative cystic duct cholangiography is also done through cystic duct which needs cholecystectomy. It demonstrates the CBD scolices, site of leak. But it is not mandatory, often may not be sufficient. ERCP or intraoperative ultrasound (IOUS) is very useful in identifying the CBD scolices. Scolices in gallbladder are very rare.

Commonly such cystobiliary communications are of peripheral duct branches and small; just secure suturing of the minute orifice using 4-0 vicryl or PDS is sufficient. In biliary tree, bile enters into scolices existing there resulting in death of parasite and so CBD scolices are rare **(Fig. 23-44)**.

If cholangiogram or on table IOUS shows hydatid debris, then choledochotomy is done and debris is removed; choledochoscope is done; T tube is placed while closing the CBD. T tube is also often placed when there are communications (which are sutured accordingly) to have assured decompression of the biliary tree so that sutures will not disrupt. Once T tube is placed per operative T tube, cholangiogram is done.

In case if suturing of the leaking orifice is impossible, then combined external drainage of the pericyst by placing a drain on pericyst and drainage of extrahepatic biliary apparatus is done (either external or internal). This method of draining both pericyst and biliary apparatus is called as bipolar drainage. External biliary apparatus drainage is achieved by placing a T tube into CBD. Often a multiperforated drain is passed through the orifice to drain fistula across the parenchyma; another such drain is placed into the cyst cavity; T tube is placed in the CBD—*Perdomo procedure*.

Internal drainage of biliary tree can be achieved by *ERCP sphincterotomy* or transduodenal sphincteroplasty or bilioenteric anastomosis (Roux-en-Y choledochojejunostomy or duodenostomy). Bilioenteric drainage is done when there are many daughter cysts in CBD or dilated CBD or when there is cholangitis.

Cystobiliary communication into a major biliary ductal system if sutured may obliterate ductal drainage partially which is dangerous. Here Roux-en-Y cystojejunostomy or intracystic hepaticojejunostomy or intracystic bile duct repair is done. These procedures are often technically difficult and liver resection may be final answer in these patients.

Residual cavity of the cyst often needs obliteration by different methods. This cavity may be superficial or anterior or posterior or superior or inferior; it can have large opening with large capacity or small opening with large capacity. Residual cavity can be managed by—(1) Leaving cyst open; (2) With rim oversewn on the entire edge—marsupialisation; (3) Small cyst can have simple closure; (4) Placing drainage tube into the cyst cavity as external drainage; (5) Introflexion by infolding edge of the cyst inward with taking bites from overlying liver tissue; (6) Capitonage—redundant pericyst is infolded from depth to outwards by consecutive interrupted layer of sutures or by continuous spiral suture bites taken from pericyst wall at alternative sides; this is difficult in large or calcified cysts; deep bites may injure liver parenchyma or hepatic veins underneath or stiff cyst wall may get avulsed off from the liver tissue causing severe haemorrhage; (7) Omentoplasty—viable omental pedicle is placed into the cavity and fixed with absorbable sutures; drain is placed adjacent to the omental flap; omentum obliterates the cavity but will not prevent bile leak; omentoplasty can be combined with partly capitonage; (8) Roux-en-Y cystojejunostomy not commonly used; (9) Rectus abdominis and diaphragm myoplasty **(Figs. 23-45 to 23-48)**.

Radical Surgical Procedures for Hydatid Liver Disease

It is done if conservative surgery is impossible; already done conservative surgery has failed; lobe involved is irreversibly damaged; adequate biliary drainage if cannot be achieved. Every patient with hydatid disease is not an indication for radical procedure. Closed pericystectomy; open pericystectomy; near total cystectomy; subadventitial cystectomy; non-anatomical liver resection and anatomical liver resections are different procedures done. In closed pericystectomy, cyst is not opened, instead entire pericyst is removed carefully and gently. In open pericystectomy after opening, the cyst is entirely removed by similar methods. Near total pericystectomy is done when pericyst is adherent to IVC and major hepatic veins where a part of pericyst is left behind after sterilisation with hypertonic saline but remaining part of the pericyst and scolices are completely removed. Pericyst is the outer most layer which is adherent to the liver tissue including vasculobiliary structures which may get damaged even by careful dissection as adhesions are very often strong. Inner avascular granulomatous exocyst layer is separated from pericyst along the subadvential plane. If dissection is done little away from pericyst, it becomes non-anatomic liver resection. Hepatectomy is done only if entire right or left liver is involved.

Pericystectomy for Hydatid Liver Cyst

There is controversy regarding optimal treatment for this parasitic disease. Options of deroofing and content evacuation is considered suboptimal and pericystectomy may be too radicle a procedure for some cases. The main principle of the surgery is to eradicate the parasite and prevent intraoperative spillage of cyst contents thus avoiding peritoneal spread. Preoperatively 10–14 mg/kg/day of albendazole is administered orally for a period of 4 weeks.

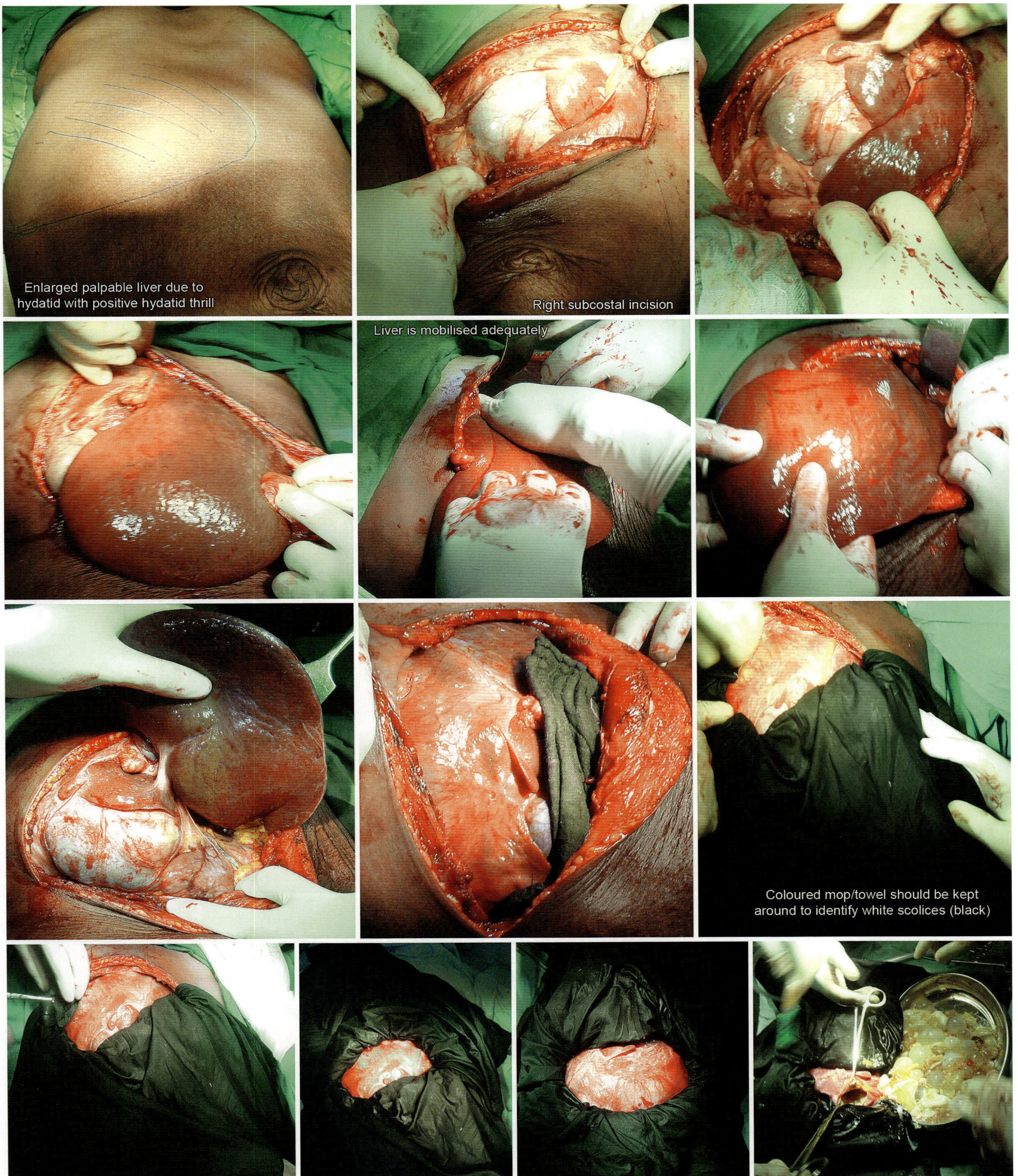
Enlarged palpable liver due to
hydatid with positive hydatid thrill
Right subcostal incision
Liver is mobilised adequately
Coloured mop/towel should be kept
around to identify white scolices (black)

Figs. 23-44(1)

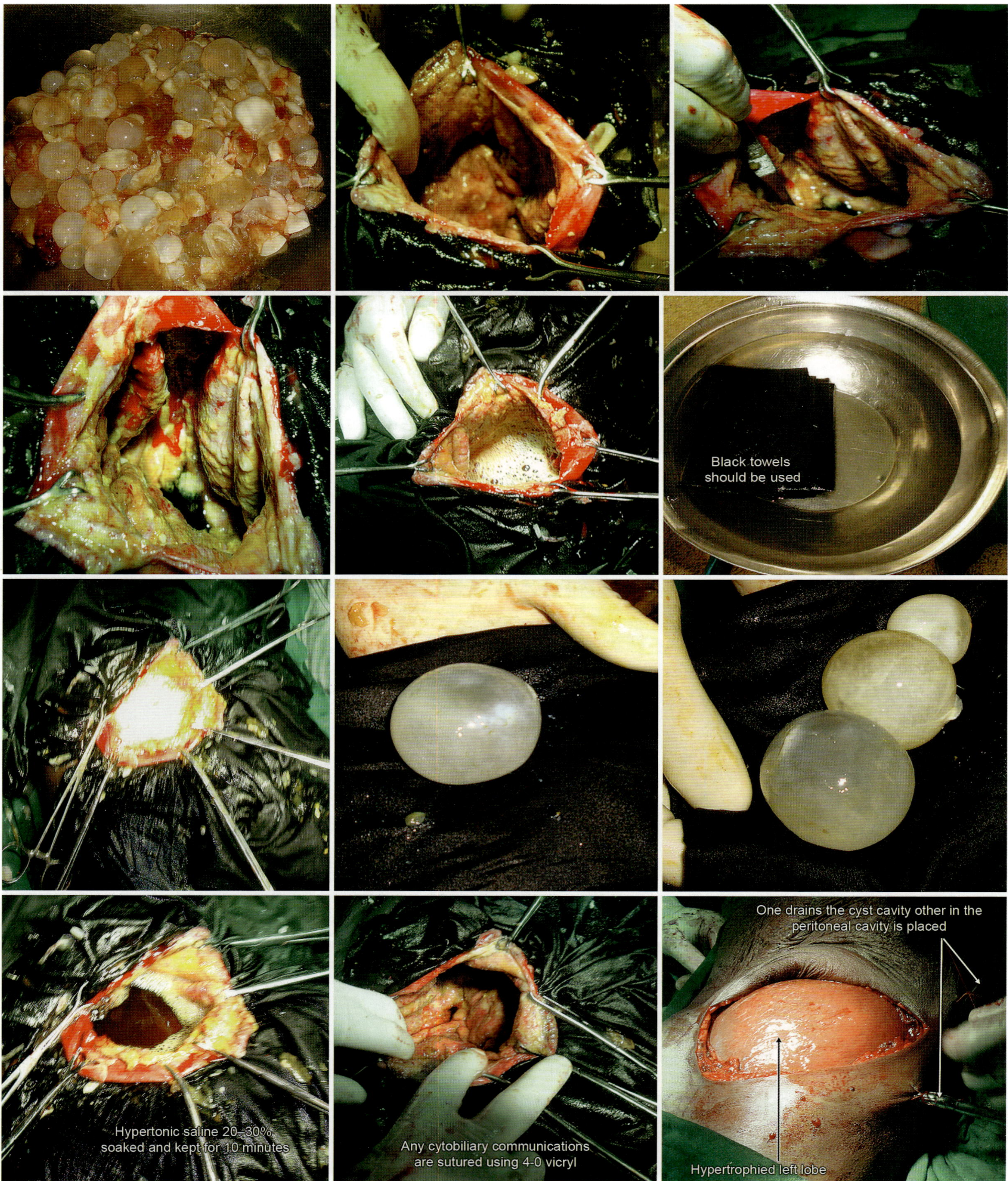
Black towels
should be used
Hypertonic saline 20–30%
soaked and kept for 10 minutes
Any cytobiliary communications
are sutured using 4-0 vicryl
One drains the cyst cavity other in the
peritoneal cavity is placed
Hypertrophied left lobe

Figs. 23-44(2)

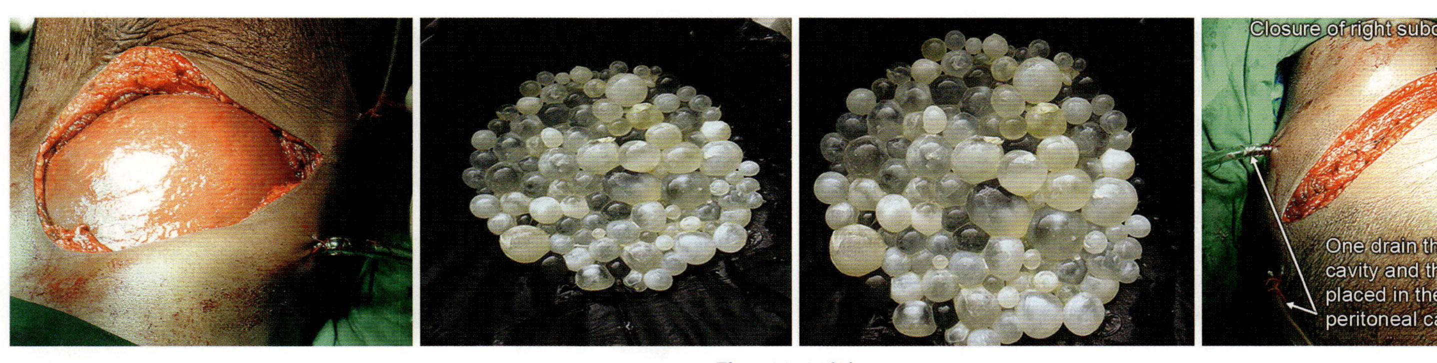

Figs. 23-44(3)

Figs. 23-44(1 to 3): Hydatid cyst—conservative decompression—drainage procedure; it is commonly advocated, reasonably safe, simple and easier than radical surgeries for hydatid cyst of liver.

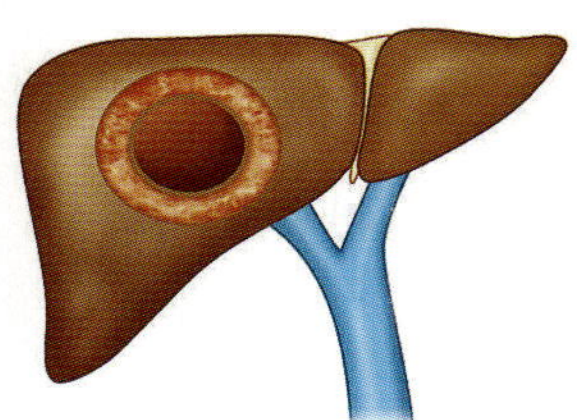

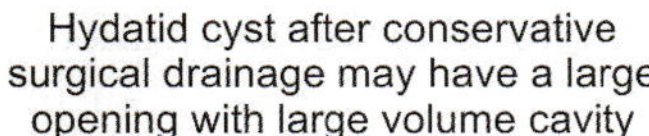

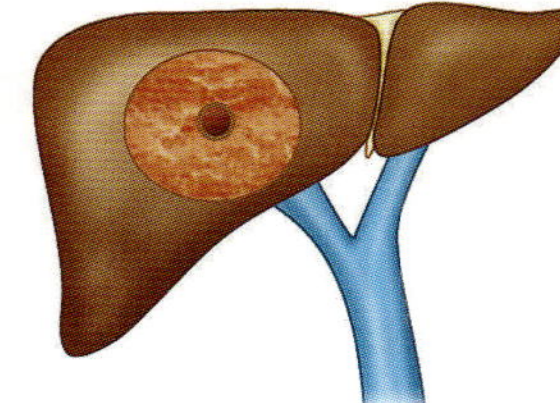

Fig. 23-45: Large and small opening of large volume/cavity hydatid cyst.

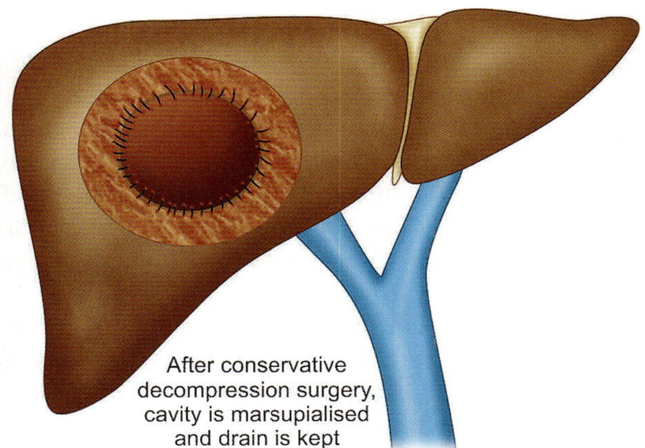

Fig. 23-46: Hydatid cyst—marsupialisation of the cyst wall and cavity.

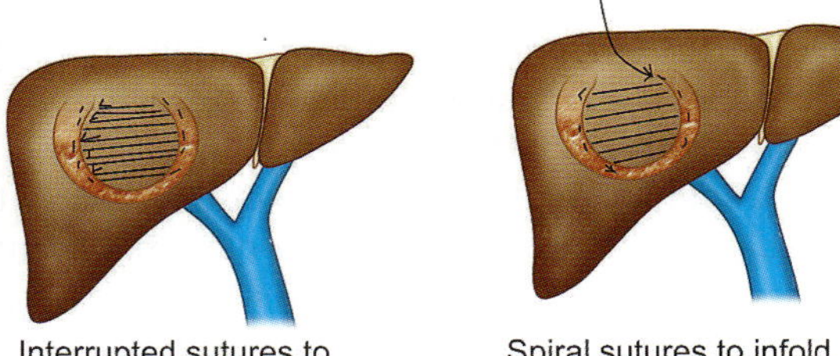

Fig. 23-47: Hydatid cyst—cavity obliteration by capitonage.

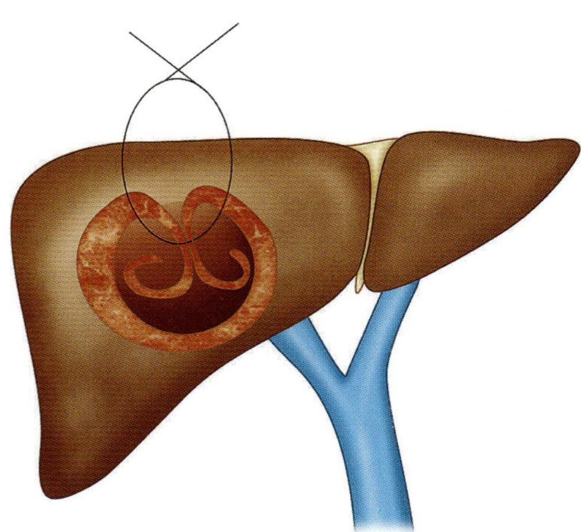

Fig. 23-48: Hydatid cyst—obliteration of cavity by introflexion.

Deep seated cysts and those close to major veins may not be candidates for pericystectomy and formal hemihepatectomy may be indicated. Access to the abdomen is gained like for any major liver surgery. Abdomen is carefully explored for presence of any extrahepatic disease. Povidine-iodine soaked mops need to be kept ready in case of spillage of the cyst contents. Intraoperative ultrasound is helpful to determine the relation of the cyst to the hepatic veins and vena cava. The cyst on the surface are separated from the under surface of the diaphragm. The central venous pressure is kept under 5 mmHg to decrease the intraoperative blood loss. The portal inflow is taped and kept ready in case there is need for inflow occlusion due to bleeding. Stay sutures are placed in the liver parenchyma around the emerging part of the cyst to enable traction and better exposure during resection. The liver capsule is incised using diathermy. The identification of the right plane around the cyst capsule is important to decrease intraoperative blood loss. The parenchyma around the cyst is dissected out using Kelly clamp method or any available energy source. Attention must be paid to identify any biliary radicles communicating with the cyst. In case of difficulty, the procedure can be abandoned in favour of deroofing of the cyst and evacuation of the contents. After giving good wash inside a careful inspection is done to identify biliary communications if any and they are underrun. Omentum can be used to plug the cyst cavity.

Complications of Surgery

Biliary leak is the most important complication in large hydatid disease surgeries. Causes are—persistent cystobiliary communications; biliary tree injury; retained debris in CBD; calcified cyst. Conservative treatment with or without ERCP and sphincterotomy is usually sufficient.

Infection is one of the most common complications after hydatid cyst surgery; often patient develops septicaemia. Subphrenic abscess, liver abscess formation are not uncommon which should be addressed accordingly by antibiotics and guided external drainage using a tube.

Liver failure is the most dreaded complication especially very large cyst. Often patient succumbs to liver failure.

Respiratory problems like bronchopneumonia and ARDS can occur which should be addressed accordingly with ICU care.

Recurrences during long-term follow-up can also occur due to retained scolices or part of the germinative membrane. Progression of disease at different sites as secondary hydatids can occur which should be addressed depends on the site of the cyst. Recurrence rate is 1-30% in different studies. Initial surgical precision plays a major role in recurrence incidences.

B. GALLBLADDER WITH EXTRAHEPATIC BILIARY TREE

SURGICAL ANATOMY

Gallbladder

It is a pear-shaped (size is 5–12 cm) reservoir, located in a fossa on the inferior surface of the liver. Four parts of gallbladder are fundus, body, infundibulum and neck. *Hartmann's pouch* is pathological one located in the infundibular region created by gallstones. The hepatic surface is attached to liver by connective tissue of liver capsule; non-hepatic surface and fundus is covered by peritoneum. Body of the gallbladder is covered by peritoneum on the non-hepatic surface and is related to transverse colon, and 1st and 2nd portions of the duodenum. In 4% of individuals body has got its own mesentery. Such gallbladder is called as *floating/roving gallbladder* and is prone for torsion and gangrene. Body of the gallbladder is related to transverse colon and 1st and 2nd part of the duodenum.

Gallbladder drains through cystic duct into common hepatic duct to form common bile duct. It is supplied by cystic artery, a branch of right hepatic artery. *Calot's triangle* is (Calot, 1891; cholecystohepatic triangle) formed by common hepatic duct on the left, cystic duct and gallbladder below, and inferior surface of liver above. Cystic artery originating from right hepatic artery passes behind the common hepatic duct enters the Calot's triangle to reach the gallbladder. It contains lymph node of *'Lund' (Fred Bates Lund)*. Often cystic artery, hepatic artery, cystic duct have anomalous positions and anomalous origins. Both gallbladder neck and cystic duct contain mucosal fold called *valves of Heister*. Gallbladder is pear-shaped with 50 mL capacity. *Fundus* is in the summit like a dome and is covered fully by peritoneum; it projects beyond the liver margin. It contains smooth muscle. This part is anastomosed to small bowel while doing cholecystojejunostomy. *Body* contains mainly elastic tissue which is a storage part; in deeper plane it is attached to liver and outer part is attached to peritoneal cavity. Body tapers into *neck* like a funnel lying on the free border of hepatoduodenal ligament; its distended convexity is called as *infundibulum*/Hartmann's pouch (pathological). *Lining* of the gallbladder is columnar epithelium which contains cholesterol and fat globules. The *mucus* secreted into the gallbladder originates in the globular cells of tubuloalveolar glands lining the mucosa of infundibulum and neck **(Figs. 23-49 to 23-52)**.

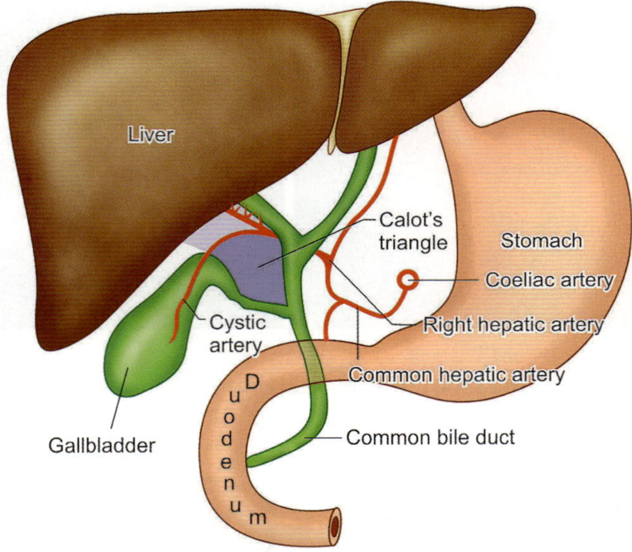

Fig. 23-49: Anatomy of gallbladder and Calot's triangle.

Extrahepatic Biliary Tree

The left hepatic duct is formed by the ducts draining II, III, IV segments of the liver. The right hepatic duct is formed by the ducts draining V, VI, VII, VIII segments of the liver. Both join to form the *common hepatic duct (CHD)*, which joins with the cystic duct to form the *common bile duct (CBD)*. Junction of right and left hepatic ducts to form common hepatic duct is 0.25–2.5 cm from the surface of the liver. Left duct is longer (about 1.7 cm) than right hepatic duct which is 0.9 cm. Occasionally this junction may be intrahepatic due to enlargement of the liver. Common hepatic duct is variable in length from 1.5 cm to 3.5 cm. When cystic duct joins the junction of the right and left hepatic ducts then common hepatic duct is considered as absent. Cystohepatic junction may be angular, parallel and spiral.

Cystic duct is 3 mm in diameter and 2–4 cm in length. Variations are common. During surgery these variations should be remembered to avoid inadvertent injury to common bile duct.

Common bile duct is normally 5–12 cm in length and 6–8 mm in diameter. Length depends on the position where cystic duct joins. It has got 4 parts—(1) *Supraduodenal* with a length of 2 cm; (2) *Retroduodenal* part with a length of 1.5 cm; (3) *Pancreatic part* with a length of 3.0 cm; (4) *Intramural/intraduodenal* part with a length of 1.1 cm. Length of each part is variable. Supraduodenal portion lies in the two leaves of the hepatoduodenal ligament, in front of the portal vein to the right of the proper hepatic artery. Retroduodenal part runs from the superior margin of the 1st part of the duodenum to upper margin of the head of the pancreas. Gastroduodenal artery is left of the duct; posterior superior pancreaticoduodenal artery crosses the duct first in front of the duct later behind it just before it joins the duodenum. Common bile duct may be covered partly by pancreas (44%) or fully (embedded in the pancreas—30%) or not covered by pancreas (16%) or covered by two leaves. It joins the major pancreatic duct in the wall of the 2nd part of duodenum to form the *ampulla of Vater*. Intraduodenal part of common bile duct (CBD) is surrounded by smooth muscle fibres called as *sphincter of Oddi*. CBD if more than 8 mm diameter is pathological. Pancreatic CBD is palpable from behind after Kocher's duodenal mobilisation. Intraduodenal part is oblique in the duodenal wall running for 1.5 cm. Here CBD diameter reduces from 5.5 to 3.5 mm. Pancreatic and bile ducts are initially separated by a septum with a common adventitia for 5–10 mm which then eventually forms a confluence of ducts **(Figs. 23-53 and 23-54)**.

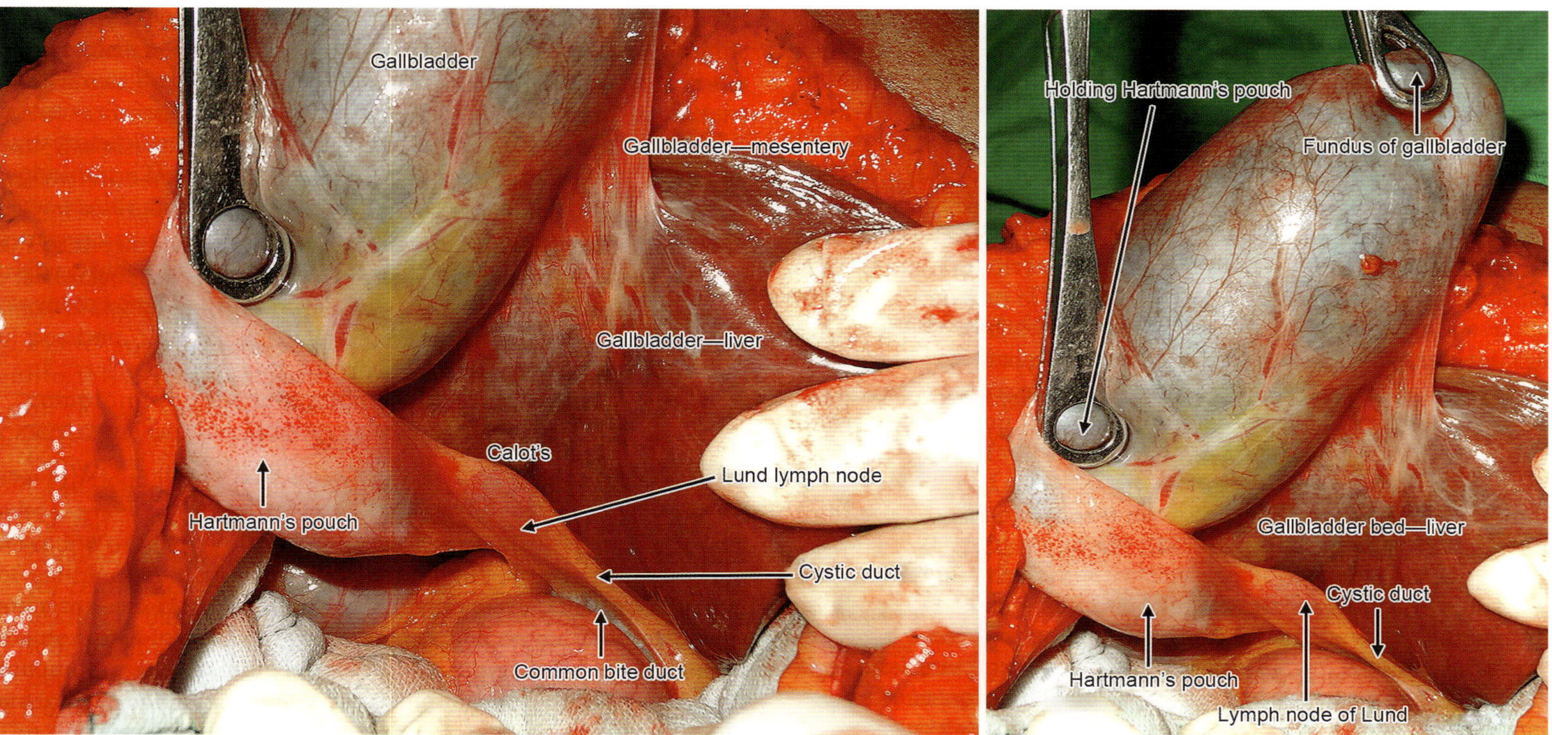

Fig. 23-50: Gallbladder—surgical anatomy as it looks in open method.

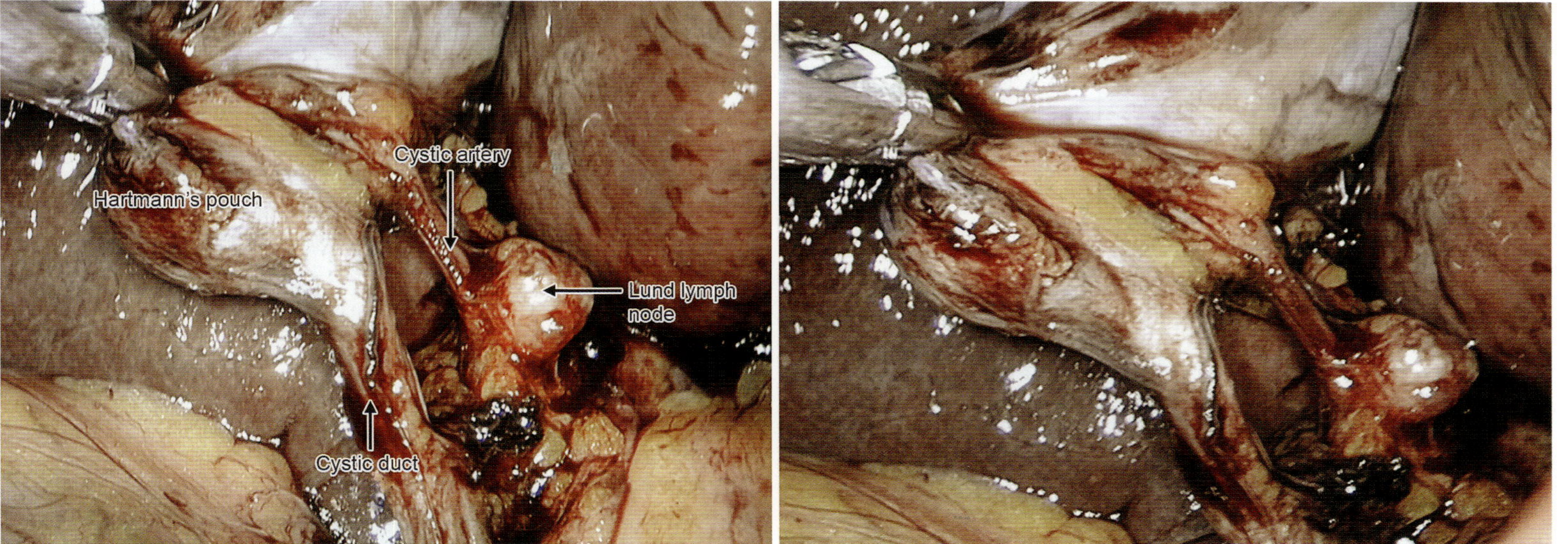

Fig. 23-51: Laparoscopic view of the Calot's triangle with lymph node of Lund.

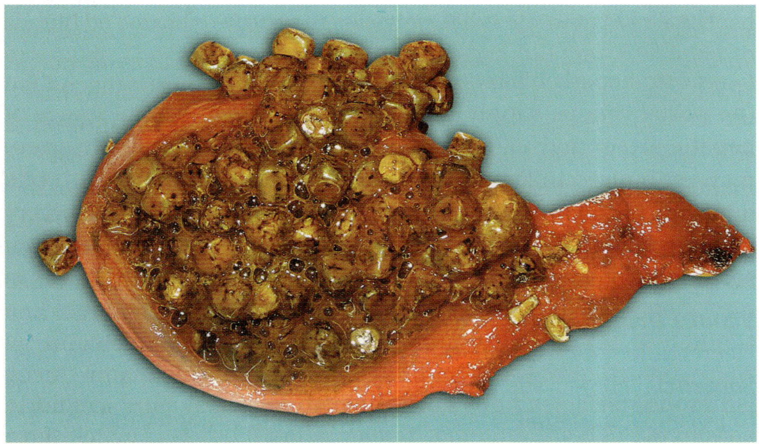

Fig. 23-52: Gallbladder stones—multiple—after removal.

Blood Supply

Arterial Supply

Gallbladder receives its blood supply from cystic artery which is a branch of right hepatic artery or aberrant hepatic artery. Right hepatic artery runs behind the common hepatic duct (87%), often it may be in front of common hepatic duct (13%). Incidence of aberrant right hepatic artery is 15–20%; cystic artery arises from this (in 80% cases) when it is present.

Aberrant right hepatic artery may replace right hepatic artery (12–16%) or may be accessory to existing right hepatic artery (4–5%). Aberrant/accessory right hepatic artery arises from superior mesenteric artery.

Anomalies of left hepatic artery is important. Left hepatic artery may originate from left gastric artery in 5% of cases. In such patients

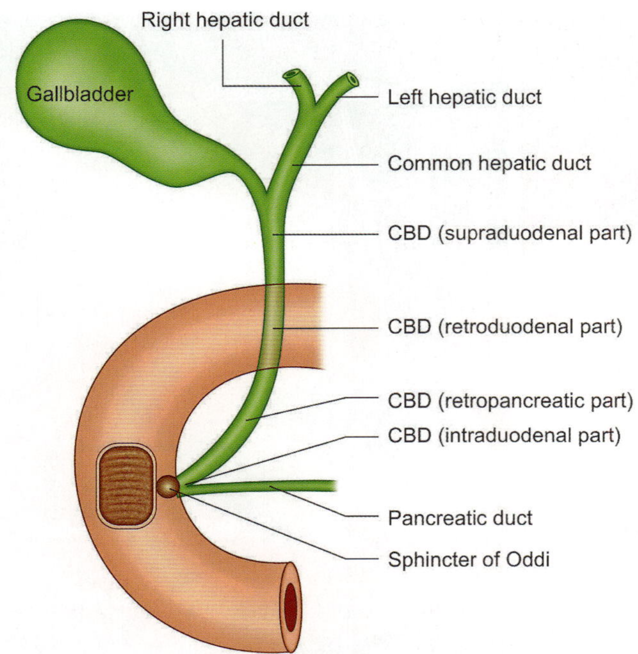

Fig. 23-53: Parts of common bile duct.

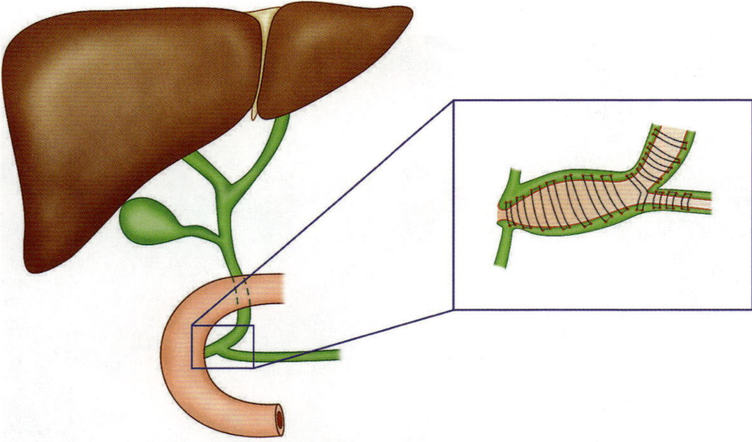

Fig. 23-54: Sphincter of Oddi—surgical anatomy.

during gastrectomy, while dissecting and ligating this, *aberrant left hepatic artery* may get ligated causing devascularisation of the left lobe of the liver. Often normal left hepatic artery is present originating from common (proper) hepatic artery as usual; but additionally an *accessory left hepatic artery* arising from left gastric artery may also be present (5%).

Cystic artery after its origin, runs towards the neck of the gallbladder where it divides into superficial (anterior) and deep (posterior) branches. Cystic artery as *variation* may arise from left hepatic or proper hepatic or common hepatic or gastroduodenal arteries.

Bile and hepatic ducts are supplied by gastroduodenal, retroduodenal, right and left hepatic and posterosuperior pancreaticoduodenal arteries. One should not devascularise more than 3 cm of the surface of the common bile duct. Supraduodenal bile duct derives its blood supply from retroduodenal artery (60% from below and 38% from above) through right hepatic artery. Bile duct ischaemia should be avoided while doing choledochojejunostomy or choledochoduodenostomy. Two arteries run parallel in the common bile duct at 3 and 9 o'clock position. Interruption of these two arteries lead into bile duct stricture.

Afferent arteries supply the bile duct. Bile duct is not supplied by portal venous system unlike liver. Afferent arteries are gastroduodenal, retroduodenal, right and left hepatic and posterosuperior pancreaticoduodenal arteries. Afferent arteries empty into the marginal arteries which run at 3 and 9 o'clock positions longitudinally along the common bile duct and common hepatic duct. Hilar marginal artery is located at the upper angle of the confluence of right and left hepatic ducts. These marginal arteries form fine network of epicholedochal plexus on the surface of the bile duct, common, right and left hepatic ducts. At the confluence of right and left hepatic ducts confluence it forms hilar plexus. These plexus will not extend above beyond the fibrous sheath of the hilar plate. So dissection above hilar plate should be done with the sheath itself, not between sheath and hepatic ducts **(Fig. 23-55)**.

Transection of the bile duct at superior most part makes lower cut edge ischaemic; transection at inferior part close to duodenum makes upper cut edge ischaemic. So in bile duct transection (traumatic/iatrogenic), primary anastomosis (choledochocholedochal) is not safer and is not practiced.

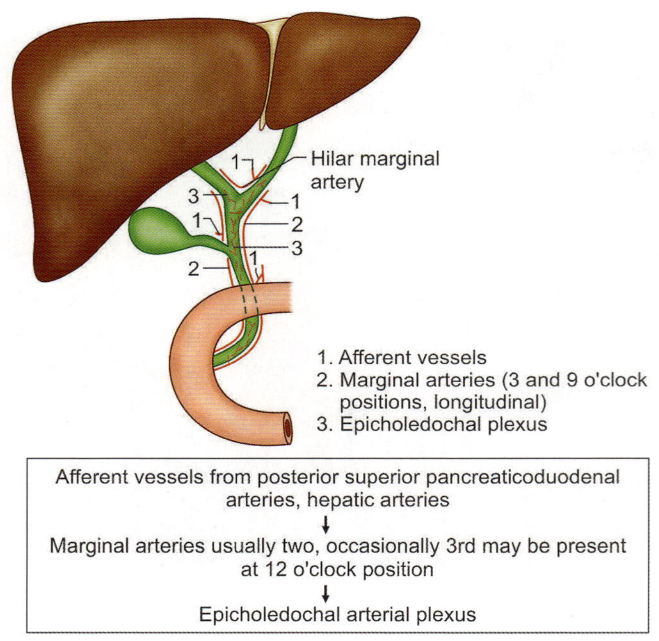

Fig. 23-55: Pattern of blood vessels in extrahepatic biliary apparatus.

As extrahepatic biliary tree is supplied by hepatic arterial system (no portal venous supply) unlike dual supply of liver, blockage of hepatic artery may cause bile duct necrosis. Right hepatic artery may get injured in laparoscopic cholecystectomy along with bile duct injury. It may cause ischaemia of bile duct also. During surgery bile duct should be divided sharply; it should not be dissected from surrounding tissue to main epicholedochal plexus.

Venous Drainage

Deep cholecystic veins in the gallbladder bed drains into the liver. Superficial cholecystic veins drain upwards to liver and downwards to portal vein. Usually these veins are less prominent and will not cause significant bleeding after division. But in portal biliopathy gallbladder and choledochal varices will develop which may cause torrential bleeding on dissection **(Fig. 23-56)**.

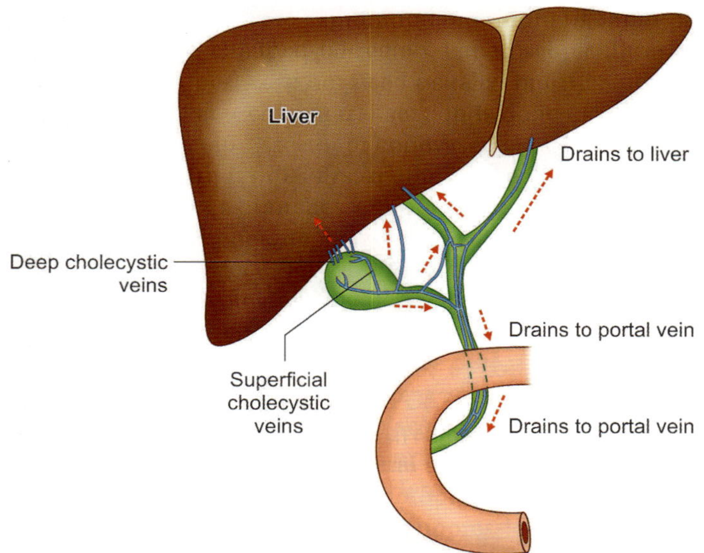

Fig. 23-56: Veins in biliary system—extrahepatic.

Lymphatic Drainage

Gallbladder drains into the cystic node at the junction of the cystic and common hepatic ducts (lymph node of *Lund*); from here to the '*node of the hiatus*' and posterior pancreaticoduodenal nodes. The *pericholedochal nodes* get their afferent lymphatics from extrahepatic bile duct and right lobe of the liver **(Fig. 23-57)**.

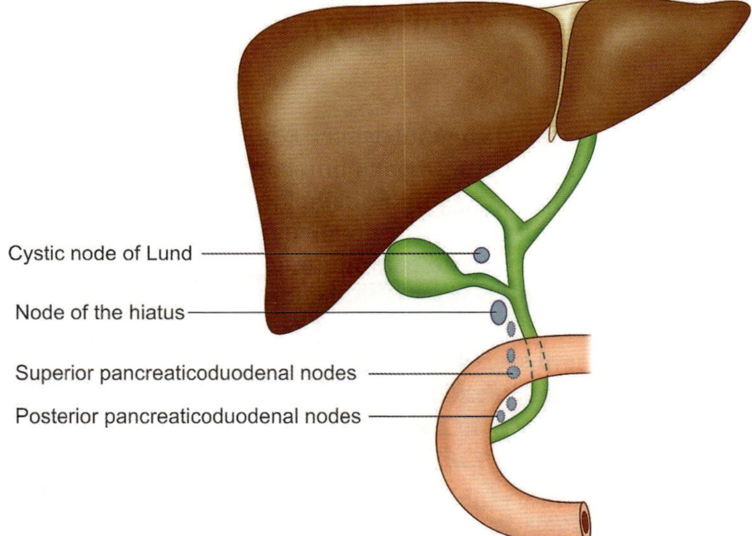

Fig. 23-57: Lymphatics of biliary system.

Bile

Daily up to 1000 mL of bile is secreted from the liver which contains water (98%), bile salts, bile pigments, fatty acids, lecithin, cholesterol, and electrolytes (sodium, potassium, chloride, bicarbonate, calcium, magnesium) with a pH more than 7.0. Main function of gallbladder is to concentrate and store the bile. Capacity of gallbladder is 40–50 mL. Bile salts form micelle which makes cholesterol soluble. Bile salts (i.e. salts of cholic and chenodeoxycholic acids) with formed deoxycholic acid (in the bowel) enter the enterohepatic circulation to get resecreted in the bile. Bilirubin conjugated in the liver is secreted into the bile, which in the bowel is converted into urobilinogen by bacteria. Urobilinogen gets absorbed in the bowel, enters the liver for resecretion again and part of it is excreted in the urine. Absence of urobilinogen in the urine signifies obstructive jaundice. In the absence of gallstones or any other disease, bile is sterile. Symptomatic gallstone disease shows positive culture for bacteria, commonest being *E. coli* and *Klebsiella*.

Congenital Anomalies of Gallbladder and Extrahepatic Biliary Tree

Anomalies of gallbladder may be in number; form; position.

Absence of gallbladder—rare.

Phrygian cap: A cap-like projection and bend over the fundus of the gallbladder (*Phrygia* is an ancient Asian country—Mongolia) (Liberte cap of French revolution). It is identified in cholecystogram. It is 6% common.

Double/triple gallbladder: Additional one may be intrahepatic. Cystic ducts may join to form a common cystic duct which joins the CBD, or cystic duct of each gallbladder may join separately into the CBD.

Mobile/floating/mesenteric gallbladder: Gallbladder has a long mesentery attached. It may cause torsion. It can cause recurrent abdominal pain. It is also called as gallbladder ptosis. Its incidence is 5%. There are three types of floating gallbladder. (1) Gallbladder is completely invested by peritoneum without mesentery and only attachment between liver and gallbladder is cystic duct and artery. (2) Gallbladder is having complete mesentery. (3) Cystic duct and neck of the gallbladder have mesentery with fundus and body are free hanging and ptosed. Such a ptosed gallbladder can position in iliac fossa, lumbar or pelvic region. Torsion is common in elderly, thin people. Its removal is easier through laparoscopic or open method **(Figs. 23-58A and B)**.

Long cystic duct with low insertion of the cystic duct into CBD near the ampulla is possible. This is important in all pancreatic/biliary/laparoscopic biliary surgeries.

Absence of cystic duct with gallbladder directly entering the CBD through a wide opening near infundibulum.

Accessory cholecystohepatic duct (duct of Luschka) may be present (10%) which if not identified and ligated during cholecystectomy will cause biliary fistula/peritonitis due to continuous leak.

Cystic artery may originate anteriorly (15%) from right hepatic artery/from common hepatic artery.

Very tortuous hepatic artery in front of the origin of the cystic duct is called as *Moynihan's caterpillar hump*. It is important cause of bleeding in cholecystectomy.

There may be *double cystic duct* or cystic duct may insert high into the common hepatic duct or right hepatic duct.

Aberrant hepatic duct is a normal segmental duct that joins the biliary tract just outside the liver instead of just within. It drains normal portion of the liver but travels hepatocystic triangle and may get injured during cholecystectomy **(Figs. 23-59 to 23-82)**.

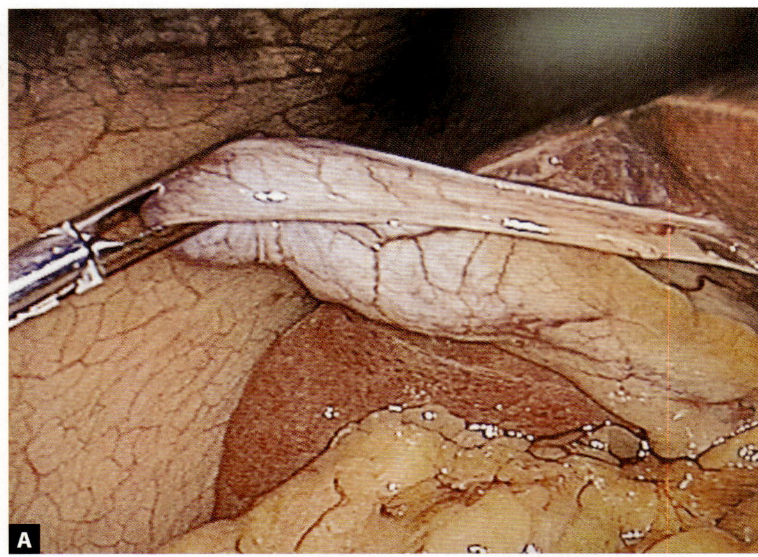

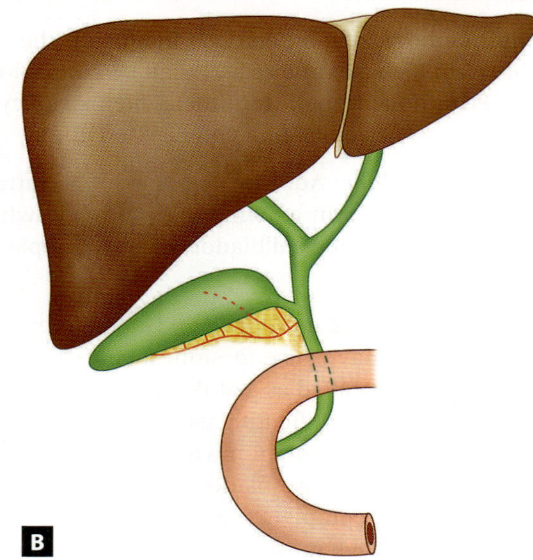

Figs. 23-58A and B: (A) Laparoscopic view of gallbladder mesentery; (B) Diagrammatic look.

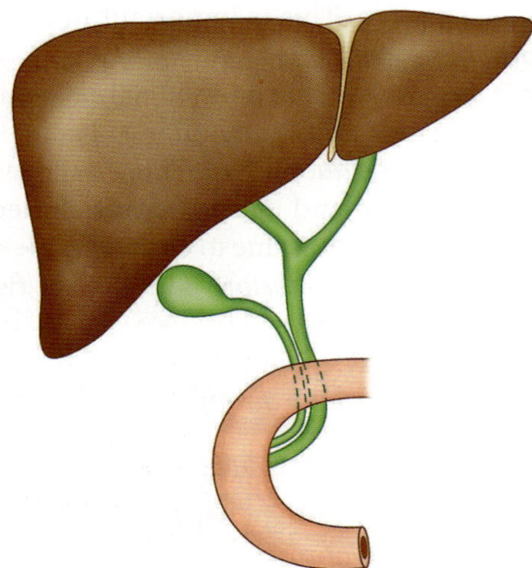

Fig. 23-59: Absence common bile duct; here cystic duct joins duodenum separately.

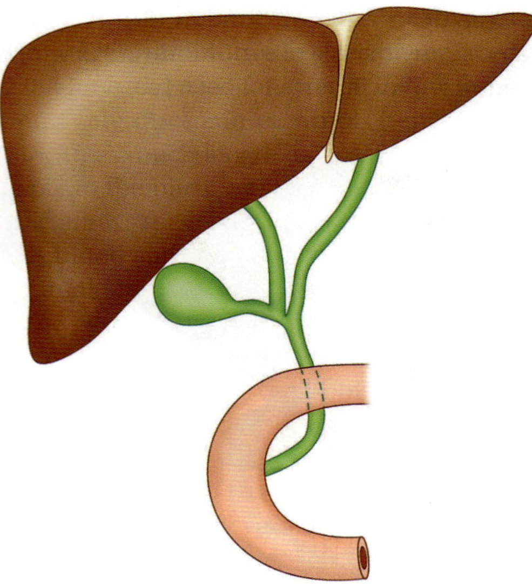

Fig. 23-60: Absence common hepatic duct; here right and hepatic ducts join at the confluence where cystic duct joins the bile duct.

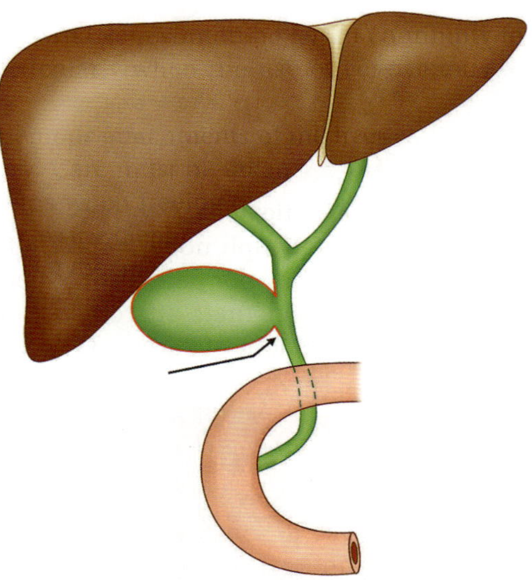

Fig. 23-61: Cystic duct is absent with wide communication into CBD. There is higher chance of CBD injury here.

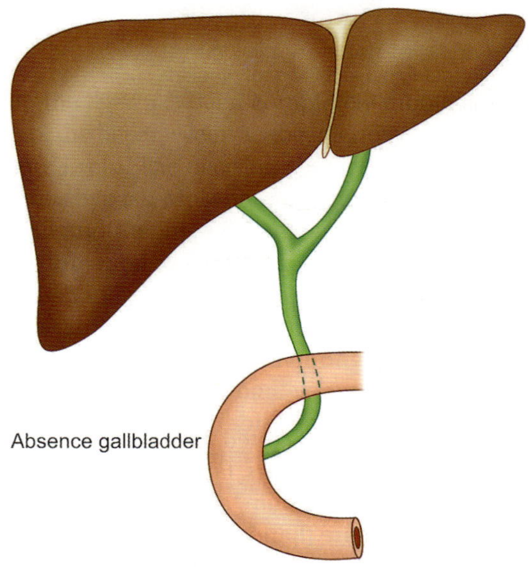

Fig. 23-62: Absent gallbladder.

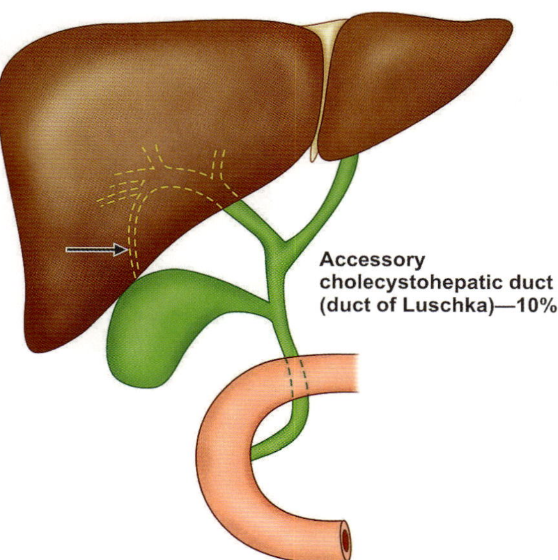

Fig. 23-63: Accessory cholecystohepatic duct (duct of Luschka—10%). It may cause bile leak postoperatively if it is not ligated during cholecystectomy.

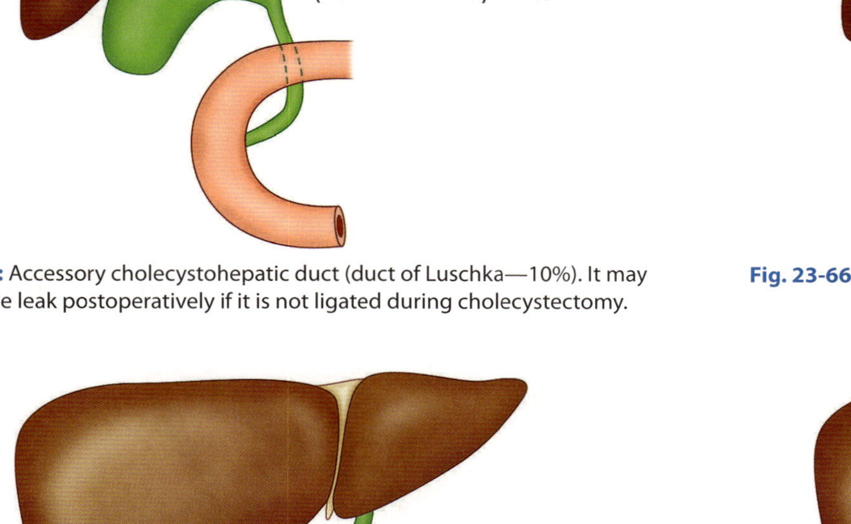

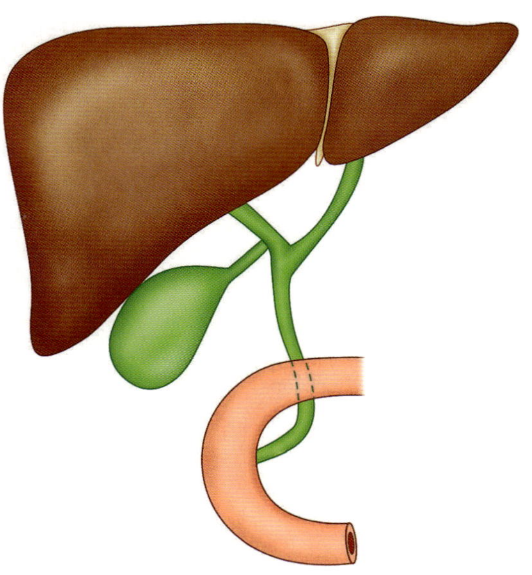

Fig. 23-66: Cystic duct joining the right hepatic duct—a variation.

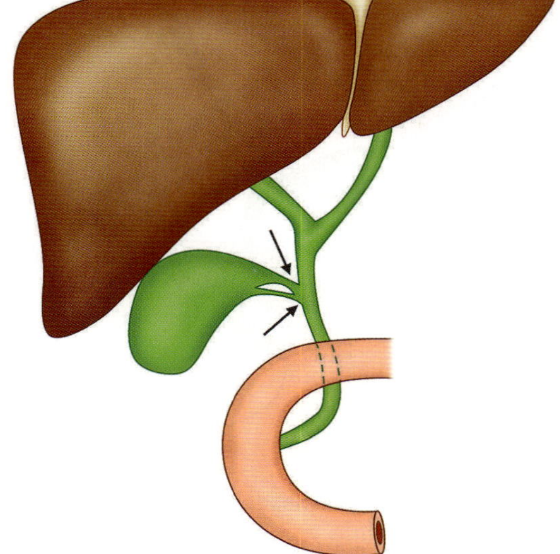

Fig. 23-64: Double cystic ducts from the gallbladder joining the CBD.

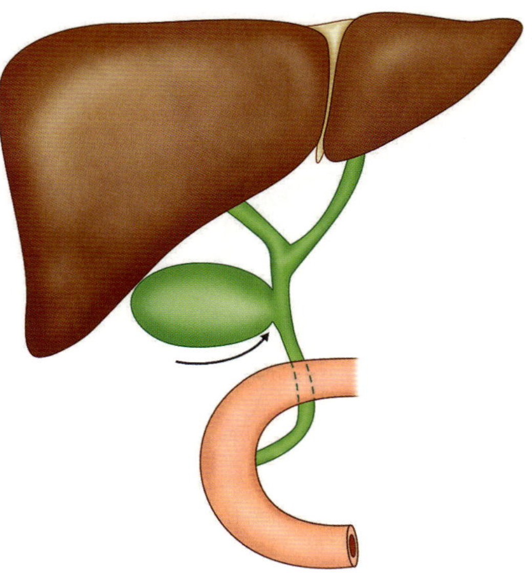

Fig. 23-67: Cystic duct with wide opening into CBD.

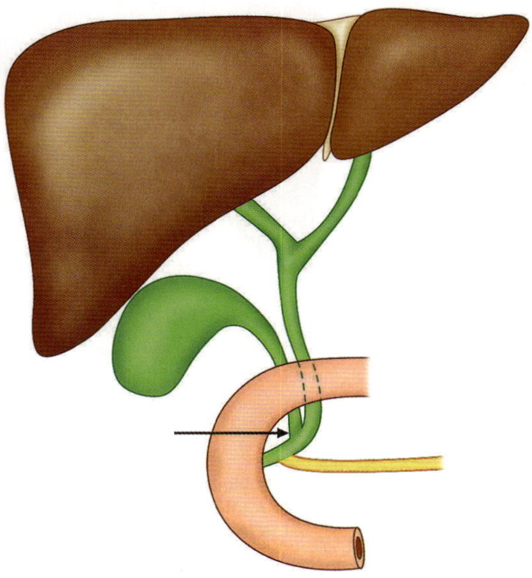

Fig. 23-65: Long cystic duct joining the CBD very low.

PREOPERATIVE PREPARATION AND ASSESSMENT

Outcome in hepatobiliary surgery depends on many factors. (1) *Hepatobiliary function*—Low pressure biliary system with obstruction to all functions of liver cells (synthetic, metabolic, secretory) will be affected. Secretion gets reduced due to increased pressure. If bilirubin is less than 1.5 mg%, mortality is less than 3%; if it becomes more than 20 mg% mortality raises up to or more than 30%. Metabolisms of many drugs are also affected. Bile acid serum level raises and inhibits cytochrome 450 enzymes reducing the oxidation. Albumin, coagulation factors and immunoglobulin synthesis is affected. (2) 50% of obstructive patients have *higher endotoxin level* in blood; it is due to reduced bile salts in intestinal lumen which normally prevents absorption of endotoxins from intestine and bile salts also inhibit anaerobic bacterial growth. So reduced bile salt causes sepsis and endotoxaemia. That also causes acute tubular necrosis, and *renal failure*. Sludging of bile salts in the renal tubules reduces the tubular function by blockage and aggravates the problem.

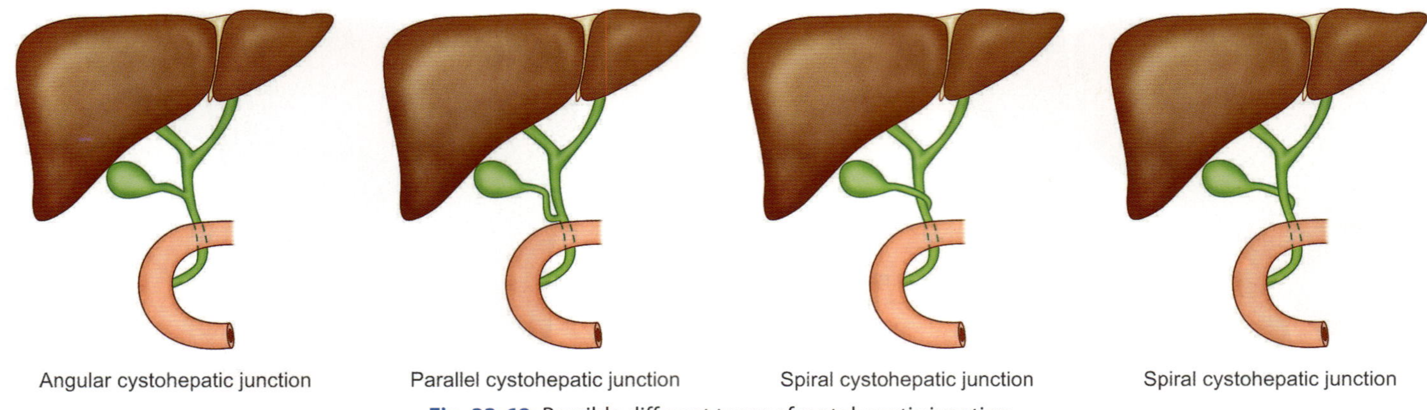

Fig. 23-68: Possible different types of cystohepatic junction.

Fig. 23-69: Phrygian (cap) gallbladder.

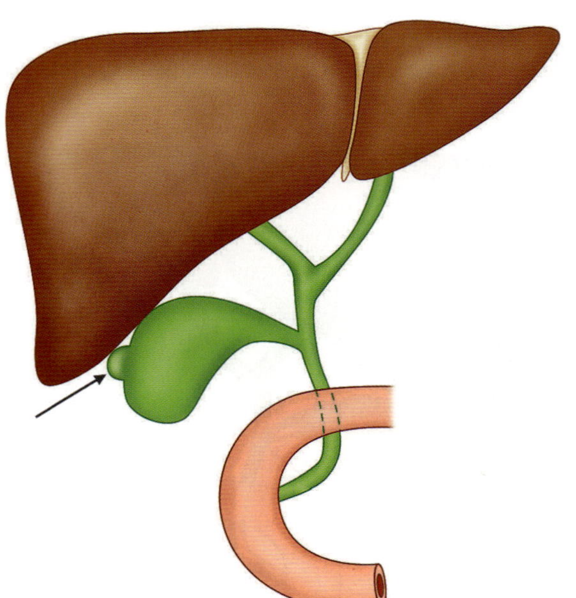

Fig. 23-70: Gallbladder diverticulum.

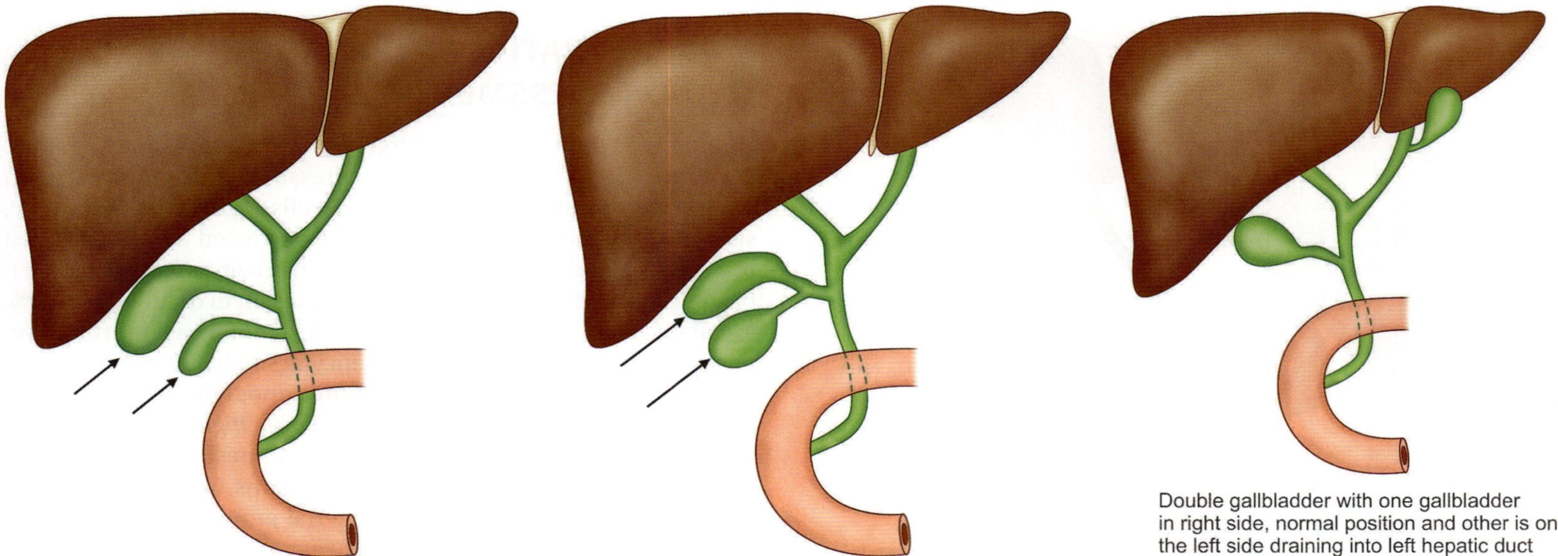

Fig. 23-71: Double gallbladder. One may be intrahepatic. It may have separate cystic ducts joining common bile duct (CBD) or two cystic ducts join to form single duct to join the CBD. One gallbladder may be on right side, other one on left side.

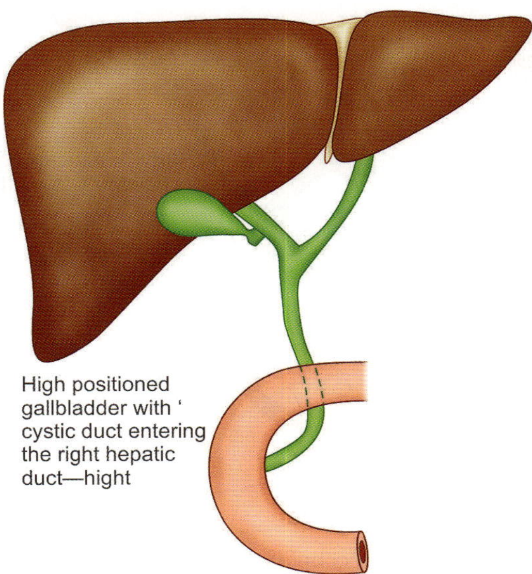

Fig. 23-72: High position gallbladder.

Mannitol probably and also proper hydration prevents this problem in tubules. (3) *Bleeding tendencies*—Vitamin K absorption from the intestine is reduced due to decrease in bile acids in the lumen. It prolongs the prothrombin time. This can be corrected by giving IM or IV vitamin K. Endotoxin absorption is increased due to reduced bile acids in the gut which causes recurrent mild disseminated intravascular coagulation (DIC) and raise in fibrin degradation products. It causes tendency for bleeding during surgery and postoperative period. Additionally defective coagulation factor synthesis, hypersplenism (if there is cirrhosis) and fibrinolysins in circulation aggravates the thrombocytopaenia. (4) *Nutritional deficiencies*—Obstructive jaundice causes severe malnutrition with anorexia and weight loss. Pancreatic head or periampullary pathology causes duodenal obstruction and also poor exocrine and endocrine function of the pancreas. (5) *Altered body resistance and immunity with sepsis*—Obstructive jaundice causes defect in T cell proliferation, phagocytosis, delayed hypersensitivity reaction. It reduces the defensive function of the Kupffer cell to phagocytose and neutralise endotoxins. (6) *Gut endotoxins* are increased due to reduced gut bile acids (bile acids emulsify endotoxins);

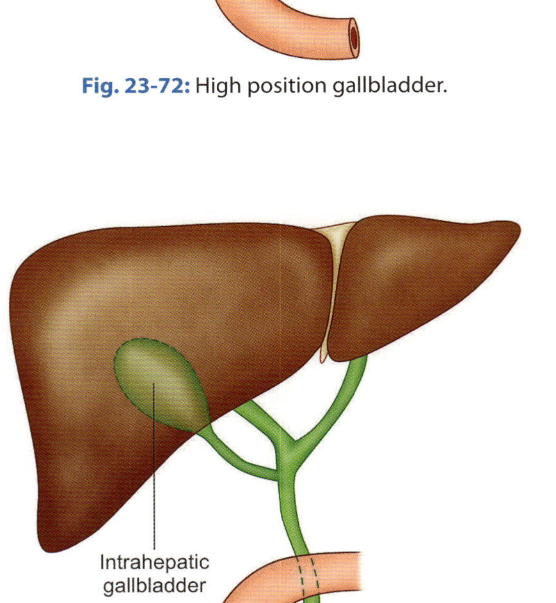

Fig. 23-73: Intrahepatic gallbladder.

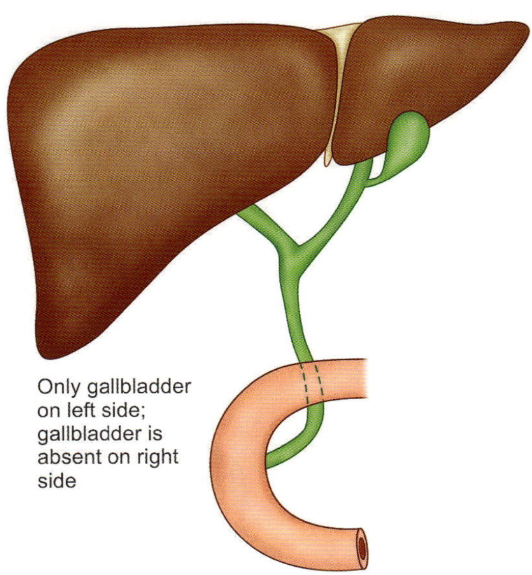

Fig. 23-74: Gallbladder is present only on left side joining left hepatic duct.

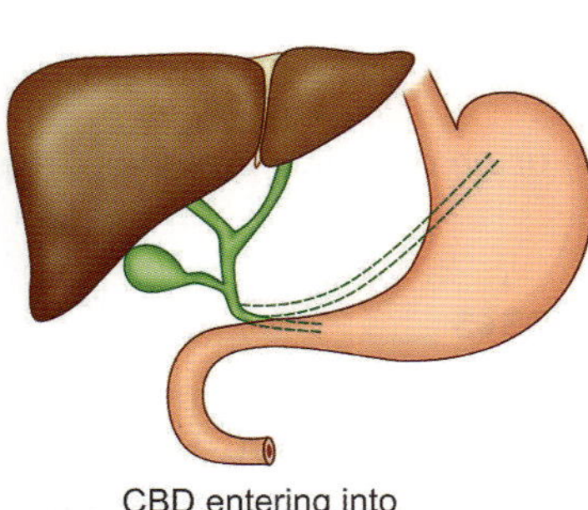

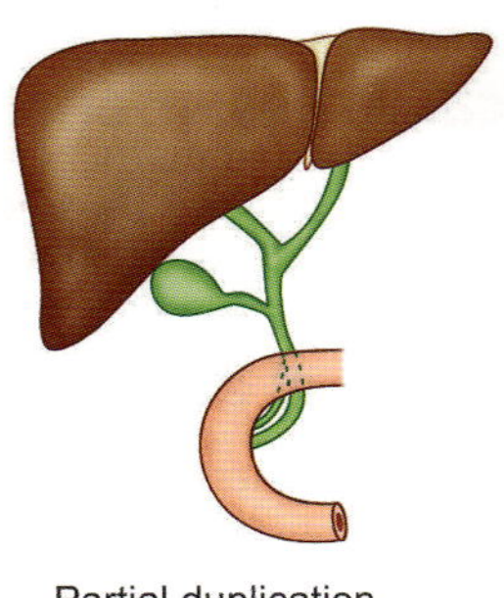

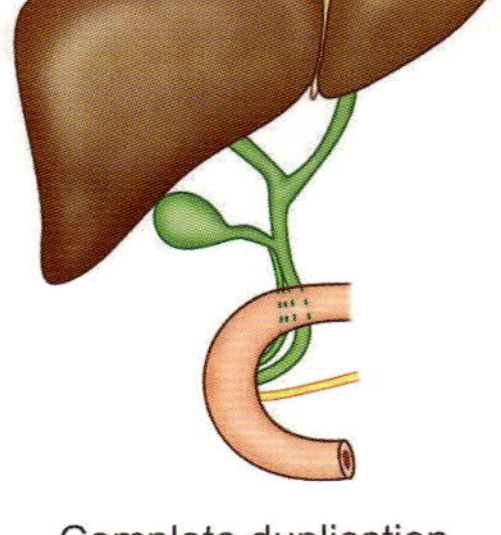

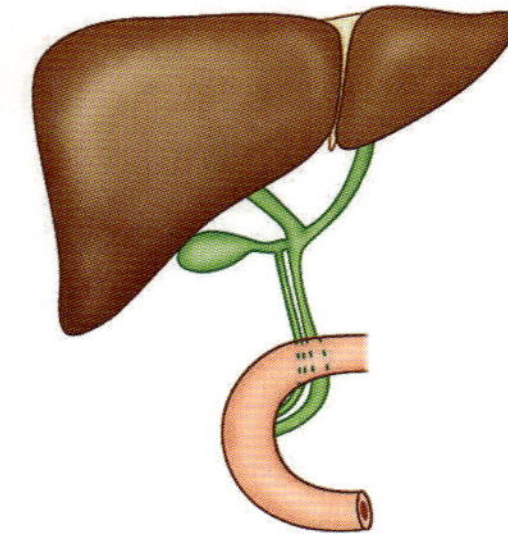

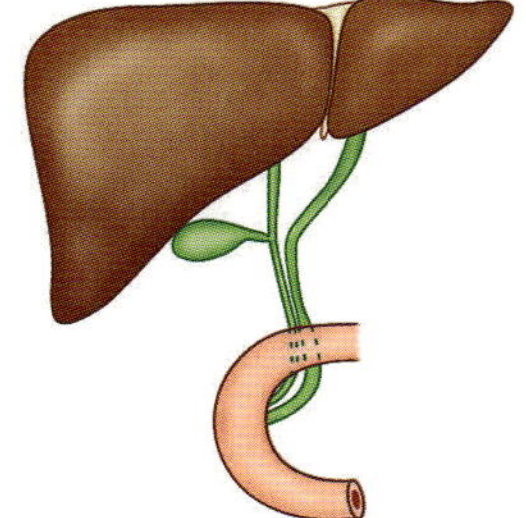

Fig. 23-75: Duplications of common bile duct.

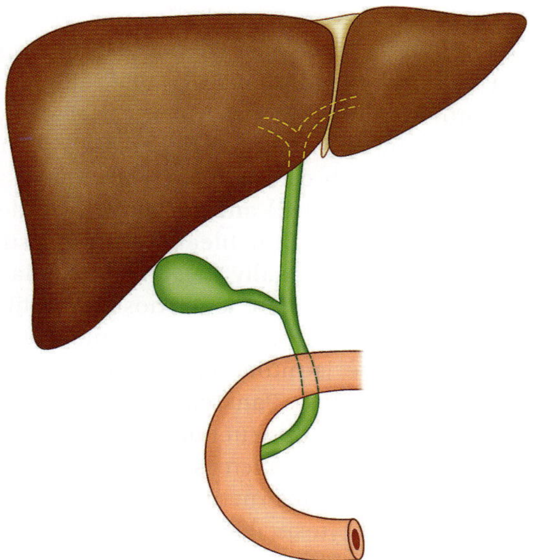

Fig. 23-76: Right and left hepatic duct junction is intrahepatic deep to hepatic plate/hilum.

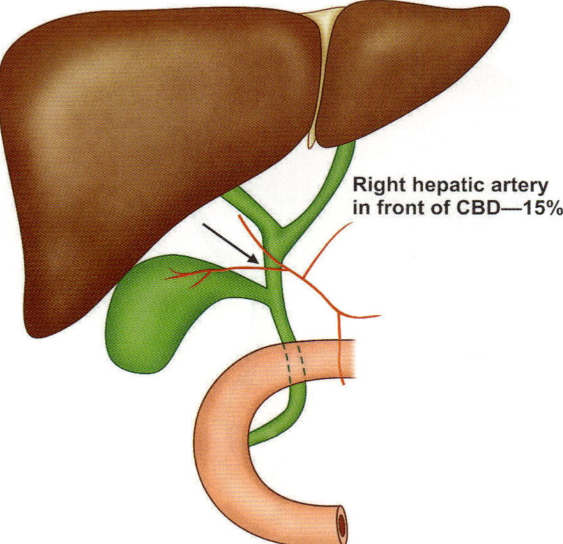

Fig. 23-78: Cystic artery originates from right hepatic artery which is anterior to common bile duct.

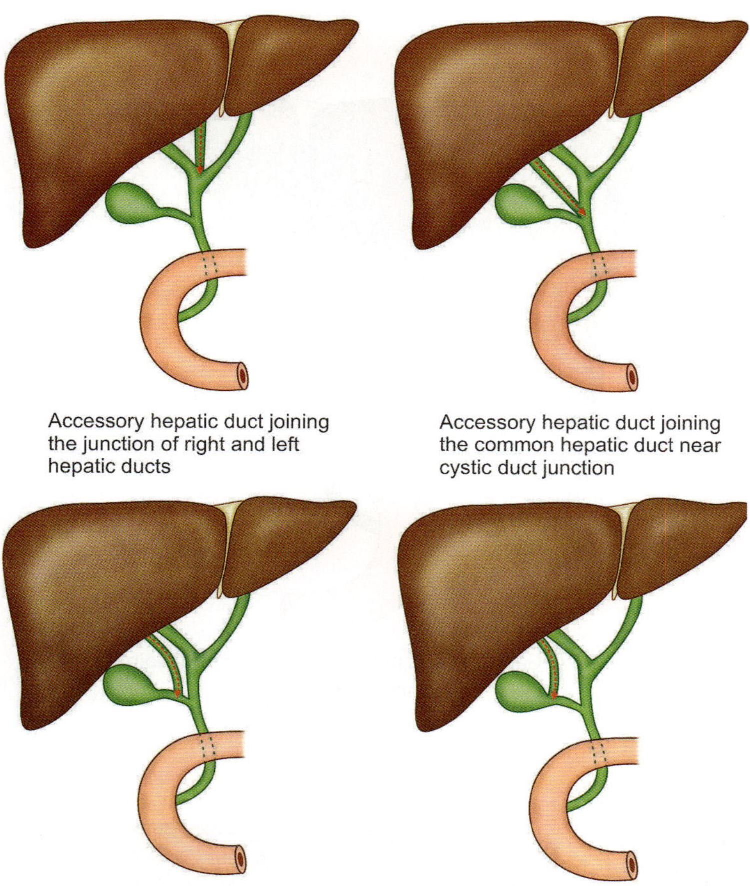

Fig. 23-77: Different types of multiple hepatic ducts.

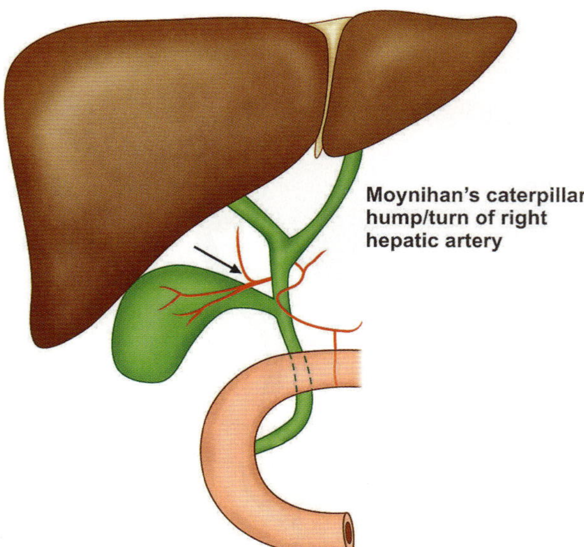

Fig. 23-79: Moynihan's caterpillar turn/hump is bending of right hepatic artery in front of/close to cystic duct. It may get injured during cholecystectomy causing torrential haemorrhage.

there will be increased bacterial translocation across the gut; this overall will increase the sepsis rate in obstructive jaundice patient. (7) Obstructive jaundice reduces the *activity of propylhydroxylase enzyme* in the skin (enzyme helps proline attachment to collagen) and so diminishes the effective collagen formation and its strength. So burst abdomen and incisional hernia is common. (8) *Cardiac problems*—Obstructive jaundice causes decreased contractility; poor response to drugs; decreased peripheral vascular resistance; hypovolaemia. Raised serum bile acids cause diuresis and natriuresis.

ASSESSMENT

Clinical Assessment

Jaundice **(Fig. 23-83)**, fever, chills, urine output, weight loss, mass abdomen to be looked for.

Biochemical and Blood Tests

Liver function tests; serum amylase, lipase; renal function tests; coagulation profile (V, VII, IX, X, prothrombin, fibrinogen); prothrombin time (INR); platelet count; urine-bilirubin, urobilinogen, bile salts; reticulocyte count, osmotic fragility test, Coomb's test. In obstruction—direct bilirubin and serum alkaline phosphatase (very sensitive indicator of obstruction) is raised. But serum alkaline phosphatase is raised in bone diseases also; 5'-nucleotidase and

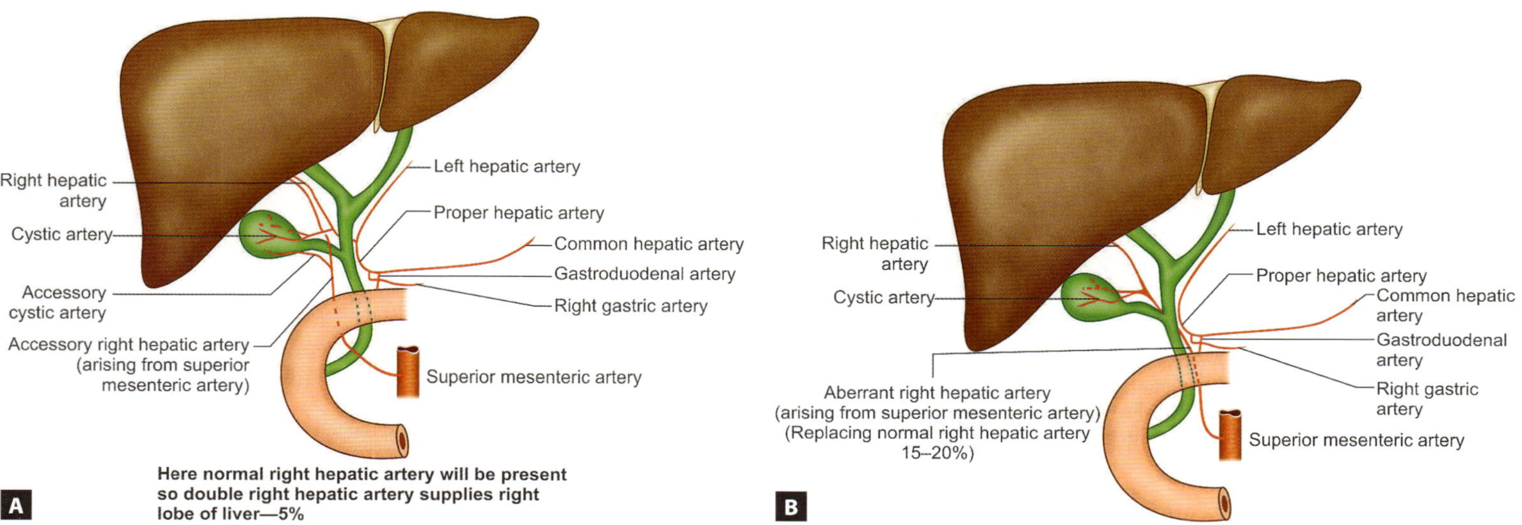

Figs. 23-80A and B: Accessory right hepatic artery originates from superior mesenteric artery additional to normally located right hepatic artery; aberrant right hepatic artery arising similarly from superior mesenteric artery but replacing the normal right hepatic artery.

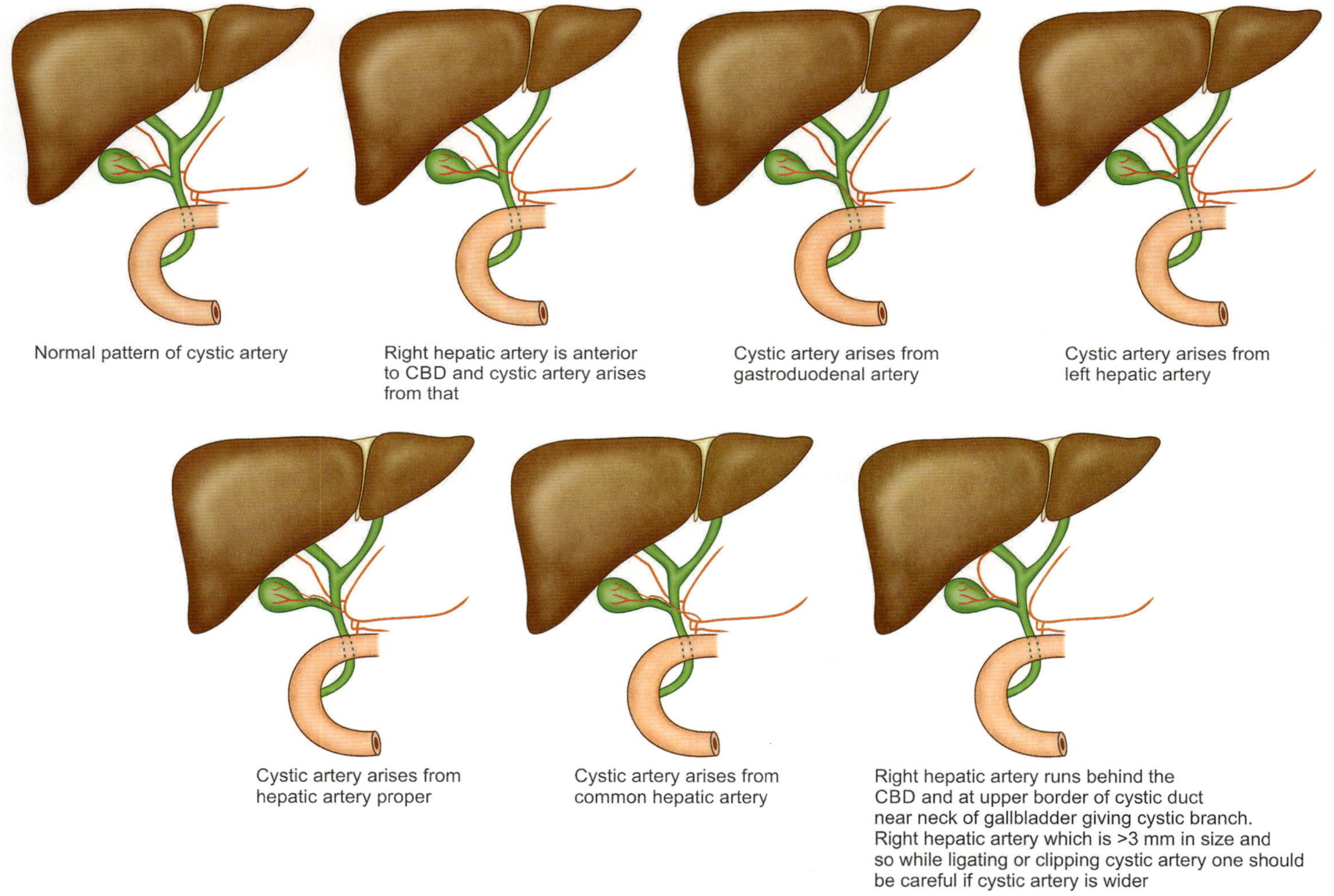

Normal pattern of cystic artery

Right hepatic artery is anterior to CBD and cystic artery arises from that

Cystic artery arises from gastroduodenal artery

Cystic artery arises from left hepatic artery

Cystic artery arises from hepatic artery proper

Cystic artery arises from common hepatic artery

Right hepatic artery runs behind the CBD and at upper border of cystic duct near neck of gallbladder giving cystic branch. Right hepatic artery which is >3 mm in size and so while ligating or clipping cystic artery one should be careful if cystic artery is wider

Fig. 23-81: Variations in cystic artery—different from normal.

serum γ-glutamyl transferase level raise are specific for hepatocytes as they are not found in bone. Serum alanine aminotransferase (ALT; it is predominantly found inside hepatocytes), raise suggests liver injury; degree of liver injury is assessed by serum albumin and prothrombin time. High levels of direct bilirubin more than 20 mg% may suggest malignant obstruction.

Imaging

Plain X-ray abdomen is of less use in identifying the gallstones (10%). It is useful to diagnose biliary fistula, emphysematous cholecystitis.

Ultrasound is good investigation to detect gallstones, and biliary dilatation. Normal size of the CBD is 8 mm; more than 10 mm

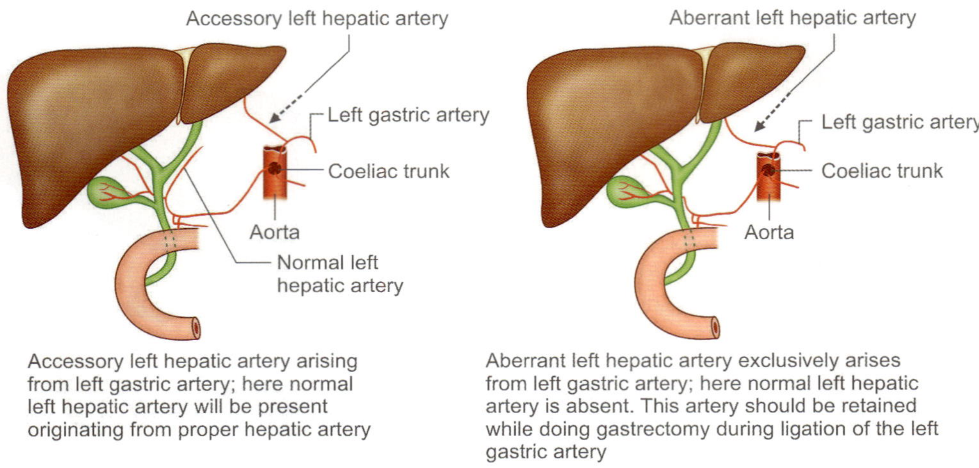

Fig. 23-82: Anomalies of left hepatic artery.

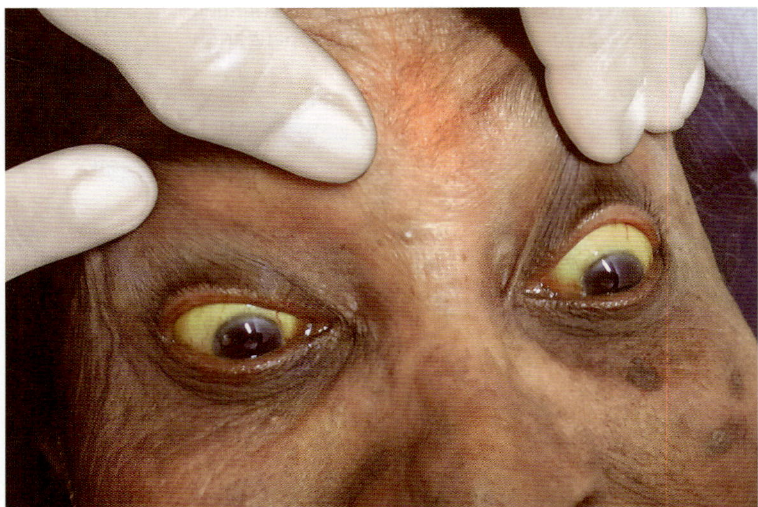

Fig. 23-83: Typical obstructive jaundice.

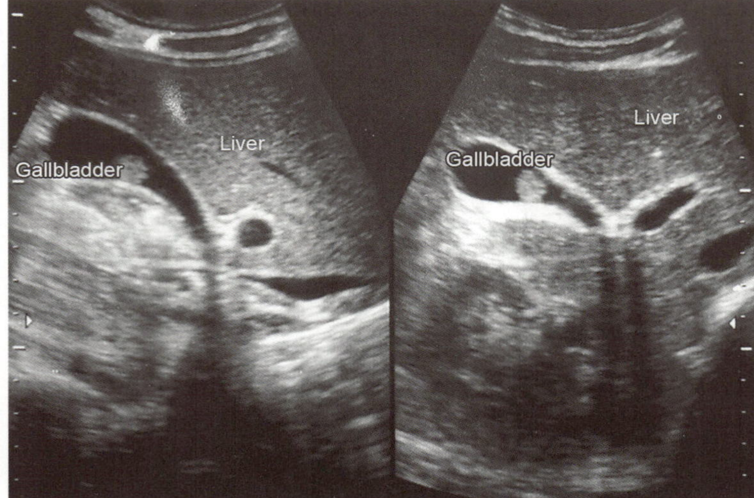

Fig. 23-84: Ultrasound abdomen showing gallbladder stone and normal sized CBD.

suggests dilatation. However, its accuracy rate is only 80%. Stones in CBD and hepatic ducts are difficult to identify by ultrasound. Ultrasound cannot pick up malignancy which is a differential diagnosis for obstructive jaundice **(Fig. 23-84)**.

CT scan is effective in identifying non-dilated ducts and stones within. Anatomy is better seen with 90% accuracy. CT is better to rule out malignancy in head of pancreas or periampullary region **(Figs. 23-85A and B)**.

MRI and **MRCP** are better to identify the biliary tree. It gives idea about venous anatomy and parenchymal status **(Fig. 23-86)**.

Endoscopic retrograde cholangiopancreatography (ERCP): Through a side viewing gastroduodenoscope, sphincter of Oddi is cannulated, and dye is injected. Biliary and pancreatic trees are visualised. It is done under C-arm guidance and sedation like midazolam or propofol anaesthesia. Patient is placed in prone position with the head turned towards right. After passing gastroduodenoscope, sphincter is identified and cannulated. Under visualisation 3 mL of water-soluble iodine contrast is injected into the bile duct and pancreatic duct. When cannula goes upwards beside vertebra, it signifies that it is in bile duct; and if cannula goes across the vertebra, it is in pancreatic duct. ***Indications:*** Malignancy—irregular filling defect;

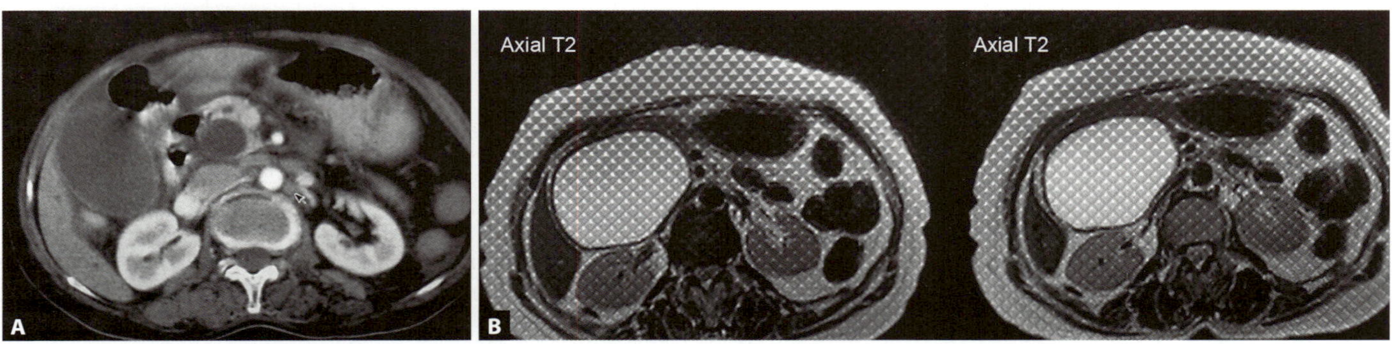

Figs. 23-85A and B: (A) CT scan showing dilated CBD; (B) CT scan showing choledochal cyst.

chronic pancreatitis—*'chain-of-lakes'* appearance; congenital anomalies; stones; stricture of biliary tree; choledochal cyst; for sampling of biliary and pancreatic juices for analysis and cytology; brush biopsy from tumour site. ***Therapeutic uses:*** Extraction of stone from biliary duct; nasobiliary drainage; stenting of tumour in the CBD or in the pancreas; dilatation of the biliary stricture; endoscopic papillotomy **(Fig. 23-87)**.

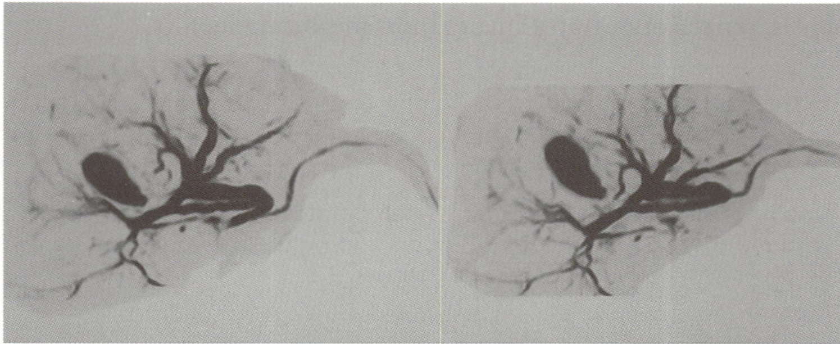

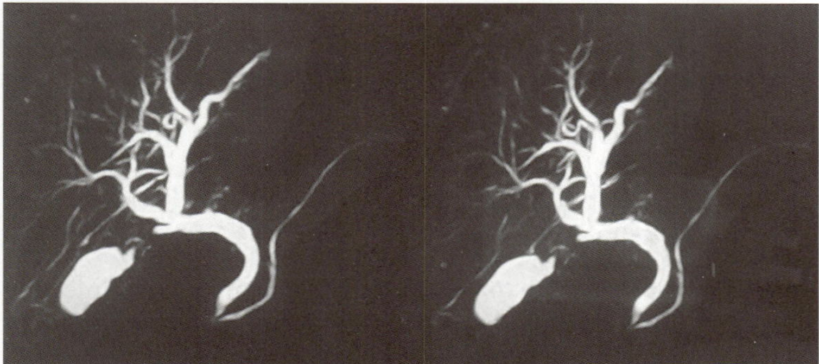

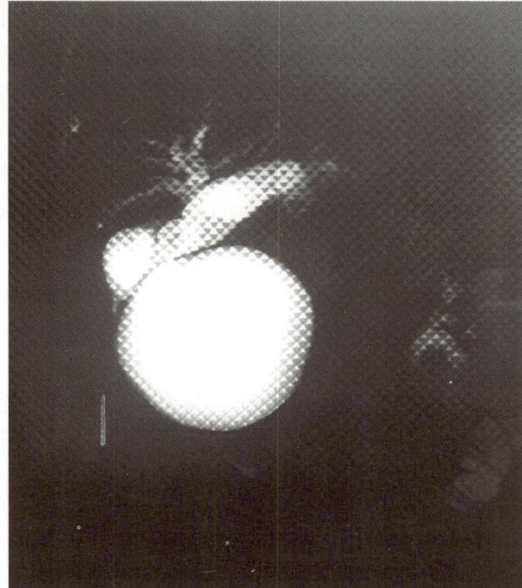

Fig. 23-86: MRI is a useful method to assess biliary anatomy.

Complications: Pancreatitis; duodenal injury, perforation; cholangitis; bleeding from pancreaticoduodenal artery; sphincter stenosis. ***Relative contraindications:*** Acute pancreatitis; previous gastrectomy.

Percutaneous transhepatic cholangiography (PTC): It is done in case of severe obstructive jaundice under cover of antibiotics and after control of any bleeding tendency—by giving injection vitamin K or FFP transfusion. ***Indications:*** Failure of ERCP; high biliary strictures; Klatskin tumour; high blocks when external catheter drainage is needed; stenting in high tumours with the help of fluoroscopy (C-arm)/US/CT guided, *Chiba* or *Okuda needle* which is long, flexible, thin, blunt, without a bevelled end (15 cm long and 0.7 mm in diameter) is passed into the liver through right 8th intercostal space in midaxillary line. Once needle is in the dilated biliary radicle, bile is aspirated (sent for culture, cytology, analysis) and then water-soluble iodine dye is injected into the same so as to visualise the dilated biliary radicles, also the site and extent of the obstruction, i.e. tumour, stricture. Procedure can be used for therapeutic stenting across the biliary tree through the obstruction either in the hepatic ducts or in the CBD into the duodenum. It is used whenever ERCP fails, in high strictures (in CHD), in Klatskin tumour, in catheter drainage (external) in high blocks, in stenting high tumours. ***Prerequisites for PTC:*** It should have normal prothrombin time (or should be made normal by injection vitamin K or FFP); should be a last and final inevitable method for evaluation; or therapy; blood for transfusion in case of bleed, consent for intervention in need, antibiotic prophylaxis—are a must prior to PTC. ***Complications:*** Bleeding, biliary leak and biliary peritonitis and septicaemia. PTC has got 95% accuracy rate. It confirms the diagnosis; site and cause of obstruction is determined; specific anatomy is identified.

Note:
Chiba is a university in Japan. Okuda is the name of person.

PTBD is percutaneous transhepatic biliary drainage. It can be *external or internal.* It is done through PTC.

Preoperative cholangiogram: It is done during CBD exploration for stricture, residual CBD stones, atresia, choledochal cyst, cholangitis. Fine polythene catheter is passed into the CBD through cystic duct

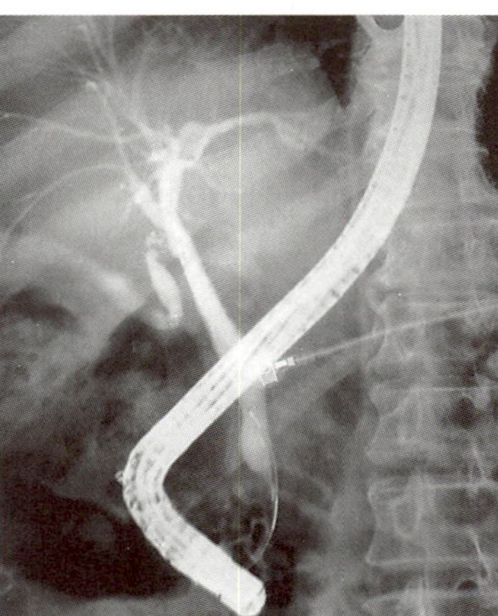

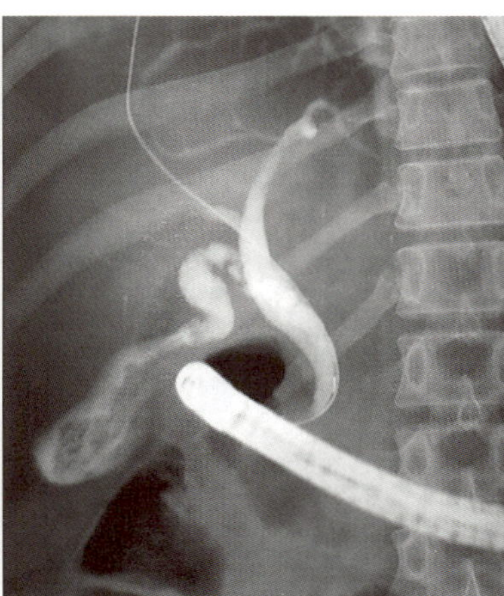

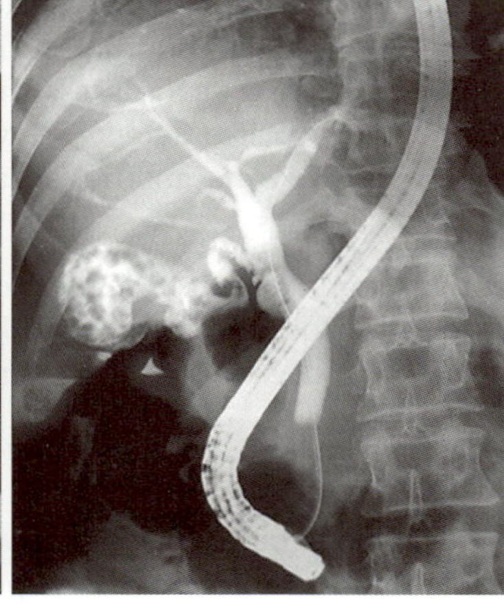

Fig. 23-87: Endoscopic retrograde cholangiopancreatography (ERCP).

and dye is injected. *Under C-arm image-intensifier*, any block or stricture can be identified and completion of the procedure can be confirmed. ***Complications:*** Infection; bile leak. ***Precaution:*** Air should not be present in the syringe, as it may mimic stones **(Fig. 23-88)**.

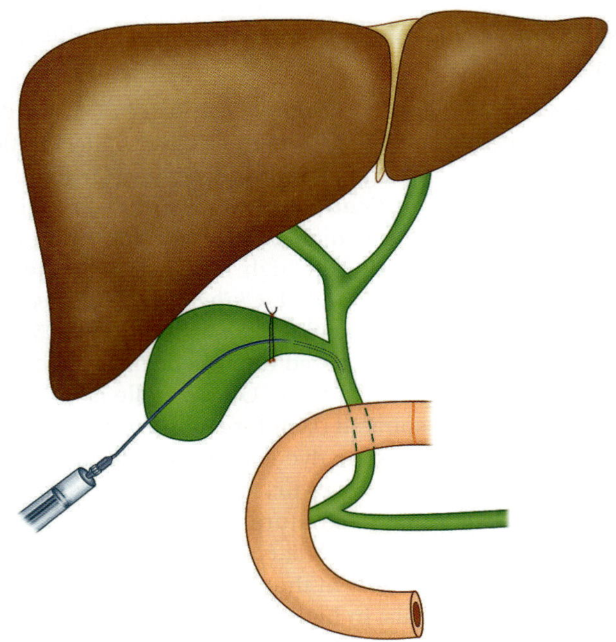

Fig. 23-88: Preoperative cholangiogram. Fine catheter is passed through cystic duct into the CBD. Care should be taken to avoid air getting into the CBD (it will mimic stone). Dye is injected under C-arm guidance.

Postoperative T-tube cholangiogram: After choledochotomy, *Kehr's T-tube* is *placed in CBD for 14 days* and then water soluble dye is injected into the tube and X-ray is taken. Complete free flow of dye into the duodenum indicates that there is no blockage. T-tube can then be removed safely. Block indicates residual CBD stones. **Residual CBD stones are removed by:** Dormia basket; Fogarty's catheter; choledochoscope; ERCP.

Biliary scintigraphy: Technetium 99m labelled iminodiacetic acid is (HIDA/PIPIDA) injected IV; it is secreted in bile to give functional nature. It is used in neonatal jaundice, biliary fistulas, acute cholecystitis. It assesses the patency of bile flow like in biliary enteric anastomosis.

Coeliac and superior mesenteric angiography: It is useful in bleeding varices in cirrhosis. It is done prior to porta systemic shunt surgery; therapeutic vasopressin injection; diagnosis of hemobilia; during selective embolisation in haemobilia and hepatic artery pseudoaneurysm (postoperative). It can assess the resectability of biliary cholangiocarcinomas. It also detects the vascularity and encasement of the major vessels like mesenteric vein and portal vein.

Endoscopic ultrasound (EUS): It detects tumour, its infiltration, lymph node status. Normal lymph node is hyperechoic and indistinct; metastatic lymph nodes are hypoechoic and well-defined. Needle aspiration cytology of lymph node can be done through the EUS.

Laparoscopy

Laparoscopy and laparoscopic ultrasound is very useful for on-table staging of cancer and determine the encasement, operability, vessel invasion, peritoneal deposits.

Risk Factors in Obstructive Jaundice

Age >60 years; temperature; haematocrit <30%; leucocytosis; hypoalbuminaemia; raised serum bilirubin, alkaline phosphatase, blood urea nitrogen, serum creatinine; malignant obstruction. Sepsis, renal status, nutrition are most important factors.

Little's mortality index

Mortality score = (0.0016 × serum creatinine in µmol/L)—(0.0227 × albumin g/L) + (0.0641 × cholangitis score) + 0.6935.

Cholangitis score: 0—afebrile; 1—temperature <37.5°C; 2—>37.5°C without rigors; 3—> 37.5°C with rigors and right upper quadrant pain; 4—fever with shock and or mental changes.

Note: An index of 0.5 or more is associated with high risk of death.

PREOPERATIVE PREPARATION

Preoperative hyperalimentation is required if serum albumin is less than 3 gram%; weight loss of 20% serum transferrin level less than 200 mg%. Adequate hydration either orally or intravenously using normal saline is a must.

Prolonged prothrombin time is common; it is corrected by injecting vitamin K 10 mg IV or IM once a day daily for 5 days; prothrombin time is repeated after 5 days; often fresh frozen plasma is needed to correct the prothrombin time. Platelet infusion is also required often if DIC is anticipated. Epsilon amino caproic acid (EACA) may be useful with shortened clot lysis time and hypofibrinogenaemia.

Renal function should be maintained properly in obstructive jaundice patients by adequate hydration; mannitol therapy; oral bile salts may reduce endotoxin absorption from gut and so its toxic effects on kidney.

Sepsis with cholangitis is a real threat in obstructive jaundice. Such patient (toxic cholangitis—with mental changes and hypotension) requires higher generation antibiotics and emergency decompression of biliary system by ERCP and stenting; otherwise it is life-threatening. Normally bile and biliary systems are sterile. Stasis, obstruction, enteric anastomosis, foreign body precipitates biliary sepsis. *E coli*, *Klebsiella*, *Enterococcus* and *Bacteriodes fragilis* are common organisms found in biliary tree with sepsis. Bile culture, ability of antibiotics to excrete in bile, concentrations in liver and blood; toxic effects are the parameters to decide type of antibiotics chosen. Piperacillin and tazobactum is quiet effective. Prophylactic antibiotics should be given if patient is undergoing surgery or ERCP or otherwise.

Preoperative biliary drainage through transhepatic route in obstructive jaundice routinely is not necessary but in selected patients with severe obstructive jaundice, it may be beneficial.

Cardiac and respiratory problems can occur; detailed cardiac and respiratory evaluations are needed with respiratory physiotherapy.

CHOLECYSTECTOMY

In 1743, Jean Louis Petit did first cholecystostomy for gallstones. Until 1882, cholecystostomy was the procedure used to be practiced for gallstones. In 1882, Carl von Langenbeck did first cholecystectomy. In 1985, Prof Erich Muhe of Boblingen from Germany did first laparoscopic cholecystectomy which he presented in congress of

German surgical society. In 1987, Mouret of Lyon, France reported first laparoscopic cholecystectomy. Jacques Perissat (France) presented first paper on laparoscopic cholecystectomy.

Indications

Gallstones—symptomatic; cholecystitis—acute, chronic; acalculous cholecystitis; empyema gallbladder; mucocoele of gallbladder.

Prophylactic cholecystectomy is done in diabetic patients; congenital haemolytic anaemia; patients who has underwent bariatric surgery; while giving intra-arterial chemotherapy through hepatic artery.

Approaches

Open Method

Different incisions are—right subcostal incision (Kocher's); Kehr hockey stick modification (medial end is extended upwards towards xiphisternum); upper midline incision; right paramedian; horizontal incision; Mayo-Robson incision. Right subcostal incision is commonly used.

Open approach is done when laparoscopic approach is not possible; or during laparoscopy difficulty arises and so conversion has been done to open method (failed laparoscopy); or if patient is not fit for general anaesthesia or for pneumoperitoneum **(Figs. 23-89 and 23-90)**.

Laparoscopic Approach

Laparoscopic cholecystectomy has become standard and ideal **(Fig. 23-91)**.

Preoperative Preparation

Evaluation by liver function tests, prothrombin time, diabetes, ultrasound (CBD should be assessed properly including its diameter); CT scan when needed to assess the biliary tree, pancreas; gastroduodenoscopy if hiatus hernia, oesophageal varices (portal hypertension) is suspected. If CBD stone is present, ERCP and stenting should be done prior to laparoscopic cholecystectomy. If open cholecystectomy is planned then CBD exploration should also be planned in these patients. Preoperative antibiotics are also necessary in cholecystectomy. Cardiac and respiratory assessment is required in these patients. Heparin as a prophylaxis for deep vein thrombosis may be a need.

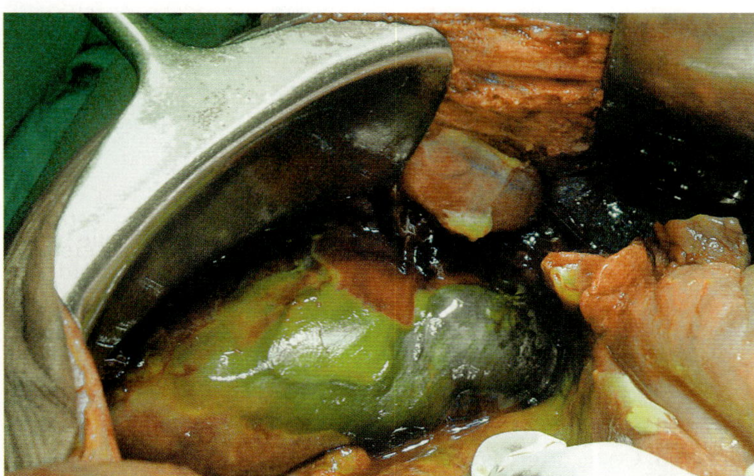

Fig. 23-89: Gangrene of gallbladder is probably a sure indication of open cholecystectomy. But presently even such gallbladders can be removed laparoscopically by an experienced skilled laparoscopic surgeon only. Learner should convert such gallbladder into open method rather than inviting trouble.

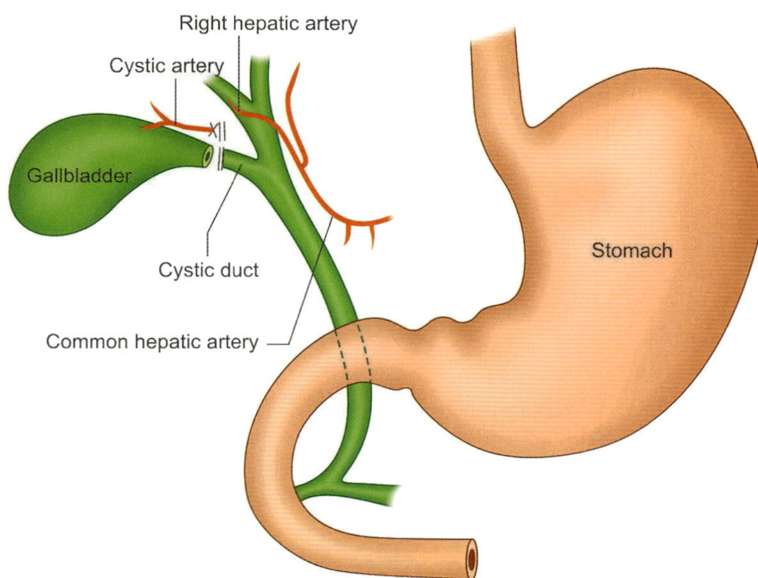

Fig. 23-90: Technique of open cholecystectomy.

TECHNIQUE OF OPEN CHOLECYSTECTOMY

General anaesthesia or epidural anaesthesia is used. Nasogastric tube and urinary catheterisation is passed. Patient is in supine position. C-arm image intensifier/fluoroscopy should be kept in place or cassette changer should be placed underneath the patient at the level of surgical field. Preoperative antibiotics are given—tazobactam or amoxicillin as common organisms are *Escherichia coli* and *Streptococcus faecalis*. Heparin should be injected subcutaneously to prevent formation of deep venous thrombosis. Cleaning of entire abdomen is done; draping is done in the incision area. Surgeon stands on the right side; two assistants on left side; during retraction of right costal margin, if needed, one assistant may have to come to right side towards left of the operating surgeon.

Incision: Right subcostal incision is used—2 cm below the right costal margin. Skin, subcutaneous tissue, external oblique, internal oblique and transverse abdominis muscles are cut (transverse abdominis is often thin and can be split also). Medially rectus sheath is incised up to the midline; a haemostat is passed underneath the rectus muscle and is cut using monopolar cautery. 9th intercostal nerve is divided where it emerges lateral to the rectus muscle border. It causes only slight skin hypoesthesia but not muscle weakness (if possible it can be retained). Vessels underneath should be fulgurated. Rectus muscle after dividing will not retract in upper abdomen due to presence of tendinous intersections. Peritoneum is opened. Peritoneal cavity is explored. Oesophageal hiatus, gallbladder, pancreas, duodenum should also be palpated **(Fig. 23-92)**.

Retraction: Right hand is placed between liver and diaphragm to retract liver downward and allow air to enter above the liver causing downward displacement of liver to make gallbladder more visible.

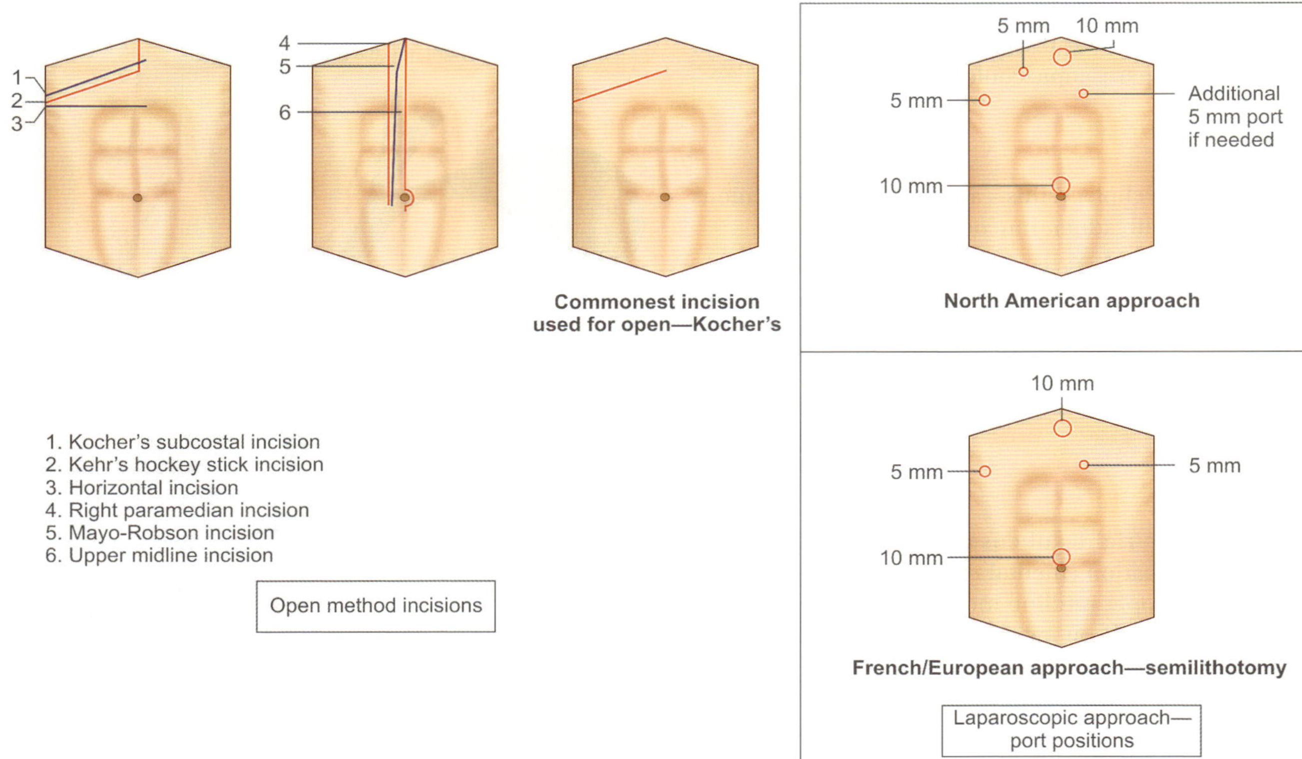

Fig. 23-91: Incisions for open and laparoscopic cholecystectomy.

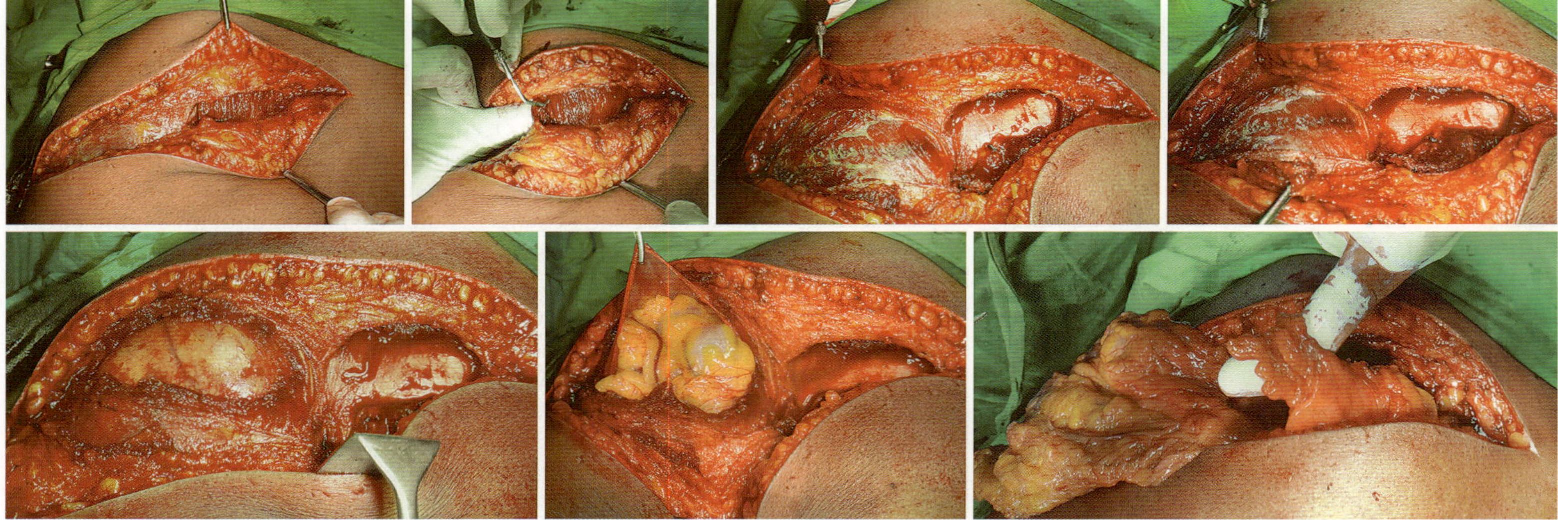

Fig. 23-92: Kocher's right subcostal incision for cholecystectomy.

Often colon and duodenum may be adherent to the gallbladder, they should be dissected by sharp and finger dissection. Colon is pushed downwards; duodenum and stomach medially. Care should be taken not to injure the colon or duodenum. Moist mops are kept on the colon and it is retracted downwards using a Deaver's retractor; another moist mop is kept on the stomach and duodenum and is retracted medially towards left using another Deaver's retractor. Right costal margin is retracted upwards using an abdominal wall Morris retractor with a moist mop underneath. Liver is often retracted upwards from left of the falciform ligament or medial to the gallbladder using another Deaver's retractor **(Figs. 23-93A to C)**.

Often gallbladder is very tense due to mucus or pus or bile which needs aspiration so that gallbladder is made easier to hold and handle **(Fig. 23-94)**.

Two Methods Used for Cholecystectomy

Duct—first method (Calot's first method): Here *Calot's triangle* is dissected. Cystic artery is identified and ligated. Cystic duct is ligated close to the gallbladder. Gallbladder is separated from gallbladder fossa and removed. Haemostasis is maintained. Usually Calot's first method is used.

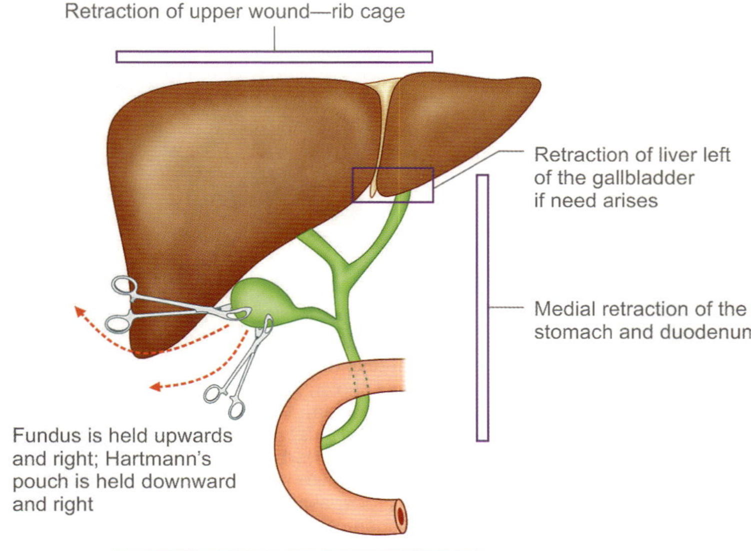

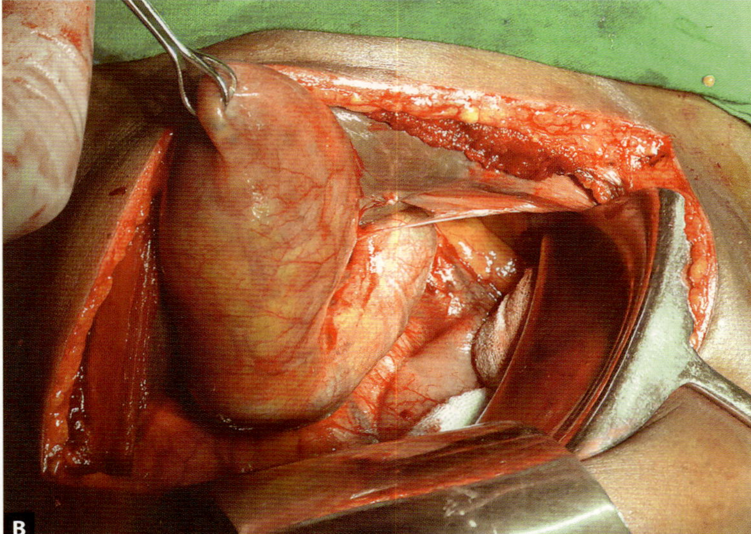

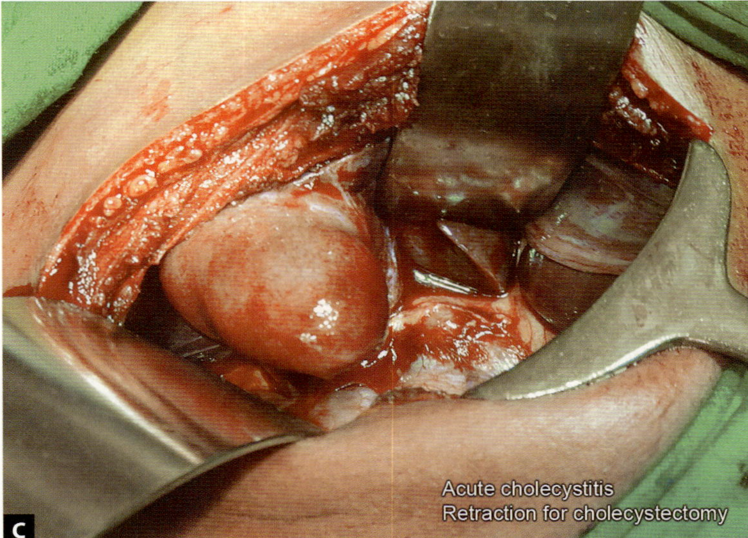

Figs. 23-93A to C: (A) Method of retraction in open cholecystectomy and CBD exploration—below to the colon; (B) Medially to stomach and duodenum; (C) Above towards left of gallbladder on liver.

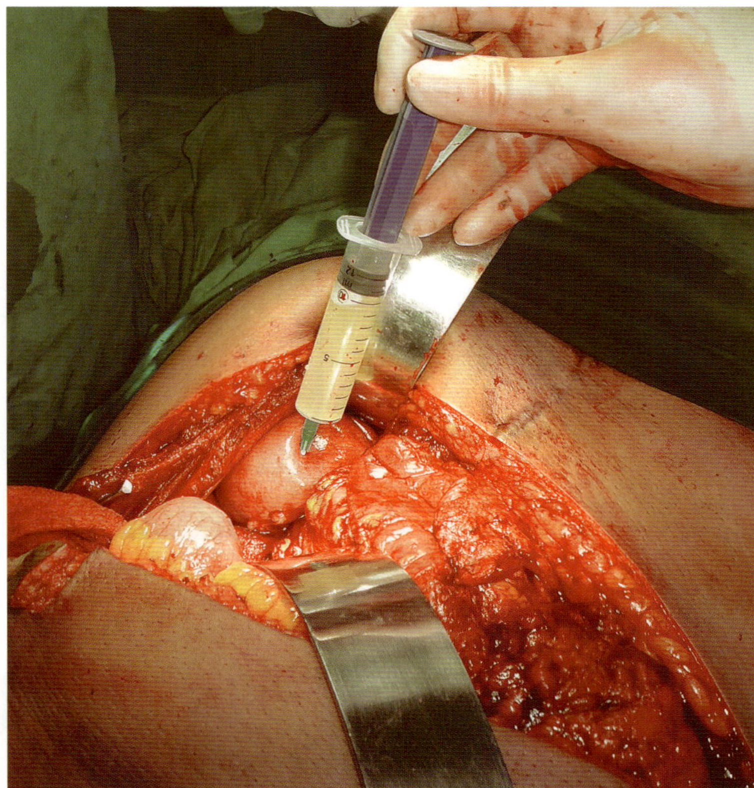

Fig. 23-94: Aspiration of the gallbladder is done if gallbladder is tense.

Fundus—first method: It is done in difficult gallbladder due to dense adhesions. Fundus is separated from the liver bed. Dissection is carried proximally until cystic duct and cystic artery are identified, which are then ligated.

Calot's First (Conventional; Below Upward) Method

Fundus of the gallbladder is held with Babcock's or sponge holding forceps or gallbladder holding forceps. Traction is given to fundus upwards and towards right (outwards). Hartmann's pouch is held with another Babcock's or sponge holding forceps and traction is given downwards and outwards.

In the Calot's triangle, peritoneum is incised using long curved scissor to expose the cystic duct and artery. With fine dissection using peanut (pledget in haemostat), haemostat and right angle clamp Calot's triangle is dissected to identify the cystic artery, cystic duct, and junction where cystic duct joins the common bile duct. Cystic duct lymph node of Lund will be seen in Calot's triangle lying on the top of cystic artery.

Two silk or vicryl ligatures are passed around the cystic duct. Any stones in the cystic duct are felt and milked proximally into the gallbladder. Entire length of the cystic duct is dissected using sharp and finger dissection. Ligature close to the Hartmann's pouch is ligated **(Fig. 23-95)**.

Technique of cystic duct cholangiography: Distal ligature is not ligated instead is held apart with stretching. Cystic duct is incised near its beginning close to the gallbladder just distal to the tied ligature. A fine plastic tube (or infant feeding tube no. 5-8 or ureteric catheter) or cholangiogram catheter (which has got a bead at the tip)

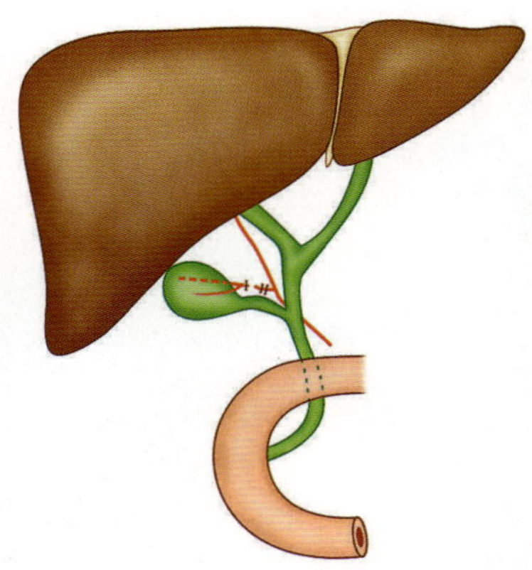

Cystic artery and duct are dissected meticulously. Anomalies should be kept in mind. Cystohepatic junction should be identified. Cystic artery is ligated first (proximally double)

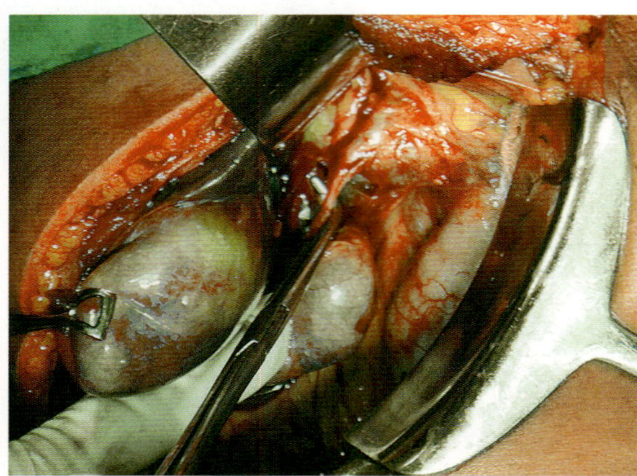

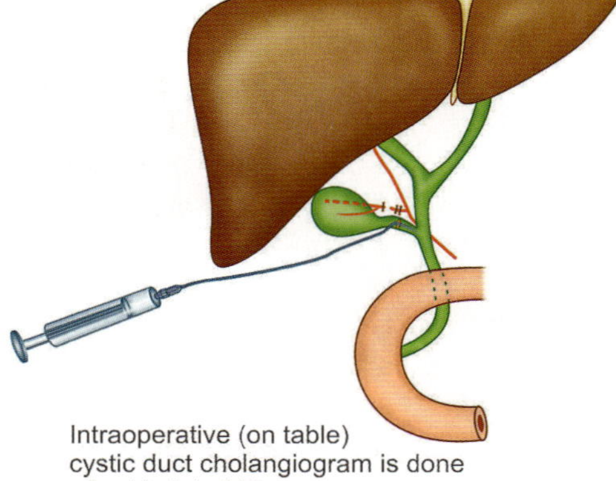

Intraoperative (on table) cystic duct cholangiogram is done
- Avoid air bubble
- 1:1 sodium diatrizoate with warm saline 50 mL
- Avoid concentrated dye
- Assure that entire biliary tree is filled with dye
- If sphincter spasm is present nitroglycerin or glucagon can be injected

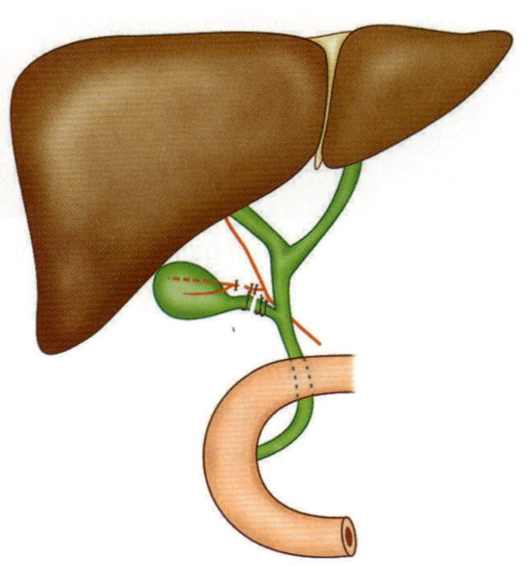

Cystic duct is doubly ligated. Care should be taken to avoid inadvertent placing of the ligature on to the CBD due to traction or kink

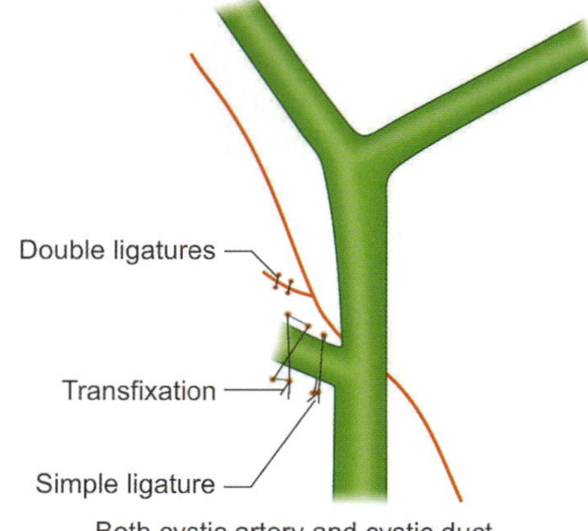

Both cystic artery and cystic duct are doubly ligated
- Cystic duct is often tansfixed towards stump side; proximally simple ligature is applied

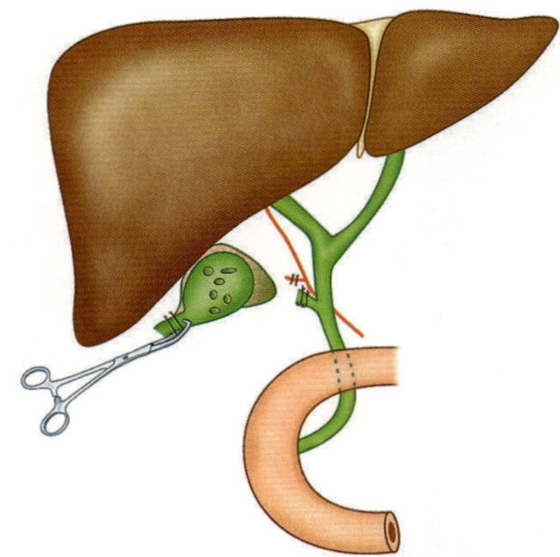

Neck of the gallbladder is held laterally
Gallblader is dissected off from the liver bed using cautery, scissor and finger dissection
One should avoid opening the liver parenchyma
Bipolar cautery may be used

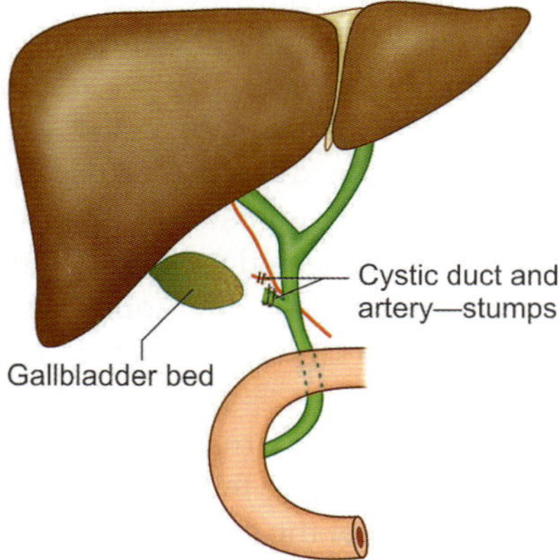

Gallblader bed after removal of gallbladder is inspected for bleeding; small bleeders are fulgurated; often surgicel, if needed, may be placed on the bed. Safety of CBD is again confirmed. Mops are removed with proper count. Tube drain may be placed if indicated. Wound closed in layers using no. 1 vicryl

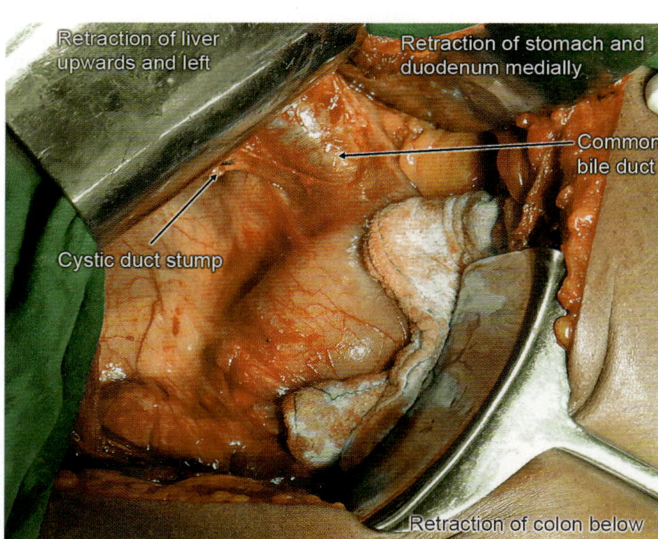

Fig. 23-95: Calot's first method of open cholecystectomy.

of 2 meter length with 50 mL syringe filled with dilute sodium diatrizoate is taken (1:1 with normal saline; 25 mL saline + 25 mL dye). Entire syringe and plastic tube should be devoid of air bubble—very important. Plastic tube negotiated across the cystic duct for 5 mm close to bile duct. Narrow lumen or valve of Heister in the cystic duct may cause difficulty in negotiating the tube. Distal ligature is tied on the catheter with cystic duct. Bile should not be aspirated into the tube to prevent air bubble formation; if surgeon wants to confirm that tip is inside the lumen small quantity can be aspirated gently with care. Left side of the theatre table is tilted upwards for 10 cm to avoid superimposition of the bile duct image with vertebrae. If C-arm is available, dye is injected and under fluoroscopy guidance; bile duct is visualised and also the flow into the duodenum. A radiolucent area is identified as common bile duct stone. Often dye may not enter the duodenum due to sphincter spasm; in such situations small dose of nitroglycerin or 1 mg of glucagon intravenously will relieve the spasm to allow the dye to pass into the duodenum. Even with this, if the dye has not entered the duodenum, then bile duct exploration is indicated. *Findings* to be observed in the cholangiogram are—diameter of the bile duct, any radiolucent area in the biliary tree, status of hepatic ducts, smooth tapering at ampulla of Vater and free flow of dye into the duodenum. Cystic duct cholangiogram ensures and confirms ductal anatomy, may aid in limiting the ductal injury (even though it may not prevent) and decides need for common bile duct exploration.

If C-arm image intensifier is not available, initially 4 mL of dye is injected to take first X-ray film; 2nd X-ray film is taken after injecting remaining part of the dye.

Intraoperative cholangiogram

- Cystic duct cholangiogram—commonly used
  - Real time fluoroscopy—ideal
  - Static film technique—two films should be taken
  - Needle technique in laparoscopic cholecystectomy percutaneous needle is used
- Gallbladder cholangiography
- Infundibular approach (Kumar's)

Precautions while doing cystic duct cholangiography are—avoiding injecting more quantity and more concentrated contrast material as this will cause missing of small calculi and duodenum will be flooded with dye; air bubble should be avoided compulsorily; entire biliary system should be visualised including hepatic ducts; correction of sphincter spasm by drugs while doing the study if needed.

Cystic artery is doubly ligated using silk and divided. Usually cystic artery is above the level of cystic duct and in slight posterior plane than the cystic duct. Cystic artery is in close proximity to liver. Cystic artery should be adequately dissected for about 1 cm using right-angled Mixter instrument; often its branches may need to be ligated independently. Any variations, if possible, should be kept in mind. In adhesions, dissection of artery may take time; artery should be dissected and ligated as far as possible. Occasionally, in dense adhesions where dissection is not possible, then mass ligation may be done if it seems mandatory; but it carries higher chance of ligating or injuring right hepatic artery or hepatic duct. While dissecting the cystic artery, artery may get torn inadvertently; then blind clamping the area with haemostat should be avoided; instead a mop is kept in the place with pressure and with proper retraction and lighting, mop is gently removed to identify the bleeding point of proximal end of cystic artery which is held with right angle and carefully ligated. Often in such situation, bipolar cautery fulguration helps in controlling the bleeding. If identification of cut end of cystic artery is still difficult, the incision should be extended medially or upward medially towards xiphisternum to get adequate exposure. Too large a cystic artery, if present, it is unlikely to be; rather it could be right hepatic artery (3 mm or more in diameter). *Cystic artery should be ligated first* to allow subsequent Calot's dissection easier; to make cystic duct straight by eliminating the convolutions; to avoid its tearing due to traction on the gallbladder. Accessory cystic artery may be present in anomalous position.

Bile duct should not be extensively dissected unnecessarily; but cystohepatic junction should be delineated properly. Monopolar cautery should be avoided close to bile duct; bipolar cautery is suitable.

Once bile duct exploration is not under strategy, then *cystic duct is doubly ligated* proximally after removing cholangiogram catheter. Simple ligature is placed using vicryl or silk close to cystohepatic junction; just distal to its transfixation suture. Cystic duct is divided. It is *ideal* to place ligatures and then divide the cystic duct rather than clamping, dividing and then ligating the duct. Many feel that cystic duct ligation is done only after complete mobilisation of the gallbladder from liver bed. However, if dissection is adequate in Calot's then cystic duct can be ligated safely prior to dissection of gallbladder from liver bed.

Dissection of the gallbladder from the liver bed: Usually it is easier to dissect the gallbladder from the liver by giving traction to fundus and Hartmann's pouch. Cystic duct stump is held with a haemostat to give outward traction to make peritoneal fold between gallbladder and liver stretched and fold is incised to proceed with the dissection. Dissection should be close to the gallbladder wall without injuring the liver tissue. Dissection begins from Calot's area towards fundus. Dissection is done using scissor or monopolar cautery or using peanut. Plane of dissection is deep to mucosa of the gallbladder. All small bleeders from the liver surface should be fulgurated. Care is taken to look for direct entry of accessory duct from liver to gallbladder; if present, should be ligated securely to prevent bile leak. After removal of gallbladder, mop is kept in place for few minutes. Often gelfoam or surgical may be kept to prevent oozing from the liver bed. Occasionally *under running of the bleeding point* using 4-0 vicryl may be useful. Catching with a haemostat and ligating should not be attempted in liver bed.

Complete haemostasis is achieved. Common bile duct is again palpated for confirmation that stones are not missed. It is done by palpating supraduodenal portion of the common bile duct and also pancreatic portion by placing fingers behind the second part of the duodenum. Mops are removed; counts should be checked **(Figs. 23-96 and 23-97)**.

Tube or Jackson Pratt closed suction drain is placed when there is acute cholecystitis or in difficult gallbladder surgery. Abdominal wall is closed as single or two layers using vicryl. Skin can be approximated using stapler or nylon.

Fundus First Method (Above Downward)

Here after opening the abdomen and exposure with proper retraction instead of dissecting the Calot's, fundus of the gallbladder is held with sponge holding forceps. Using sharp scissor or monopolar cautery, fundus and body of gallbladder is dissected from its liver bed from fundus, to begin with, towards neck and Calot's triangle.

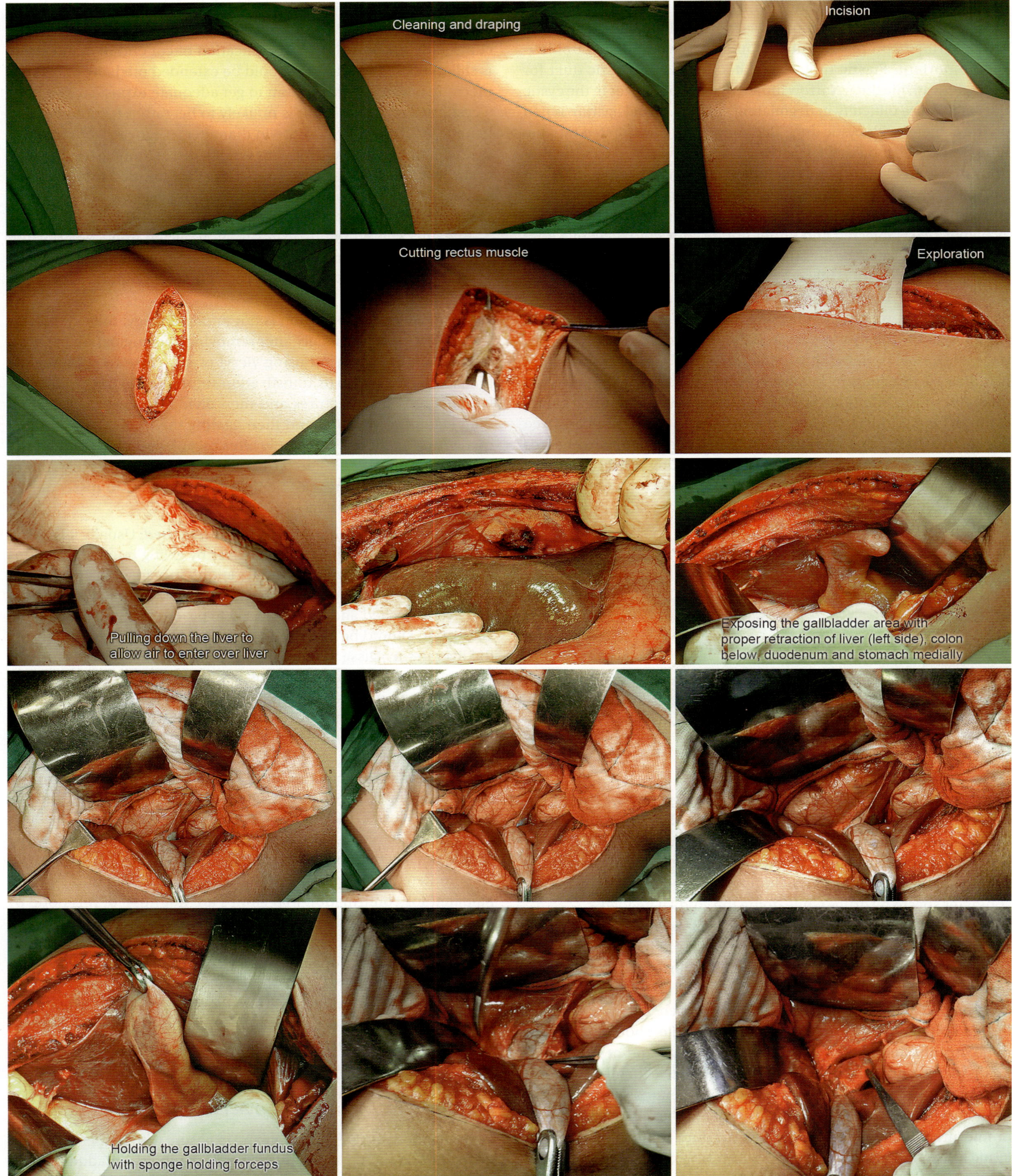
Cleaning and draping
Incision
Cutting rectus muscle
Exploration
Pulling down the liver to allow air to enter over liver
Exposing the gallbladder area with proper retraction of liver (left side), colon below, duodenum and stomach medially
Holding the gallbladder fundus with sponge holding forceps

Figs. 23-96(1)

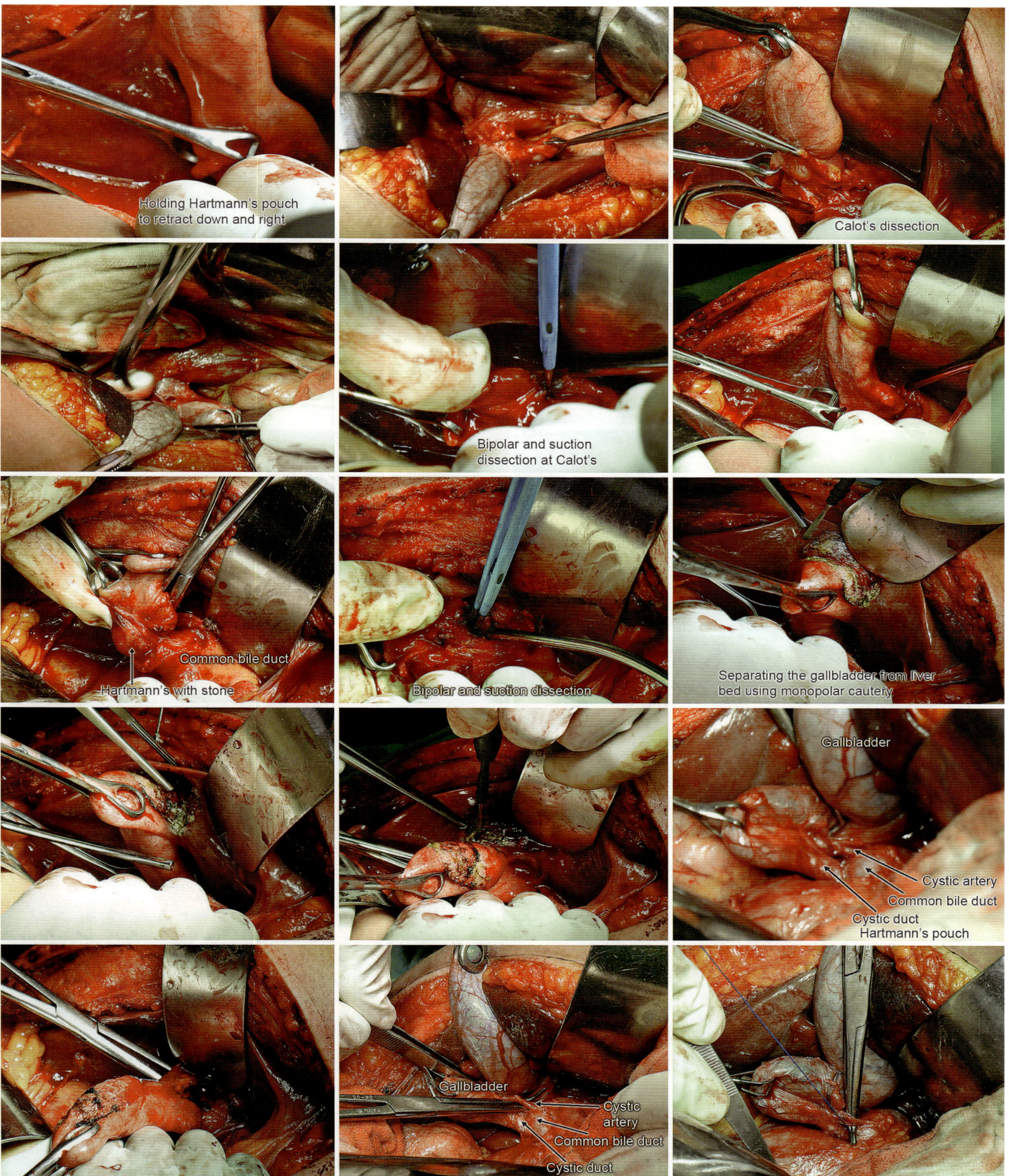
Holding Hartmann's pouch
to retract down and right
Calot's dissection
Bipolar and suction
dissection at Calot's
Common bile duct
Hartmann's with stone
Bipolar and suction dissection
Separating the gallbladder from liver
bed using monopolar cautery
Gallbladder
Cystic artery
Common bile duct
Cystic duct
Hartmann's pouch
Gallbladder
Cystic
artery
Common bile duct
Cystic duct

Figs. 23-96(2)

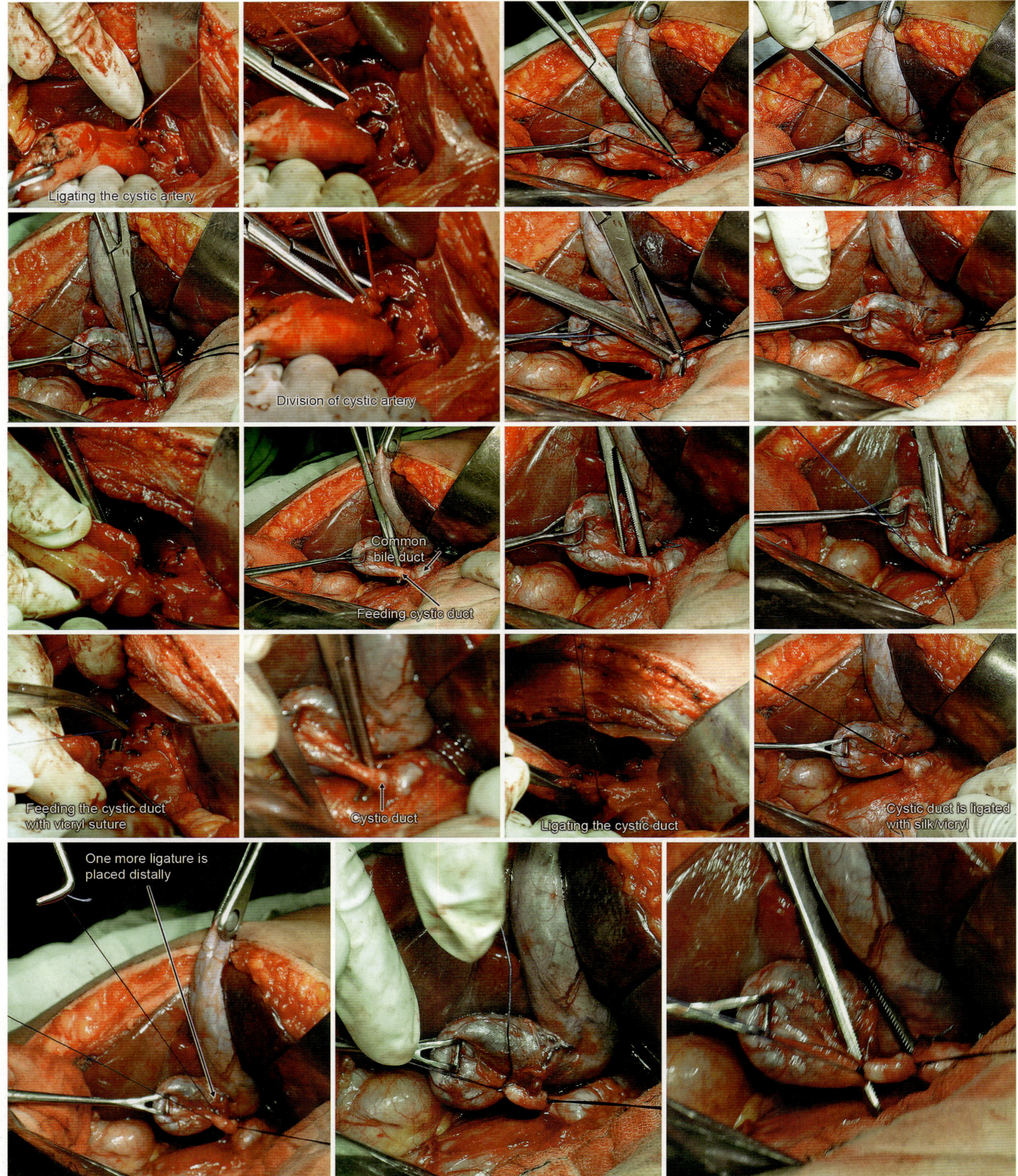
Ligating the cystic artery
Division of cystic artery
Common bile duct
Feeding cystic duct
Feeding the cystic duct with vicryl suture
Cystic duct
Ligating the cystic duct
Cystic duct is ligated with silk/vicryl
One more ligature is placed distally

Figs. 23-96(3)

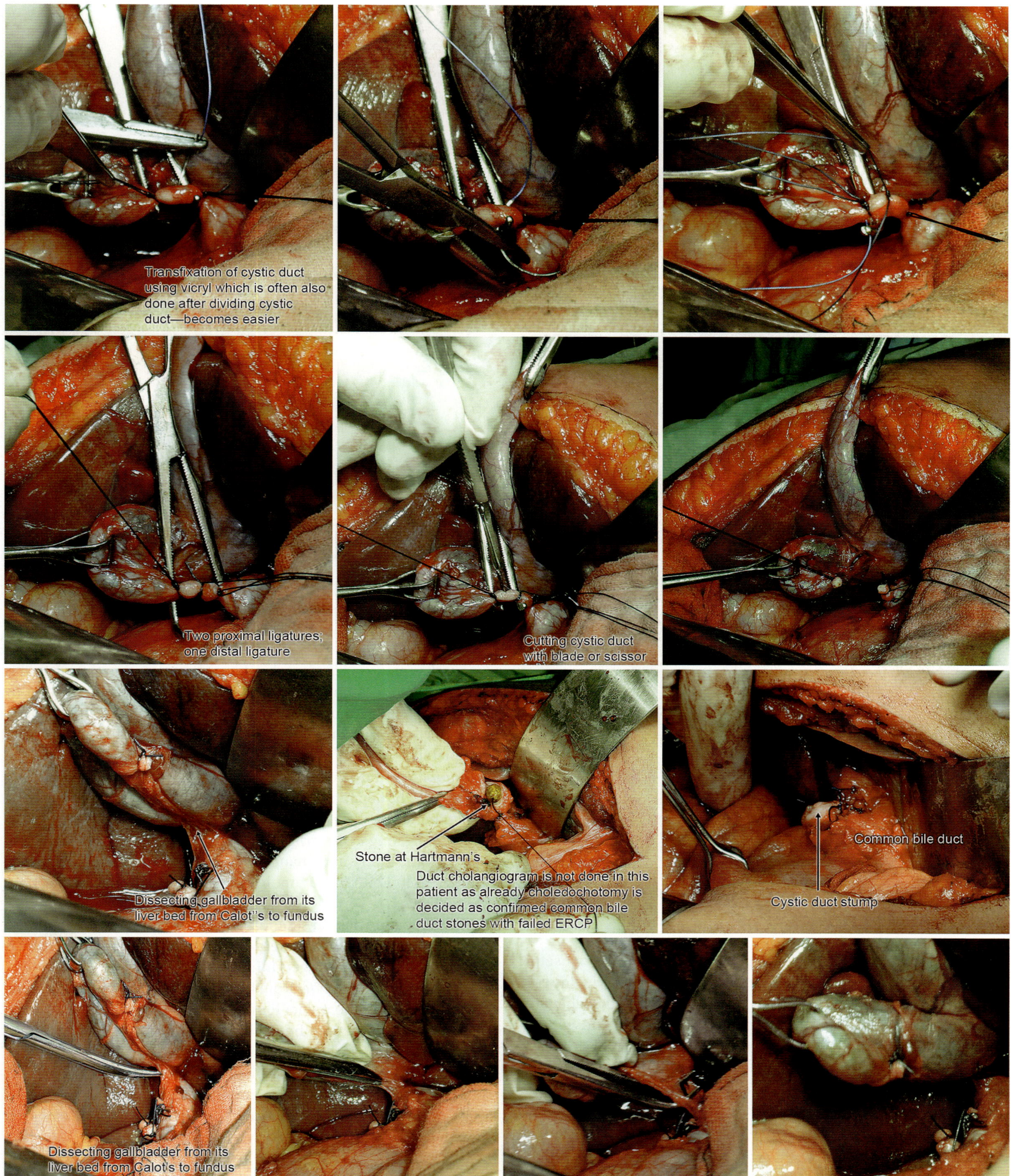
Transfixation of cystic duct using vicryl which is often also done after dividing cystic duct—becomes easier
Two proximal ligatures; one distal ligature
Cutting cystic duct with blade or scissor
Dissecting gallbladder from its liver bed from Calot's to fundus
Stone at Hartmann's
Duct cholangiogram is not done in this patient as already choledochotomy is decided as confirmed common bile duct stones with failed ERCP
Common bile duct
Cystic duct stump
Dissecting gallbladder from its liver bed from Calot's to fundus

Figs. 23-96(4)

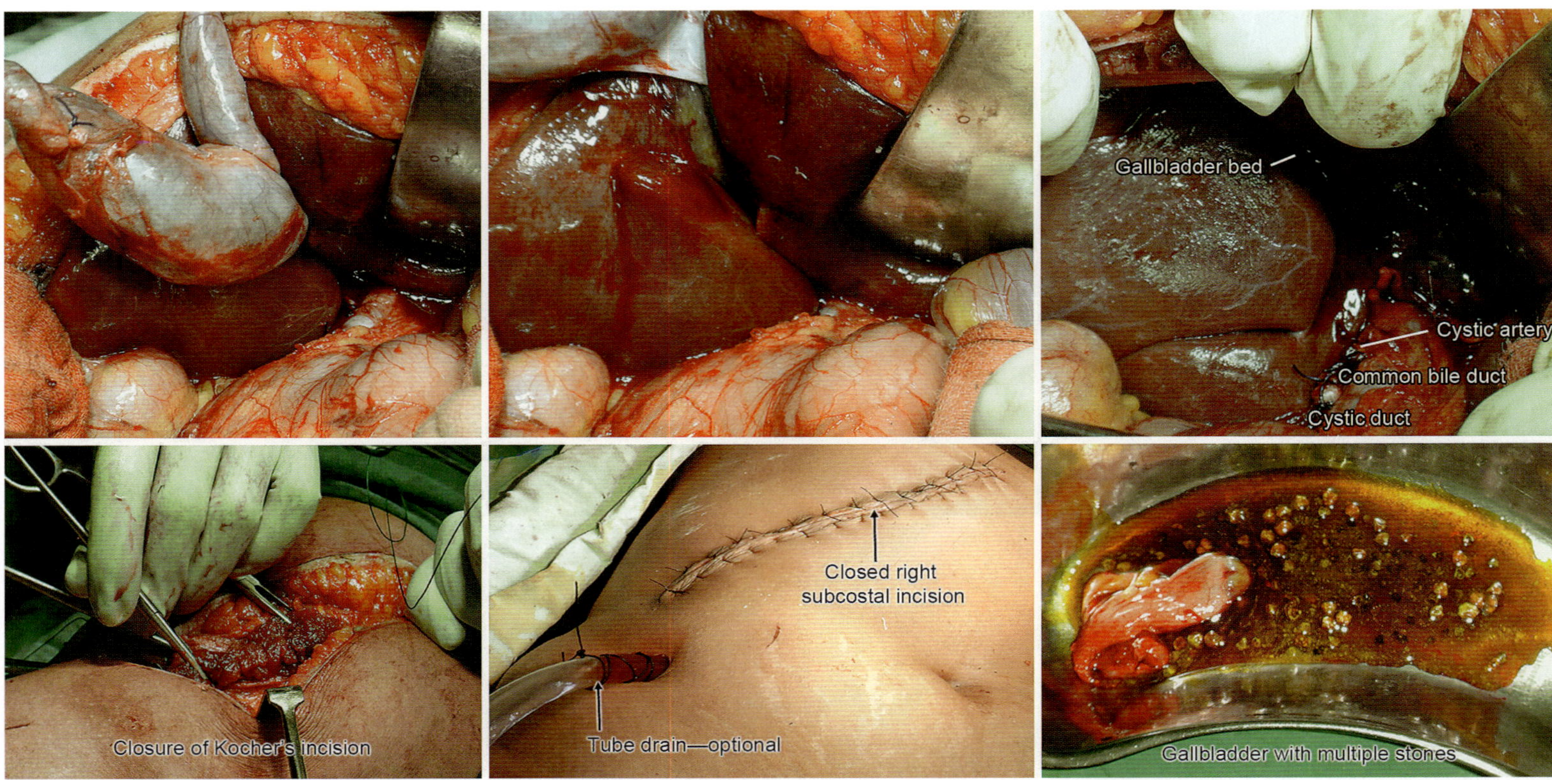

Figs. 23-96(5)

Figs. 23-96(1 to 5): Open cholecystectomy—steps. In one patient after difficult Calot's dissection, gallbladder is separated from liver bed from fundus towards Calot's then cystic duct is ligated. In another patient, Calot's is addressed with ligation of cystic artery and duct, and gallbladder is separated from Calot's towards fundus (from its liver bed).

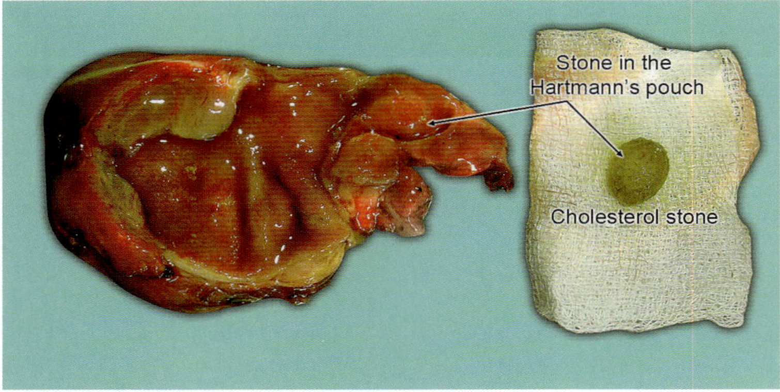

Fig. 23-97: Specimen of gallbladder with cholesterol stone.

Blunt dissection using peanut or suction apparatus is very useful. One should avoid entering the parenchyma of liver. It is done in difficult cases wherein dissection at Calot's is difficult to begin with. Fundus first method ensures that common bile duct and hepatic ducts will not be injured. But oozing from the liver bed makes further dissection cumbersome. Once Calot's is reached, cystic artery is ligated and divided. Cystic duct is ligated doubly after doing cystic duct cholangiography by similar method.

Postoperative Care

Nasogastric tube is removed within 24 hours unless there is paralytic ileus. In infected gallbladder, antibiotics are continued. Drain when kept is removed in 4 days.

Precautions

Size of the common bile duct should not be overestimated; often it is small enough to mimic the cystic duct and inadvertent ligation by mistake is known to occur. Kinking at cystohepatic junction due to traction can cause clamping the junction with bile duct partially and completely.

Anomalies of cystic duct (short or long; may enter right hepatic duct), of right hepatic duct; presence of accessory ducts should be remembered.

While ligating *cystic artery* care should be taken of variations of right hepatic artery and chances of ligating the right hepatic artery. Any artery if more than 3 mm in size, one should suspect it as right hepatic artery.

Cystohepatic junction should be identified and dissected prior to ligation of the cystic duct. Caterpillar hump of right hepatic artery is known to exist and easily gets injured while dissecting.

Dissection of gallbladder from liver bed often may be troublesome and is also should be meticulous. It is often observed that surgeon relaxes while dissecting the gallbladder from its bed once Calot's is addressed properly.

Blind clamping and ligation should not be undertaken.

If needed, incision should be *extended* accordingly.

Cystic duct cholangiogram ideally should be done in all cases even though it is not practiced by many surgeons routinely.

Cholecystitis in pregnancy: Ideally if possible cholecystectomy should be postponed and is done 3 months after delivery. If there is secondary choledocholithiasis or if it becomes inevitable then ideal timing to do surgery is 2nd trimester. Cholecystectomy is safer.

But if bile duct exploration is needed whether cholangiogram to be done or not is a debate. It is said that X-ray is safer after 1st trimester. Even then uterus shield should be used if cholangiogram is done. Bile duct stone after choledochotomy can be removed using choledochoscope. CT imaging should be avoided in pregnancy. Ultrasound is the main imaging modality in pregnancy. MRI is safer. Laparoscopic cholecystectomy is becoming an accepted method in 2nd trimester but needs expertise; open trocar placement; low pressure surgery and keeping PCO_2 less than 40 mmHg are the essential measures to be taken. Fetal monitoring during surgery, obstetrician help and follow up fetal monitoring in immediate postoperative period are essential measures.

Cholecystectomy in cirrhotic patients: In cirrhotics, selection of the patient is important. Liver will be nodular. All adhesions are vascular and often bleed profusely. Dissection of the gallbladder from the liver bed may create technical problems. Preoperative preparation should be adequate like—injection vitamin K; fresh frozen plasma transfusion, platelet transfusions, antibiotic therapy. Even then *laparoscopic cholecystectomy is better than open approach in cirrhotics.* Fundus first method should be used in cirrhotics; harmonic scalpel or other energy sources should be used. Doing partial cholecystectomy by ligating at the of Hartmann's pouch is much safer than dissecting Calot's. Often conversion is needed; still often limiting the procedure towards cholecystostomy may be a compulsion due to technical hurdles. In cirrhotics, one should avoid placing T tube as localisation and track formation is poorer and chances of biliary peritonitis are higher. If at all. T-tube is placed then critical postoperative care is needed. T tube should be removed only after 4 weeks. Profuse bleeding from the liver bed in cirrhotics is a real matter of concern. Often it is difficult to achieve adequate required haemostasis and keeping a pack/mop in the bed to achieve compression for 24–48 hours is the only choice; such packs should be removed in 48 hours under anaesthesia gently with all precautions. Posterior part of the gallbladder can be left alone removing only the remaining parts. Mucosa of such left out difficult gallbladder is ablated using ideally argon laser or bipolar cautery. Opening of the cystic duct is invaginated using absorbable 3-0 suture material like vicryl.

In patients with coagulative disorders, cholecystectomy should be done by keeping ready adequate number of units of frozen plasma or platelets or factor VIII depending on the type of coagulopathy patient harbours.

Complications

Injury to colon, duodenum and mesentery can occur whenever there are adhesions.

Bile leak: It is the most distressing complication surgeon faces. Small bile leak through the drain is probably due to either cystic duct stump disruption or accessory duct leak. Usually it is 100–200 mL/day. It usually subsides in 7–10 days. If leak persists ERCP and stenting is needed; it also identifies the bile duct and hepatic duct status. If bile leak is more than 400 mL/day it means probably it is bile duct or hepatic duct injury. It needs proper evaluation with CT scan/MRCP. It is addressed only at a later period once inflammation subsides after 3 months. Nutrition during this period should be maintained adequately. It needs expertise work and needed proper

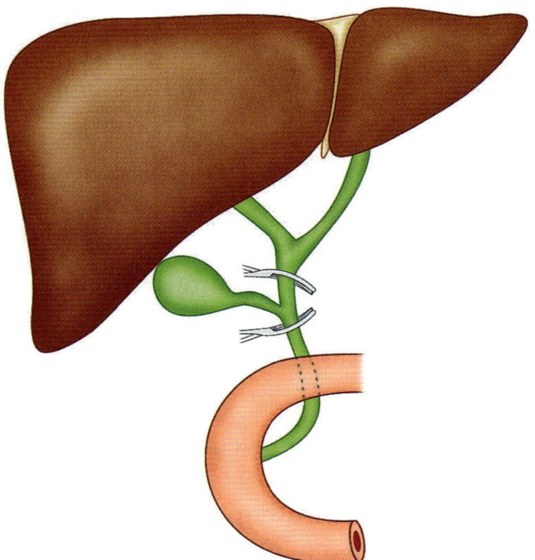

Fig. 23-98: Injury to bile duct can occur if inadvertent clamping has occurred.

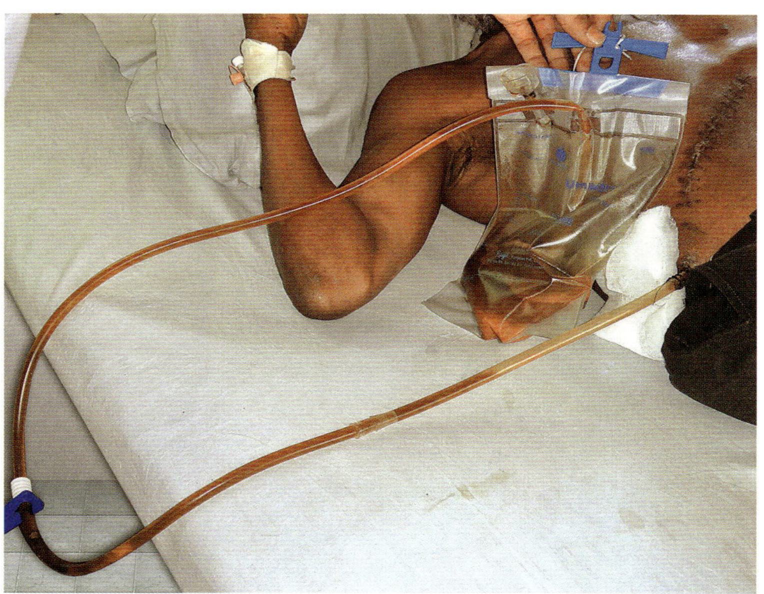

Fig. 23-99: Bile leak after open cholecystectomy.

identification, dissection of biliary tree and hepaticojejunostomy **(Figs. 23-98 and 23-99)**.

Post-cholecystectomy jaundice may be due to cholangitis, missed bile duct stones, bile duct stricture due to trauma or ligation of bile duct or hepatic duct. ERCP, liver function tests proper imaging to identify the problem are needed to plan the eventual surgical correction.

Postoperative bleeding is not common. But can occur if cystic artery ligature is slipped or if there is sepsis at the gallbladder bed. Occasionally it could be due to anomalous right hepatic artery which is injured due to inability to identify the vascular anomaly. Infection may cause hepatic artery pseudoaneurysm which may often be life-threatening. It needs CT angiogram and intervention radiology to address the feeding artery of the pseudoaneurysm by glue or other embolisation devices. However, inadvertent embolisation or gluing of the right hepatic artery may cause acute fulminant hepatic necrosis of the liver and may kill the patient. Hogarth Pringle's manoeuvre is ideal to control bleeding on table by applying pressure using thumb and fingers over the Foramen Winslow.

Sepsis: Subphrenic, pelvic, hepatic abscess can occur occasionally when there is cholangitis, immunosuppression or if surgery done in a badly infected gallbladder. Blood culture, blood count, clinical assessment is a must. Higher generation antibiotics should be started to prevent septicaemia. Abscess can be addressed usually by image guided catheter drainage or aspiration. Open drainage is needed only rarely.

Biliary stricture can occur as late sequelae after cholecystectomy due to bile duct injury. 80% of biliary strictures are postoperative. After cholecystectomy [open or laparoscopic, more common following laparoscopic (0.8%) than open method (0.35%)]. ***Clinical features are:*** Obstructive jaundice; pain abdomen; features of ascending cholangitis; profuse persistent bile leak.

Waltmann Walter syndrome: It is compression of IVC due to collection of fluid in gallbladder fossa and subphrenic space after cholecystectomy; it mimics coronary artery thrombosis.

Bismuth classification of biliary stricture (Fig. 23-100)

I. Low CBD stricture with stump (proximal to stricture) >2 cm
II. Middle CBD stricture with proximal stump <2 cm
III. Hilar: Confluence of right and left hepatic ducts is intact
IV. Separated right and left hepatic ducts
V. Stricture involving intrahepatic ducts

Causes of postoperative stricture

- Too much traction to the GB during 'Fundus first cholecystectomy'
- Blind application of artery forceps in Calot's to control bleeding
- Anomalies of biliary tree
- Inflammatory adhesions at Calot's triangle
- Injury during other surgery like gastrectomy

Management

Liver function test (LFT), prothrombin time, endoscopic retrograde cholangiopancreatography (ERCP), computed tomography (CT), magnetic resonance cholangiopancreatography (MRCP); choledochoduodenostomy or choledochojejunostomy.

Minilaparotomy Cholecystectomy

Here incision of 5 cm length is made lateral to the right rectus in subcostal region. It was done in olden days in thin individuals where easy retraction makes Calot's dissection possible. In present era

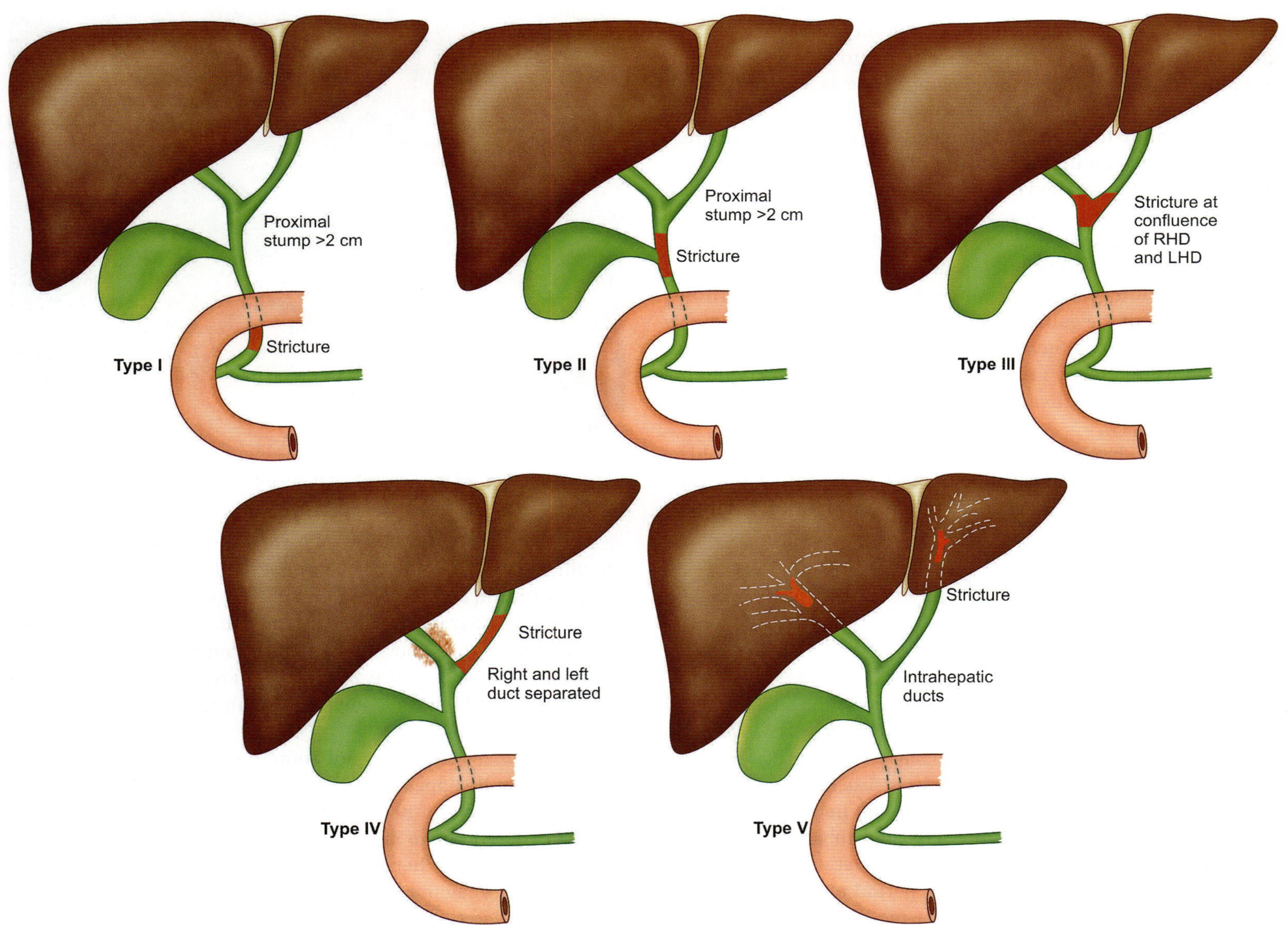

Fig. 23-100: Bismuth classification of biliary stricture.

of laparoscopic surgery, minilaparotomy cholecystectomy or any other surgeries should not be done. When open surgery is done, adequate incision with adequate exposure of the dissecting surgical field should be the approach. Hence minilaparotomy has become a surgical legacy.

Partial Cholecystectomy

It is done in severely adherent Calot's triangle which is difficult for dissections and biliary tree cannot be delineated. It is also useful in cirrhosis with portal hypertension. Here gallbladder is removed distal to the Calot's triangle at Hartmann's pouch level. When there is dense adhesion in the Calot's and dissection is impossible, it is better to do partial cholecystectomy than injuring the bile duct or hepatic artery that leads to dreaded complications. Fundus first dissection is done carefully. When reaching towards the Calot's, care should be taken not to meddle and create complications. Hartmann's pouch is held with Babcock's forceps. Tissue just behind the Hartmann's is ligated and divided. Hartmann's pouch is divided. Gallbladder is removed. Any stones in the Hartmann's are removed; warm saline wash is given. Usually in such situations, cystic duct will already be sealed without communicating into the bile duct. Mucosa of the retained part of the Hartmann's pouch is fulgurated using bipolar cautery or argon laser. Hartmann's pouch on the cystic duct side is transfixed and ligated using vicryl **(Fig. 23-101)**.

Subtotal cholecystectomy is a similar procedure but it is divided still further away from the Hartmann's pouch at the beginning of the body of the gallbladder. Technically there is hardly any difference.

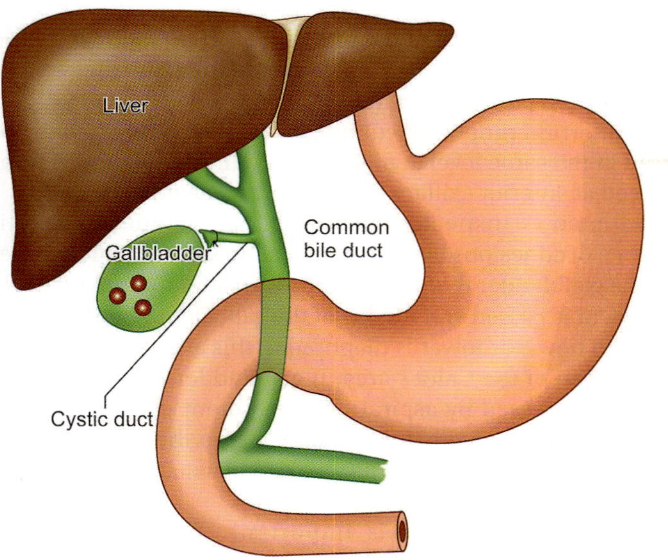

Fig. 23-101: Partial cholecystectomy.

CHOLECYSTOSTOMY

It is the drainage of the gallbladder exteriorly. It is only a life-saving procedure; not a definitive procedure.

Indications

It is done during process of surgical cholecystitis if cholecystectomy seems not possible with acute cholecystitis or empyema gallbladder or on table anaesthetic problem causes compulsion to terminate the definitive procedure. After cholecystostomy, once patient recovers, definitive procedure of cholecystectomy should be done at later period.

Cholecystostomy is done only in critically ill patients who are on severe sepsis and renal failure **(Fig. 23-102)**.

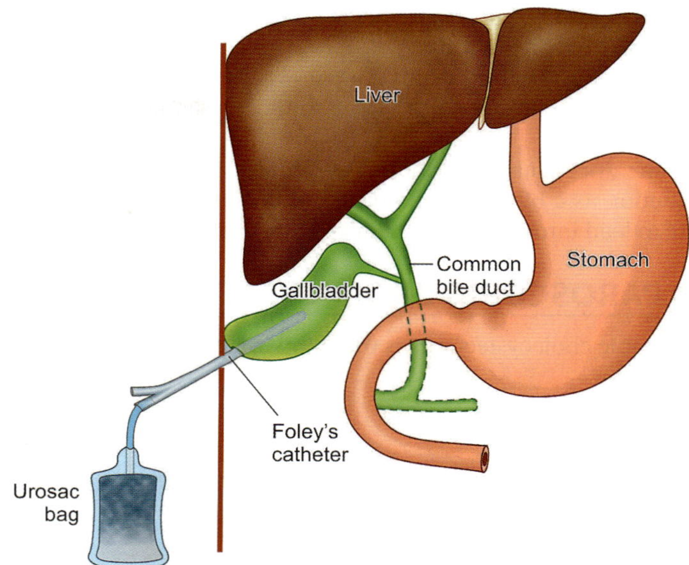

Fig. 23-102: A Foley's or Malecot's catheter is placed in severely ill patients with acute cholecystitis to drain pus initially, and later elective cholecystectomy is done. Procedure is done in elderly, severely ill, empyema GB, emphysematous GB, perforation of GB (cholecystostomy).

In olden days, in periampullary carcinoma or carcinoma head of the pancreas with severe obstructive jaundice with bilirubin as high as 30 mg% and in really poor general condition and when eventual definitive resectable procedure like Whipple's is feasible, cholecystostomy was done as initial decompression procedure. But nowadays, in carcinoma pancreas, if operable, Whipple's operation is done otherwise bypass is done. Because of the availability of ERCP, cholecystostomy is rarely done nowadays.

Technique

If cholecystostomy is not decided on table during laparotomy, then right subcostal incision of 5 cm length is made under general or local anaesthesia; abdomen is opened; liver is pushed down by placing hand over the liver; gallbladder is identified and felt; it is held with Babcock's forceps. If gallbladder is tense it should be aspirated; otherwise using trocar and cannula contents are decompressed. Fluid should be collected for culture.

Two stay sutures are placed on the fundus of the gallbladder. Gallbladder is incised for about 1 cm in between stay sutures. Contents are aspirated after collecting for culture. All stones are removed using stone removal instruments (Randall stone removal forceps). Warm saline wash is given thoroughly into the gallbladder. Finger is passed into the gallbladder to milk out all stones and contents. Foley's or Malecot's or de Pezzer catheter 22–24 sized is passed into the gallbladder. Purse string suture is passed around the tube by taking bites through the fundus of the gallbladder all around the gallbladder. Additional interrupted sutures if needed should be placed. Tube can be brought out through the omentum or omentum may be wrapped around it to reduce the chance of leak. Through a separate stab wound tube is brought out of the abdominal wall. Often tube is also fixed to abdominal wall from inside by placing interrupted sutures between parietal peritoneum and fundus of the gallbladder. Tube is fixed outside using skin suture.

Problems

If there is necrosis or gangrene of the gallbladder then cholecystostomy is contraindicated as necrosed part will disrupt and cause biliary peritonitis.

It is totally contraindicated in acute cholangitis where, when there is obstruction ERCP is a must.

Perse cholecystostomy is not done nowadays as in these patients alternatively percutaneous drainage under guidance serves same purpose.

If cystic duct is already blocked by fibrosis cholecystostomy will not function as a bile drainage system. But sepsis will come under control to lead into eventual definitive cholecystectomy.

LAPAROSCOPIC CHOLECYSTECTOMY

Laparoscopic cholecystectomy is the standard technique for removal of gallbladder.

Indications

- Symptomatic gallstone diseases—pain, mucocoele, cholecystitis acute or chronic.
- Acalculous cholecystitis.
- Asymptomatic gallstones—when patient is undergoing bariatric surgery, diabetics, renal transplantation, haemolytic diseases, in children.
- Complications of the gallstones like gallstone ileus, empyema, and perforation also can undergo laparoscopic cholecystectomy; but conversion rate may be more. If during laparoscopic procedure, when dissection becomes difficult surgeon should not be hesitant to convert into open cholecystectomy to avoid serious complications.
- Gallstone dyspepsia where biliary pain is present without the presence of gallstones. Here patient may get relieved of the symptoms by laparoscopic cholecystectomy. Biliary dyskinesia may be an indication.
- Gallbladder polyps—if polyps are multiple, if they are increasing in size, if size is more than 1 cm then laparoscopic cholecystectomy is indicated.

Contraindications

There is a debate about absolute contraindication for laparoscopic cholecystectomy. Patients who are unfit for general anaesthesia is a contraindication. In patients with portal hypertension and coagulopathy laparoscopic cholecystectomy is still better than open but adequate precautions should be taken including correction of coagulopathy, need for plasma or platelet transfusions. Proven gallbladder cancer is a sure contraindication for laparoscopic cholecystectomy. Multiple earlier laparotomies, severe dense adhesions in cholecystitis, acute pancreatitis, anomalies in the biliary system, cirrhosis, pregnancy, obesity are the real challenging situations while doing laparoscopic cholecystectomy. Need for a conversion and non-hesitant to convert at right time prior to creation of critical problem are to be kept in mind by surgeons.

Technique

Patient is placed in 15° head up anti-Trendelenburg position with 15° right upward tilt. Probably, this is done after insertion of the first camera port in supine position. Nasogastric tube should be passed to decompress the stomach. Urinary catheter is placed otherwise bladder should be emptied before patient is brought into the operation theatre table. It is required in difficult cases or complications are suspected or when prolonged anaesthesia is needed.

After clearing and draping, monitor is kept on the right side facing towards the table; surgeon stands on the left side; camera assistant on the left of the surgeon; scrub nurse on the right side near foot end of the patient. Ideally two monitors on right and left sides should be kept. What is commonly practiced is North American approach with the position explained as above. Radiolucent table is essential to do fluoroscopy whenever needed like on table cholangiogram.

Instruments (Fig. 23-103)

1. Veress needle
2. 10 mm port—2 in no.
3. 5 mm port—2 in no.
4. Maryland forceps.
5. Atraumatic (Universal) grasper.
6. Toothed grasper 5 mm.
7. Gallbladder extracting forceps 10 mm.
8. Clip applicator.
9. Suction irrigation.
10. Scissors.
11. Hook/spatula dissector.
12. Endo bag.

Alternatively patient may be kept in semilithotomy position with anti-Trendelenburg tilt; thighs should be kept parallel to ground. Surgeon stands in between legs. Port placements are almost similar but right hand working port is placed in the left hypochondrium to achieve triangulation. This position is called as French or European position.

Camera port (10 mm) is placed at upper umbilical crease line. But position can be at changed depending on obesity, previous surgery. Open or closed method can be used. A 10 mm working port is placed in the epigastrium just below the xiphoid process in the subcostal region. After initially puncturing the rectus sheath, it is directed towards right to avoid entering through the falciform ligament. If it passes through the falciform ligament then bleeding may occur as falciform ligament is vascular; falciform ligament may act as a flap to interrupt proper functioning of the port. Third (5 mm) port is placed in the same level at midclavicular line; 4th lateral 5 mm port is placed at anterior axillary or still lateral depending on need.

Abdomen is inspected all round. Gallbladder is identified; presence of adhesions by omentum, colon, stomach and duodenum over the gallbladder is identified. Through lateral 5 mm port toothed instrument is passed and fundus of the gallbladder is held firmly and is pushed upwards towards diaphragm; this allows the opening and visualisation of the Calot's area. If gallbladder is found tense then it is decompressed by aspirating the content using a long needle passed directly through abdominal wall into the gallbladder under vision. Fine trocar and cannula also can be used but usually needle aspiration is sufficient.

Release of adhesions is important. Through epigastrium port Maryland instrument is passed using a reducer. Through midclavicular port 5 mm non-toothed atraumatic grasper is passed. Omentum is pulled down from the gallbladder by holding the edge using Maryland very close to the gallbladder. Cautery and blunt traction separates the omentum. Similarly colon, stomach and duodenum are released from the field. Monopolar cautery may injure these structures due to heat generated and so should be used judiciously. Once adhesions are released, infundibulum is held using the midclavicular port instrument. Infundibulum is held downwards and towards right.

Calot's triangle is dissected using Maryland forceps. In infundibular technique, cystic duct is dissected carefully both in front and behind and traced towards infundibulum to visualise typical flare when cystic duct joins the infundibulum and with a funnel shape. Cystic duct is further dissected from infundibulum towards the cystohepatic junction; i.e. from safety zone to danger zone.

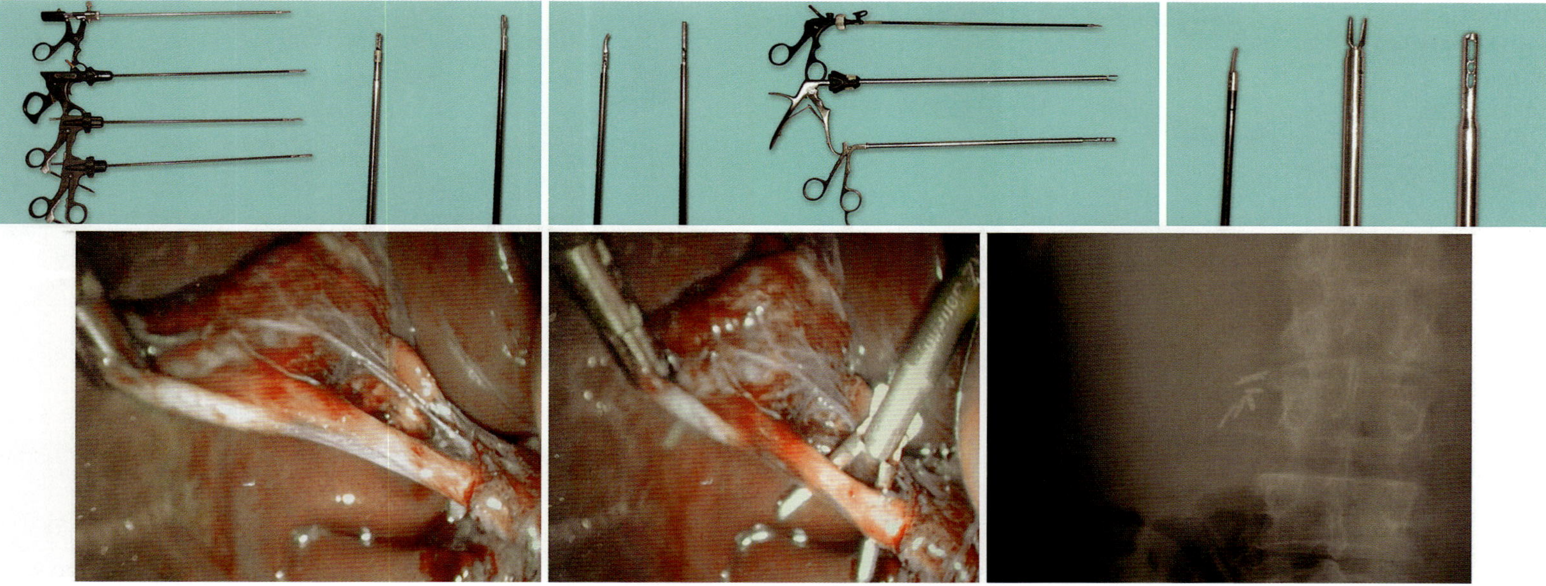

Fig. 23-103: Laparoscopic cholecystectomy instruments and Calot's triangle dissection and X-ray view of the clips placed.

Bipolar cautery should be used rather than monopolar cautery. Entire Calot's should be dissected including cystic artery. It should be made sure that only two structures enter the gland. Lymph node of Lund is a good marker to dissect cystic artery; node is anterior to the artery. Calot's dissection should not extend posterior to a constant landmark on the inferior surface of the liver—*Rouvier sulcus* **(Fig. 23-104)**. This oblique sulcus usually is present in the liver; dissection should be in front of it; never extend to posterior level of this landmark.

Another technique is '*critical view of safety*' in which entire Calot's triangle including Hartmann's pouch is dissected off from the liver bed to identify the cystic duct and artery. *Strasberg (Steven S Strasberg) critical view of "Safety"* is the technique of identifications of cystic artery and cystic duct with three elements: (1) To clear hepatocystic triangle of fat and fibrous tissue; (2) To take the lower part of the gallbladder off the cystic plate; (3) To see/confirm that two and only two structures are entering the gallbladder.

Cystic artery is dissected using Maryland forceps and isolated. Any anomalies should be identified. Lymph node of Lund is a good marker to identify, which lies in front of the artery. Often anterior/superficial and posterior/deep branches are identified. After dissecting entire Calot's and confirming only two structures are entering the gallbladder, cystic artery is clipped on both sides and divided with curved scissor. Harmonic scalpel can also be used to divide the cystic artery. Cystic artery is usually divided prior to cystic duct.

Then cystic duct is clipped using 10 mm clip applicator through epigastric port. Two clips are applied proximally and one clip distally and divided in between. Blind application of clip should be avoided; clip applied should be away from bile duct. Undue traction during clipping should be avoided. Before clipping, if any stone is present in cystic duct, they are milked into the gallbladder.

Gallbladder is detached from the liver using various instruments. Spatula with monopolar cautery is commonly used and safer. Monopolar hook can also be used; its bend is commonly used; to cut peritoneal edge sharp tip is hooked and fulgurated. Harmonic scalpel is an excellent tool for this. Hartmann's pouch is held using the 5 mm grasper (dolphin nosed) and alternatively its position is changed according to its need. Undue deeper fulguration may open up the liver tissue. It is safer to keep the instrument closer to the gallbladder than liver bed. When small peritoneal fold attachment is left near the fundus, bed is retracted to inspect the Calot's and gallbladder bed properly for the clip placement and to see if there is any oozing. Often gallbladder may get opened to spilling the stones and bile. Bile should be sucked out properly and stones should be extracted or kept in an extracting bag placed in the peritoneal cavity.

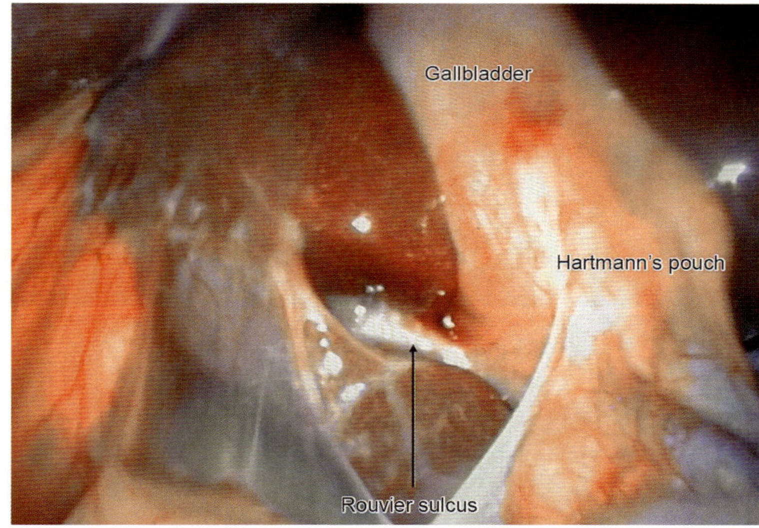

Fig. 23-104: Laparoscopic view of Rouvier sulcus.

Gallbladder is extracted through the epigastric port; 10 mm stout gallbladder holding instrument (claw-shaped) is used to hold at neck of the dissected gallbladder; instrument with 10 mm port is removed with the gallbladder. Often rectus sheath and skin incision at port site may need to be widened by few mm. Gallbladder neck when once comes out of the wound can be opened and all bile is sucked out. Stones in the gallbladder can be removed using an artery forceps to make its removal easier. Gallbladder can be held by passing curved Kocher's clamp through the epigastric port site wound after removing the port temporarily. Retrieval bag can be used to remove the gallbladder and is probably ideal.

Once gallbladder is removed, gallbladder is checked for its opening and contents. Port is placed again. Gallbladder bed and Calot's triangle is checked again. Bed is irrigated and inspected before the final closure.

Usually closure is not necessary. When there is difficulty in dissection or if sepsis is present, then drain is kept. A 14 French nasogastric tube is passed through the lateral 5 mm port and placed in gallbladder bed **(Fig. 23-105)**.

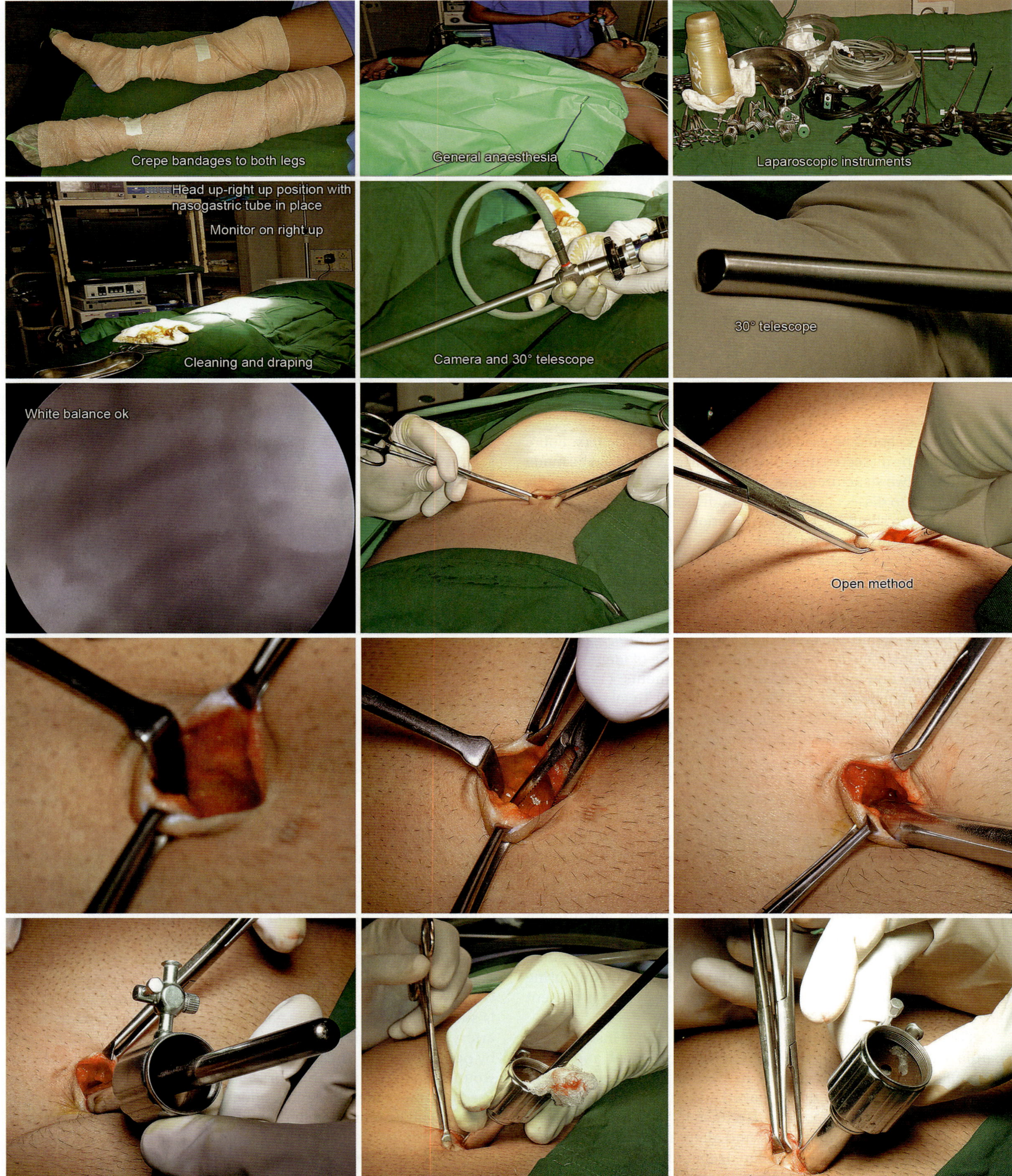
Crepe bandages to both legs
General anaesthesia
Laparoscopic instruments
Head up-right up position with nasogastric tube in place
Monitor on right up
Cleaning and draping
Camera and 30° telescope
30° telescope
White balance ok
Open method

Figs. 23-105(1)

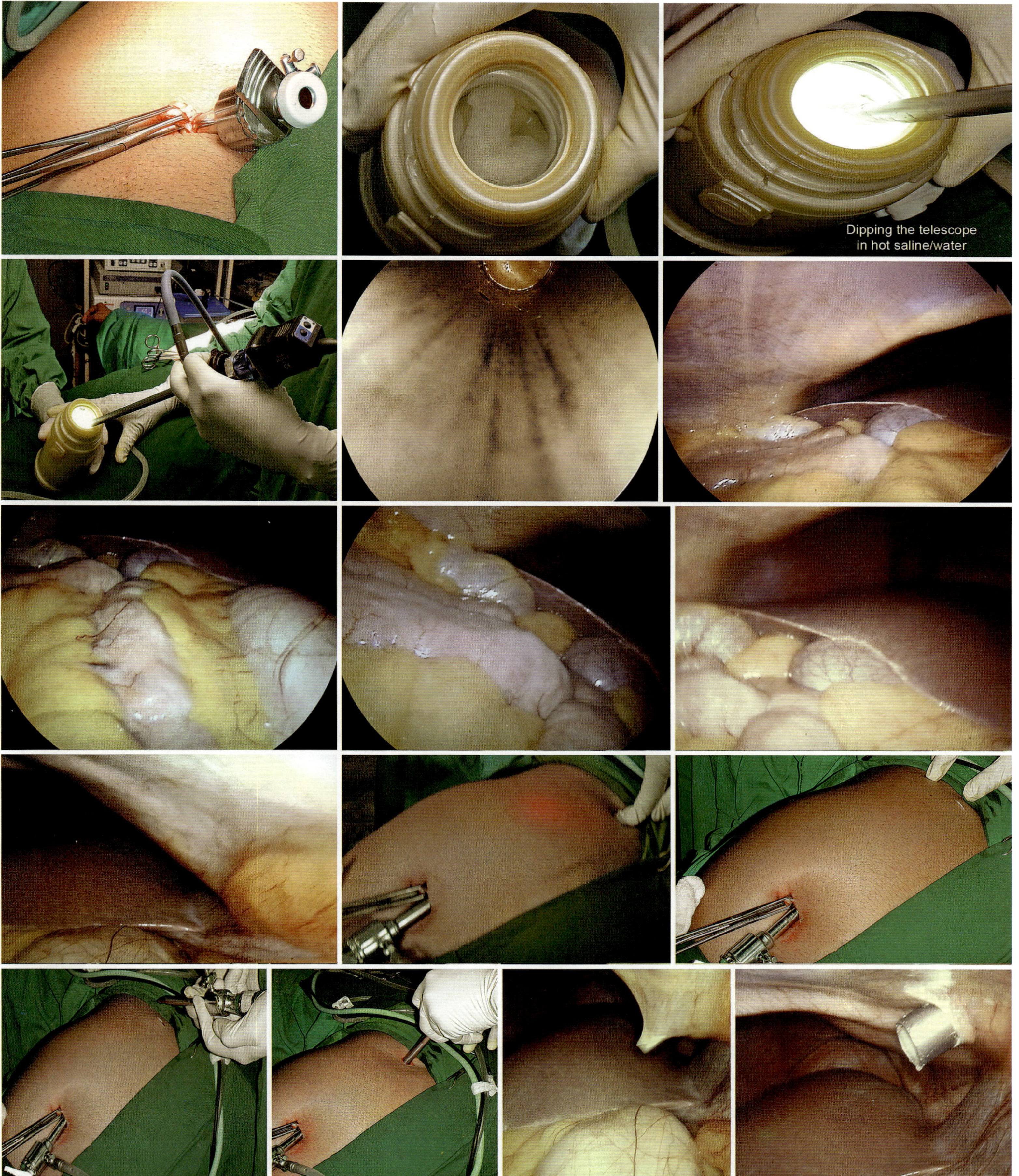

Figs. 23-105(2)

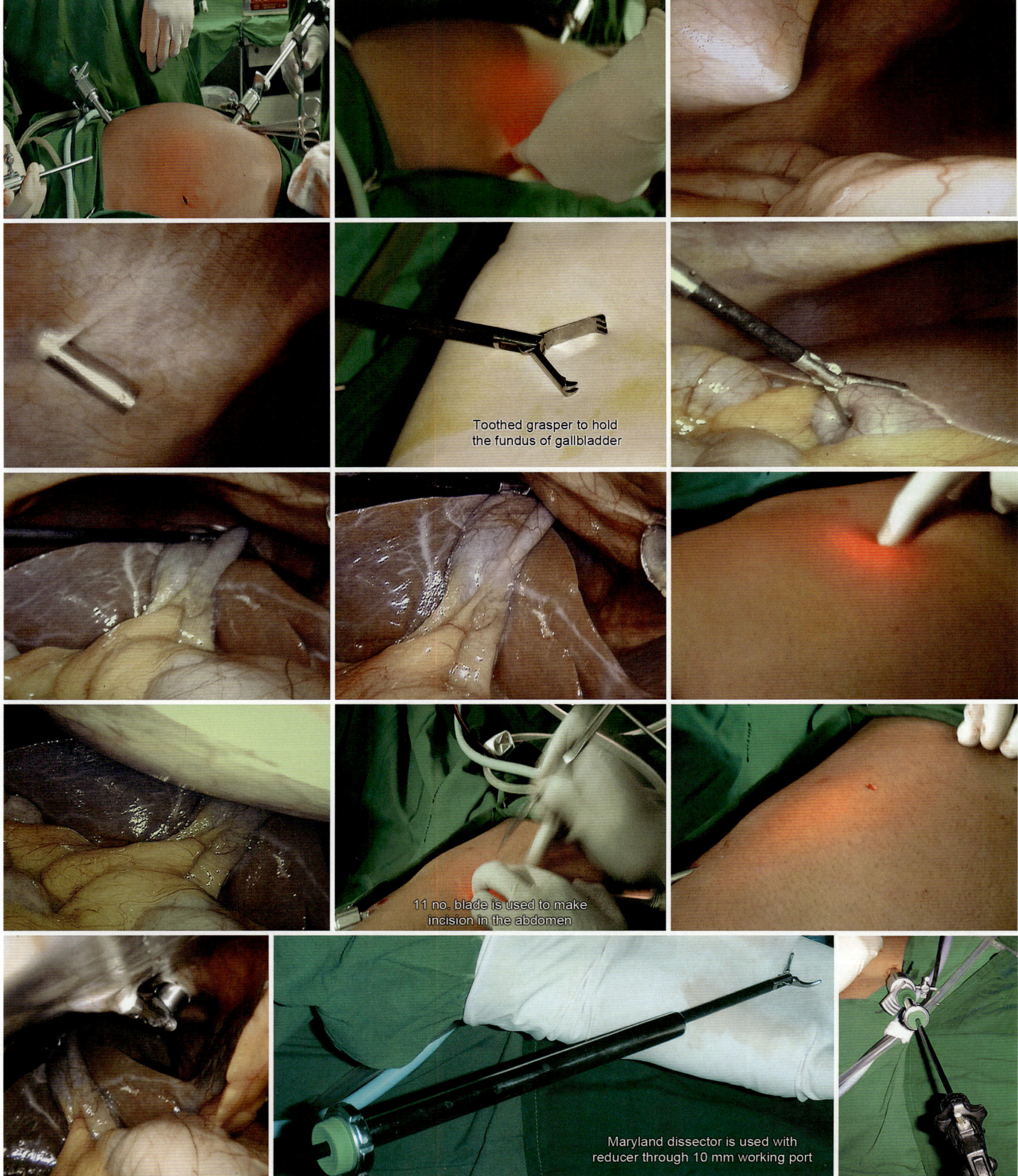
Toothed grasper to hold
the fundus of gallbladder
11 no. blade is used to make
incision in the abdomen
Maryland dissector is used with
reducer through 10 mm working port

Figs. 23-105(3)

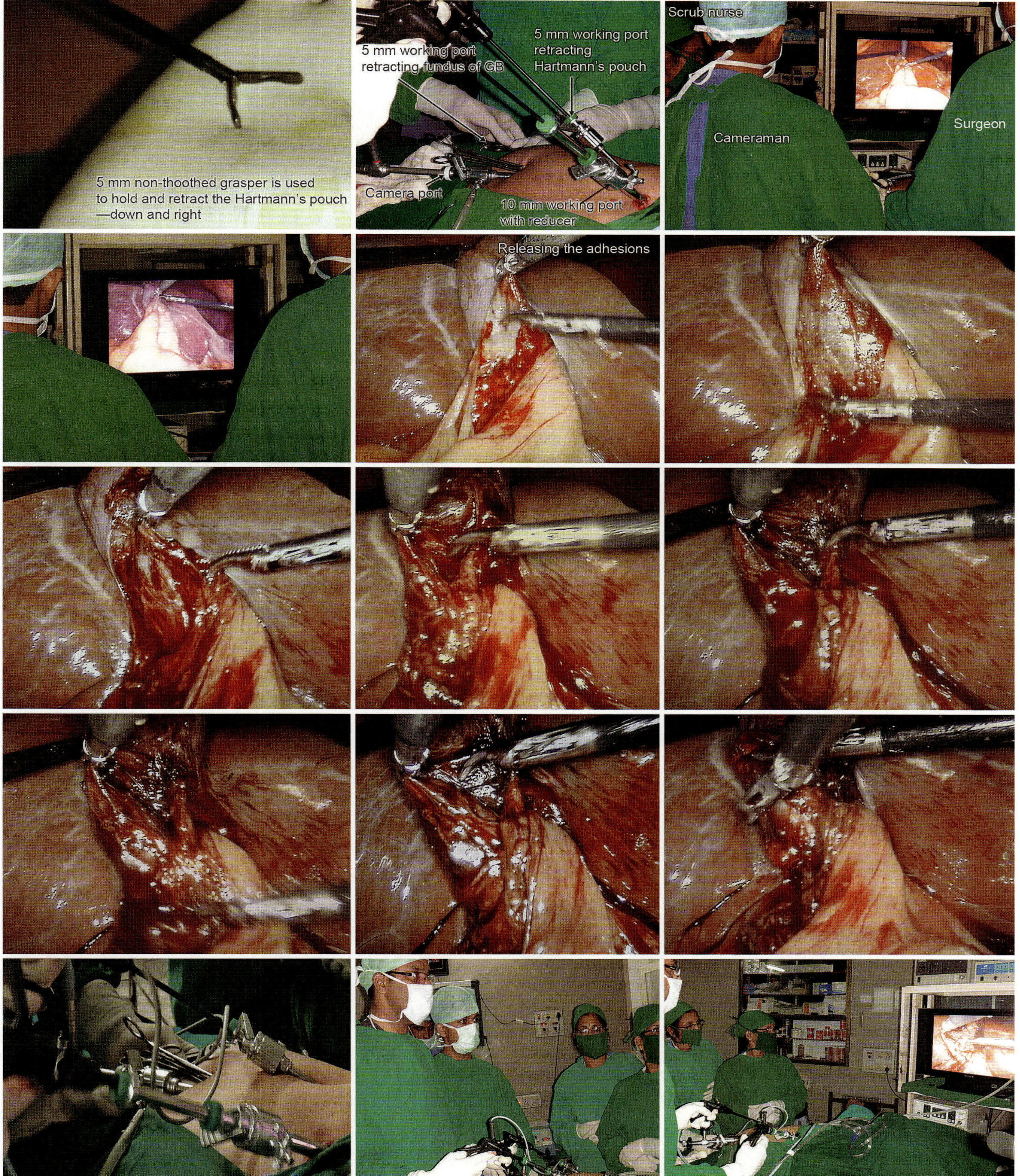
5 mm non-thoothed grasper is used
to hold and retract the Hartmann's pouch
—down and right
5 mm working port
retracting fundus of GB
5 mm working port
retracting
Hartmann's pouch
Camera port
10 mm working port
with reducer
Scrub nurse
Cameraman
Surgeon
Releasing the adhesions

Figs. 23-105(4)

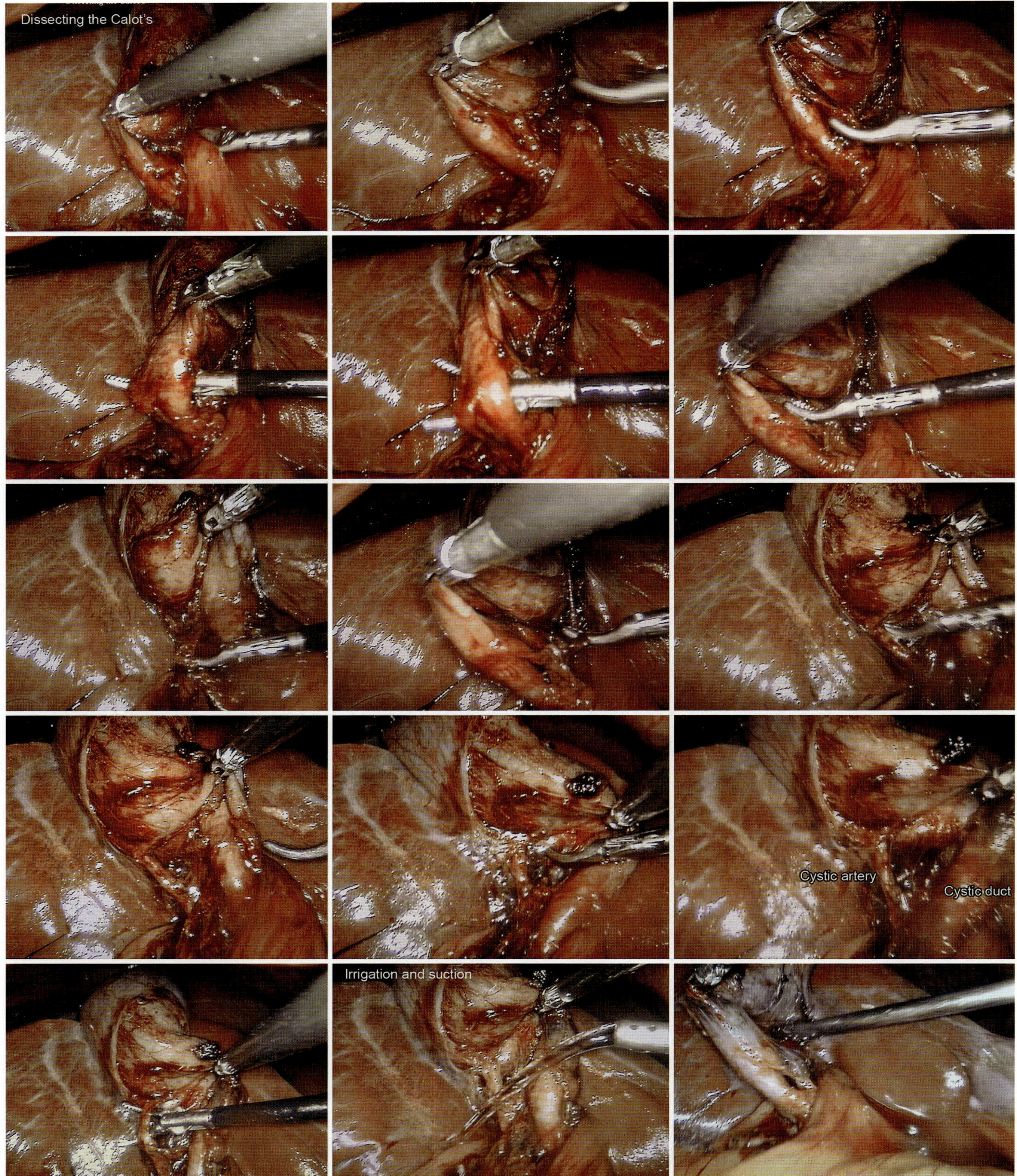
Dissecting the Calot's
Cystic artery
Cystic duct
Irrigation and suction

Figs. 23-105(5)

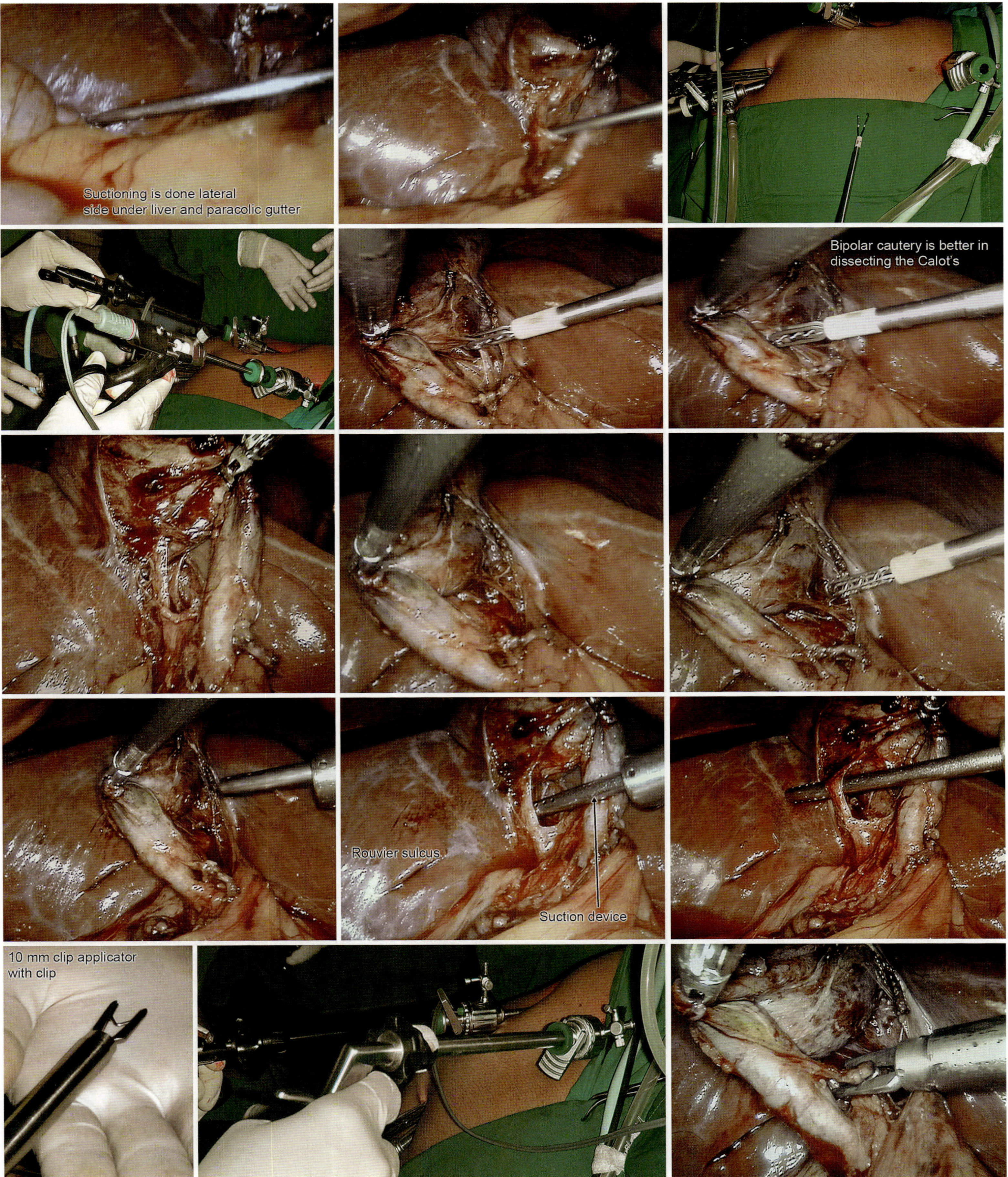
Suctioning is done lateral
side under liver and paracolic gutter
Bipolar cautery is better in
dissecting the Calot's
Rouvier sulcus
Suction device
10 mm clip applicator
with clip

Figs. 23-105(6)

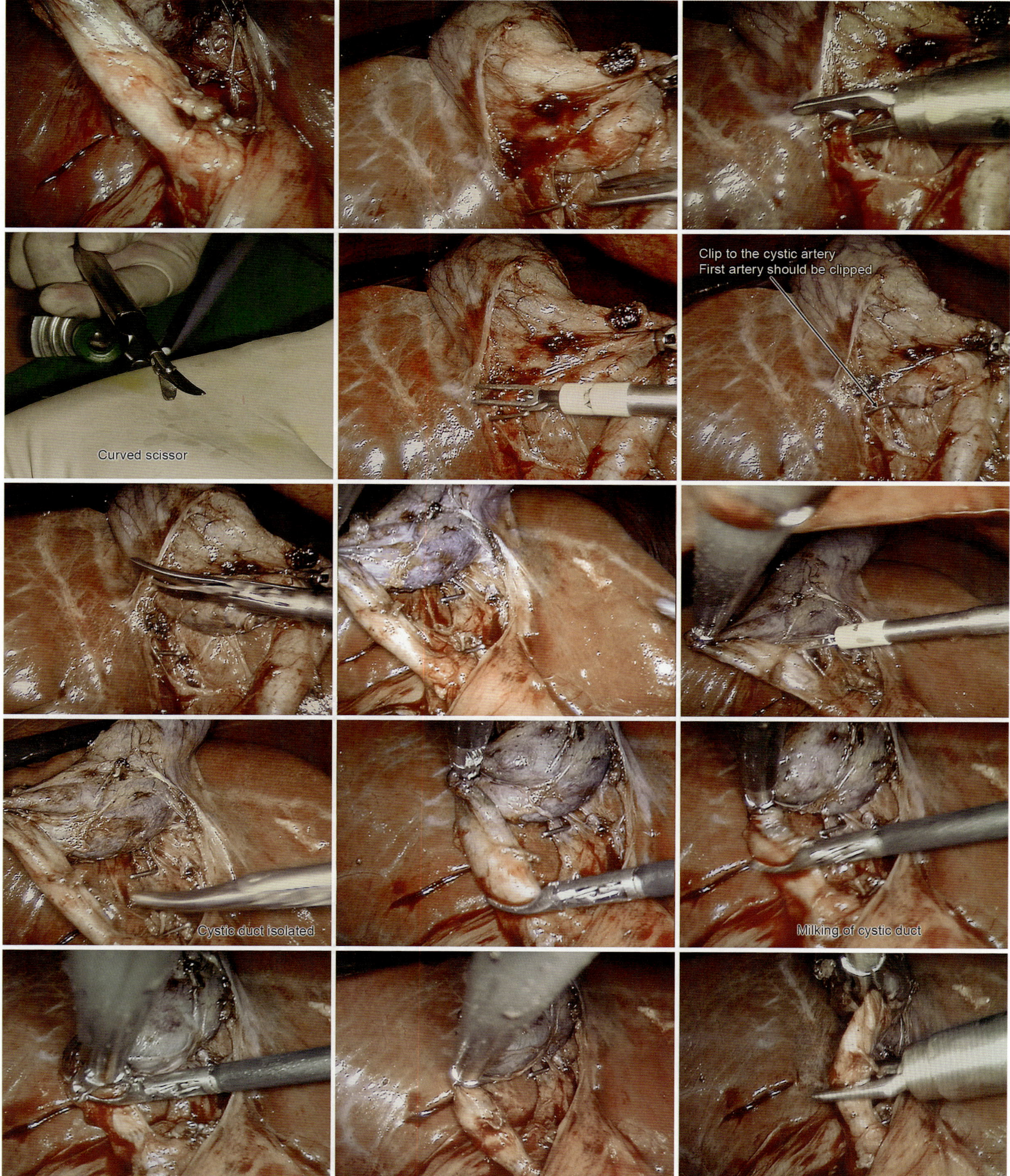
Curved scissor
Clip to the cystic artery
First artery should be clipped
Cystic duct isolated
Milking of cystic duct

Figs. 23-105(7)

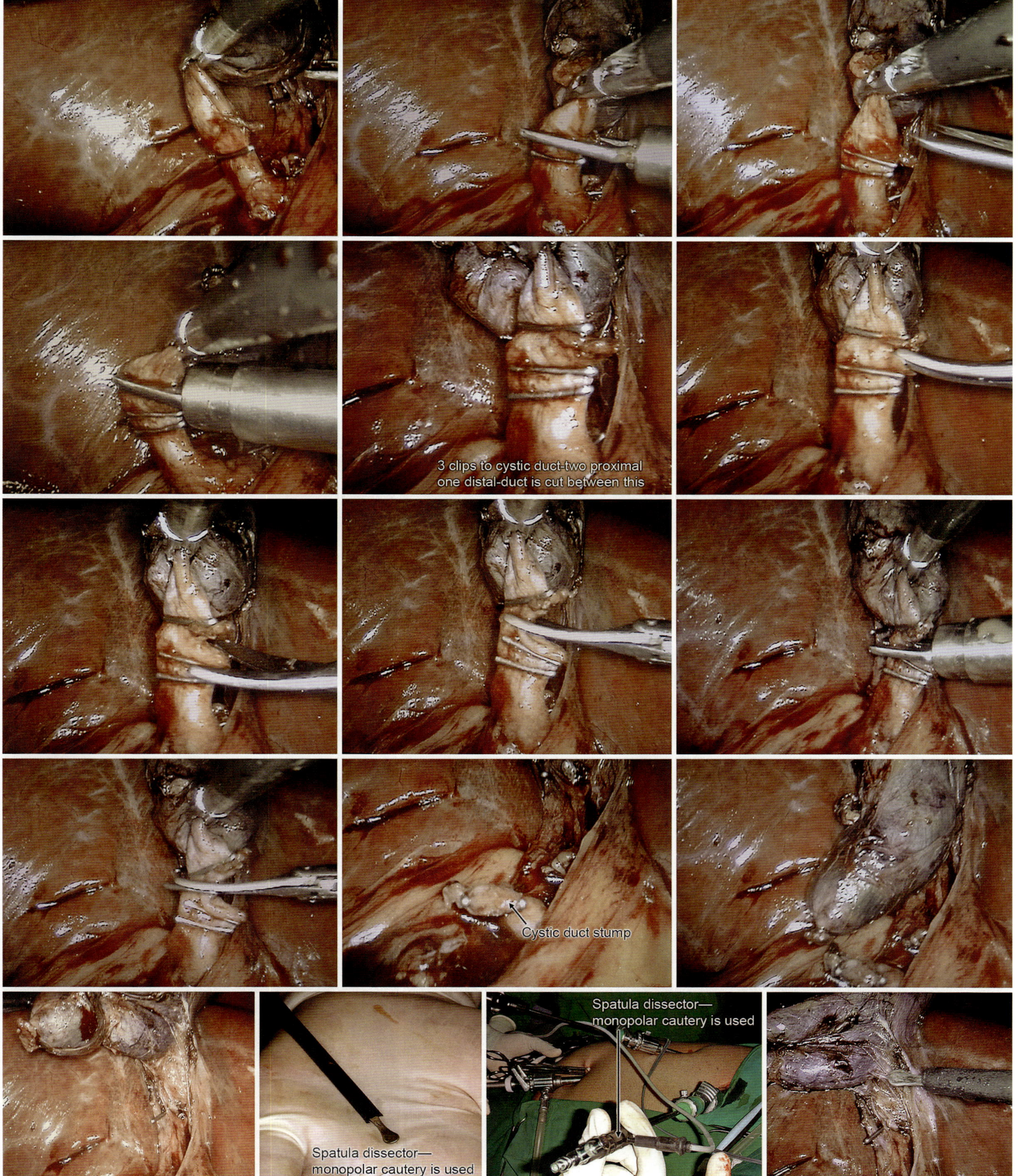
3 clips to cystic duct-two proximal one distal-duct is cut between this
Cystic duct stump
Spatula dissector—monopolar cautery is used
Spatula dissector—monopolar cautery is used

Figs. 23-105(8)

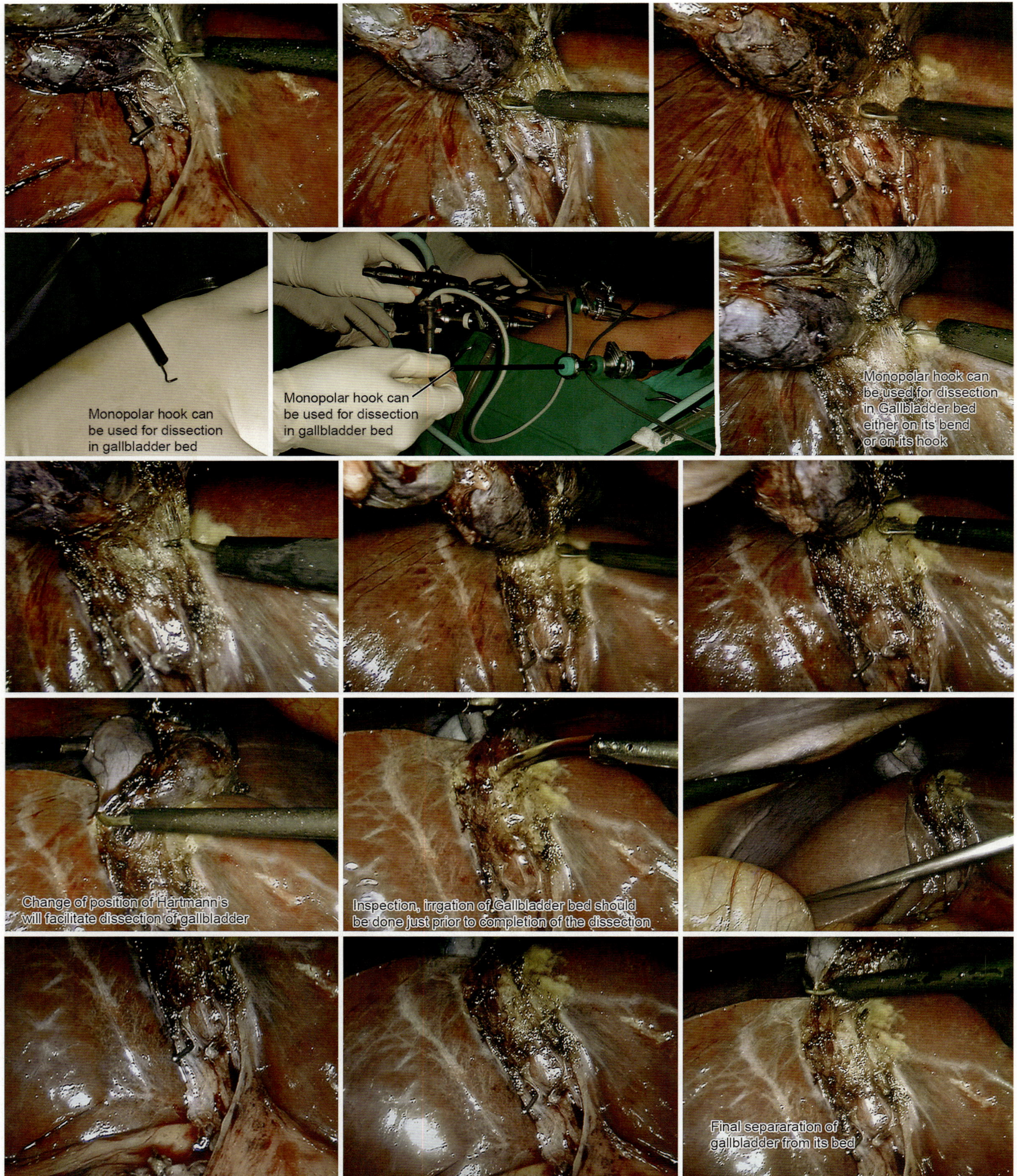
Monopolar hook can be used for dissection in gallbladder bed
Monopolar hook can be used for dissection in gallbladder bed
Monopolar hook can be used for dissection in Gallbladder bed either on its bend or on its hook
Change of position of Hartmann's will facilitate dissection of gallbladder
Inspection, irrgation of Gallbladder bed should be done just prior to completion of the dissection
Final separaration of gallbladder from its bed

Figs. 23-105(9)

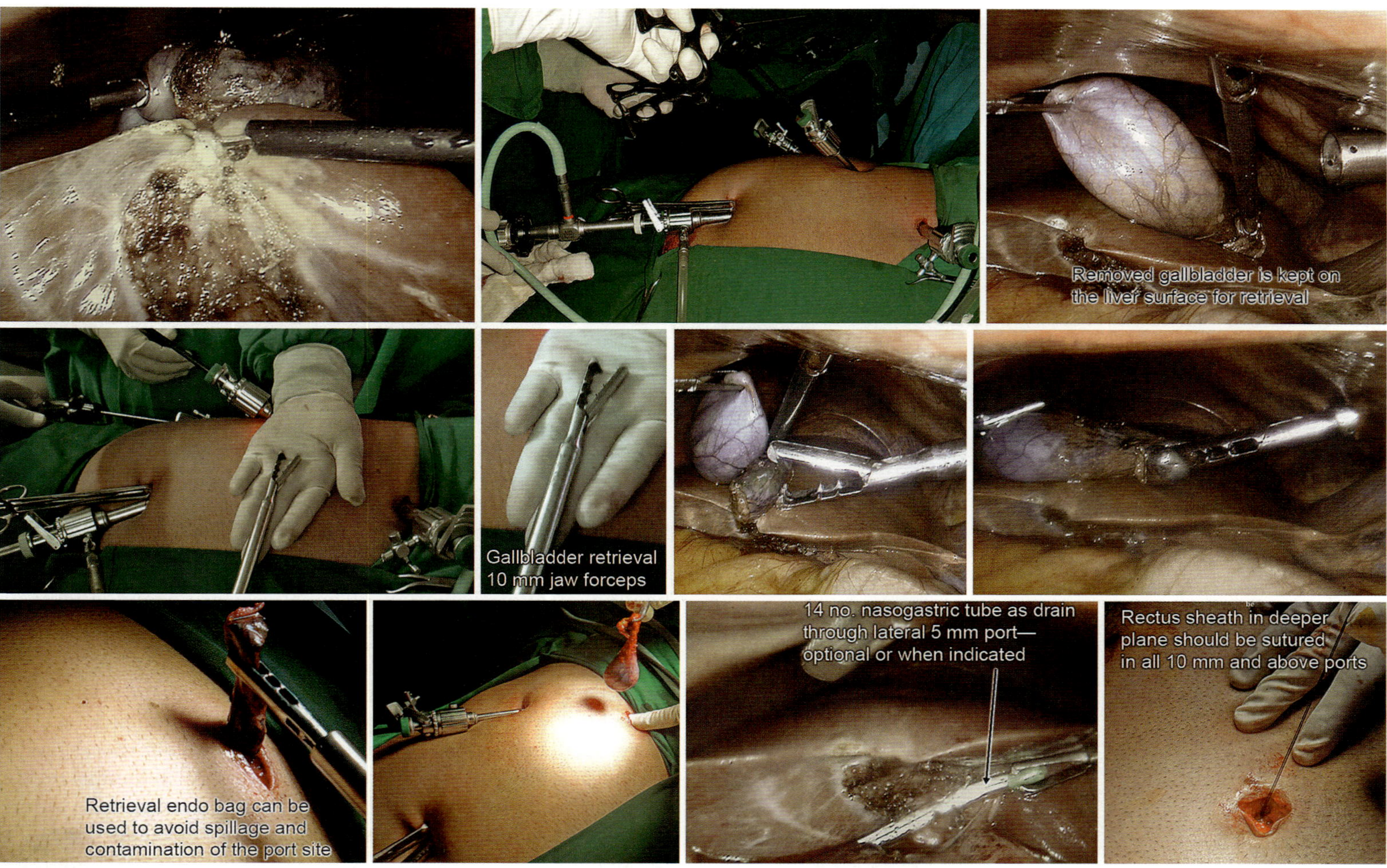

Figs. 23-105(10)

Figs. 23-105(1 to 10): Technique of laparoscopic cholecystectomy in detail.

Key steps

1. Place four standard ports.
2. Right up and head up position.
3. Maintain adequate traction on the gallbladder at all times.
4. Posterior dissection at Calot's triangle.
5. Cystic artery and duct are identified dissected properly from safe distal zone (infundibular) to danger proximal zone (CBD level)
6. Clip application after confirming anatomy.
7. Clip artery first then only duct.
8. Dissect gallbladder close to the wall.
9. Inspect gallbladder fossa.
10. Drain the gallbladder bed.
11. Fascial sheaths of all 10 mm port sites should be closed securely.

Trocars are removed, rectus sheaths are closed in 10 mm ports. Skin is sutured or sealed with cyancrylate glue **(Figs. 23-106 to 23-108)**.

The drain is removed after 24 hours and oral diet is started. The patient is mobilised as early as possible and discharged after 48 hours.

Difficult Gallbladder

The safest thing to do when the anatomy of the Calot's triangle is not defined is to convert to open surgery. Conversion should not be taken as a failure but as a wise decision in the interest of the patient. At times, the Calot's triangle is adherent and all planes are lost. In such cases, the suction irrigation device can be used as a blunt dissector and dissection can be done using jet of saline through the channel. One should always be aware of the position of the duodenum and the CBD as they are likely to be damaged. A gauze piece can be used to keep the field clean provided utmost care is given and the same is retrieved at the end of the procedure. It is easy to lose track of the small piece and later struggle to find it. Retrograde dissection can be done provided the surgeon is experienced but for the majority of us it may be safe to convert into an open surgery. Subtotal cholecystectomy is an alternative which can be undertaken. Additional instrument using additional port can be tried like fan liver retractor.

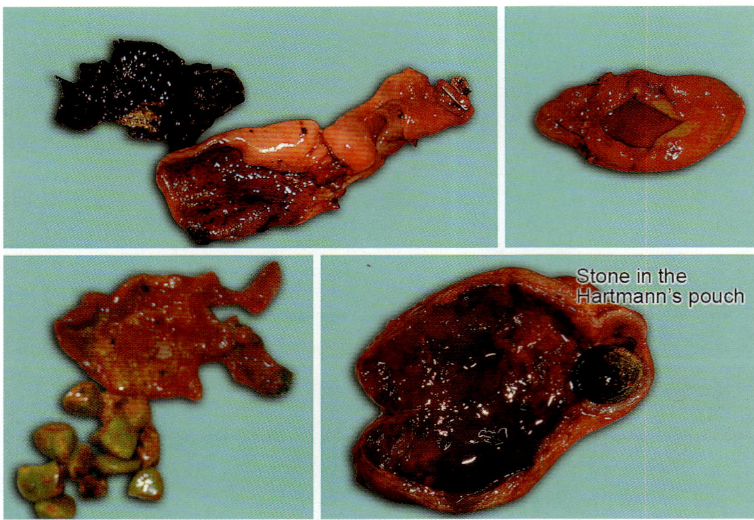

Fig. 23-106: Gallbladder specimens removed in different patients—through laparoscopy.

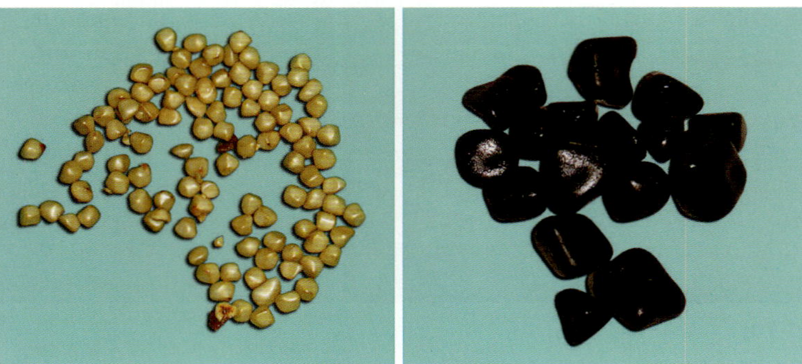

Fig. 23-107: Different gallstone—types.

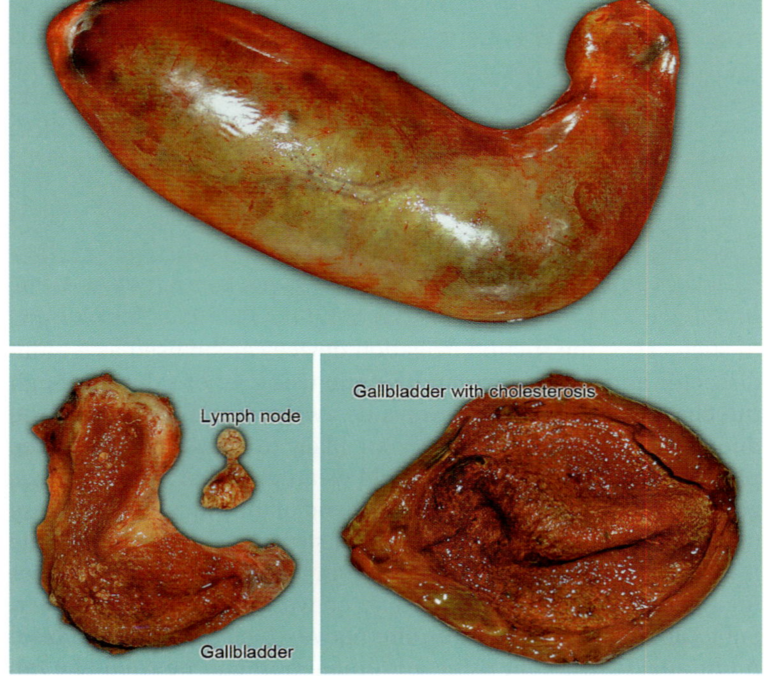

Fig. 23-108: Gallbladder specimens with different pathological look.

Trouble Shooting

1. Difficulty in visualising the Calot's triangle	♦ Reposition the patient. ♦ Apply the traction cranially. ♦ Clear the viscera away from the operative field. ♦ Aspirate the Ryle's tube to deflate the stomach. ♦ Apply lateral traction to the Hartmann's pouch.
2. Bleeding at Calot's triangle	♦ Try to perform posterior dissection. ♦ Apply compression using gauze piece and wait for 5 minutes. ♦ Do not dissect the area blindly which you cannot visualise.
3. Short cystic duct	♦ Confirm the anatomy. ♦ Apply intracorporeal knots using silk or vicryl
4. Bleeding from liver bed	♦ Take the gallbladder on the spot and apply pressure keeping the gallbladder on it. Wait for 5 minutes. ♦ Stay close to the gallbladder while dissecting.

Complications of Laparoscopic Cholecystectomy

Haemorrhage: It can be from liver bed, or slippage of cystic artery ligation or after formation of hepatic artery pseudoaneurysm **(Fig. 23-109)**. Trocar site bleeding can also cause significant difficulty in controlling.

Spillage of stones: They should be extracted carefully. Often it is left behind as stone gets migrated and it is difficult to pick up every stone. Such unidentified stone may cause real problem occasionally. It can cause abscess in subphrenic space or intra-abdominal region; can cause sinus formation, granuloma formation. It can erode various vital structures in the peritoneal cavity causing colocutaneous fistula, duodenal fistula, intestinal obstruction, major vessel thrombosis (middle colic artery), haematuria, and septicaemia.

Biliary tree injuries are due to missed anatomy, over traction on the CBD, anomalies, adhesions, etc. If biliary tree (bile duct or hepatic duct) injury occurs conversion should be done. Type of injury is identified and classified. ERCP stenting may be tried on table. Otherwise choledochojejunostomy should be done. It is unwise to repair a completely transected common bile duct as stricture will develop eventually **(Fig. 23-110)**.

Injury to colon, stomach, and duodenum can occur. Complications specific to laparoscopy should be kept in mind.

Wound infection, incisional hernia can occur.

Pancreatitis, retained stones, biliary stricture are other complications.

SINGLE INCISION LAPAROSCOPIC SURGERY IN CHOLECYSTECTOMY (FIG. 23-111)

Single incision laparoscopic surgery (SILS) is an advanced minimally invasive surgical procedure wherein surgeon operates exclusively through a single umbilical entry port. It is also called as single port access surgery (SPA), one port umbilical surgery (OPUS), and single port incision less conventional equipment utilising surgery (SPICES), natural orifice transumbilical surgery (NOTUS).

Whales did tubal ligation in 1969 through single incision; Pelosi did SIL appendicectomy in 1992; Navarra et al. did SIL cholecystectomy in 1997; Pishkun et al. did SIL cholecystectomy in 1999.

It needs general anaesthesia, specialised umbilical large trocars which accommodates working instruments, flexible laparoscope, rotatable instruments, articulating handles and harmonic scalpel.

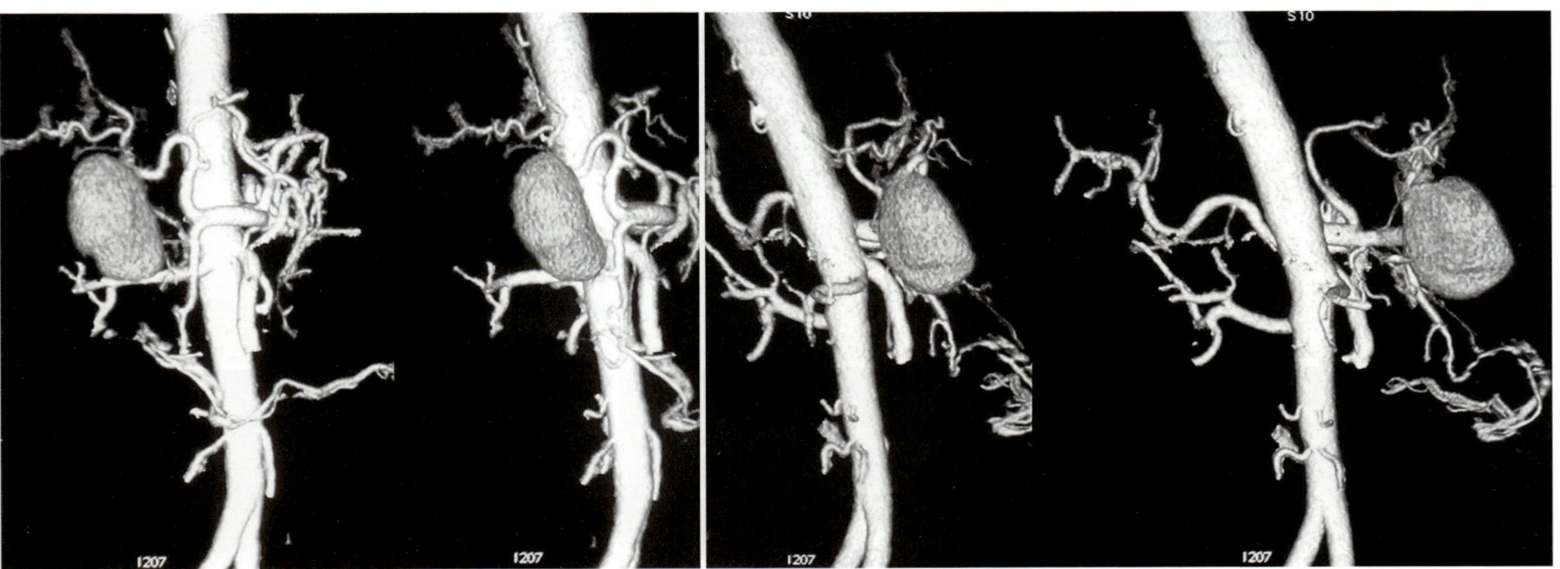

Fig. 23-109: Hepatic artery pseudoaneurysm after laparoscopic cholecystectomy; it is treated successfully by injection of glue and coils through intervention radiology.

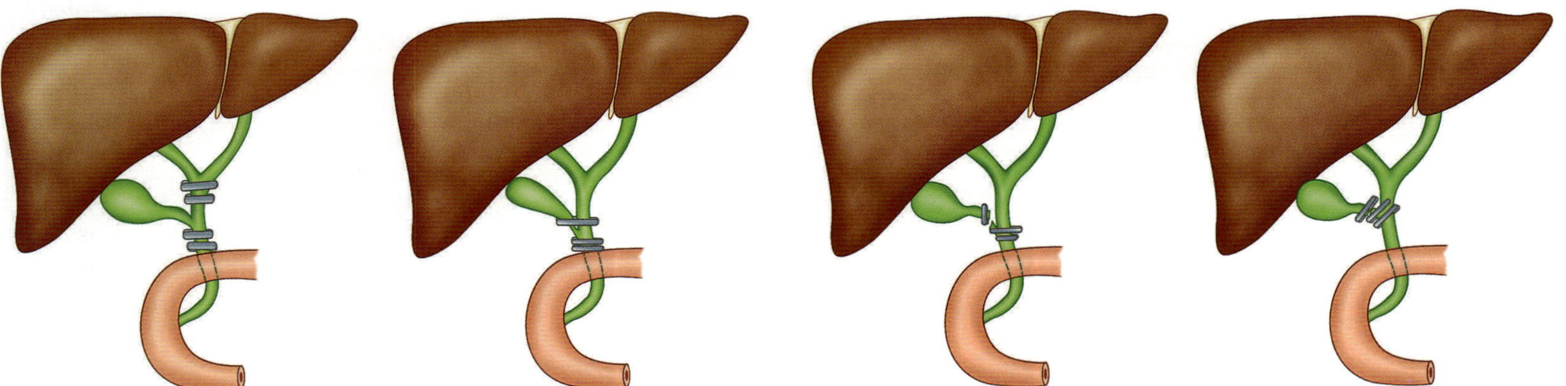

Different ways where bile duct and hepatic duct can get injured during laproscopic surgery—during clipping of the cystic duct

Fig. 23-110: Possible ways by which common bile duct and right hepatic duct can get injured while doing laparoscopic cholecystectomy.

Here through a large 2.5 cm umbilical vertical incision dissection is done by open method to reach peritoneal cavity. Specialised port in which one can pass 10 mm telescope and two 5 mm instruments for work. Instruments are angled and flexible to meet the ergonomic principles to certain extent. Dissection of gallbladder is done in similar fashion like four port technique. Specimen is easily retrieved through umbilical port as it is wider enough. If difficulty arises any time one can add additional ports as required.

Advantages

There is no visible scar like a traditional multiport, faster recovery time, early return to work and cosmetically better.

Disadvantages

Expensive trocars and instruments, skilled work, learning curve, dissection against normal surgical ergonomics. Coaxial orientation of optics and instruments, loss of triangulation—'Azimuth angle', sword fighting of instruments inside; nutcracking outside—are real problems.

Complications

Umbilical wound pain, infection, umbilical hernia, time consuming because of limited visibility during learning curve complications of cholecystectomy and conversion rate may be more, selection of case is very important.

COMMON BILE DUCT EXPLORATION

It is done to remove the CBD stones after open cholecystectomy. In this present era of ERCP with laparoscopic cholecystectomy its indications are not that common unlike as in olden days. However, failed ERCP patients needs open choledochotomy and extraction of the biliary tree stones. In olden days, it is indicated if intraoperative duct cholangiography shows stones in CBD; recent history of jaundice; palpable stones in the CBD; CBD diameter more than 10 mm; if ultrasound shows stones in CBD; and when in doubt. Many times even if ultrasound is normal with altered liver function in blood parameters one should suspect the presence of CBD stones; CT abdomen or MRI is ideal in such situation. One has to remember that without confirming the presence or absence of CBD stones,

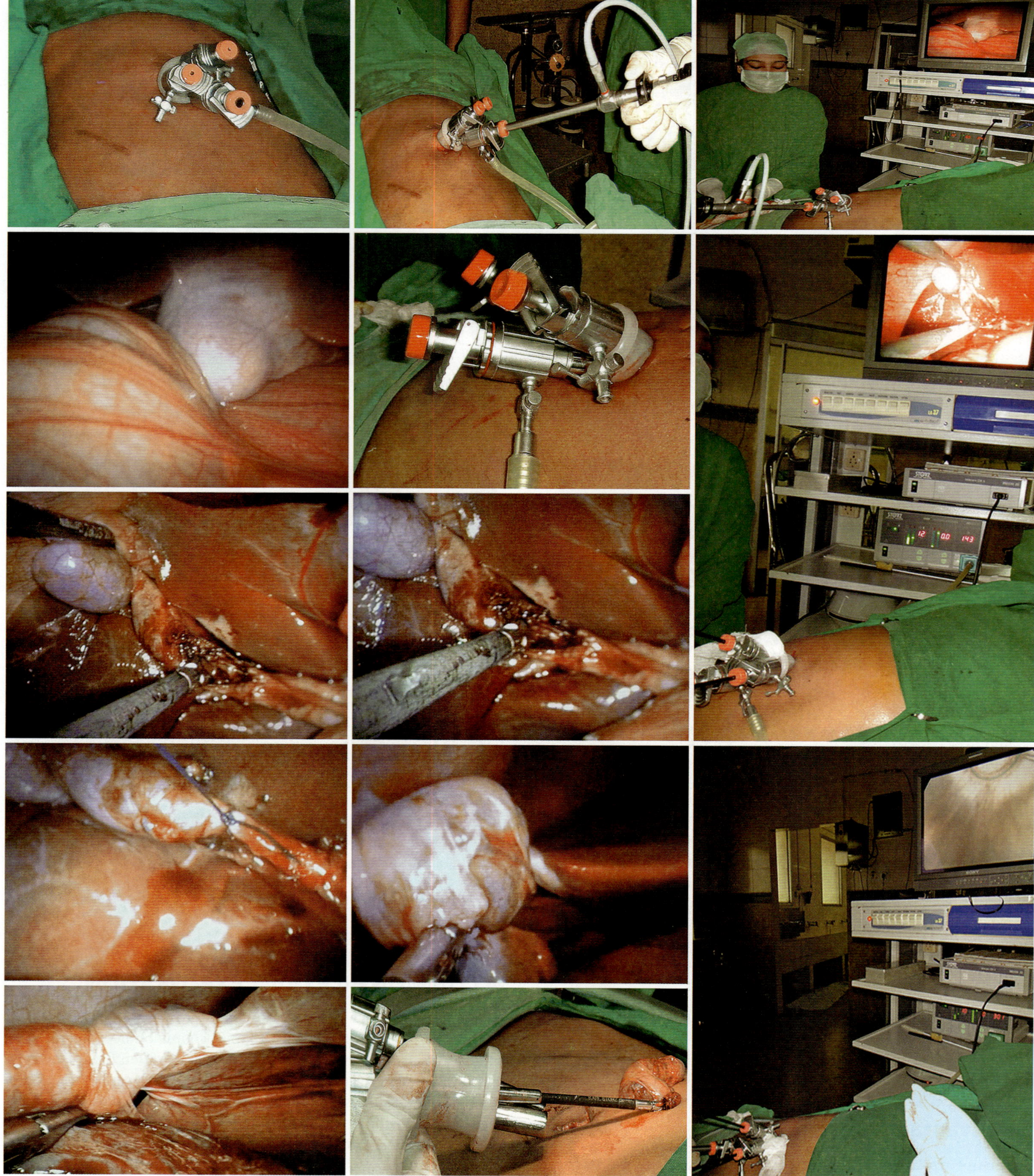

Fig. 23-111: Single incision laparoscopic surgery (SILS) for cholecystectomy.

if cholecystectomy is done either by open or laparoscopic approach and if on table cholangiogram is not done, it will definitely trouble the surgeon in postoperative period.

It is now usual in specified center that by a skilled authentic laparoscopic surgeon, duct cholangiogram and CBD exploration can be done through laparoscopy without opening.

If ERCP has failed or on table duct cholangiogram during open approach which is mandatory shows stones in the CBD, then CBD exploration is indicated **(Fig. 23-112)**.

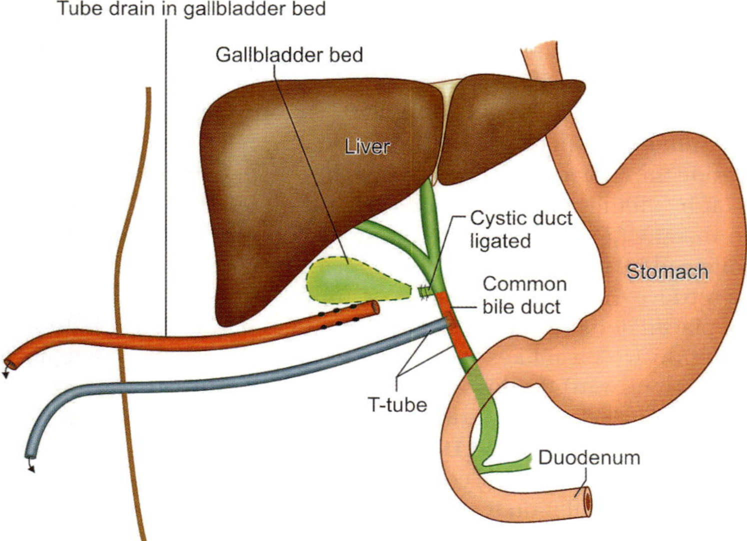

Fig. 23-112: Placement of T-tube in CBD after choledocholithotomy. Note the separate drain placed in the cholecystectomy bed to drain fluid, blood and bile.

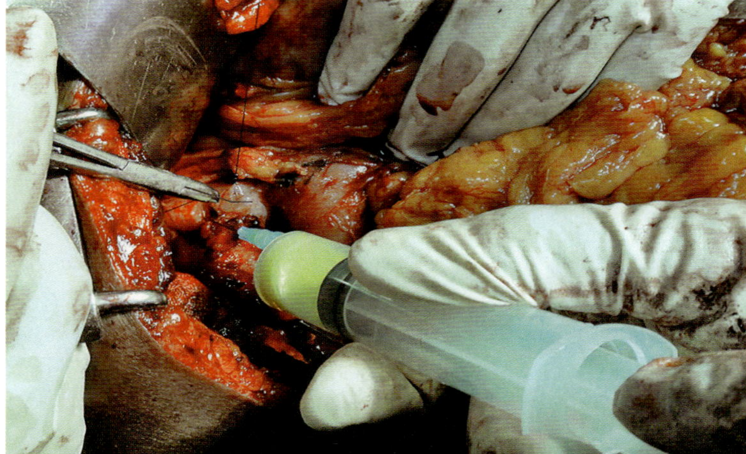

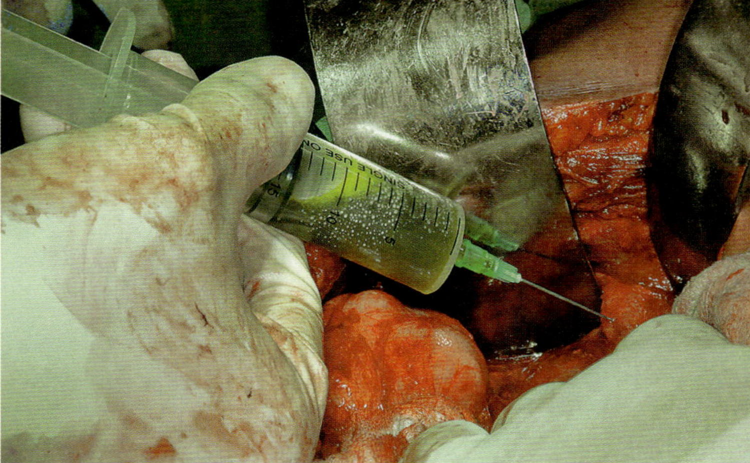

Fig. 23-113: Needle aspiration of common bile duct is done to aspirate bile which often may be infected.

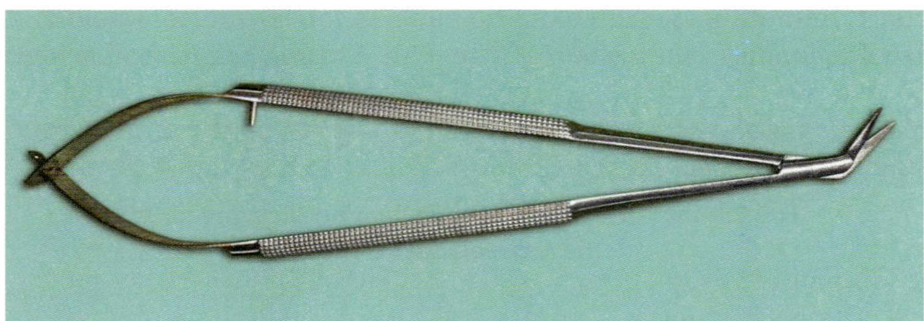

Fig. 23-114: Pott's scissor is better to cut and extend the incision in the common bile duct after making incision using no. 15 blade.

Technique

Incision is same as Kocher's incision but may require upwards extension towards xiphisternum or towards left side as partly bucket handle. After exploring the abdomen, cholecystectomy is done in usual manner with on table duct cholangiogram. Kocherisation of the duodenum is a must. Peritoneum on the anterior part of the CBD is incised to expose the CBD for 2–3 cm; small bleeders are cauterised using bipolar cautery; monopolar cautery should not be used. Two stay sutures are placed on the CBD using 3-zero vicryl; one just above the duodenum; another just below the level of the joining of cystic duct. Stay sutures are placed on the anteromedial surface of the CBD. Needle with syringe is passed into the CBD to aspirate bile which is collected for cytology and culture **(Fig. 23-113)**.

Incision is made vertically in the CBD on its anteromedial surface between stay sutures for 1.5–2 cm using no. 15 blade **(Fig. 23-114)**; incision begins at its upper hepatic side downwards towards duodenum just up to upper level of the duodenum; care should be taken not to pass across the posterior wall and so into the portal vein even though it is very rare; suctioning of bile is done (Incision should not be done on the lateral right side of CBD as cystic duct and CBD may have a common channel for 2 cm).

Mobilised 2nd part of the duodenum is held with thumb and fingers of one hand. Any stones if felt is carefully milked upwards towards choledochotomy wound. Stones are removed by different means—pituitary scoop of proper size; Randall's stone forceps; Fogarty catheter; Dormia basket; *choledochoscope (ideal)*; Desjardin's choledocholithotomy forceps; Bake's CBD dilator (malleable no. 3) are used. One should not force the stiff instrument downwards towards the ampulla as it may perforate the pancreatic part of the CBD causing fatal pancreatitis or bleeding or sepsis. 10 F catheter or infant feeding tube can be gently passed through the ampulla and if it is so that means ampulla is adequately patent without obstruction. Repeated warm saline irrigation both below through the CBD and above through the hepatic ducts should be done. First retrograde exploration is done; then downwards. It is easier to negotiate the tube and flush the left hepatic duct. One should be careful in passing tube into the right hepatic duct as it may get injured causing haemobilia **(Figs. 23-115 to 23-118)**.

Fogarty catheter when used is negotiated into the duodenum and confirmed by feeling the duodenum. It is only partially inflated and allowed just to pass through the ampulla proximally; then it is fully inflated to gently pull upwards towards choledochotomy to retrieve the stone along with that.

Ideally choledochoscope is best to visualise and retrieve the stones. Both rigid and flexible choldochoscopes are available. Both are

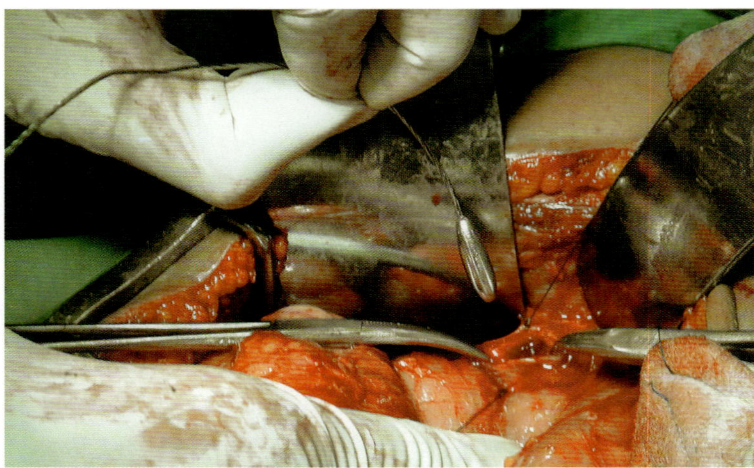

Fig. 23-115: Bakes dilator no. 3 F is used; one should be gentle while using it as forcible push may damage pancreas due to bile duct perforation.

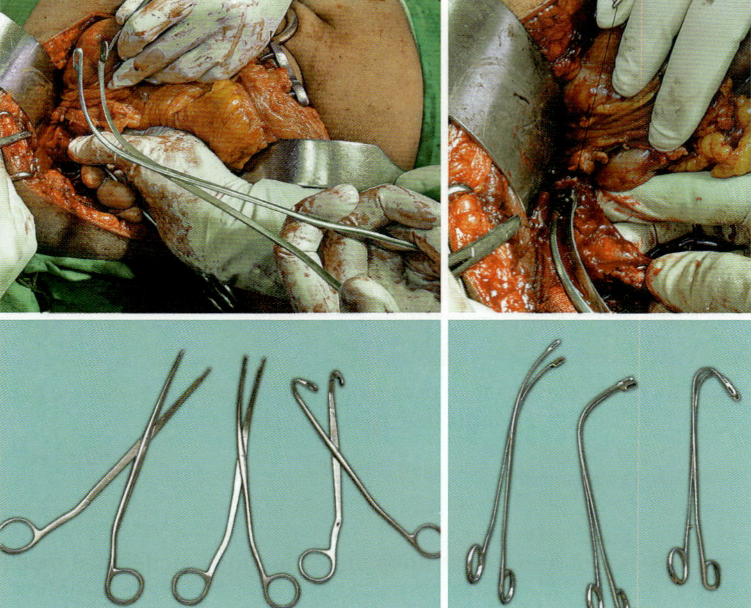

Fig. 23-116: Desjardin's choledocholithotomy forceps to retrieve gallbladder stones.

sterilised by ethylene oxide for repeated uses. Flexible scope has got poorer quality of image, costly, damageable, less life-span than rigid one even though it is safer easily negotiable into the CBD and hepatic ducts to retrieve the stones. Rigid scope is commonly used; 4 cm and 6 cm rigid scopes are available with 5 (outer) × 3 (inner) mm diameter. If size of the CBD in lesser than this instrument which is unlikely, is a contraindication for choledochoscope. Warm saline irrigation is done through the choledochoscope (rigid choledochoscope needs continuous saline irrigation like in cystoscope done by urologists otherwise mucosa cannot be seen). Choledochoscope is done with surgeon standing on the left side of the patient. Scope can be carefully negotiated proximally up to often tertiary ducts. Distally choledochscope is passed with guidance of other hand under Kocherised duodenum. If stones are visualised in distal CBD they are removed using different flexible instruments which are passed beside the choledochoscope so that their retrieval will be easy.

If by all these means, stones are still retained due to impaction in distal CBD, then duodenotomy in 2nd part of the duodenum followed by sphincterotomy is done at 11 o'clock position for 1 cm to retrieve the stone; later sphincteroplasty is done. T-tube should be placed; it has got vertical and horizontal part with a soft flexible junction which makes its removal safer. 16 French size is used (diameter 5 mm). As this size facilitates passage of choledochoscope later through the track formed after 21 days in case if there are any retained stones **(Fig. 23-119)**.

T-tube (Kehr's T tube) comes in different sizes; 16 F size is usually used. Horizontal limb is cut shorter; each horizontal limb should be

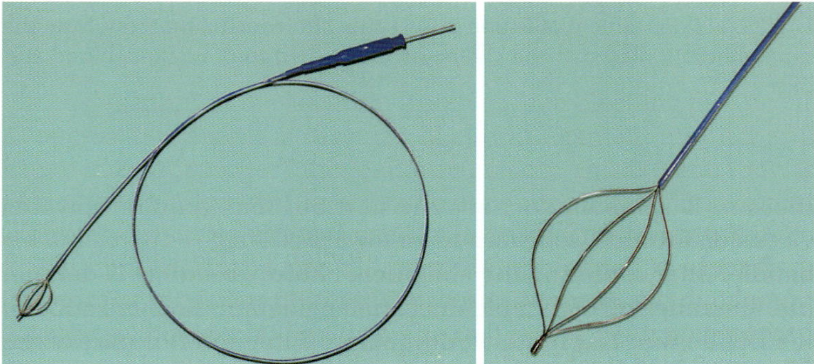

Fig. 23-117: Dormia basket to retrieve stones from CBD.

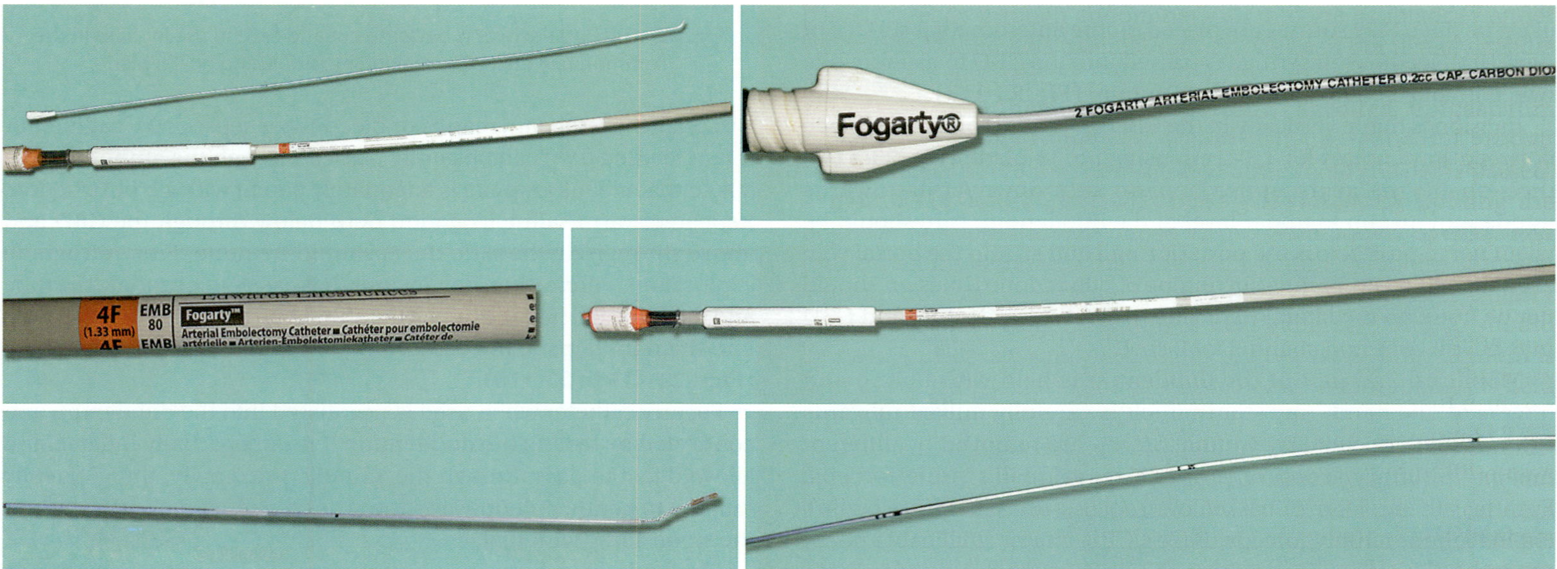

Fig. 23-118: Fogarty catheter often used to retrieve the CBD stones.

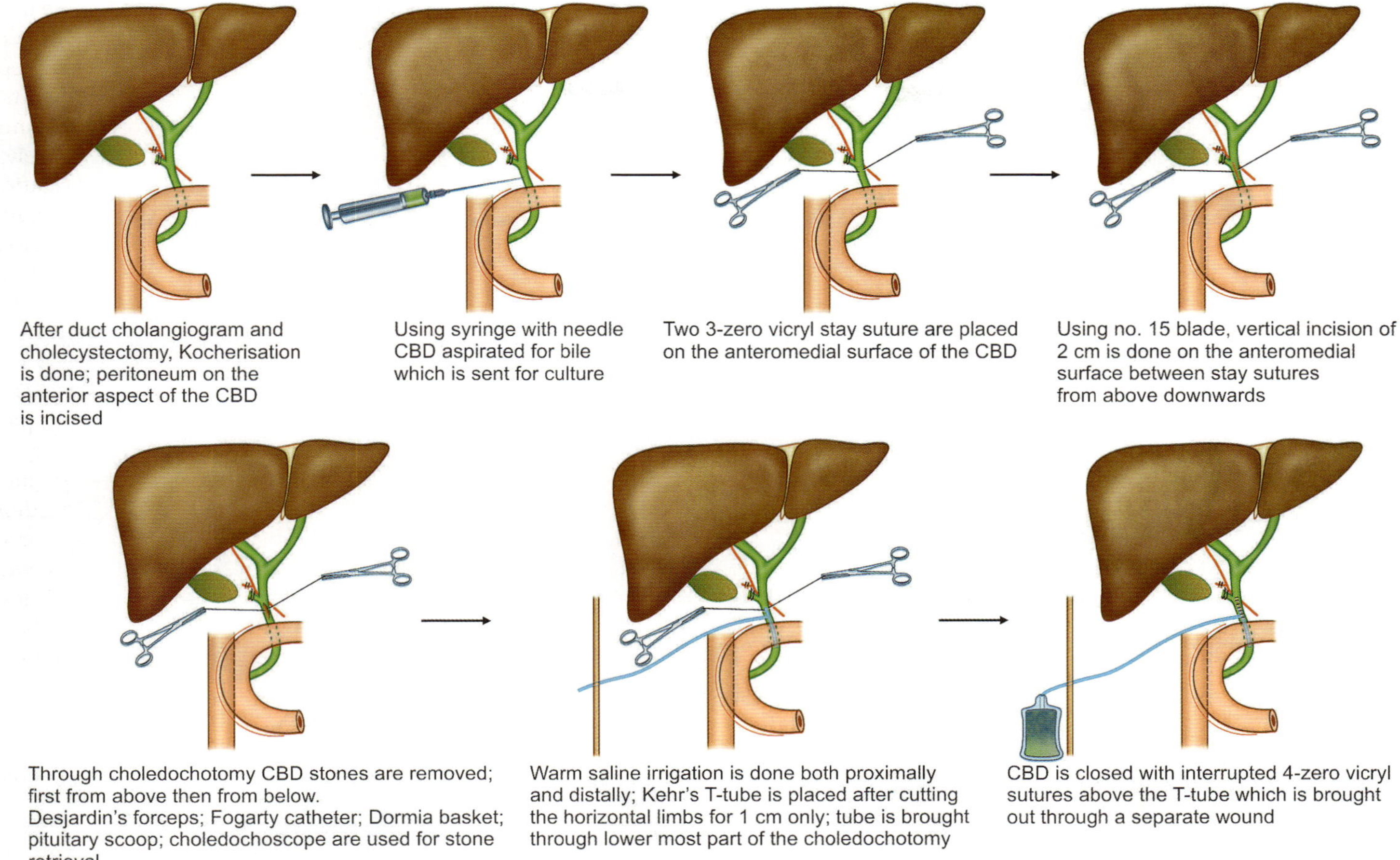

Fig. 23-119: Technique of common bile duct exploration and placement of T-tube.

1 cm; lengthy tube inside CBD may precipitate pancreatitis or may traumatise during its removal after 14–21 days. T-tube should be brought out at the lower most part of the choledochotomy incision to avoid the disruption of the suture line while removal. T-tube should be ideally made up of latex rubber, not of plastic or polyvinyl. Latex causes extensive reaction to create a track prevents bile leak into peritoneal cavity and so biliary peritonitis. Different modifications are available. Maingot's split type is also available with a slit on the opposite side of the junction. CBD is closed above the T-tube keeping T-tube at the lower most part of the CBD. Interrupted 3-zero vicryl or 4-zero PDS is used. Patency of the tube should be checked by saline infusion.

Completion on table T-tube cholangiogram is a must. T-tube is brought out of the abdomen through a separate stab incision at anterior axillary line. Tube drain is placed at gallbladder bed **(Fig. 23-120)**.

Postoperative Care

Antibiotics are continued. Nasogastric tube can be removed in 48 hours. Drain is removed in 5–7 days. Postoperative T-tube cholangiogram is done in 1–14 days. In doubtful cases T-tube should be kept in place for 21 days more. Prior to removal, one should confirm that there are no residual stones. Often T-tube is clamped for 24 hours; if patient develops pain, vomiting, pain abdomen, bile leak from side of T-tube, it is probable that there are retained stones.

Problems and Complications

Haemorrhage during surgery may be due to oozing from gallbladder bed, hepatic artery injury, portal vein injury even though it is rare.

Postoperative pancreatitis due to CBD perforation by forcible negotiation of the tube across the ampulla into the duodenum.

Bile leak and bile peritonitis is equally dangerous and life-threatening.

Haemobilia may be due to intrahepatic injury while retrieving the stones from hepatic ducts. Plasma, vitamin K injection is usual treatment. Hepatic angiography confirms the diagnosis. Therapeutic embolisation may be required.

Septicaemia, subphrenic abscess can develop mainly in diabetic and old aged.

Residual bile duct stones: It is confirmed by T-tube cholangiogram. Its incidence is 3%; but less if choledochoscope is used. Small stones less than 1 cm is retrieved by saline (1 litre) in heparin (5000 units) infusion into the T-tube. In 5 days often, stone reduces in size. Patient is discharged with T-tube with an advice of daily infusion of 50 mL of saline into the T-tube. Patient is asked to come after 8 weeks for further management of retained stones. During this period, so as track, has formed well. It is managed by Burhenne (radiologist, Canada) method. Under fluoroscopic guidance after removal of T-tube, flexible catheter is passed into the track to reach the duodenum across the stone; Dormia basket is passed through the flexible catheter; under guidance it is gently manipulated to trap the stones into the basket for retrieval. Repeated attempts will clear all the stones. It has got 90% success rate. Flexible choledochoscopy can be passed (not rigid) through the track to visualise and retrieve the stone. Repeat ERCP, sphincteroplasty, re-exploration, choledochoduodenostomy or choledochojejunostomy are other methods in these patients **(Fig. 23-121)**.

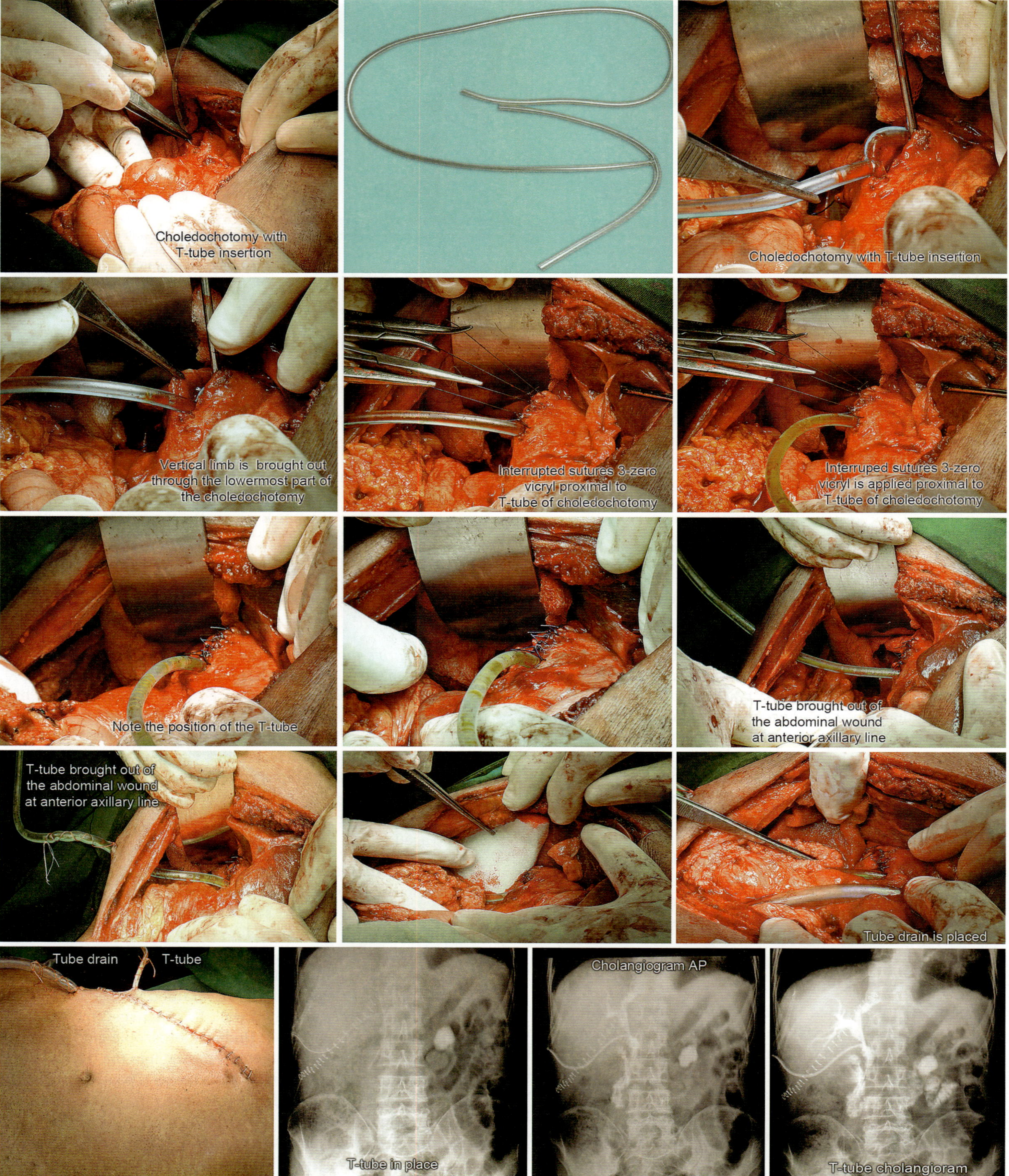

Fig. 23-120: Placement of T-tube after CBD exploration and removal of the CBD stone. It is done in secondary CBD stone where stones have slipped from the gallbladder into the CBD.

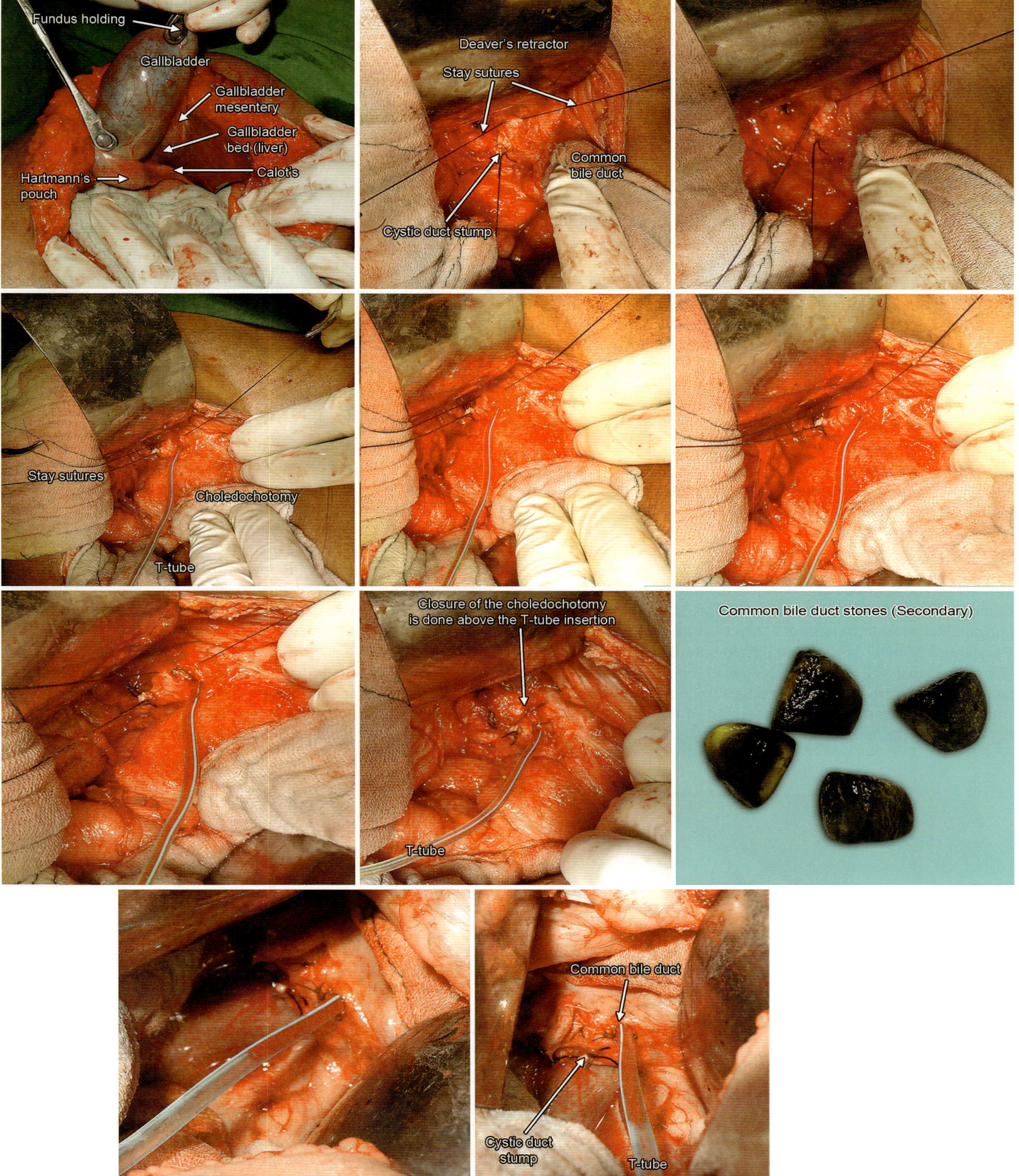

Fig. 23-121: Placement of T-tube. Note that CBD should be closed above the T-tube insertion site using interrupted 3-zero/4-zero vicryl. T-tube should come out at the lowest part of the choledochotomy wound (*not at upper part*).

CHOLEDOCHODUODENOSTOMY

Riedel in 1881 did first choledochoduodenostomy.

Indications

- Stones still remained in CBD after CBD exploration for multiple CBD calculi. It could be with primary CBD stones or secondary stones. But commonly such stones are primary one. Retained stones in the hepatic ducts are also indication.
- ***Papillary stenosis:*** It is often known to occur. It is diagnosed by failure of the dye reaching the duodenum during operative cholangiography and inability to pass 3 mm dilator across CBD into the duodenum.
- Impacted distal CBD stone wherein removal is impossible.
- Intrahepatic calculi, residual stones after removal of T-tube in earlier operation, diverticula in the duodenum causing CBD obstruction and cholangitis, benign stricture of the distal CBD.

Prerequisite

Common bile duct (CBD) should be more than 1.5 cm to do choledochoduodenostomy.

Contraindications: CBD if not dilated significantly, sclerosing cholangitis, chronic pancreatitis which needs surgical decompression, malignant obstruction, duodenal oedema.

Technique (Fig. 23-122)

Preparation anaesthesia and position is same as cholecystectomy. Cholecystectomy is done. Kocherisation should be done adequately. Longitudinal choledochotomy of 2.5 cm in length is made on the CBD. Duodenum is incised on its first part longitudinally around 2.2 cm (3 mm lesser than CBD incision). Through the opening ampulla is again palpated to avoid any missing of malignancy; often choledochoscope can be done to confirm that. Distal end of the choledochotomy is brought to the middle of the lower leaf of the duodenotomy. Middle points of the edges of the choledochotomy is brought towards the ends of the duodenotomy incision; stay sutures are placed using 3-zero vicryl. Further 3-zero vicryl interrupted sutures are placed initially to complete the posterior layer (knots should be outside ideally); then anterior layer done. Finally funnel-shaped choledochoduodenostomy anastomosis is completed. Stoma should be at least 2.5 cm. Abdomen is closed with a tube drain.

Problems

- ***Sump syndrome:*** It is due to creation of blind segment/pouch at distal CBD causing stasis and cholangitis. This pouch contains infected bile, food, calculi **(Fig. 23-123)**.
- Bile leak due to anastomotic disruption can occur.
- Recurrent cholangitis is another problem.

TRANSDUODENAL SPHINCTEROPLASTY

Indications are same as choledochoduodenostomy.

Technique (Fig. 23-124)

After cholecystectomy through Kocher's incision, Kocher's manoeuvre is done; common bile duct is explored. No. 3 Bake's dilator is passed into the CBD but not across the ampulla of Vater. Tip of the dilator is palpated through the anterior duodenal wall which allows the proper placement of the sphincterotomy incision.

Duodenotomy of 4 cm length is made in the 2nd part of the duodenum centering at the level of the ampulla. Retractors are placed into the cut edges of the duodenotomy to expose the ampulla adequately. It is better to place four stay sutures to retract edges at four corners.

Incision is made at 11 o'clock position. It keeps incision away from pancreatic duct entry and also is relatively avascular. With tip of Bakes's dilator as a guide using no. 15 blade or Pott's scissor, incision is made along the orifice. After cutting partially, 4-zero vicryl sutures are placed on either sides of the opened ampulla and

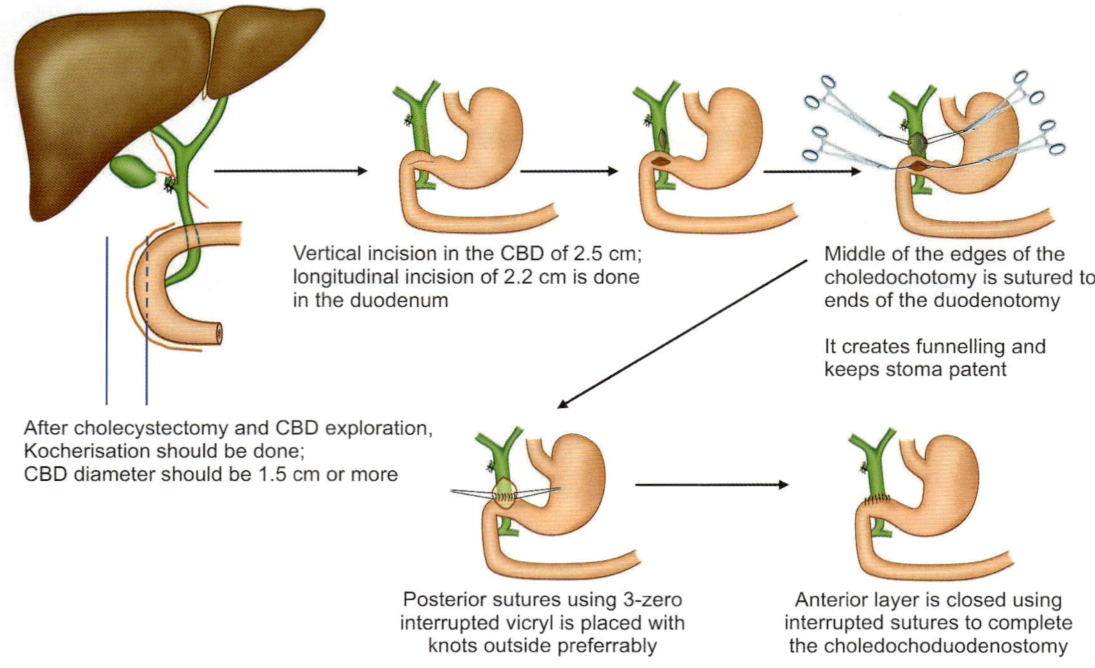

Fig. 23-122: Choledochoduodenostomy—technique.

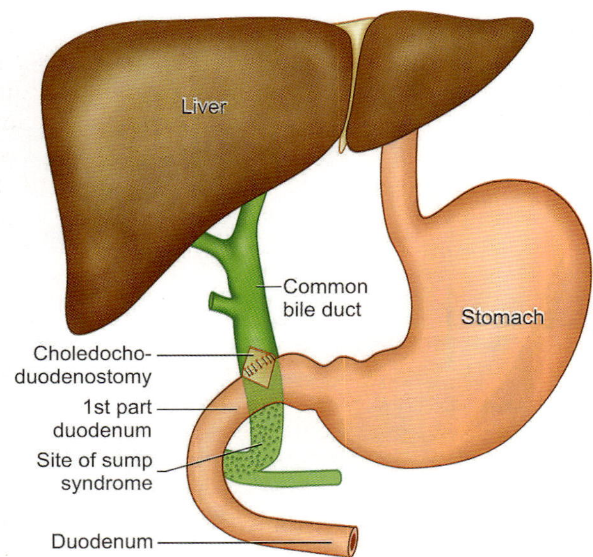

Fig. 23-123: Technique of choledochoduodenostomy for CBD stones. Note the site of possible occurrence of sump syndrome.

held apart to give traction. Pancreatic duct orifice is identified at 5 o'clock position on the posterior aspect. Incision is further extended for 3 mm and additional stay sutures are placed. Pancreatic ductal orifice may be better visualised by injecting secretin one unit/kg IV which stimulates the flow of pancreatic juice across the orifice. Incision is continued sequentially every time for 3 mm with a pair of vicryl stay sutures. Sphincterotomy of entire sphincter of Oddi needs 2 cm length of incision along the ampulla. Otherwise length of the sphincterotomy should be length of the CBD diameter. At the apex, figure of eight suture should be placed.

If there is associated chronic pancreatitis and stenosis of the pancreatic duct, if no. 3 Bake's dilator is not negotiable, then pancreatic ductoplasty also should be done. Probe is passed into duct. Duct is incised at its anterior wall for 10 mm using Pott's scissor at 5 o'clock position; technique is as similar as sphincteroplasty of sphincter of Oddi; i.e. for every 3 mm incision paired 4-zero vicryl stay sutures placed; sequentially until adequate ductoplasty (of Wirsung) is achieved.

Choledochotomy is closed with a T-tube; duodenotomy is closed; tube drain is placed. Abdomen closed in layers **(Fig. 23-125)**.

Postoperatively antibiotics are given; nasogastric tube is removed in 48 hours and oral feeding is started. Liver function, serum amylase levels are estimated during feeding in postoperative period. Tube drain is removed in 5 days. T-tube is removed in 2 weeks.

Complications

Duodenal fistula, sepsis, subphrenic abscess formation, and pancreatitis are complications.

CHOLEDOCHOJEJUNOSTOMY/ BILIARY ENTERIC ANASTOMOSIS/ HEPATICOJEJUNOSTOMY

Indications

Major ductal injury, inoperable tumour (palliative bypass), chronic pancreatitis; biliary stricture are indications.

Side-to-side or side-to-end choledochojejunostomy can be done. Unless CBD is completely transected and distally ligated in definitive resections like Whipple's operation, end-to-side type is usually not necessary **(Fig. 23-126)**.

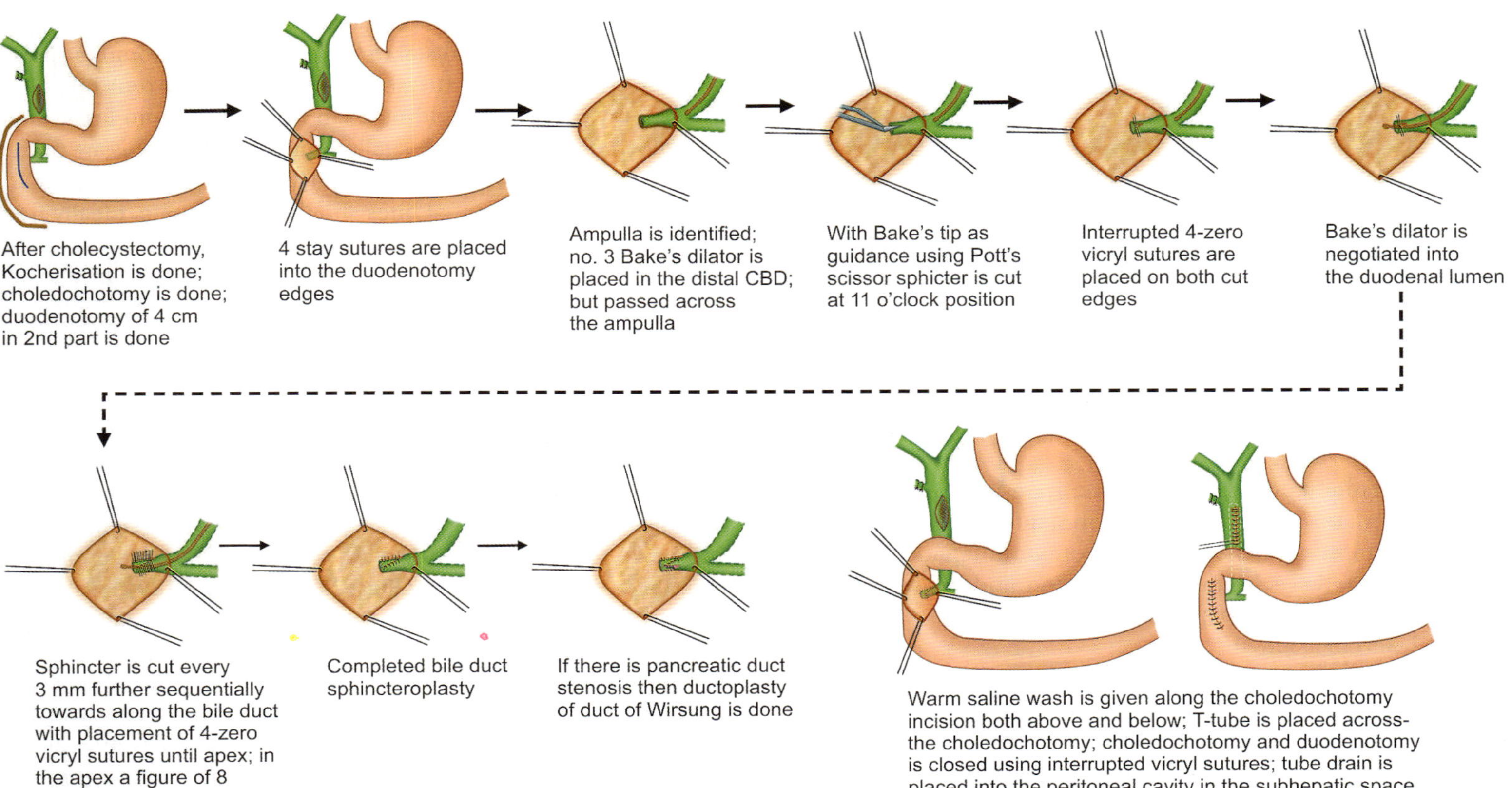

Fig. 23-124: Technique and steps of transduodenal sphincteroplasty.

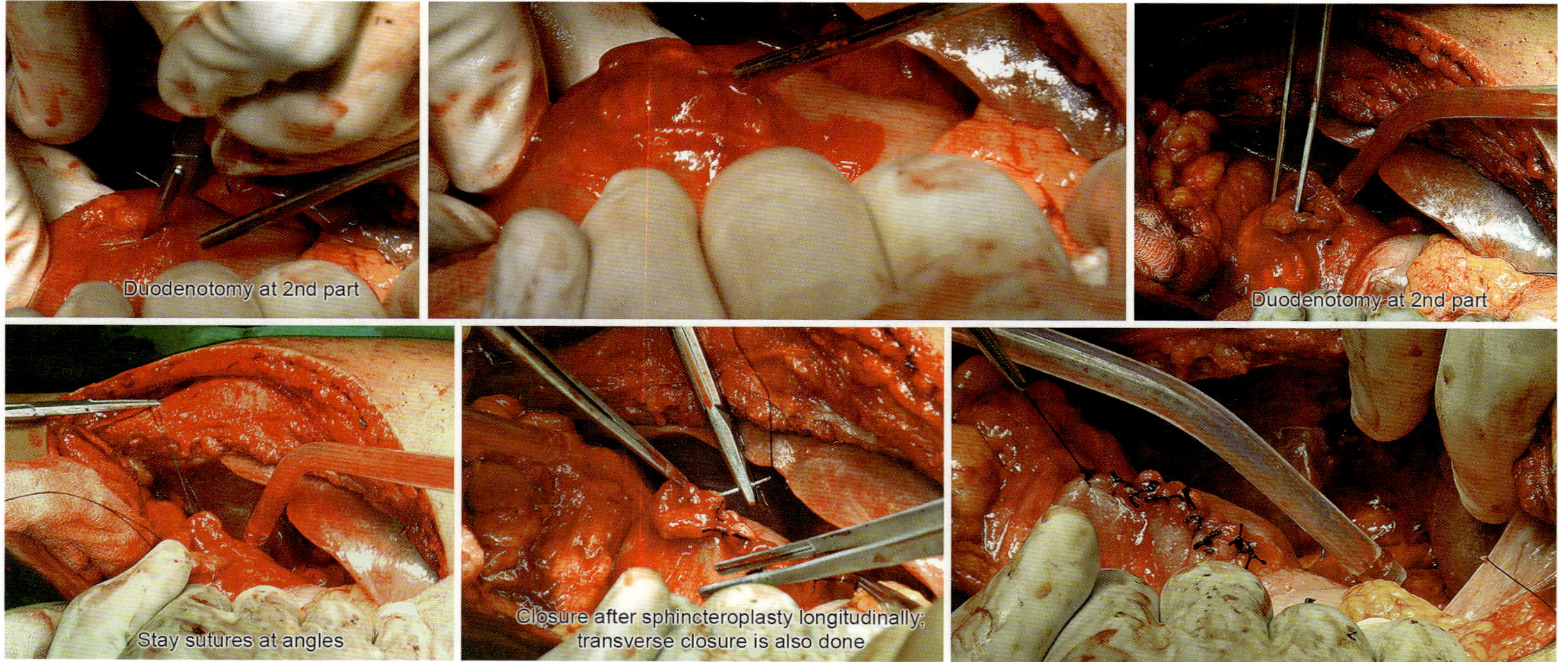

Fig. 23-125: Duodenotomy in transduodenal sphincteroplasty and closure of duodenum ideally transverse; here longitudinal closure was done which is also accepted.

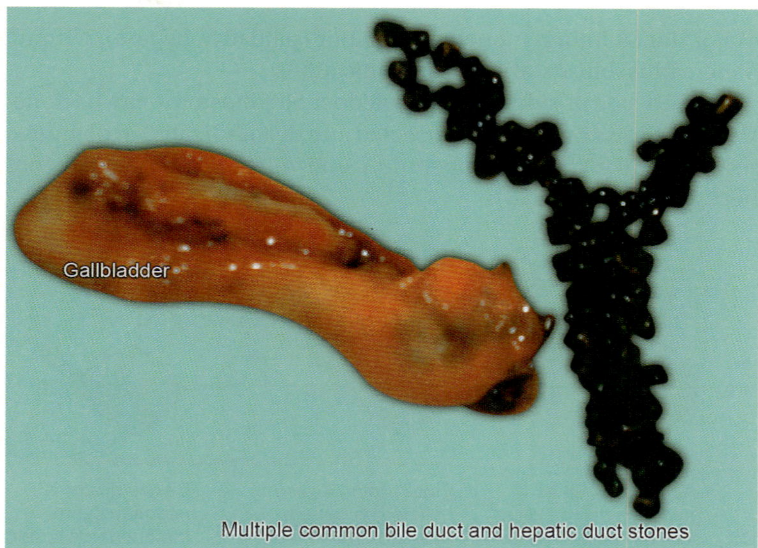

Fig. 23-126: Primary biliary stones in common bile duct and hepatic ducts. It needs choledochojejunostomy.

Technique

After doing cholecystectomy (it facilitates the approach and visualisation and avoids later development of cholecystitis) and choledochotomy or incision on the common hepatic duct, Roux limb is prepared. Technique of dissection and choledochotomy is same as for bile duct exploration. Choledochotomy should be around 2–2.5 cm in length.

Duodenojejunal junction is identified by ligament of Treitz and inferior mesenteric vein. After 2nd arcade of the blood supply in the mesentery, through transillumination arcades are identified and divided using small haemostats. Bipolar or harmonic scalpel can be used. 20 cm from the duodenojejunal junction is the site taken for Roux limb. Jejunum is cut with no. 15 blade between occlusion clamps; or stapler transection can be done. Roux limb is passed across the transverse mesocolon through a rent which is to right of the middle colic artery to reach the CBD area. Antecolic placement loop can be done if there are lot of adhesions and if there are infiltrations in case of malignancy at mesocolon level. Blood supply of the Roux limb is assessed by its colour and pulsation at its mesentery **(Figs. 23-127 and 23-128)**.

In *side-to-side anastomosis*, 4-zero vicryl sutures are used. Jejunum is incised over its antimesenteric border 1 cm proximal to the stapled end. Lengthy distal part distal to the proposed anastomosis should not be kept as it may cause blind loop and recurrent infection. Jejunotomy incision should be 2 cm in length (3 mm lesser than choledochotomy incision). Usually 4 interrupted sutures are placed between jejunum (posterior cut edge) and right margin of the CBD with 3–4 mm apart. Jejunal bites should be adequate. Ideally from CBD outside in, then from jejunum inside out bites are taken so that knots are placed outside; but posterior knots can be placed inside by taking bites from inside out and outside if technical difficulty arises. All sutures are placed and kept long with haemostats; only after placing all posterior sutures jejunum is pushed gently into the choledochotomy and knots are tied; all threads are kept long and cut at the end. Anterior sutures are taken similarly with knot placement outside. After taking all bites, knots are tied sequentially at the end. It is logically better to take bite from the middle of the choledochotomy cut edge on both sides to the ends of the jejunostomy so that stoma will be kept patent; however, both ways are adequate enough to maintain the stomal patency **(Figs. 23-129 and 23-130)**.

It is often practice that both posterior and anterior suture bites are taken together and kept aside using haemostats. With *parachute technique* (railroading, *Voyles-Blumgart technique*, 1982) jejunum is pushed and posterior and anterior knots are placed sequentially. However, it is often technically difficult especially to identify the corresponding sutures to put knots and may create problem while knotting. If surgeon is not well-practiced with this technique, he should avoid it to prevent problems thereafter.

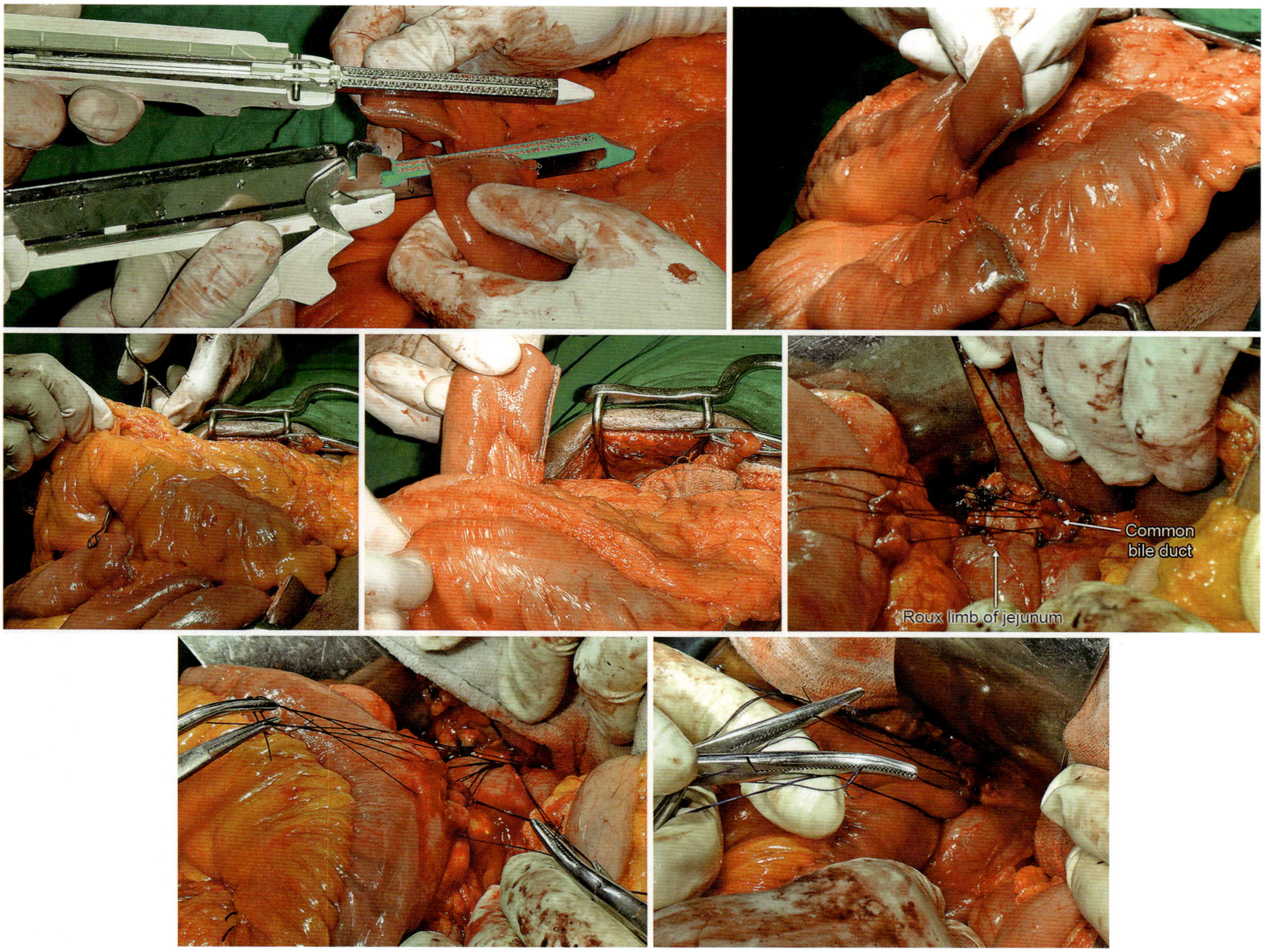

Fig. 23-127: Creation of Roux jejunal loop.

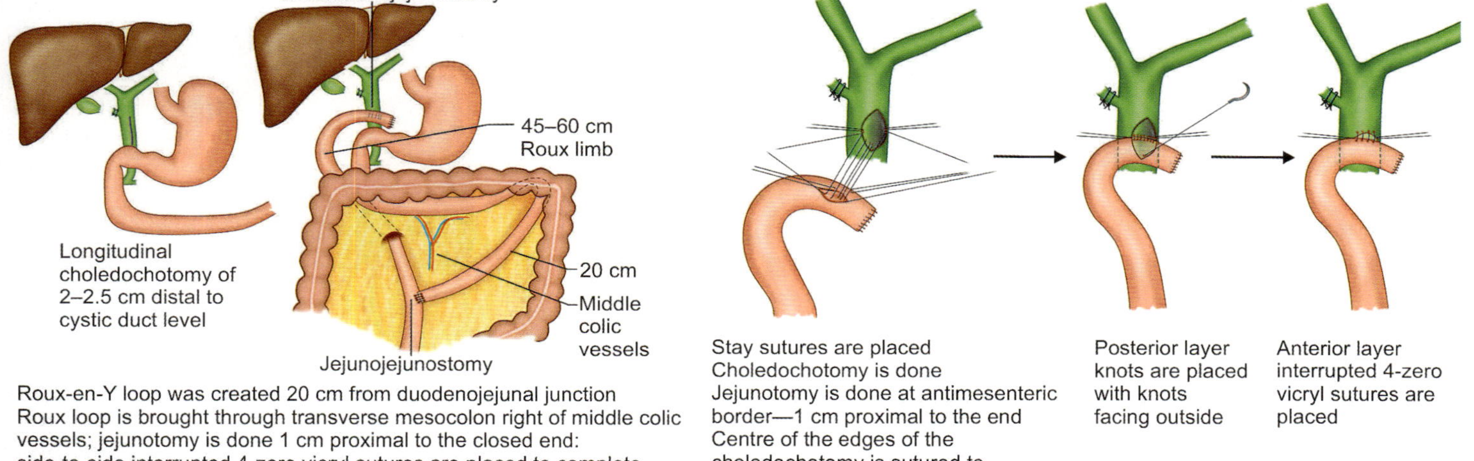

Fig. 23-128: Choledochojejunostomy technique.

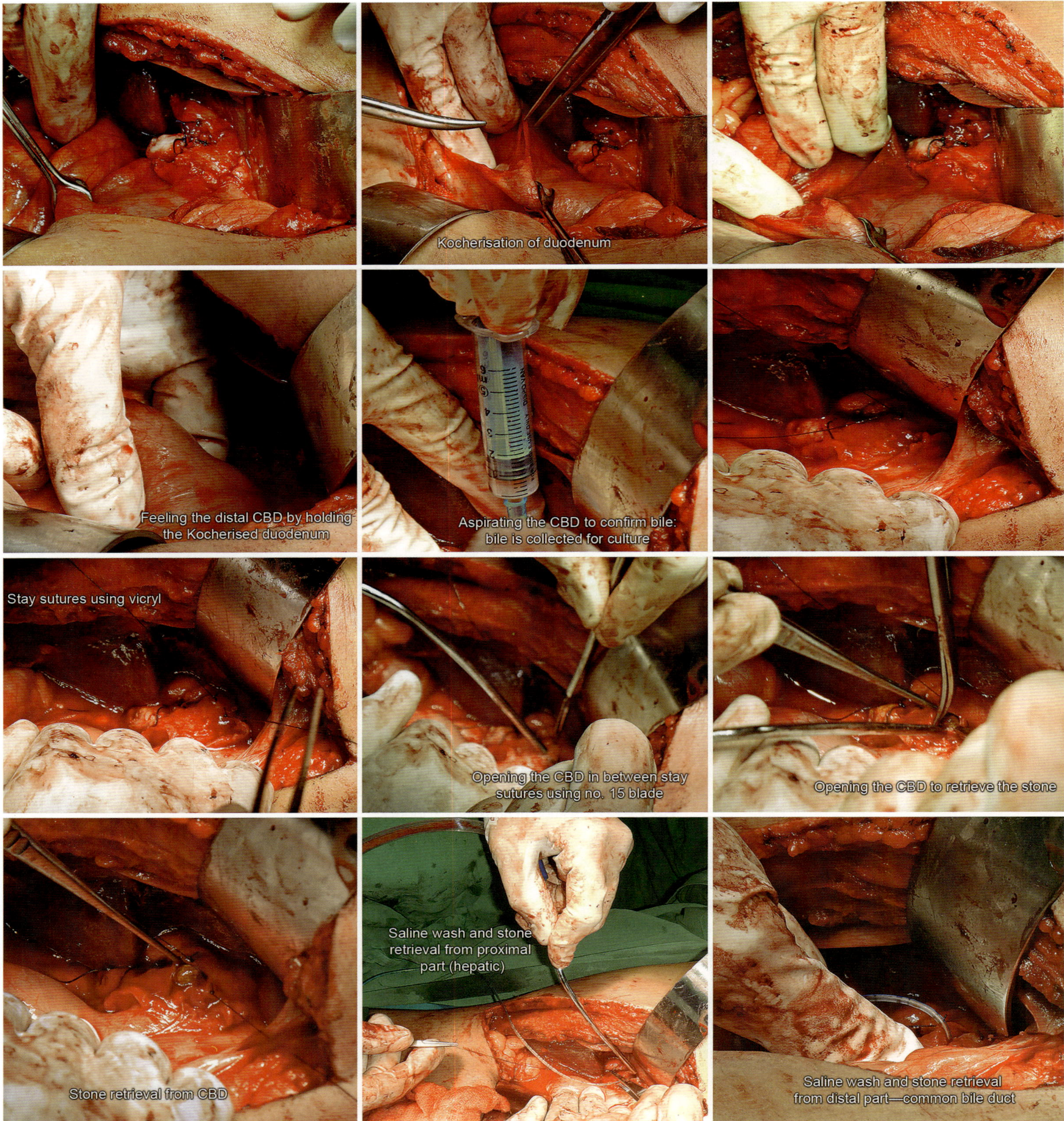
Kocherisation of duodenum
Feeling the distal CBD by holding the Kocherised duodenum
Aspirating the CBD to confirm bile: bile is collected for culture
Stay sutures using vicryl
Opening the CBD in between stay sutures using no. 15 blade
Opening the CBD to retrieve the stone
Stone retrieval from CBD
Saline wash and stone retrieval from proximal part (hepatic)
Saline wash and stone retrieval from distal part—common bile duct

Figs. 23-129(1)

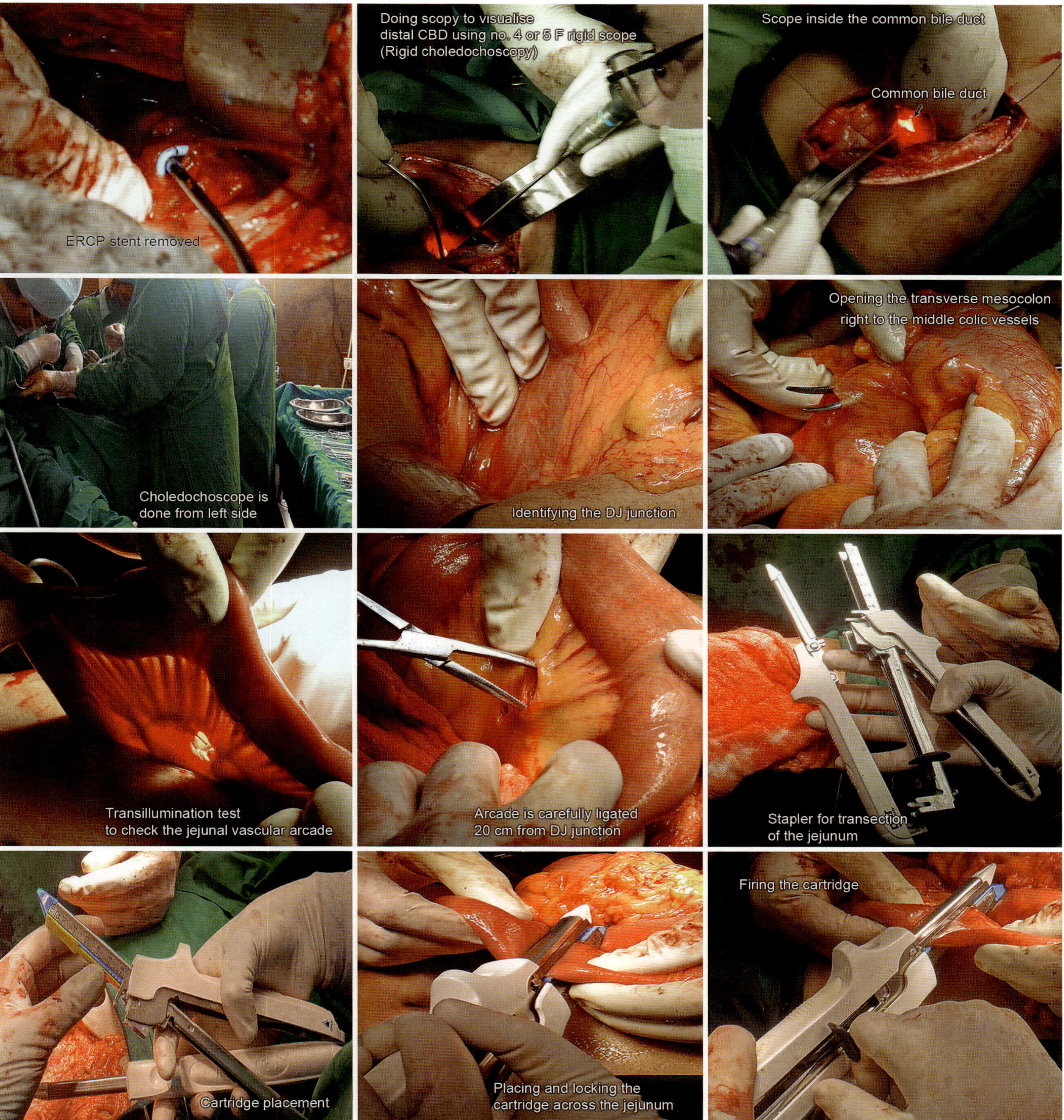
ERCP stent removed
Doing scopy to visualise distal CBD using no. 4 or 5 F rigid scope (Rigid choledochoscopy)
Scope inside the common bile duct
Common bile duct
Choledochoscope is done from left side
Identifying the DJ junction
Opening the transverse mesocolon right to the middle colic vessels
Transillumination test to check the jejunal vascular arcade
Arcade is carefully ligated 20 cm from DJ junction
Stapler for transection of the jejunum
Cartridge placement
Placing and locking the cartridge across the jejunum
Firing the cartridge

Figs. 23-129(2)

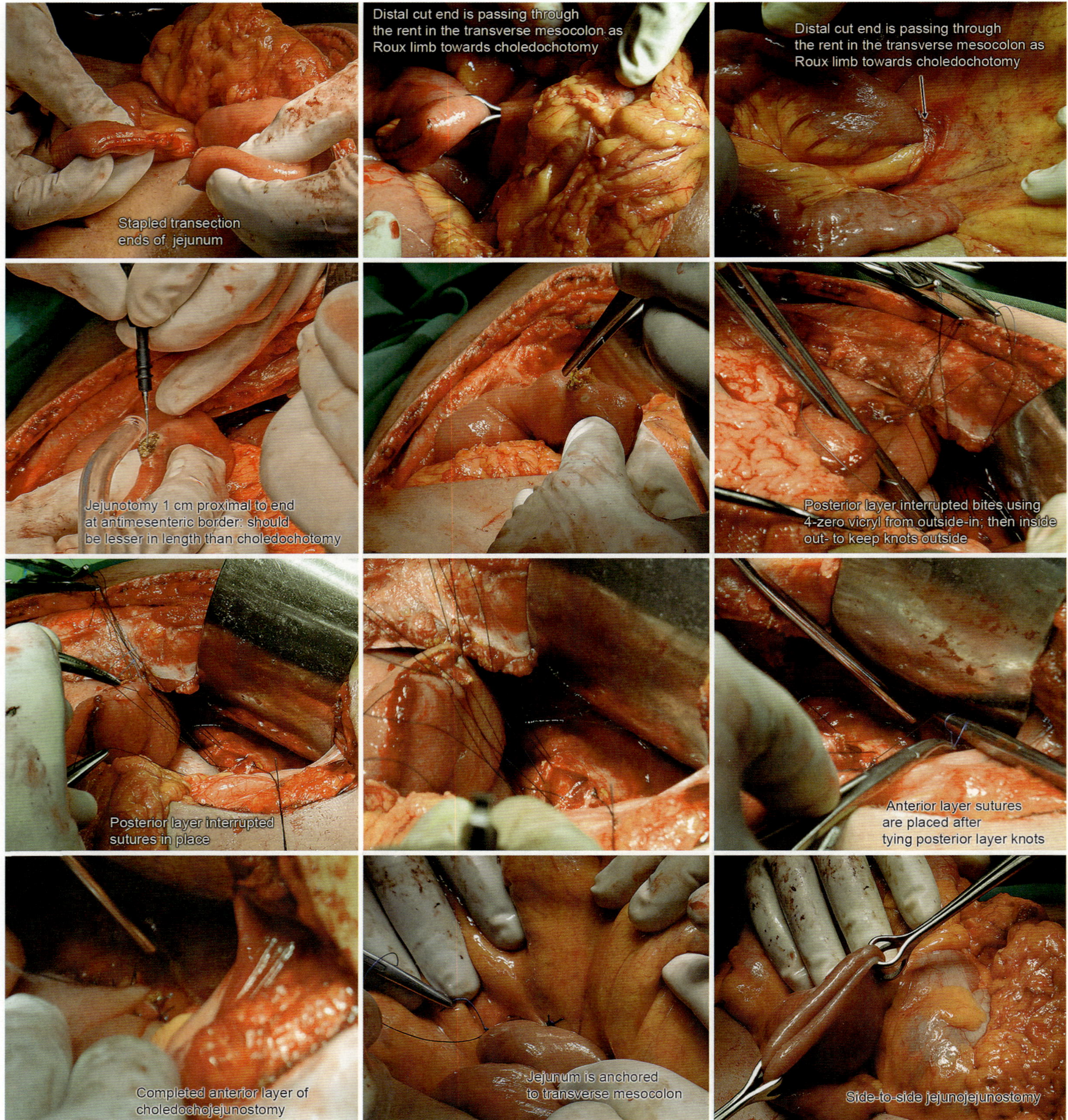
Stapled transection
ends of jejunum
Distal cut end is passing through
the rent in the transverse mesocolon as
Roux limb towards choledochotomy
Distal cut end is passing through
the rent in the transverse mesocolon as
Roux limb towards choledochotomy
Jejunotomy 1 cm proximal to end
at antimesenteric border: should
be lesser in length than choledochotomy
Posterior layer interrupted bites using
4-zero vicryl from outside-in; then inside
out- to keep knots outside
Posterior layer interrupted
sutures in place
Anterior layer sutures
are placed after
tying posterior layer knots
Completed anterior layer of
choledochojejunostomy
Jejunum is anchored
to transverse mesocolon
Side-to-side jejunojejunostomy

Figs. 23-129(3)

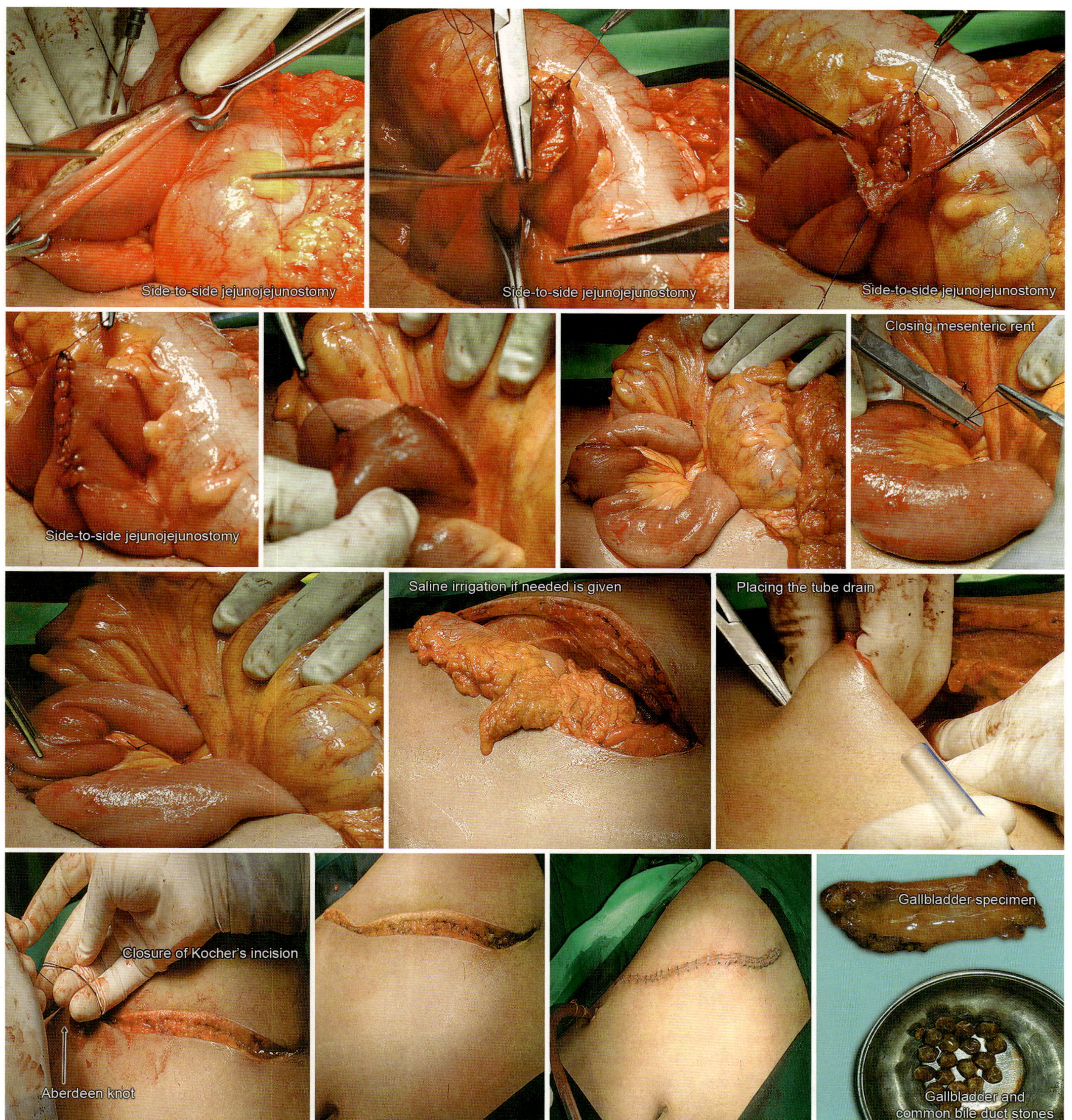

Figs. 23-129(4)

Figs. 23-129(1 to 4): Choledochotomy, choledochoscopy, Roux-en-Y side to side choledochojejunostomy with side-to-side enteroenterostomy. Here stapler is used initially to transect the jejunum.

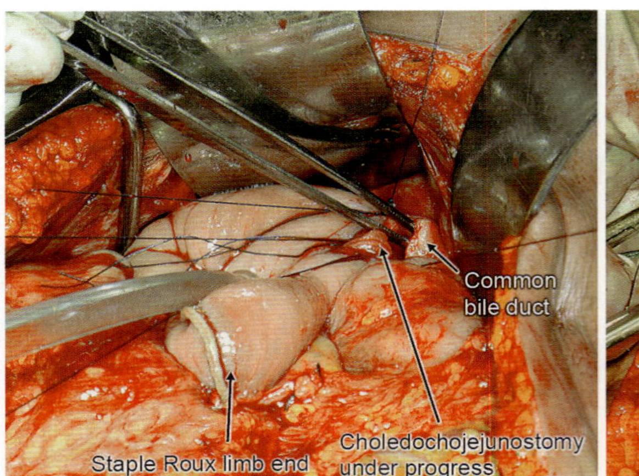

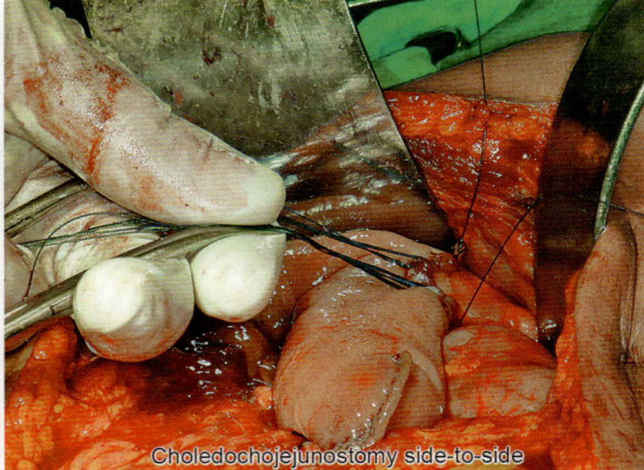

Fig. 23-130: Roux-en-Y side-to-side choledochojejunostomy.

End-to-end anastomosis can be done if CBD diameter is wider. It is done in malignancy with obstruction either after resection or as palliative procedure. Technique is similar like end-to-end anastomosis. Knots are placed outside. Interrupted vicryl sutures are placed.

Side-to-end anastomosis also can be done between side of bile duct to end of Roux limb provided bile duct is sufficiently dilated **(Fig. 23-131)**.

Stenting of the choledochojejunostomy or hepaticojejunostomy is done often by many but is not mandatory. When it is done, it is brought out through the Roux jejunal limb outside and then through a stab wound through abdomen. T-tube may be passed which is brought out through bile duct proximally. It is usually not necessary. Stenting across the stoma through as biliary radicle across the liver to be brought out through the abdominal wall is also practiced but may damage biliary tree and may cause bleeding or haemobilia.

Enteroenterostomy is done 60 cm distal to the stoma to complete the Roux-en-Y anastomosis. This is usually end-to-side either hand sewn or stapler. If initial transection was stapler one; then without dismantling original one, a side to side enteroenterostomy can be done **(Figs. 23-132 and 23-133)**.

There is usually not necessary to keep a stent through the choledochojejunostomy. If needed no 8 French tube can be passed

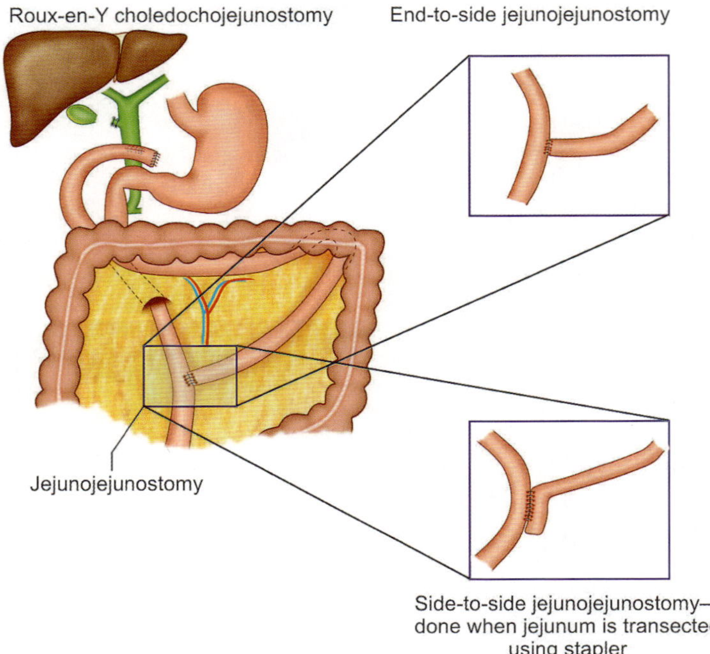

Fig. 23-132: Types of jejunojejunostomy done in Roux-en-Y anastomosis—side-to-side or end-to-side.

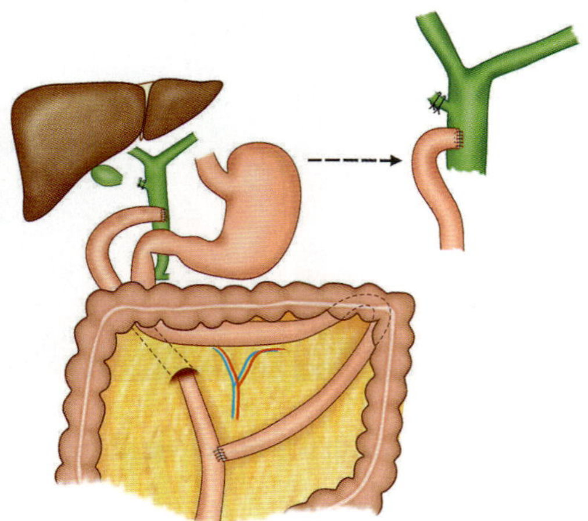

Fig. 23-131: Choledochojejunostomy side-to-end.

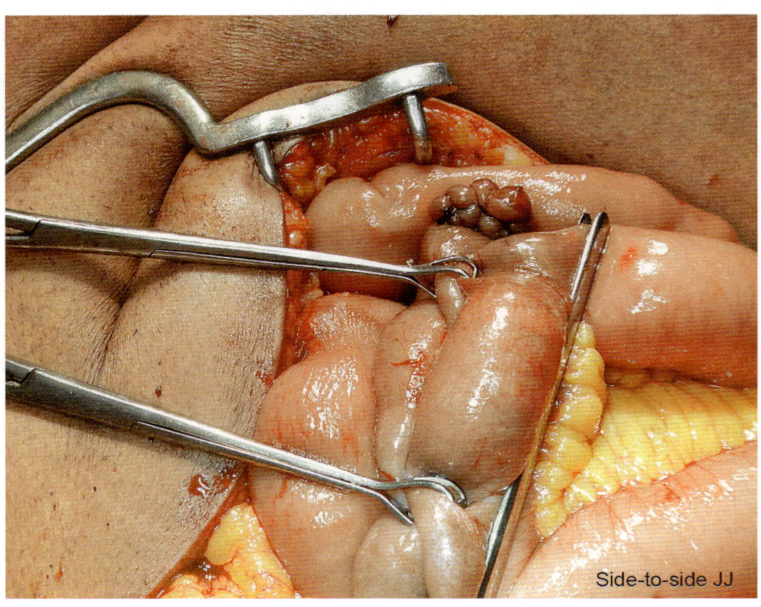

Fig. 23-133: Side-to-side jejunojejunostomy.

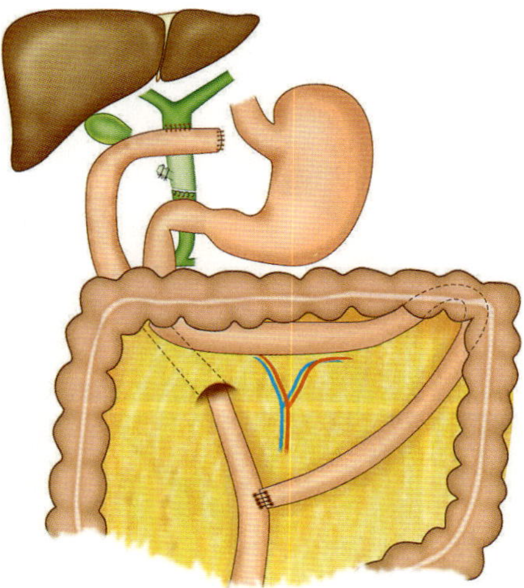

Fig. 23-134: Hepaticojejunostomy Roux-en-Y anastomosis.

across the stoma to reach the efferent loop and is brought out through a small stab incision in the antimesenteric border which is fixed to parietal wall. Finally tube is brought out through a separate stab wound on the abdominal wall. But displacement, falling of the tube is common.

Hepaticojejunostomy after resection is usually end-to-side of Roux loop **(Fig. 23-134)**. It is also often used in trauma. Here biliary enteric anastomosis is achieved by anastomosing into the right and left hepatic ducts. Often confluence of the right and left hepatic ducts to form common hepatic duct is intrahepatic; it is approached at the base of the segment four by cutting the bridging liver tissue between umbilical fissure and segment 4 liver lobe (quadrate). Through same approach left hepatic duct is approached. Technique of anastomosis is similar—interrupted 4-zero vicryl or PDS posterior layer knots will come outside; as well as anterior layer knots. It is always better to keep the knots outside rather than inside even though many contemplate that inside knots are safer. Approaching left hepatic duct is called as Hepp-Couinaud technique **(Fig. 23-135)**.

If there is duodenal obstruction, gastrojejunostomy also should be done to prevent gastric outlet obstruction which may call for 2nd surgery at a later period. Duodenal obstruction occurs especially when there is associated pancreatitis **(Fig. 23-136)**.

Access loop: Often access loop is used to reach the biliary system. It is done by keeping more length of the distal blind end of the Roux limb to bring close to the abdominal wall and fix it; whenever needed this can be opened and stoma and biliary system can be reached through endoscope. Alternatively Roux blind end can be anastomosed to pylorus near lesser curve which can be used as access to biliary system through endoscope **(Fig. 23-137)**.

Loop choledochojejunostomy with enteroenterostomy (Braun) is not commonly advocated. It is technically easier; there is no transection of the jejunum and dissection of mesenteric arcade. It was the common procedure in olden days. Often when it is done few plication sutures are placed to afferent limb to prevent entry of food into the biliary system (to avoid cholangitis)—Kenneth Warren stitch. Loop anastomosis is done nowadays to gallbladder while doing cholecystojejunostomy in advanced malignancies with dilated patent gallbladder **(Fig. 23-138)**.

RADICAL/EXTENDED CHOLECYSTECTOMY

It is done in operable cases of carcinoma of gallbladder.

Cholecystectomy with resection of liver segments IV and V—*extended cholecystectomy with perihepatic nodal clearance*. At least 2 cm margin in the liver from the gallbladder bed should be cleared. All pericholedochal lymph nodes should be removed. Frozen section biopsy from cystic duct stump should be done to identify for the existence of microscopic tumour. If present, CBD resection and hepaticojejunostomy is done. *Open approach* rather than laparoscopic is ideal for carcinoma gallbladder. Hemihepatectomy with cholecystectomy with nodal clearance is done.

If patient has undergone laparoscopic cholecystectomy and histology has confirmed carcinoma, then staging should be done. All port areas should be reexcised to prevent *port site recurrence*. Often extended resection of segment IV and lymph nodes may be needed. Spillage of bile during laparoscopic cholecystectomy is common (30% in non-malignant GB, 50% in carcinoma GB).

Kocher's incision is put with extension upwards on its medial aspect or towards opposite side. Initial exploration is done for tumour extent, nodal status, and liver secondaries. Once felt that it is operable extended cholecystectomy is done. Here approach is totally different from traditional approach of cholecystectomy. Marking is done on the surface of the liver, 2 cm away from gallbladder bed; stay sutures are placed on this line and away correspondingly on the liver side. Liver is dissected between these two parallel stay sutures with classic methods—finger reaction, bipolar, ligating or clipping the biliary ductules. Ductules are ligated using 4-zero polypropylene sutures. It is deepened towards the neck of the gallbladder and Calot's triangle. One should not injure posterior sectional/sectorial duct which may come on its way. All lymph nodes are cleared at Calot's, perihepatic and on the bile duct. Cystic artery and duct is ligated close to right hepatic artery and bile duct. Duct margin is sent for frozen section biopsy. If negative wound is closed with a tube drain. If positive then common bile duct is excised (resection of CBD) along with hepaticojejunostomy **(Fig. 23-139)**.

TREATMENT OF BILE DUCT CARCINOMA/ CHOLANGIOCARCINOMA

When operable (only 5%), portal region clearance with hemihepatectomy can be done. *Intrahepatic type* is treated with hemihepatectomy. *Perihilar* is treated with hemihepatectomy or extensive bile duct resection, nodal clearance, caudate lobe removal, cholecystectomy. Distal tumour is treated with Whipple's pancreaticoduodenectomy.

Staging laparoscopy with a laparoscopic ultrasound is done. Laparotomy is done if operable with bilateral subcostal with xiphisternum extension (Mercedes Benz incision); on table ultrasound and Doppler is needed to rule out liver metastases and vascularity of the tumour. Coeliac axis and hepatoduodenal lymph node dissection is done; CBD is resected distally and frozen section of the distal margin is done; if positive then pancreaticoduodenectomy is added. Hemihepatectomy is often added. Hepatic artery or portal vein involvement needs its resection and vascular grafts for reconstruction with saphenous or external iliac vein. Remnant hepatic duct is sutured to jejunum as Roux-en-Y hepaticojejunostomy using 7-zero PDS.

Most often it is inoperable. Stenting can be done to relieve jaundice, through PTC or ERCP or on table. Chemotherapy—5 FU; gemcitabine,

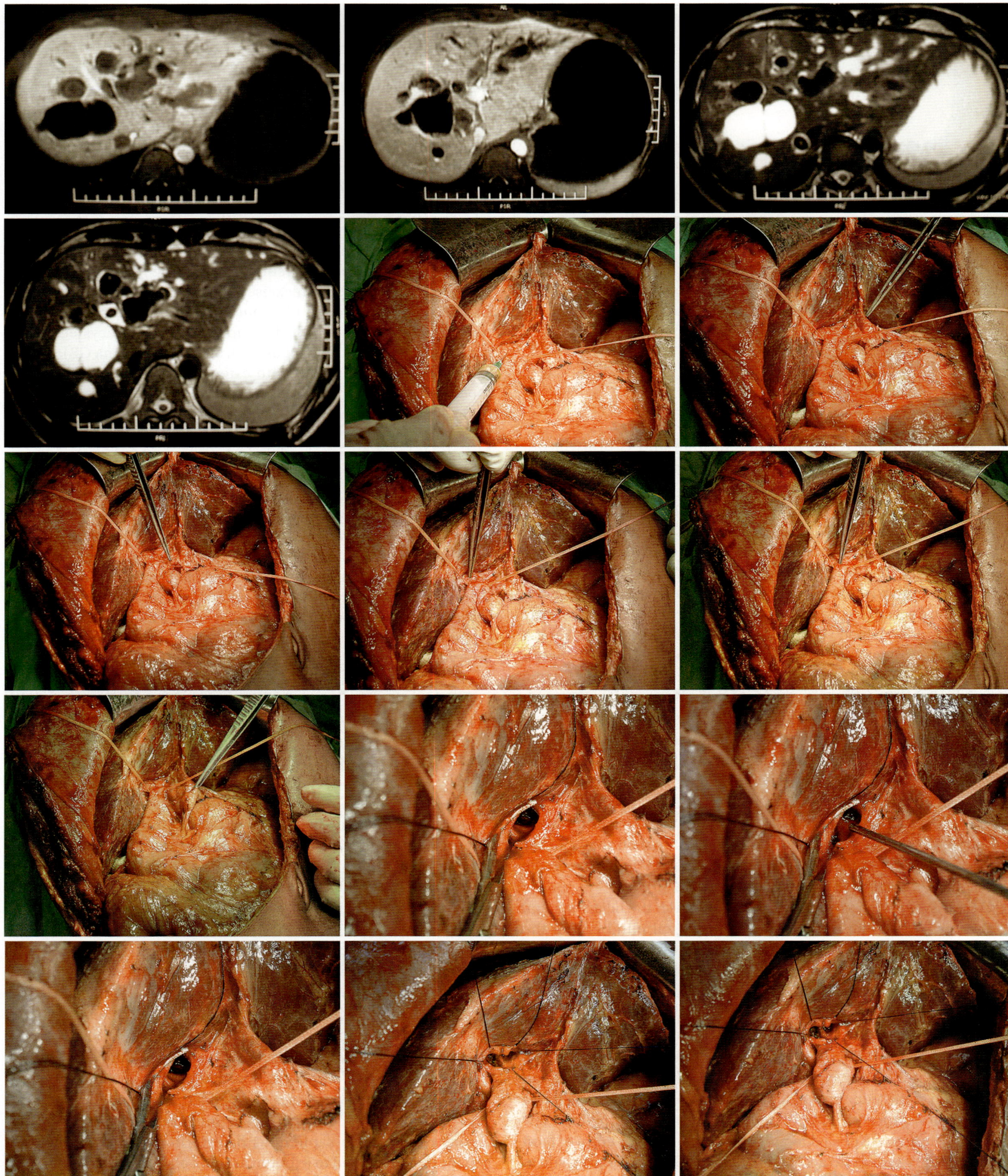

Figs. 23-135(1)

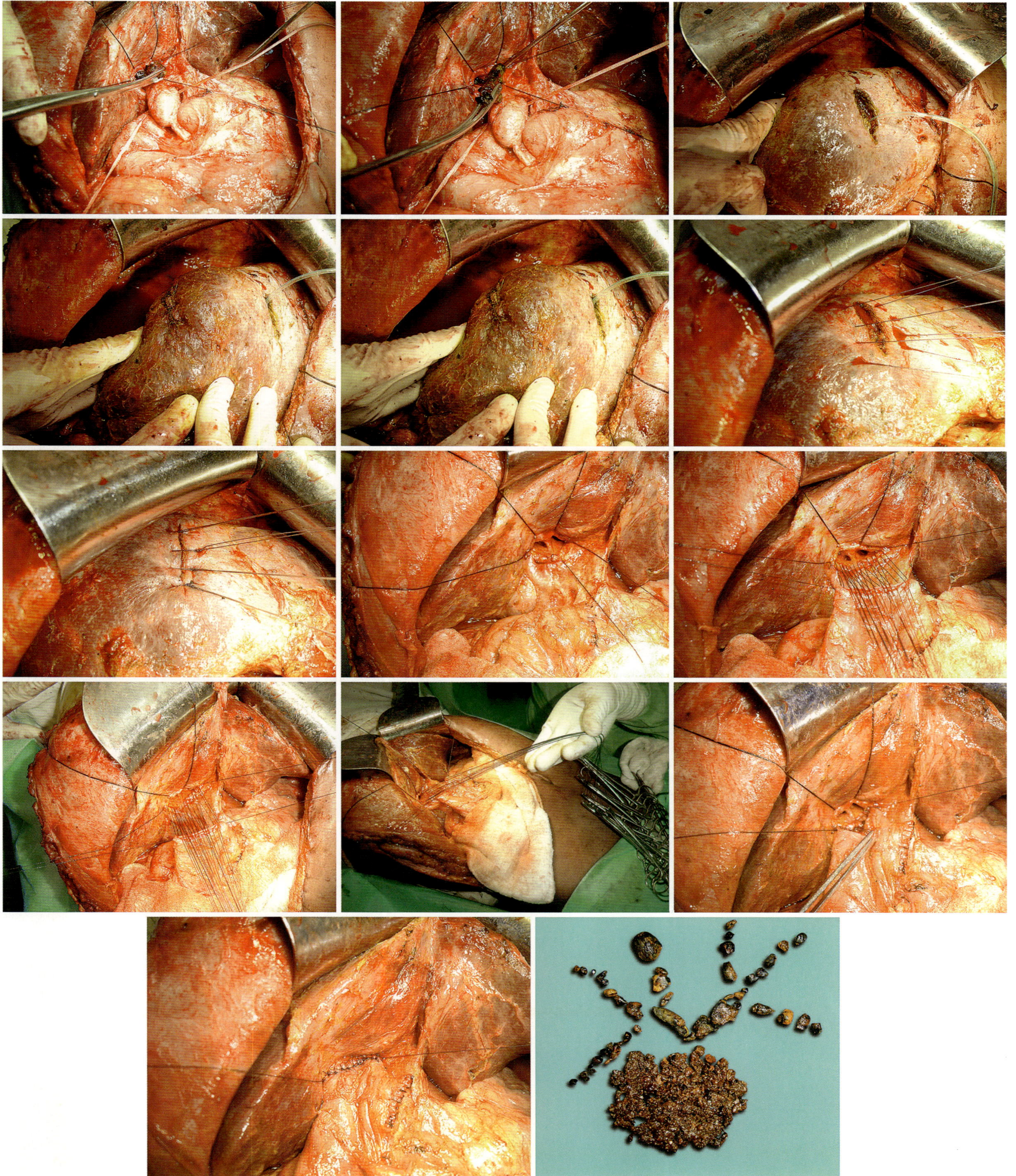

Figs. 23-135(2)

Figs. 23-135(1 and 2): Redoing of hepaticojejunostomy for retained stones in the hepatic ducts and intrahepatic biliary system.
Courtesy: Dr Arunkumar, MCh, Gastrointestinal surgeon.

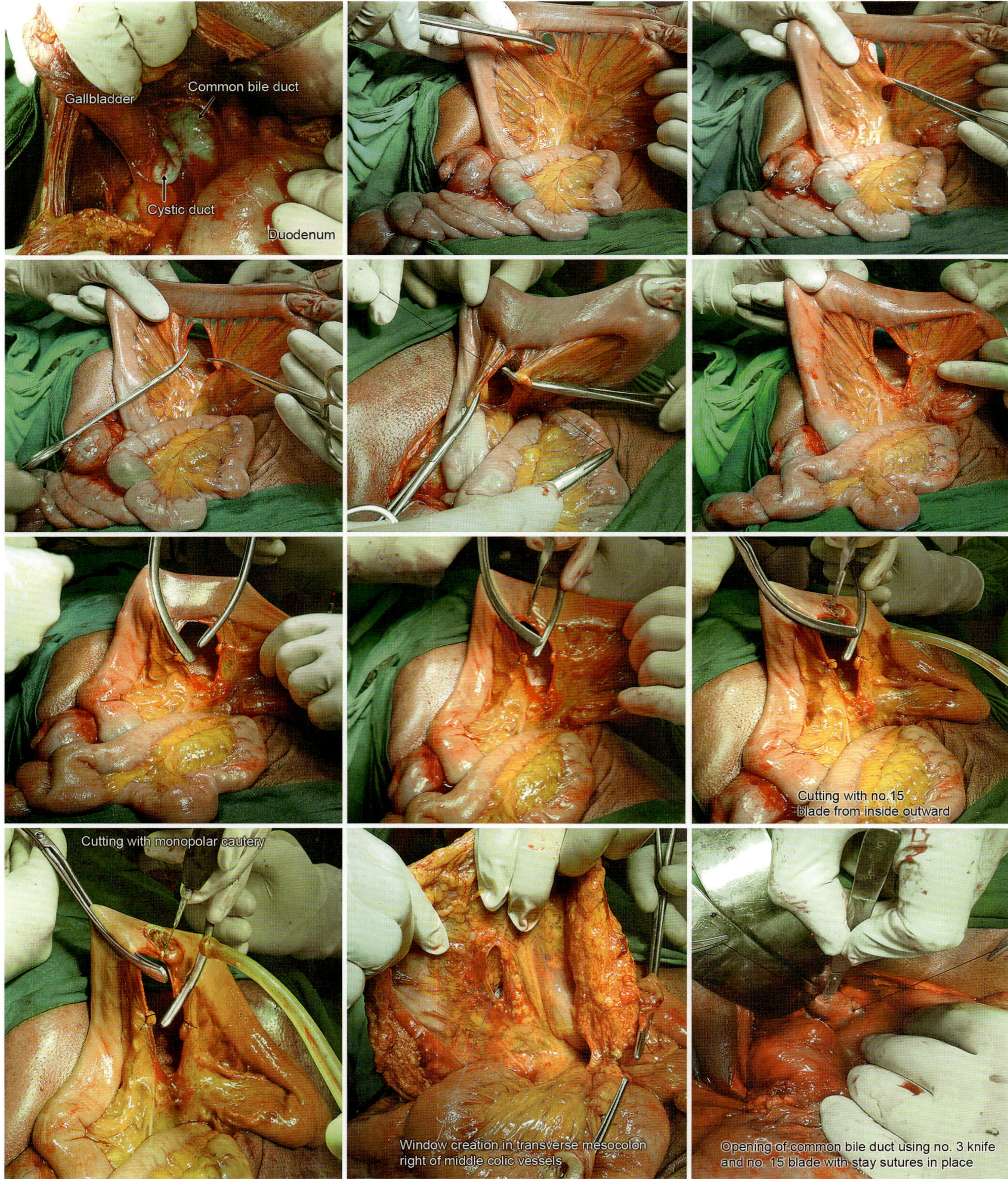
Gallbladder
Common bile duct
Cystic duct
Duodenum
Cutting with no.15
blade from inside outward
Cutting with monopolar cautery
Window creation in transverse mesocolon
right of middle colic vessels
Opening of common bile duct using no. 3 knife
and no. 15 blade with stay sutures in place

Figs. 23-136(1)

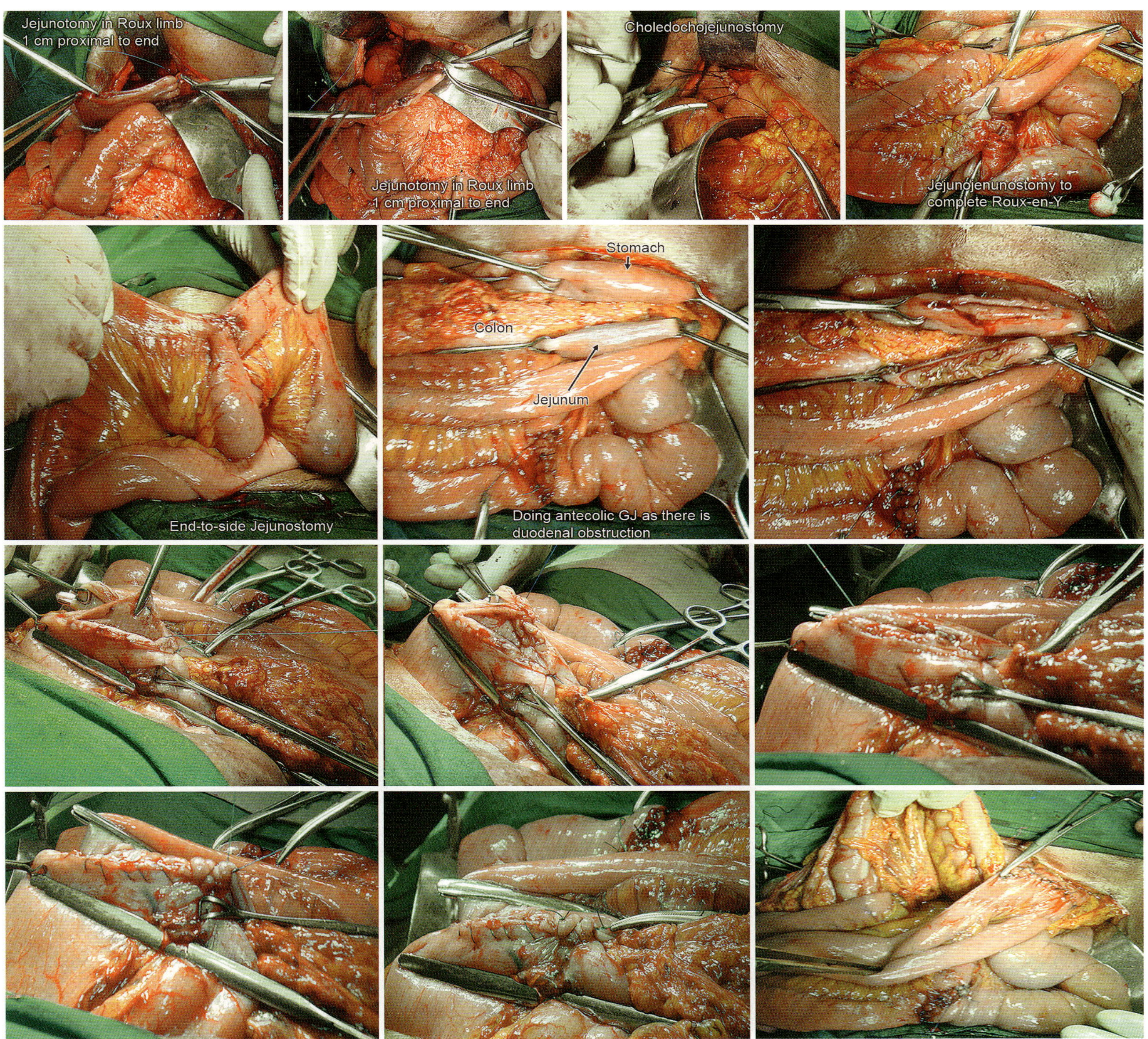

Figs. 23-136(2)

Figs. 23-136(1 and 2): Choledochojenunostomy (Roux-en-Y) with gastrojejunostomy (GJ) for duodenal obstruction.

cis platin; chemotherapy with external beam radiotherapy (ERBT) are other options.

Klatskin Tumour

It is cholangiocarcinoma at the confluence of the hepatic ducts and common hepatic duct above the level of the cystic duct (20% of cholangiocarcinomas). *It causes obstructive jaundice with hydrohepatosis without enlargement of gallbladder.* Management is like cholangiocarcinoma. Hilar resection with hepaticojejunostomy; segment III left hepaticojejunostomy—Blumgart's; Longmire's left hepaticojejunostomy after left liver lobe resection; Cattell's hepaticojejunostomy; Smith's mucosal graft hepaticojejunostomy; Palliative PTC with stenting/ERCP stenting, intraoperative stenting. Metal stents show long period of patency (12 months) than polyethylene stents (4 months) **(Figs. 23-140A and B)**.

BILE DUCT INJURIES

Causes

Cholecystectomy—open or laparoscopic; trauma; instrumentation—ERCP, baby endoscope, choledochoscope; other surgeries—pancreatic, duodenal, gastric; anomalous biliary system increases the risk of injury.

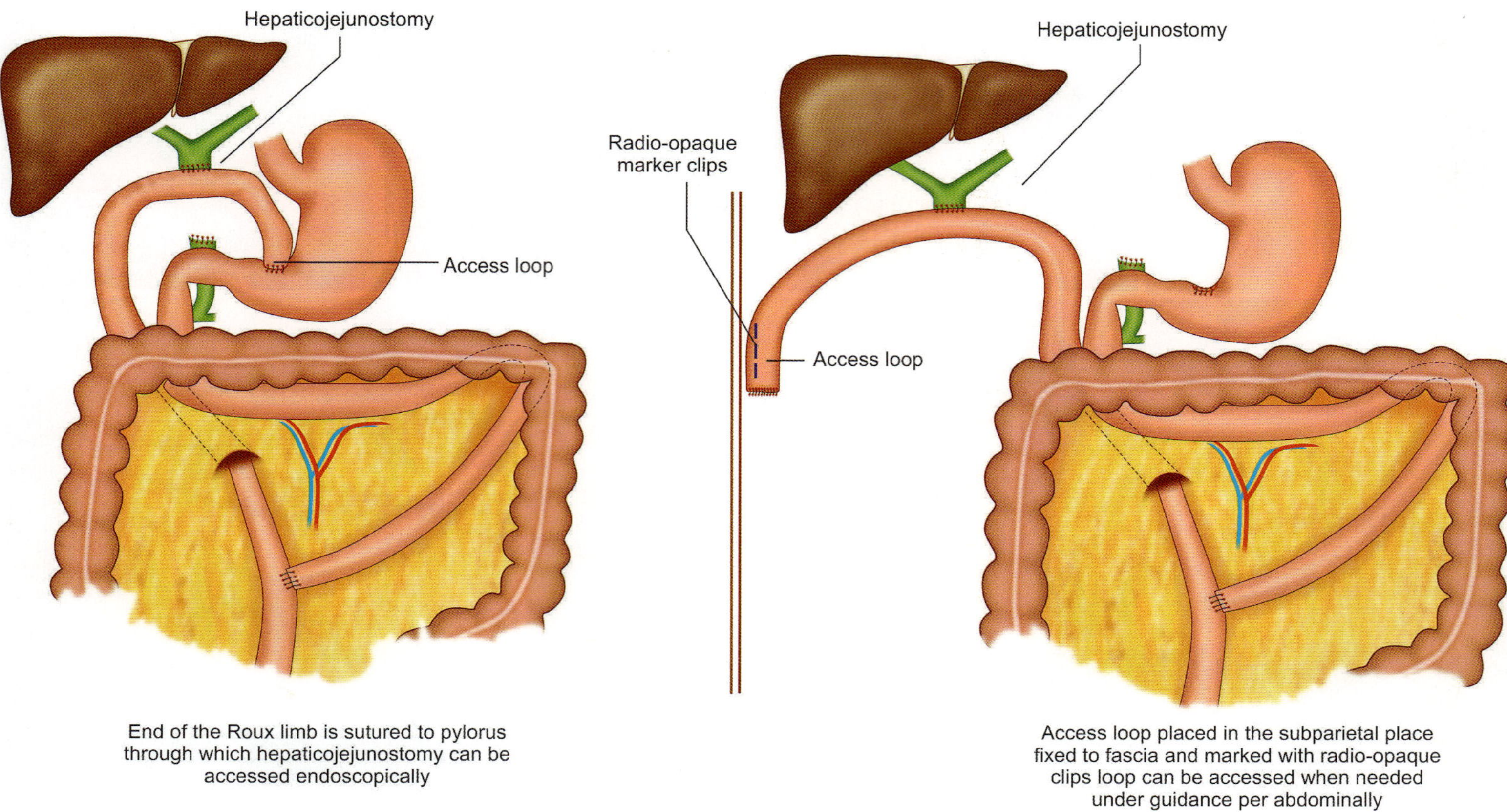

Fig. 23-137: Hepaticojejunostomy access loop—two approaches.

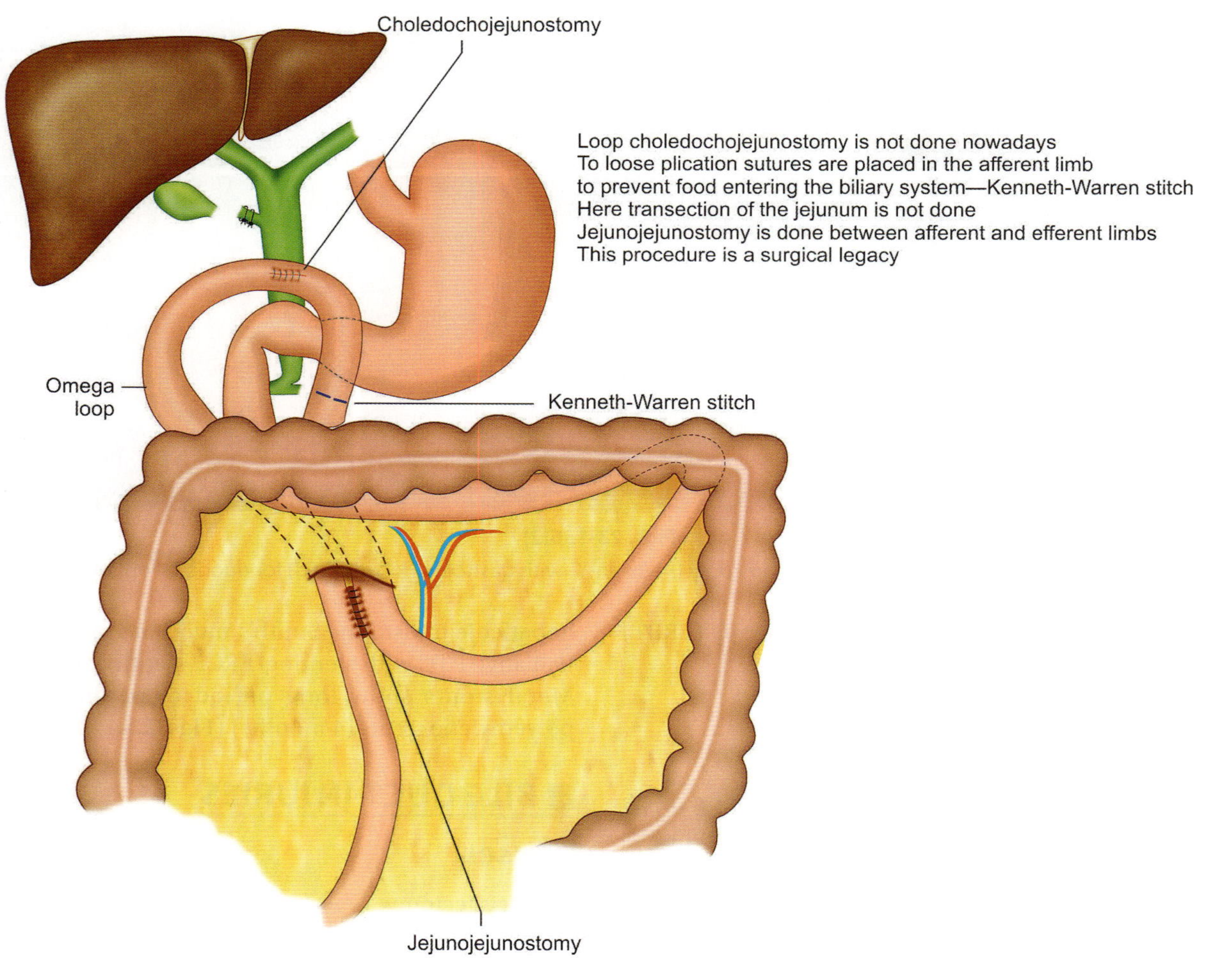

Fig. 23-138: Loop choledochojejunostomy with enteroenterostomy. It is not advocated commonly now.

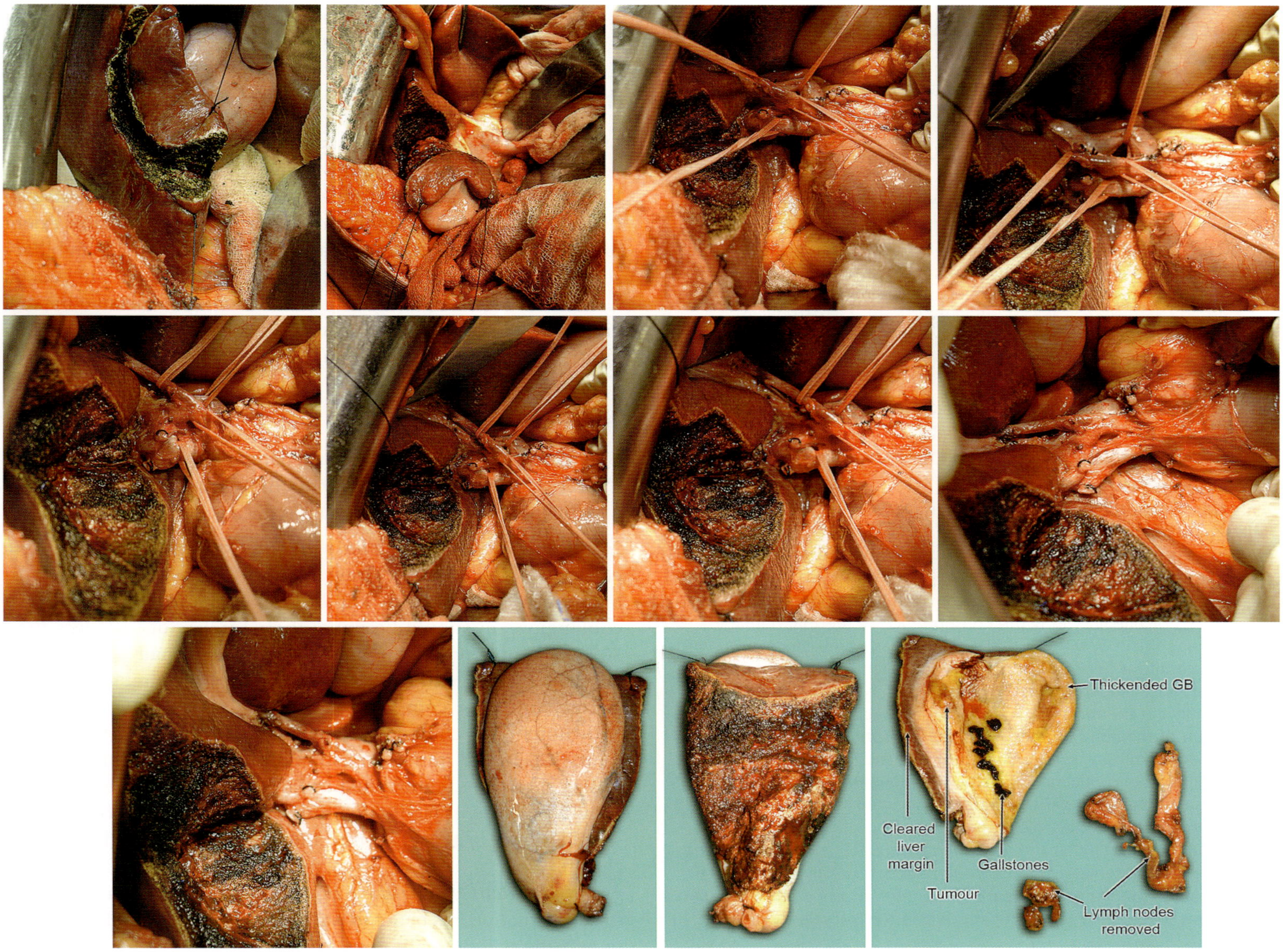

Fig. 23-139: Extended cholecystectomy for gallbladder carcinoma.
Courtesy: Dr Arunkumar, MCh, Gastrointestinal surgeon.

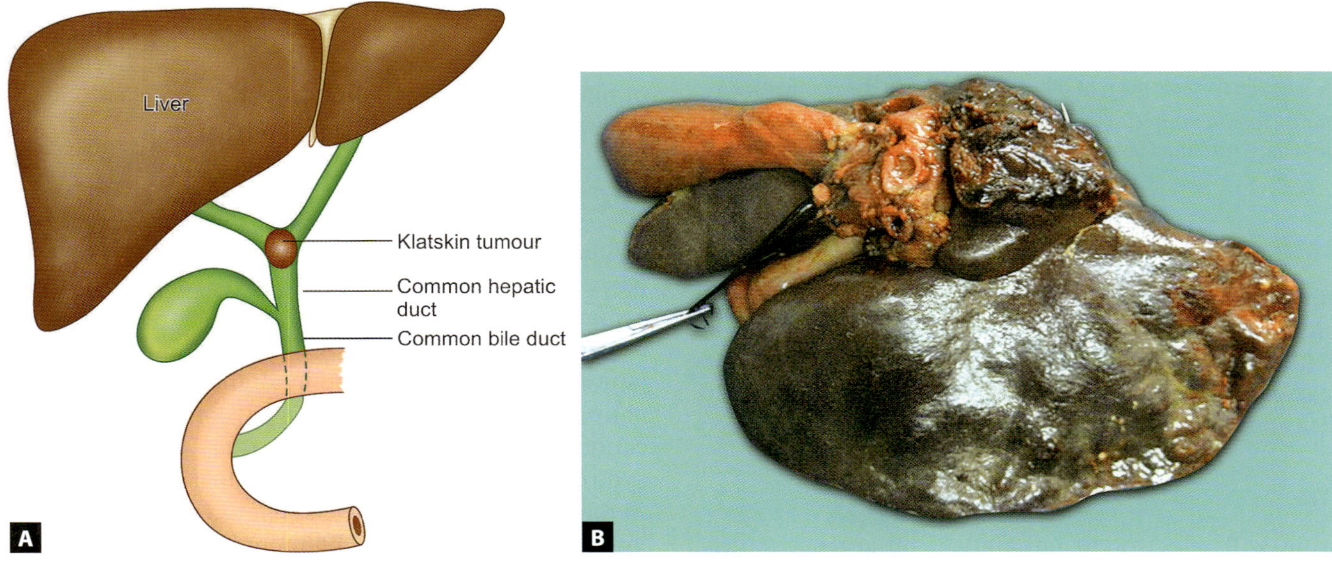

Figs. 23-140A and B: Klatskin tumour; its location (A), and resected specimen (B).

Classifications

Strasberg classification

- Class A: Bile leak from the cystic duct or an accessory duct showing continuity with the common bile duct.
- Class B: Section/injury of an accessory duct/sectorial ducts/aberrant right hepatic duct with no continuity with the common bile duct with occlusion.
- Class C: Leak/open drainage from a sectorial duct/aberrant right hepatic duct with no continuity with the common bile duct.
- Class D: Partial section/lateral injury of an extrahepatic duct/bile duct with no complete loss of continuity with the rest of the bile duct system.
- Class E: Complete section/circumferential injury of the bile duct with subtypes according to the length of the stump at various levels.
  - E1–Stricture/injury at more than 2 cm distal to bifurcation.
  - E2–Stricture/injury at less than 2 cm distal to bifurcation.
  - E3–Stricture/injury at bifurcation.
  - E4–Stricture/injury involving right and left hepatic ducts.
  - E5–Complete obstruction of entire bile duct.

Note: Only right and left partial injuries are not included in this classification.

Stewart-Way classification

This classification involves four strata based on the mechanism and anatomy of injury.

- Class I: It refers to the incomplete section of bile duct with no loss of tissue. It has a prevalence rate of 8%.
- Class II: It is a lateral injury of the common hepatic duct that leads to stenosis or bile leak. It is the consequence of thermal damage and clamping the duct with surgical staples. It has a prevalence of 2% with a concomitant hepatic artery injury in 20% of cases. T-tube related injuries are included within this class.
- Class III: It is the most common (60%) type represents the complete section of the common hepatic duct. It is subdivided in to type IIIa, remnant common hepatic duct; type IIIb, section at the confluence; type IIIc, loss of confluence; and type IIId, injuries higher than confluence with section of secondary bile ducts. Associated injury of right hepatic artery occurs in 25% of cases.
- Class IV: It is right (65%) and accessory right (25%) hepatic duct injuries with associated injury of the right hepatic artery (60%). Occasionally, it includes the common hepatic duct injury at the confluence (5%) besides the accessory right hepatic duct lesion (prevalence of 10%).

Hannover classification (2007)

It classifies injuries in relationship to the confluence and also includes vascular injuries.

- Type A: It refers to cystic and/or gallbladder bed leaks.
- Type B is a complete or incomplete stenosis caused by a surgical staple.
- Type C represents lateral tangential injuries.
- Type D refers to complete section of the common bile duct emphasising their distance to the confluence as well as the hepatic artery and portal vein concomitant injuries.
- Type E is late bile duct stenosis at different lengths to the confluence.

Note: *Bismuth classification* (for open surgery/prelaparoscopic era) is discussed in biliary stricture topic earlier.

Presentations

Fever, pain, bile stasis features like cholangitis, jaundice; 10% of laparoscopic bile duct injuries are identified on table; 30% with bile leak; 25% with obstructive jaundice; 30% with cholangitis. Patients with bile leak present early; with formed biliary stricture presents with jaundice and cholangitis months or years later.

Problems

Biliary fistula with electrolyte imbalance; biliary peritonitis, septicaemia; subphrenic abscess formation; *Biloma* formation; severe malnutrition, deficiencies; late—biliary cirrhosis, portal hypertension.

Investigations

Liver function test (LFT), coagulation profile; US abdomen, fistulogram; Dynamic CT scan will delineate the anatomy of injury; ERCP is useful if injury is only partial where stenting can also be done. PTC is the *investigation of choice* to identify site, nature, extent of stricture. It also facilitates drainage and stenting. Hepatobiliary scintigraphy may be useful. MRCP may be useful to identify ductal anatomy. CT arteriography is useful to identify associated hepatic artery or portal vein injury which is 20% in association with CBD injury.

Management

General: Antibiotics, nutrition, total parenteral nutrition (TPN).
Conservative: Small partial injury to CBD may resolve spontaneously or with the help of ERCP, sphincterotomy and stenting is done.

Management of on table biliary duct injury (during ***laparoscopic cholecystectomy***/open): Conversion into open procedure with a lengthy subcostal/bucket handle incision. Intraoperative cholangiogram should be done. Partial injury of CBD less than 30% of circumference is treated with primary repair with a T-tube in place. Extensive injury more than 30% of the circumference or cautery injury or complete CBD transection should be treated with Roux-en-Y choledochojejunostomy. Isolated hepatic duct injury less than 3 mm in size should be ligated. More than 3 mm in size should be reimplanted or Roux-en-Y hepaticojejunostomy should be done. If facility for surgical repair is available, patient should be sent to a higher centre after placing a drain with abdomen closure.

Management of bile duct injury identified at a later period: In such situation it is better to wait for 6 weeks for the inflammation to subside which facilitates easier proximal CBD identification. After proper assessment of injury, Roux-en-Y choledochjojejunostomy or *Roux en Y hepaticojejunostomy* is done.

Hepp-Couinaud approach: Here hilar plate is meticulously dissected; left hepatic duct is anastomosed to Roux jejunal loop to create hepaticojejunostomy often with creation of proximal 'access loop' for future endoscopic approach. Complications are—recurrent cholangitis, bile leak from stoma, haemobilia, stenosis of biliary enteric anastomotic site (10%; occurs often after many years).

CHOLECYSTOJEJUNOSTOMY

It is not commonly advocated now. It is indicated in advanced pancreatic malignancy as a bypass as life expectancy in these patients is short. It is often combined with gastrojejunostomy whenever there is duodenal obstruction. It is a palliative procedure in obstructive jaundice due to advanced malignancy in head of pancreas or periampullary carcinoma. It is not done in benign disease and in conditions where long-term results are anticipated. It is possible to do only if there is patency of cystic duct and the common bile duct so that obstructive jaundice is relieved through patent cystic duct into jejunum. Additional enteroenterostomy is also done (Braun) **(Fig. 23-141)**.

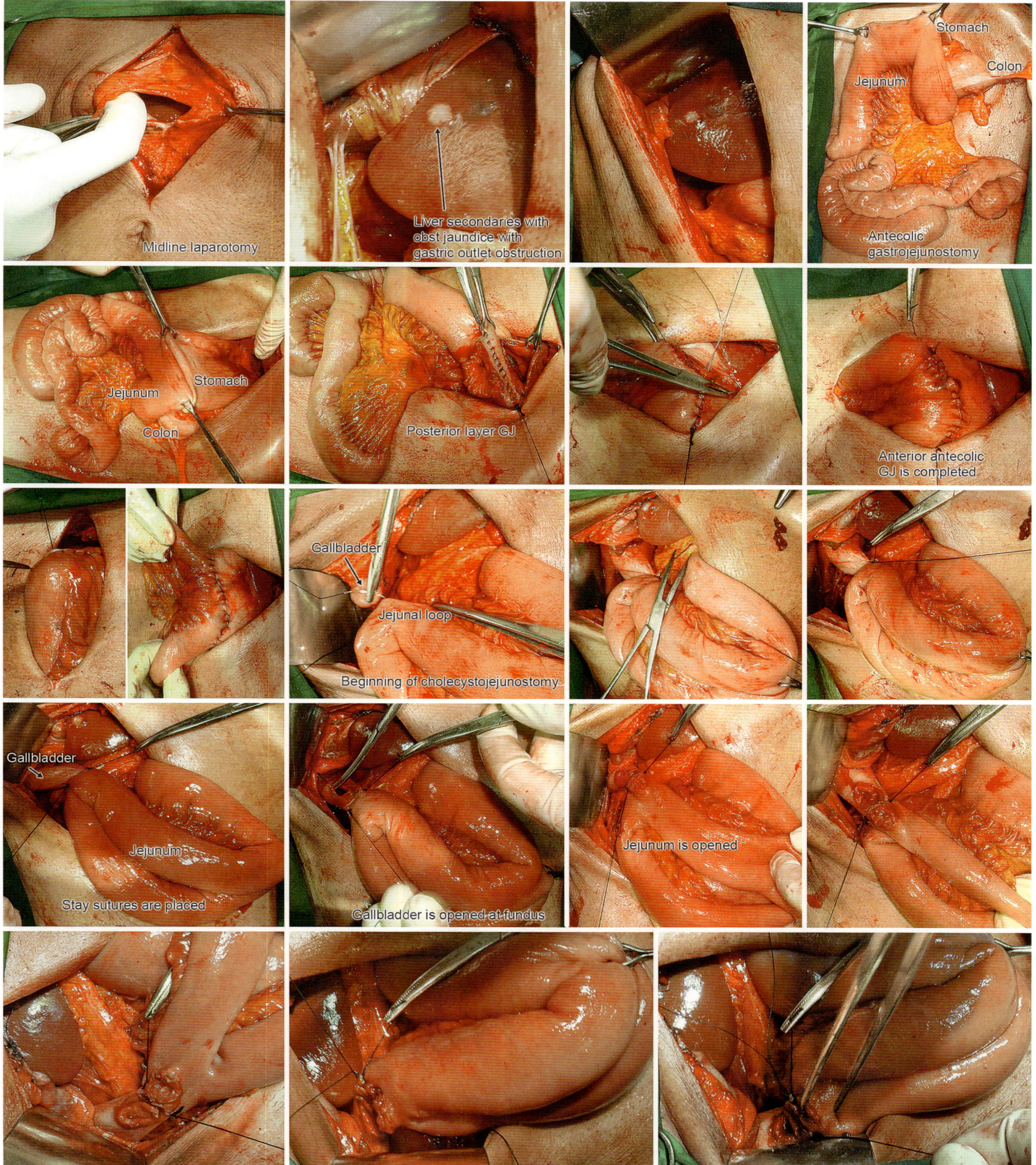
Midline laparotomy
Liver secondaries with obst jaundice with gastric outlet obstruction
Stomach
Colon
Jejunum
Antecolic gastrojejunostomy
Stomach
Jejunum
Colon
Posterior layer GJ
Anterior antecolic GJ is completed
Gallbladder
Jejunal loop
Beginning of cholecystojejunostomy
Gallbladder
Jejunum
Stay sutures are placed
Gallbladder is opened at fundus
Jejunum is opened

Figs. 23-141(1)

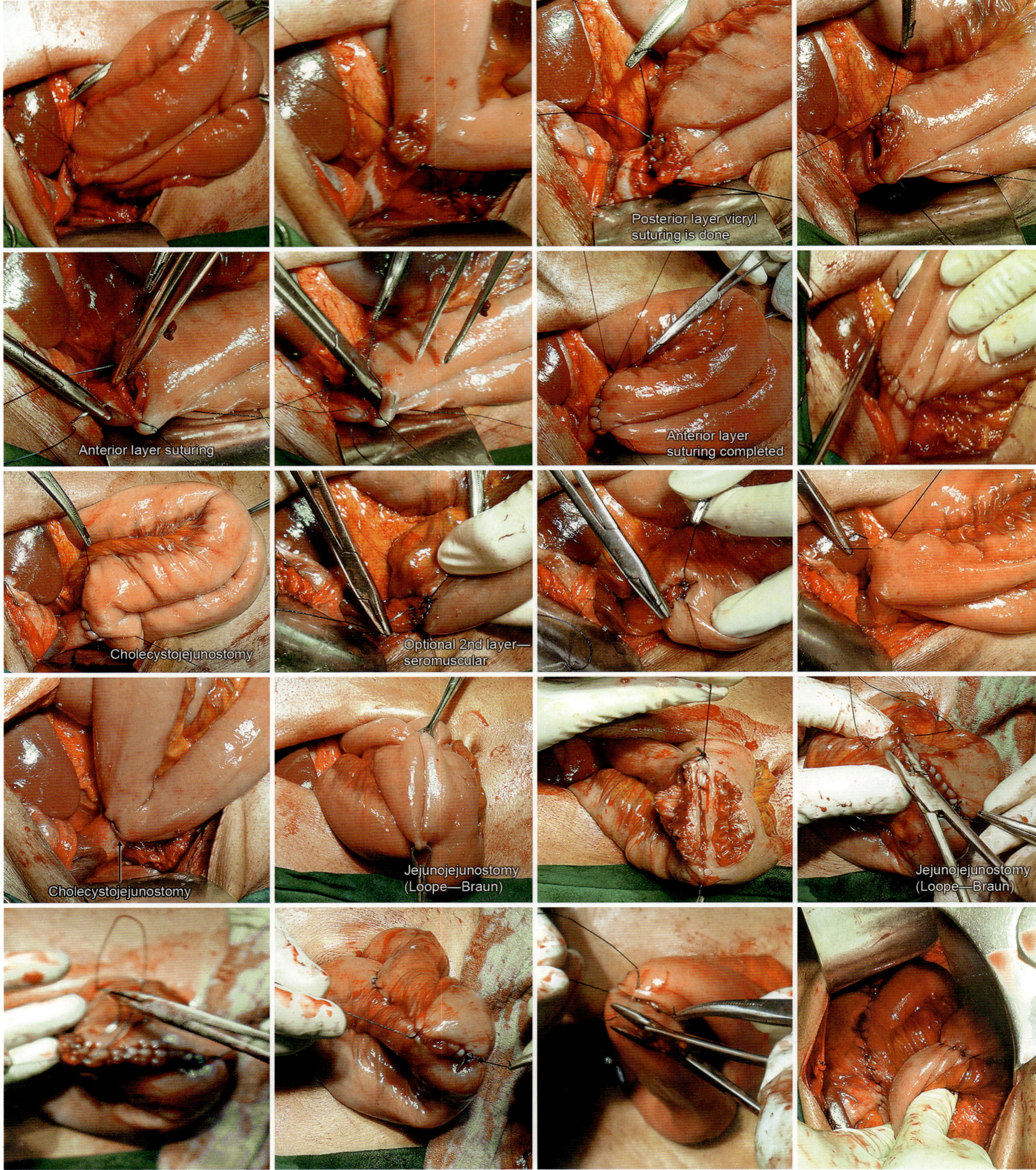

Figs. 23-141(2)

Figs. 23-141(1 and 2): Technique of palliative gastrojejunostomy and loop cholecystojejunostomy with jejunojejunostomy (Braun) as a palliative procedure. Patient has got liver metastasis.

Technique: Midline laparotomy is sufficient. First antecolic gastrojejunostomy is done to anterior wall of the stomach. Then jejunal loop is selected for anastomosing into the fundus of the gallbladder. Gallbladder is aspirated to confirm presence of bile. Preoperative CT may be useful to assess cystic duct patency. It also can be confirmed by on table dye study. Stay sutures are placed between fundus of gallbladder and jejunal loop. Fundus is opened horizontally; jejunum is opened on its antimesenteric border little lesser size than that of fundus of gallbladder. Usually single layer is sufficient. However, if two layer anastomosis is planned, posterior seromuscular layer is placed using interrupted silk or vicryl sutures. Full thickness posterior seromucosal 2nd layer is sutured using continuous or interrupted 3-zero vicryl. Third layer full thickness anterior seromucosal layer is placed similarly; finally anterior seromuscular interrupted sutures are placed. Between afferent and efferent limb of the anastomosis enteroenterostomy is done using single layer continuous vicryl suture. Abdomen is closed in layers without drain. Nasogastric tube is removed after 72 hours. Jaundice will reduce in 10 days; patient can eat food as palliation.

Complications: Cystic duct may get blocked and jaundice will reappear. Severe cholangitis may develop.

TREATMENT OF CHOLEDOCHAL CYST

Types of choledochal cysts (Todani modification of Alonso-Lej classification) **(Fig. 23-142)**.
Type I: Dilatation of extrahepatic biliary tree (60%).
Type Ia: Cystic.
Type Ib: Focal segmental (saccular).
Type Ic: Fusiform.
Type II: Diverticulum of extrahepatic biliary tree (5%).
Type III: Choledochocoele—cystic dilatation of intraduodenal part of CBD (5%).
Type IV: Dilatation of extra- and intrahepatic or multiple parts of extrahepatic biliary tree (30%).
Type IVa: Dilatation of extrahepatic and intrahepatic biliary tree. It is 2nd most common.
Type IVb: Dilatation of multiple sections of the extrahepatic bile duct.
Type V: Dilatation of the only intrahepatic biliary tree (*Caroli's disease*) **(Figs. 23-143 and 23-144)**.

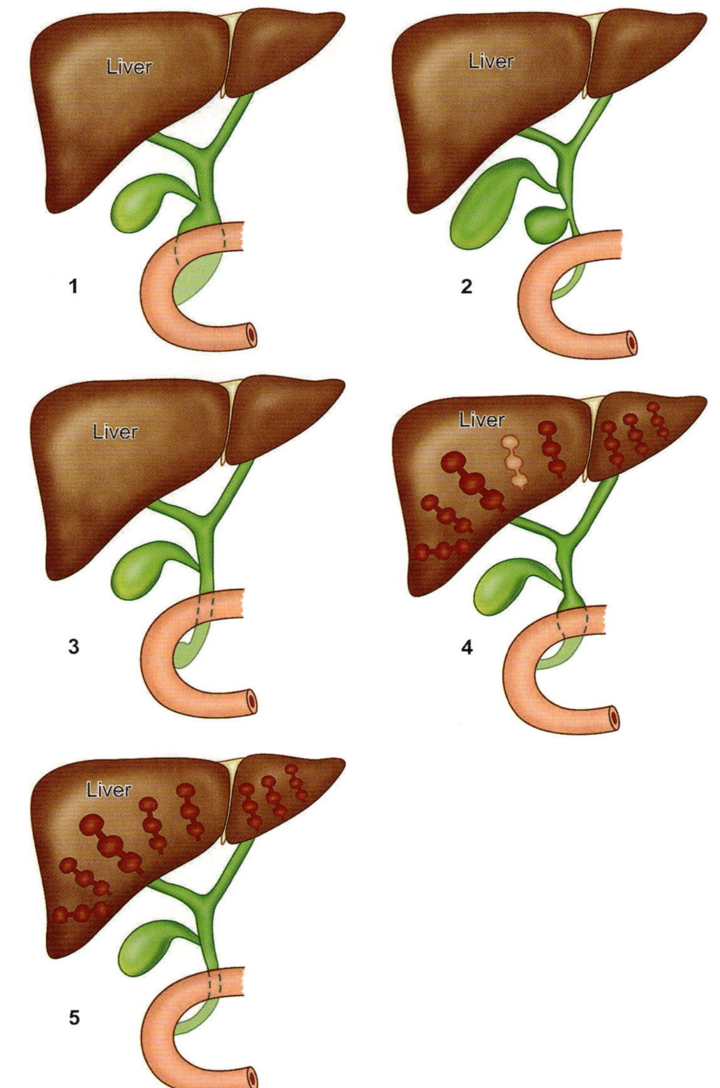

Fig. 23-142: Different types of choledochal cysts—(1) Fusiform type, (2) Saccular type, (3) Choledochocoele, (4) Fusiform + Intrahepatic type, (5) Intrahepatic type.

Treatment

Choledochal cyst should be treated to avoid possible late complications of the cyst—cirrhosis, portal hypertension, abscess formation, malignant changes (cholangiocarcinoma).

Resection of extrahepatic biliary tree with removal of choledochal cyst along with cholecystectomy and Roux-en-Y hepaticojejunostomy is the ideal treatment for choledochal cyst especially in types I, II and IVb. In Type I—excision of cyst with its mucosa and reconstruction by Roux-en-Y hepaticojejunostomy is done. In Type II—excision of the diverticulum and suturing of the CBD wall is done. In type III—endoscopic sphincterotomy is done. Excision is also often needed. Intrahepatic dilatation is difficult to treat. If it is localised, hepatectomy is sufficient, but if it is diffuse, liver transplantation may be required. In type IV if cyst is adherent to portal vein posteriorly, that part of the cyst wall over the portal vein is left behind. But mucosa of the part should be removed (*Lily's operation*). Liver resection is often necessary in type IV. Frozen section biopsy of

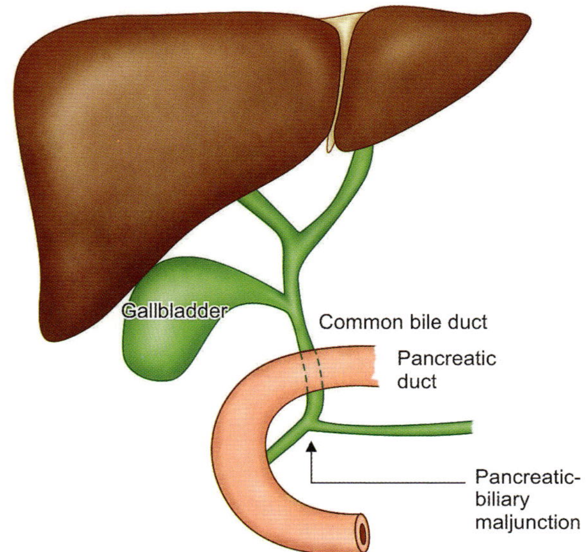

Fig. 23-143: Pancreaticobiliary maljunction. Here pancreatic duct joins CBD more proximally than normal causing reflux of pancreatic enzymes into the CBD. It leads into weakening, dilatation and choledochal cyst.

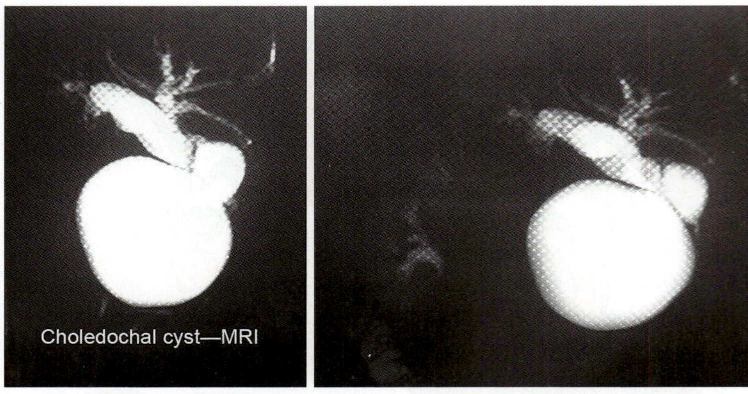

Fig. 23-144: MRI of choledochal cyst.

the choledochal cyst should be done for possible chances of existing cholangiocarcinoma; if biopsy becomes positive then hepatic resection along with bile duct resection is needed. Caroli's disease needs liver transplantation.

When CBD excision with cholecystectomy is done; distal CBD is washed using cystoscope to remove all stones, debris. Level I excision will retain cyst mucosa; level II will be adequate; level III is likely to damage the pancreatic duct as there will be biliopancreatic malposition with pancreatic duct joining the bile duct much more proximally than normal **(Figs. 23-145 and 23-146)**.

Note: Cystoenterostomy should not be done for choledochal cyst.

Complications

Ascending cholangitis; formation of intrahepatic biliary stones; pancreatic stones formation; malignancy—cholangiocarcinoma; pancreatitis; liver disease and failure.

BILIARY ATRESIA—TREATMENT

Classification

Correctable—10%; Non-correctable—90%.

Biliary Atresia

Type I: Atretic CBD—10%
Type II: Atretic CBD and common hepatic duct
Type III: Atretic CBD, common hepatic duct and right and left hepatic ducts—88% **(Fig. 23-147)**.

Biliary atresia can be:
Perinatal acquired (70%) type is not associated with congenital anomalies. *Fetal/embryonic* (30%) is associated with congenital anomalies. It may be associated with other congenital anomalies (20%) of the GIT—(malrotation, annular pancreas duodenal atresia) and congenital heart diseases, polysplenia, situs inversus, absent vena cava, preduodenal portal vein.

Treatment

In correctable cases: Roux-en-Y jejunal anastomosis is done; In non-correctable cases, hepaticoportojejunostomy (*Kasai's operation*). Liver transplantation is becoming more popular in biliary atresia—ideal.

Presently *Kasai (1974) hepatoportoenterostomy* (Kasai and Susuki, 1959) is done (in 8 weeks) as a preliminary procedure followed by liver transplantation eventually. After opening the abdomen, gallbladder is cannulated and on table cholangiogram is done to confirm atretic segment. Liver biopsy should also be done at the same time **(Fig. 23-148)**.

If biliary patency is found procedure is abandoned. In atretic biliary tree, gallbladder is dissected off the liver and by applying traction to it; fibrotic atretic biliary tree is felt and dissected up to intrahepatic segment (up to the segmental branches of portal vein). Atretic extrahepatic tissue is removed to open up the microscopic ductules. Portal plate (edge of the dissected fibrous mass in portal plate)/hepatic hilum is anastomosed to Roux-en-Y part of the small bowel. Postoperatively, antibiotics, intravenous corticosteroids initially, later orally (for 6–12 weeks), ursodeoxycholic acid (for 1 year), nutrition, medium chain and essential fatty acids, essential elements supplementation is given. Success of procedure depends on age of the patient; presence of cholangitis; ductule size (more than 200 μm is better); bridging fibrosis; type of atresia; bilirubin level. Eventually cholangitis, portal hypertension, variceal bleeding will develop.

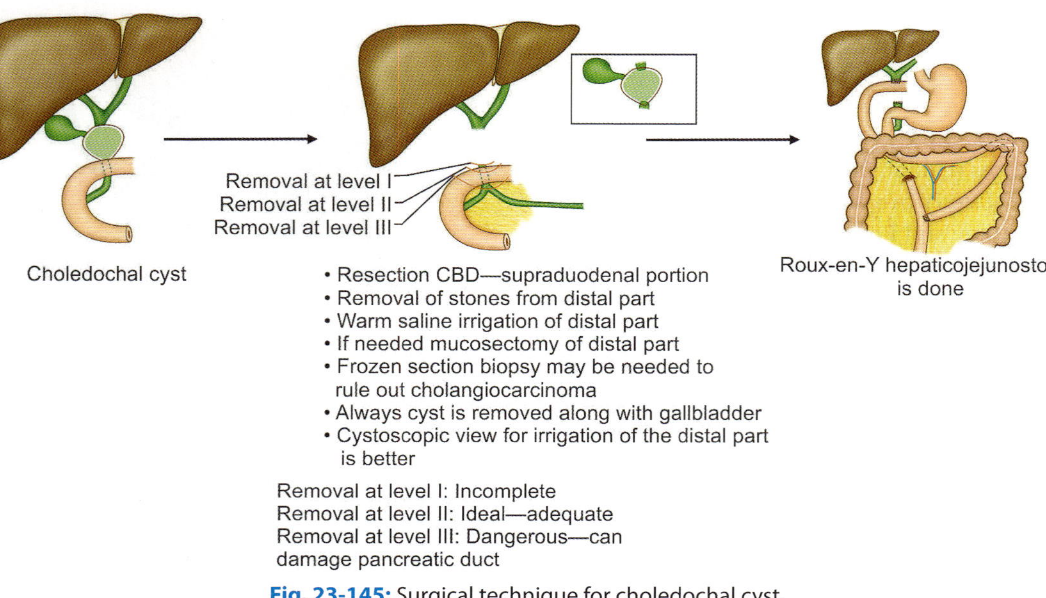

Fig. 23-145: Surgical technique for choledochal cyst.

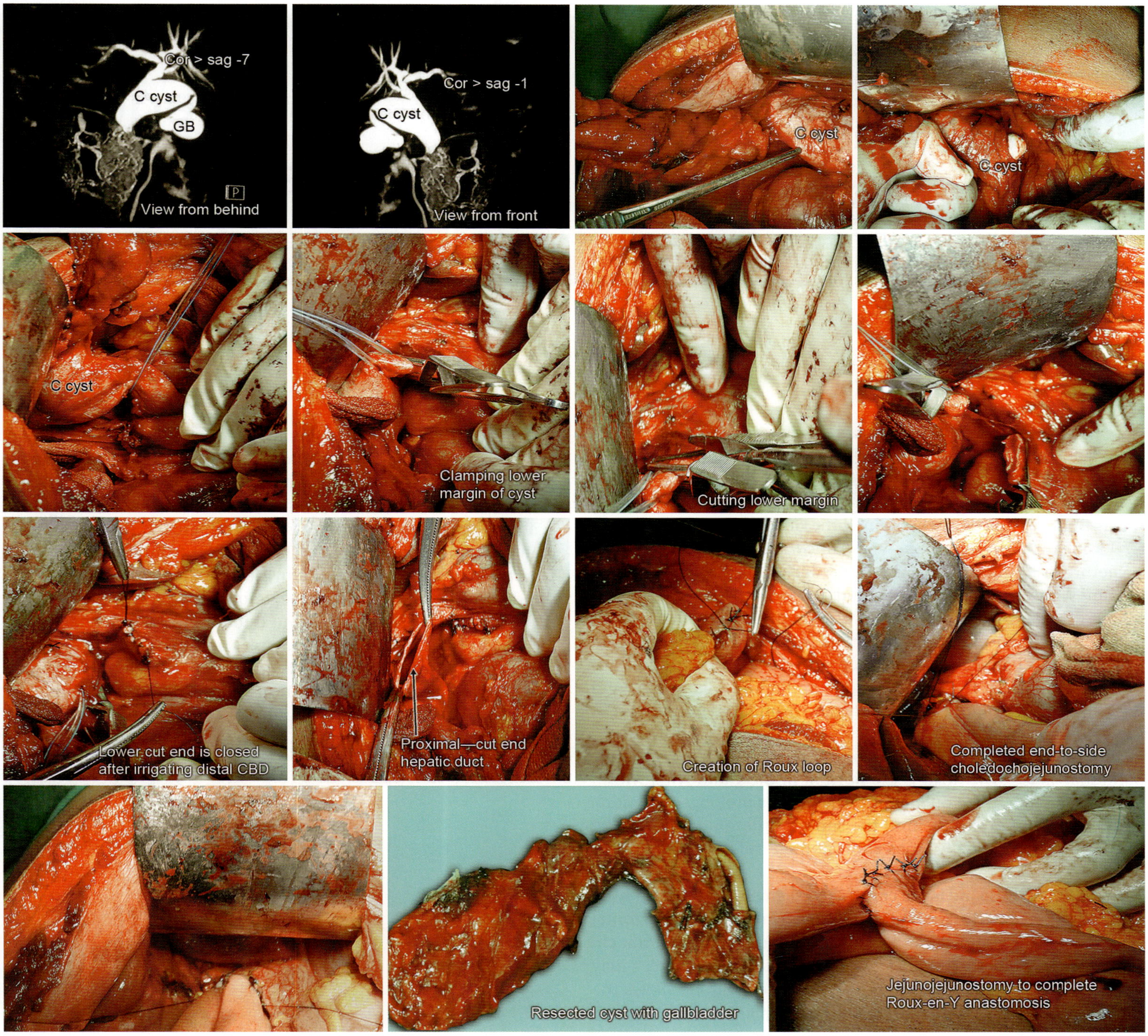

Cor > sag -7
C cyst
GB
View from behind
Cor > sag -1
C cyst
View from front
C cyst
C cyst
C cyst
Clamping lower margin of cyst
Cutting lower margin
Lower cut end is closed after irrigating distal CBD
Proximal—cut end hepatic duct
Creation of Roux loop
Completed end-to-side choledochojejunostomy
Resected cyst with gallbladder
Jejunojejunostomy to complete Roux-en-Y anastomosis

Fig. 23-146: Operative technique of choledochal cyst excision.

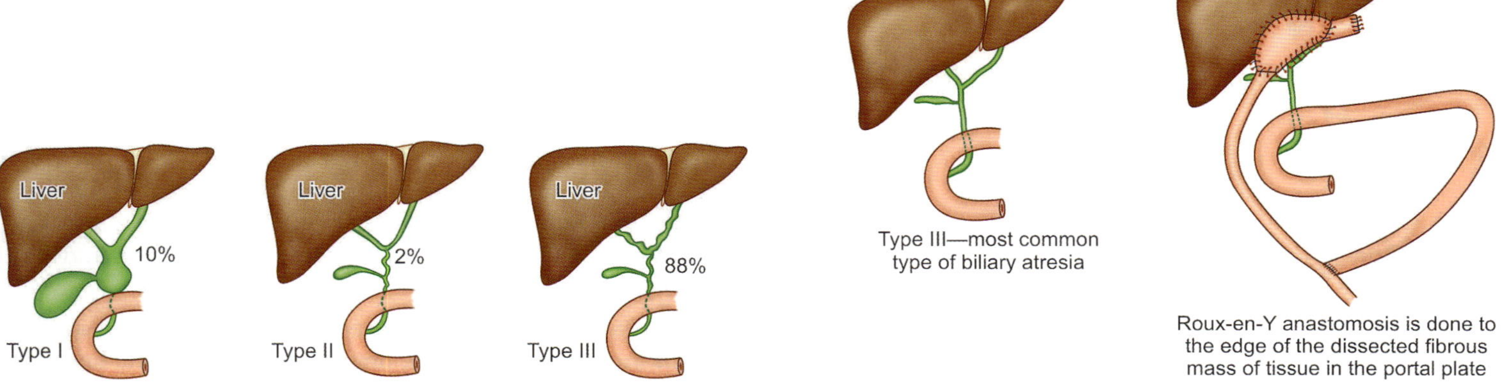

Fig. 23-147: Biliary atresia—types.

Fig. 23-148: Kasai hepatoportoenterostomy.

24 CHAPTER

Surgeries of Pancreas and Spleen

A. THE PANCREAS

SURGICAL ANATOMY

It was Rufus of Ephesus who named the organ 'pancreas', which in Greek means *Pan*—all; *Kreas—flesh/meat*. Homer used the word 'sweetbread' to describe it as animal flesh; but the fact is that it becomes bitter to the surgeons and not sweet when it develops major disease like pancreatitis. Moynihan described pancreas as an 'abdominal tiger'. The pancreas is a gland located deep in the abdomen between the stomach and the spine (2nd and 3rd lumbar vertebrae). The liver, intestine and other organs surround the pancreas. It extends on the right side from duodenum towards spleen on the left side.

The pancreas lies in the retroperitoneum within the anterior pararenal space. The head is the portion of the gland lying within the C-loop curve of the duodenum. The head is prolonged inferiorly and medially to extend behind the superior mesenteric vein. The uncinate process usually stops short at the level of the right renal hilum inferiorly.

The neck of the gland is the constricted segment of the gland lying anterior to the superior mesenteric vessels. The body is a horizontal segment of the gland lying behind the lesser sac and stomach. Dorsal to the body runs the splenic vein. The tail of pancreas may be inclined slightly cephalic to the level of the head. It follows the splenic vessels into the splenic hilum **(Fig. 24-1)**.

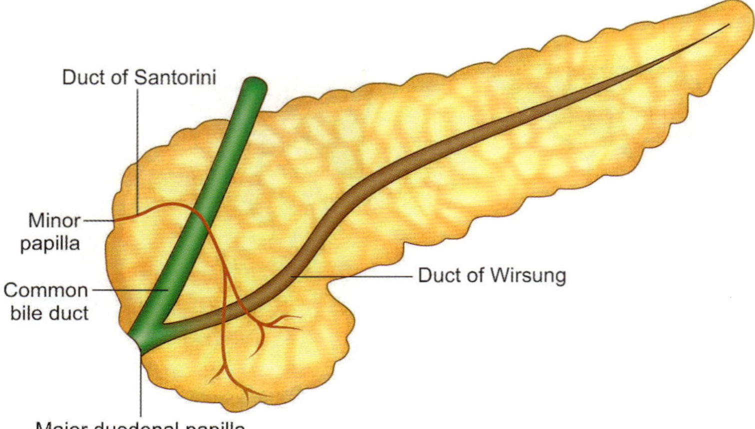

Fig. 24-1: Ductal parts of the pancreas.

The pancreas is about 15 cm long, 3 cm broad and 1.5 cm thick and is flat pear/retort shaped. It weighs around 100 g. The widest part of the pancreas is the head, the middle section is the body, and the thinnest part is the tail. Pancreas is a fixed organ. Omental bursa is above; transverse mesocolon is in front; greater sac is below the pancreas. Above it is related to 1st part of the duodenum, pylorus, stomach, liver and spleen. Below it is related to 3rd part of the duodenum, jejunum, transverse colon and spleen. Inner part of the 1st, 2nd and 3rd parts of the duodenum is closely adherent to the corresponding parts of pancreas and duodenum here is not having peritoneal coverage and is called as bare area of duodenum. Posteriorly pancreas extends from hilum of kidney to hilum of spleen. It is related behind to hilum of kidney, inferior vena cava (IVC), superior mesenteric vein and portal vein, aorta, left kidney and hilum of spleen **(Fig. 24-2)**.

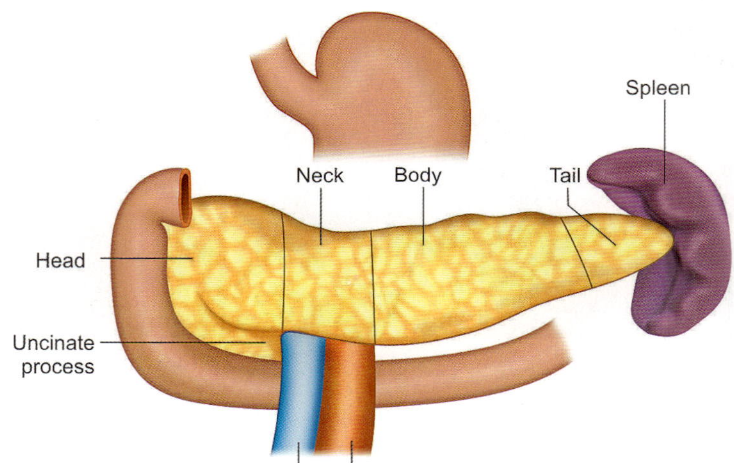

Fig. 24-2: Parts of the pancreas.

Head lies to the right of the superior mesenteric vessels. It is adherent to the inner part of the C-loop of the duodenum. Posteriorly, it is related to the hilum and adjacent right kidney, right renal vessels, IVC, left renal vein entering IVC, right crus of the diaphragm, posterior pancreaticoduodenal arcade, right gonadal vein and distal common bile duct (CBD).

Neck is 1.5 cm in length; lies between coeliac trunk above and superior mesenteric vessels below. Its junction with the head is at an imaginary line from the portal vein to the superior mesenteric vessels below. At this junction anterior superior pancreaticoduodenal artery originates from the gastroduodenal artery near the upper part of the neck of the pancreas. Behind, the superior mesenteric vein joins the splenic vein to form portal vein. Small veins may enter the portal vein and the superior mesenteric vein directly from the neck of the pancreas. Short and often stout lateral veins may enter it from its lateral part to portal vein; left gastric, splenic and rarely inferior mesenteric vein may enter the portal vein from the left side.

Lower posterior part of the head of the pancreas extends behind the superior mesenteric vessels and in front of IVC and aorta is known as ***uncinate process***. It gets blood supply from the superior mesenteric vessels through very short vessels. One should ligate these vessels carefully while dissecting the uncinate process, otherwise tear of these vessels may lead into torrential bleeding. Occasionally, this process may be absent or encircle superior mesenteric vessels completely. Left renal vein is above it; duodenum is below it. An anomalous right hepatic artery may pass through the uncinate process after originating from the superior mesenteric artery.

Pancreas lying towards the left of the neck/superior mesenteric vein is known as ***body of pancreas***. It is related to the 4th part of the duodenum, suspensory ligament of Treitz, first part of jejunum, left side transverse colon. Superior mesenteric vein and artery run between head and uncinate process to run in front of the duodenum. Vein is towards the right of the artery. Above body of the pancreas is related to coeliac axis, common hepatic artery and splenic vessels from right to left. In front, it is covered by posterior wall of the omental bursa which has got two layers of the peritoneum. Stomach covers in front of it. Transverse colon with its two leaves is also in front of it. Middle colic vessels are connected here. Middle colic artery after originating from superior mesenteric artery runs between two leaves of mesocolon. Inferior mesenteric vein runs close to inferior border of the distal part of the body of pancreas to join splenic vein. Posteriorly, it is devoid of peritoneum and is related to aorta, origin of superior mesenteric artery, left crus of diaphragm, left suprarenal gland, left kidney, left renal vessels and splenic vein **(Fig. 24-3)**.

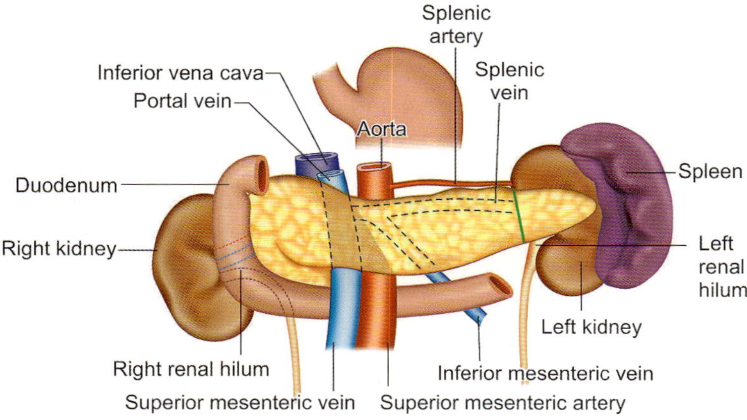

Fig. 24-3: Posterior relations of the pancreas.

Tail of the pancreas is the distal most part of the pancreas; its tip is related to spleen; it is enveloped within two layers of splenorenal ligament along with the splenic vessels. Tail of the pancreas may be mobile.

Pancreas is long, flat and irregularly prismatic in shape; its right extremity, being broad, is called the head, and is connected to the main portion of the organ, or body, by a slight constriction, the neck; while its left extremity gradually tapers to form the tail. It is situated transversely across the posterior wall of the abdomen, at the back of the epigastric and left hypochondriac regions. Conventionally it shows two segments; cephalocervical right segment is supplied by gastroduodenal and superior mesenteric arteries. Left-sided corporocaudate segment is supplied by splenic and dorsal pancreatic arteries. Junction of two segments is relatively avascular.

The main pancreatic duct (duct of Wirsung) opens at the major duodenal papilla, measuring 3–4 mm in diameter in adults. It enlarges slightly with advancing age. The diameter of the duct tapers to 1-2 mm toward the tail. A slight narrowing at the head and body of the pancreas is a normal variation. The accessory pancreatic duct (duct of Santorini) opens at the minor duodenal papilla, proximal to the major duodenal papilla. Both bile and pancreatic ducts open into the duodenum in 60% of individuals; in 30%, duct of Santorini ends blindly and duct of Wirsung carries the secretion; in 10%, duct of Wirsung may be small or absent and duct of Santorini secretes entirely.

On cross-sectional images, the measurements of normal pancreas diameters generally are as follows: head of the pancreas, 3 cm; neck and body of the pancreas, 2.5 cm; and tail, as long as 2 cm.

The position, size and shape of the pancreas vary among patients. The pancreas gradually diminishes with advancing age, sometimes becoming more marked beyond the seventh decade. The surface of the pancreas is smooth in 80% of patients and lobulated in approximately 20%. Ampulla of Vater is situated on the posteromedial wall of the 2nd part of the duodenum; right of 2nd and 3rd lumbar vertebrae (commonly at the level of spine of 2nd lumbar vertebra). Muscular sphincteric complex (Sphincter of Oddi, 1887; sphincter of Boyden) of 6–30 mm in length is obliquely placed, contains four separate sphincters—superior bile duct sphincter, inferior submucosal bile duct sphincter, pancreatic sphincter and ampullary sphincter. Papilla is found in the mucosa (on endoscopy) where longitudinal mucosal fold meets the transverse fold like a 'T'. Papilla is nipple-like projection of duodenal mucosa; major duodenal papilla is located on the posteromedial wall of the 2nd part of the duodenum 10 cm from pylorus (but may vary); minor duodenal papilla is located 2 cm proximal to major papilla **(Figs. 24-4 and 24-5)**.

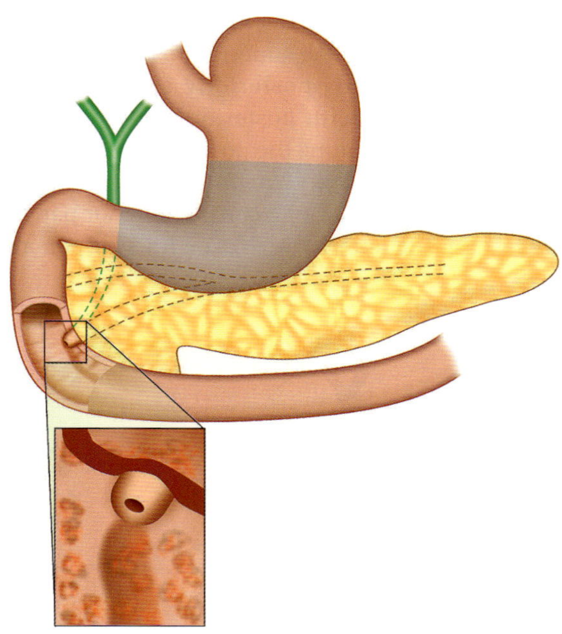

Fig. 24-4: Orifice of ampulla of Vater in the duodenal mucosa.

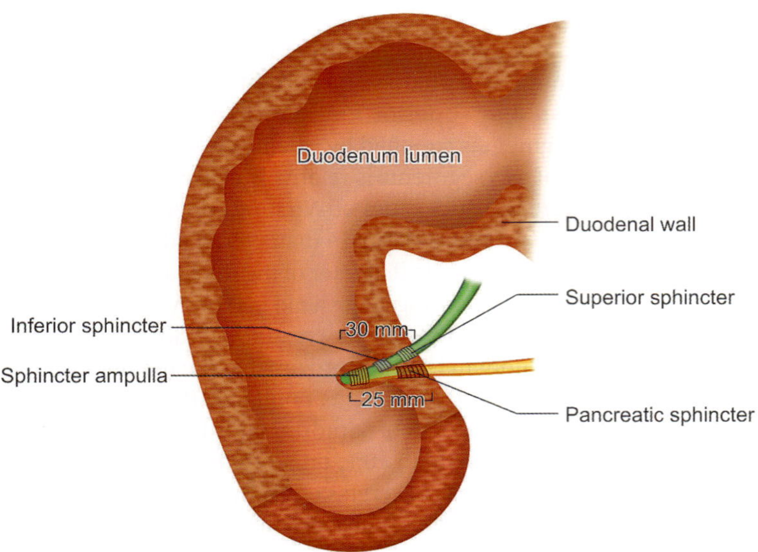

Fig. 24-5: Sphincter complex of ampulla of Vater.

Ampulla (ampulla of Vater; Abraham Vater, 1684) is slightly widened part of common pancreaticobiliary channel beyond the septum. Ampulla will not be obvious if septum between bile duct and pancreatic duct extends up to the orifice. Variations are—I: The pancreatic duct joins bile duct at a variable distance; II: The pancreatic and bile ducts open separately on the major duodenal papilla (5%); and III: Both ducts open into the duodenum at separate points (10%) **(Figs. 24-6A to C)**.

The pancreas produces insulin and other hormones—exocrine and endocrine both. The pancreas also produces pancreatic enzymes that help to digest food. The pancreas releases the juices into a system of ducts leading to the pancreatic duct. The pancreatic duct empties into the second part of the duodenum through the ampulla of Vater.

Blood Supply

Arterial Supply

The gastroduodenal artery is the descending branch of common hepatic artery which courses in front of the portal vein. The first branch of this artery is the superior posterior pancreaticoduodenal artery which descends posteriorly along the common hepatic duct to anastomose with posterior branch of inferior pancreaticoduodenal artery forming the posterior arch. The superior anterior pancreaticoduodenal artery runs in the curve of the duodenum down to anastomose with anterior branch of inferior pancreaticoduodenal artery to form the anterior arch. The inferior pancreaticoduodenal artery begins behind the uncinate process of the pancreas as the first right branch of the **superior mesenteric artery (SMA)** and divides after a short distance into an anterior and a posterior branch. *Arteria pancreatica magna* takes off from the splenic artery and joins into the glandular parenchyma at the level of the passage from the middle part to the left third of the tail of the pancreas. Arteria pancreatica magna also known as great pancreatic artery after originating from splenic artery anastomoses with inferior pancreatic artery **(Figs. 24-7A to C)**. The artery of the tail of the pancreas is represented by four arterial trunks which surrounds the pancreatic tail. They originate from the left gastroepiploic artery or from the so-called main inferior trunk of the splenic artery. Dorsal pancreatic artery arises from splenic artery at the neck of the pancreas close to its origin from coeliac trunk. Right branch of dorsal pancreatic artery supplies head of pancreas after joining posterior superior pancreatic arcade; its left branch runs in a groove on the inferior margin of the pancreas known as transverse or inferior pancreatic artery which supplies body and tail of the pancreas. Dorsal pancreatic artery may arise from the coeliac trunk or common hepatic artery. Major arteries of pancreas lie posterior to pancreatic duct. Splenic artery runs tortuously towards left along the upper and posterior surface of the body and tail of the pancreas. Splenic artery gives branches which communicate with inferior pancreatic artery.

Caudal pancreatic artery is often present; originates from splenic artery or left gastroepiploic artery (is a branch of splenic artery); communicates with transverse pancreatic artery and arteria pancreatica magna. It also supplies accessory spleen when present. Anomalous right hepatic artery is a common variation observed which arises from SMA which runs behind the CBD or portal vein; it may be accessory to normally existing right hepatic artery (a branch of common hepatic artery) or replacing the right hepatic artery, in which case it is the only supply to the right liver. Occasionally aberrant left hepatic artery may arise from SMA or gastroduodenal artery. These variations are important while doing Whipple's pancreaticoduodenectomy or total pancreatectomy. Middle colic artery may arise from dorsal pancreatic or inferior pancreaticoduodenal arteries instead of SMA. Middle colic artery is usually close to uncinate process but it may pass through the head of pancreas or run close to the 2nd part of the duodenum as variation in pathway. Body and tail of pancreas usually derive their arterial supply from branches of both splenic artery and dorsal pancreatic artery (50%); but dorsal pancreatic artery may be entirely absent and body and tail of pancreas are exclusively supplied by splenic artery (25%); or there may not be any branches from the splenic artery to the body and tail of the pancreas and blood supply is exclusively from the dorsal pancreatic artery (25%).

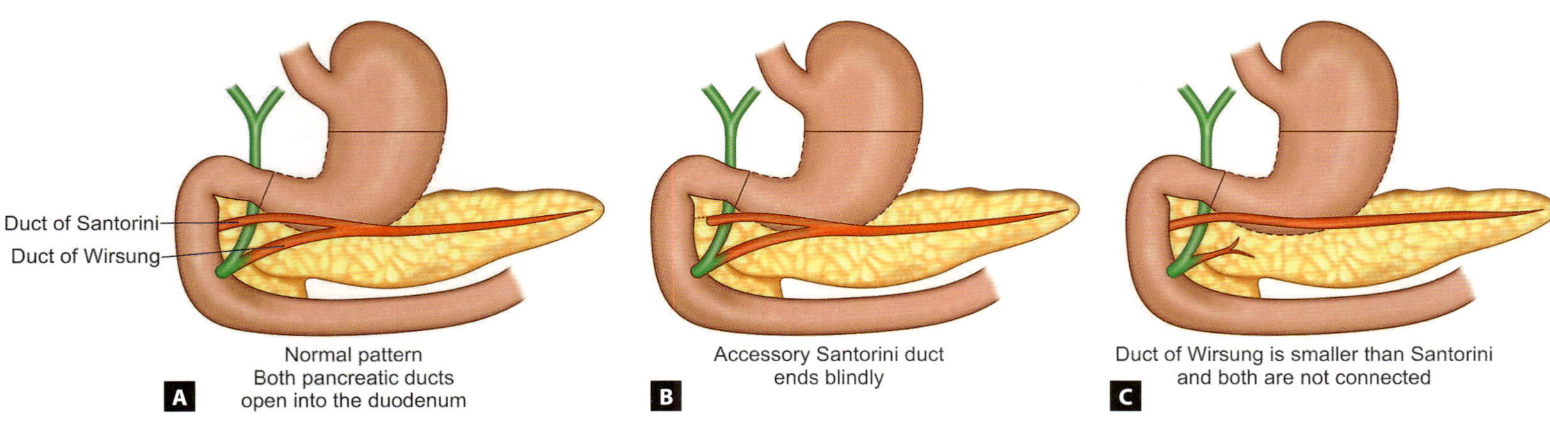

Figs. 24-6A to C: Different duct patterns in pancreas.

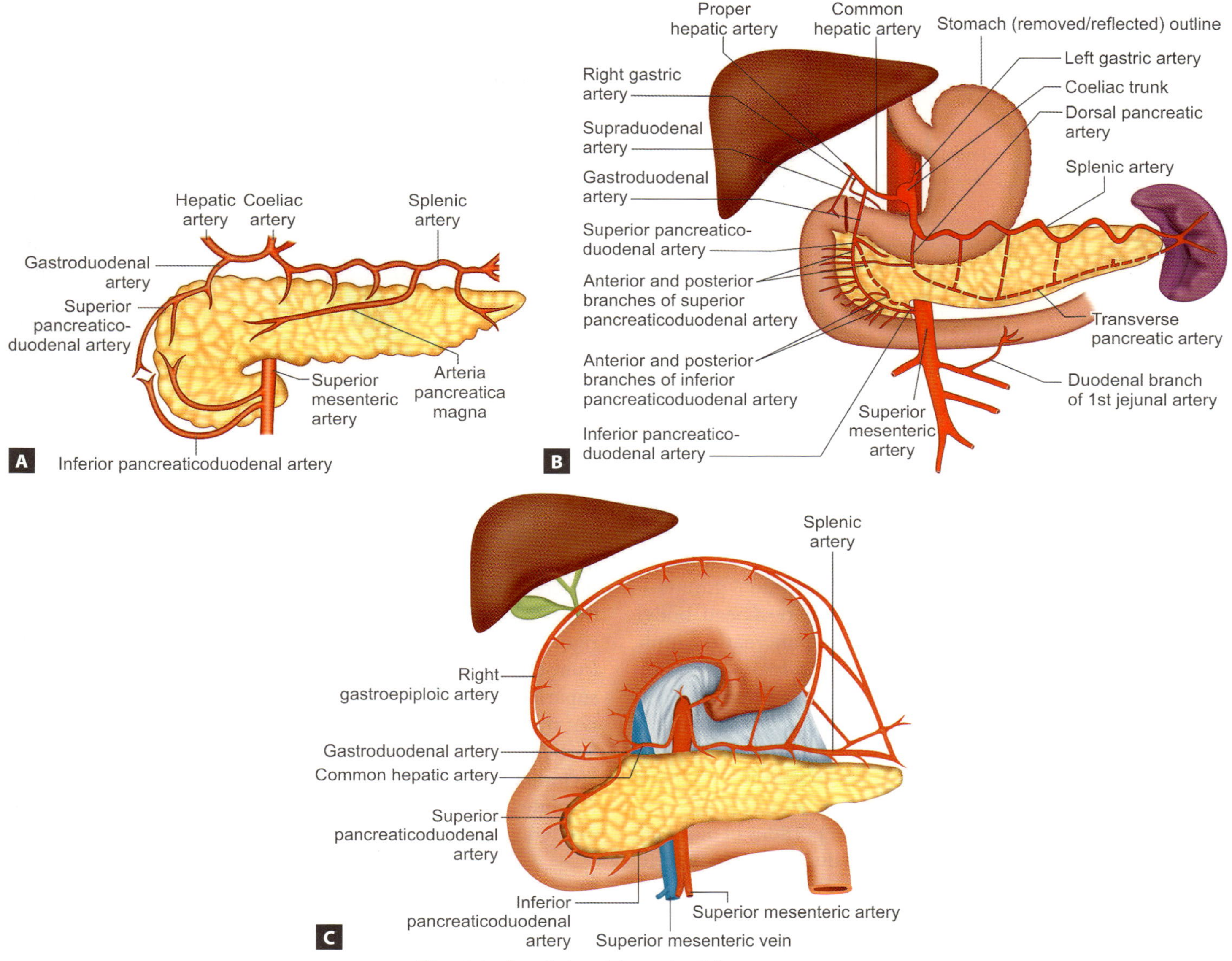

Figs. 24-7A to C: Arterial supply of the pancreas.

Ampulla is supplied by posterosuperior pancreaticoduodenal artery through epicholedochal plexus. Anterosuperior pancreaticoduodenal artery may get injured in pancreaticojejunostomy as drainage procedure for chronic pancreatitis.

Venous Drainage

The venous drainage from the head of the pancreas drains into the portal vein *via* pancreaticoduodenal veins and several small veins which drain directly into the portal vein in the medial and inferior aspect. The inferior pancreatic vein courses along the inferior margin of the pancreas and receives different small veins. It flows into the inferior or the superior mesenteric vein. Veins are superficial to arteries; both arteries and veins are deep to the pancreatic duct system. Duct → veins → arteries—is the pattern from front to back. Anterior superior pancreaticoduodenal vein and/or right gastroepiploic vein may join with a colic vein to form a common short gastrocolic trunk which joins the superior mesenteric vein (SMV) on its right side. This trunk should be ligated in pancreatic resections. Posterior superior pancreaticoduodenal vein joins portal vein on the upper margin of the pancreas **(Figs. 24-8A and B)**.

Posterior inferior pancreaticoduodenal vein joins SMV. Small branches enter the right side of the SMV and portal vein from head of the pancreas which should be ligated in Whipple's operation. Usually there are no branches in front of the SMV and portal vein underneath the neck of the pancreas, but as a variation, veins can be present. SMV joins splenic vein behind the neck of the pancreas to form portal vein. Inferior mesenteric vein usually joins splenic vein but may join portal vein or SMV directly. CBD is on the right side of the portal vein; common hepatic artery on the left side and IVC behind it. Right gastric vein joins portal vein above the joining of the left gastric vein (coronary vein); left gastric vein may join portal or splenic vein.

Lymphatic Drainage

The lymphatic ducts which drain the pancreas course towards the lymph nodes situated near the gland following the artery. The first tier of lymph nodes are situated on the surface of the pancreas and

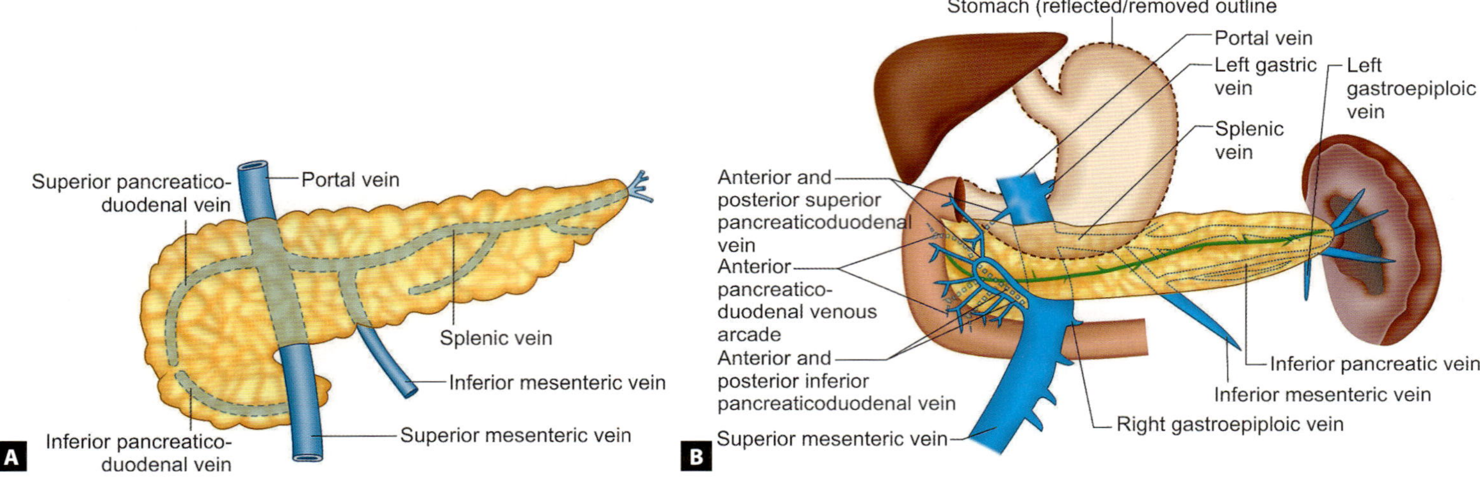

Figs. 24-8A and B: Venous drainage of pancreas.

the second tier of lymph nodes are situated along the gastroduodenal and hepatic vessels near the head and along the splenic artery in the region of the body and tail of the pancreas. Drainage is centrifugal. Cubilla et al. classified lymphatic drainage nodes into 5 groups—superior, anterior and posterior part of superior part of head, body, gastric → superior nodes drain into the suprapancreatic lymph nodes along the upper border of the pancreas; *inferior*—anterior and posterior parts of inferior part of head, body → inferior nodes drain into the inferior pancreatic group of lymph nodes which drain into the superior mesenteric nodes, left lateral aortic lymph nodes and may reach lumbar lymphatic trunk through a collecting duct; *anterior*—anterior pancreaticoduodenal, pyloric and mesenteric—drains anterior part of both superior and inferior portions of the head of pancreas—anterior nodes → 2 collecting ducts → infrapyloric and anterior pancreaticoduodenal nodes → nodes in the root of the mesentery; *posterior*—posterior pancreaticoduodenal, along common bile duct—drains from posterior surface of the superior and inferior parts of the head of the pancreas → reaches right lateral aortic nodes and nodes at origin of the superior mesenteric artery and lymphatics from bile duct and ampulla reaches to posterior pancreaticoduodenal lymph nodes; *splenic*—along its hilum and tail of the pancreas. Lymph flow is from pancreas to duodenum **(Fig. 24-9)**.

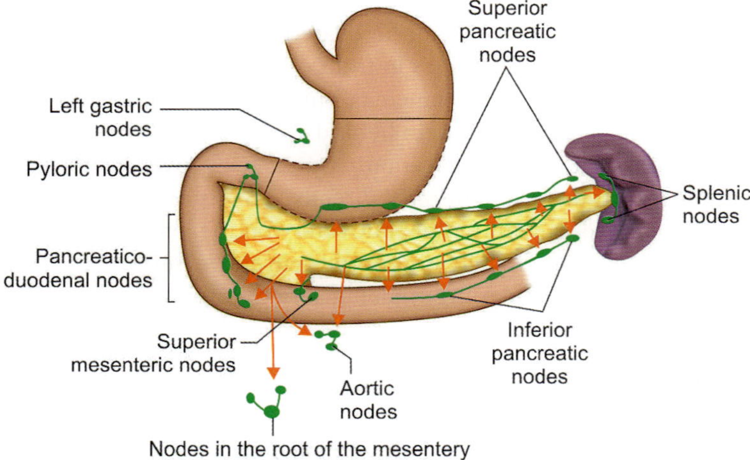

Fig. 24-9: Lymphatic drainage of pancreas.

There are no lymphatic communications between pancreatic nodes and gastric nodes. So, omentectomy is not necessary in pancreatic resections for malignancies. Lymphatics from head of the pancreas may reach hepatic nodes along the bile duct and common hepatic artery. Lymphatics of the head finally drain into nodes right of the coeliac and superior mesenteric arteries. Lymphatics from the body and tail drain to the nodes left of the coeliac and superior mesenteric arteries. Lymphatics from the head usually will not travel towards the body and tail. All drain finally towards the aortic nodes. Proper Whipple's pancreaticoduodenectomy should include removal of 35 nodes; total pancreatectomy should include 70 nodes. For adequate staging of pancreatic cancer, 15 nodes are needed.

Nerve Supply

Preganglionic sympathetic supply is derived from preganglionic efferent fibres of 5th to 9th thoracic segments to form greater splanchnic nerve. Fibres from 10th and 11th segments form lesser splanchnic nerve. Occasionally some fibres form the least splanchnic nerves. These nerves pass across the crura of diaphragm to supply coeliac and superior mesenteric ganglia. Postganglionic branches from these ganglia reach the pancreas through its arterial branches. Cell bodies of efferent fibres are interconnected with the cell bodies of the dorsal root ganglia of spinal nerve of the same level; hence pancreatic pain refers to the abdominal wall. Parasympathetic supply is by coeliac division of the posterior vagus. Efferent fibres from the brain reach coeliac ganglion and then reach ganglion cells in the pancreas; their postganglionic fibres supply islet of Langerhan cells. Surgical significance of coeliac ganglion is for managing the pancreatic pain by coeliac plexus block, splanchnicectomy, and guided coeliac injection, etc. Pain in chronic and relapsing pancreatitis is due to raised intraductal pressure (ductal hypertension), fibrosis of pancreas, multiple strictures, pancreatic ischaemia, multiple pseudocysts and pancreatic neuropathy. Pancreatic neuropathy is due to neural and perineural inflammation of intrapancreatic nerves with infiltration of immune cells. In carcinoma pancreas, through initially tumour is painless then typical pain develops once perineural invasion by tumour cells occurs.

GENERAL PRINCIPLES IN PANCREATIC SURGERIES

Pancreas is an organ located deep in the retroperitoneum extending from right to left side. Its clear anatomy, vasculature and relations are to be known while doing pancreatic surgery. Variations and major vessels should be tackled carefully. 60% of the gland is in the body and tail of the pancreas. Only 40% of the gland will be removed in Whipple's operation.

Preservation of duodenum in surgeries of pancreatic head is difficult due to strong attachment of pancreas and vascular arcade. Preoperative imaging is essential. Helical CT scan with contrast to arterial and portal venous phase is needed. ERCP, endoultrasound (EUS), MRI may be needed in selected patients. Liver function tests, prothrombin time, coagulation profile, adequate hydration is needed preoperatively. Laparoscopic assessment prior to opening the abdomen is better to assess the final operability **(Figs. 24-10A to C)**.

Pancreas is reached by dividing gastrocolic ligament (greater omentum). It can be reached through hepatogastric ligament (lesser omentum) also. Vagus is usually preserved.

Hepatic flexure is better to be mobilised to reach and expose the head of pancreas adequately—**Cattell-Braasch** manoeuvre; ***Kocherisation of the duodenum*** is a must in all pancreatic surgeries in relation to head. In Whipple's operation and total pancreatectomy, extended Kocherisation is needed wherein 2nd part of the duodenum is mobilised beyond the left margin of the aorta. Peritoneum lateral to the 2nd part of the duodenum is incised above and below; posteriorly IVC with its fascial covering is seen; plane is loose areolar and is relatively avascular; left index and middle fingers are placed behind the duodenum through the incision; left thumb is placed in front; it allows proper palpation of head of the pancreas to assess the size and possible operability. But this will not clearly indicate the portal vein invasion.

Left hand index finger is passed from above underneath the neck gently downwards in front of the portal vein; right hand index finger is passed similarly in front of SMV from below upwards to reach the opposite finger. Care should be taken to keep the fingers strictly in front which is usually avascular (laterally draining veins enter SMV and portal vein and so finger should not pass laterally). Even though it is crude it reasonably confirms the operability. But always it is better to do preoperative dynamic imaging with arterial phase to confirm the operability. Gastrocolic omentum and splenic flexure should be mobilised downwards adequately to expose the body and tail of the pancreas.

It is the invasion or encasement of the SMA or coeliac trunk precludes the resection in malignancy. Portal vein/SMV invasion is not considered as unresectable. It is still resectable with resection of segment of vein with later placement of patch graft over it. These invasions can be assessed properly by endoultrasound, MRI, arteriogram or venous and arterial phase in CT.

Once operability is confirmed in Whipple's operation, only then superior and inferior pancreaticoduodenal arteries should be ligated; as their ligation causes necrosis of duodenum and pancreatic head.

In pancreaticoduodenectomy, bile duct is usually resected above the level of cystic duct, and cystic duct and hepatic duct margins should be sent for frozen section biopsy **(Fig. 24-11)**.

Presently pylorus preserving pancreaticoduodenectomy is favoured. Duodenum is transected just distal to the pylorus. But cut margin should be sent for frozen section biopsy prior to proceeding with the further steps of pylorus preserving pancreaticoduodenectomy **(Figs. 24-12 and 24-13)**.

In distal pancreatectomy, ligation of splenic artery and vein leads into splenectomy. If short gastric vessels are preserved, spleen can be salvaged even though splenic vessels are ligated; it is called as ***Warshaw procedure***; but late development of splenic congestion and gastric varices can occur.

Portal vein anomaly and right hepatic artery anomalies should be remembered while doing pancreatic resection.

Secure anastomosis, patience and postoperative care are needed in all patients. Sepsis, bile and pancreatic leak, pancreatic pseudoaneurysm, renal failure, liver failure, disseminated intravascular coagulation, postoperative haemorrhages are the possible different complications which can occur in pancreatic surgeries. Daily monitoring—clinically, biochemically, often imaging are needed during postoperative care **(Fig. 24-14)**.

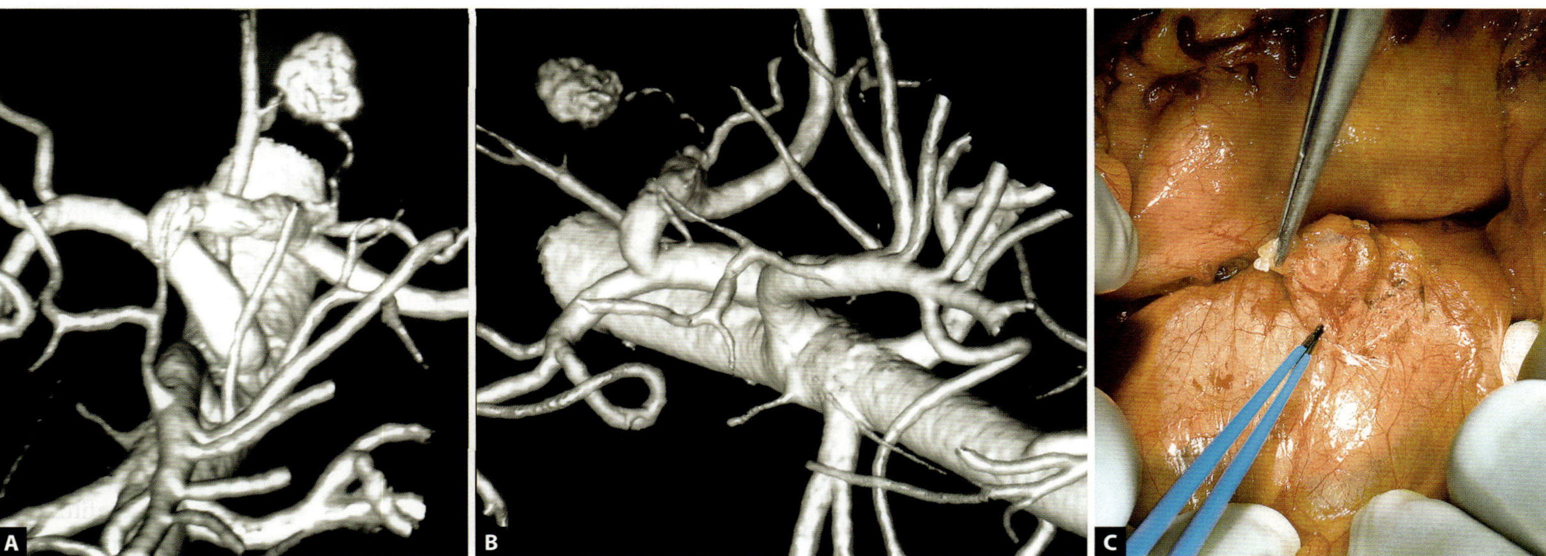

Figs. 24-10A to C: Insulinoma in the body of pancreas. Enucleation can be done; but if multiple in the body and tail of the pancreas, distal pancreatectomy is needed.

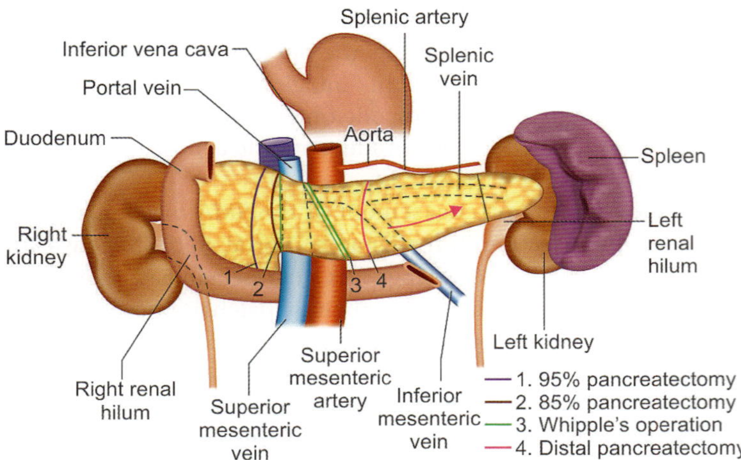

Fig. 24-11: Partial pancreatectomies—types—95% subtotal; 85% subtotal; Whipple's; distal.

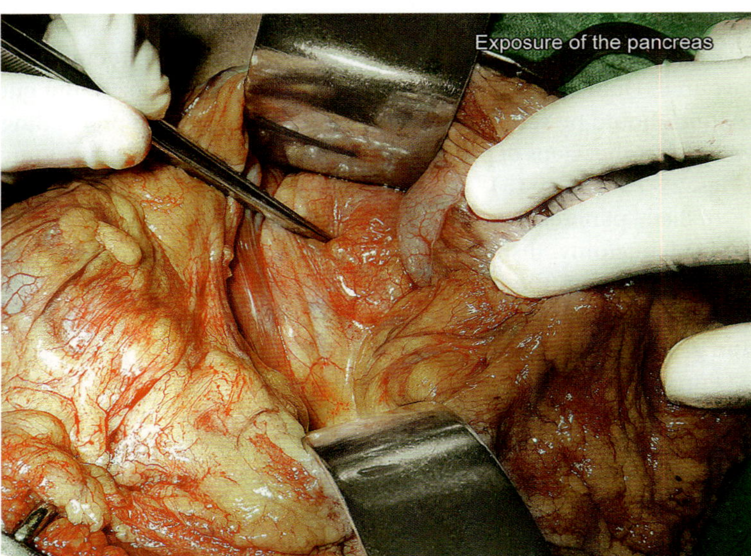

Fig. 24-12: Exposure of the pancreas. It needs mobilisation of the right flexure of colon and transverse colon, often leaves flexure also.

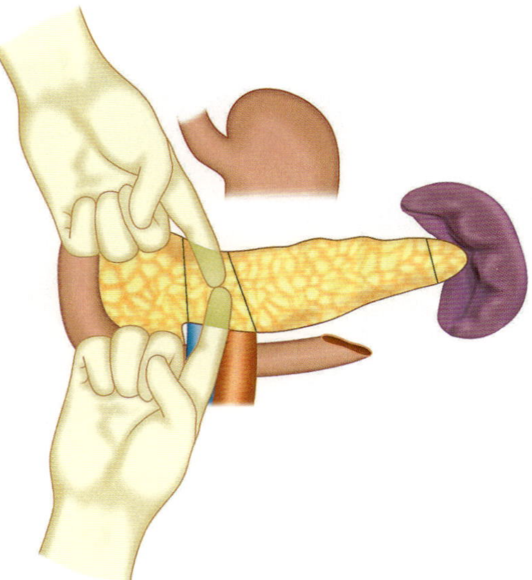

Fig. 24-13: In pancreaticoduodenectomy, whether portal vein and SMV are free of tumour (not adherent to portal vein) is assessed by placing left index finger between neck of pancreas and portal vein; right index finger between neck and SMV; both fingertips if felt easily and freely to be in contact with each other, then portal invasion/adhesion is not present.

SURGICAL TREATMENT FOR CHRONIC PANCREATITIS

Indications for Surgery

Persisting pain is the main indication; severe malabsorption; suspicion of malignant transformation; multiple relapses; complications like pseudocyst, segmental portal hypertension; biliary obstruction (*Wadsworth syndrome*); pseudocyst; pancreatic ductal dilatation >5 mm; pancreatic ascites/fistula; pancreatic ductal stenosis.

Objectives of Surgery

Pain relief when endotherapy has failed; management of complications; procedure is selected which shows less morbidity and mortality; Quality of life (QOL) should be preserved.

Problems and Limitations of Surgery

Disease is irreversible parenchymal and ductal damage and so surgery *cannot cure* or reverse completely. Disease progression cannot be prevented or arrested by surgery. Risk of development of cancer continues. Complications of surgery are a drawback.

Benefits of Surgery in Relation to Pain Relief and Obstruction

It relieves intraductal, interstitial, intracellular hypertension through drainage procedures. Entrapped nerves are released and reduction in pancreatic enzyme reduces nerve irritation—resectional methods. *Pacemaker*—head of pancreas is removed in head-coring procedure (Frey's) to relieve pain. It is less morbid and acceptable method. Resection is better than the drainage procedure but technically demanding and has got higher mortality.

Principles of Surgery

Pancreatic duct decompression (drainage) reduces the pain and retains the existing exocrine and endocrine functions. But chances of malignant transformation are still high. In significant number of patients, recurrence of symptoms (50% recurrence of pain in 5 years) and progression of the disease pathology occur and it does not give a complete cure. Normal diameter of pancreatic duct is 4 mm in head; 3 mm in body; 2 mm in tail of the pancreas. *Pancreatic duct diameter more than 5-7 mm is an indication for surgery (pancreaticojejunostomy). Pancreatic resection* (total pancreatectomy) is the actually ideal technique which relieves pain, removes entire diseased tissue. But technical difficulty; high surgical mortality (21%); and severe exocrine and endocrine deficiency (brittle diabetes) are the drawbacks. Head of pancreas is considered as pacemaker and origin of the pancreatitis disease and so pancreaticoduodenectomy (*Whipple's*) is the other option to give adequate relief. It is preferred in patients who are having relatively normal body and tail of the pancreas. Occasionally when the disease is limited to tail and body, then *distal pancreatectomy* with or without splenectomy often with distal pancreaticojejunostomy may be done. But it is not beneficial if disease is extensive and diffuse. Resection is the main method of treatment if ductal dilatation is not adequate. *Combined resection and drainage procedures* are also done. Head is decored at various levels and decompressed duct is anastomosed to jejunum.

Patient should completely stop alcohol and smoking after surgery. Nutrition should be reasonably adequate; serum albumin should be more than 3 g%. Otherwise surgery is done after improvement of nutrition. Proper preoperative evaluation is a must.

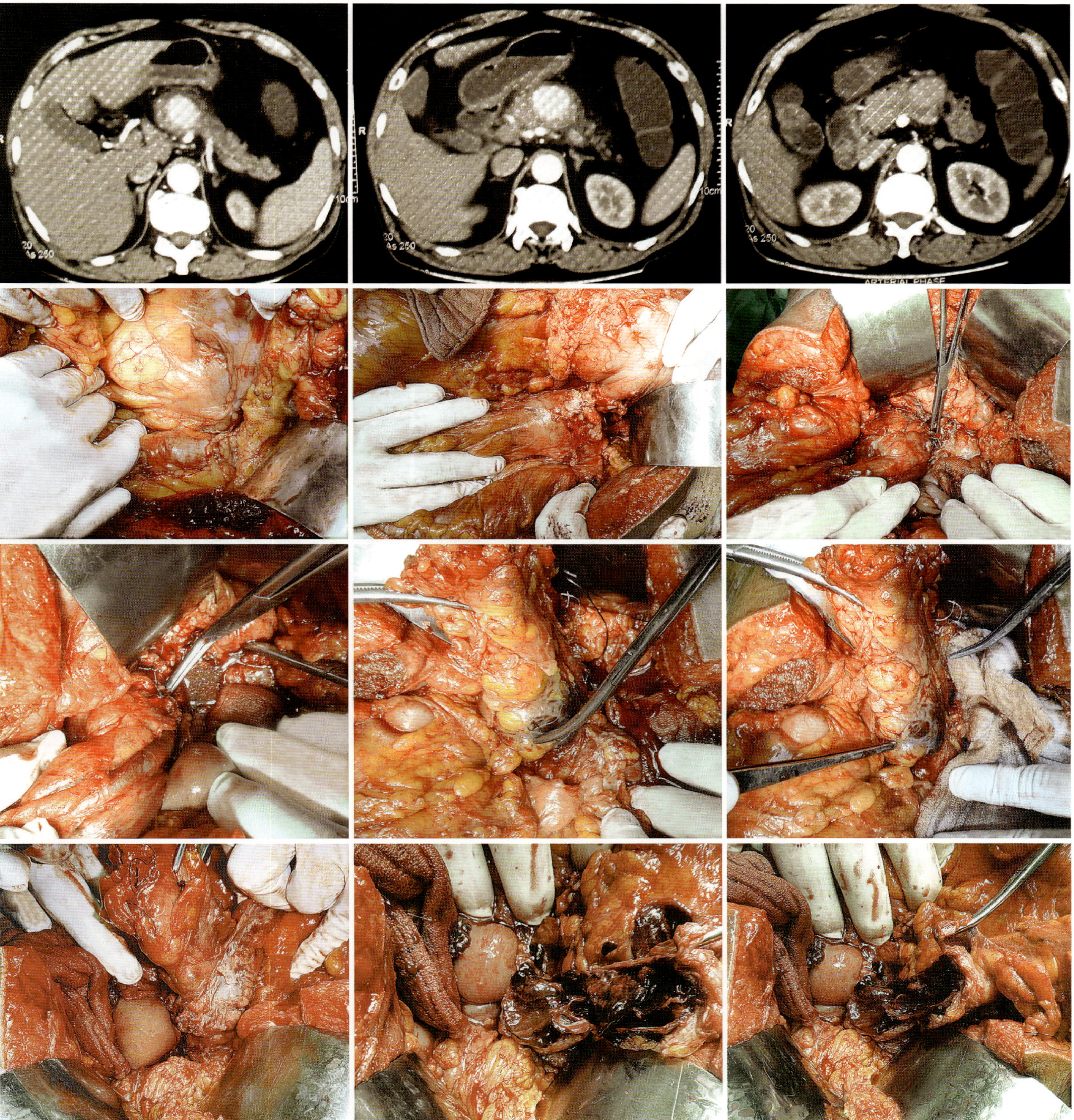

Figs. 24-14(1)

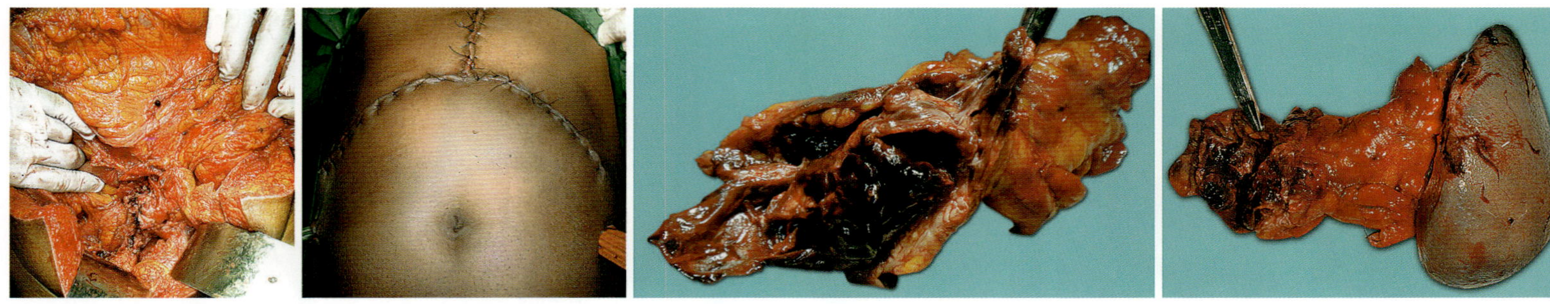

Figs. 24-14(2)

Figs. 24-14(1 and 2): Pancreatic pseudoaneurysm—patient underwent removal of pseudoaneurysm and distal pancreatectomy. Intervention radiology is ideal; but when it fails surgery is the option.

Proper preoperative evaluation, assessment of variations in portal vein and arterial pattern, frozen section biopsy are important in all pancreatic surgeries.

Exposure of pancreas needs mobilisation of the right flexure of colon (Cattell-Braasch) transverse colon and often left flexure also; extended Kocherisation (duodenal mobilisation), separation of stomach from anterior part of the pancreas, separation of spleen and tail of the pancreas from left adrenal gland, left kidney and left renal vessels.

Meticulous dissection, control of bleeding by using bipolar cautery or other energy sources minimises the bleeding and improve and hastens the dissection.

Anastomosis in pancreatic surgery should be careful, skilled and meticulous as leak from pancreas will be disastrous **(Figs. 24-15 to 24-17)**.

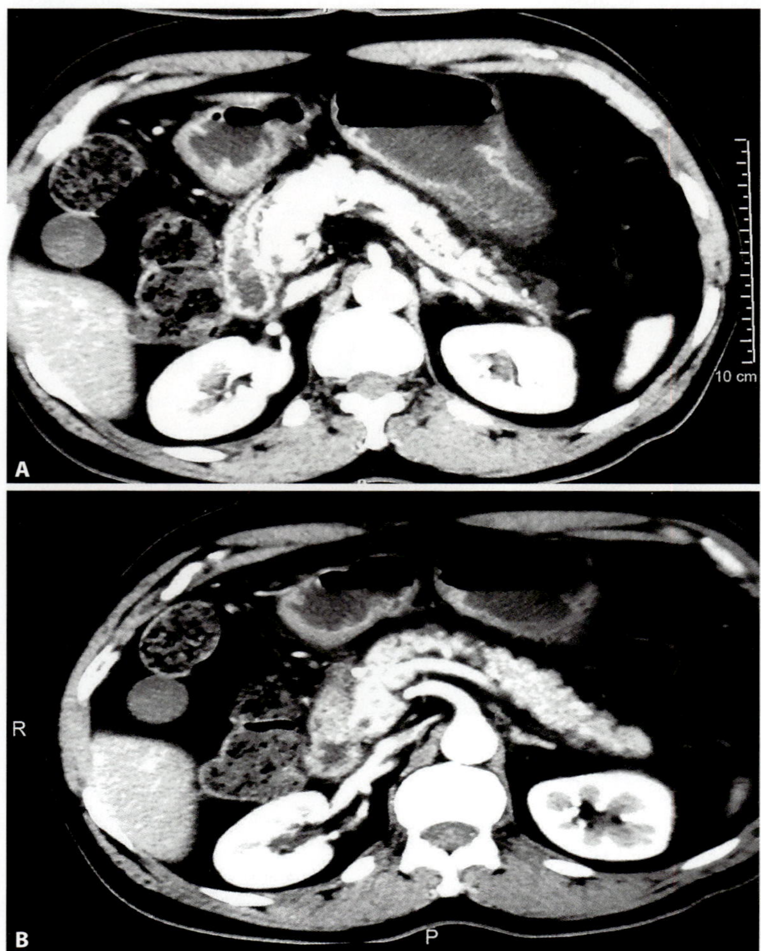

Figs. 24-15A and B: CT scan of chronic pancreatitis.

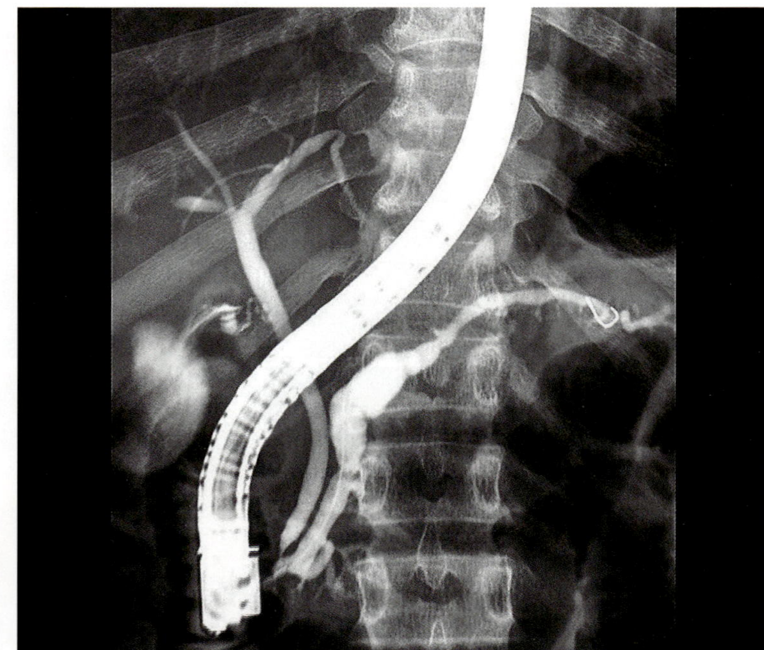

Fig. 24-16: ERCP showing pancreatic duct pathology with strictures.

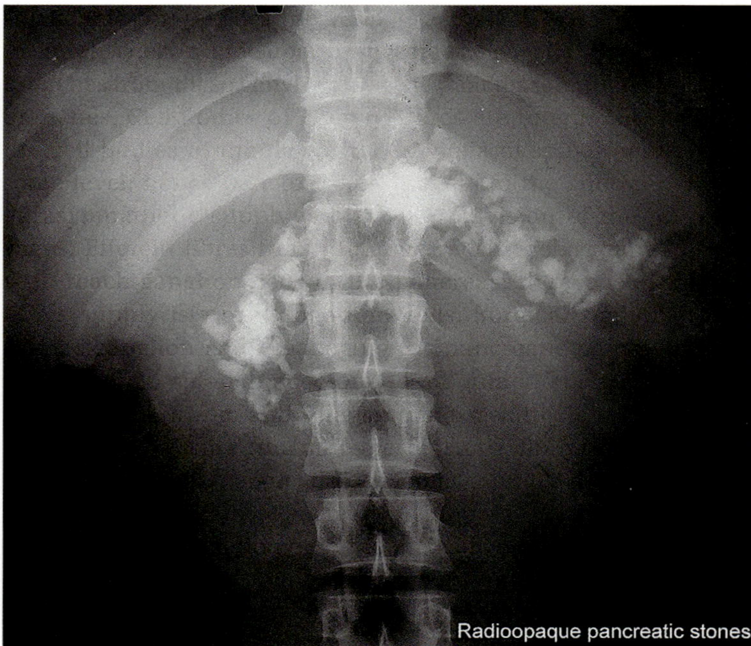

Fig. 24-17: X-ray showing multiple pancreatic stones.

Surgeries

1. *Puestow's operation* [*Puestow-Gilesby* (1958)]: As the duct is dilated more than 7–8 mm, duct can easily be opened longitudinally. After removing all stones from the duct, it is anastomosed to the jejunum as *Roux-en-Y anastomosis*. In Puestow's operation, spleen is removed **(Fig. 24-18)**.
2. *Partington-Rochelle operation/Modified Puestow's operation (1960):* Here longitudinal pancreaticojejunostomy is done using almost entire laid open pancreatic duct. Spleen is retained in this procedure. This is now a commonly done procedure **(Fig. 24-19)**.

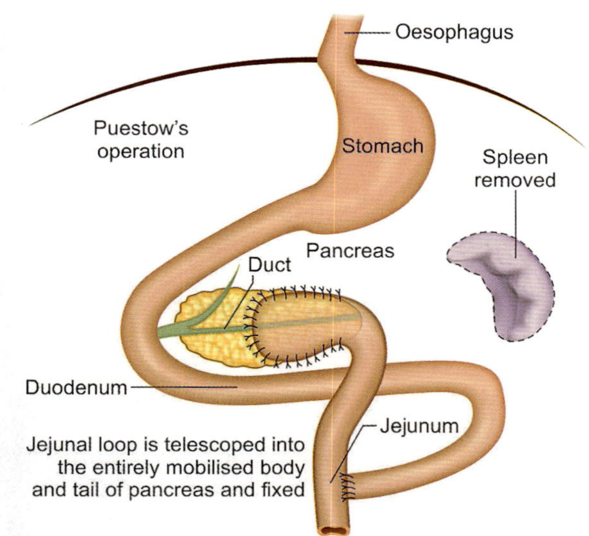

Fig. 24-18: Puestow's pancreaticojejunostomy. Here spleen is removed. Entire length of dilated duct is opened. Distal pancreas is mobilised up to the superior mesenteric vessels. Pancreas with opened duct is telescoped into the Roux loop of jejunum and anastomosed.

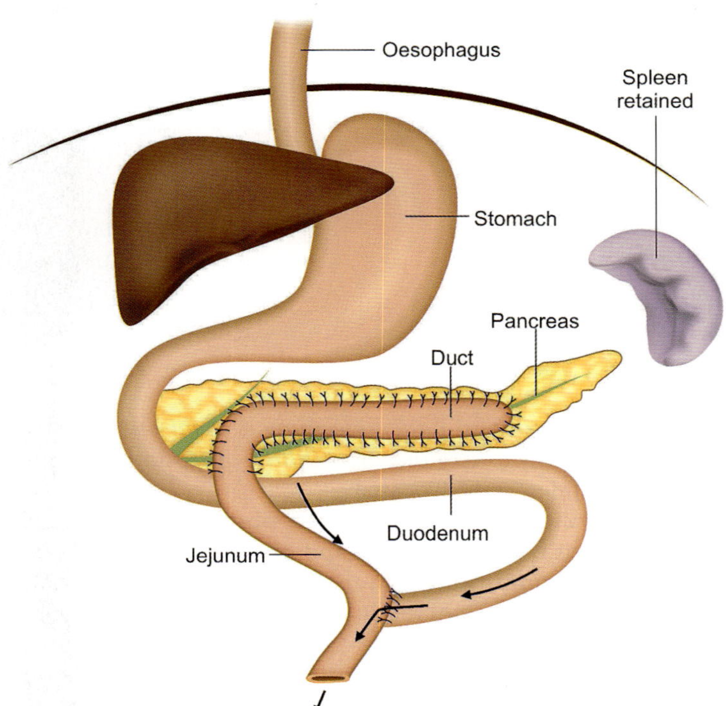

Fig. 24-19: Partington-Rochelle operation. Here spleen is retained and longitudinal pancreaticojejunostomy is done to the opened duct from the front.

3. Duodenal preserving with resection of head of pancreas in front of portal vein with jejunal loop anastomosis to the transected neck of pancreas—*Beger procedure (Hans Beger from Ulm, Germany, 1980)*. Here extensive resection of head (than Frey's) is done. It addresses the inflammatory mass present in the head of pancreas by resecting it but preserving the blood supply of duodenum and bile duct. Here two anastomoses are present; one proximal over the extensive decored area; another on to the distal pancreas to its ductal system. Sleeve of pancreas is left behind with duodenum to preserve the blood supply. It is less radical resection; but it needs transection of the neck of pancreas and double separate anastomoses; one at the decored transected part of the head; another at distal cut end of the body with laid open duct. Pancreaticojejunostomy is done at two sites of the Roux limb. It is also known as *duodenal preserving pancreatic head resection (DPPHR)*. Pain relief is 94%; insulin secretory capacity and glucose tolerance improve in this **(Figs. 24-20 and 24-21)**.
4. *Berne modification of Beger procedure:* This modification spares the dissection of the pancreatic body from the portal vein. After the resection of pancreatic head, a single cavity results which can be anastomosed end to side with a Roux-en-Y jejunal loop. If stenosis of the intrapancreatic part of the common bile duct cannot be resolved by decompression and resection of the surrounding pancreatic tissue, or if the intrapancreatic portion of the common bile duct is opened accidentally during pancreatic head resection, the wall of the opened bile duct is fixed with single stitches to the surrounding tissues and is included in the same anastomosis. Complete transection of the neck is not done here.
5. *Longitudinal pancreaticojejunostomy* after excision of peripancreatic duct tissue: Here superficial part of the head of pancreas is removed to achieve improved drainage—*Frey procedure (Frey and Smith, 1987)*. It is done when ductal dilatation is not adequate; head is more than 4 cm thick. Head coring is done with retaining 5 mm thick tissue in front of veins, close to duodenum. It shows 75% pain relief in 3 years. Here procedure is similar but decoring is done up to duct of Wirsung and Santorini and single longitudinal pancreaticojejunostomy is done **(Fig. 24-22)**.

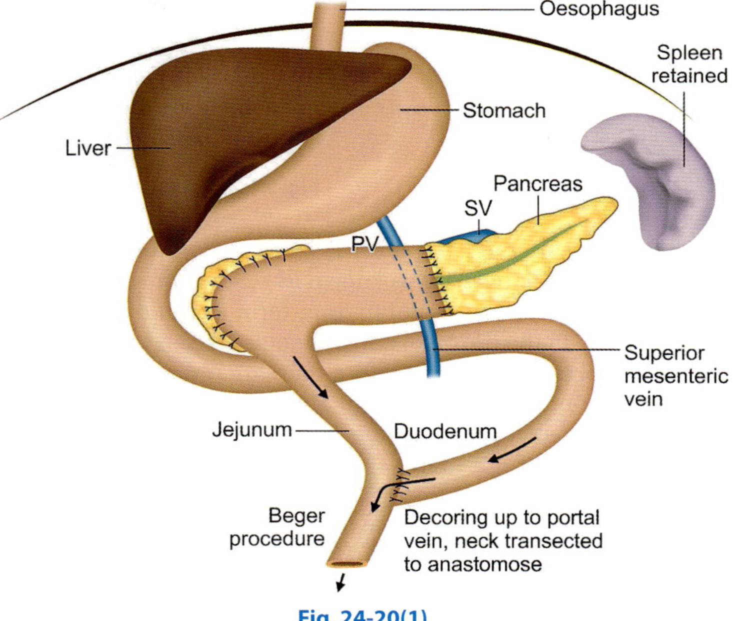

Fig. 24-20(1)

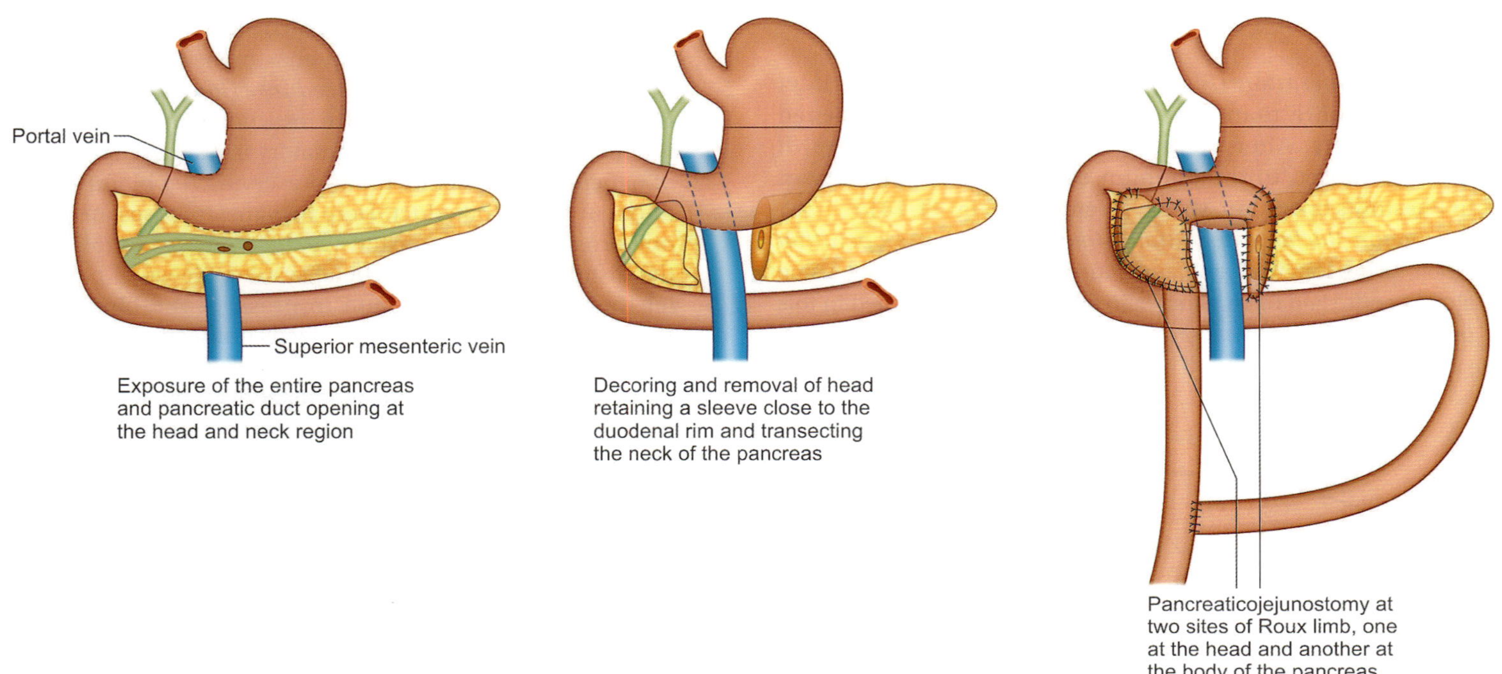

Figs. 24-20(2)

Figs. 24-20(1 and 2): Beger procedure. Here head is decorated up to the visible portal vein. Neck is transected. Distal end of the pancreas with retained part is anastomosed to Roux loop of jejunum.

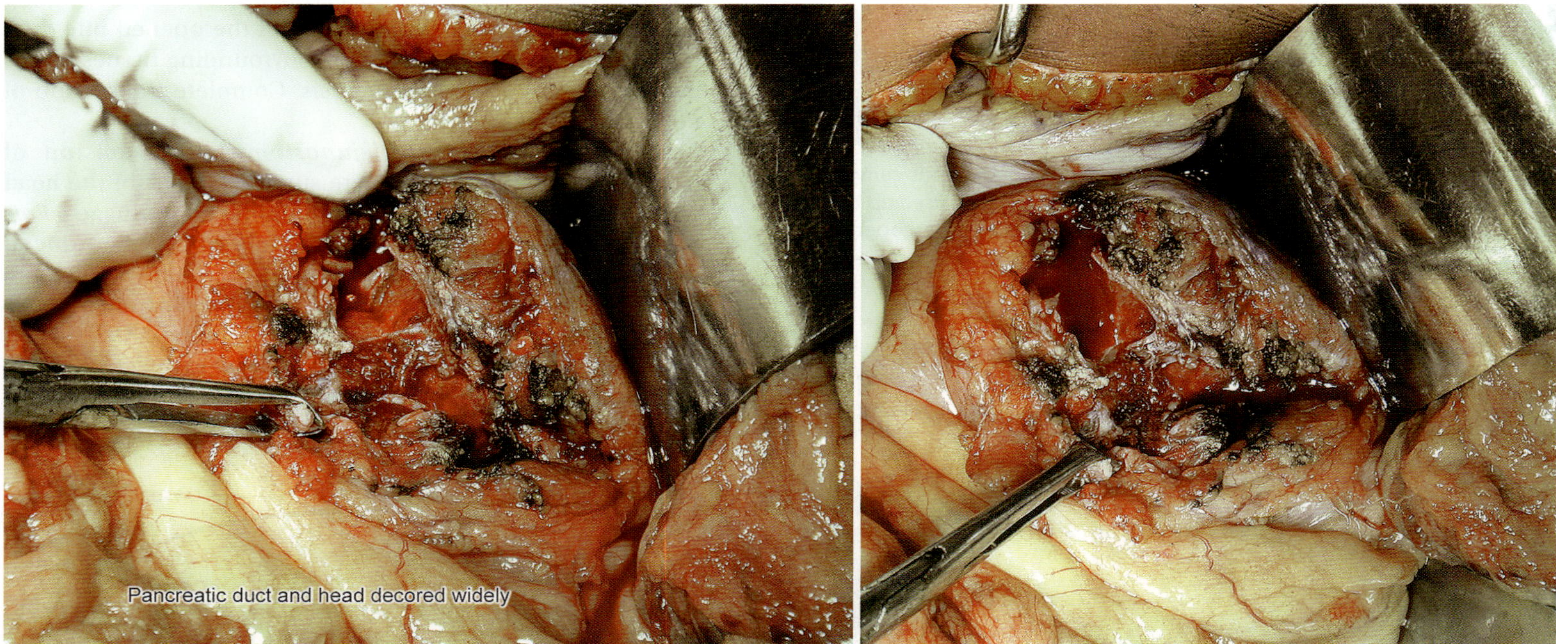

Fig. 24-21: Decoring of the pancreatic duct and head in Beger technique.

6. Resection of tail of pancreas with retrograde Roux-en-Y pancreaticojejunostomy is known as—*Duval procedure (1954).* It was not very successful in long-term as multiple strictures especially in the proximal part are not laid open and addressed. Decompression of the main pancreatic duct is achieved by resection of the pancreatic tail and retrograde drainage of the pancreatic duct via a termino-lateral pancreaticojejunostomy. It may be useful if there is single stricture, which is unlikely **(Figs. 24-23 to 24-26)**.
7. If disease mainly involves head of the pancreas, then pancreaticoduodenectomy can be done—*Whipple's procedure.*
8. *Subtotal pancreatic resection:* Here spleen, body and tail of the pancreas are removed entirely, retaining the head of pancreas.
9. About 95% *subtotal pancreatectomy is ideal but technically not feasible and demanding—Child's operation.* It is never recommended and advocated.
10. *Total pancreatectomy* is indicated when the entire gland is diseased. It relieves the pain and also prevents the diseased pancreas from turning into malignancy. Patient has to take insulin and oral pancreatic enzymes permanently (*brittle diabetes*).
11. The cause is treated like cholecystectomy for gallstones. Therapeutic ERCP is useful in removal of stones in dilated duct.
12. When duodenal, biliary and pancreatic obstruction is present—choledochojejunal, pancreaticojejunal and gastrojejunal anastomosis may be needed—*triple anastomosis.*

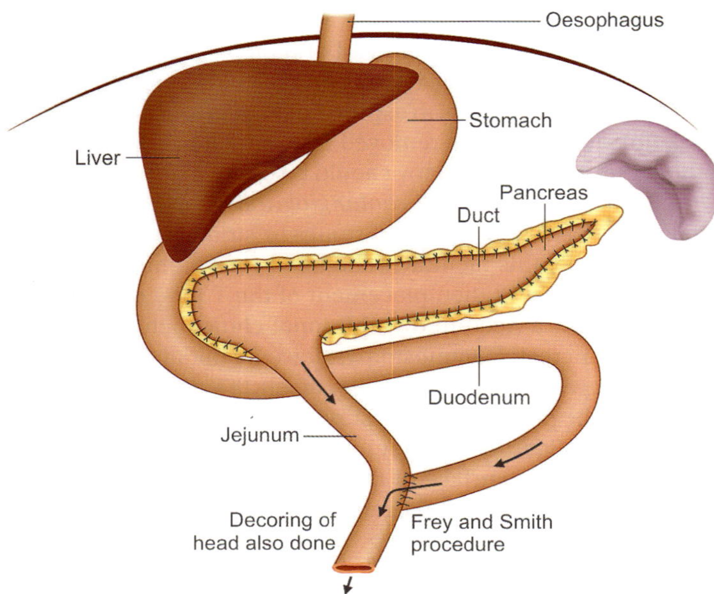

Fig. 24-22: Frey's procedure. Here head of pancreas is decorated and opened duct with decored head is anastomosed to Roux loop of jejunum.

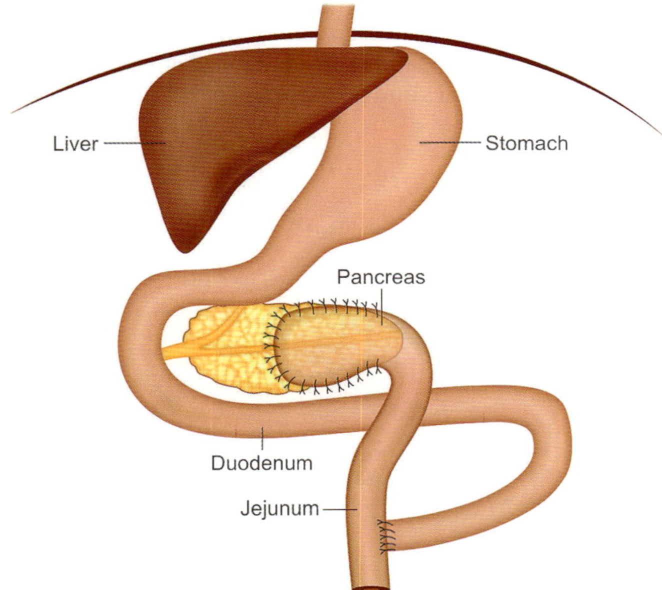

Fig. 24-23: Retrograde pancreaticojejunostomy after resection of the tail of the pancreas (Duval).

13. Only biliary stricture which cannot be managed by ERCP needs choledochojejunostomy.

Technique of Longitudinal Pancreaticojejunostomy—(Partington-Rochelle Operation—LPJ)

Longitudinal pancreaticojejunostomy is commonly done as drainage procedure as it is technically easier with reasonable good results with minimum morbidity and mortality. Preoperative CT scan to assess the ductal pattern diameter and splenic vein status is important. Duct dilatation more than 5–7 mm is better for pancreaticojejunostomy to drain the pancreas; it is also now done in non-dilated or less dilated duct system as it acts like a permanent fasciotomy on the pancreas which allows significant decompression. Splenic vein thrombosis when present, patient will have varices which are tortuous and dilated and so may cause troublesome bleeding during surgery. ERCP is essential to assess ductal anatomy, strictures ('chain of lakes' appearance), and stones. Pancreatic malignancy and chronic pancreatitis are difficult to differentiate grossly and on table biopsy is a must. Chronic pancreatitis itself predisposes malignancy **(Fig. 24-27)**.

Under general anaesthesia, patient is in supine position, lengthy midline incision is placed. In obese patients, bilateral subcostal or upper transverse incision may be needed. After thorough exploration,

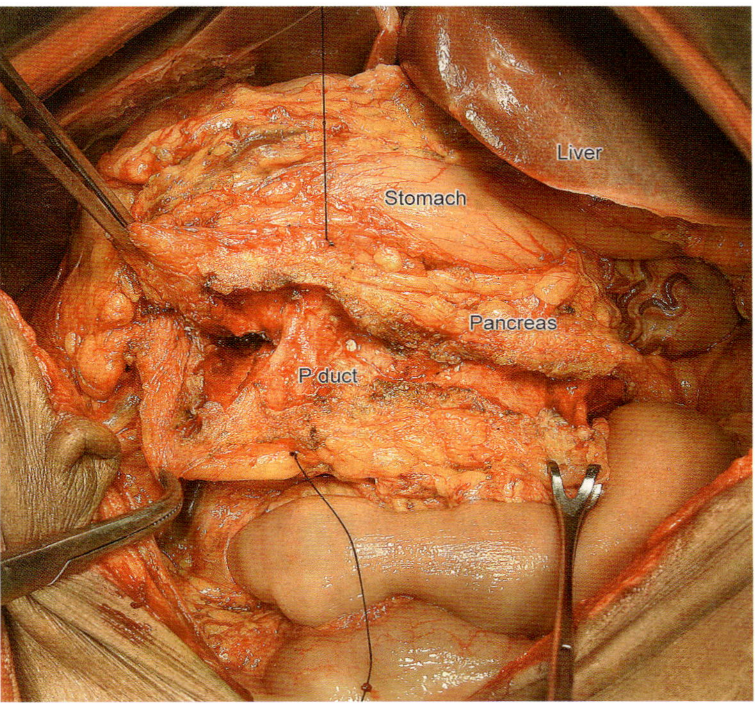

Fig. 24-24: Dilated pancreatic duct is laid open; multiple stones are removed and duct is ready for longitudinal pancreaticojejunostomy (LPJ).
Courtesy: Dr Arunkumar, MCh, Gastro, Kochi.

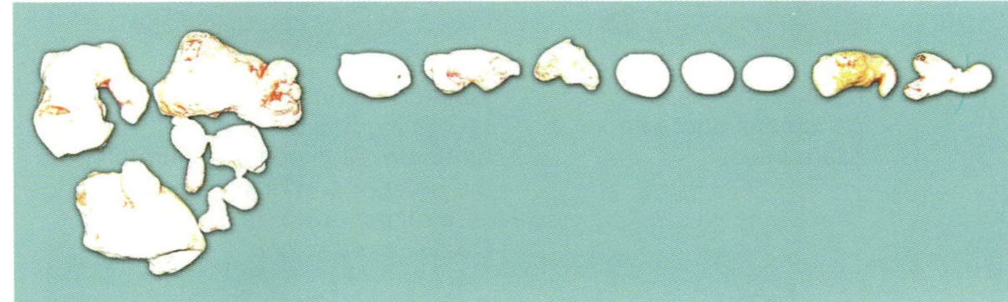

Fig. 24-25: Pancreatic duct stones—removed during pancreaticojejunostomy.

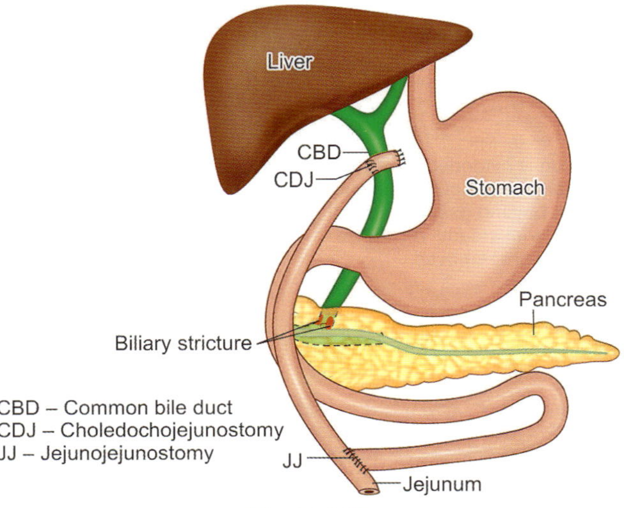

Fig. 24-26A

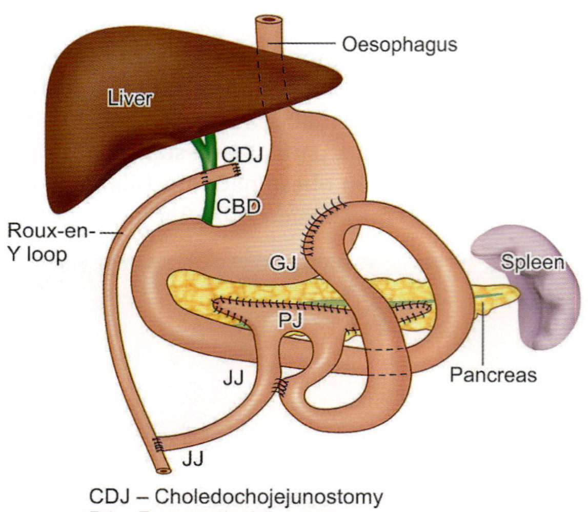

Fig. 24-26B

Figs. 24-26A and B: *Choledochojejunostomy*. It is Roux-en-Y anastomosis. It is done whenever there is complication of biliary stricture after pancreatitis. Often triple anastomosis may be required—pancreaticojejunostomy, choledochojejunostomy and gastrojejunostomy. It is done whenever there is duodenal obstruction, biliary block and pancreatic duct dilatation (drainage procedure).

self-retaining retractor is placed. Usually Kocherisation is not essential but it is done to feel head of pancreas and if decoring is planned. It is better to release transverse colon on right side and hepatic flexure downwards to expose field adequately.

If gallbladder is not yet removed earlier by laparoscopy or open method, then cholecystectomy should be done.

It is better to do on table cholangiogram by injecting dye and confirm the possible presence of stones or strictures using a C arm image guidance; this facilitates the need for opening of the CBD to remove stones and then placement of the T tube or if there is a stricture there is a need to do additional choledochojejunostomy along with pancreaticojejunostomy. However initial CT or MRCP or ERCP might give a clear idea preoperatively the status of the CBD as such to plan the possible need of surgical intervention of the CBD.

Gastrocolic ligament is opened and transversely divided to expose the anterior surface of the pancreas. Omentum is held in between clamps, divided and ligated; alternatively harmonic scalpel or ligaseal can be used here to hasten the technique. Stomach is retracted upwards using a wide Deaver retractor. All adhesions between the posterior surface of the stomach and pancreas should be released over the head, uncinate process, body and tail of the pancreas **(Fig. 24-28)**.

Transverse colon and small bowel are retracted downwards. Peritoneal attachment on the front of the pancreas may be incised but not necessary. Entire gland from head to tail is carefully palpated for location of duct, stones and possible site of malignancy.

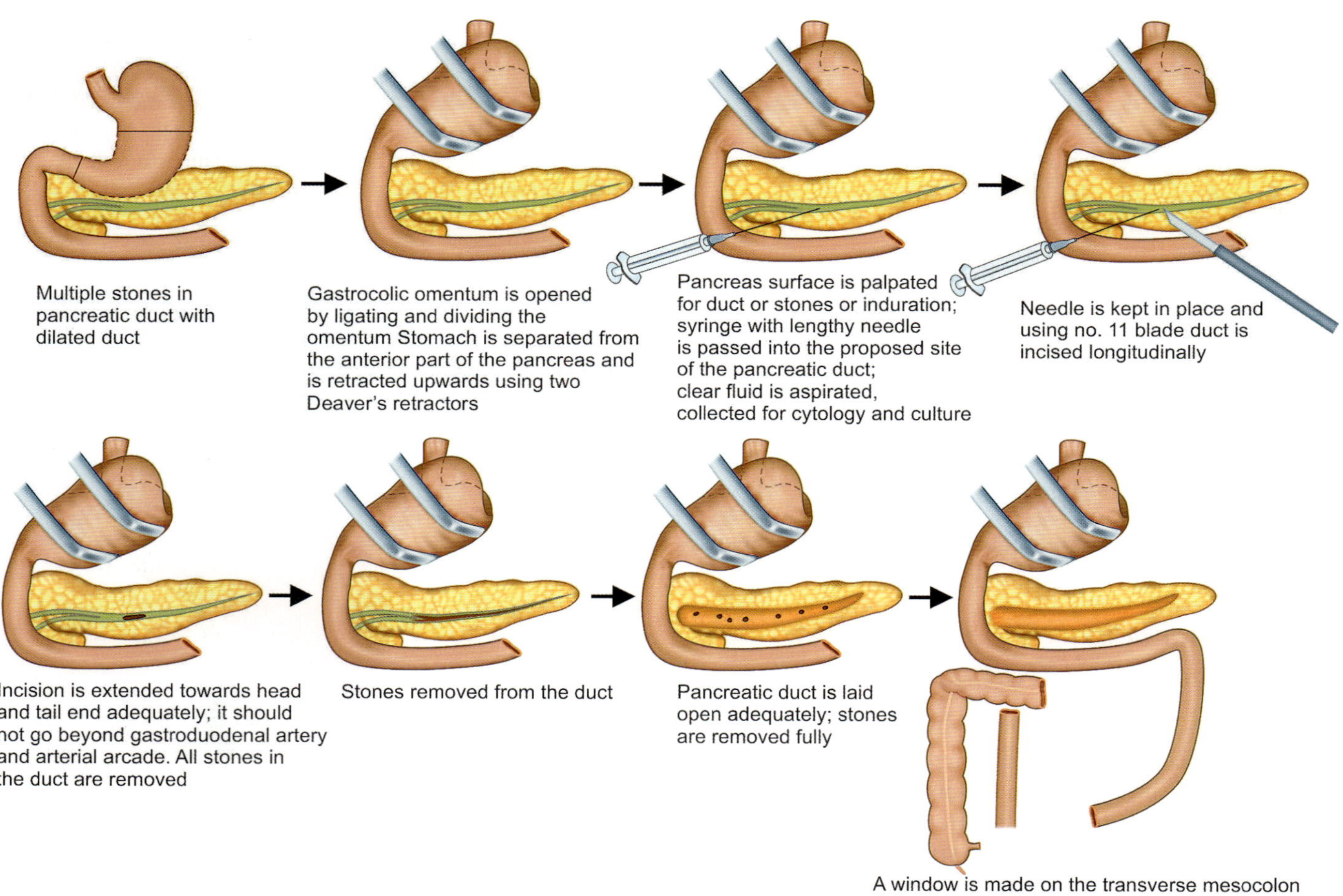

Figs. 24-27(1)

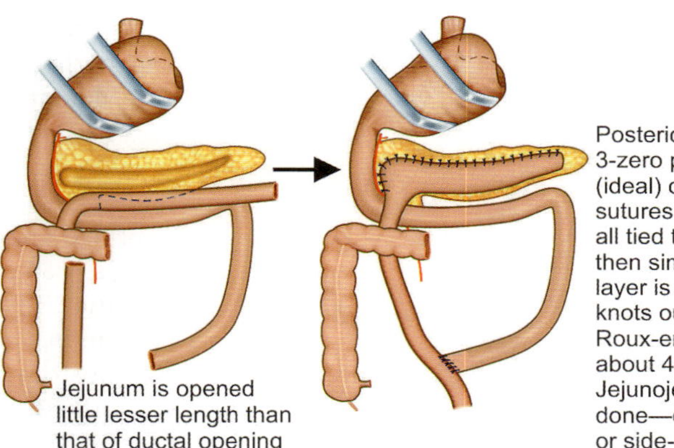

Figs. 24-27(2)

Figs. 24-27(1 and 2): Technique of longitudinal pancreaticojejunostomy.

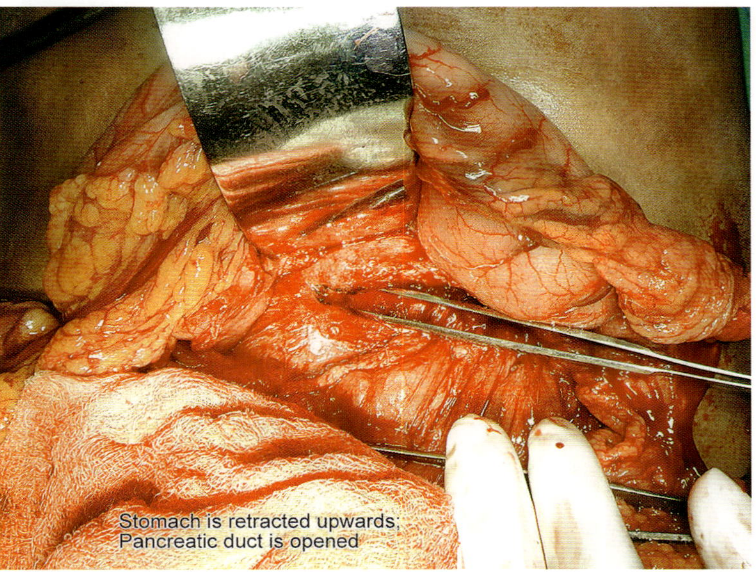

Fig. 24-28: Stomach is retracted upwards.

A 21-gauge needle with syringe is taken; suspected site of the duct usually in lower part of the gland is pricked; by trial and error method usually dilated part of duct can be reached; clear pancreatic fluid is aspirated; fluid is collected for culture, analysis and cytology. With the needle in place no. 11 blade is passed adjacent to the needle to enter into the duct. It can also be done using a cautery **(Fig. 24-29)**.

After the needle aspiration of the pancreatic duct, if dye is injected then it is possible to delineate the ductal anatomy precisely on table which will make opening the pancreatic duct easier; duct is usually located near superior part of the pancreas and not very inferiorly as often surgeons think; dense fibrosis due to chronic inflammation makes it difficult to identify the duct even if it dilated significantly due to thickened pancreatic tissue in front. It is also important to maintain the absolute haemostasis during opening of the duct either by bipolar cautery or using fine vicryl ligatures. While opening the duct over the head of the pancreas one should be careful for torrential bleeding. Usually 8–10 cm length of the pancreatic duct is opened.

Once duct is visualised, a Bake's dilator or any probe or infant feeding tube is passed to locate the duct direction and stones. If identification of the duct system has failed by repeated needle punctures which is not uncommon, then on table ultrasound is very useful to identify the duct. If it is not available, then carefully millimetre by millimetre pancreatic tissue is cut near the neck of the pancreas towards body side until duct is reached. In olden days tail used to be transected often with splenectomy to identify the duct and proceeded with standard old Puestow Gilesby technique—but

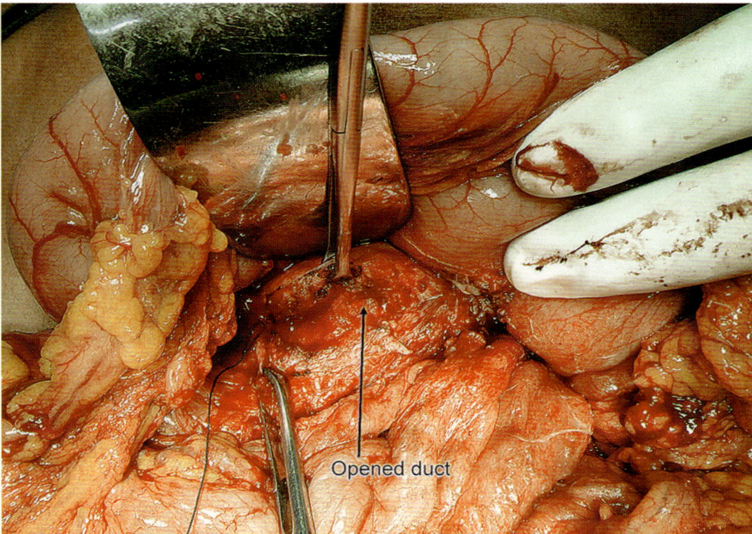

Fig. 24-29: Pancreatic duct is opened for adequate length from head to tail, minimum of 8 cm.

nowadays it is not necessary to change to Puestow. Any bleeders in the cut edge of the duct are controlled using bipolar cautery. Duct is incised towards head up to the gastroduodenal artery not beyond; distally it is opened up to the end of the duct as much as possible. All stricture parts should be laid open; all stones should be removed. Minimum 8 cm duct length should be opened. Venous plane is deeper to ductal system. Deep incision across the posterior wall of the duct may injure the splenic vein. In the head, there are chances of injuring anterior pancreaticoduodenal vessels; one should be careful to preserve them. After passing the needle, intraductal pressure can be measured; or another fine needle can be inserted into the parenchyma to measure interstitial pressure of the pancreas. Entire duct of Wirsung, duct of Santorini and duct of uncinate process should be laid open; but should limit within the anterior pancreaticoduodenal arcade **(Fig. 24-30)**.

If Frey's procedure is undertaken, entire pancreatic tissue in front of these ducts should be excised and laid open. It is done by placing series of consecutive stay sutures using silk or vicryl and cutting the pancreatic tissue using tough curved scissor (Pott's scissor or another one). Bleeders are addressed with suture ligation using 3-zero silk or vicryl. Monopolar cautery should not be used. Bipolar cautery is safer.

Roux limb is prepared 20 cm from the ligament of Treitz. Jejunal vessels are ligated. Small bowel is transected between two occlusion clamps; proximal end is left like that to do later end-to-side jejunojejunostomy later. Alternatively stapler transection of the jejunum can be done. A window is created in the transverse mesocolon to the right of the middle colic artery. Distal Roux limb is brought through it to reach supracolic compartment. Loop is brought towards the tail end of the pancreas so that anastomosis becomes isoperistaltic in relation to the ductal drainage. If loop end is brought towards the head part of the pancreas it will become antiperistaltic, still can drain the duct adequately. Usually 45–50 cm Roux loop is sufficient **(Fig. 24-31)**.

Entire pancreatomy on the duct is anastomosed to the jejunum. Jejunotomy/enterotomy is done on the antimesenteric border of the jejunum just 1 cm proximal from the distal end of the Roux loop. Enterotomy should be 5 mm lesser than the ductal opening. Side-to-side pancreaticojejunostomy is done. Posterior layer is sutured first. Interrupted 3-zero polypropylene (ideal) or 3-zero silk sutures are used. All suture bites should be taken first. While taking bites from pancreatic side full thickness bite including fibrous peripancreatic tissue should be taken. Few advocate that mucosal bite should be avoided. But usually it does not cause any problem.

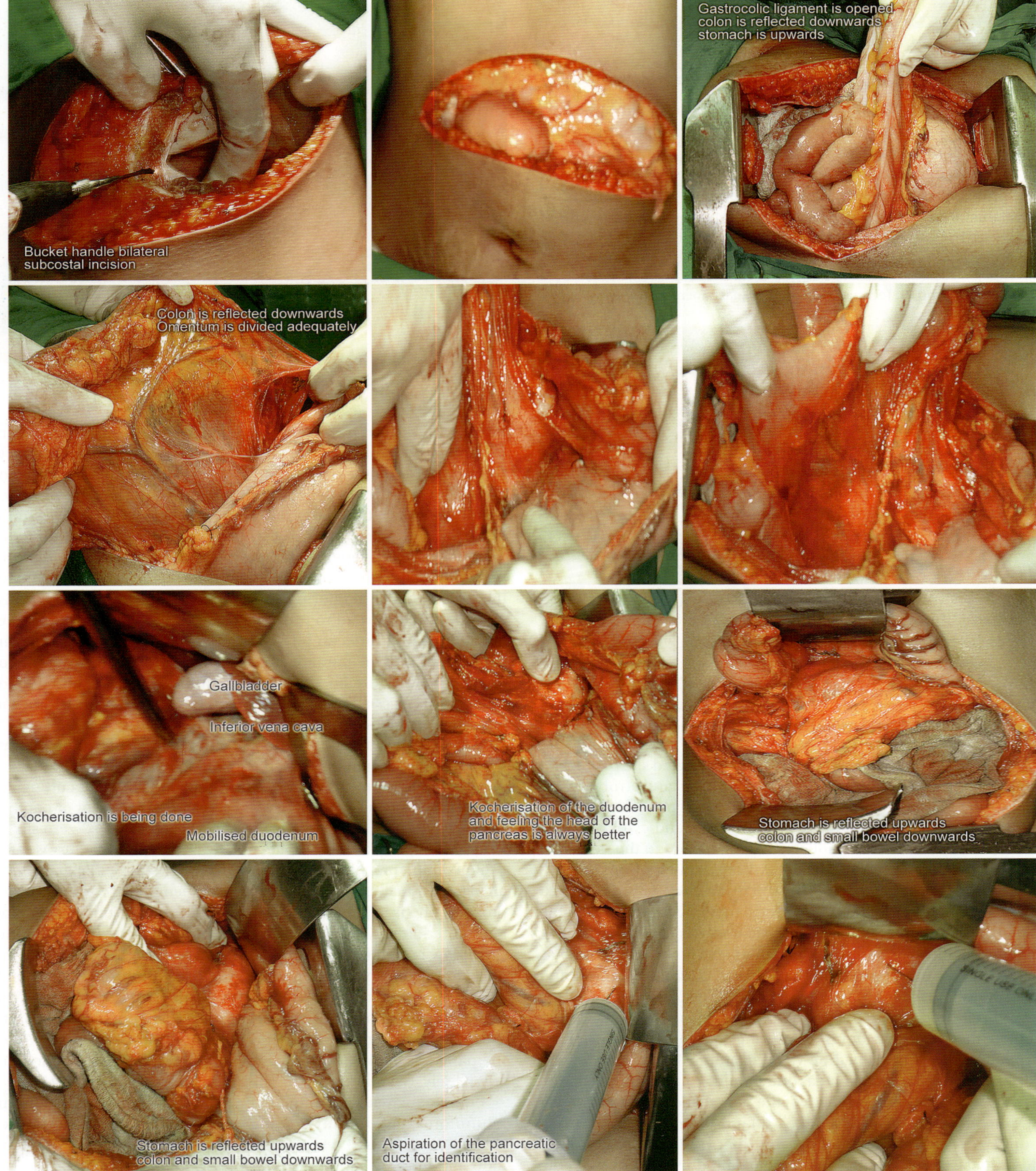
Bucket handle bilateral
subcostal incision
Gastrocolic ligament is opened
colon is reflected downwards
stomach is upwards
Colon is reflected downwards
Omentum is divided adequately
Gallbladder
Inferior vena cava
Kocherisation is being done
Mobilised duodenum
Kocherisation of the duodenum
and feeling the head of the
pancreas is always better
Stomach is reflected upwards
colon and small bowel downwards
Stomach is reflected upwards
colon and small bowel downwards
Aspiration of the pancreatic
duct for identification

Figs. 24-30(1)

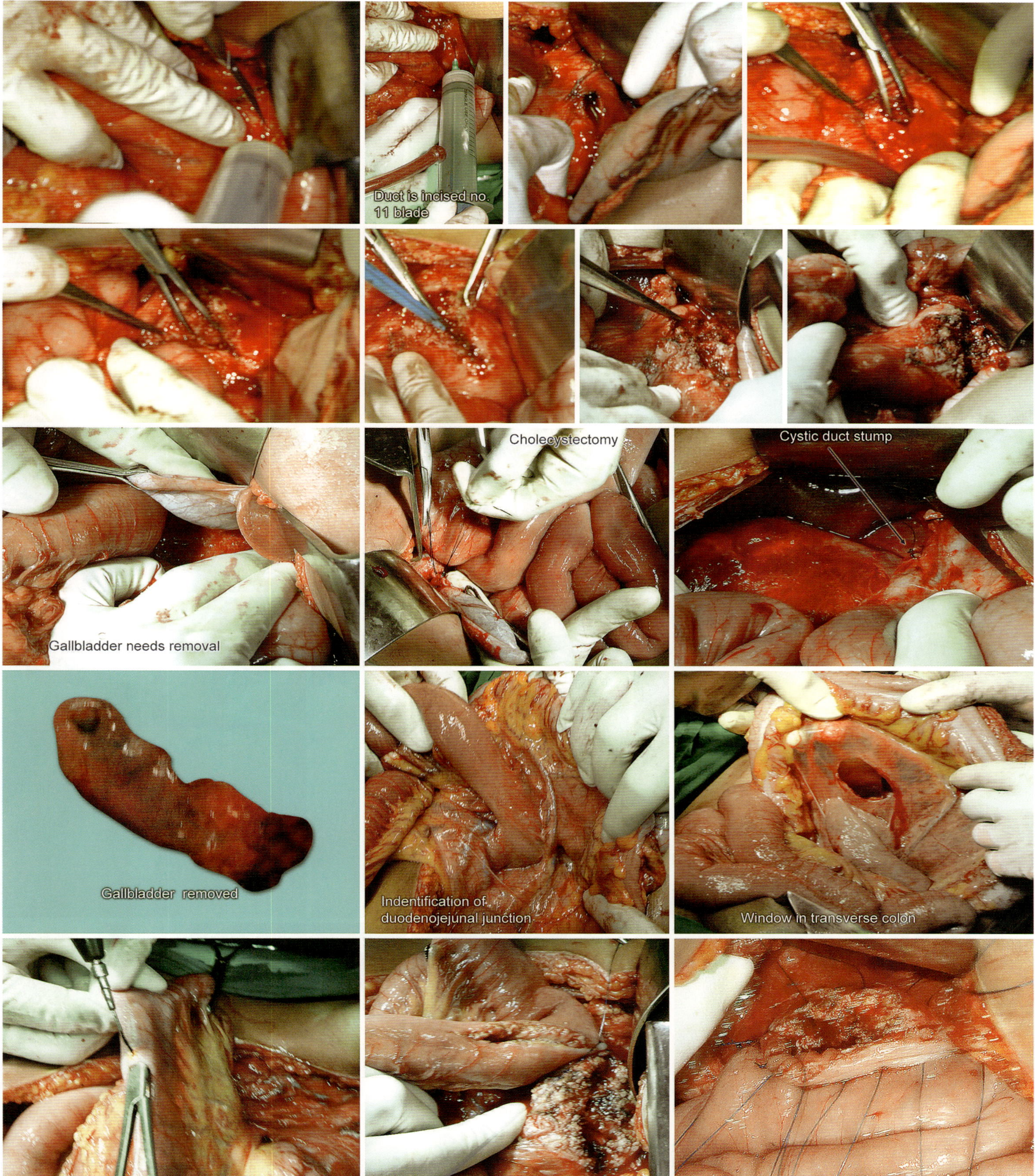

Figs. 24-30(2)

Figs. 24-30(1 and 2): Initial steps in longitudinal pancreaticojejunostomy.

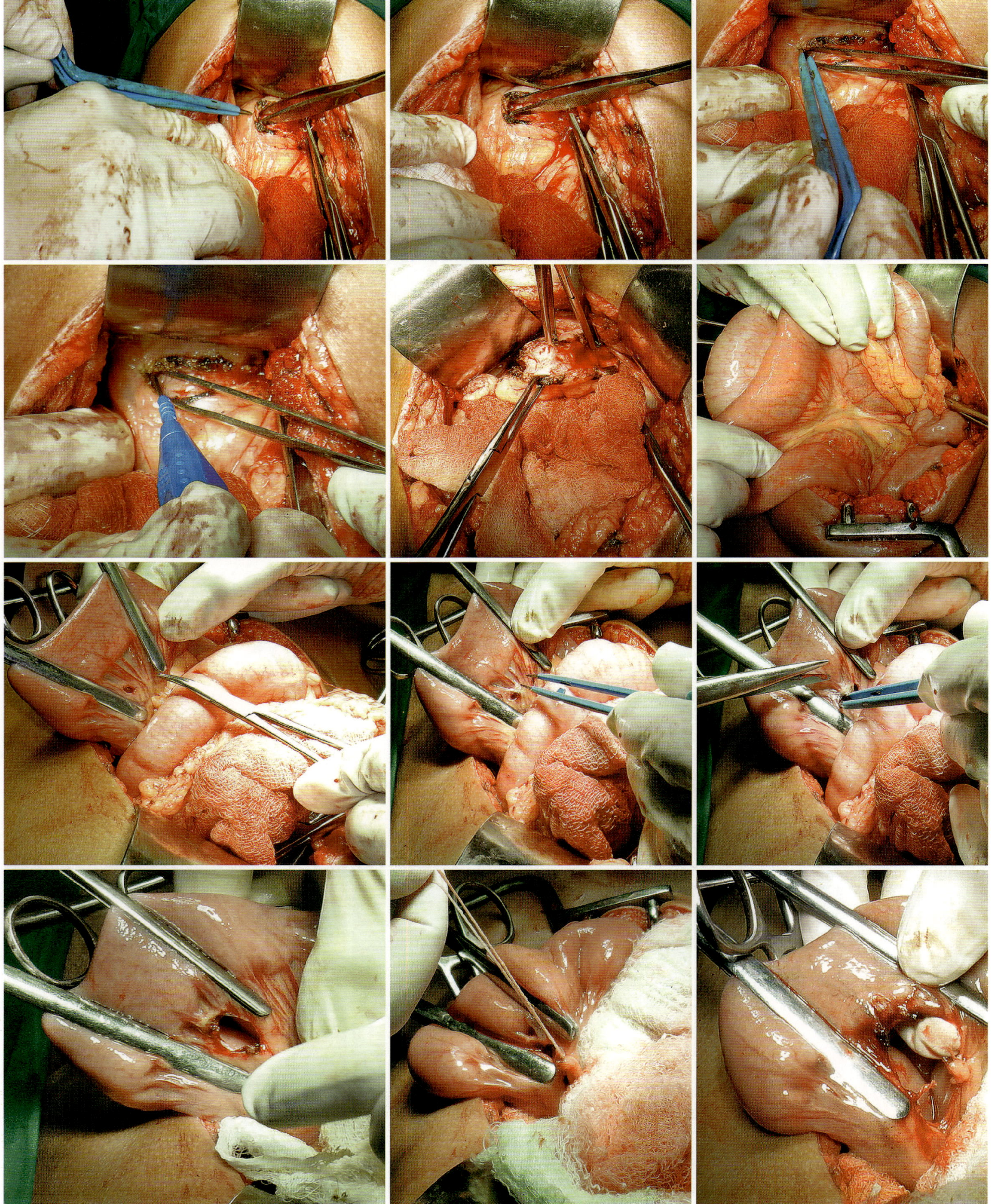

Figs. 24-31(1)

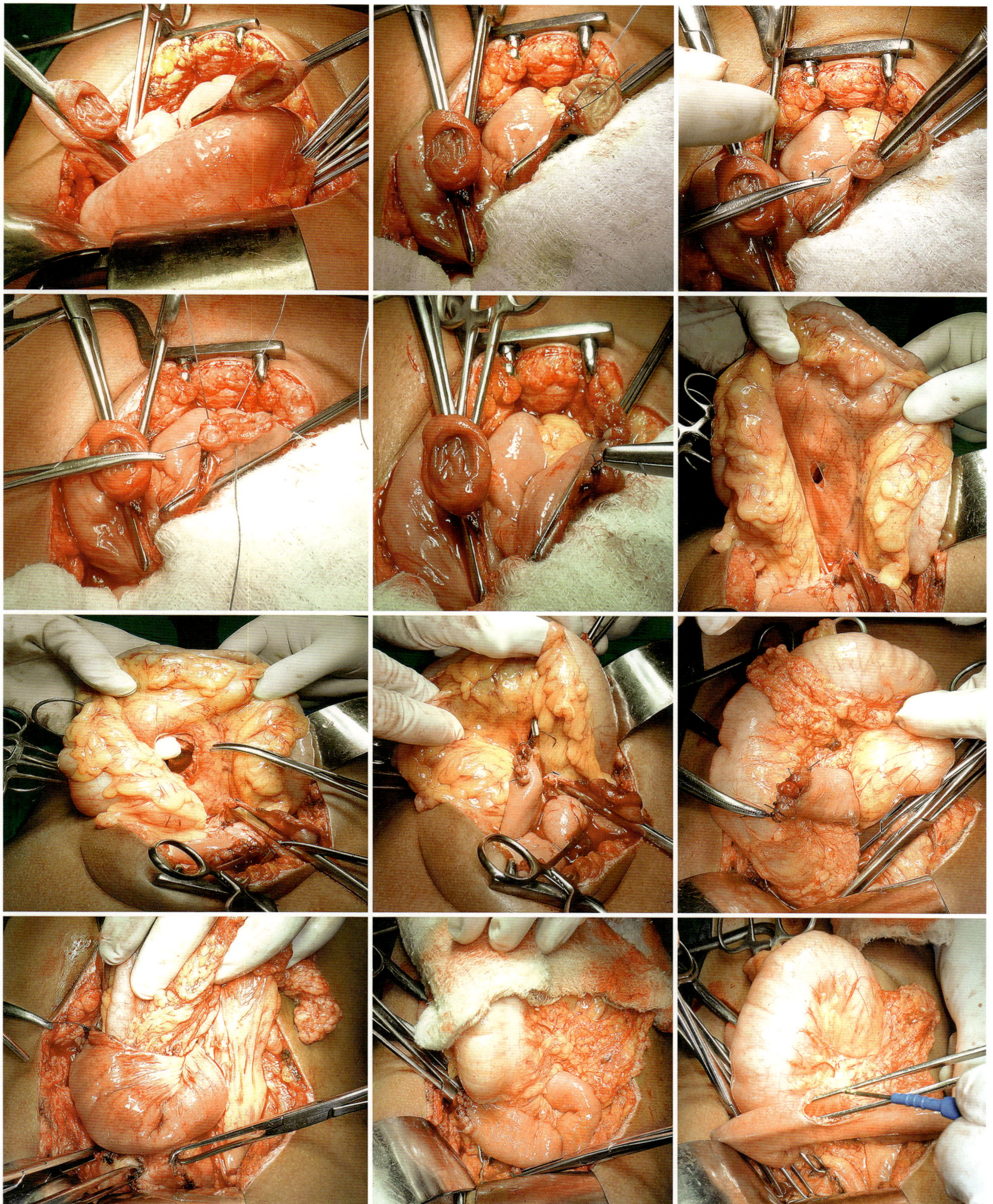

Figs. 24-31(2)

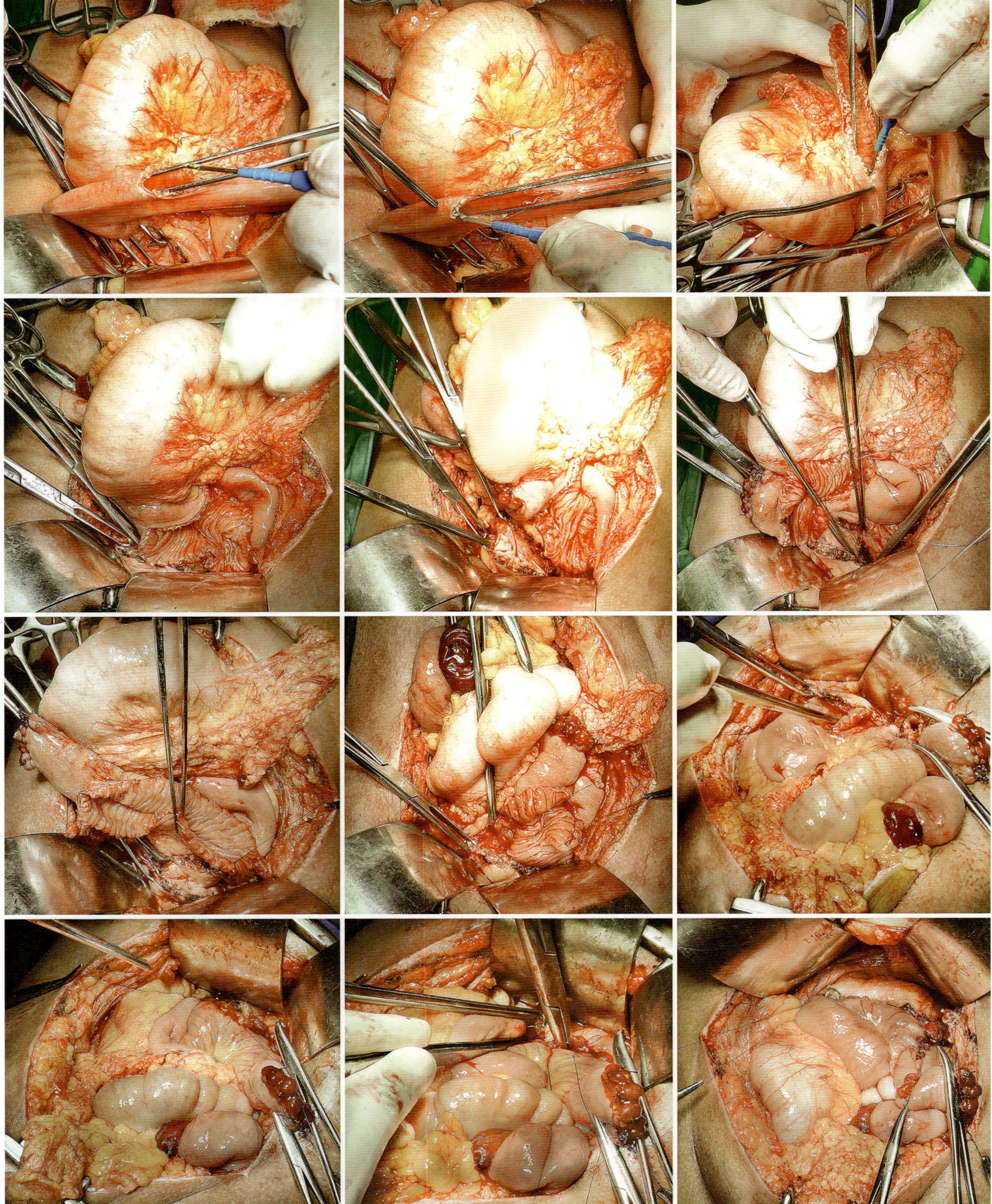

Figs. 24-31(3)

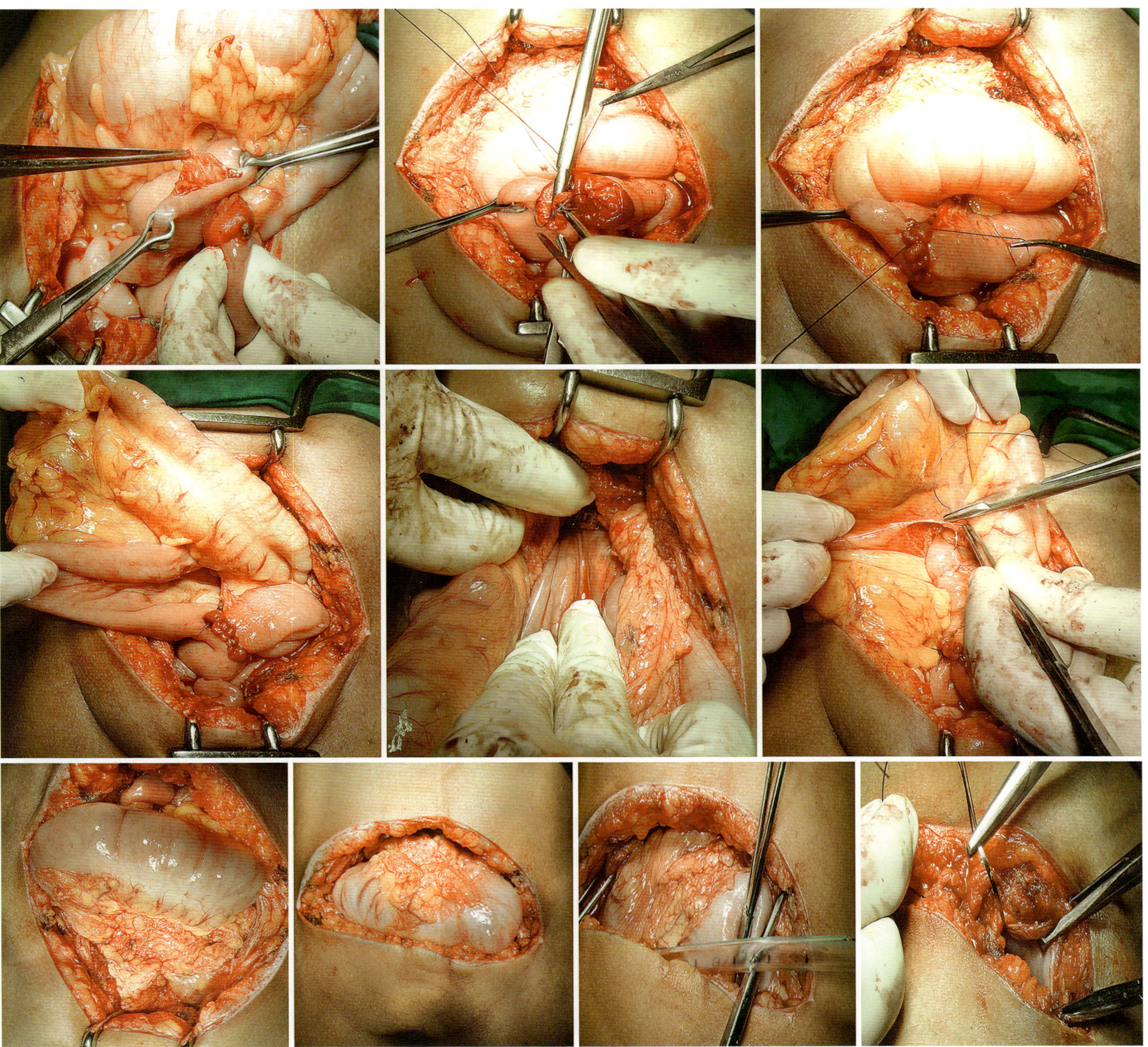

Figs. 24-31(4)

Figs. 24-31(1 to 4): Longitudinal pancreaticojejunostomy procedure.

Logic again is—it is sufficient enough if proper fibrous peripancreatic tissue bites are taken as it holds very well with very minimal chances of disruption and also facilitates the better drainage from the ductular openings of the pancreatic duct as mucosa and ductular openings are spared from getting blocked by sutures. Anastomosis can be done with cut end of the jejunal Roux loop either towards tail end or towards head end depending on the feasibility of the vascular arcade and length. Continuous suturing should be avoided as it will block endings of the small ducts into the main pancreatic duct. After taking all bites, posterior layer knots are placed one after other. Ties on either side (one on each end) are kept long. Knots are placed inside. It is also often practised that knots are placed outside in posterior layer; if it is so, bites should be taken from outside to inside of the duct and then inside to outside of the jejunum to place the knots at end. Placing knots inside the pancreaticojejunostomy is very well accepted. Anterior layer anastomosis is done by taking series of interrupted bites from anterior edge of the duct opening to anterior edge of the jejunal incision. Here also all bites are taken, tied one by one later and then ends are cut. Knots are placed outside in anterior layer. Single layer is sufficient in pancreaticojejunostomy even though few practice double-layer anastomosis which is technically difficult and not essential as such. Roux limb may be fixed to anterior pancreatic tissue to prevent kinking proximal to lengthy anastomosis **(Fig. 24-32)**.

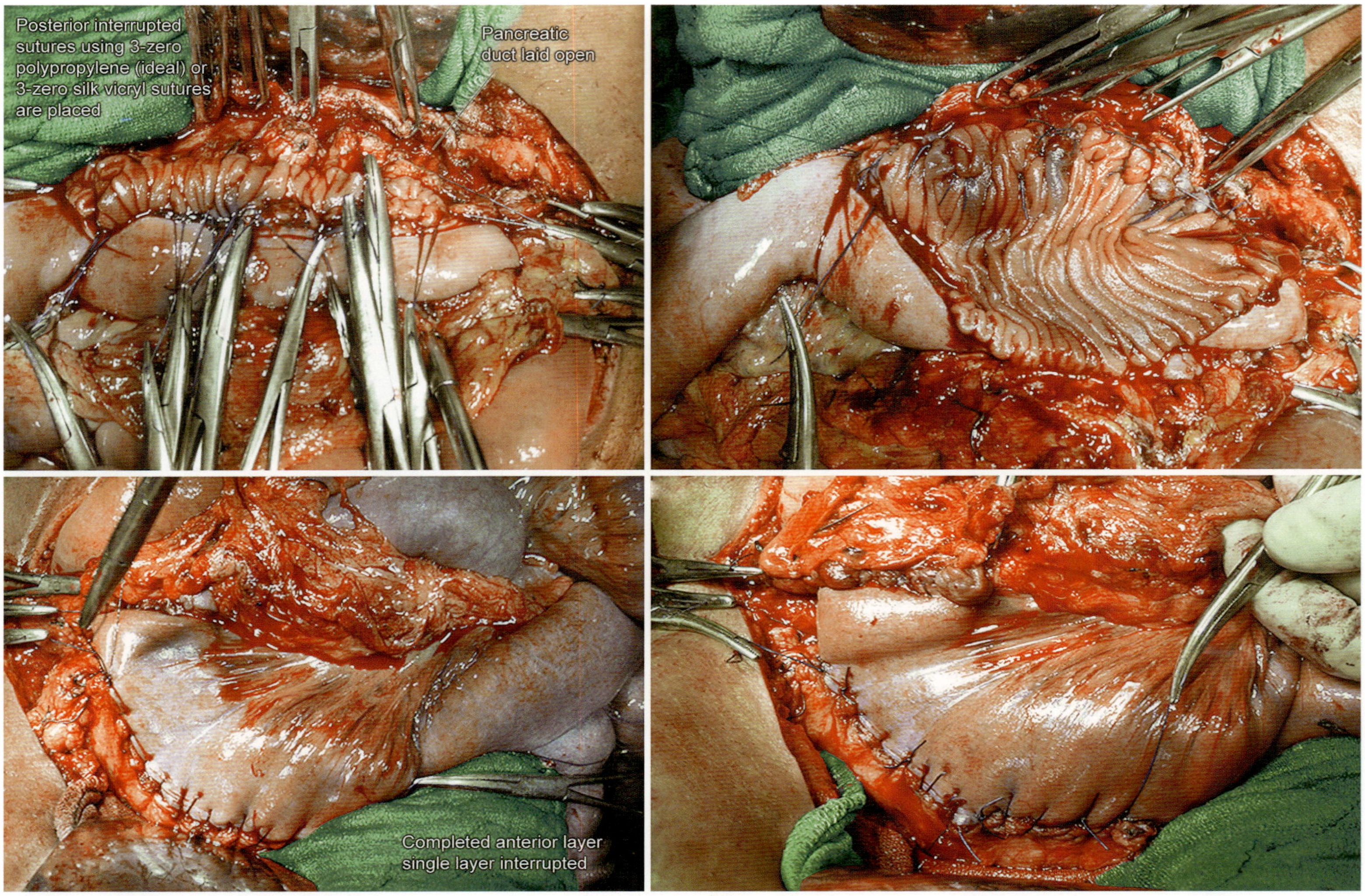

Fig. 24-32: Longitudinal pancreaticojejunostomy.

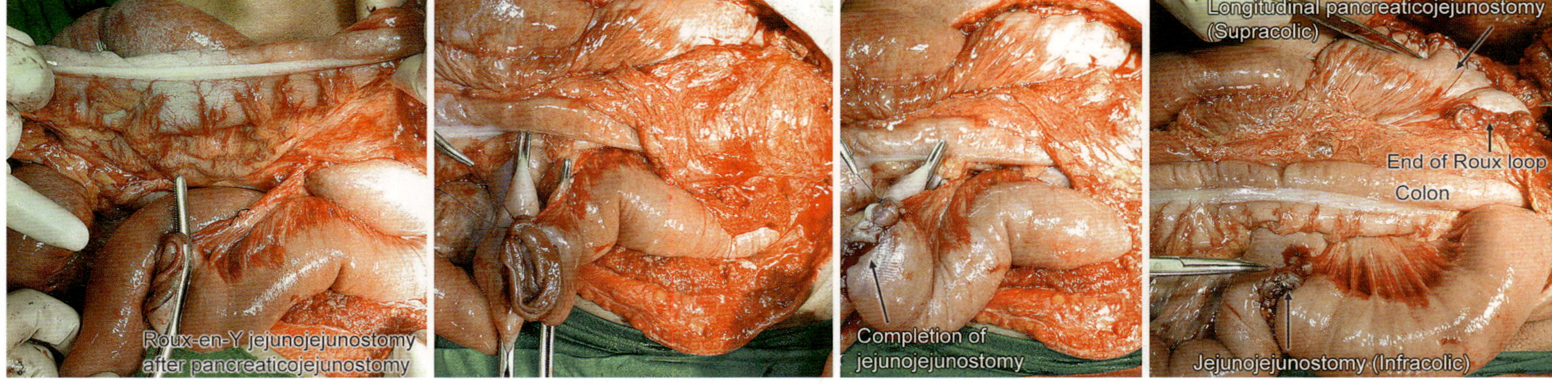

Fig. 24-33: Jejunojejunostomy in Roux-en-Y pancreaticojejunostomy.

End-to-side jejunojejunostomy is done to maintain the bowel continuity (45–50 cm from pancreaticojejunostomy site). If stapler transection is done, side-to-side anastomosis can be undertaken. Single layer continuous or interrupted 3-zero vicryl sutures are used for the same. Second layer 3-zero silk interrupted seromuscular sutures can be added **(Fig. 24-33)**.

Different Methods of Doing Pancreaticojejunostomy

Lateral fish mouth anastomosis: After opening the pancreatic duct, 20 cm from duodenojejunal junction Roux limb is selected and arcades are ligated; jejunum is transected; distal cut end will be proximal end of the Roux limb which is not sutured but left open; its antimesenteric border is marked for the adequate length needed for anastomosis with pancreatic duct. It is opened longitudinally in the antimesenteric border from the cut end of the Roux limb of the jejunum either using monopolar cautery or using stapler device. In this type cut end usually comes towards the duct over the pancreatic head (right side). Posterior layer is sutured between peripancreatic fibrotic tissue with or without mucosal bites as interrupted sutures using 3-zero polypropylene or silk sutures. Cut circumferential margin of the Roux jejunal limb is sutured to duct margin on the right side (over the head of the pancreas).

A. Drainage procedure

- *Partial:* Draining the duct partially
  - a. Sphincterotomy and sphincteroplasty
  - b. Duval procedure
  - c. Puestow-Gillesby procedure
  - d. Leger's procedure: Here splenectomy; opening of the duct; retrograde loop pancreaticojejunostomy is done instead of Roux-en-Y.
  - e. Marcadier procedure: Only duct in the body is drained through a side-to-side loop pancreaticojejunostomy.
- *Complete:* Draining the main duct completely
  - a. Pancreaticojejunostomy
    - Partington-Rochelle procedure
    - Bapat's (India, 1997) modification of Partington's procedure: Here end of Roux loop is not closed but fish mouth is created by giving a cut at antimesenteric border and entire part is anastomosed to side of the duct.
    - Moreno Gonzales procedure: Pancreatic and bile duct drainage is established into an isolated vascularised loop of jejunum which is then anastomosed to the duodenum.
  - b. Pancreaticogastrostomy

    It is technically found easier; however, it is not practised usually. Patients developed steatorrhoea because of the inactivation of the pancreatic enzymes by gastric acid.

B. Resectional procedures

a. Whipple's operation.

b. Traverso-Longmire procedure: pylorus preserving pancreaticoduodenectomy, 1978.

c. Beger's procedure: Decoring of head with transection of the neck and two anastomoses are done—one at head and another at cut end of the body of pancreas to a single Roux loop. In Berne's modification, head is decored but neck is not transected and a single cavity created is anastomosed to a Roux jejunal loop; CBD when opened here, its edge is also involved in stitches so that bile is also made to drain into the Roux loop.

d. Denervated pancreatic flap: Warrens denervated pancreatic flap: The pancreas is divided over the portal superior mesenteric vein after ligation of the splenic artery and vein. The pancreatic head is excised leaving a thin rim. The remaining pancreas is not drained. Ligation of splenic vein and artery is probably denervate the gland.

Shires' denervated splenopancreatic flap: Complete mobilisation of the pancreas from the retroperitoneum, resection of the head and the uncinate process leaving a thin rim of pancreas adjacent to the duodenum, division of the splenic vein at its junction with the SMV and drainage of the distal pancreatic remnant into a Roux-en-Y limb of jejunum.

e. Subtotal pancreatic resection: body and tail of pancreas is removed. Disease in the body and the tail is often secondary to disease in the head of the pancreas, thereby limiting its role. This procedure is still indicated when the disease is confined to body and tail, e.g. pseudocyst, failed pancreaticojejunostomy, non-dilated duct, pseudoaneurysm and when there is disease beyond the neck of pancreas, and the pancreatic duct is oversewn. A concomitant splenectomy is unavoidable in the majority of patients because of dense fibrosis precluding the isolation of the splenic vessels.

f. Child's procedure: 95% distal pancreatectomy. The spleen, the tail, body and uncinate processes are completely removed. The small cuff of the head that is preserved protects the vascularity and common bile duct during surgery. This procedure is performed when lesser procedures have failed or when the entire pancreas is severely diseased.

g. Total pancreatectomy: With duodenal preservation (Russel, 1987); without duodenal preservation.

C. Extended drainage procedure

a. Rumpf's extended drainage (1983): This is a combination of Partington's procedure with a transduodenal pancreatic sphincteroplasty. It is indicated when there is a prepapillary obstruction to the drainage of pancreatic duct due to stones or stricture.

D. Resection with extended drainage

a. Extended Beger procedure: In addition to the duodenum preserving head resection, a side-to-side lateral pancreaticojejunostomy is performed after slitting open the main pancreatic duct.

b. Frey's procedure.

c. Izbicki V-shaped ventral pancreatic excision. In this procedure, a long V-shaped excision of ventral aspect of the pancreas is done with a lateral pancreaticojejunostomy by a mucosa to capsule anastomosis. This procedure drains the main as well as the second and third order ducts. This is an ideal procedure for small duct disease with a maximum diameter of the Wirsung's duct less than 3 mm.

E. Pancreatic denervation alone

a. Left splanchnicectomy with coeliac ganglionectomy: Mallet Guy (1983) advocated an extraperitoneal approach through the 12th rib for left splanchnicectomy with coeliac ganglionectomy. This is done after correcting the extrapancreatic pathology.

b. Left splanchnicectomy, coeliac ganglionectomy with bilateral vagotomy.

c. Complete pancreatic denervation: Hirokawa described a more extensive denervation procedure, which includes freeing the pancreas from the posterior abdominal wall and resection of all postganglionic pancreatic nerve plexus including those surrounding the common hepatic and splenic arteries (1986).

d. Transthoracic/videothoracoscopic pancreatic denervation: The greater splanchnic nerves are responsible for pain in supramesenteric viscera and the nerve trunks lie above the level of the 10th thoracic vertebra and descend along the spine to end in the coeliac plexus, similarly the lesser splanchnic plexus. Transthoracic division of the splanchnic nerves with bilateral vagotomy performed through a left thoracotomy. Procedure can be performed using a videothoracoscopic technique [Makarewicz W et al. (2003)].

F. Pancreatic autotransplantation

a. Islet cell transplantation

b. Segmental pancreatic transplantation.

Procedure is completed by anastomosing the anterior part of the jejunum to superior margin of the cut part of the remaining pancreatic duct. 45 cm of Roux limb is maintained. Proximal jejunal cut end is sutured to Roux limb using vicryl or silk single or double layered. Opening in the mesocolon is sutured to Roux jejunal limb with circumferential 2-3 sutures; mesentery of the jejunum is sutured similarly using interrupted silk sutures to ascending limb of the Roux—to prevent formation of internal hernia.

Full width side to side lateral pancreaticojejunostomy *(Partigton Rochelle operation):* Here cut end of Roux limb is closed either using stapler or by hand suturing using vicryl or silk by two layered closure technique.

Pancreatic implantation into the Roux jejunal loop *(original Puestow's technique):* When pancreatic duct is unable to be identified during dissection then distal pancreas including both body and tail are mobilised completely after doing splenectomy. Splenic artery is ligated near its origin; splenic vein is ligated close to inferior mesenteric vein. Tip of the tail end of the pancreas is transected to identify the duct opening through which a probe is passed (or a fine polythene tube/catheter). Pancreas in front of the duct including anterior wall of the duct is opened longitudinally over the probe which acts as a guide (or using polythene tube as a guide); Pott's scissor or monopolar cautery or no 15 blade can be used carefully to open the duct. Duct is opened adequately up to the mobilised head of the pancreas. Often existing strictures are also opened, stones if present in the duct are also removed. Haemostasis is achieved using bipolar cautery or fine vicryl sutures. Two silk traction sutures (2-zero silk) are placed on the superior and inferior borders of the distal cut ends of the tail end of the pancreas. Needles of the sutures are kept intact. Needles of the traction sutures placed earlier to the pancreas tail borders are carefully passed across the open end of Roux limb of the jejunum along the lumen; once adequately needed length is passed using long needle holder; it is penetrated across the wall of the bowel outside. Roux limb is telescoped across the tail and body of the pancreas up to the right end of the opened duct; bowel is sutured to the pancreatic capsule circumferentially using interrupted polypropylene sutures. Both traction silk sutures which are brought out from the pancreatic tail and bowel wall are tied each other to secure the tail distally. Distal jejunojejunostomy is completed; mesenteric defect in the mesocolon is sutured; small bowel mesentery of the limb is sutured to the ascending limb.

If coeliac ganglion block is needed, it can be given on table by direct palpation of aorta. 20 mL of 50% ethanol is injected along each side of the aorta using 21-gauge spinal needle.

Jejunum is fixed to the mesocolon by few interrupted silk sutures to prevent herniation. Jejunostomy, if needed, is done. Drain is placed. Abdomen is closed in layers.

Problem with this procedure (LPJ) is failure to identify the portal hypertension and dilated veins in the pancreas, and possible occult carcinoma of the pancreas.

Complications of Surgery

Pancreatic leak/fistula (10%); infection; bleeding; recurrence; brittle diabetes in total pancreatectomy.

Pain/relief in chronic pancreatitis is achieved by drugs; decompression/drainage surgeries, resection surgeries, epidural analgesia, coeliac ganglion block, operative chemical splanchnicectomy, extra/intraperitoneal right and left splanchnicectomy, transhiatal bilateral splanchnicectomy, thoracoscopic splanchnicectomy. 5-year pain-free period in decompression surgery is 70%.

Postoperative Care

Nutrition: TPN/jejunostomy feed; fluid and electrolyte management; prevention/control of sepsis; proper monitoring; Octreotide on table and postoperatively—regular intervals or slow infusion—5 days. Nasogastric tube is removed in 48 hours. Oral fluid is started in 4–5 days. Drain is removed in 5–7 days.

Surgery for Chronic Pancreatitis

Drainage: Technically easier; Less mortality <2–5%; Adequate pain relief; Recurrence of pain in 5 years—50%. But diseased tissue is left behind; Disease progression and fear of existing occult carcinoma (17%) or later onset.

Resection: Technically demanding; Mortality is 8–21%—very high; done when carcinoma is suspected or localised disease. Head is the pacemaker of the disease. Whipple's is preferred. Total pancreatectomy, though ideal, it is not done commonly. It causes brittle diabetes and has high mortality.

Islet Cell Autotransplantation

The Mirkowitch technique: Partially purified islet produce a fairly large volume of minced digested islet cell tissue which is then injected into a portal vein very slowly. But portal pressure is markedly raised several fold. *Let preparation technique (Hinshaw et al)—* 5 mL tissue pellet is produced containing 500,000–2000,000 islets for transplantation, portal pressure remained essentially unchanged. Total pancreatectomy and islet autotransplantation are done for chronic pancreatitis with intractable pain when other treatment measures have failed, allowing insulin secretory capacity to be preserved, minimising or preventing diabetes, while at the same time removing the root cause of the pain. Pain relief is obtained in most patients, and insulin independence preserved long-term in about a third, with another third having sufficient beta-cell function so that the surgical diabetes is mild. Islet autotransplantation has been done with partial or total pancreatectomy for benign and premalignant conditions. Islet autotransplantation should be used more widely to preserve beta-cell mass in major pancreatic resections [Blondet JJ et al. (2007)].

Segmental Pancreatic Transplantation

Autotransplantation of the resected body and tail of the pancreas is done into the thigh following near total pancreatectomy. The splenic vessels are anastomosed to the femoral vessels. The divided end of the pancreas is closed and the duct is ligated or injected with synthetic polymers (e.g. prolamine or neoprene). Duct obliteration is thought to cause rapid and permanent atrophy of the exocrine pancreas but preserves endocrine function. Still it is found that duct obliteration does not prevent relapse or progression of chronic pancreatitis in the preserved pancreatic segment. Internal drainage of the duct into a Roux-en-Y limb of jejunum has also been reported.

Laparoscopic Pancreatic Resection

Laparoscopic resection of the pancreas is technically quite demanding. It is technically feasible. The benefit of the laparoscopic approach may not be as apparent as that of a less complex laparoscopic procedure. The use of laparoscopy for distal pancreatic resection with splenic preservation is beneficial. Optimal closure of the cut edge of the pancreas and preservation of the spleen and its main vessels are the most important aspects of this operation. Laparoscopic longitudinal pancreaticojejunostomy and laparoscopic Whipple's procedures are done now in specified centres by skilled laparoscopic surgeons with same principles and technique as open surgery.

SURGICAL TREATMENT FOR PSEUDOCYST OF PANCREAS

It is a localised collection of sequestered pancreatic fluid, usually 3 weeks after an attack of acute pancreatitis. It can occur after trauma and recurrent chronic pancreatitis. Collection usually occurs in the lesser sac in relation to stomach, but can occur in relation with duodenum, jejunum, colon and splenic hilum. About 50% of acute pancreatitis leads to pseudocyst formation, but among that 20–40% will resolve spontaneously. **Sites**—lesser sac—commonest, i.e. between colon and stomach; can occur in relation to duodenum, jejunum, colon and splenic hilum. **Types**—depending on whether it communicates with pancreatic duct or not is classified as: 1. *Communicating pseudocyst,* and 2. *Non-communicating pseudocyst. Pseudocyst can also be acute pseudocyst or chronic pseudocyst.*

Initially, cyst wall is thin *(unformed)*, but later it gets fibrosed and thickened *(formed)* (matured). It is lined by fibrin layer but no endothelium, hence known as pseudocyst. It contains typically brownish fluid with sludge-like necrotic material. It can get infected to form *infected pseudocyst* or *pancreatic abscess.* Amylase level in the cyst fluid is very high (>5000 units/mL).

Complications of pseudocyst: Rupture—3%—into bowel or peritoneum; bleeding from the splenic vessels—7%; cholangitis; duodenal obstruction; portal/splenic vein thrombosis and segmental portal hypertension; cholestasis due to CBD block.

D'Egidio's classification of pseudocyst

Type I: After an attack of acute pancreatitis; Normal duct anatomy; no fistula/communication.

Type II: After an attack of acute on chronic pancreatitis; Abnormal duct anatomy without stricture; 50% chances of fistula.

Type III: After an attack of chronic pancreatitis, abnormal anatomy with stricture; always communicating. It appears like retention cyst.

Investigations

Ultrasound abdomen (commonly done procedure), reveals the size and thickness of the pseudocyst. Size less than 6 cm indicates that one can wait for spontaneous resolution. Ultrasound also shows the presence of gallstones. Endosonography (EUS) is very useful. CT scan is ideal and study of choice. It is two times more sensitive than ultrasound. It demonstrates size, shape, number, wall thickness, contents, pancreatic duct size, and extent of necrosis in pancreas, calcification and atrophy in chronic pancreatitis, regional vessels, pseudoaneurysm, and splenic/portal vein thrombosis. Splenic artery CT angiography is very relevant in suspected cases of pseudoaneurysm. MRCP delineates the ductal anatomy and its abnormality. ERCP can be done to find out the communication **(Fig. 24-34)**.

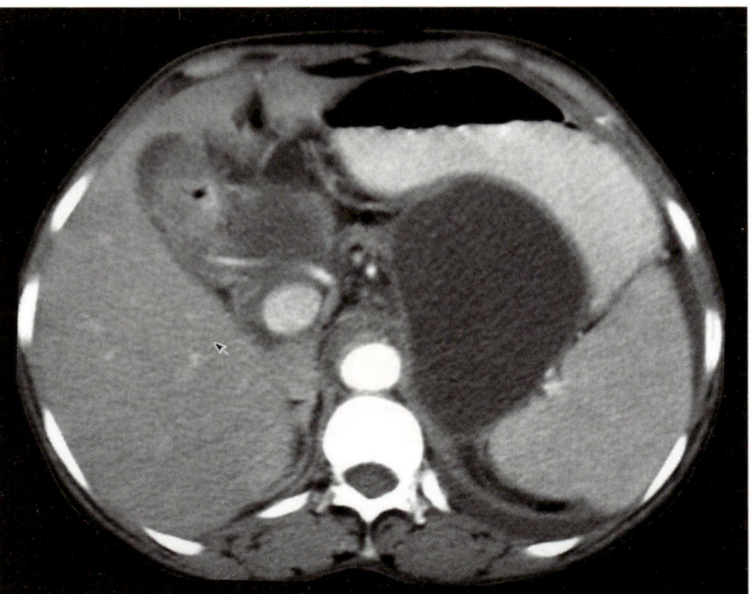

Fig. 24-34: CT scan of pseudocyst of pancreas.

Indications for Surgery/Intervention

Size more than 6 cm; formed pseudocyst; infected pseudocyst; cyst persisting after 6 weeks/progressive cyst; multiple cysts/cyst due to trauma; communicating cysts/cyst with severe pain; thick-walled pseudocyst.

Cystogastrostomy

Procedure is done under general anaesthesia. Preoperative antibiotics are given. Nasogastric tube is passed. Cyst should be firmly attached to the wall of the stomach to do cystogastrostomy. Cyst wall should be thick to do cystogastrostomy otherwise only external drainage is possible **(Figs. 24-35 and 24-36)**. *30 degree head up position* will expose the cyst better. On table cystogram and cholangiogram if needed should be done and facility for that should be kept ready.

On laparotomy, cyst is palpated. Any undue pulsation more than usual should one suspect pseudoaneurysm. Anterior wall of the stomach is easily exposed. Gastrostomy on the anterior wall of the stomach is made—6–8 cm on its most prominent part. Posterior wall of the stomach is opened after confirming that cyst wall is adherent to the stomach. Anterior wall is retracted by placing two Deaver's retractors inside anterior wall; or 4 stay sutures can be placed on 4 points. Long needle with syringe is passed into the cyst; brownish coloured fluid is aspirated. If blood is aspirated, pseudoaneurysm is suspected. Fluid is sent for cytology and biochemical assessment (amylase level). Aspiration is often done prior to gastrotomy but usually done after gastrotomy. Posterior wall of the stomach with an elliptical incision is excised along with similar sized anterior cyst wall. This cyst wall is sent for histology. The thick capsule of pseudocyst is opened. All fluid with necrotic material is sucked. Fluid should be sent for cytology, culture and sensitivity and amylase estimation. Cyst wall always should be biopsied—ideally frozen section biopsy. Cyst cavity should be washed with warm normal saline after breaking septae. Cut edge of the stomach is anastomosed to the cut edge of the cyst wall using

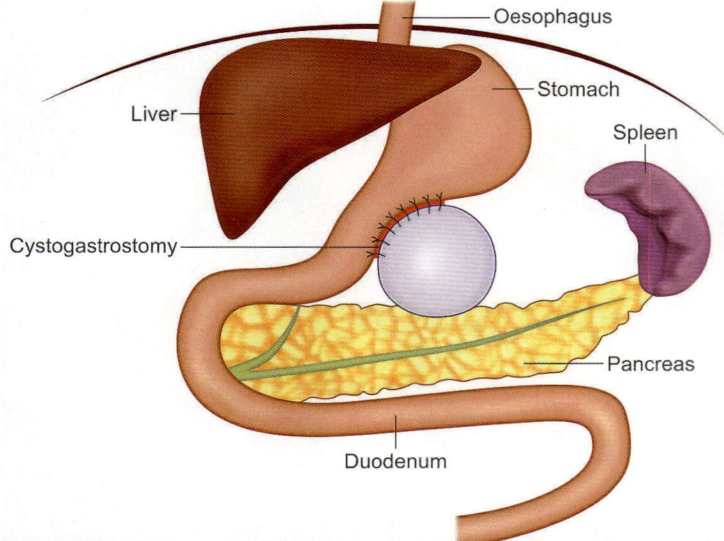

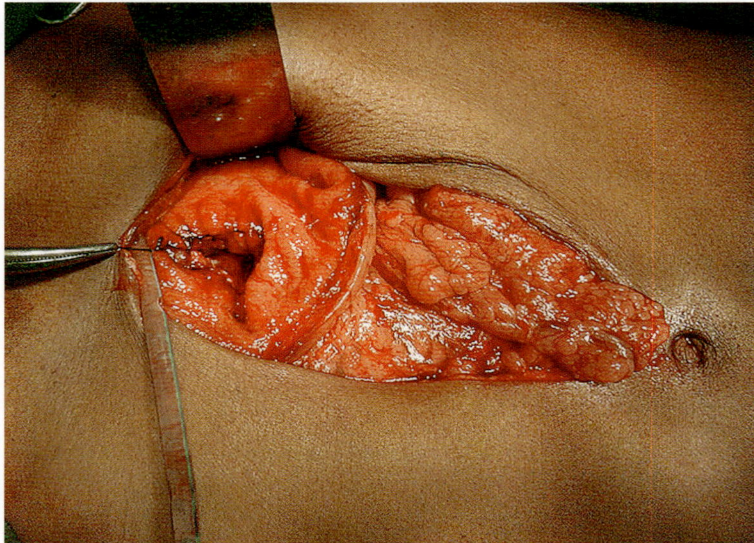

Fig. 24-35: Cystogastrostomy.

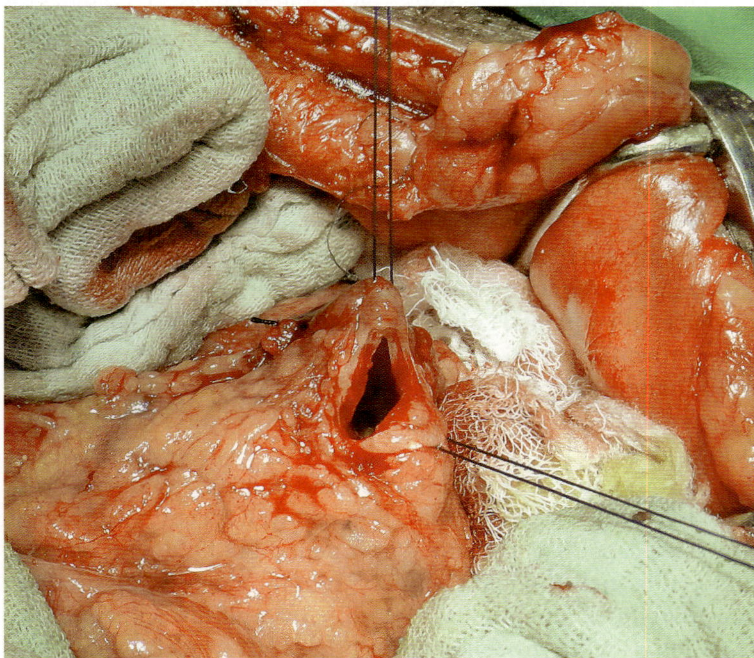

Fig. 24-36: Opened pseudocyst wall. Always collect fluid for amylase which will be very high; and also for CEA; take frozen section biopsy from the edge.

continuous or interrupted vicryl sutures. *Necrosectomy* can be done but gently as aggressive approach may cause torrential bleeding. This pseudocapsule which is anastomosed to posterior wall of the stomach is known as *Jurasz operation.* Anterior wall gastrostomy is closed with continuous single layer vicryl sutures. Stapler closure also can be done. Usually peritoneal drainage is not necessary. Nasogastric tube is kept for 48 hours. Oral started in 72 hours **(Fig. 24-37)**.

If stomach is not adherent to cyst wall, then cystojejunostomy is done; if cyst wall is found not thick on table, then only external drainage should be done.

If cyst contains pseudoaneurysm, then on table ultrasound should be done; here it is better to do distal pancreatectomy with the removal of cyst and ligation of splenic artery **(Figs. 24-38 and 24-39)**.

Note:

Feel for pulsation to rule out pseudoaneurysm and needed adhesion between stomach and cyst; aspirate to rule out blood and to confirm brownish-black fluid of cyst; do always frozen section biopsy of cyst wall to rule out cystadenocarcinoma. Cyst fluid is sent for amylase and CEA.

On table cholangiogram can be done if need arises. If patient general condition is optimum cholecystectomy can be added if there are gallstones.

Other Procedures

1. ***Cystoduodenostomy:*** It is similar to stomach technically; but duodenum is opened and anastomosis is done. It is commonly not used as duodenum healing is not as good as cystogastrostomy and leak may occur. Cystoduodenostomy needs *proper Kocherisation* of the duodenum. Ampulla should be identified after opening the duodenum. Sphincterotomy can be added if needed which is an additional advantage of this procedure.
2. ***Cystojejunostomy:*** It is done in large cyst and recurrent cyst. Roux-en-Y cystojejunostomy is better with lesser recurrence rate than cystogastrostomy. Upper midline incision is used; laparotomy exploration is done. Cholecystectomy, if needed, is done. Anterior wall of the cyst is exposed by releasing the omental adhesions using sharp and bipolar cautery dissection. Cyst is aspirated in similar way and collected for culture, cytology and biochemical analysis. 4 cm cyst wall is excised elliptically; tissue is sent for frozen section biopsy. Jejunum is transected 20 cm from the ligament of Treitz; distal Roux limb is brought upwards through a created window in the transverse mesocolon. End of the Roux loop is anastomosed to the cyst wall as end-to-end using interrupted 3-zero vicryl or silk sutures. Rent in the mesocolon is sutured to the jejunum. Divided proximal cut end of the jejunum is anastomosed to the antimesenteric side of the Roux limb 50 cm from the cystojejunostomy site. Defect in the jejunal mesentery is closed with interrupted sutures **(Figs. 24-40 and 24-41)**.
3. If infected, cystogastrostomy with external drainage is done using Malecot's catheter (*Smith operation*) **(Fig. 24-42)**.
4. ***Laparoscopic cystogastrostomy*** is becoming popular, effective and less invasive.
5. ***Distal pancreatectomy*** with pseudocyst removal if cyst is in distal part or if there is a pseudoaneurysm **(Fig. 24-43)**.

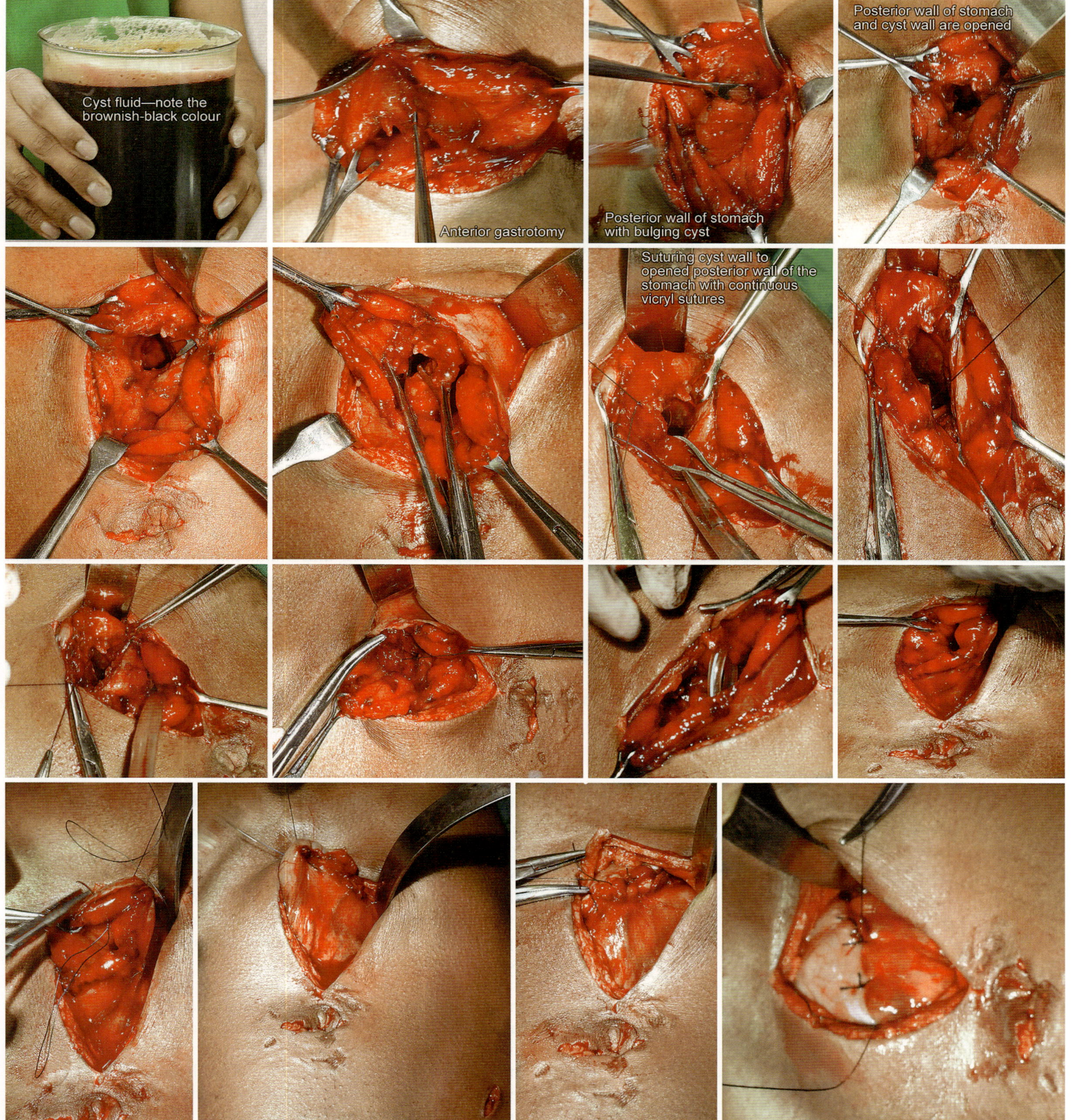

Fig. 24-37: Pseudocyst with cystogastrostomy.

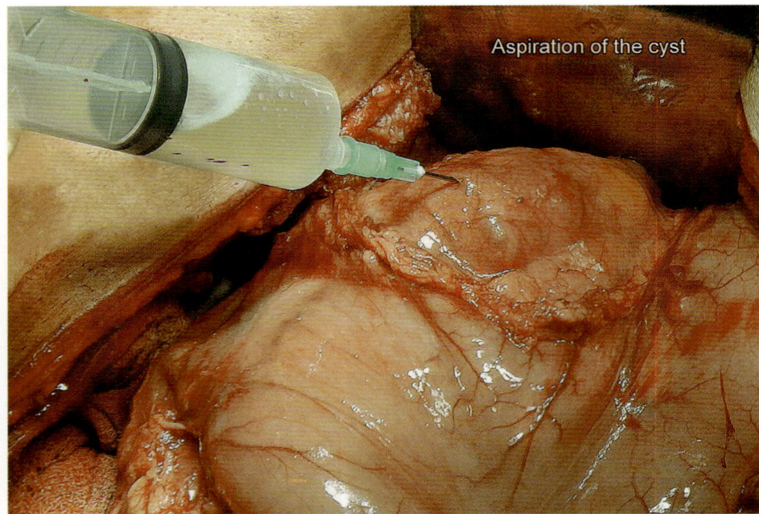

Fig. 24-38: Aspiration of the cyst.

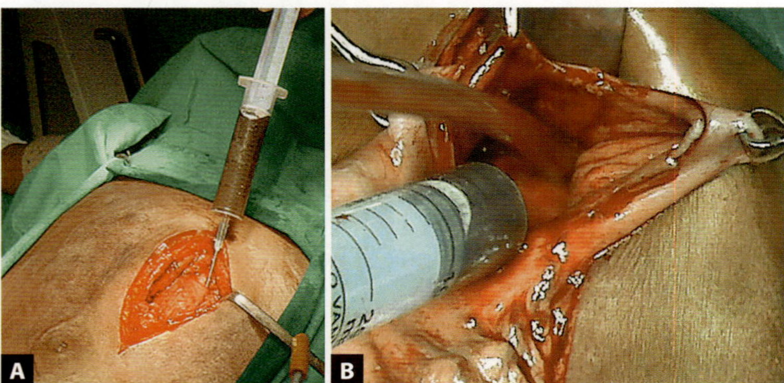

Figs. 24-39A and B: Aspiration of pseudocyst of the pancreas.

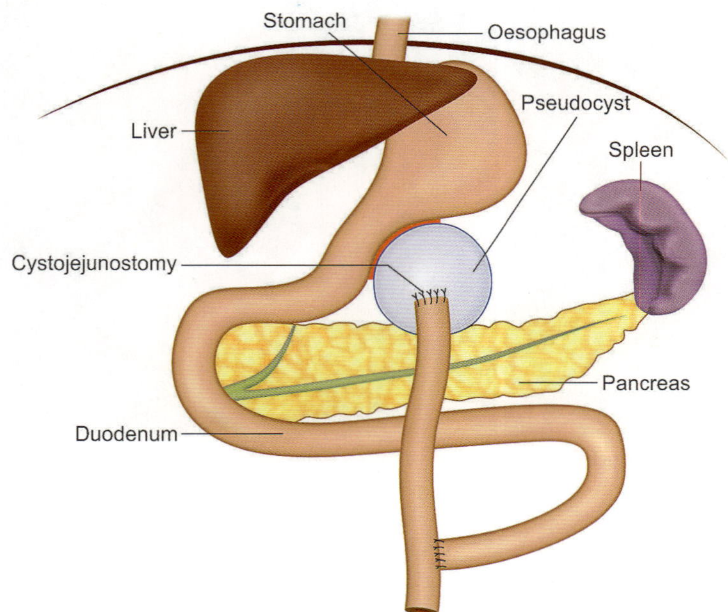

Fig. 24-40: Cystojejunostomy is better. If cyst is not adherent to stomach with thick cyst wall, cystojejunostomy is done.

PANCREATICODUODENECTOMY (WHIPPLE'S OPERATION/PARTIAL PANCREATICODUODENECTOMY)

The standard surgical treatment for pancreatic cancer remains the pancreaticoduodenectomy, first described by Whipple (Allen Oldfather Whipple) in 1935. Initially he did two staged procedure and in 1942 he modified into one stage procedure. High operative morbidity and mortality rates led to technical modifications of the operation which, combined with improvement in anaesthesia and critical care, have resulted in current perioperative mortality rate of 2% or less **(Fig. 24-44)**.

Indications

Periampullary carcinoma, carcinoma of 2nd part of the duodenum, ampulla, distal CBD are traditional indications. Chronic pancreatitis with disease involving mainly head of pancreas with severe pain is also an indication **(Fig. 24-45)**.

Contraindications

Liver and peritoneal secondaries; coeliac lymph node involvement; involvement of the SMA or root of the mesentery. Significant deep infiltration of portal vein precludes the resection, even though resection of portal vein with graft is done.

Preoperative staging and evaluation with CT, MRI, ERCP, EUS, liver function tests, prothrombin time, and coagulation profile are needed. Adequate hydration in preoperative period is needed. Preoperative antibiotic may be needed if cholangitis is suspected. Malignant obstructive cholangitis, if present, is a high-risk, may require an initial decompression by ERCP and then proceed with pancreaticoduodenectomy. However, routine preoperative decompression is not practised nowadays **(Fig. 24-46)**.

Risks are—intraoperative bleeding; anomalies of vessels; pancreatic and biliary leak; infection; acute pancreatitis; postoperative bleeding.

Technique of Whipple's Operation

The current practised technique utilises a *bilateral subcostal incision (Chevron incision)*. The liver and peritoneal surface is carefully examined to exclude the presence of metastatic disease, and intraoperative ultrasonography of liver and pancreas is performed. Random lymph node sampling is not done however; suspicious lymph nodes found during the operation are subjected to frozen section analysis.

In an operable case, it is often practised to go ahead with pancreaticoduodenectomy without biopsy. Ideally on table fine needle aspiration cytology (FNAC) of the tumour directly or transduodenal needle tissue biopsy or choledochotomy with choledochoscopic biopsy in case of CBD tumour is preferable; however preoperative endoscopic biopsy of periampullary carcinoma or ERCP biopsy is also commonly advocated.

Adequate exposure is essential for proper Whipple's operation. Good retraction with self-retaining retractor makes assistant's hands free to help the surgeon during surgical procedure. Bipolar cautery, ligaseal, harmonic scalpel are of benefits including staplers to divide stomach and duodenum. Initial mobilisation is done by reflecting the hepatic flexure and transverse colon downwards; then extended Kocherisation is done by lateral duodenal ligament which exposes SMV, IVC and aorta partly. Invasion or encasement of these vessels

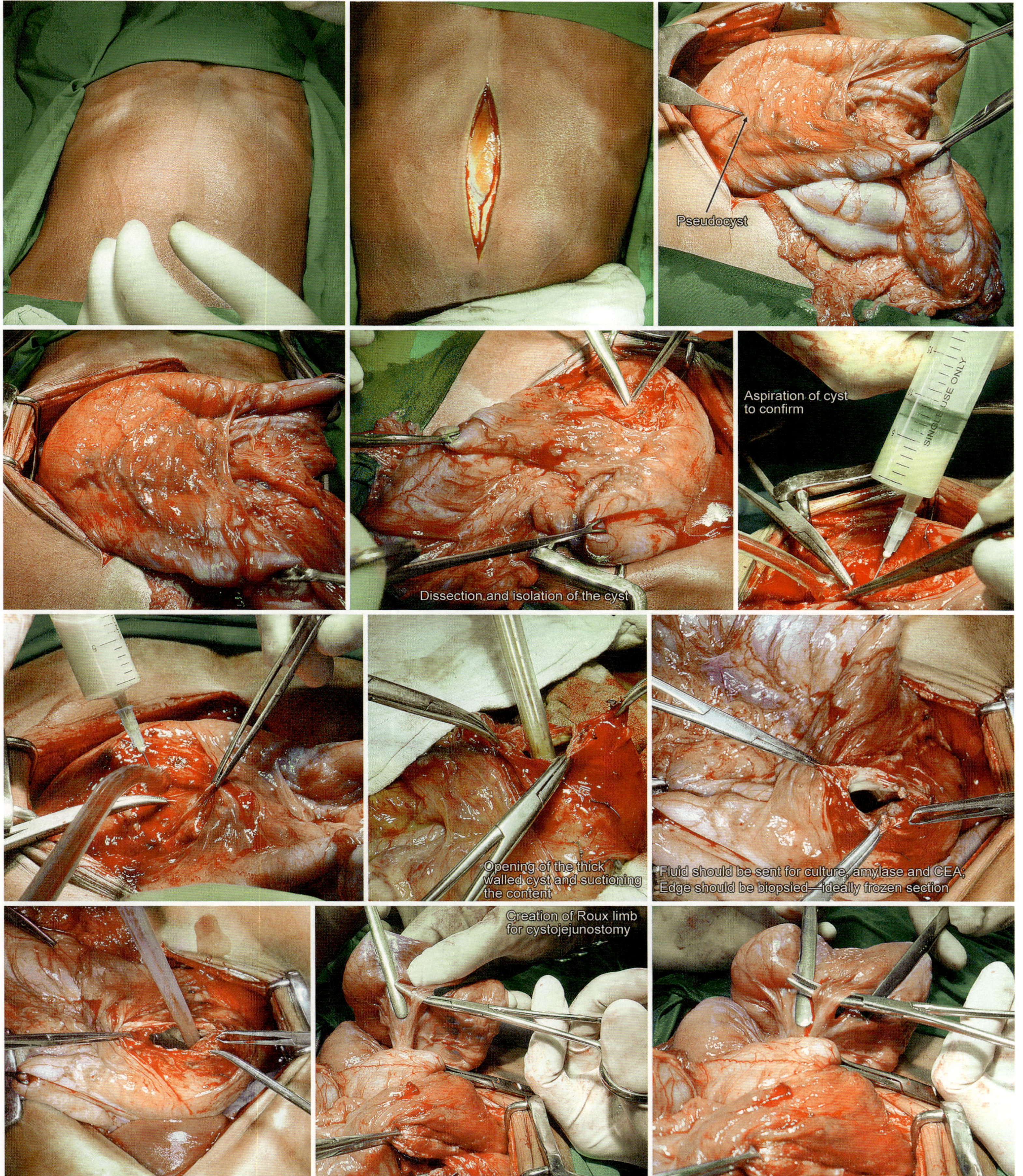
Pseudocyst
Aspiration of cyst to confirm
SINGLE USE ONLY
Dissection and isolation of the cyst
Opening of the thick walled cyst and suctioning the content
Fluid should be sent for culture, amylase and CEA; Edge should be biopsied—ideally frozen section
Creation of Roux limb for cystojejunostomy

Figs. 24-41(1)

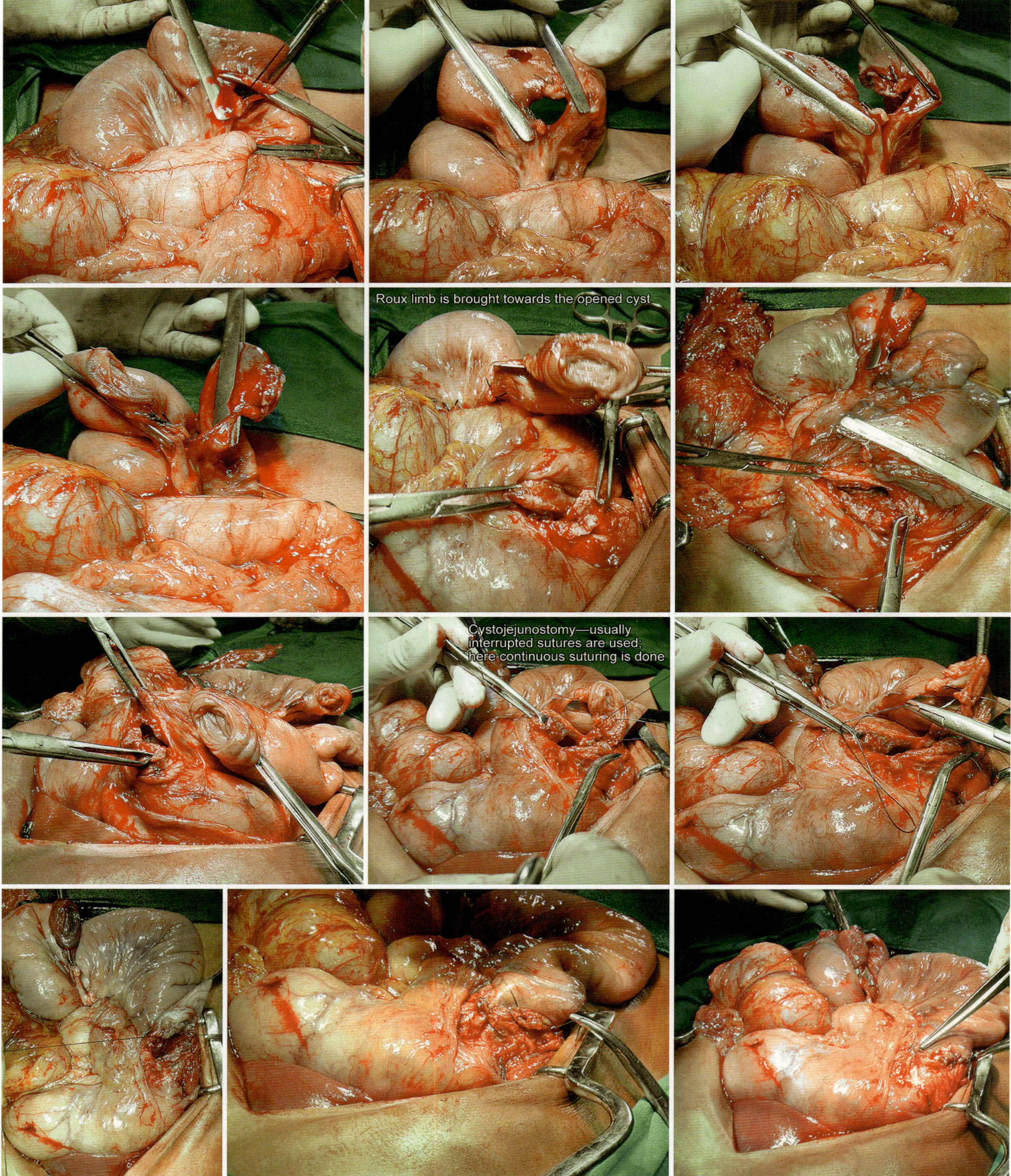
Roux limb is brought towards the opened cyst
Cystojejunostomy—usually interrupted sutures are used; here continuous suturing is done

Figs. 24-41(2)

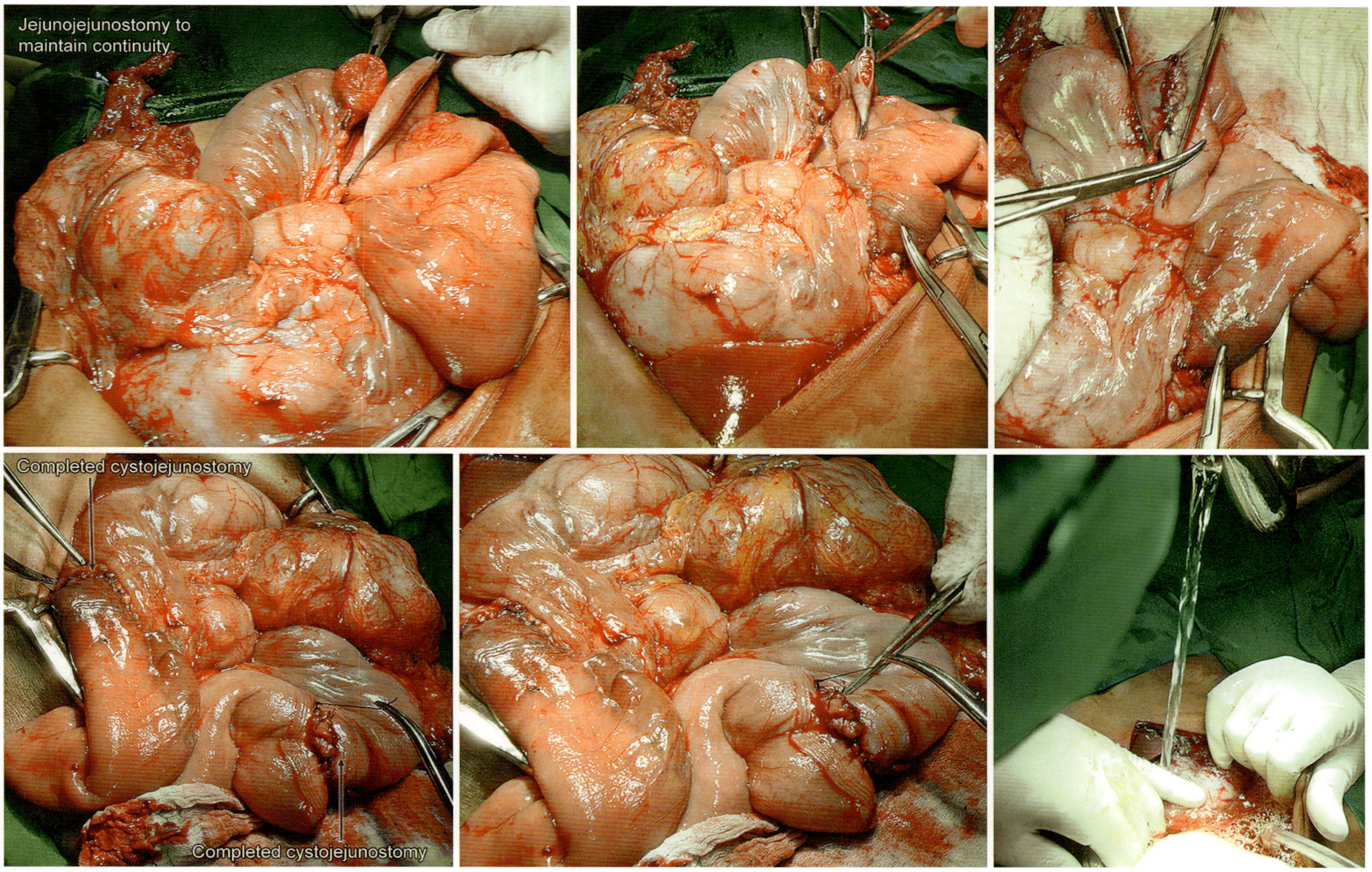

Figs. 24-41(3)

Figs. 24-41(1 to 3): Technique of cystojejunostomy for pseudocyst of pancreas.

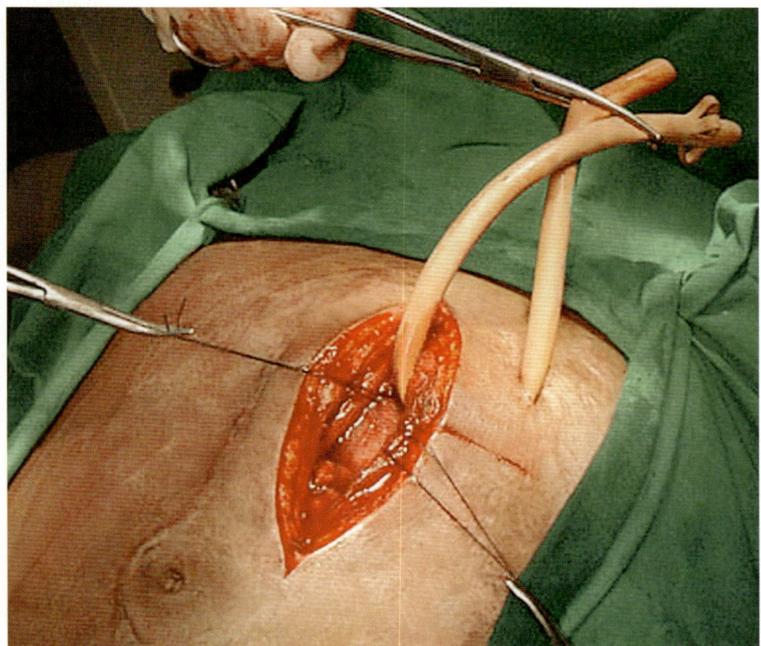

Fig. 24-42: When infected pseudocyst should be drained externally along with internal drainage (Smith).

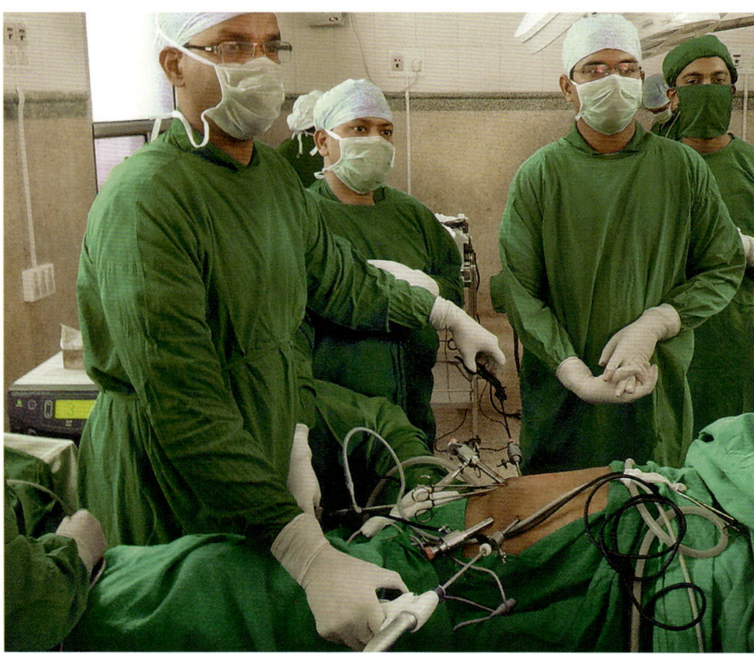

Fig. 24-43: Laparoscopic cystogastrostomy is a safe and effective method; technique and principles are the same. Intracorporeal suturing is needed.

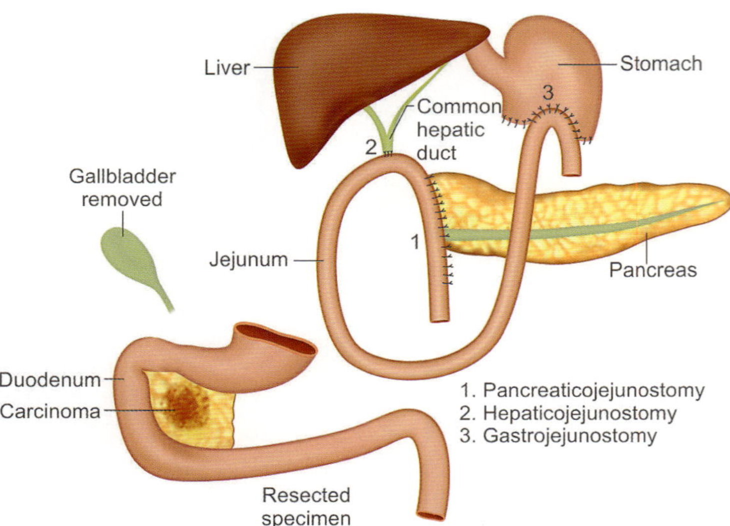

Fig. 24-44: Configuration of Whipple's operation.

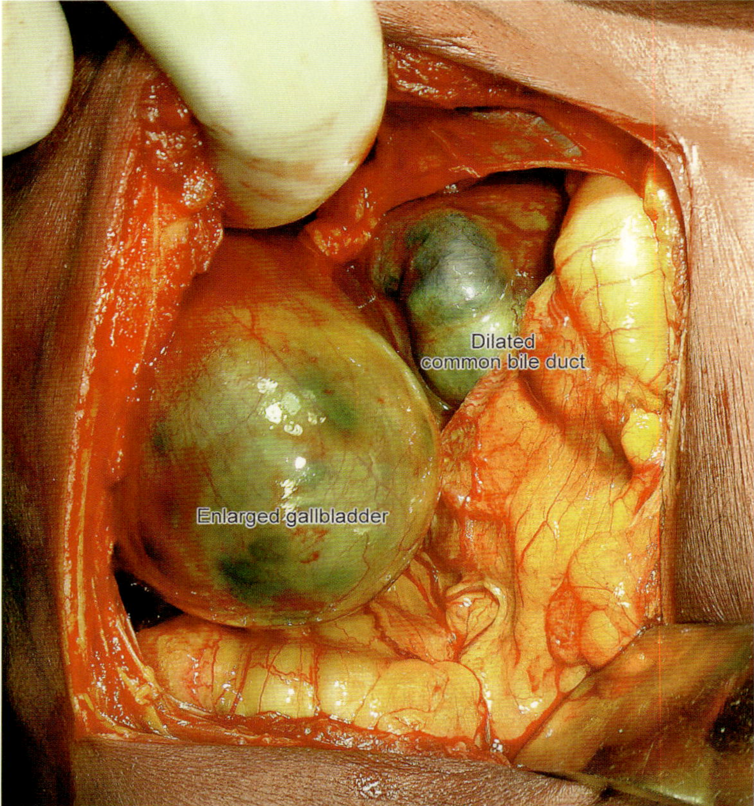

Fig. 24-45: Periampullary carcinoma with dilated CBD and gallbladder.

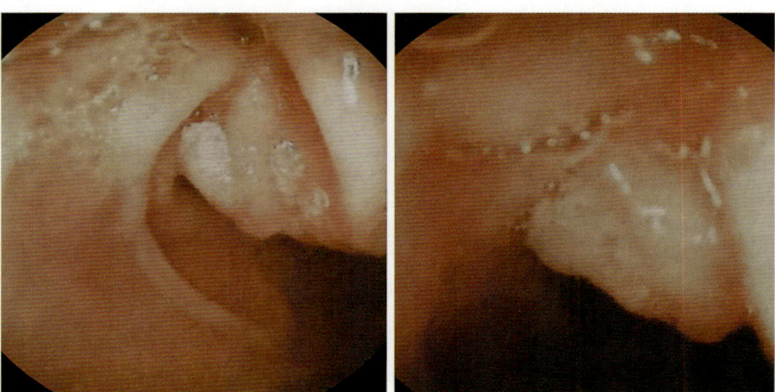

Fig. 24-46: Endoscopic view of periampullary carcinoma.

will prevent from proceeding with resection; just essential bypass will be sufficient. Middle colic vein when traced will help in identifying the SMV **(Figs. 24-47 and 24-48)**.

Dissection in this area should be careful and gentle as venous tear causes torrential bleeding and becomes time consuming to control bleeding. Duodenum is freed above up to foramen Winslow. Gastrohepatic ligament is dissected to identify proper hepatic artery after incising the peritoneum over it. Any lymph nodes identified are brought down towards the specimen. Gastroduodenal artery is identified which is a branch of common hepatic artery. It runs downwards under the 1st part of the duodenum on the surface of the head of the pancreas to divide into right gastroepiploic artery and superior pancreaticoduodenal artery. Gastroduodenal artery is divided between double silk ligatures. Once dissection proceeds medially, anterior surface of the portal vein is identified; anterior surface usually being avascular is dissected gently between it and neck of the pancreas downwards; similarly another index finger is passed from below between SMV and neck of the pancreas upwards to feel the other finger from above. But this is not sufficient to confirm the invasion; finger has to be passed under the 2nd part of the Kocherised duodenum with thumb in front to feel for invasion of the uncinate process and posterior wall of the portal vein and superior mesenteric vessels. Right gastric artery is also divided which is much smaller than the gastroduodenal artery. Incision of the peritoneum over the CBD allows clearing of the lymph nodes in the porta hepatis. Hepatic artery and CBD should be visualised properly after this part of the dissection. Cholecystectomy is performed. Common hepatic duct (CHD) is transected just above the joining of the cystic duct. CHD is temporarily occluded with a soft camp. It is a routine to do frozen section biopsy of the edge of the CHD and cystic duct in all patients whenever facilities are available. Antrectomy (with vagotomy if desired) is done now **(Figs. 24-49 to 24-52)**.

Division of the pancreas can be done now or after the mobilisation of the duodenojejunal loop and bringing the loop towards right underneath the superior mesenteric vessels. Pancreas is carefully mobilised towards the left of the portal vein and SMV at least for 3 cm. Small vessels entering the splenic vein should be carefully

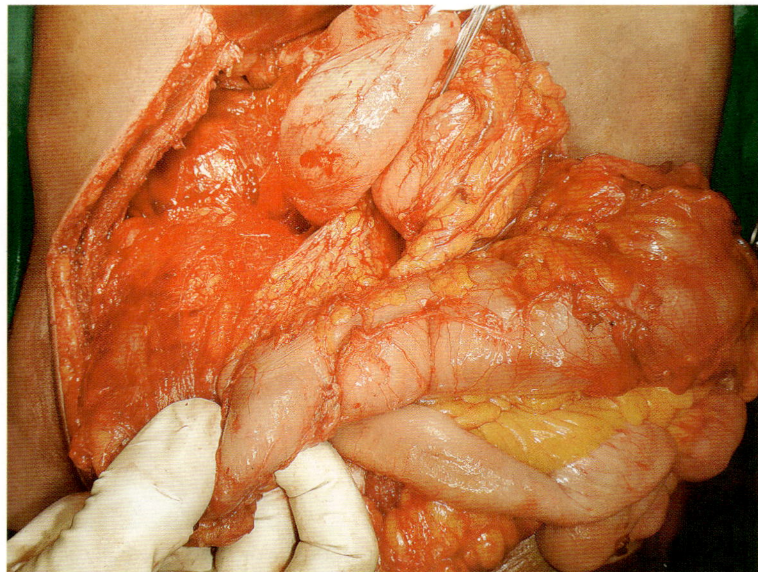

Fig. 24-47: Kocher's manoeuvre and Cattell-Braasch manoeuvre to mobilise the duodenum and right-sided colon.

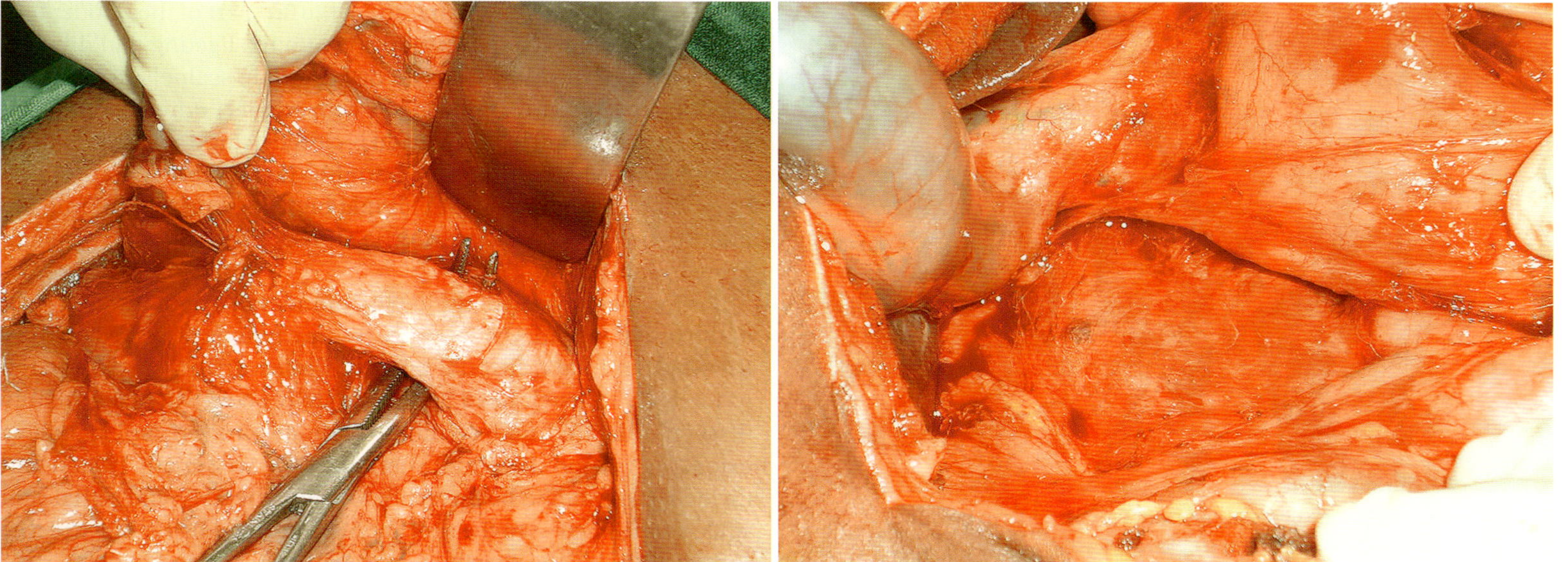

Fig. 24-48: Mobilisation of duodenum and colon in Whipple's operation.

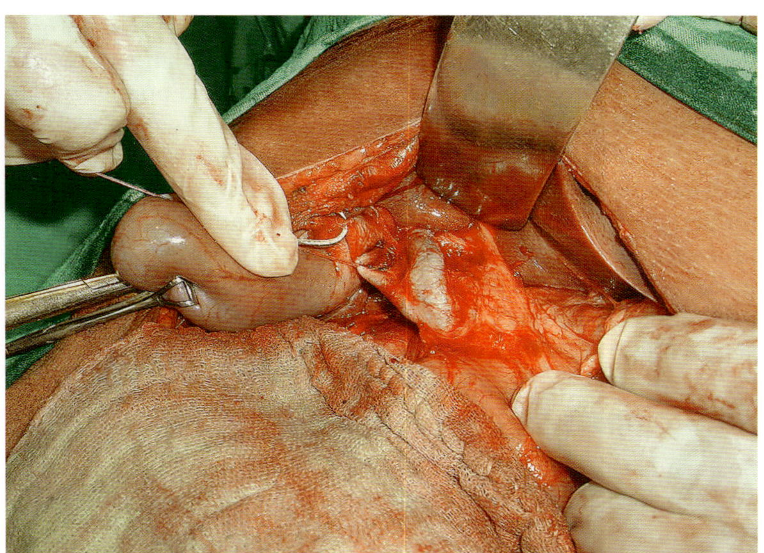

Fig. 24-49: Cholecystectomy is done during portal dissection in Whipple's operation.

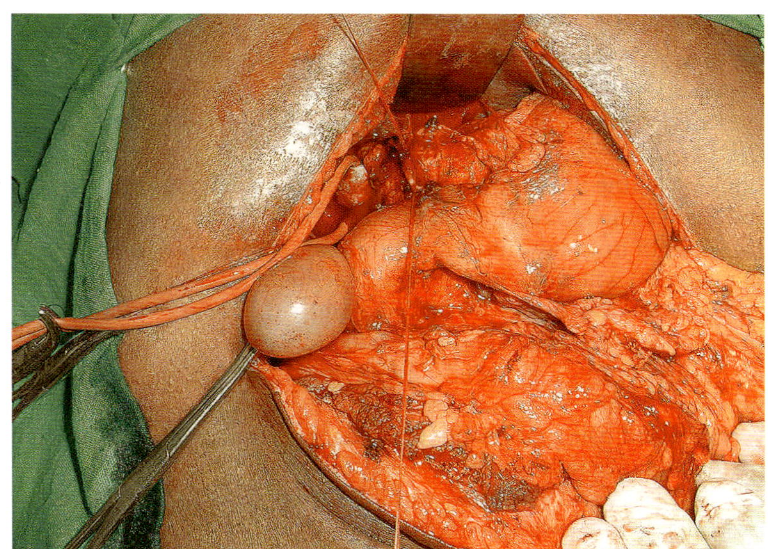

Fig. 24-50: Transection of bile duct and ligation of the gastroduodenal artery in Whipple's operation.

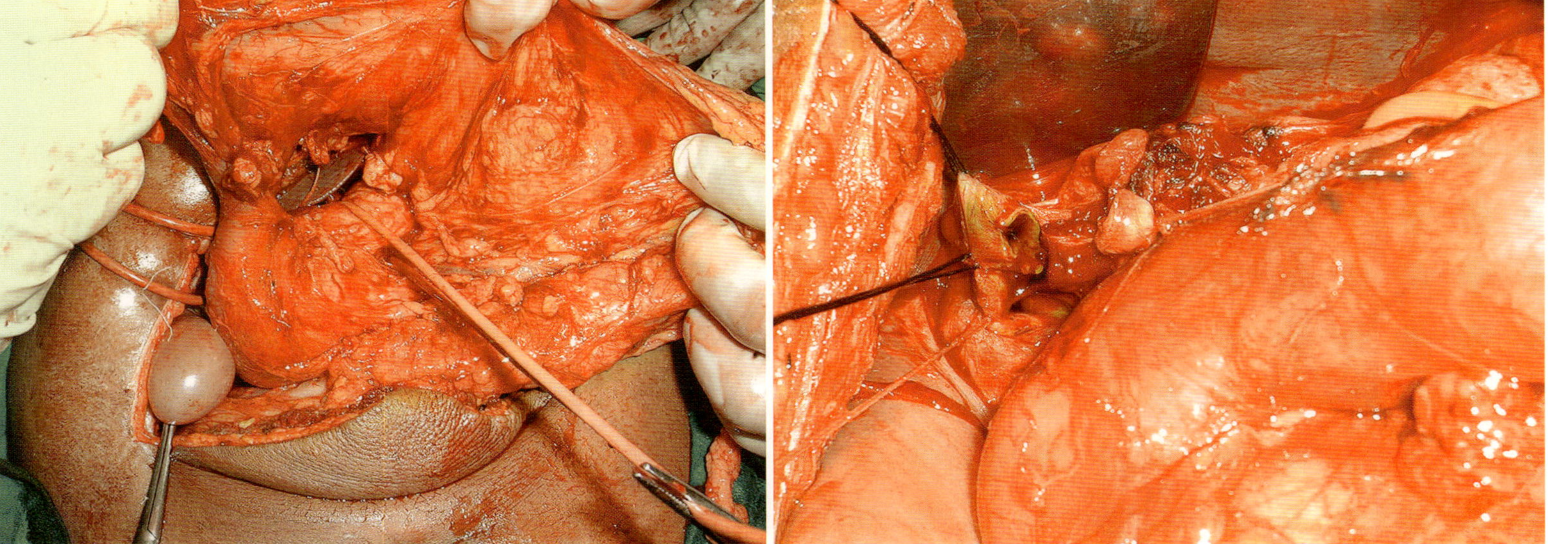

Fig. 24-51: Portal dissection in Whipple's operation.

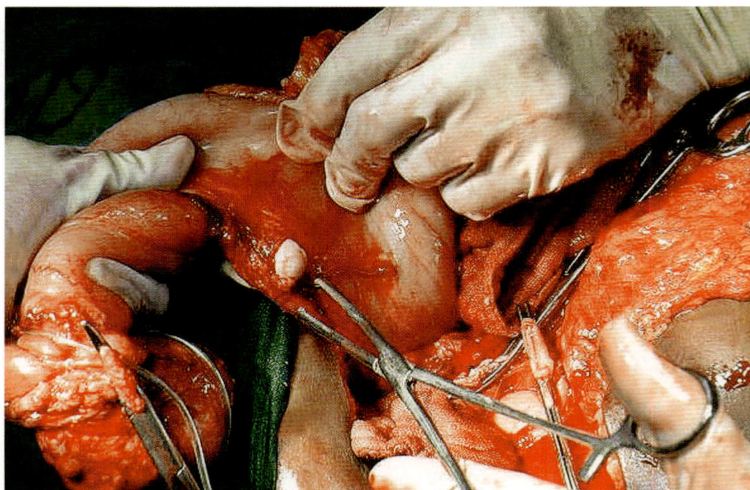

Fig. 24-52: Antrum is transected. Transection can be done using stapler device.

divided after ligation. Splenic vein located on undersurface of the distal pancreas should not be injured but should be separated for adequate length so that safe anastomosis of pancreas into the jejunum can be undertaken. Ligation of the superior and inferior pancreatic artery in the pancreas is needed prior to transecting the pancreas. Stapler transection of the neck of pancreas can be done left of the SMV level; pancreas need to be divided again left of the stapler line to keep the cut distal end open for later anastomosis. Cut margin from left side should be sent for frozen section biopsy. Stapled part will come towards the specimen. Alternatively two stay sutures using 3-zero vicryl is placed on the superior and inferior parts of the neck of the pancreas towards left and held apart and forward; often stay sutures are placed—2 front and 2 behind; flat instrument like scalpel knife is placed underneath to guard the portal vein; neck is transected using no. 15 blade under vision from below upwards; finger guidance underneath is also useful. Duct distally when dilated will be visible and is stented with a fine plastic tube temporarily to prevent it getting entangled with sutures **(Fig. 24-53)**.

Proximal 6 cm of the jejunum is dissected by separating it from jejunal vessels extending proximally along the ligament of Treitz towards the superior mesenteric vessels on the right side; SMV (right) and SMA (left) pass in front of the 3rd part of the duodenum; duodenojejunum is freed by serial clamping, ligating and dividing the vessels of this part; ligaseal or harmonic scalpel saves time if used here. Jejunum is transected with stapler; otherwise divided between clamps and proximal end is closed using 3-zero continuous or interrupted single layer or double layer sutures. 1st jejunal branch arising from the SMA should be ligated prior to sliding the duodenojejunum underneath the superior mesenteric vessels to bring towards right.

Entire specimen with duodenojejunum has come towards right of the portal system. Uncinate process is carefully dissected off from the SMA and SMV. Arterial branches often arise from SMA deep to the SMV to reach head and uncinate process which is carefully dissected, ligated and divided. Uncinate process and pancreas extending behind the portal vein and SMV are serially ligated and divided. Care should be taken not to injure the SMV and portal vein while giving traction to the specimen. Often it is a better practice that a surgeon holds the specimen with his left hand and with his right hand, he dissects, allowing the assistant to pass a polypropylene or silk ligature through a right-angled Mixter forceps and ligate it towards left side; opposite specimen side can be divided without ligature as surgeon is holding it firmly. All veins draining from the pancreas towards the right margin of the SMV and portal vein are ligated similarly and divided. Dividing without ligation will end with unnecessary bleeding and as such delays the procedure rather than hastening it. SMV should be retracted using gentle curved vein retractor towards left to visualise the SMA under which uncinate process ends. This dissection is carried out from below upwards. It is again better to do frozen section biopsy of the uncinate process to confirm the adequacy of resection as far as clearance is considered **(Fig. 24-54)**.

Anastomoses Parts

First pancreaticojejunal anastomosis is done usually as end to side; *then* hepaticojejunostomy is done; *later* antecolic gastrojejunostomy is done.

Distal transected jejunal loop is brought through the transverse mesocolon window towards pancreatic region. *Pancreaticojejunostomy* is done by different methods—(1) When pancreatic

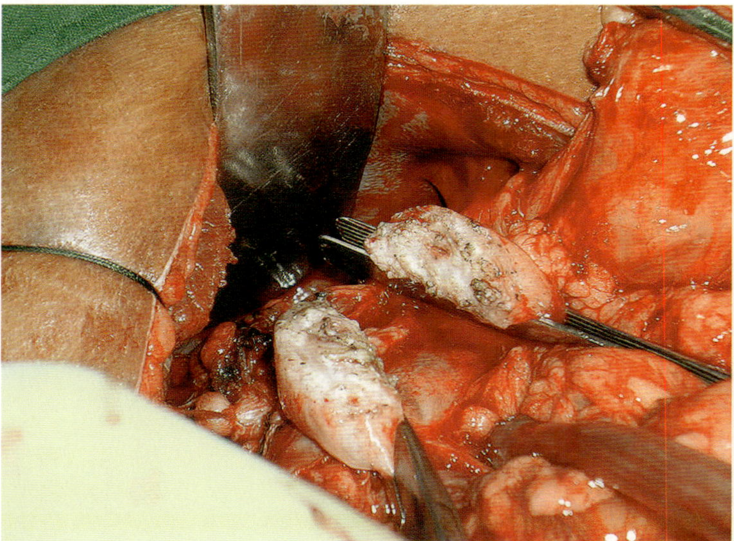

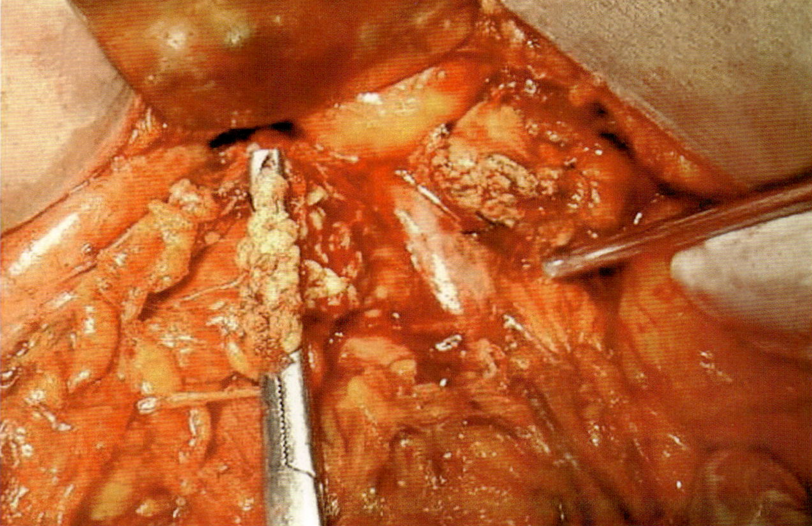

Fig. 24-53: Transection of the neck of pancreas in Whipple's operation.

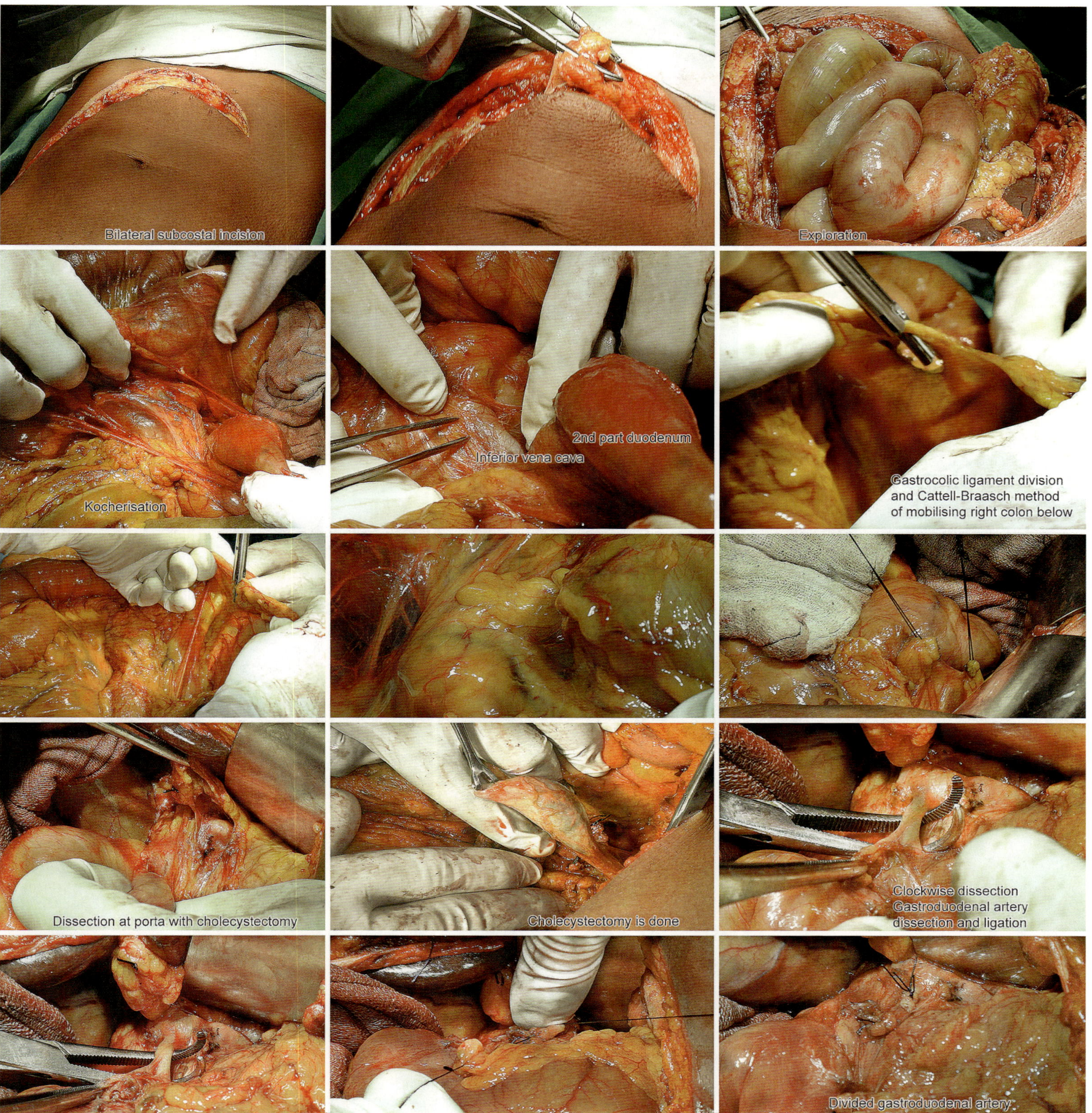
Bilateral subcostal incision
Exploration
Kocherisation
2nd part duodenum
Inferior vena cava
Gastrocolic ligament division
and Cattell-Braasch method
of mobilising right colon below
Dissection at porta with cholecystectomy
Cholecystectomy is done
Clockwise dissection
Gastroduodenal artery
dissection and ligation
Divided gastroduodenal artery

Figs. 24-54(1)

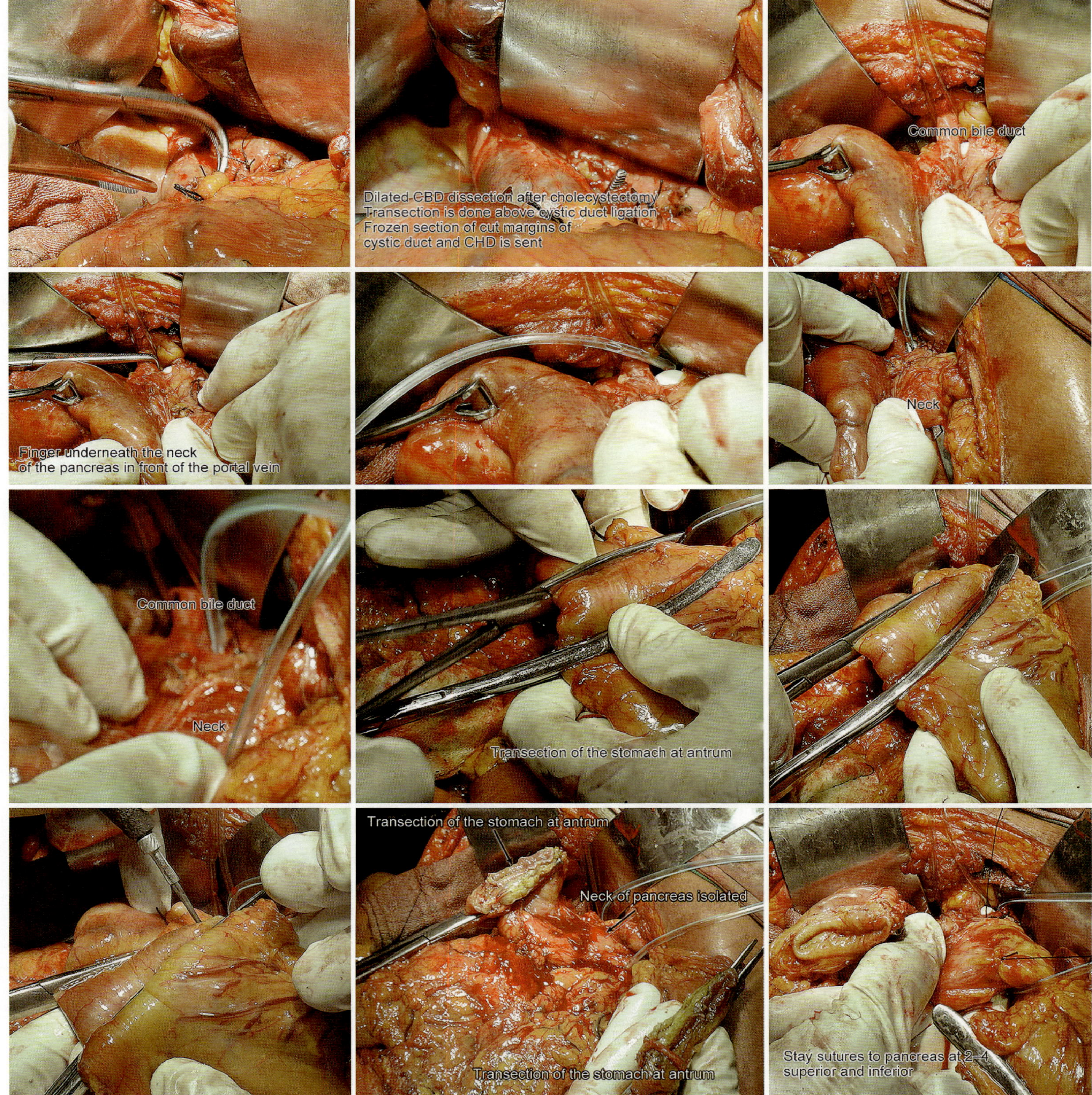
Dilated CBD dissection after cholecystectomy
Transection is done above cystic duct ligation
Frozen section of cut margins of cystic duct and CHD is sent
Common bile duct
Finger underneath the neck of the pancreas in front of the portal vein
Neck
Common bile duct
Neck
Transection of the stomach at antrum
Transection of the stomach at antrum
Neck of pancreas isolated
Transection of the stomach at antrum
Stay sutures to pancreas at 2–4 superior and inferior

Figs. 24-54(2)

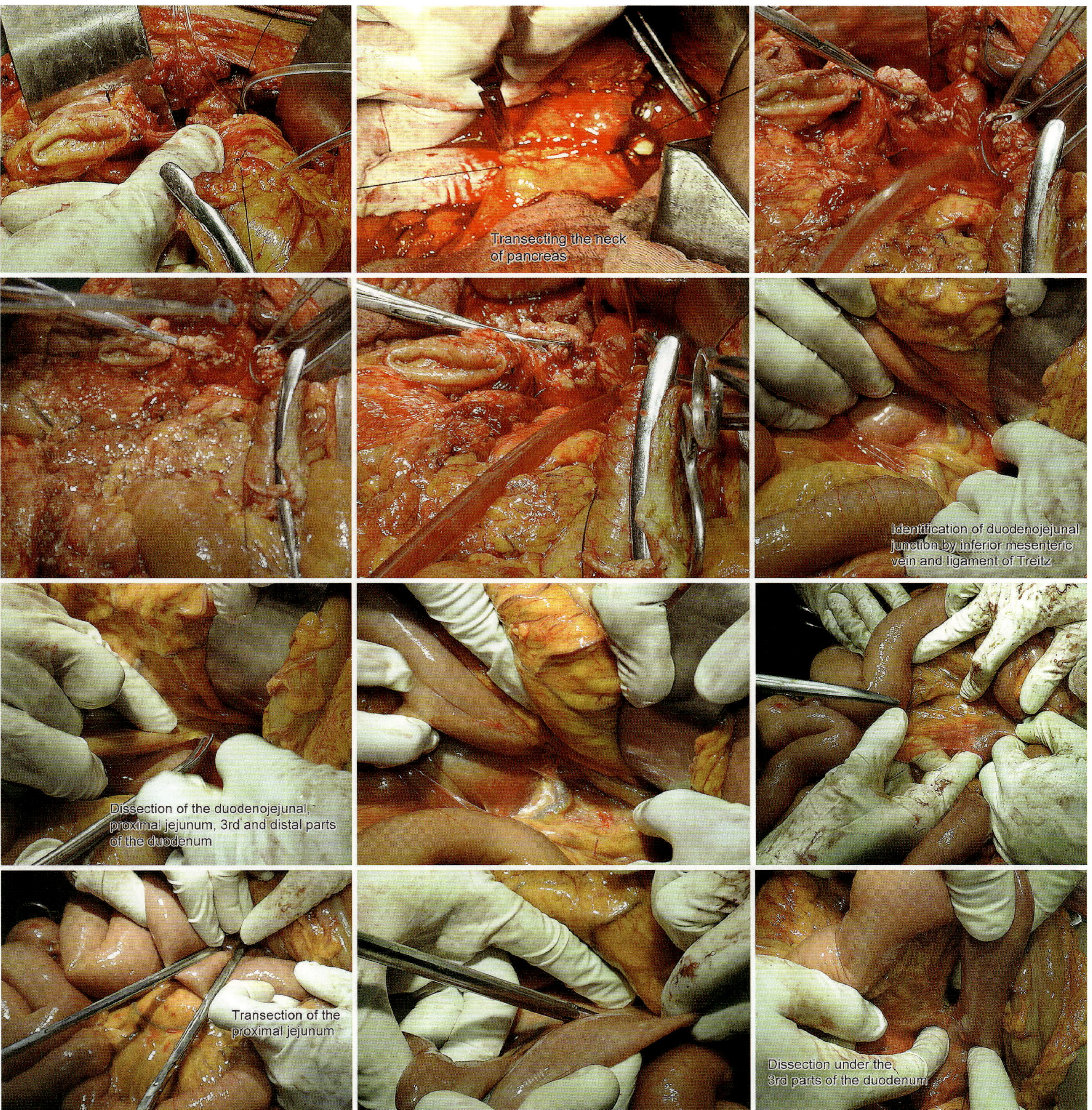
Transecting the neck of pancreas
Identification of duodenojejunal junction by inferior mesenteric vein and ligament of Treitz
Dissection of the duodenojejunal, proximal jejunum, 3rd and distal parts of the duodenum
Transection of the proximal jejunum
Dissection under the 3rd parts of the duodenum

Figs. 24-54(3)

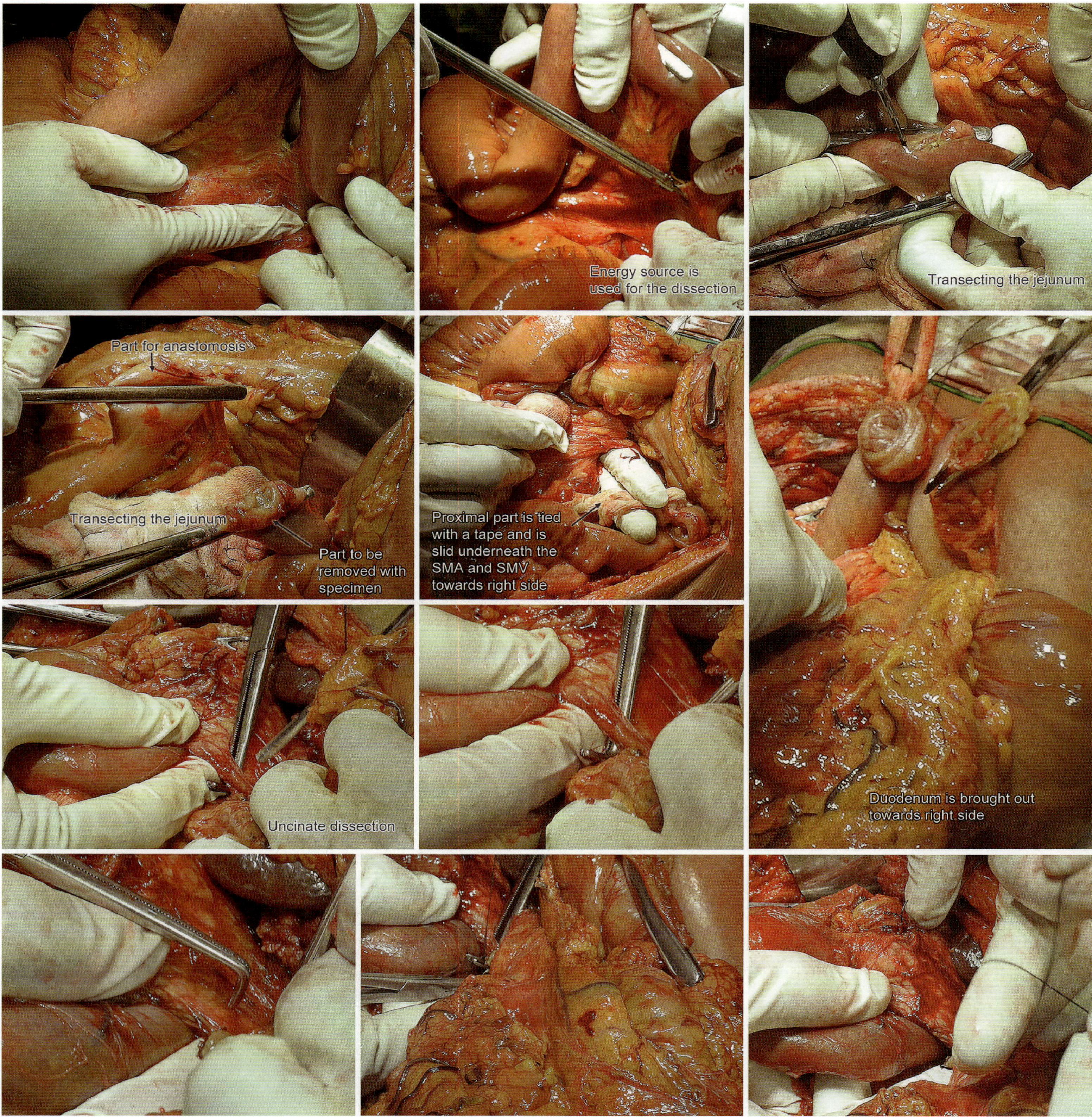
Energy source is
used for the dissection
Transecting the jejunum
Part for anastomosis
Transecting the jejunum
Part to be
removed with
specimen
Proximal part is tied
with a tape and is
slid underneath the
SMA and SMV
towards right side
Uncinate dissection
Duodenum is brought out
towards right side

Figs. 24-54(4)

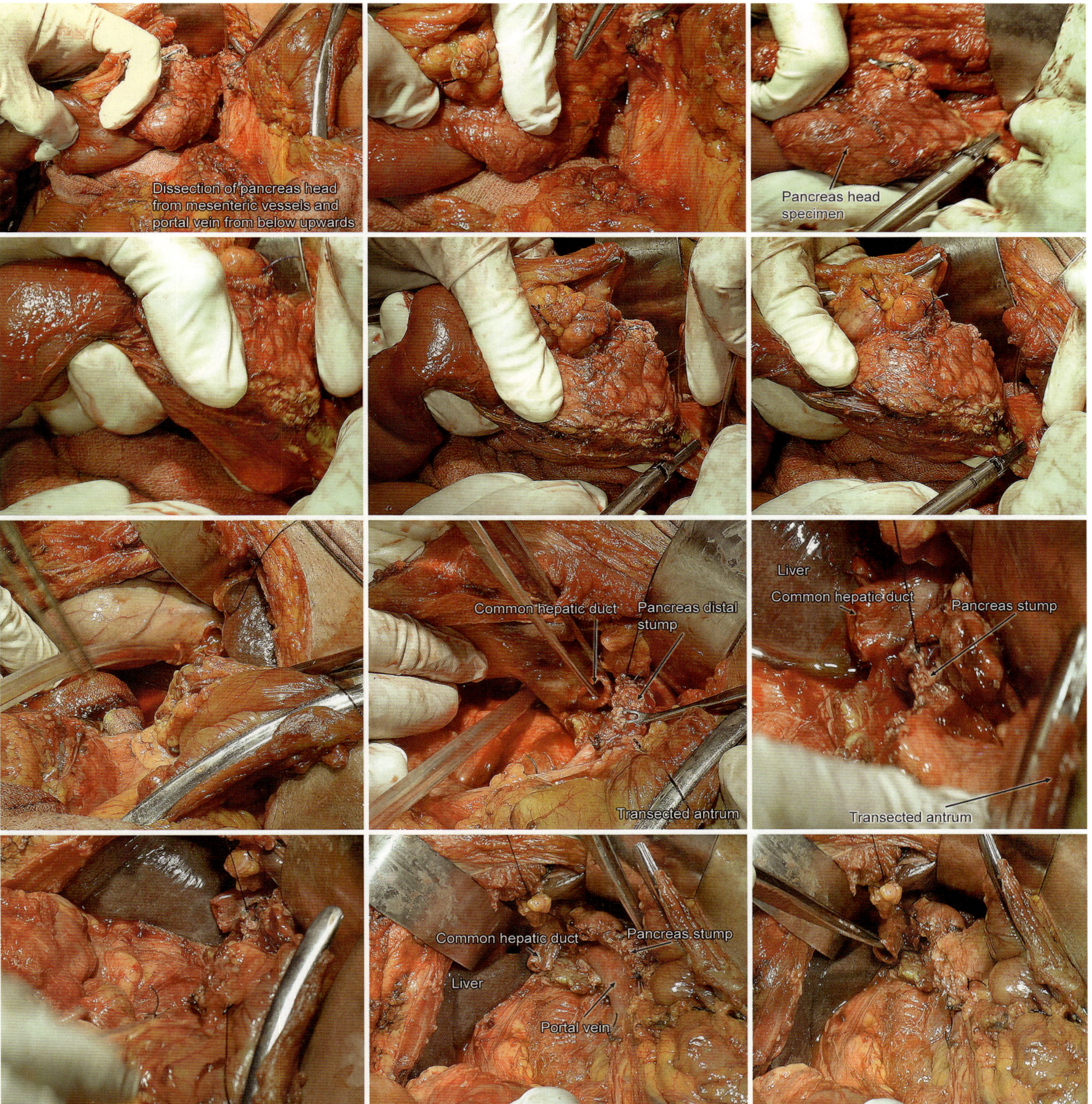

Dissection of pancreas head from mesenteric vessels and portal vein from below upwards
Pancreas head specimen
Common hepatic duct
Pancreas distal stump
Transected antrum
Liver
Common hepatic duct
Pancreas stump
Transected antrum
Common hepatic duct
Pancreas stump
Liver
Portal vein

Figs. 24-54(5)

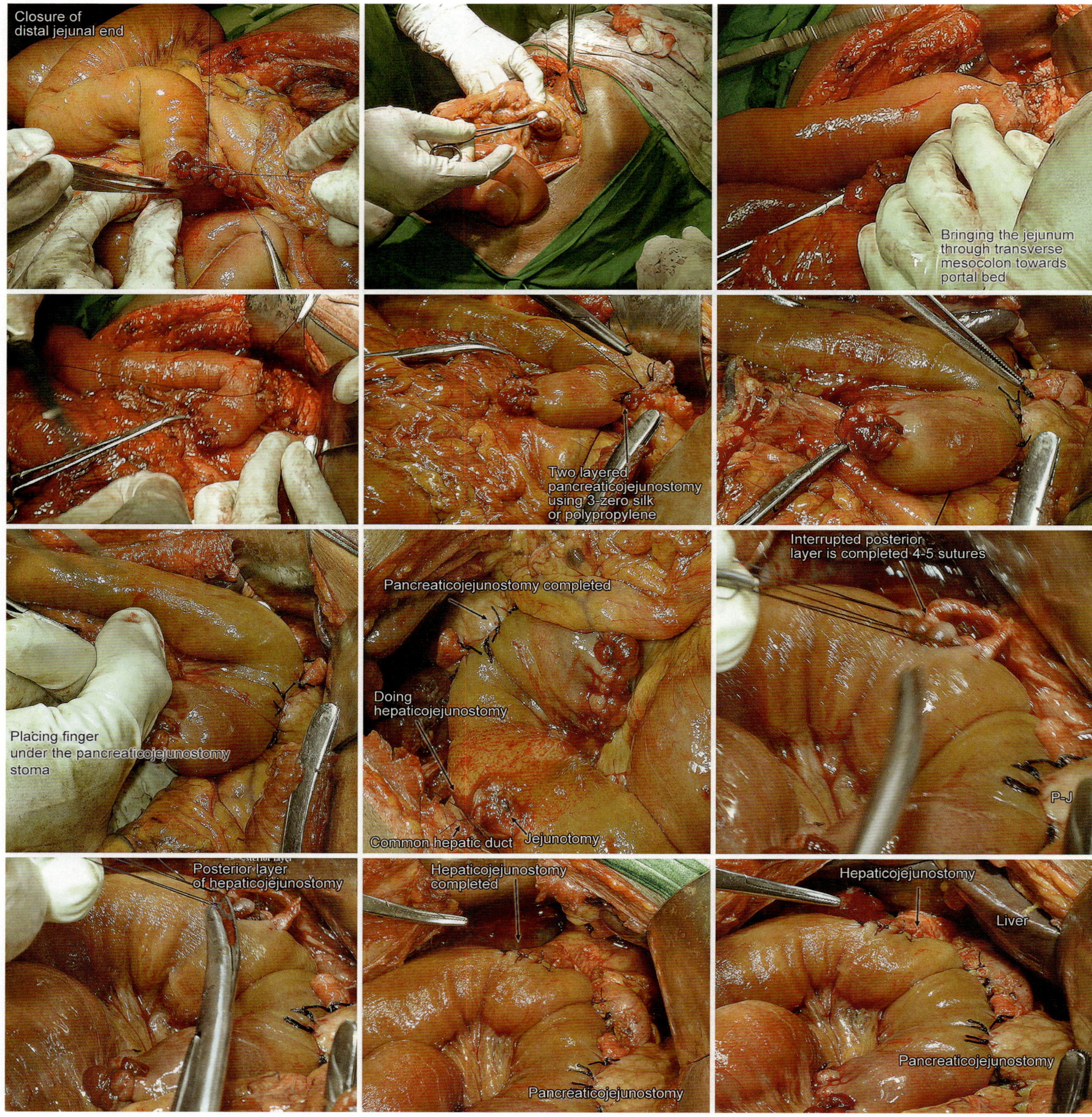
Closure of
distal jejunal end
Bringing the jejunum
through transverse
mesocolon towards
portal bed
Two layered
pancreaticojejunostomy
using 3-zero silk
or polypropylene
Placing finger
under the pancreaticojejunostomy
stoma
Pancreaticojejunostomy completed
Doing
hepaticojejunostomy
Common hepatic duct
Jejunotomy
Interrupted posterior
layer is completed 4-5 sutures
P-J
Posterior layer
of hepaticojejunostomy
Hepaticojejunostomy
completed
Pancreaticojejunostomy
Hepaticojejunostomy
Liver
Pancreaticojejunostomy

Figs. 24-54(6)

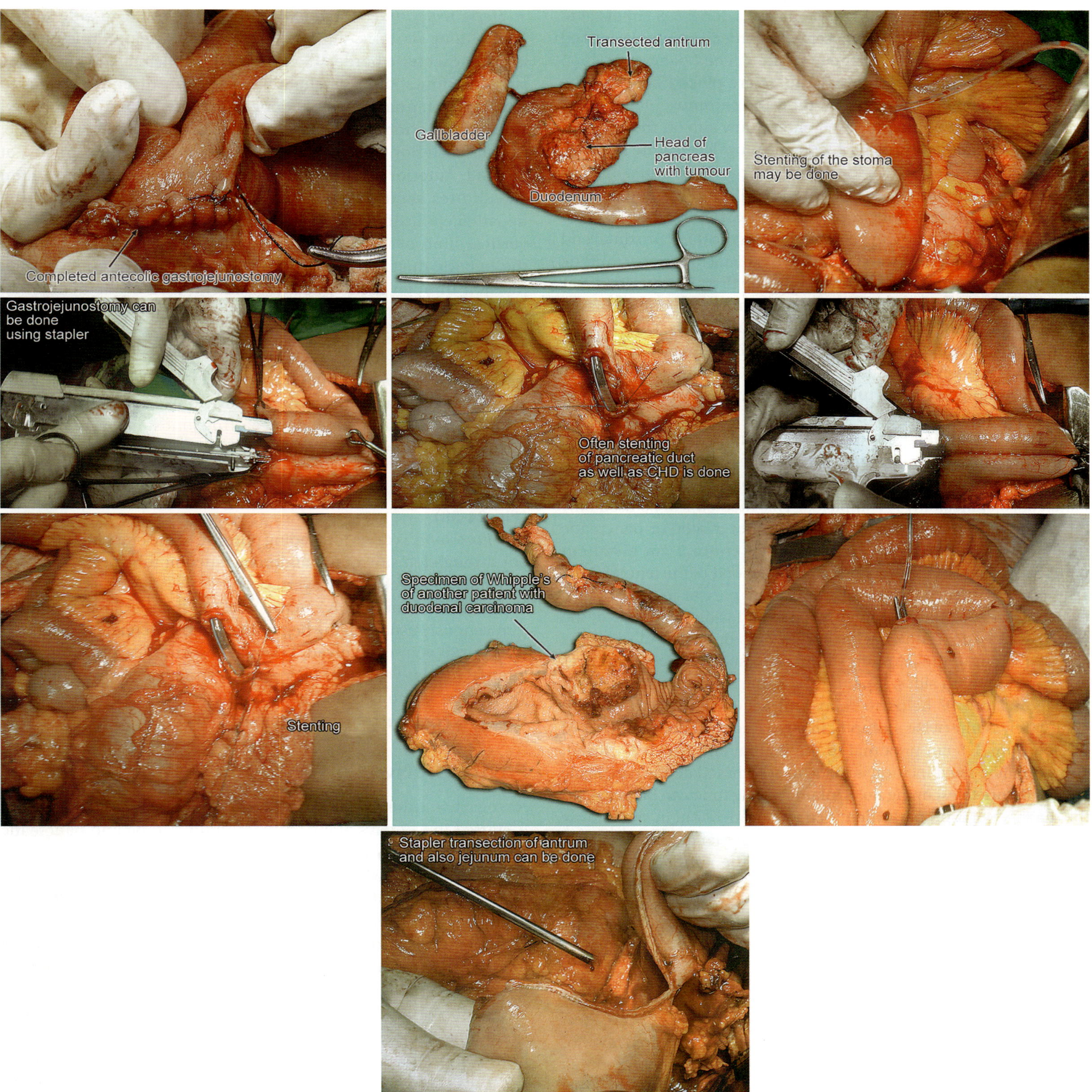

Figs. 24-54(7)

Figs. 24-54(1 to 7): Technique of pancreaticoduodenectomy—steps.

duct is dilated duct to mucosa anastomosis is done; 3–5 cm distal to the stapled line along the antimesenteric border, jejunum is opened slightly lengthier than the diameter of the opened pancreatic duct; prior to enterotomy interrupted sutures are placed between the posterior capsule of the pancreas and the seromuscular layer of the posterior part of the proposed enterotomy site on the jejunum (posterior to enterotomy) using 4-zero polypropylene suture material. 5-6 such sutures are needed. Posterior layer pancreatic duct mucosa is sutured to the full thickness jejunum with interrupted sutures using 5-zero or 6-zero polypropylene or PDS suture material. Fine no. 8 infant feeding tube can be passed across the duct; proximal end is brought out through a stab wound 10 cm distal to the anastomotic site and also brought out of the abdominal wall; anterior layer duct mucosa full thickness jejunum anastomosis is done similarly; magnifying lens may be useful for ductal anastomosis. Duct may be fixed to pancreas and jejunal edge by a single 6-zero vicryl. Anterior pancreatic capsules to seromuscular jejunal interrupted sutures are placed. Stenting of ductal tube done which was brought out and fixed to jejunum with 5-zero vicryl sutures and this jejunal point is fixed to the parietal abdominal wall with 4-zero silk sutures. This stent also can be brought out through the proximal cut end of the jejunal stump through a separate stab incision similarly. End-to-side pancreaticojejunostomy is completed. This method can be used only for end-to-side anastomosis. (2) If duct is not dilated or pancreatic tissue is friable to take suture bites, then entire 2 cm distal cut pancreatic stump is invaginated into the cut end of the jejunal limb. Telescopic sutures are passed from outer part of jejunum 2 cm from the cut edge into its lumen, then from inside to outside of the pancreatic tissue; returning back from outside inside of pancreas and inside out of the jejunum stump. Two such telescopic sutures are placed on both sides. If pancreatic stump is too bulky, injection glucagon 1 mg IV helps to relax and accommodate the stump adequately. Otherwise stump is invaginated to the lateral part of the jejunum 3–5 cm proximal to the jejunal end which is closed; corresponding sized incision is made to accommodate the pancreatic stump. Before telescoping no. 8 infant feeding tube can be placed in the duct if duct is properly identified and brought out in similar way 10 cm proximally. If duct is too small, it is not mandatory to stent or suture the duct as proper telescoping of the pancreas with two layers of interrupted, sutures both posteriorly and anteriorly, is sufficient without any problem. When these telescopic sutures are pulled in, pancreatic stump gets invaginated automatically into the jejunum; these telescoping sutures are not tied. Cut edge of the pancreas telescoped inside is sutured again to the bowel wall at 2 cm distance with interrupted polypropylene 4-zero sutures—circumferentially. All sutures round are placed then later tied together. Telescoping sutures are tied now. Next layer of the anastomosis is done between the cut edge of the jejunum as full thickness and the pancreatic capsule as interrupted sutures. This method is used for either side or end of the jejunal limb. (3) Another method is to place the posterior seromuscular layer of the jejunum to the pancreatic capsule 2 cm away from the cut margin; then 2nd posterior full thickness jejunum to the pancreatic cut edge with or without including the posterior edge of the duct; 3rd layer is anterior full thickness bowel wall to the cut edge of the pancreatic stump with or without taking bites from anterior part of the duct; 4th layer is seromuscular bite from the bowel 2 cm from the earlier layer and from the pancreatic capsule at corresponding distance. This method is used for either side or end of the jejunal limb **(Fig. 24-55)**.

Hepaticojejunal anastomosis is done as end-to-side of the jejunal loop on to its antimesenteric border. Jejunum is opened at antimesenteric border 15 cm from the pancreaticojejunostomy site; incision should be slightly lesser than or equal to that of hepatic duct. Anastomosis is done using interrupted 4-zero vicryl sutures; posterior layer sutures are placed first with knots outside; first all posterior suture bites are taken and then knots are tied at the end. Anterior layer is sutured with knots outside. Every 3 mm gap sutures should be placed. If surgeon wants stenting of the hepaticojejunostomy, then prior to placing sutures, longitudinal/vertical limb of no. 14 F 'T' tube is passed through cut end of the hepatic duct proximally and is brought out through a small incision through the hepatic duct outside and of the abdominal wall through a separate stab wound. This drains bile outside and also promotes healing of the pancreaticojejunostomy **(Figs. 24-56 and 24-57)**.

Gastrojejunostomy is done 20 cm distal to the hepaticojejunostomy as an antecolic anastomosis. As already stomach is transected with stapler earlier during procedure, gastrojejunostomy is done using linear stapler device just proximal and posterior to the stapled line. Single layer 3-zero vicryl hand sewn anastomosis also can be done after doing gastrotomy and corresponding jejunotomy **(Fig. 24-58)**.

Jejunostomy is done for feeding purpose at the end and is brought out through left side of the abdomen. Suction tube drain is placed and abdomen is closed in layers.

On table intraoperative octreotide 100 micrograms is injected intravenously usually at the beginning of the pancreatic resection.

If portal vein is involved, vascular resection can be done with internal jugular vein *(IJV) interposition graft*; usually from left side. Technique is often called as ***extended Whipple's operation or Fortner's regional pancreatectomy***.

Postoperative Care

Nasogastric tube is removed in 5–7 days; jejunostomy feeding is started in 5–7 days along with oral fluid. T-tube and pancreatic tube are kept for 21 days. Antibiotics are given. TPN may be needed. Daily monitoring with liver function, renal function, haemogram (with platelet count) and prothrombin time is needed. CVP line is better for all these purposes, as hypotension is common in immediate postoperative period despite less bleeding on table, which is due to lot of fluid loss into 3rd space. So patient needs adequate fluid therapy to combat this. Intravenous octreotide is given daily either as infusion or at regular intervals for 5 days to reduce pancreatic secretions. Pancreatic leak can be identified as clear fluid leak from the drain. It may subside spontaneously; but often needs 1-2 litres saline wash daily. If it persists and condition of patient deteriorates, then relaparotomy may be done to remove the remaining pancreas including spleen to save the life of the patient **(Figs. 24-59 and 24-60)**.

The Surgical Resection is Divided into the following Six Clearly Defined Steps

1. ***A Cattell-Braasch* manoeuvre** is performed by mobilising the right colon and incising the visceral peritoneum to the ligament of Treitz. When complete, this manoeuvre allows retraction of right colon and small bowel downward and towards right exposing

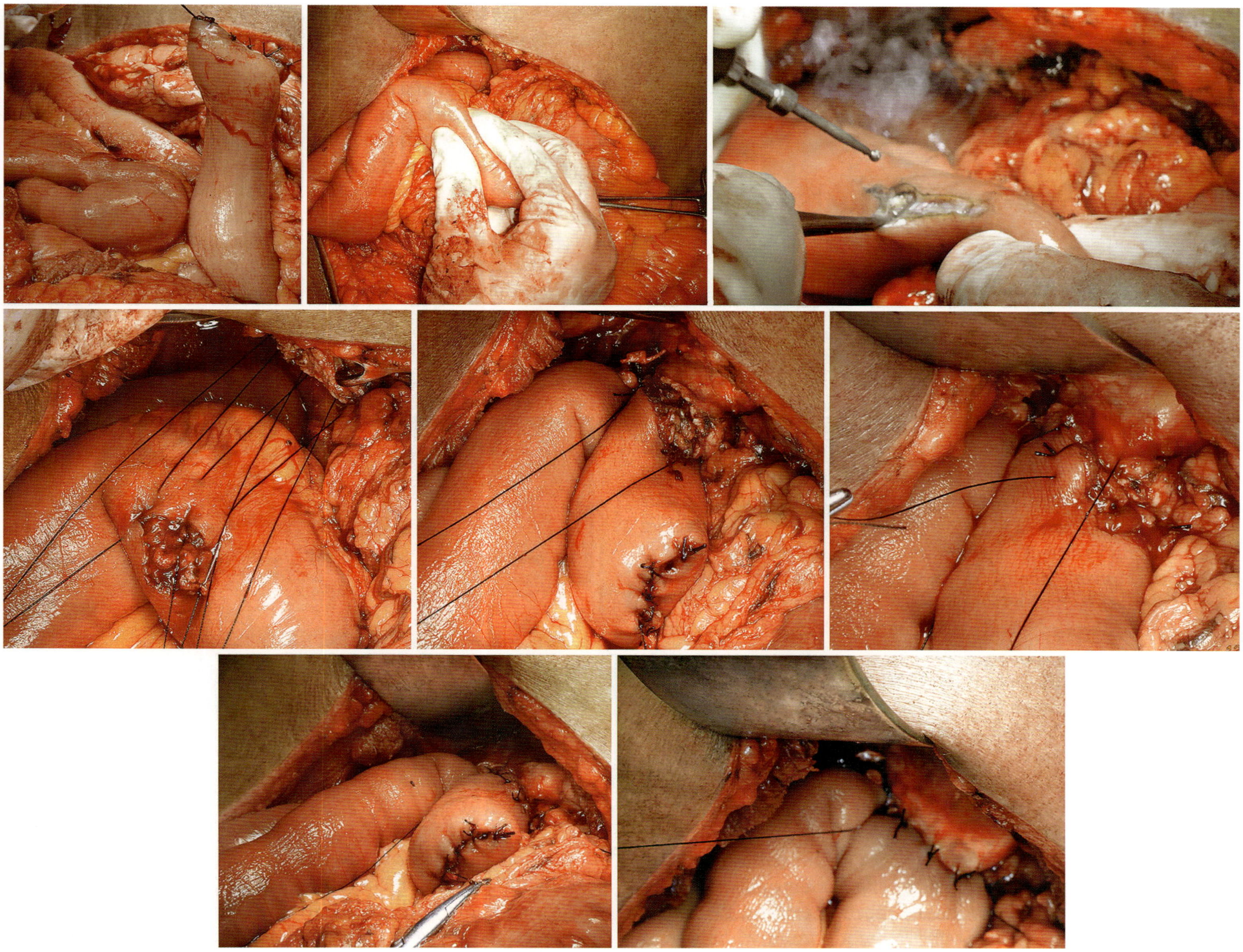

Fig. 24-55: Pancreaticojejunostomy in Whipple's operation.

the third and fourth parts of duodenum. The omental bursa is entered by taking the greater omentum from the transverse colon. The middle colic vein is identified, ligated and divided before its junction with the SMV. This allows greater exposure of the infrapancreatic SMV and prevents iatrogenic injury during dissection of the middle colic vein—MV junction.

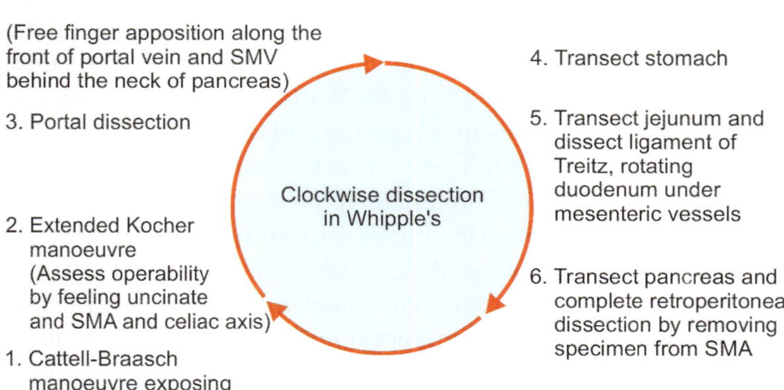

2. ***The Kocher's manoeuvre*** is begun at the junction of the ureter and the right gonadal vein. The right gonadal vein is ligated and divided, and all fibro fatty and lymphatic structures overlying the medial aspect of the right kidney and inferior vena cava is removed with the specimen. The Kocher's manoeuvre is continued to the lateral edge of the aorta (extended Kocher manoeuvre), carefully identifying the left renal vein. Traditionally, the relation of the tumour to the SMA is assessed by manual palpation following a complete Kocher manoeuvre.
3. ***The portal dissection*** is initiated by exposing the common hepatic artery proximal and distal to the gastroduodenal artery. The gastroduodenal artery is then ligated and divided. Two large lymph nodes are commonly encountered during portal dissection, removal of this en-block with the specimen is necessary to adequately mobilise the hepatic artery and portal vein. The gallbladder is dissected out of the liver bed and the common bile duct transected just cephalad to its junction with the cystic duct. The anterior wall of the portal vein is easily exposed following division of common hepatic duct and medial retraction of the

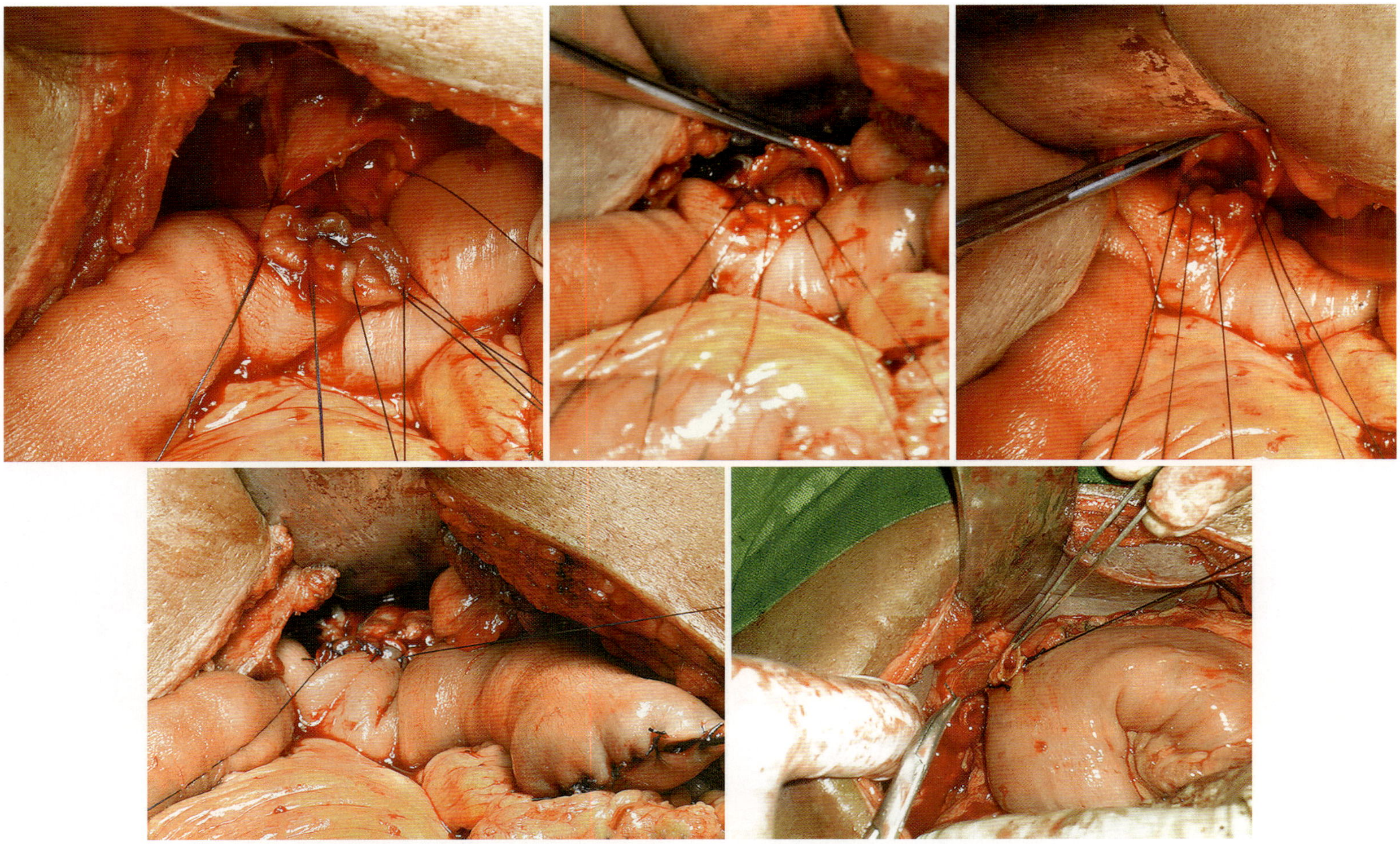

Fig. 24-56: Hepaticojejunostomy in Whipple's operation.

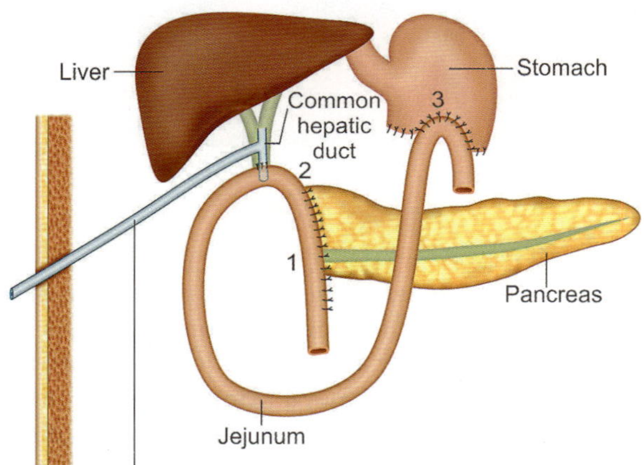

T-tube is placed along the CHD if needed
1. Pancreaticojejunostomy
2. Hepaticojejunostomy
3. Gastrojejunostomy

Fig. 24-57: T-tube may be placed in the CHD and across the hepaticojejunostomy if needed; but it is not mandatory.

common hepatic artery. Bleeding caused by injury to posterior superior pancreaticoduodenal vein may be difficult to control at this point in the operation. Portal vein should be mobilised after stomach and pancreas have been divided as in step 6. The portal dissection is made more difficult in the presence of anomalous hepatic arterial circulation, particularly in reoperative cases when preoperative arteriography is of help.

4. The stomach is transected at the level of third or fourth transverse vein on the lesser curvature and at the confluence of the gastroepiploic veins on the greater curvature. The omentum is divided at the level of the greater curvature transection.
5. The jejunum is transected approximately 10 cm distal to the ligament of Treitz, and its mesentery is sequentially ligated and divided. The duodenal mesentery is similarly divided to the level of aorta, and duodenum and jejunum are then reflected beneath mesenteric vessels.
6. After traction sutures are placed on the superior and inferior borders of the pancreas using 2-zero silk (this is important to reduce bleeding from marginal vessels during transection), the pancreas is transected with an electrocautery at the level of portal vein. If there is an evidence of tumour adherence to the portal vein or the SMV, the pancreas can be resected at a more distant location in preparation for segmental venous resection. The specimen is cleared from SMV and often SMA depending on its posterior extension by ligating and dividing small venous tributaries to the uncinate process and pancreatic head. Complete resection of the uncinate process along with medial retraction of the superior mesenteric-portal vein confluence facilitates exposure of the SMA, which is then dissected out to its origin at the aorta. Frozen section analysis of the pancreatic and common hepatic duct transection margin is obtained. Positive resection margins mandate further resection until clear margins are achieved.

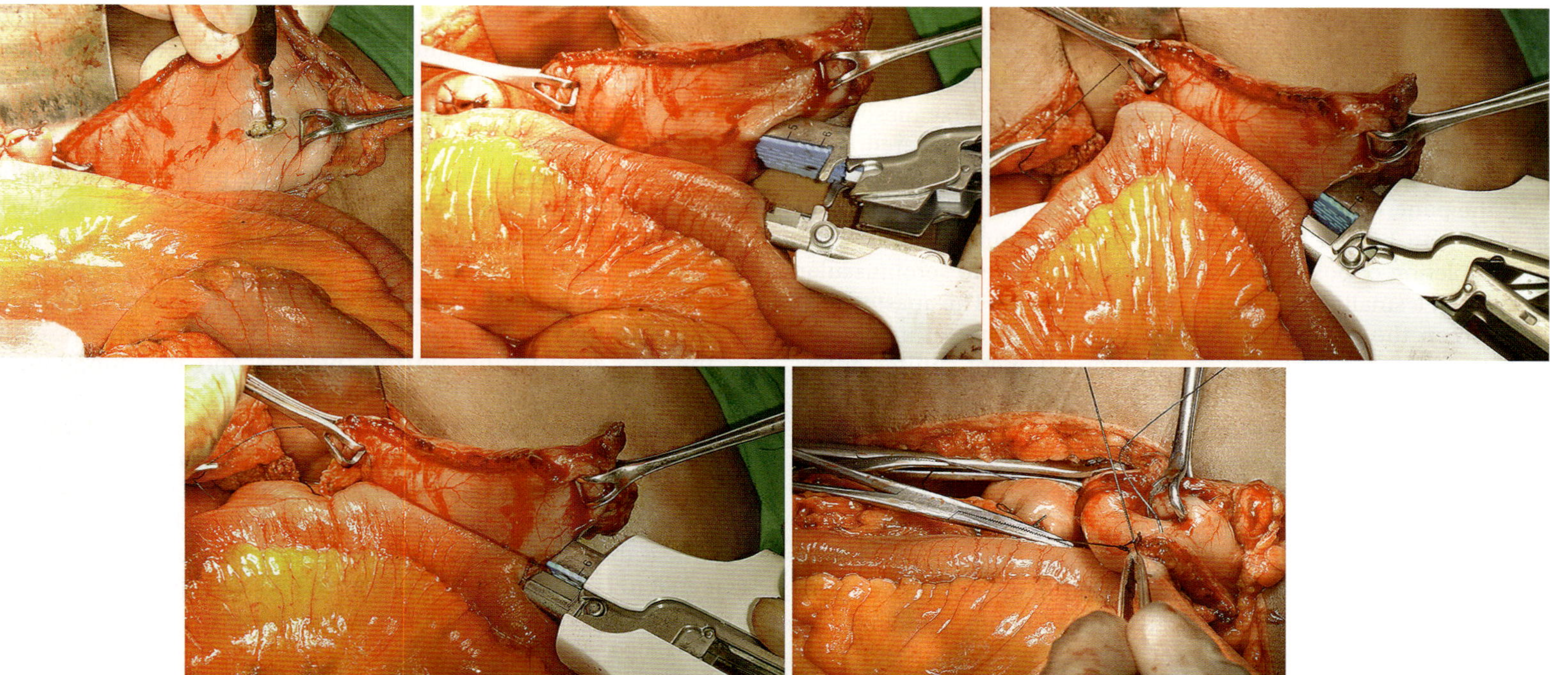

Fig. 24-58: Gastrojejunostomy in Whipple's operation. It can be hand-sewn or by using stapler on the posterior surface of the earlier transected part of the stomach.

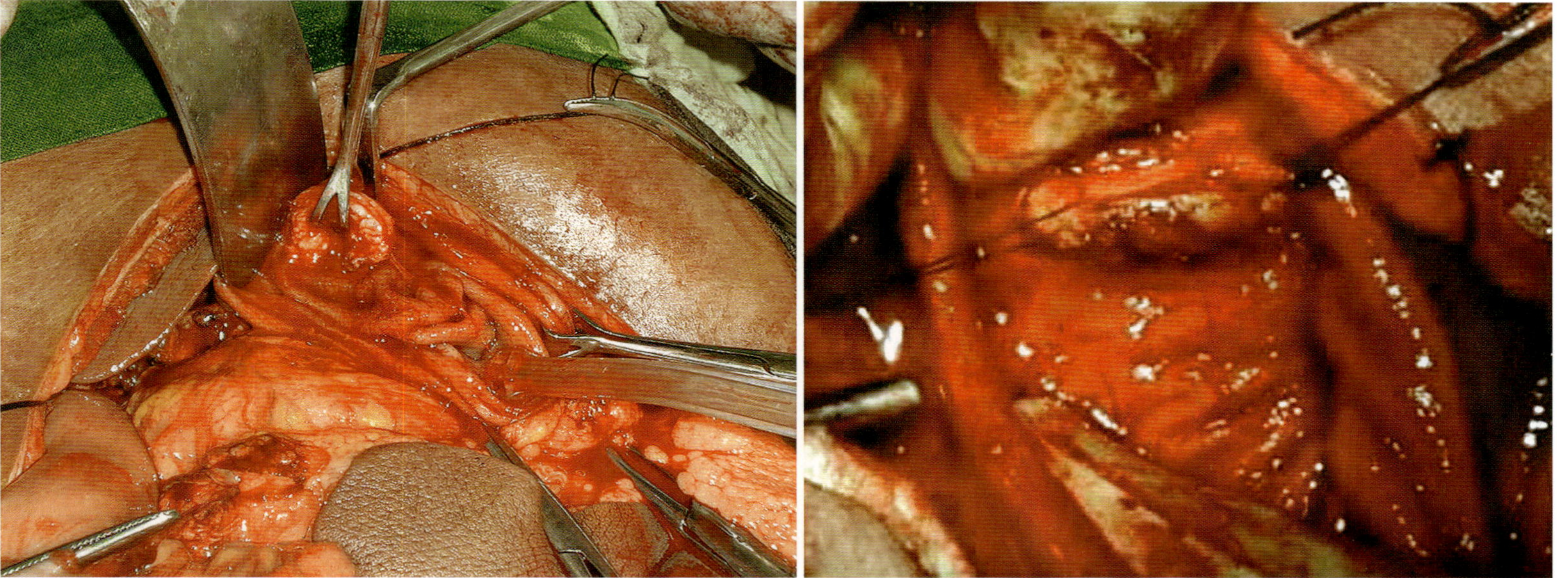

Fig. 24-59: Pancreaticogastrostomy in Whipple's operation. Pancreatic secretion is neutralised in gastric acid pH.

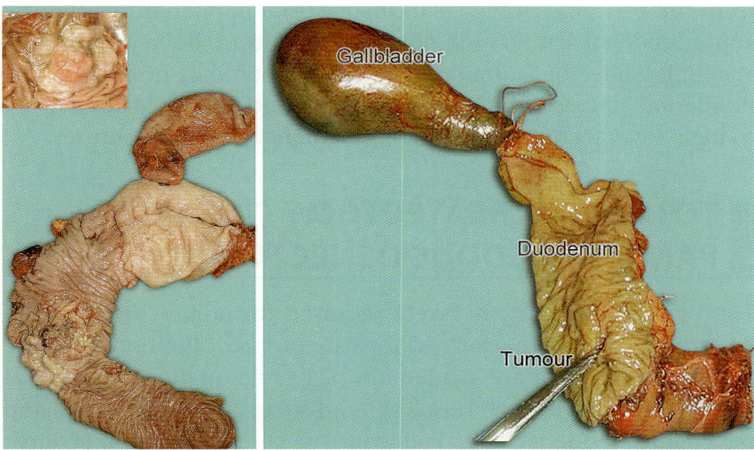

Fig. 24-60: Periampullary carcinoma of pancreas—gross look in two different patients.

Pancreatic, Biliary and Gastrointestinal Reconstruction

Reconstruction proceeds in the counterclockwise direction and again in a stepwise and orderly fashion.

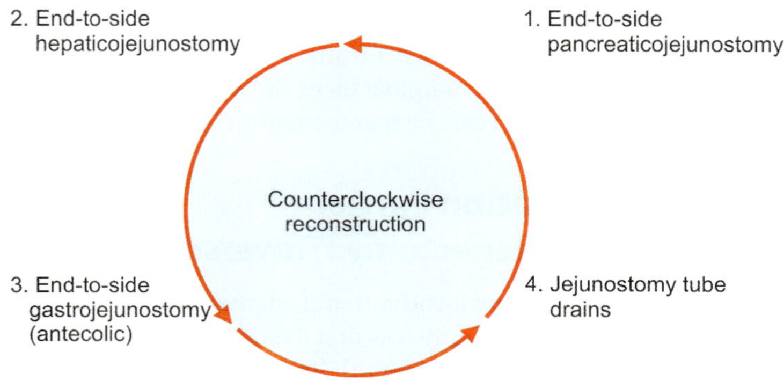

1. ***Pancreaticojejunal anastomosis***
   The pancreatic remnant is mobilised from retroperitoneum and splenic vein for a distance of 2 to 3 cm. The transected jejunum is brought through a small incision in the transverse mesocolon to the right or left of middle colic vessels. A two-layered, end-to-side, duct-to-mucosa pancreaticojejunostomy is performed. If the pancreatic duct is small (<4 mm), a small silastic internal stent can be left behind under the anastomosis. Following completion of posterior row of interrupted 3-zero seromuscular sutures, a small full thickness opening is made. The anastomosis between the pancreatic duct and the small bowel mucosa is completed with 4-zero or 5-zero monofilament sutures either vicryl or prolene depending on the centre preference. The anastomosis is completed with placement of anterior row of 3-zero seromuscular sutures.
   Pancreaticogastric anastomosis
   The advantage claimed in this type of anastomosis is that there are lesser chances of pancreatic fistulae formation due to the good blood supply of the stomach and the presence of acidic environment that prevents activation of pancreatic enzymes causing less autodigestion at anastomosis site. The anastomosis is technically simple because the stomach is right in front of the cut remnant of the pancreas. The remnant is mobilised off the bed for 2–3 cm and brought into the stomach through an opening in the posterior wall of stomach. The pancreas is anastomosed using single layer of suture running from the pancreatic capsule to the gastric serosa using prolene 3-zero suture. Internal stent can be left in situ if the pancreatic duct is very small.
2. A single-layer biliary enteric (***hepaticojejunostomy***) anastomosis using interrupted, 4-zero absorbable monofilament sutures (PDS). It is important to align jejunum with the bile duct to avoid tension on the pancreatic and biliary anastomosis. A stent is rarely used in the construction of the hepaticojejunostomy.
3. An antecolic, and end-to-side ***gastrojejunostomy*** is constructed in two layers. A posterior row of silk sutures is followed by a running, monofilament, full-thickness inner layer; the anterior row of silk sutures completes the anastomosis. The distance between the biliary and gastric anastomosis should allow the jejunum to assume its antecolic position (for the G-J) without tension. There is no harm in making a long (25-30 cm) afferent limb.
4. ***Feeding jejunostomy*** tubes are placed using the Witzel technique, and then two closed suction drains are placed. Enteral feeding via a jejunostomy tube avoids a delay in the hospital discharge due to poor oral intake.

Complications of Whipple's Operation

Pancreatic fistula, biliary fistula, sepsis, subphrenic abscess, respiratory complications, cholangitis and hepatic failure, renal failure, anastomotic dehiscence of any stomas, bleeding, post-operative acute pancreatitis, marginal ulcer, SMA or SMV thrombosis, portal vein thrombosis, gastric bezoar formation.

Pylorus Preservation Partial Pancreaticoduodenectomy (Traverso Longmire)

Preservation of the antropyloroduodenal segment in combination with pancreaticoduodenectomy was first described by Traverso and colleagues in 1978 (Traverso Longmire). Proponents of the technique argue that preservation of the antropyloric pump mechanism results in long-term upper gastrointestinal tract function with associated salutary nutritional squeal. Published data to date involve a retrospective comparison that has yielded mixed results.

Nevertheless, most pancreatic surgeons agree that pylorus preservation should not be performed for patients with bulky tumours of the pancreatic head, duodenal tumours involving first or second part of the duodenum, or lesions in which pyloric and peripyloric lymph nodes are grossly positive.

The steps in pylorus preserving pancreaticoduodenectomy are identical to that of standard pancreaticoduodenectomy, except in the approach to the antrum, pylorus and the duodenum. Preservation of sufficient blood supply to the proximal duodenum and preservation of vagal innervation to the antrum and pylorus are critical. Therefore, appropriate caution must be exercised during the portal dissection to avoid unnecessary division of the right gastric artery or injury to the nerves of Latarjet. This is the fundamental technical difference in the pylorus-preserving procedure and is essential to facilitate a well-vascularised duodenojejunostomy and to avoid postoperative gastroparesis **(Fig. 24-61)**.

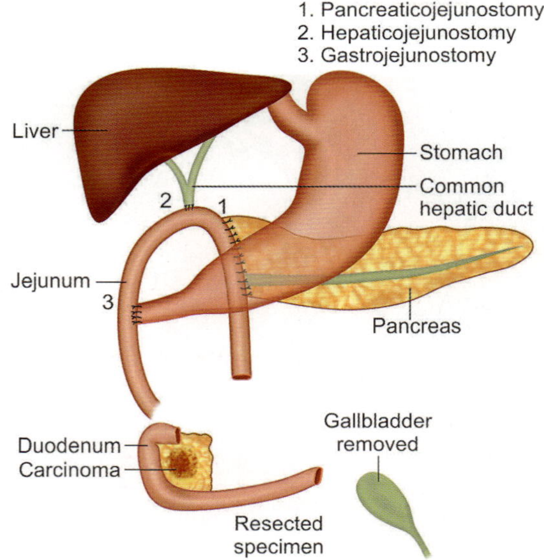

Fig. 24-61: Pylorus preserving pancreaticoduodenectomy.

The duodenum is divided approximately 2–3 cm beyond the pylorus. The blood supply to the first portion of the duodenum arises from the proximal branches of the gastroduodenal artery and the supraduodenal artery, both of which arise from the hepatic artery. When possible, the supraduodenal artery should be preserved. The duodenojejunostomy is performed in an end-to-side fashion using a single-layer technique with monofilament absorbable sutures.

TOTAL PANCREATECTOMY (TOTAL PANCREATICODUODENECTOMY)

Total pancreatectomy is rarely required for adenocarcinoma of pancreas. It can be performed for carcinoma of the body and tail that present early or are incidentally picked up on ultrasound. Total pancreatectomy is performed by modifying step 1 in the six-step pancreaticoduodenectomy. Following the completion of the Cattell-Braasch manoeuvre and identification of the infrapancreatic SMV, the greater omentum is separated from the left side of transverse colon and the splenic flexure is mobilised. The peritoneum lateral to the spleen is then incised in the cephalad direction to the gastroesophageal junction. The short gastric vessels are ligated and divided, allowing medial and cephalad retraction of the stomach. Mobilisation of the spleen and the pancreas from their retroperitoneal attachments to the kidney and the adrenals is completed. The inferior mesenteric vein is divided and the mesenteric root divided from the lateral border of the SMV to the lateral border of the aorta, staying anterior to the SMA. Division of the splenic artery and vein is delayed until steps 2 through 5 are completed. Then, in preparation for completion of the retroperitoneal dissection, the spleen and the distal pancreas are again reflected medially, exposing the origin of the splenic artery and the splenic vein—SMV junction. The splenic artery and vein are then ligated and divided. Hepaticojejunostomy and gastrojejunostomy are done similarly **(Fig. 24-62)**.

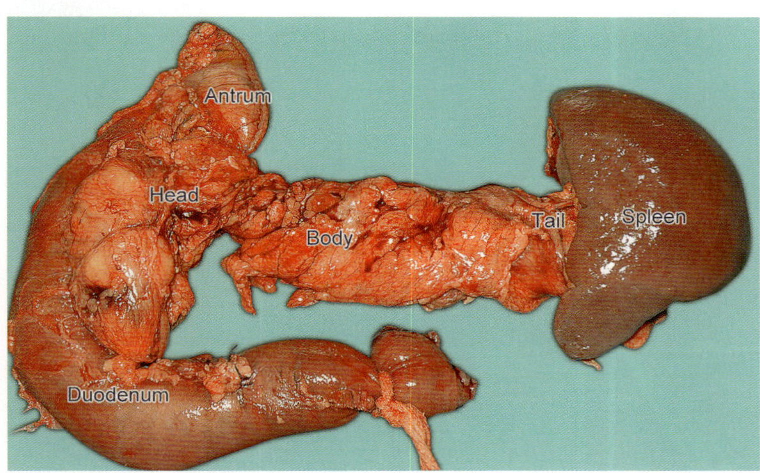

Fig. 24-62: Total pancreatectomy—specimen.

DISTAL PANCREATECTOMY

Any tumour in the body and tail of the pancreas; endocrine tumours when cannot be excised locally; trauma to the tail of the pancreas; in selected patients when chronic pancreatitis is localised to the tail of the pancreas with or without pseudocyst in the tail **(Fig. 24-63)**.

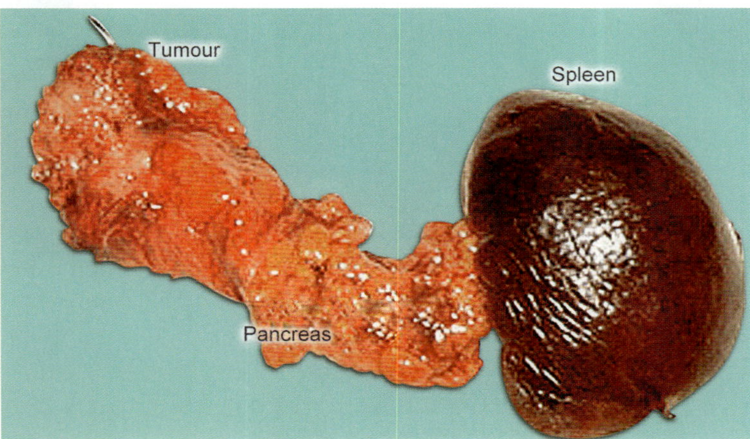

Fig. 24-63: Distal pancreatectomy specimen.

Usually distal pancreatectomy is done with splenectomy. Splenic preservation is often tried. Open and laparoscopic approaches are used for distal pancreatectomy. Invasion of the junction of splenic vein and portal vein by the tumour is an inoperable sign of the tumour. Any attempt of resection in such situation makes disastrous portal vein laceration **(Figs. 24-64A and B)**.

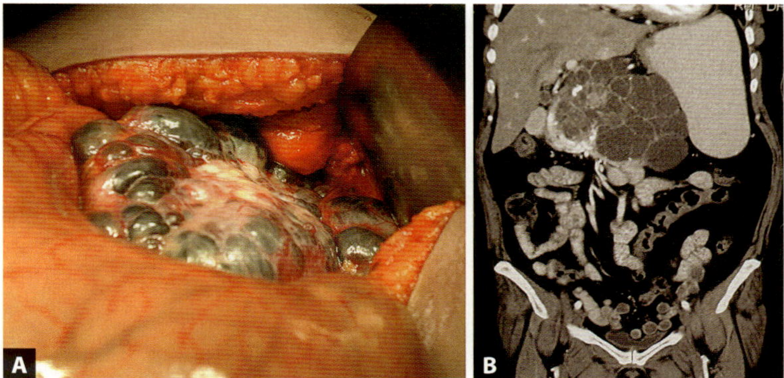

Figs. 24-64A and B: Cystadenocarcinoma of pancreas. CT picture of same patient.

Technique

Under general anaesthesia, patient is placed in supine position with left side upwards slightly. Lengthy upper midline incision or left subcostal incision is used. Abdomen is explored for operability and metastases.

Greater omentum is divided between ligatures and detached completely from the transverse colon. Splenic flexure is mobilised downwards and separated completely. Peritoneal layer is incised at the lower part of the pancreas to expose the lower margin. Care should be taken at this stage not to injure inferior mesenteric vein which will be ligated at a later period. Peritoneum along the superior margin is also incised with care as tortuous splenic artery is on the upper margin of the pancreas. Splenic artery near the neck of the pancreas is identified by feeling its pulsation. One should not get confused with the common hepatic artery. Splenic artery is dissected, isolated and ligated but divided only at later period **(Fig. 24-65)**.

Spleen is mobilised towards right of the patient by dividing splenorenal ligament. Posteriorly kidney, renal vessels and adrenal gland will be present from which tail of the pancreas is gently separated by blunt and sharp dissection as usually the plane is avascular. But if tumour is close to the tail of pancreas, there may be adhesions due to desmoblastic reaction or invasion of the tumour to these structures. Adrenal vein may be close to the dissecting area which should be safeguarded. If tumour invasion occurs into the renal vessels (which are very well identified preoperatively by proper imaging), left side nephrectomy is to be done provided opposite kidney is functioning well. Spleen with tail, body of the pancreas is lifted upwards into the wound. Left gastroepiploic vessels and short gastric vessels are carefully ligated. Further dissection and elevation of the body of the pancreas will visualise the inferior mesenteric vein joining the splenic vein. Inferior mesenteric vein is doubly ligated with silk and divided. Further dissection posteriorly with finger or peanut will show the splenic vein joining the SMV to form portal vein. 2 cm away from this junction splenic vein is gently dissected from the tissues around as often it is embedded in the pancreatic tissue. Splenic vein is encircled with a right angle and doubly ligated and divided. Previously ligated splenic artery is divided with double ligation **(Figs. 24-66 and 24-67)**.

Peripancreatic tissues are dissected to bare the neck of the pancreas. Neck is divided using stapler. Specimen is retrieved. Usually stapler transected proximal cut end of pancreas does not require any additional sutures. If stapler is not used then transected

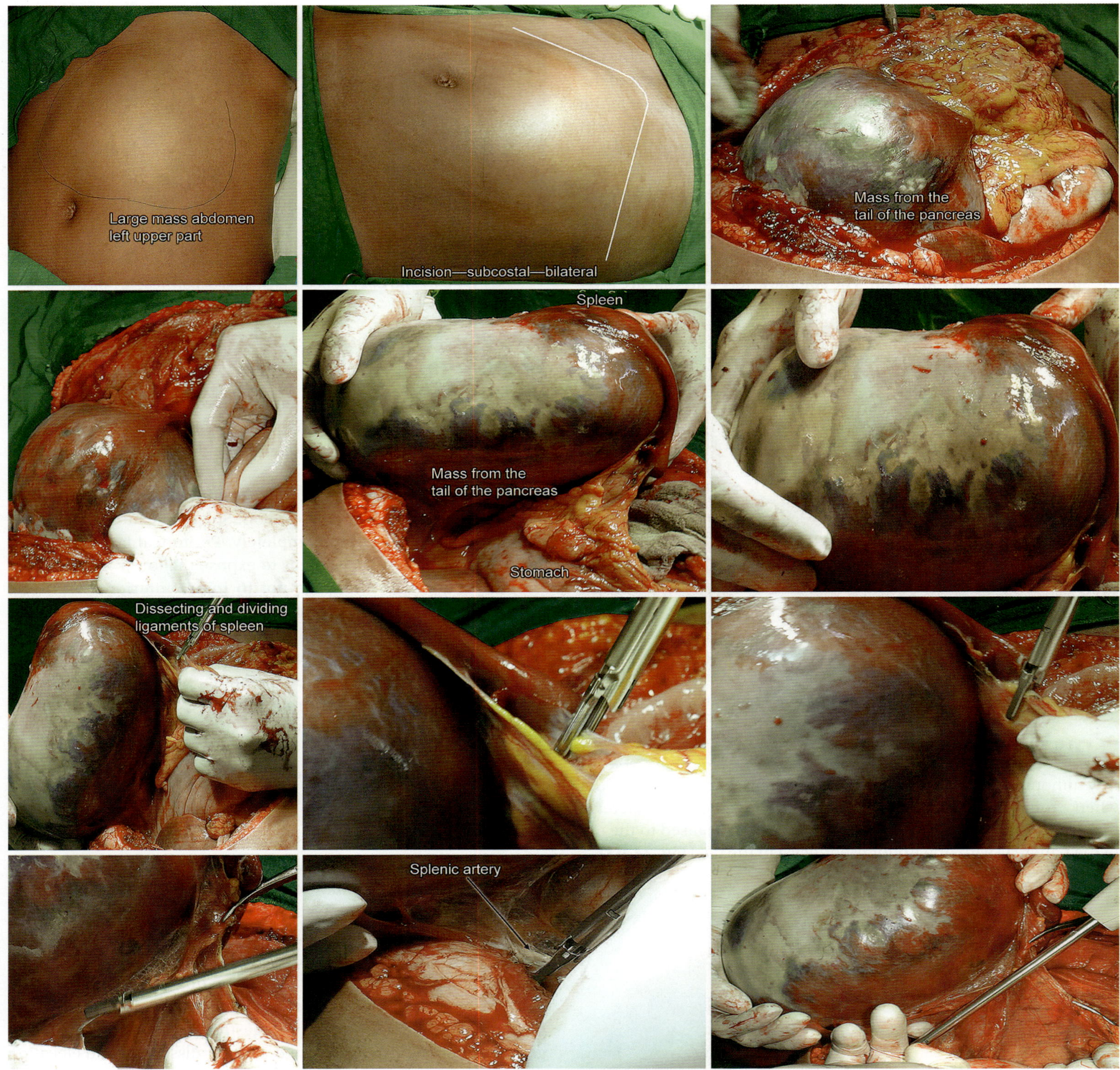
Large mass abdomen
left upper part
Incision—subcostal—bilateral
Mass from the
tail of the pancreas
Spleen
Mass from the
tail of the pancreas
Stomach
Dissecting and dividing
ligaments of spleen
Splenic artery

Figs. 24-65(1)

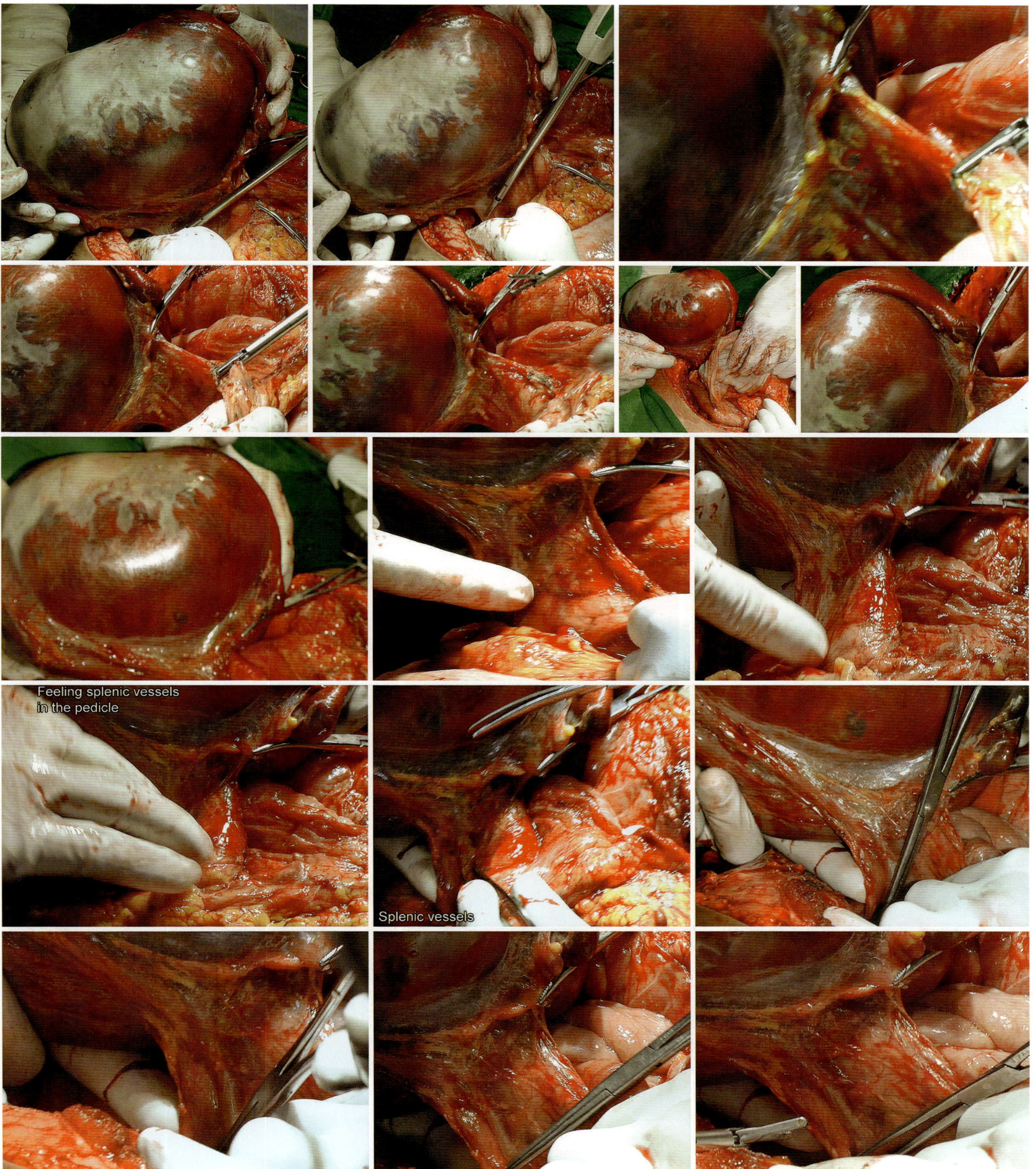

Figs. 24-65(2)

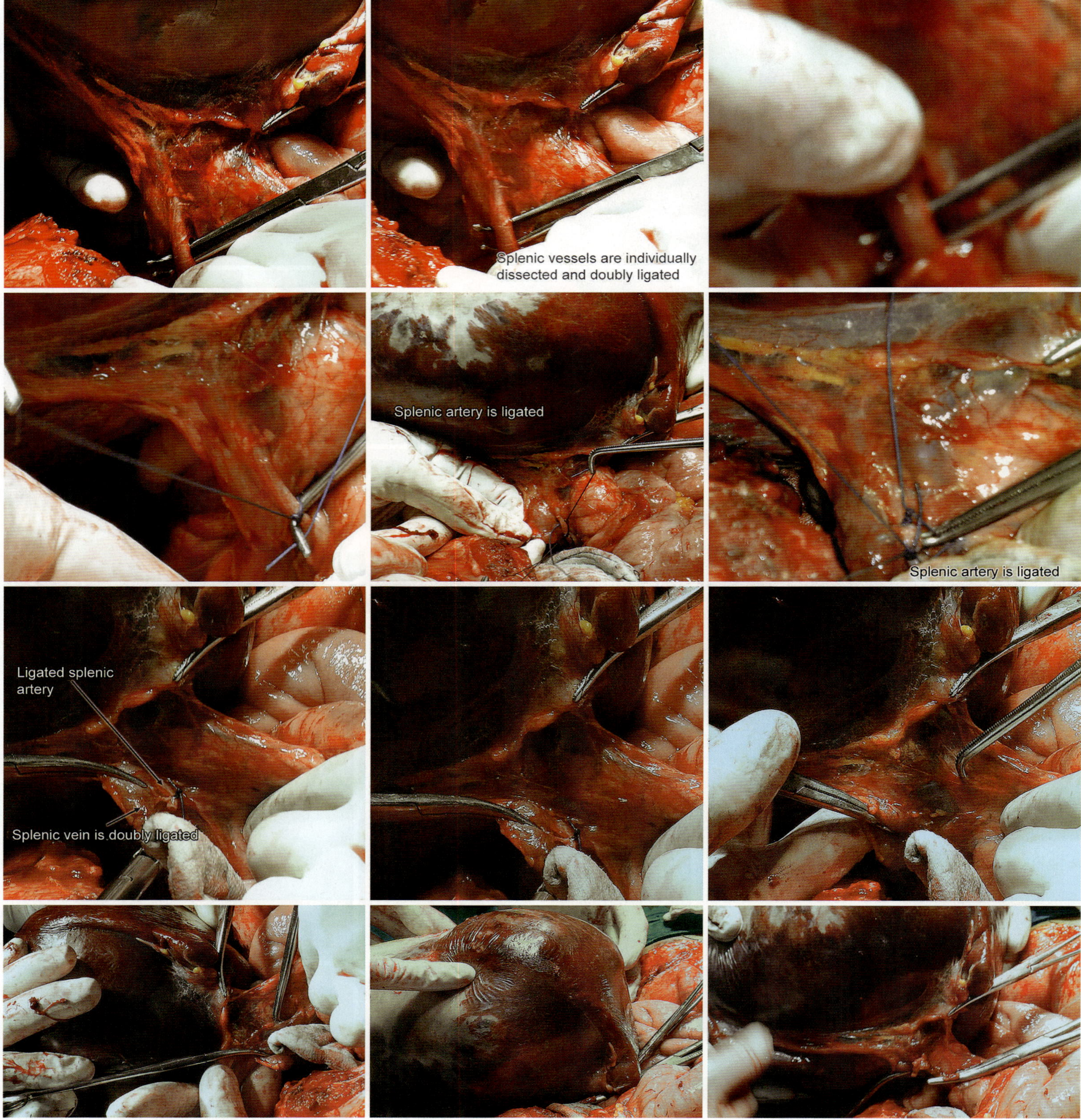
Splenic vessels are individually dissected and doubly ligated
Splenic artery is ligated
Splenic artery is ligated
Ligated splenic artery
Splenic vein is doubly ligated

Figs. 24-65(3)

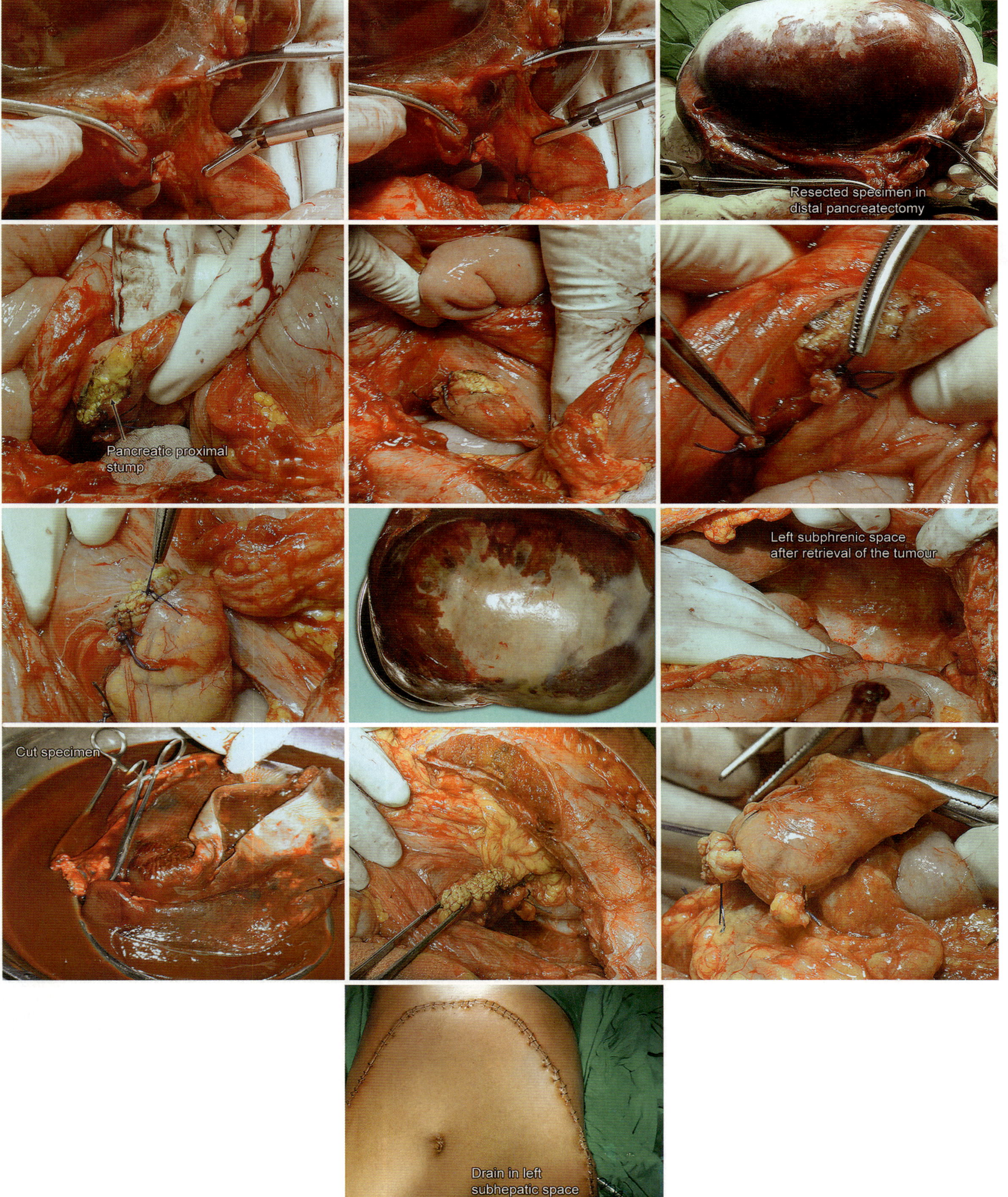

Figs. 24-65(4)

Figs. 24-65(1 to 4): Distal pancreatectomy for pancreatic tail tumour/mass.

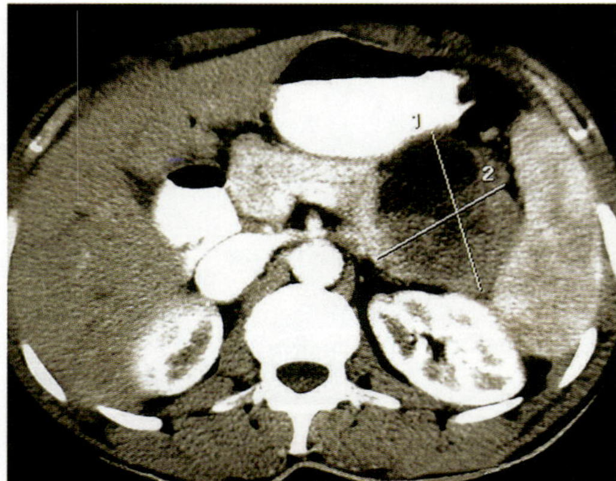
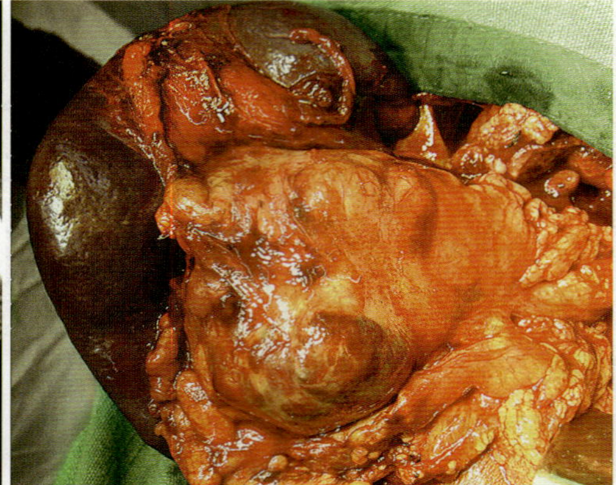
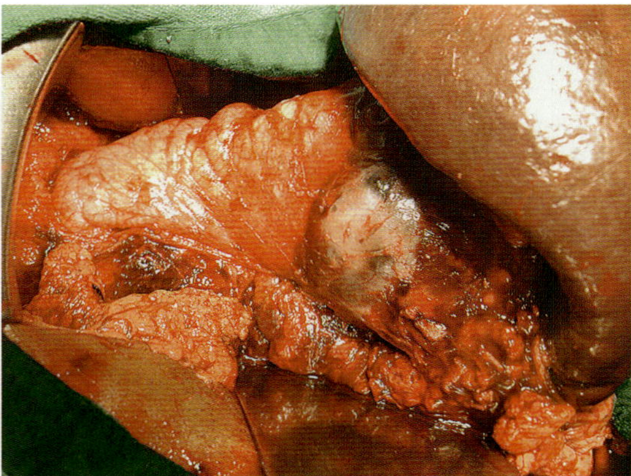

Fig. 24-66: Mucinous cystadenocarcinoma of pancreas.

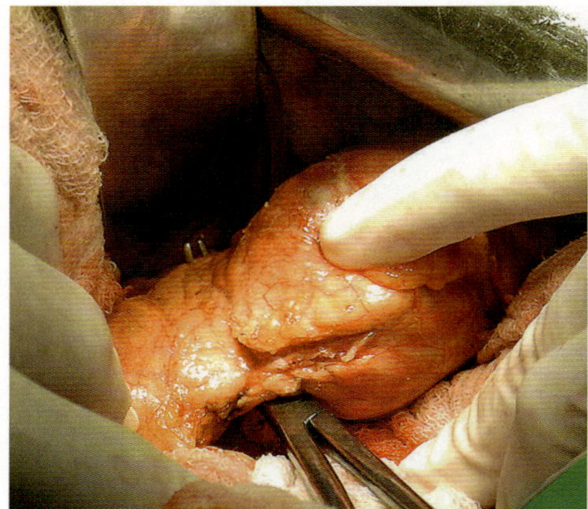
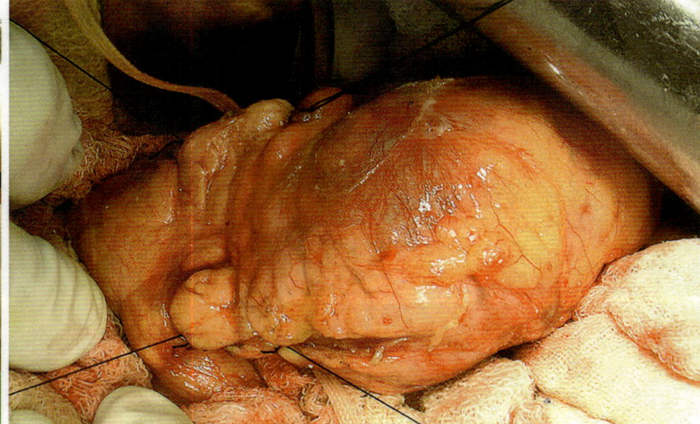
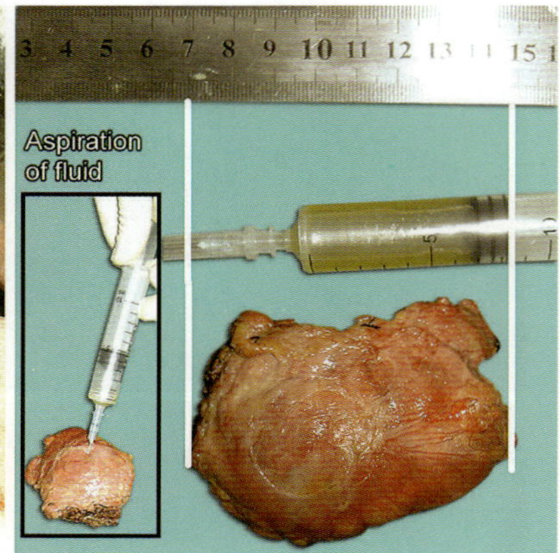

Fig. 24-67: Mucinous cystadenoma of pancreas.
Courtesy: Dr Arunkumar, MCh, Gastro, Kochi.

pancreas is closed using interrupted mattress sutures by 3-zero non-absorbable suture—polypropylene or silk. Pancreatic duct needs a separate transfixation using 3-zero polypropylene suture. Cavity is inspected for any bleeding. Sutured pancreatic stump is again inspected. Tube suction drain is placed in the left subphrenic space. Abdomen is closed in layers.

Postoperative Care

Fluid therapy is continued; nasogastric tube is removed in 72 hours; drain is kept for 5–7 days. Antibiotics may be needed as sepsis can occur. Serum amylase and lipase estimation may require to be done during postoperative period.

Complications

Pancreatic fistula can occur which usually subsides spontaneously by conservative therapy.

Subphrenic abscess formation, acute pancreatitis, left-sided pleural effusion, complications of splenectomy like OPSI, injury to left kidney, left renal vessels, diaphragm and colon can occur.

RADICAL ANTEGRADE MODULAR PANCREATOSPLENECTOMY (RAMPS)

Here distal pancreatectomy with splenectomy is done from right towards left instead of standard left to right technique. This gives early control of splenic vessels and also achieves optimum tumour clearance. It is done for tumours of body and tail of the pancreas. Nodal clearance is also important in this technique. Greater omentum is freed from colon. Short gastric vessels are ligated and divided. Right colon is mobilised, SMV is identified; portal dissection is done; gastroduodenal artery is not divided; all lymph nodes are removed and reflected towards left on the body of the pancreas. Kocherisation should be done. Portal vein and SMV are separated from the neck of the pancreas like in Whipple's operation. Neck towards left of portal vein is transected after placing 4 stay sutures. Stump towards head of the pancreas is sutured securely using non-absorbable sutures (polypropylene). Posterior peritoneum is opened; fat and lymph nodes are cleared from crus of the diaphragm, in front of the common hepatic artery; nodes adjacent to left gastric artery are dissected; left gastric vein (coronary vein) is dissected, ligated and divided. Splenic artery originating from the coeliac trunk is identified, ligated with transfixation at its origin. Spleen and tail of the pancreas is dissected off. Dissection can be done anterior to adrenal gland (anterior RAMPS) or posterior to adrenal gland if tumour has invaded adrenal gland (posterior RAMPS). Inferior mesenteric vein is ligated here where it joins the splenic vein. But renal vessels and kidney are kept away from dissection. Once final mobilisation is done, splenic vein is doubly ligated and divided. Neck is transected using stapler or hand suturing of the cut head end of the pancreas is done using 3-zero polypropylene interrupted sutures after transection. Duct may be separately sutured.

Modified Appley's (Canadian surgeon, 1954) technique is RAMPS with resection of the coeliac or common hepatic artery. Here blood supply to liver, duodenum and pancreas is achieved through inferior pancreaticoduodenal artery arising from SMA. Often an arterial (PTFE) graft from the aorta to proper hepatic artery is also done.

CHOLECYSTOJEJUNOSTOMY

Cholecystojejunostomy is occasionally done as a palliation in carcinoma of pancreas. Even though choledochojejunostomy is better and ideal for palliation and also to relieve obstruction, in advanced malignancy with involvement of mesocolon and extensive nodes, simpler surgery like cholecystojejunostomy still carries a role because of its simplicity in doing it in selected patients. However, it is useful only if cystic duct remains patent. Technique is detailed in the chapter on gallbladder **(Fig. 24-68)**.

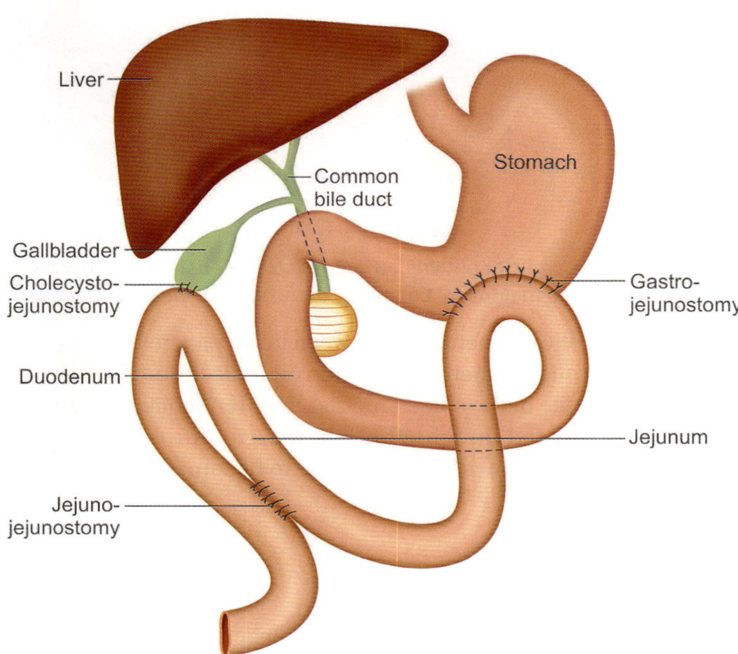

Fig. 24-68: Cholecystojejunostomy as a palliation in advanced carcinoma of pancreas is done occasionally. Gastrojejunostomy is added for possible duodenal obstruction.

B. SPLEEN

SURGICAL ANATOMY

Spleen is derived from the word *splen* in Greek; and *lien* from Latin. It is a wedge-shaped organ lying mainly in left hypochondrium, along the long axis of 10th rib. It is obliquely placed along the 10th rib downwards, forwards and laterally. It is wedged between fundus of stomach and diaphragm. Hilum of spleen transmits splenic vessels and nerves. Spleen has got anterior and posterior ends; two surfaces (parietal and visceral); three borders (superior is notched in front; inferior; intermediate) **(Fig. 24-69)**.

It is vascular purple-coloured soft organ. It is 12 cm in length; 7–8 cm in width; 2–3 cm in thickness. Normally spleen is not palpable. Its weight is 200 grams.

It is posteriorly related to left side diaphragm, diaphragmatic recess and left 9th, 10th, and 11th ribs. It is being related to left lung and pleura above these structures.

Its parietal surface is related to diaphragm; the visceral surface is related to stomach, splenic flexure of colon, pancreas and kidney. Upper pole is close to stomach and often may be fixed to stomach having short gastric vessels there. Lower pole is 4–7 cm away from the stomach **(Figs. 24-70 and 24-71)**.

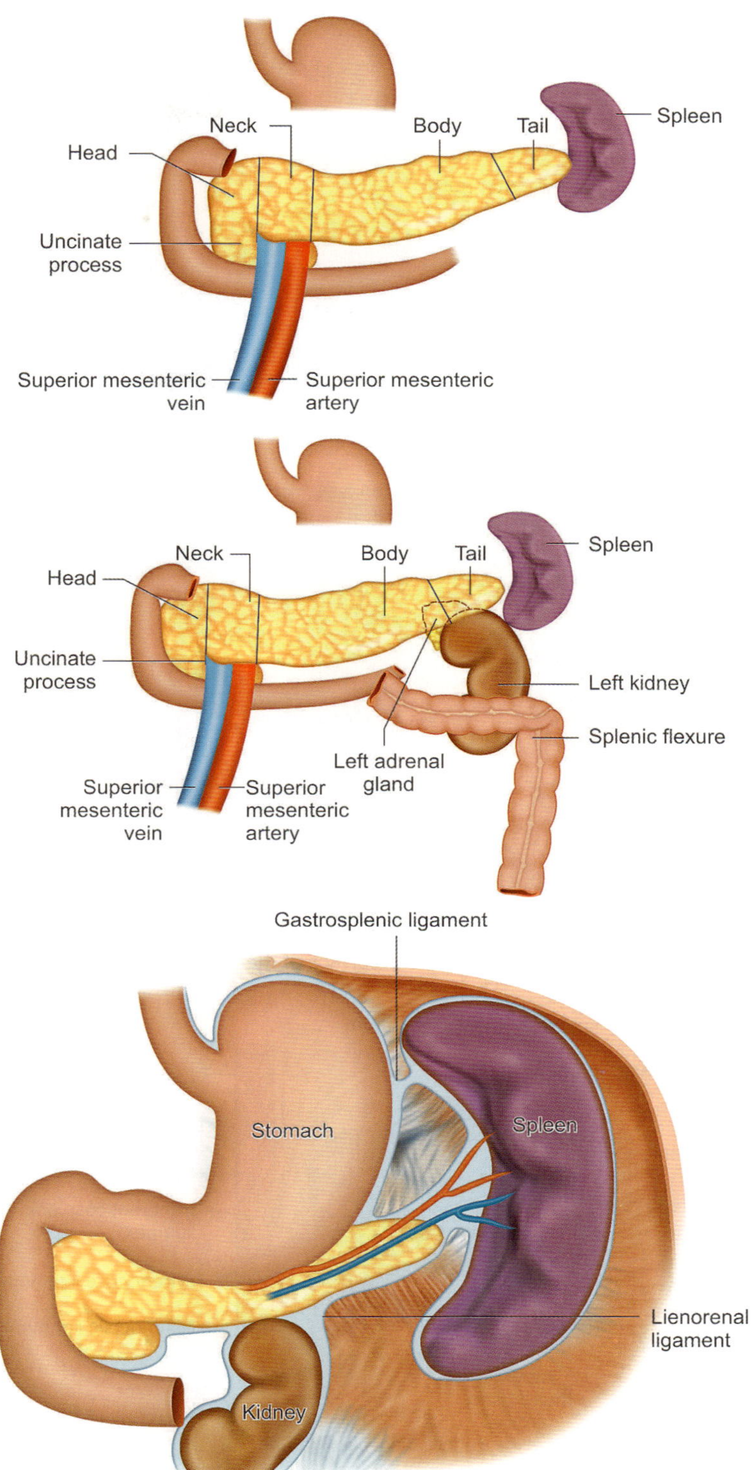

Fig. 24-69: Anatomy of spleen. Note the different relations of spleen which are surgically important during splenectomy.

Ligaments of Spleen

Spleen is suspended by two ligaments *(a) lienorenal ligament, (b) gastrosplenic ligament*. These two are main/chief splenic ligaments which form splenic pedicle. Lienorenal ligament transmits blood vessels to spleen. The tail of pancreas lies in this ligament, which can be damaged during splenectomy. Outer layer of lienorenal/splenorenal ligament forms posterior layer of gastrosplenic ligament. The gastrosplenic ligament contains short gastric vessels which

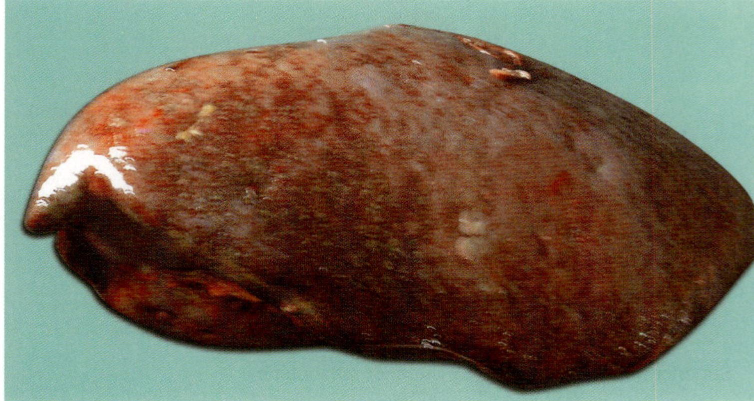

Fig. 24-70: Parietal surface of the spleen.

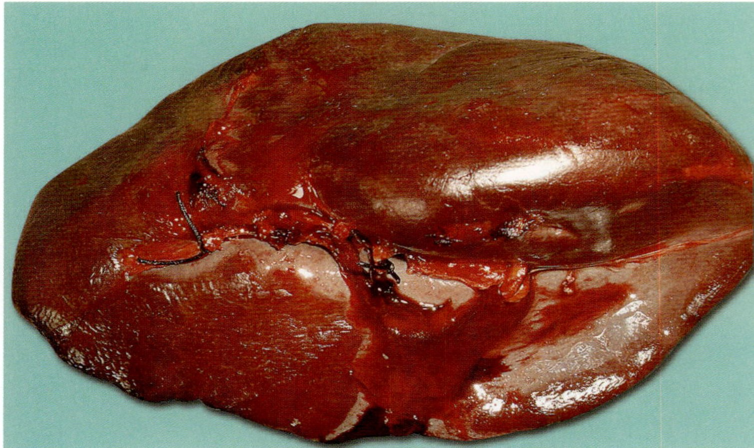

Fig. 24-71: Visceral surface of the spleen.

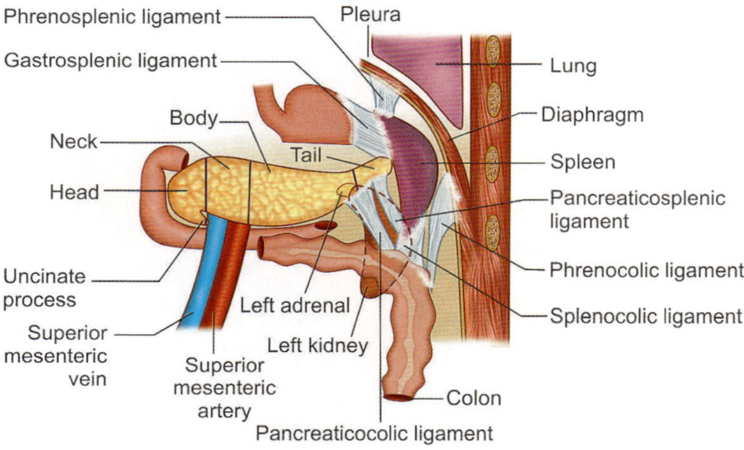

Fig. 24-72: Ligaments and relations of the spleen.

supply the left half of greater curvature of stomach. Gastrosplenic ligament also contains left gastroepiploic vessels below. Presplenic fold may be present in front of this gastrosplenic ligament which during traction may get torn and can cause bleeding from the left gastrosplenic ligament **(Fig. 24-72)**.

Phrenicocolic ligament comes in contact with lower pole of spleen, which may be damaged during mobilisation of splenic flexure of colon. It extends below from the lateral margin of the splenic flexure of the colon reflecting upwards laterally touching to the lower pole of the spleen to reach diaphragm; it is closely related to the spleen as spleen stays on its surface forming splenic floor. It is not attached to the spleen.

Splenophrenic ligament reflects between upper pole of spleen and stomach towards inferior surface of the diaphragm. Even though it is avascular, it may cause bleeding while dividing and so bipolar cautery or other energy sources should be utilised, otherwise ligation may be required **(Fig. 24-73)**.

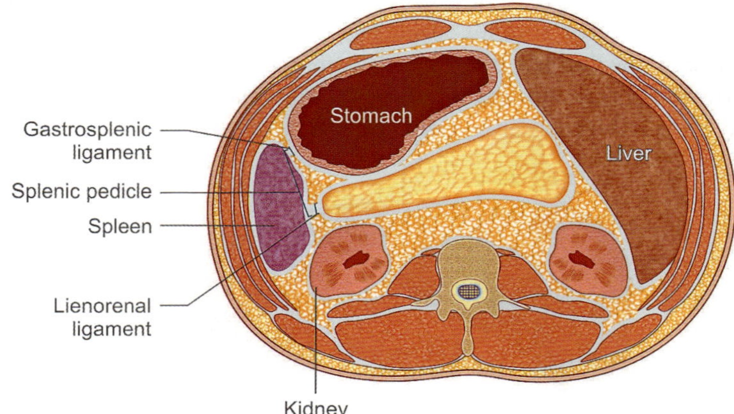

Fig. 24-73: Splenic pedicle contains lienorenal (splenorenal) and gastrosplenic ligaments; they are main/chief ligaments of the spleen (view from above).

Pancreaticocolic ligament runs between tail of pancreas and splenic flexure. Splenocolic ligament reflects from splenic flexure of the colon towards lower pole of the spleen medial to phrenocolic ligament.

Spleen is palpated under left costal margin during inspiration. It has to enlarge 2–3 times its normal size to become palpable.

Blood Supply

Arterial Supply

Splenic artery is the largest branch of coeliac artery but may arise from aorta or superior mesenteric artery, blood flow is 300 mL/min. Often it may arise from a common gastrosplenic trunk (left gastric artery and splenic artery) or common hepatosplenic trunk (common hepatic artery and splenic artery). Artery is 0.6–1.3 cm in diameter with 7–30 cm in length. It is tortuous. It runs in the upper margin of the pancreas. It initially crosses the left border of the aorta, then runs on the front of the tail of the pancreas and upper pole of kidney before reaching the splenic hilum. Tortuosity of the artery allows free movement of the spleen. Branches are dorsal pancreatic artery, posterior gastric artery, left gastroepiploic artery and arteria pancreatica magna. Artery passes through the lienorenal ligament to reach the splenic hilum where it divides into 5 or more branches. Short gastric arteries may arise from splenic artery or left gastroepiploic artery **(Figs. 24-74A and B)**.

Splenic artery shows one of the two patterns of branches towards spleen. (1) *Magistral type* where there is long main splenic artery with short terminal branches as—superior terminal artery gives superior polar artery and often short gastric arteries. Inferior terminal artery gives penultimate and an ultimate branch and other branches inside the spleen. Inferior polar artery runs downwards towards inferior pole of the spleen. (2) *Distributive type*—Here superior polar artery directly originates from the splenic artery having an anastomotic branch with inferior terminate branch.

Venous Drainage

Splenic vein joins the superior mesenteric vein at right angle behind the neck of pancreas to form the portal vein. Often 2 or more splenic vein tributaries join and form splenic vein. Its other tributaries are

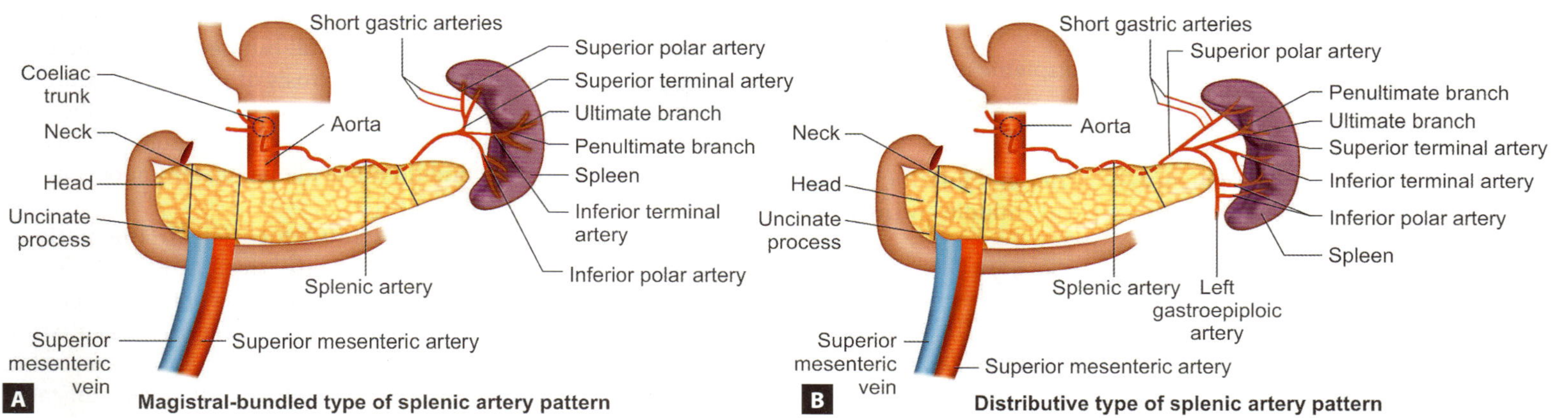

Figs. 24-74A and B: Arterial distribution of the spleen (Splenic artery).

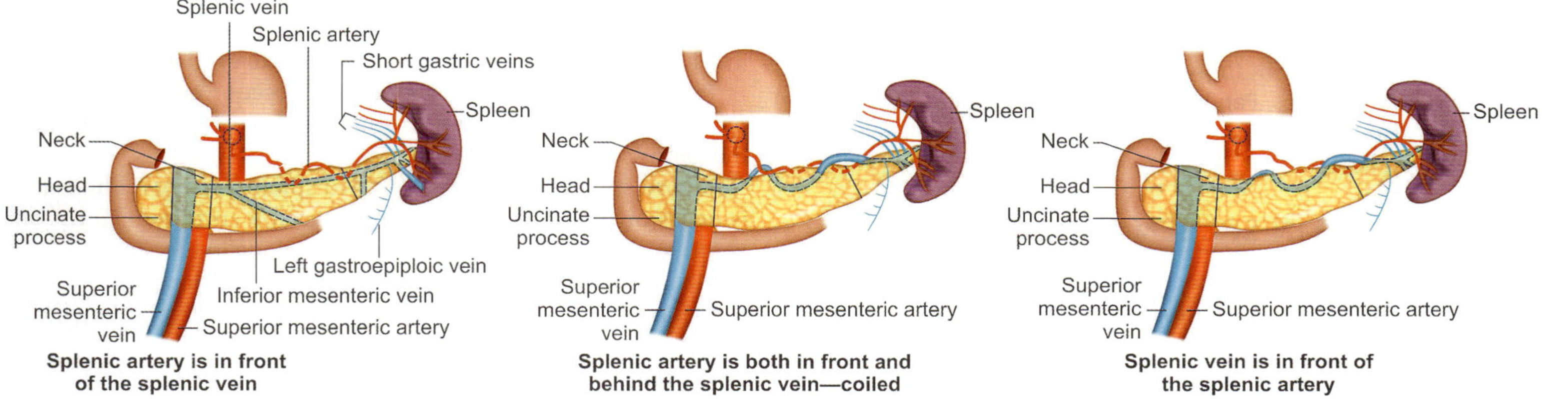

Fig. 24-75: Splenic vein tributaries and different patterns of its course.

left gastroepiploic vein, short gastric vein and pancreatic veins. Commonly inferior mesenteric vein joins splenic vein just before it joins the portal vein; but sometimes inferior mesenteric vein may join SMV or directly into the portal vein **(Fig. 24-75)**.

Splenic parenchyma contains *white pulp* and *red pulp*. *White pulp* lies in centre surrounding the central artery, which is a branch of trabecular artery. It is made up of lymphatic nodules with germinal centres and periarterial lymphatic sheaths with a network containing lymphocytes and macrophages. White pulp is surrounded by marginal zone which contains end arteries from central and peripheral peniciliary arteries **(Fig. 24-76)**.

Marginal zone contains marginal sinus which filters the materials from the white pulp. Immunoglobulins secreted by white pulp enter marginal zone and into main bloodstream. *Red pulp* is located outer to marginal zone. Red pulp contains cords and sinuses. Central artery gives reticular branches which open into these sinuses and cords wherein particles are phagocytosed. Commonly central artery eventually ends in these cords and sinuses. Few end branches of the central artery directly enter the pulp vein. Cords and sinuses eventually drain into pulp vein. Blood circulation through these cords and sinuses is known as '*open*' circulation (90%). Blood circulation through white pulp but not entering these cords and sinuses is known as '*closed*' circulation (10%).

Removal of non-deformable intracellular substances from deformable cells is known as "*pitting*". *Heinz bodies/Howell-Jolly bodies, Pappenheimer siderotic bodies* are removed by this method from RBCs. Postsplenectomy patients will show these bodies in the RBCs in peripheral smear. In splenunculi, these bodies will be absent even after splenectomy. Removal of aged/abnormal red cells is done by the process of "*culling*". RBCs which lose osmotic balance and membrane integrity are known as non-deformable and they are removed by this method. Half-life of platelets is 10 days. In splenomegaly, 80% of platelets may be sequestered in spleen causing thrombocytopenia. Normally spleen is reservoir for platelets. One-thirds of total platelet mass is present in spleen. In pathological status like immune diseases phagocytosis of platelets in spleen is accelerated by many folds. Splenomegaly and hypersplenism can cause neutropenia. Half-life of neutrophil is 6 hours. Bacterial clearance also occurs in spleen by phagocytosis. After splenectomy, patients are more prone to OPSI, *immunologic functions* like synthesis of antibody IgM; formation of lymphocytes; production of tuftsin, opsonins, properdin and interferons.

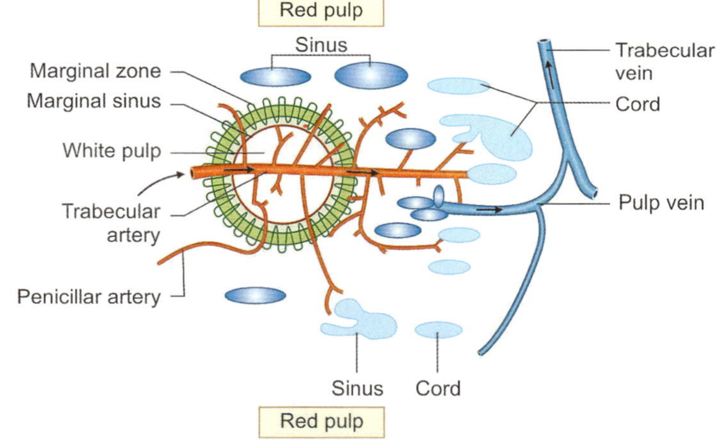

Fig. 24-76: Splenic architecture. Architecture of spleen showing red pulp (peripheral); white pulp (central); open and closed circulation; marginal zone and sinuses and trabecular artery and vein.

Lymphatic Drainage

It is to supra- and infrapancreatic nodes and splenic nodes.

Splenic Segments

Usually spleen has got two segments—superior and inferior. 15% of individuals may have three segments—superior, middle and inferior.

SPLENUNCULI (30%) (FIG. 24-77)

About 30% of individuals can have accessory spleen. These are single (60%), or two (20%) or multiple accessory spleens. Size of these accessory spleens varies from 0.5 cm to 10 cm.

Sites: Hilum of spleen (50%); near splenic vessels; tail of the pancreas (30%); splenic ligaments—gastrosplenic/splenorenal; mesocolon; greater omentum. After splenectomy, they undergo hyperplasia and lead to recurrence of the disorder for which spleen was removed. Blood peripheral smear in these patients with splenunculi *will not show* Howell-Jolly bodies, Pappenheimer siderotic bodies. Accessory spleen can also be occasionally present adjacent to left ovary or adjacent to left testis.

PRINCIPLES IN SPLEEN SURGERY

Initial immunisation for pneumococci, meningococci, haemophillus influenza by appropriate vaccines is necessary. Vaccine should be given 2 weeks prior to surgery.

Proper preoperative evaluation depending on the condition to which patient undergoes splenectomy is important. CT, peripheral smear, platelet count, osmotic fragility test, prothrombin time, coagulation profile and bone marrow aspiration, when needed, have to be done.

Splenic surgery needs proper exposure of surrounding ligaments and structures, proper dissection of the splenic vessels, avoiding trauma to pancreas, stomach, colon and left kidney.

Laparoscopic splenectomy is ideal unless spleen is massively enlarged.

Accessory splenic tissue should be identified and removed. Often it is difficult to identify these splenunculi but becomes mandatory when dealing with hereditary spherocytosis or idiopathic thrombocytopenic purpura.

Spillage of spleen during dissection or retrieval should be avoided. It will be troublesome in conditions like idiopathic thrombocytopenic purpura (ITP).

Postsplenectomy sepsis is a life time risk to the patient. Overwhelming postsplenectomy infection (OPSI) is more troublesome in splenectomy for trauma. Partial splenectomy, splenorrhaphy, mesh splenorrhaphy, splenic autotransplantation are other options that should be kept in mind. Splenic preservation in trauma is preferred unless patient is haemodynamically unstable or life-threatening haemorrhage sets in. On table Argon beam laser often helps to control bleeding from the splenic surface. Splenic salvage in splenic trauma could be non-operative and operative. Hilar injury, large splenic haematoma with a contrast splenic blush in CT are the contraindications for conservative/salvage approaches.

Postoperative sepsis like subphrenic abscess, pancreatitis, OPSI, pancreatic fistula, injury to adjacent organs, postoperative deep vein thrombosis are to be taken care of.

Before splenectomy, preoperative splenic artery embolisation is occasionally done only in very large spleen to reduce the size of the spleen; but splenectomy should be done in specified period of 7–10 days, otherwise splenic necrosis, sepsis can occur.

Laparoscopic splenectomy is ideal for elective splenectomy unless spleen is very large in size. It is ideal for ITP as spleen would not be enlarged enormously here.

Adequate exposure should be achieved through a large incision. Small incision does not have a role in open splenectomy. Thoracoabdominal incision may be needed when spleen is adherent to diaphragm or usual abdominal incision may require to be extended as thoracoabdominal if there is difficulty in dissecting the spleen.

Splenic ligaments are usually vascular; they cause troublesome oozing and so need careful dissection, ideally using bipolar cautery. Perisplenic adhesions are also vascular and need ligation prior to division. Splenic vessels at the hilum are prone to tear as they are fragile.

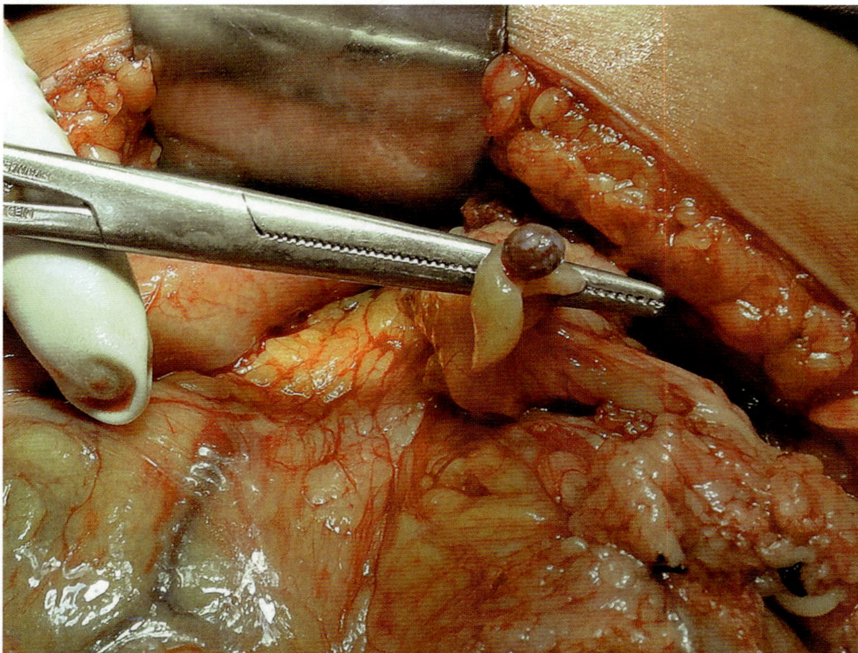

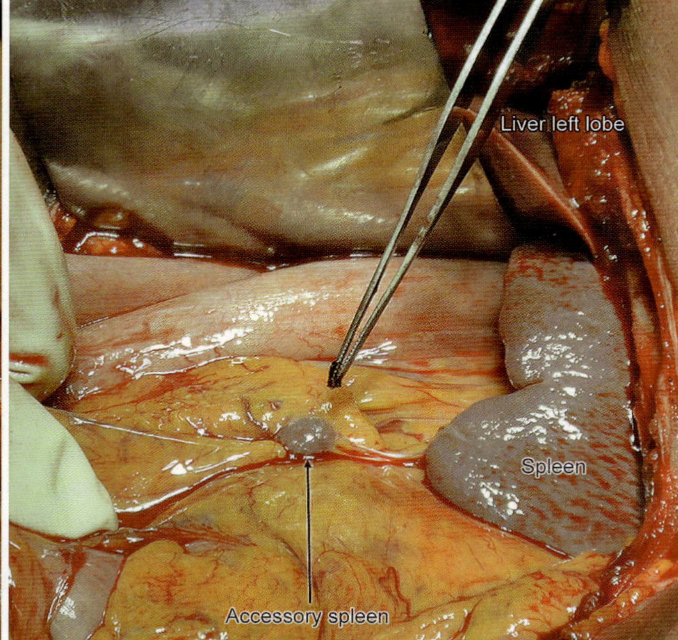

Fig. 24-77: On table photo of splenunculi with splenomegaly. Splenunculi should be removed, otherwise disease will recur.

Proximal control of the splenic artery at its origin is better in large spleen. Anatomical variation like coiling of splenic vein on the splenic artery may get injured causing torrential bleeding. In ITP splenic artery should be ligated first and platelets should be transfused only later. Even if splenic artery is ligated proximally, it should be ligated again distally at the hilum during final stage of the dissection.

Short gastric vessels should be carefully ligated and divided. Harmonic scalpel or transfixation sutures are better.

Proximal greater curvature should be invaginated using seromuscular continuous or interrupted silk sutures to avoid greater curve necrosis.

In portal hypertension and myelofibrosis and in massive spleen normal avascular splenic ligaments will be very much vascular and can cause torrential bleeding.

Blood products like fresh frozen plasma, platelets are often needed while doing splenectomy in massively enlarged spleen.

Absolute haemostasis after removal of spleen is essential; bleeding from tail of the pancreas should be suture ligated with fine polypropylene transfixation. In other areas, bipolar cautery or ligation of the bleeders should be done.

Pancreatic injury should be avoided as pancreatic fistula or pancreatitis can occur. Gastric trauma, if it occurs, can result in gastric fistula which is very difficult to manage.

SPLENECTOMY

Indications for splenectomy:

- Trauma.
- In distal pancreatectomy, total pancreatectomy, rarely radical gastrectomy—removed "*en bloc*" with stomach.
- Staging laparotomy in case of Hodgkin's lymphoma.
- Hereditary spherocytosis and other haemolytic anaemias.
- Idiopathic thrombocytopaenic purpura (ITP).
- Portal hypertension with variceal bleeding—mainly gastric varices with splenic vein thrombosis.
- Tuberculosis of spleen.
- Others:
  - Gaucher's disease.
  - Chronic myeloid leukaemia, myelofibrosis.
  - Felty's syndrome.
  - Carcinoma of tail of the pancreas during distal pancreatectomy.
  - Schistosomiasis.
  - Splenic artery aneurysm.
  - Splenic infarction.
  - Cystic disease of spleen.
  - Splenic tumours.

Elective Splenectomy

Preoperative vaccine; haemogram; Adequate blood is kept ready if need arises, antibiotics, nasogastric tube, urinary catheterisation are needed preoperatively.

Incision: Left subcostal incision is commonly used; it can be extended towards right side or upwards as Kehr's incision. Lengthy midline incision is also used but not a preferred one. In trauma lengthy midline incision is the preferred one always to explore and address other parts of the abdomen. Midline incision may be preferred when spleen extends massively towards right iliac fossa. Occasionally, thoracoabdominal incision may be needed **(Figs. 24-78 and 24-79)**.

There are two approaches for splenectomy—*anterior approach* wherein through lesser or greater omentum, splenic artery is isolated for ligation first, then dissected in front to later mobilise spleen medially to complete the splenectomy; *posterior approach* is first used in mobilising the spleen from lateral side medially, then dissection is done in the hilum of the spleen. In elective cases, anterior approach is ideal; in trauma and emergency situation, posterior approach is the preferred one **(Fig. 24-80)**.

Anterior Approach

Lesser omentum is opened to identify superior border of the pancreas. Splenic artery is identified. Peritoneum over it is opened.

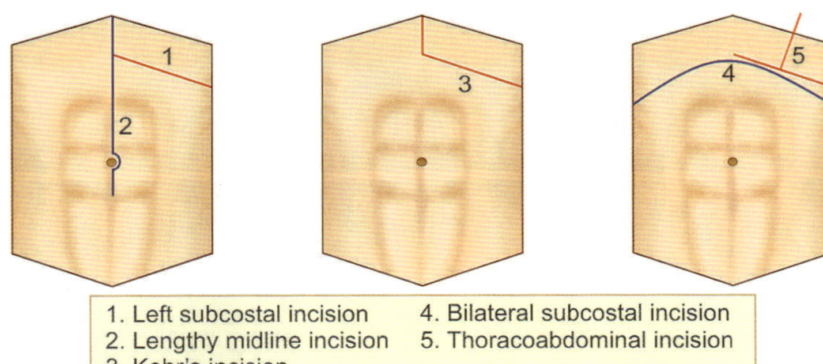

Fig. 24-78: Incisions used for splenectomy.

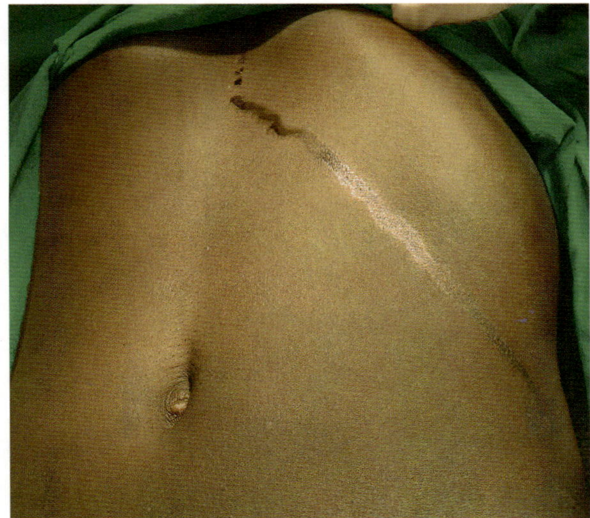

Fig. 24-79: Kehr's incision splenectomy.

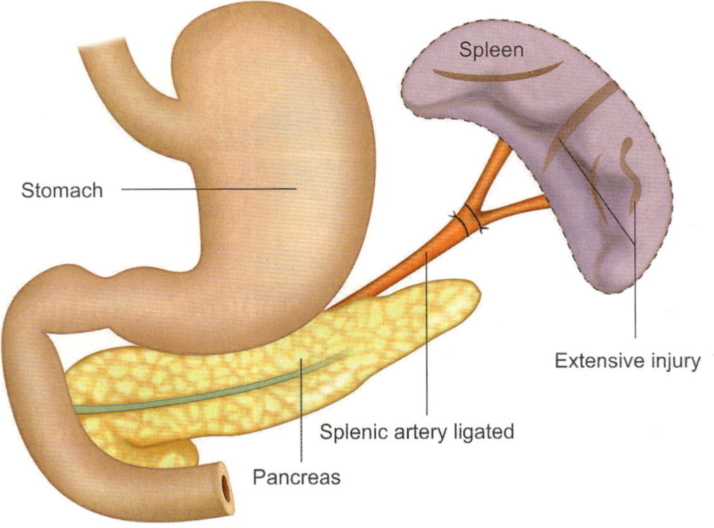

Fig. 24-80: Splenectomy.

Splenic artery at the level of the body of the pancreas is dissected, isolated and ligated. Instead of ligating it, an umbilical tape or vascular clamps can be applied to it to have a good control. Alternatively, splenic artery can be approached after opening the gastrocolic ligament greater omentum, left gastroepiploic vessels are ligated; superior margin of the body of the pancreas is dissected to identify the splenic artery which is ligated doubly using silk sutures. Short gastric vessels are ligated from below upwards along the gastrosplenic ligament; energy source like harmonic scalpel or ligaseal will be very helpful here **(Fig. 24-81)**.

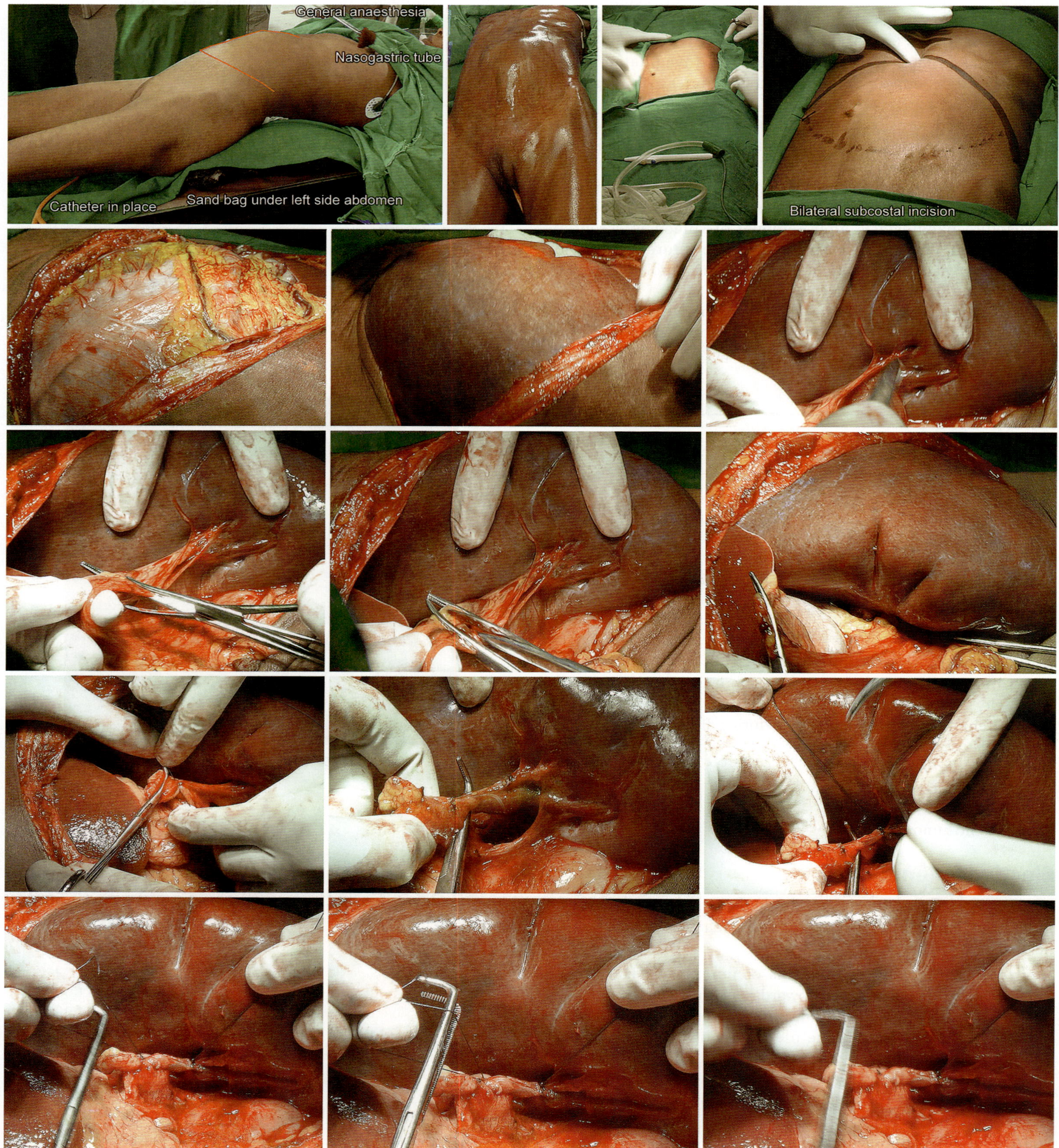

Figs. 24-81(1)

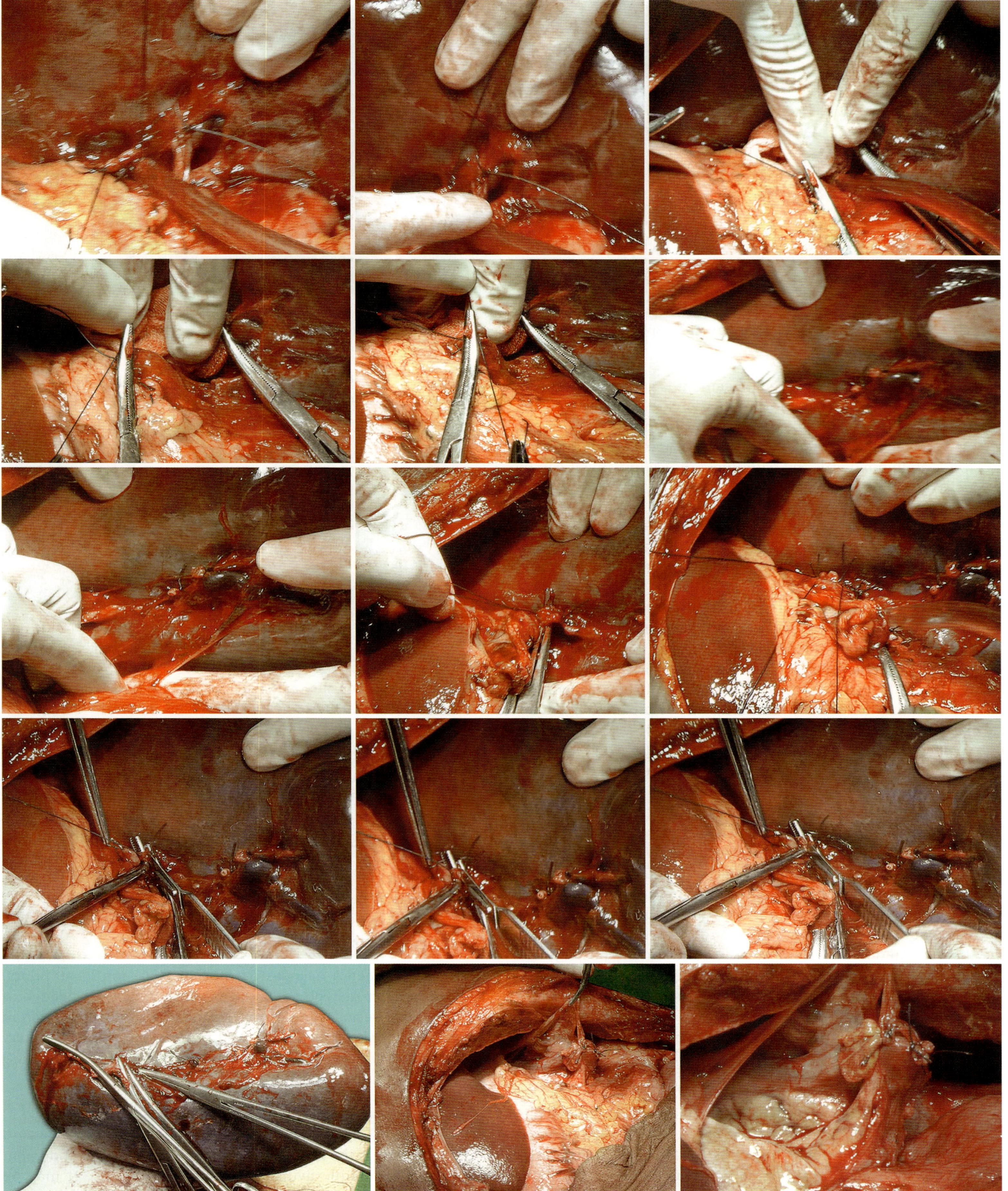

Figs. 24-81(2)

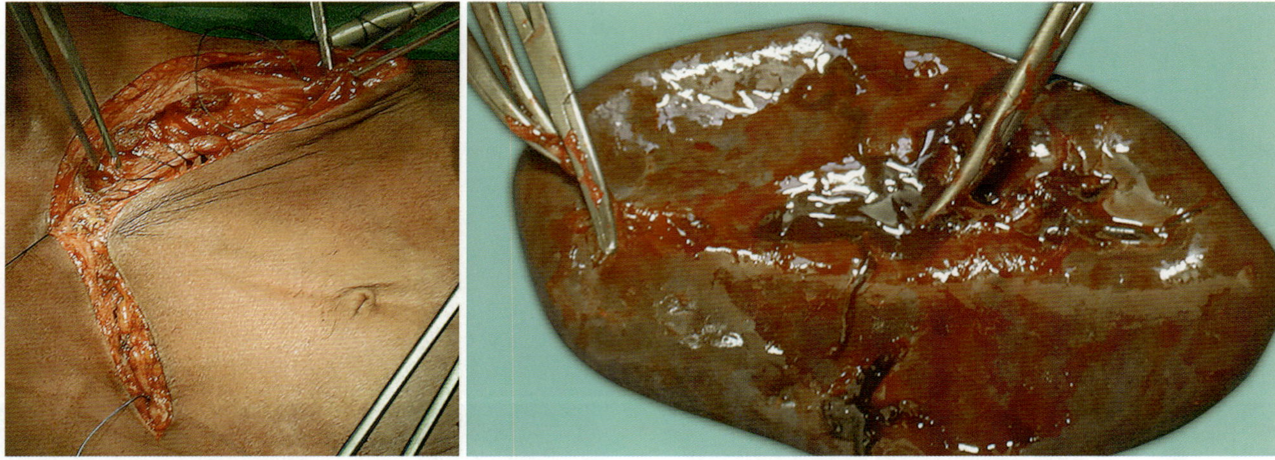

Figs. 24-81(3)

Figs. 24-81(1 to 3): Splenectomy in a large spleen through open bilateral subcostal incision.

Splenophrenic and splenorenal ligament is gently divided as it is usually avascular but ligation and division are better or by using energy sources. Spleen is dissected off from the Gerota's fascia. Plane is created between tail of the pancreas at its lower border and posterior abdominal wall and with finger dissection, finger can be encircled around.

Splenocolic ligament is divided and left flexure of the colon is released downwards. Remaining short gastric vessels and other peritoneal attachments are released using bipolar cautery and scissor or by ligation and division. Phrenicocolic ligament is also divided properly.

Spleen is elevated forward and medially to reach the splenic hilum and tail of the pancreas from behind. Splenic artery above and splenic vein below is identified and gently separated from tail of the pancreas. Splenic artery is dissected, isolated and ligated doubly using silk and divided. Branches of the splenic vein are divided after prior ligation. Splenic vein needs two or three proximal ligations; splenic vein is ligated at the end but care should be taken not to tear the vein by undue traction on the spleen towards front and medially. Splenic hilum with splenic vein is divided to get the splenic specimen out.

In elective cases for haemolytic diseases, meticulous search for accessory spleen is made and they should be removed properly. Spillage of the spleen should be avoided absolutely.

Seromuscular sutures should be placed on the greater curvature of the stomach towards fundal half side to prevent gastric necrosis or bleeding or leak. Either continuous or interrupted 2-zero silk sutures should be placed **(Figs. 24-82 and 24-83)**.

Absolute meticulous haemostasis on the surface near the tail of pancreas and in relation to different ligaments is essential. Transfixation ligatures or bipolar cautery should be used to achieve that.

Suction tube drain is placed. Abdomen is closed in layers.

Posterior Approach

Spleen is held medially towards right. Splenocolic and phrenocolic ligaments are divided to make splenic flexure of the colon descend downwards. Splenophrenic ligament is released. Splenorenal ligament is identified from behind which is incised carefully to expose the splenic vessels. In trauma where there will be continuous bleeding, assistant is made to put his thumb and index finger between the pedicle, otherwise an atraumatic occlusion clamp can be placed across the tail of the pancreas including the hilum to control the bleeding temporarily. Splenic artery is doubly ligated; branches of vein are ligated. Splenic vein is ligated doubly. Spleen is removed. Occlusion clamp is released. Any bleeding points in the pedicle are again transfixed using vicryl or silk and ligated. Tube drain is placed. Abdomen is closed in layers.

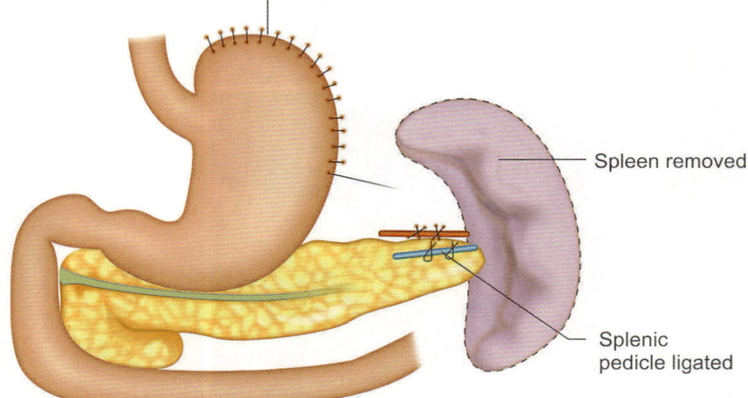

Fig. 24-82: Greater curvature of the stomach near fundus and proximal body should be invaginated using seromuscular sutures. It prevents greater curve necrosis.

Postoperative Care

It is usual to keep a nasogastric tube in place for 24–48 hours; urinary catheter may be needed. Often antibiotics are needed in postoperative period. Monitoring coagulation profile, observation for sepsis, left-sided atelectasis and pleural effusion are a must. Low molecular weight heparin, leg exercises and respiratory physiotherapy are always given.

MANAGEMENT OF SPLENIC TRAUMA

Splenic trauma is the *most common* blunt injury in the abdomen. Injury can be simple avulsion to hilar transection. It may be associated with injuries to left lobe liver, diaphragm, left lung, splenic flexure, small bowel or pancreas **(Figs. 24-84 to 24-92)**.

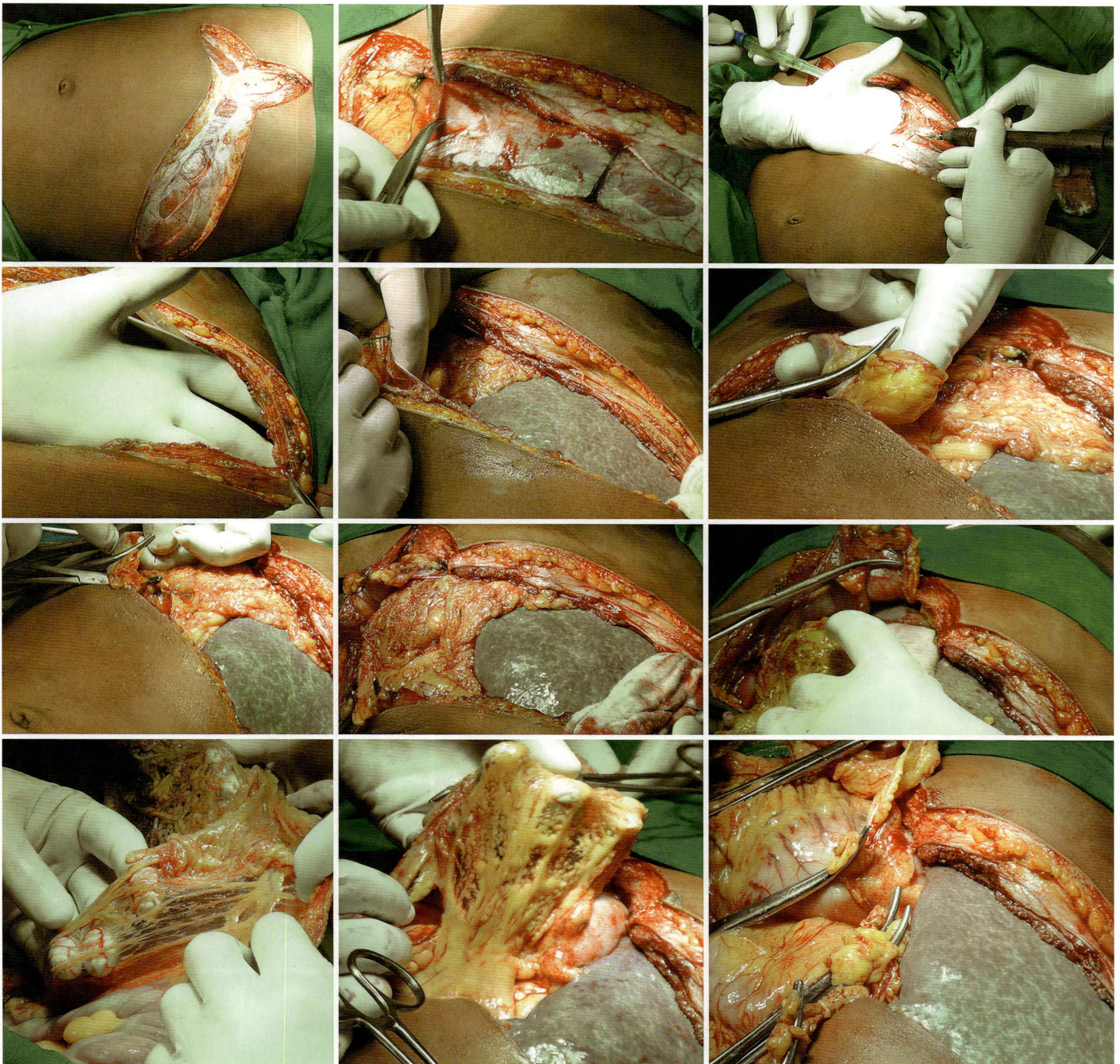

Figs. 24-83(1)

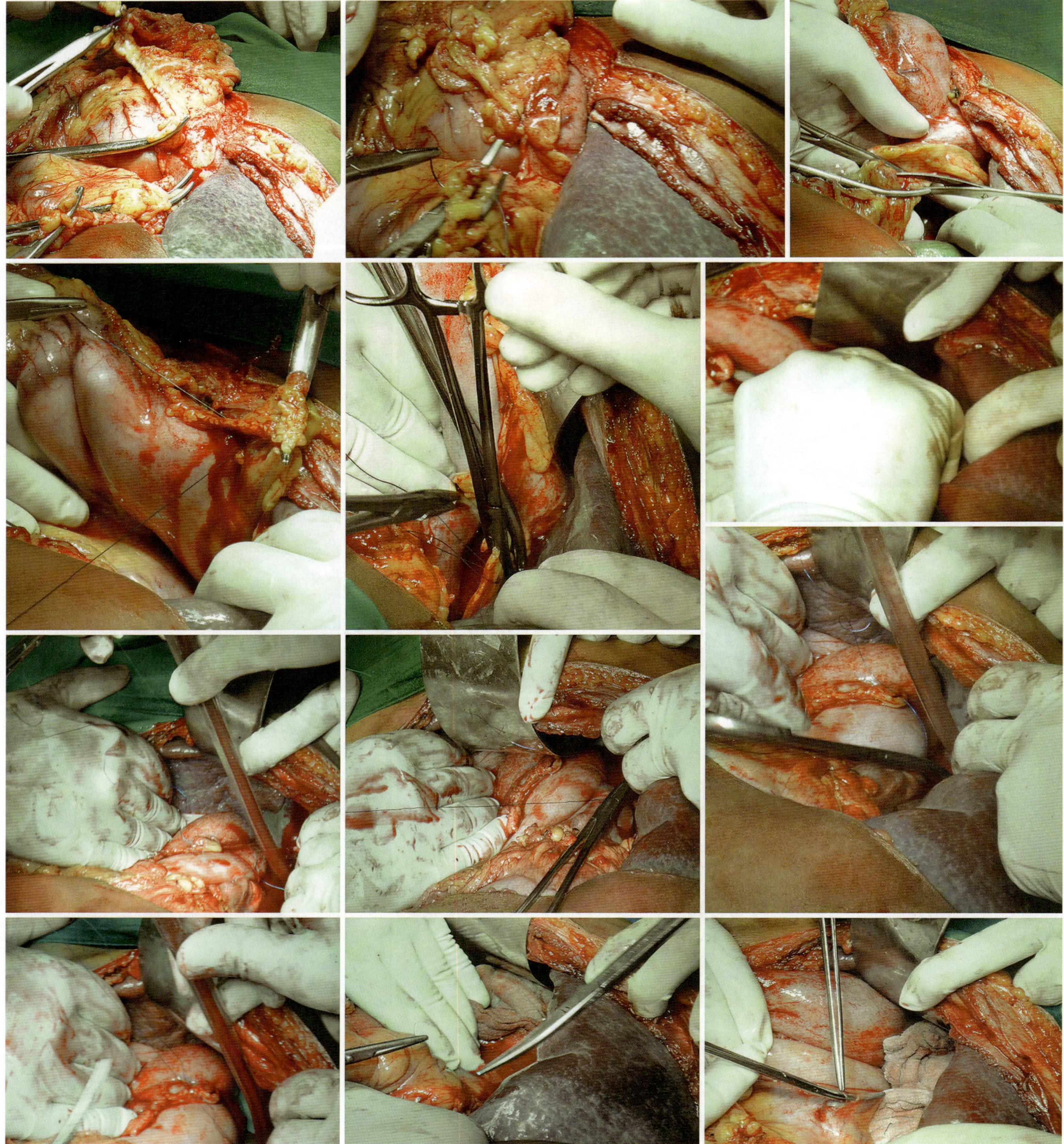

Figs. 24-83(2)

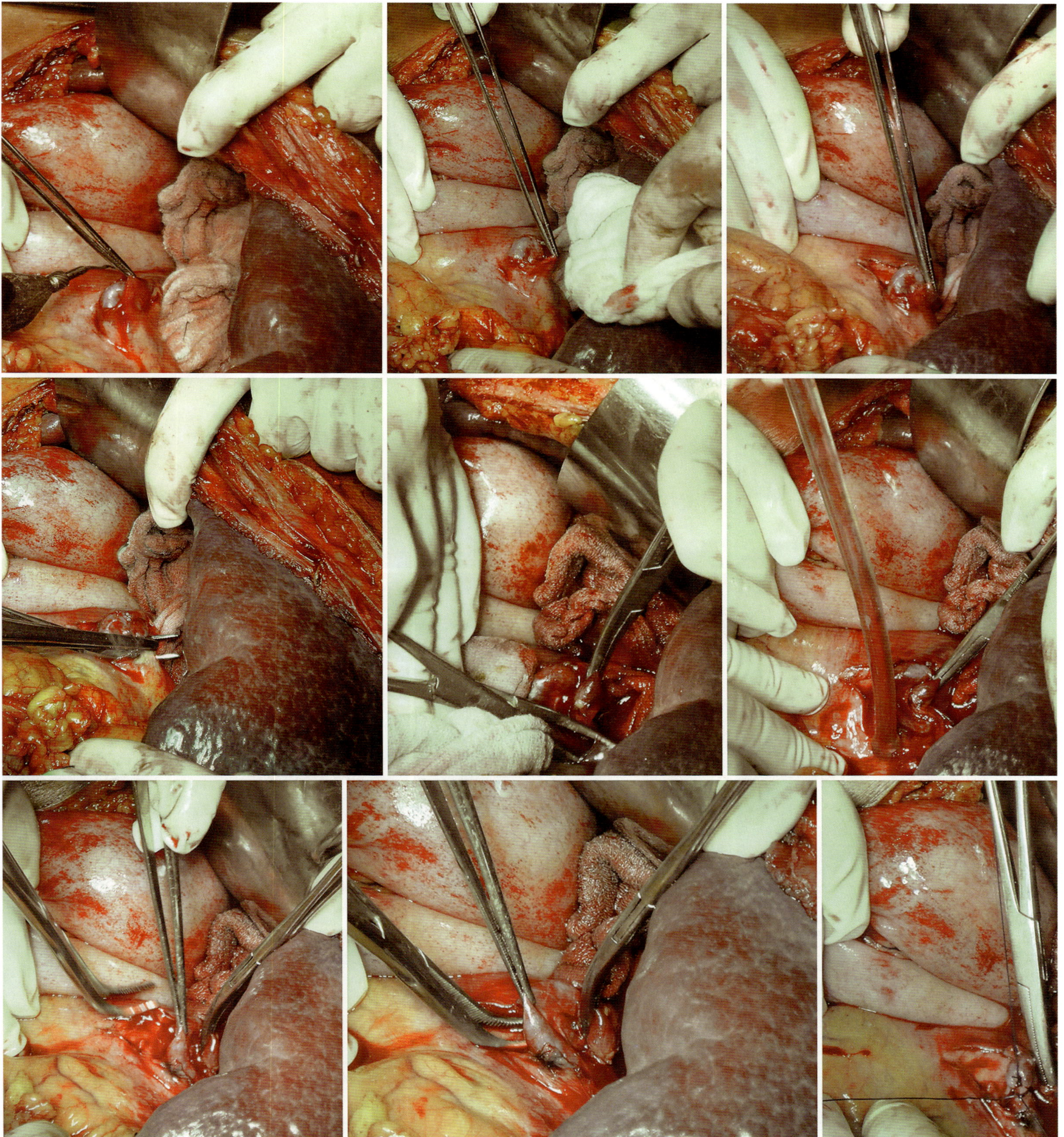

Figs. 24-83(3)

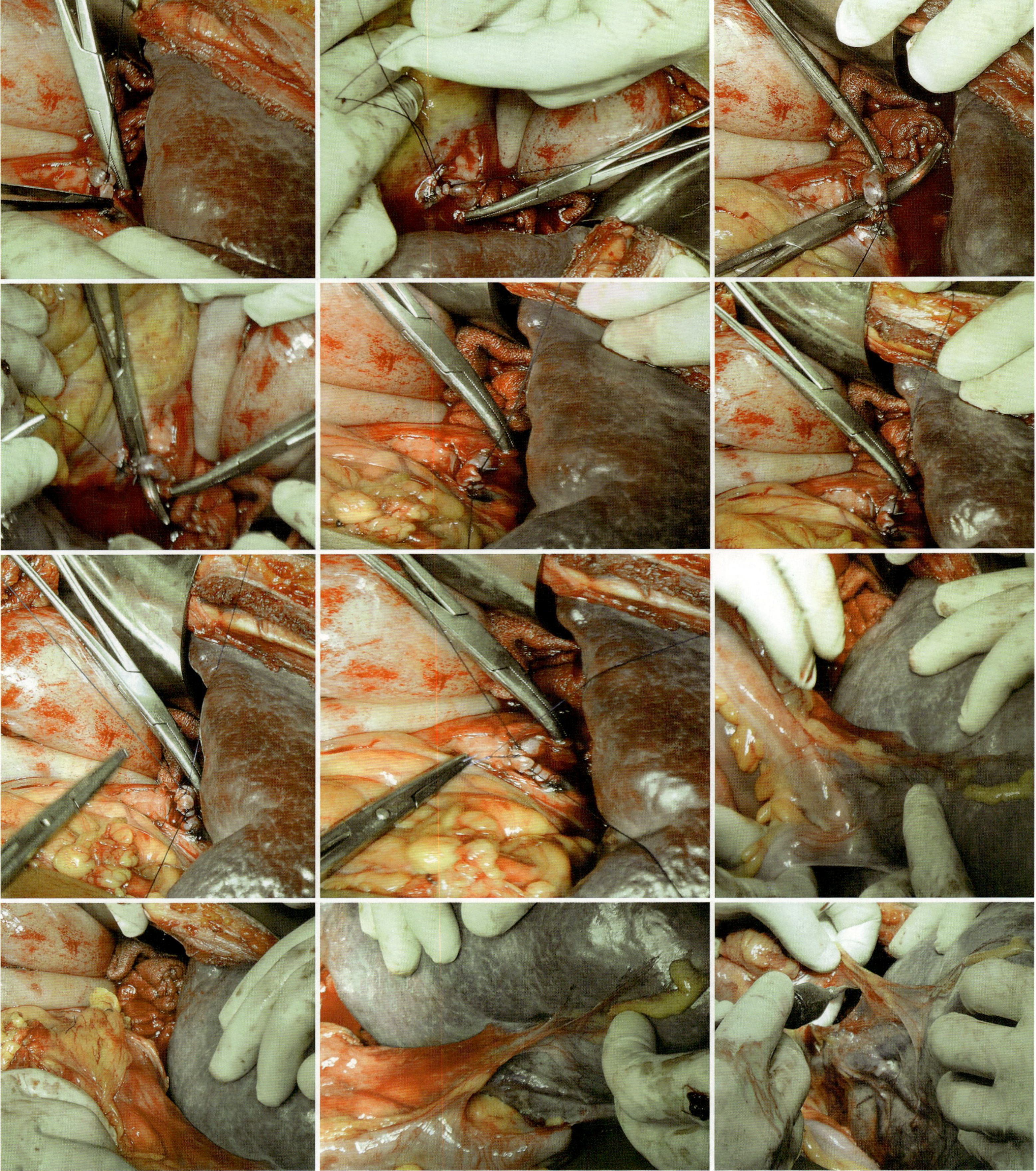

Figs. 24-83(4)

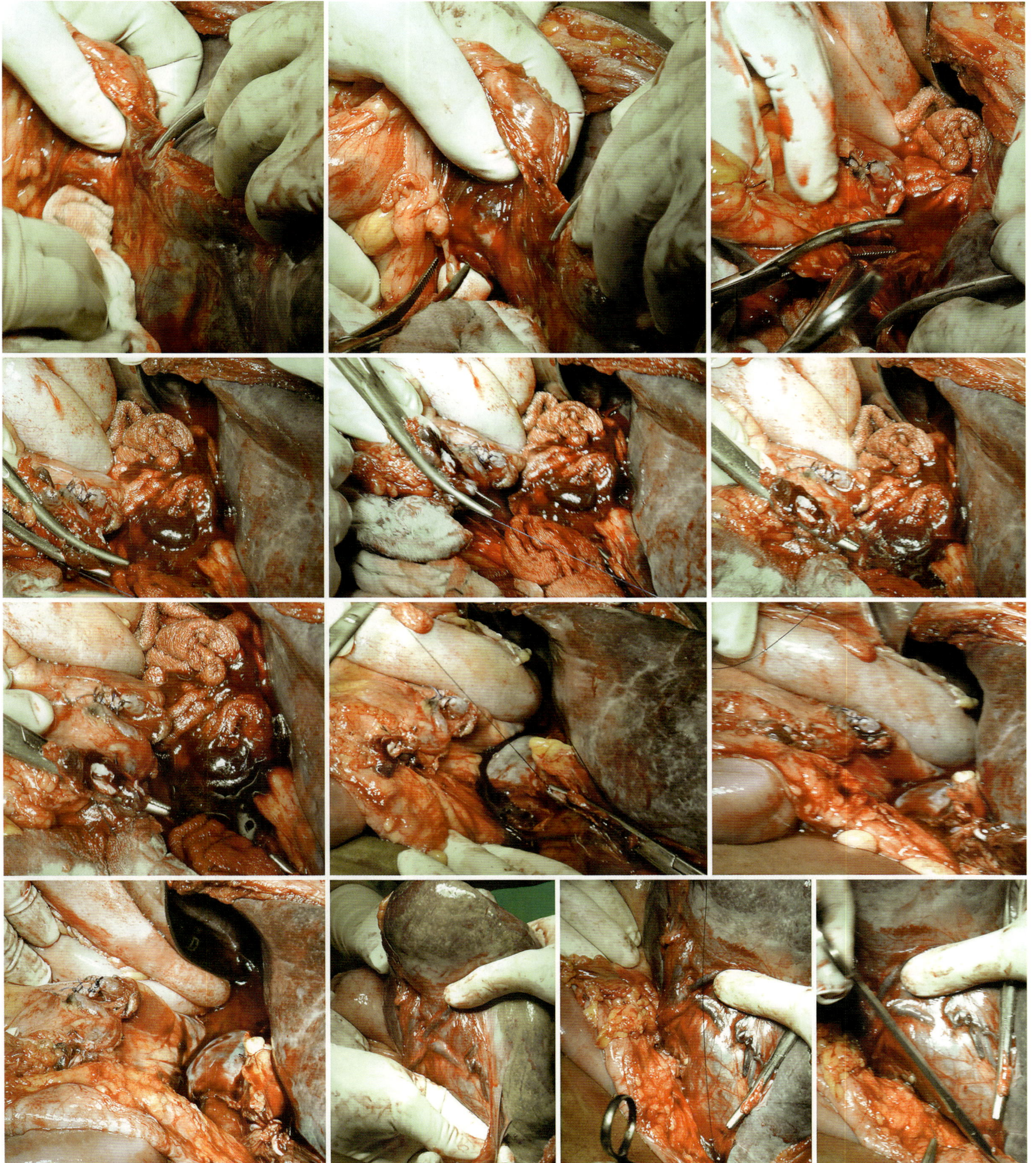

Figs. 24-83(5)

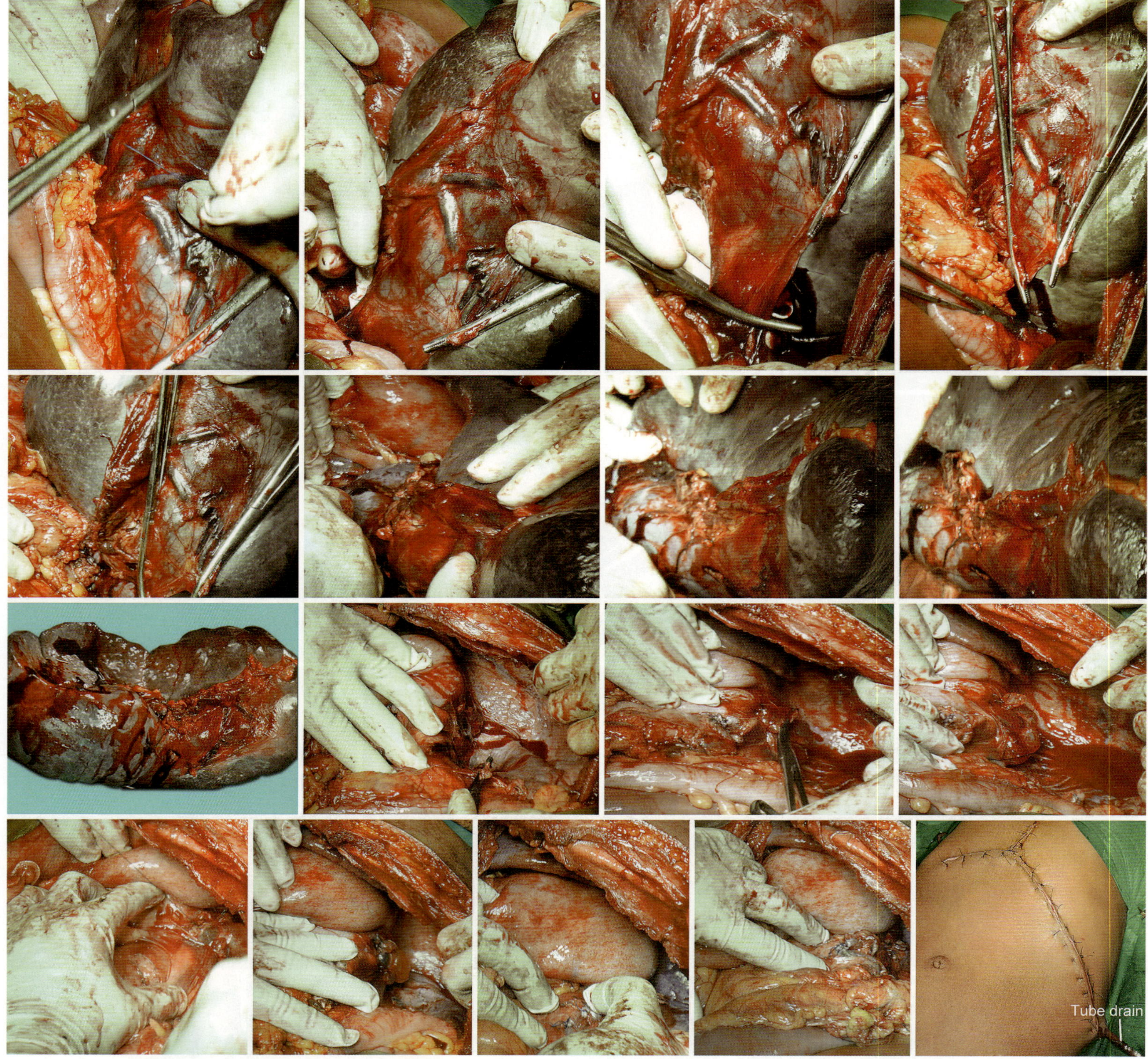

Figs. 24-83(6)

Figs. 24-83(1 to 6): Splenectomy in a massive spleen—subcostal incision extending towards right.

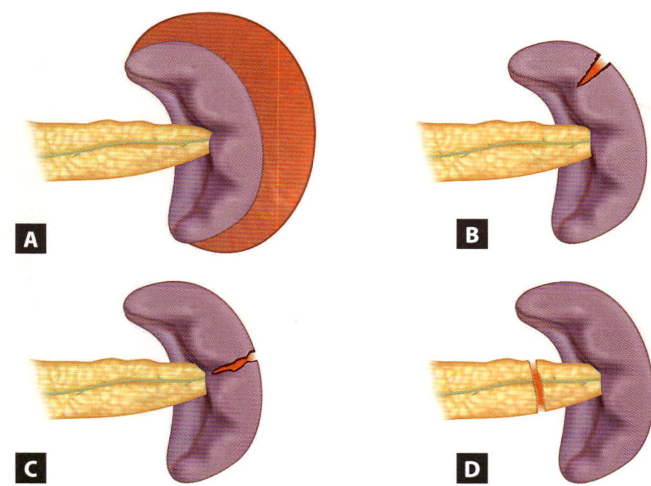

Figs. 24-84A to D: Types of splenic injury: (A) Subcapsular hematoma; (B) Incised wound; (C) Lacerated wound; and (D) Hilar injury.

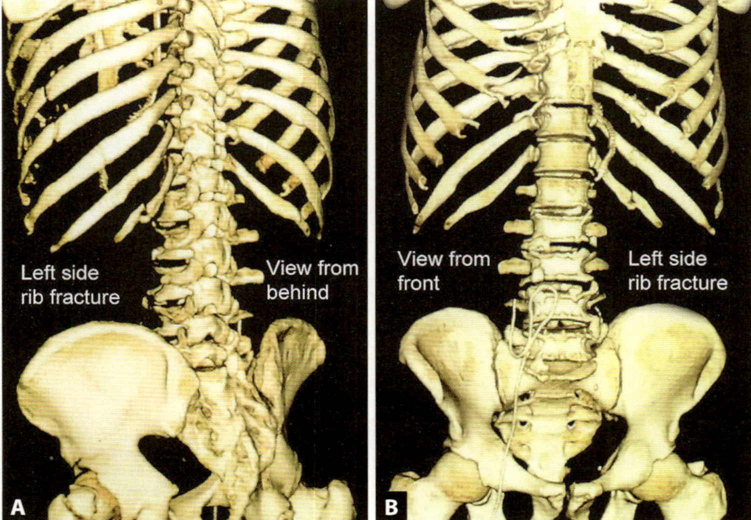

Figs. 24-85A and B: Reconstructed CT image of left lower rib fracture. It is often associated with splenic injury and left lung and diaphragmatic injuries.

Splenic organ injury scale (1994)	
Grade I	Non-expanding subcapsular haematoma <10% surface area. Non-bleeding capsular laceration with <1 cm depth
Grade II	Non-expanding subcapsular haematoma, 10–50% surface area. Non-expanding intraparenchymal haematoma <5 cm in diameter Laceration—capsular tear 1–3 cm in depth, which does not involve trabecular vessel
Grade III	Expanding subcapsular or >50% surface area or ruptured bleeding subcapsular haematoma/intraparenchymal haematoma. Intraparenchymal haematoma >5 cm or parenchymal laceration >3 cm depth involving trabecular vessels
Grade IV	Laceration involving segmental or hilar vessels with >25% devascularisation
Grade V	Shattered or avulsed spleen; hilar devascularisation with entire spleen devascularisation

Non-operative Management

Splenic trauma can be managed in majority of patients (65%) by non-operative management by observation, haemodynamic monitoring, output chart and abdominal girth measurement. Initial CT scan is a must to assess the grading of injury. Daily ultrasound monitoring and haematocrit are also important. Absolute bed rest for initial 7–10 days is needed until clot gets localised and organised. Antibiotics, blood and plasma transfusions and fluid management are needed. If any time the surgeon feels that non-operative management is not suitable, then one should go ahead for surgical intervention.

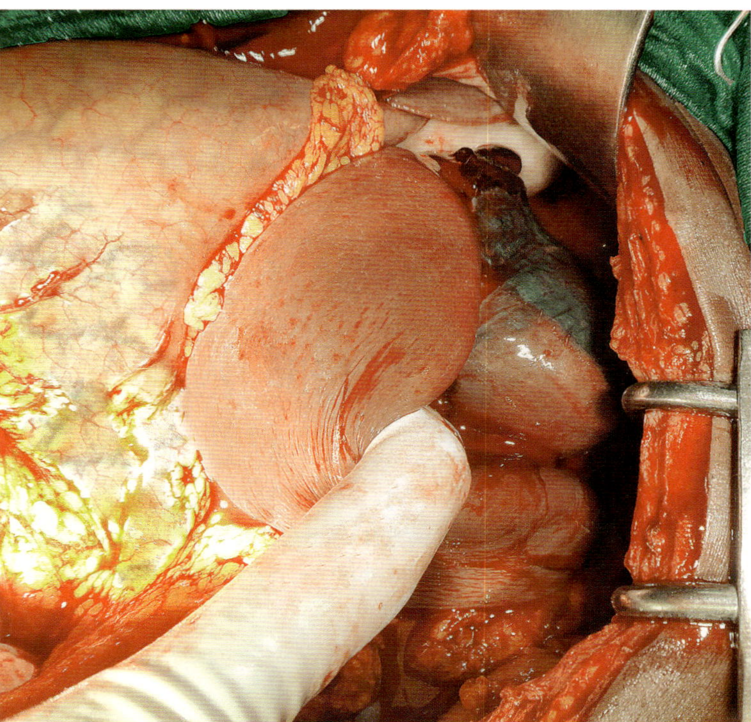

Fig. 24-86: Splenic subcapsular haematoma.

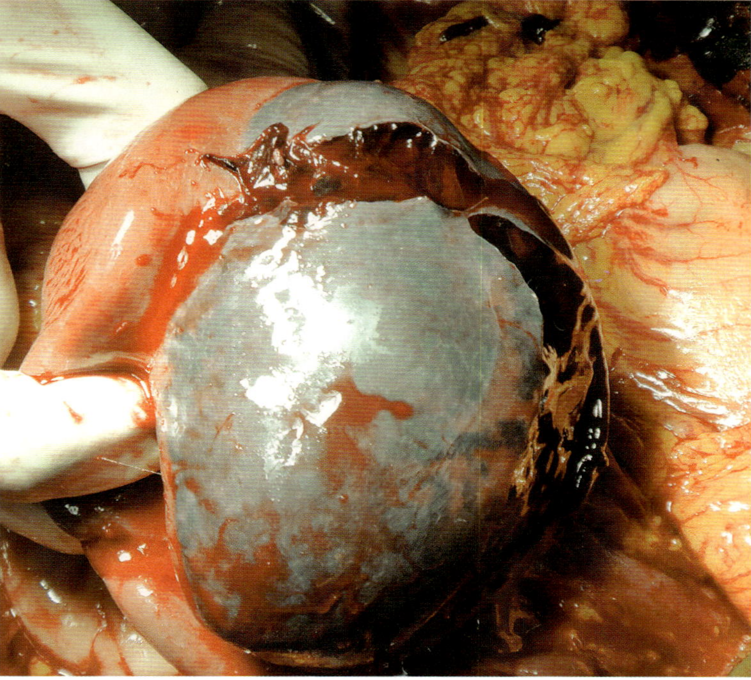

Fig. 24-87: Deep transverse splenic lacerations.

Splenic trauma may be avulsion of the capsule, superficial tears, partial transverse tears, complete transverse tears, longitudinal tears, stellate tears, subcapsular haematoma and hilar injuries.

Note:

- If patient shows features of haemodynamic instability—blood pressure below 90 mm Hg, pulse rate above 120/minute,

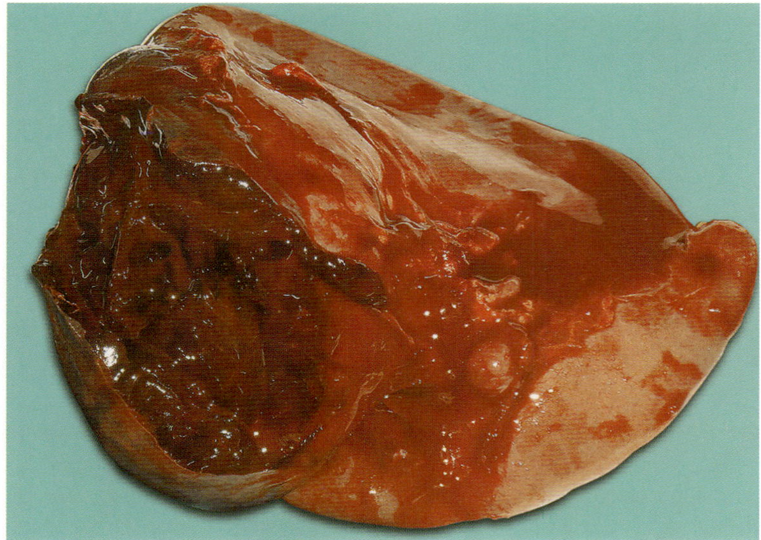

Fig. 24-88: Large splenic haematoma—splenectomy was done.

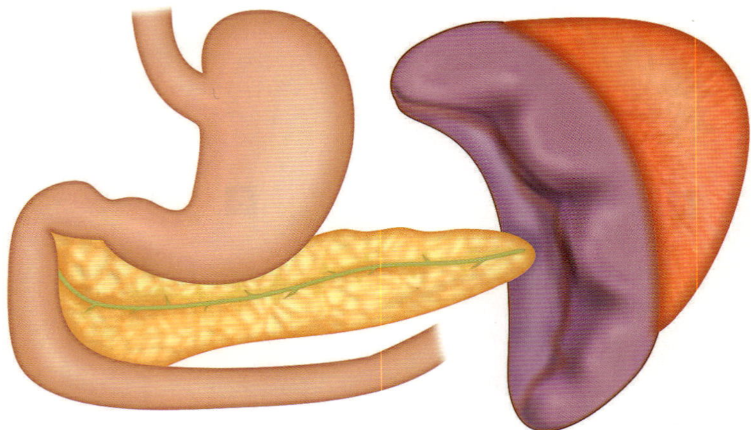

Fig. 24-91: Subcapsular haematoma. It can rupture late and can cause shock in the hospital or after discharge. Straining may precipitate rupture of the haematoma. Haematoma resolution should be confirmed by imaging prior to when the patient starts heavy straining works.

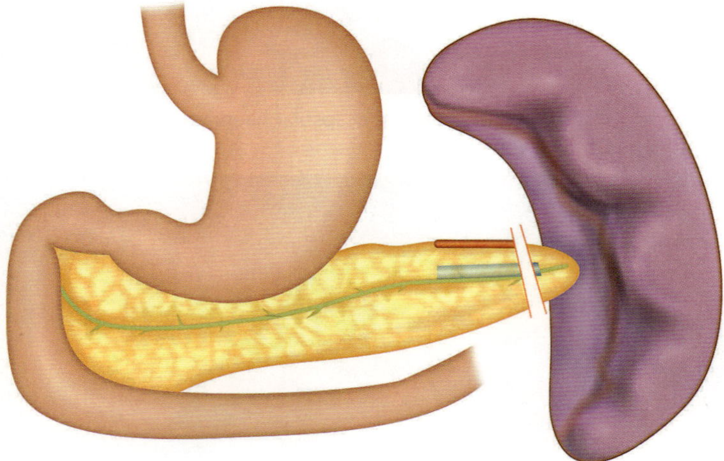

Fig. 24-89: Hilar injury—needs splenectomy.

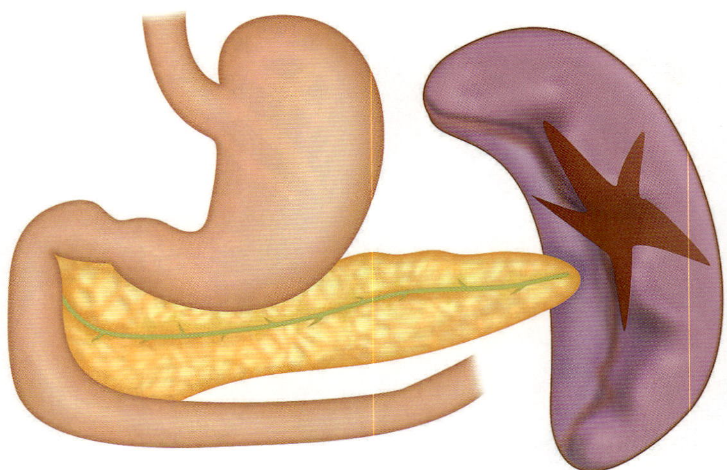

Fig. 24-92: Stellate tear in the spleen.

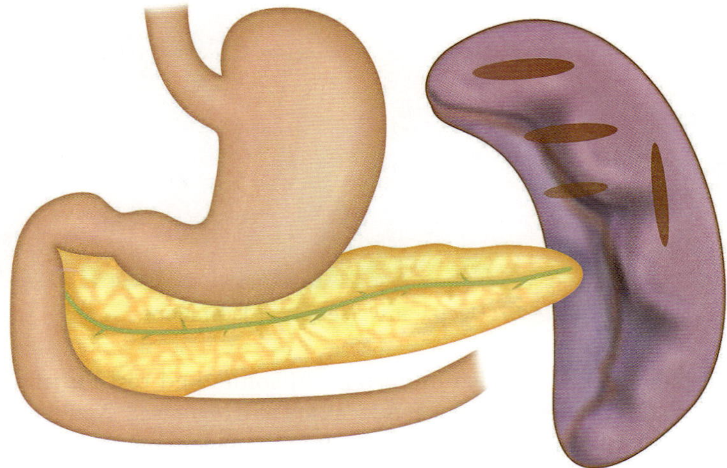

Fig. 24-90: Multiple tears often need splenectomy. If it is on to one segment, then partial splenectomy can be tried.

if patient does not show any positive response after infusion of 2 litres of crystalloid solution, then non-operative management should be abandoned.

- Non-operative approach prevents possibility of OPSI, thrombocytosis causing possible DVT.
- 80% of children (due to more elastin in spleen and complete coverage with ribs in childhood) and 50% of adult with splenic injury are treated with non-operative method.
- Failure rate in non-operative management up to grade II is 15–20% which is gradually reducing to 5% in many centres. It is more in patients with age more than 55 years.
- Delayed splenic rupture and formation of splenic pseudoaneurysm are problems in non-operative approach.
- Normal activity of the patient can be resumed only after 3 weeks following non-operative treatment in grade I and II injuries; after 8 weeks in grade III or beyond usually with a confirmation by CT scan.

Surgical Intervention

Splenectomy

Type of intervention needed is decided based on CT finding as well as on table operative findings. If there are extensive lacerations, large progressive splenic laceration with haematoma or perisplenic haematoma extending on both poles of the spleen, then splenectomy may be the only option. Splenectomy for trauma is done through posterior approach for quick reach and control. An occlusion clamp or vascular clamp is placed across the pedicle close to the tail of the pancreas initially by placing index finger underneath the pancreas. Lacerated spleen is held medially and towards right **(Fig. 24-93)**.

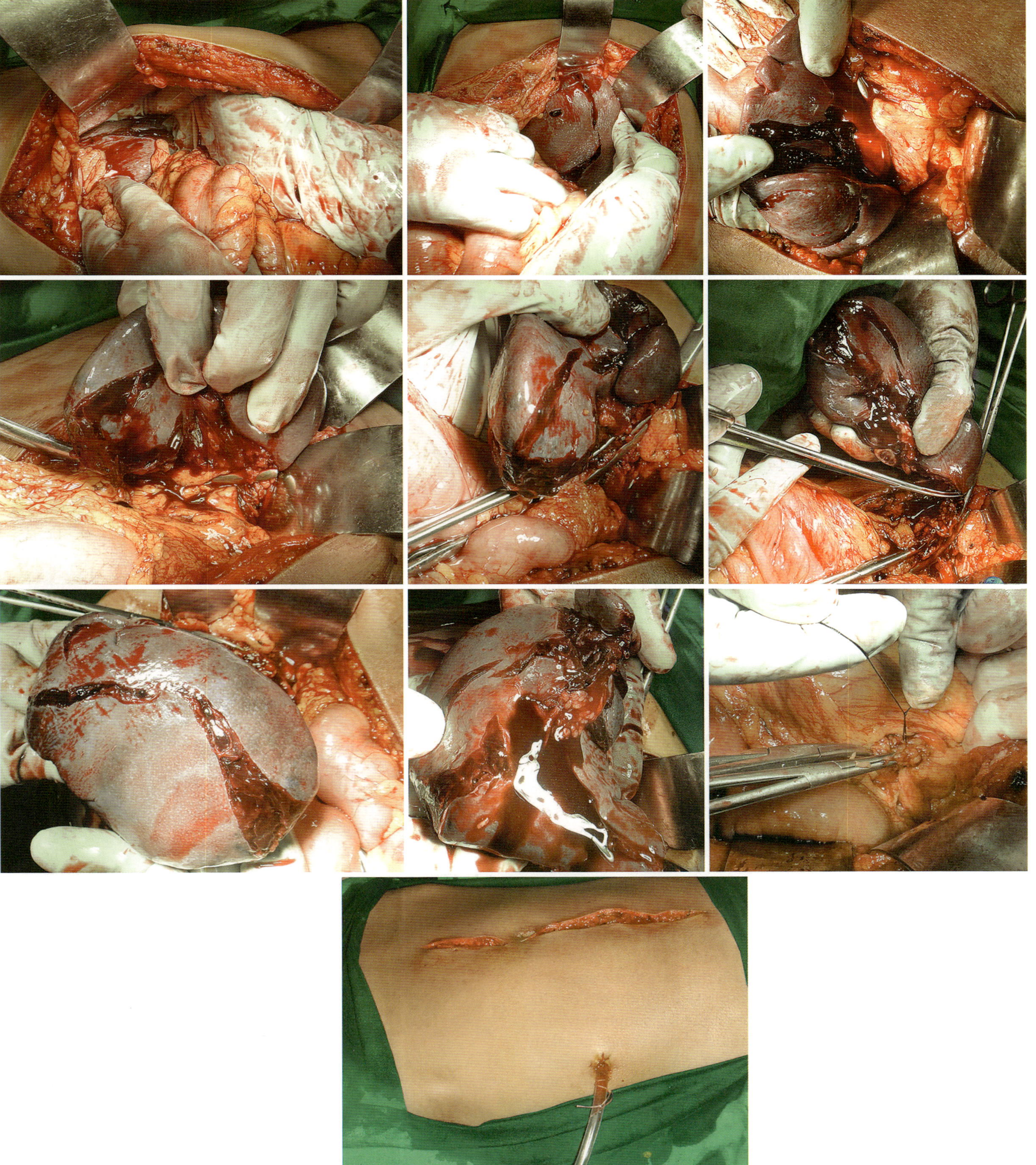

Fig. 24-93: Splenectomy in a trauma patient; lengthy midline incision is used; posterior approach is better. Soft vascular or occlusion clamp can be applied to begin with on the pedicle near the tail of the pancreas to control bleeding.

Splenophrenic, splenocolic and phrenocolic ligaments are divided to reach the splenic hilum along the lienorenal ligament. Splenic artery is identified, dissected and ligated doubly using silk. Splenic vein which is at lower part of the spleen is also ligated and divided. Rest of the attachments are also better ligated and divided. If surgeon is holding the spleen, then through right-angled Mixter instrument, dissection is done to pass ligatures and assistant will tie the knots; otherwise assistant should hold the spleen gently but firmly towards right and surgeon himself can place the ligatures. Spleen is removed. Rest of the abdomen is observed for additional injuries like that of diaphragm, liver, kidney, colon, small bowel and pancreas. Blood transfusion is done as commonly it is indicated. If there are no bowel and liver injuries, then autotransfusion of collected blood of haemoperitoneum can be done in theatre after proper filtering.

Splenic Preservation Surgeries

Small injuries like superficial lacerations which are often observed as iatrogenic injury during gastrectomy, pancreatic surgeries can be controlled by pressure, packing, haemostatic agents, surgicel, haemoclips, omental pedicle patch, suturing, etc. Argon beam laser is useful for surface oozing. These are superficial avulsions of capsule of the spleen. *Surgicel* is oxidised cellulose. Initially a gauze is placed gently but continuous firm pressure is applied for 10 minutes. Then gauze is removed; two layers of surgicel are applied again and another gauze over it; pressure is applied for 10 minutes. Gently apply pressure and outer gauze is removed to retain the surgicel at place. Avitene is another alternative to control the capillary ooze. Using forceps avitene is applied on the raw area for about 4 mm thickness; gentle pressure is applied using dry gauze for 5 minutes. Gauze is removed.

Transverse tears: Partial transverse tears can be sutured using 2-zero vicryl interrupted sutures. Initially haemostasis is required. Complete transverse tear needs partial splenectomy. Segment which is blue and dusky is removed retaining opposite one, either superior or inferior, depending on the involvement **(Figs. 24-94 and 24-95)**.

Longitudinal tears: As they cross across the segments, it is often difficult to manage and conserve. However, conservation is possible if one could be able to achieve proper haemostasis. Once it is so, omental pedicle is wrapped on the lacerated defect of the spleen and sutured over it. Further bleeding warrants splenectomy **(Fig. 24-96)**.

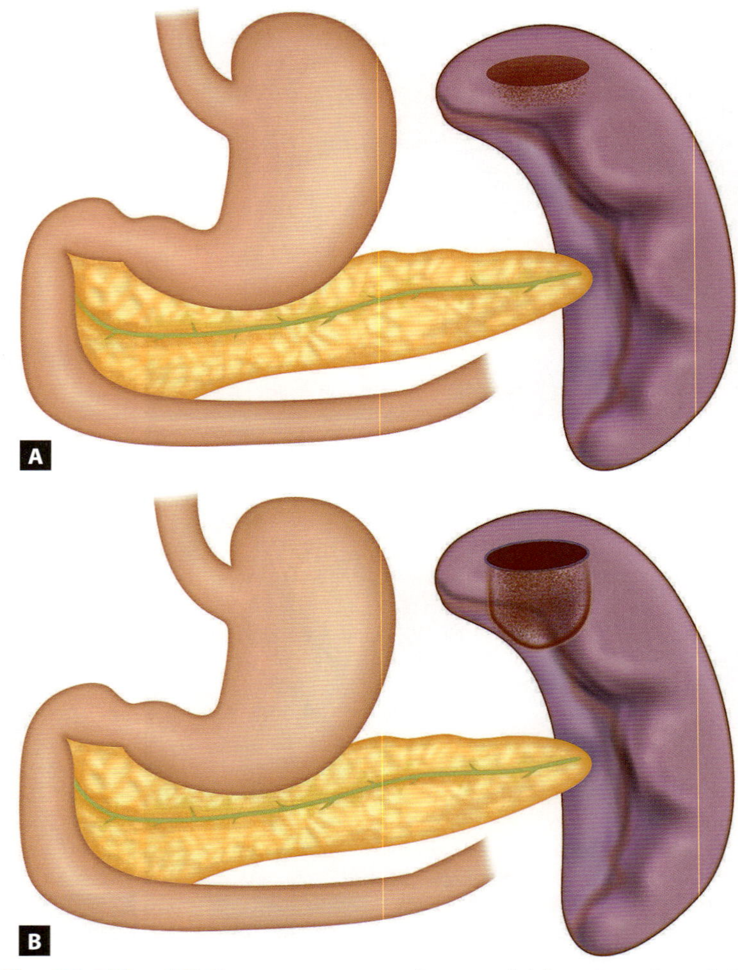

Figs. 24-94A and B: Transverse tear may be superficial or deep. Superficial tear is sutured—mattress interrupted one. Deep tear needs omental buttress or mesh wrapping; observation and repeat imaging are essential. If general condition deteriorates, partial or complete splenectomy should be done.

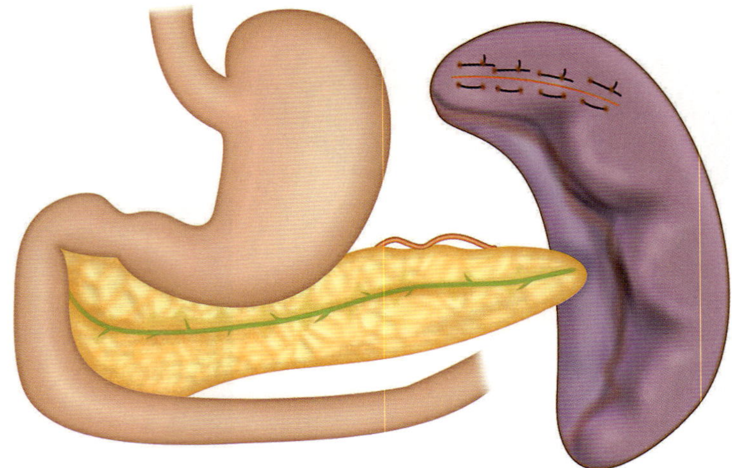

Fig. 24-95: Superficial avulsion or simple tear can be sutured by interrupted mattress vicryl 2-zero sutures.

Splenorrhaphy

Splenorrhaphy is one of the methods of splenic conservation practised. Here spleen should be carefully mobilised from the lateral aspect of the spleen and omentum. Posterior part of the spleen is packed with a mop. Assistant can gently place the thumb on the splenic artery to control bleeding. Clot on the left subphrenic area and on the lacerated wound is gently removed; care should be taken not to extend the laceration during this step. Small bleeders inside the wound are ligated using 4-zero vicryl. Wound is sutured with mattress sutures using 2-zero vicryl by taking bites from the capsule. Surgicel and Teflon pledgets can be used during capsular suturing. Just simple sutures will not hold the wound **(Fig. 24-97)**.

Splenorrhaphy by suturing is usually done for a transverse tear, usually single or often two. Longitudinal tear is difficult to appose by suturing. Multiple tears are difficult to manage. In such a situation, absorbable mesh is placed around the spleen by completely wrapping it around; a loose purse string is placed on the mesh on the inner aspect round the hilum. 2–3 plication sutures are placed on the outer surface to fix it (*mesh wrapping*).

In especially clean incised wound, spleen can be salvaged by suturing the wound carefully with placement of gel foam, topical thrombin, absorbable mesh wrap over the wound. Suture repair, oxidised cellulose and debridement of lacerated spleen—are other

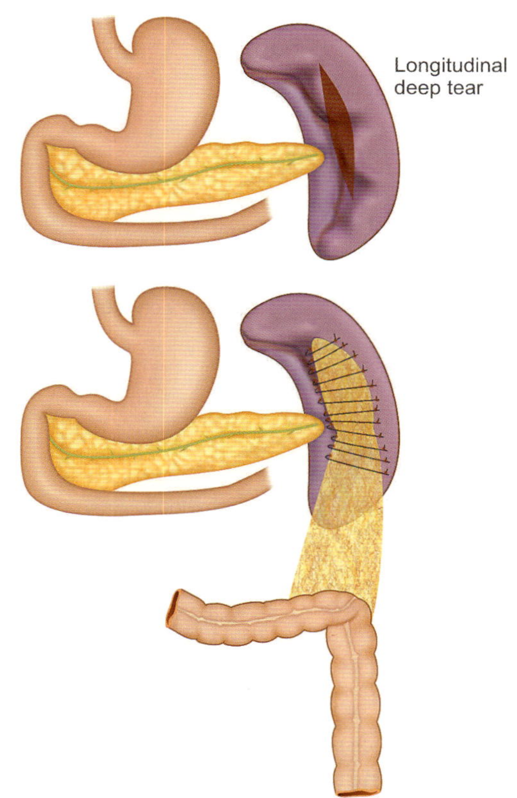

Fig. 24-96: Longitudinal tear needs omental buttressing on the wound.

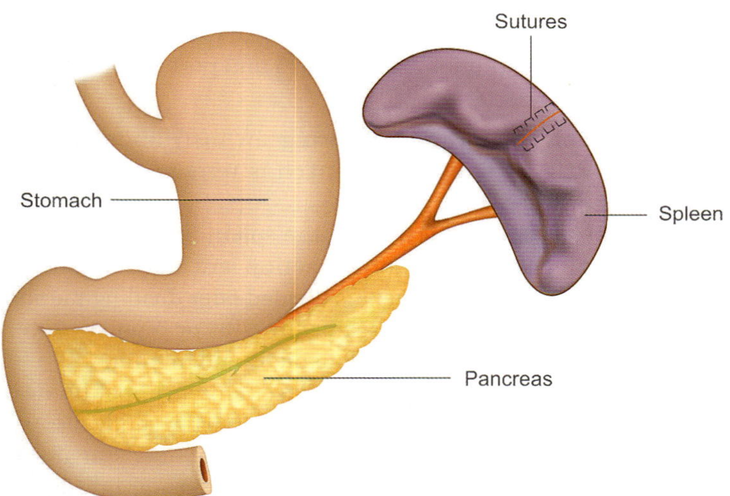

Fig. 24-97: Splenorrhaphy—diagrammatic look.

methods used. Temporary occlusion of splenic artery is often needed during splenorrhaphy. 10% of splenic injuries undergo splenorrhaphy. Its application is getting reduced due to non-operative approach in such patients. But in class IV or V injuries, splenorrhaphy is not possible.

Advantages of splenorrhaphy: It avoids OPSI; avoids dead space and so prevents potential space for subphrenic abscess; cellular components of blood are better maintained.

Partial Splenectomy (Hemi)

If deep injury to one of the segments of the spleen has occurred and if it is not possible to suture it by splenorrhaphy, then partial

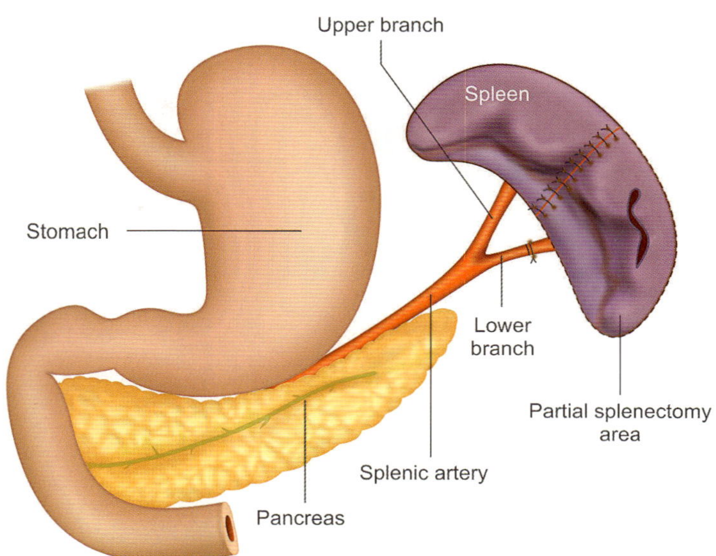

Fig. 24-98: Partial splenectomy.

splenectomy can be tried. Splenic artery is isolated proximally after initial lateral mobilisation of the spleen gently. Its branches—superior polar and inferior polar vessels are identified. Artery of the injured segment is dissected and ligated very close to the spleen in the hilum. On the other hand, without dividing the polar artery at the hilum, partial splenectomy can also be done; here splenic artery is isolated and silastic tape is placed around to control the bleeding; all bleeders on the hilum towards injured side are ligated and divided; injured spleen part is divided. Small bleeders are ligated on the surface with 4-zero vicryl. Sling on the splenic artery is released; surface is observed for any bleeding if it is so controlled with sutures. Cut edge of the partial splenectomy is sutured with mattress sutures with or without Teflon pledgets on both sides **(Figs. 24-98 and 24-99)**.

Suction tube drain is placed; wound is closed in layers. Even though the patient is undergoing conservative surgery, vaccine should be given; children should receive penicillin prophylaxis.

LAPAROSCOPIC SPLENECTOMY

First laparoscopic splenectomy was done in 1991 by Delaitre et al. He also started hanging spleen approach in 1995. Richardson adapted leaning spleen approach later.

Indications

- Haematological diseases like ITP, Felty's syndrome, thrombotic thrombocytopenic purpura, Thalassaemia and pancytopenia. ITP is the commonest indication.
- Hypersplenism, mobile spleen causing recurrent torsion, splenic cysts.
- Splenic artery aneurysm.
- Benign tumours of the spleen.
- Staging in Hodgkin's lymphoma.

Contraindications

- Massively enlarged spleen, splenic injury, splenectomy in portal hypertension, splenic vein thrombosis, pregnancy, previous upper abdominal surgery and splenic abscess are contraindications. However, these indications may be relative. in certain situations, laparoscopic splenectomy can be tried if experts are doing it.
- Obesity, spleen more than 30 cm and approximately of 3 kg weight is contraindicated.

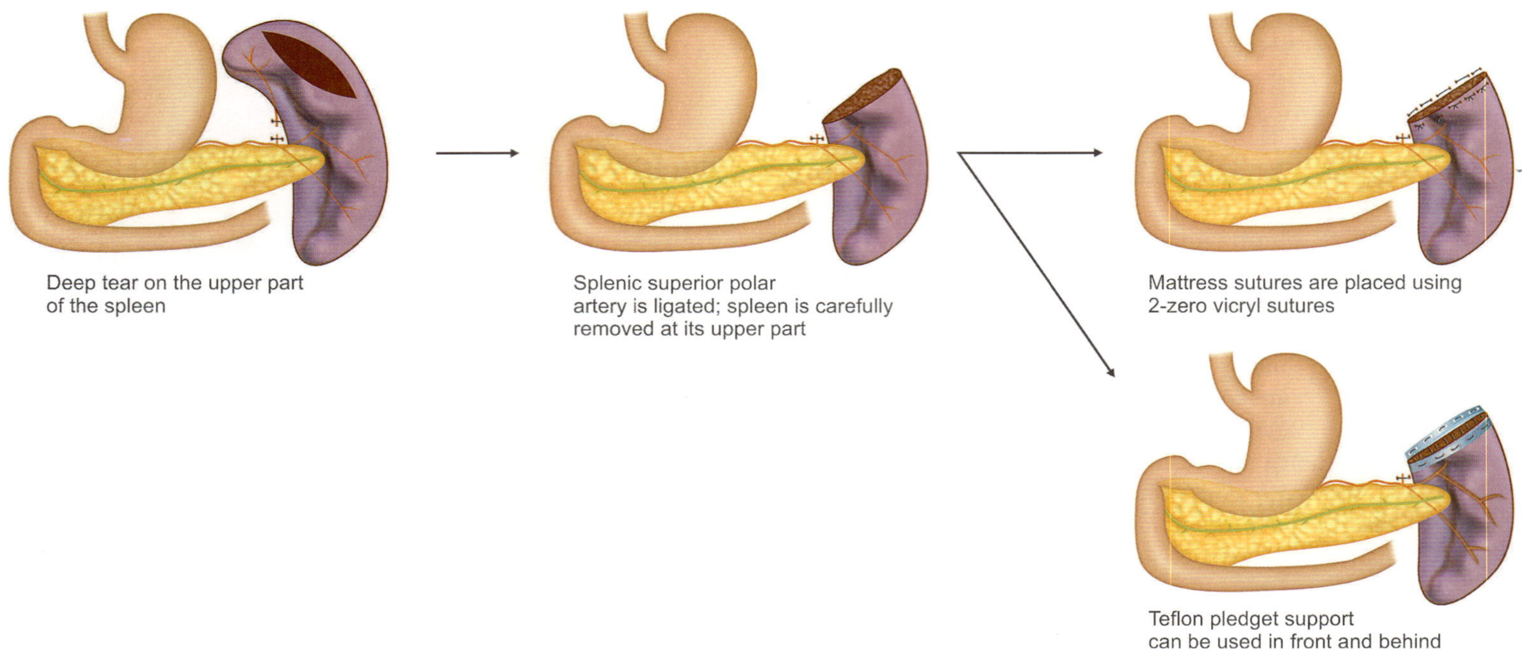

Fig. 24-99: Partial splenectomy—technique.

Preoperative Preparation

Evaluation is same as for open method. 2 weeks prior to the surgery immunisation against pneumococcal, meningococcal and haemophillus bacteria should be given.

Approaches

Anterior approach shows easier exploration for accessory spleen, and splenic artery, as well as easier rapid conversion into open midline incision, when need arises **(Fig. 24-100)**.

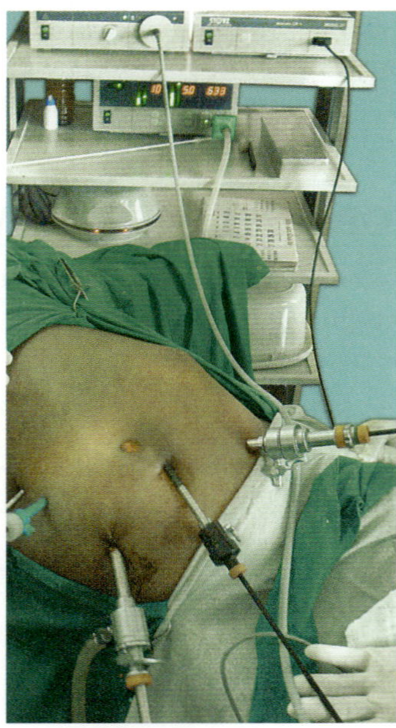

Fig. 24-100: Port positions and patient position for laparoscopic splenectomy.

Lateral approach allows easier retraction of stomach and colon; easier dissection of tail of pancreas and lower pole; splenic pedicle can be assessed and addressed easily; trocar positions are easier; operative ergonomics are better; easier control of short gastric vessels and minimum manipulation of the spleen which prevent splenic trauma and spillage.

Rotating operative table is ideal for this procedure. Right up position with surgeon standing on the right side; cameraman on the left of the surgeon on the right side of the patient. 30° telescope and harmonic scalpel are better and ideal.

10 mm port is umbilical for camera; 5 mm left hand working port is between epigastrium and camera; 10 mm right hand working port is at left midclavicuar line, if endovascular stapler is being used this port should be 12 mm; 5 mm epigastric port for retraction of the stomach; in left anterior axillary line 5 mm port when needed to retract spleen.

Technique: Spleen is retracted using an instrument through the anterior axillary line port; stomach is retracted through the epigastrium port.

Dissection starts with identifying the splenic artery. Two-hand technique, traction and counter-traction are needed for easy dissection. Gastrosplenic ligament is divided after dividing the short gastric vessels using harmonic scalpel or clips or bipolar cautery, stomach is mobilised and retracted medially and in front.

Peritoneum on the splenic artery adjacent to the upper border of the pancreas is incised to identify it. Splenic artery is gently dissected circumferentially to place a silk ligature. Ligature is tied but artery is not divided now; artery is divided only at a later period (ligation in continuity).

Splenic flexure of the colon is mobilised by dividing splenocolic, phrenocolic and other attachments; inferior pole of the spleen and lower part of the splenic hilum are visualised. Splenophrenic ligament is divided using harmonic scalpel to expose the splenorenal and retrosplenic ligaments. These ligaments are also divided to expose the hilar contents/vessels properly. Now spleen is hanging by its diaphragmatic attachment above. Splenic vein is seen in the lower part of the opened splenorenal ligament; often its wide tributaries also may be present. Ideal way to tackle these vein/veins is to pass a ligature around it using silk. Bipolar, harmonic clipping may not be adequate for this. Endostapler also sometimes may not hold. Splenic artery is doubly ligated again and divided. Splenic artery can be divided using harmonic scalpel as already once it is ligated proximally.

Once hilar vessels are divided, remaining parts of the attachment are released using harmonic scalpel. Separate upper pole vessel may be present which needs ligation, if harmonic scalpel is used.

Spleen is placed into a plastic impermeable retrieval bag; bag opening is brought through the left 10 mm port but may require lengthening of the port incision to retrieve the bag. Otherwise through bag opening, morcellator is passed to crush the spleen and retrieve the bag with specimen.

Laparoscopic splenectomy is also a good alternative in many splenectomies when splenomegaly is not massive. It is not useful in massive spleens and trauma.

Problems in laparoscopic splenectomy

In large spleen, it is difficult to manipulate and visualise; splenic artery can be approached through the lesser sac like as is done in open method after opening the lesser omentum.
Adhesions between spleen and diaphragm often may be vascular and difficult to release through laparoscopy.
Venous tear and bleeding is often difficult to control; such bleeding needs real pressure and packing and that is difficult to achieve through laparoscopy.
Spillage during dissection and retrieval of specimen may be hazardous in conditions like ITP; splenunculi might get missed, leading to failure in outcome.
Preoperative splenic artery embolisation in a large/massive spleen, splenic artery aneurysm, portal hypertension well reduce the size of the spleen which makes dissection and surgery much easier. But it is not done always as it may induce severe perisplenitis causing troublesome dissection itself.
Capsular disruption during manipulation should be avoided to prevent development of splenosis.

COMPLICATIONS OF SPLENECTOMY

Complications

1. Haemorrhage and shock
2. Haematemesis
3. Pancreatitis
4. Pancreatic fistula
5. Gastric dilatation
6. Left-sided pleural effusion
7. Left-sided colonic injury
8. Severe sepsis
9. Changes in cellular component of blood
10. Disseminated intravascular coagulation (DIC)

- *Haemorrhage*—mainly from short gastric vessels. Re-exploration and control of bleeding are needed.
- *Acute gastric dilatation*—needs nasogastric tube aspiration.
- *Haematemesis* due to mucosal congestion following ligation of short gastric vessels.
- *Left-sided pleural effusion* and left basal atelectasis (left lobe atelectasis is the commonest complication) (30%).
- *Left subphrenic abscess.*
- *Pancreatitis* following damage to tail of the pancreas and pancreatic fistula (3%).
- *Haematologic changes:* Rise in WBC and platelet count, rise in abnormal RBCs and RBC bodies.
- *Gastric fistulas*—it is better to invaginate the greater curvature using seromuscular silk or vicryl interrupted sutures.
- *Left-sided colonic injury.*
- Infection—postsplenectomy septicaemia, OPSI—most dangerous.
- *Portal vein thrombosis* can occur.
- *DVT as late sequelae* after splenectomy is often dangerous. Risk is 4 times more than non-splenectomised people and also pulmonary embolism. It is better to put them on long-term small dose of *aspirin* to reduce the incidence of thromboembolism.

Overwhelming Postsplenectomy Infection

As there is reduced IgM, tuftin, properdin and other antibodies, phagocytosis of encapsulated bacteria is defective. So, the post-splenectomised patient is more prone for *Pneumococcal septicaemia* (commonest), *N. meningitides, H. influenzae and Babesia microti* infections. Risk is more in patients on chemotherapy, radiotherapy and haemolytic diseases. Incidence is 4% or less. It is common in first two years after splenectomy. But it can occur any time. Risk persists for lifetime. Features—prodromal phase—fever, chills, sore throat; hypotension, shock; DIC; respiratory distress, coma, death. Mortality for fully developed OPSI—50–70%.

Prevention

Pneumococcal vaccine should be given to all splenectomised patients. Polyvalent pneumo-vac is given 2–3 weeks prior to surgery and soon after recovery from surgery and it is repeated once in 5 years (given to patients older than 2 years). Other vaccines advised are meningococcal vaccine (only to those who travel with high risk), *H. influenzae* 'B' vaccine (to all, whatever the age, once in 10 years). In malaria endemic areas, antimalarial prophylaxis is given for patients after splenectomy.

Treatment of OPSI: Antibiotics like cefoperazone, ceftazidime, amikacin; Ventilatory support—ICU care; blood transfusion; immunoglobulin transfusion; nutrition (TPN) and maintaining of urine output.

Prevention of OPSI: Lifelong prophylaxis using benzathine penicillin 12–24 lakh units controversial in adults (mainly it is given to children; changing concepts say it is selective in adults); pneumococcal vaccine given 2–3 weeks prior to splenectomy—gives 70% protection. *H. influenzae* B-type vaccine and meningococcal vaccine are given only to high-risk groups, as its effects are for short-term. So, it is not routinely given.

Note: Protection by vaccine is not completely guaranteed **(Fig. 24-101)**.

Note:

- OPSI is more common when splenectomy is done for malignancy or haematological diseases or when done in young individuals.
- Usage of prophylactic penicillin (benzathine) is controversial in adults even though it is beneficial in children up to 16 years.
- OPSI can occur at any time after splenectomy. Drugs like erythromycin, amoxicillin are also used as prophylactic agents.
- Mortality in fully developed OPSI (hypotension, DIC, MODS) is 60%—very high.
- Patients who survived after OPSI with therapy may develop residual problems like—gangrene of limbs, deafness, meningitis, mastoid osteomyelitis, heart valve destruction.
- About 7% of OPSI cases have *S. pneumoniae* sepsis. Others are—*N meningitidis, H. influenzae, Capnocytophaga canimorus* after dog bite.
- PPV 23 is the commonest vaccine used. Revaccination is done once in 5 years; decline in pneumococcal antibody level may be the criteria for revaccination.
- Preservation of 25% of spleen is sufficient to protect against pneumococcal infection. So, partial splenectomy is definitely helpful.
- Splenic autotransplantation into the omental pouch is under trial at present to reduce chances of OPSI.

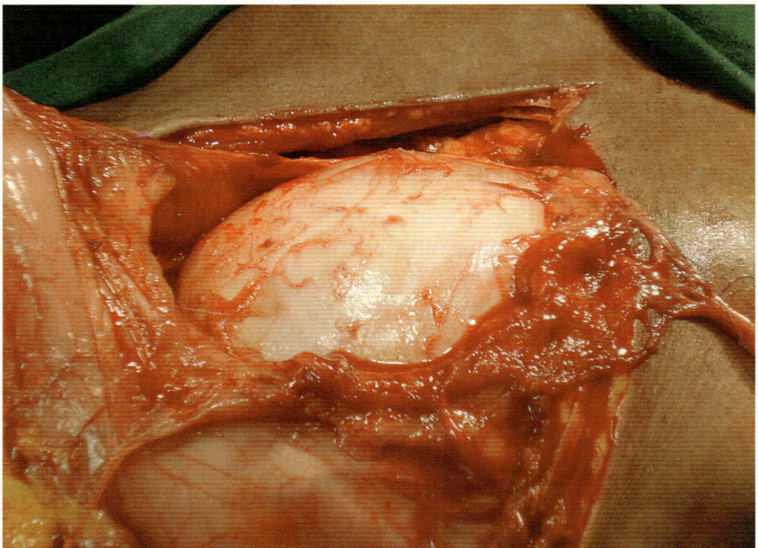

Fig. 24-101: Splenic aneurysm. It is the commonest site of aneurysm in the abdomen after aorta. Most common in women, due to atherosclerosis. Congenital splenic artery aneurysm can occur. Splenic artery pseudoaneurysm (10%) can occur after an attack of acute pancreatitis which may cause life-threatening rupture.

MESH SPLENOPEXY

It is also known as splenic mesh wrap. It is done for trauma. Electively it is often used in wandering/mobile spleen (*Splenoptosis*).

In open method in trauma, absorbable mesh is wrapped around completely. It is partly haemostatic and also creates tamponade.

Different methods are there to place the mesh as a wrap. Mesh may be wrapped around completely and at the hilar level it is bunched loosely using purse string suture. As per another method, a large absorbable mesh is taken. At its centre, a circular gap is made through which poles of the spleen are slid and mesh is wrapped from hilum outwards; mesh margins are sutured on the parietal surface of the spleen.

In wandering spleen, spleen is rotated to correct the torsion; after mobilisation, spleen is placed over one large mesh, which is fixed above and lateral to the lateral abdominal wall. Another similar mesh is placed on the front aspect of the spleen, which is also fixed to the lateral abdominal wall above and mesocolon below.

Procedure can be done in open or laparoscopic method also.

25 CHAPTER

Colonic Surgeries

SURGICAL ANATOMY

Colon extends from ileocaecal valve to rectum. It is 135–150 cm in length. Right colon is caecum, ascending colon and hepatic flexure; left colon is sigmoid colon, descending colon and splenic flexure. Transverse colon which is freely mobile joining part of right and left surgical units. Proximal colon is caecum, ascending colon and transverse colon; distal colon is descending and sigmoid colon. Large intestine is a wider terminology which includes caecum, ascending, transverse, descending, sigmoid colon and rectum and anal canal. But or convenient purpose colon is considered as large intestine. Appendix is also actually part of the large intestine.

Caecum is below the ileocaecal valve, usually of 6 cm long and 7.5 cm in width. It is situated in the lateral part of the right iliac fossa. Posteromedially there is appendix. Posteriorly caecum is related to right iliopsoas, genitofemoral, femoral and lateral cutaneous nerve of thigh, genital vessels and external iliac artery. Retrocaecal appendix will be behind it. Caecum may be of different types depending on its development (caecum develops from postarterial segment of the midgut loop as caecal bud). Usual *ampullary* type is 80% common where right caecal pouch is larger and appendix arises at its medial side. *Conical* type has appendix at its tip (12%); *intermediate* has right and left parts of the pouch of equal size with appendix coming out from its depression. Caecum gets its arterial supply from caecal branch of ileocolic artery; venous drainage into SMV. Its nerve supply is of midgut—T11; L1, parasympathetic is vagus. Ileocaecal valve opens on its posteromedial part of caecocolic junction. Ileocaecal valve has got two lips (upper lip is horizontal at ileocolic junction and lower lip is concave, is at ileocaecal junction) and two frenulae (anterior left is rounded; posterior right is narrow and pointed). When caecum distends valve closes preventing reflux of caecal contents **(Figs. 25-1A and B)**.

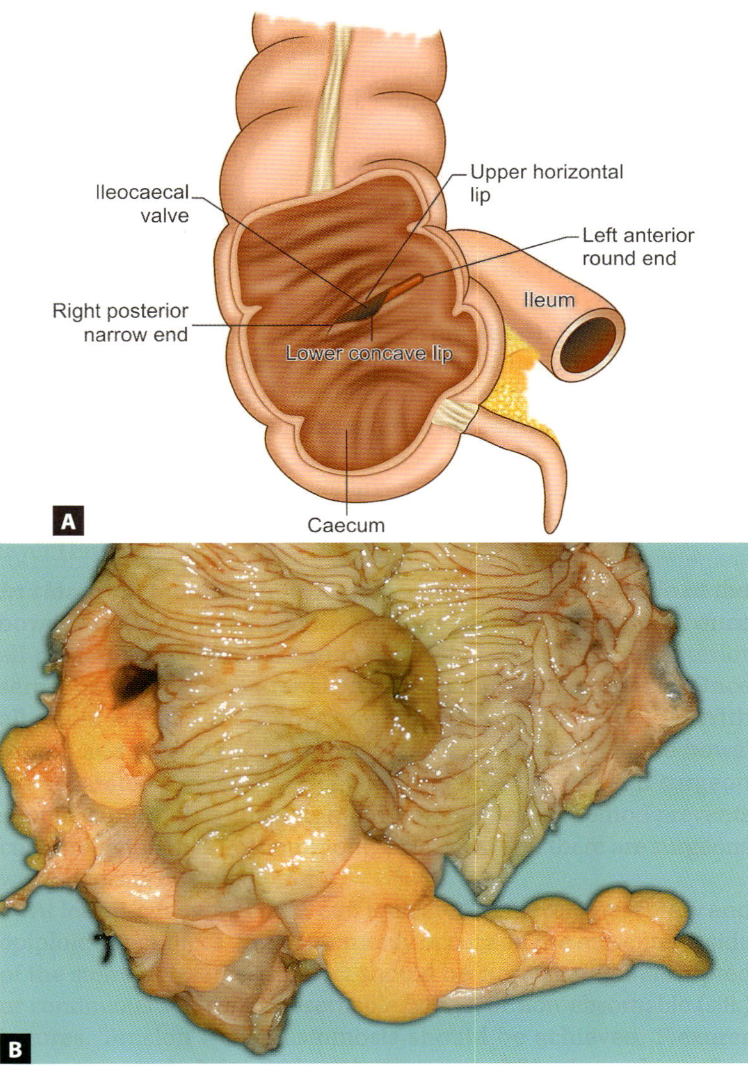

Figs. 25-1A and B: Anatomy of ileocaecal valve.

Caecum is fixed to posterior abdominal wall. In 25% of individuals, caecum is mobile. Mobility may precipitate volvulus or intussusception. Ileocolic/superior ileocaecal fossa, which opens towards left, is formed by fold of the peritoneum around anterior caecal artery. It is related to ileum and its mesentery, ascending colon and ileocaecal vessels in front. Inferior ileocaecal fossa is formed by bloodless fold of Treves extending from the terminal ileum and caecum in appendicular mesentery. It is below the ileum and its mesentery, in front of the mesentery of the appendix. Retrocaecal fossa is located behind the caecum, to the left of the right paracolic gutter, to the right of the mesentery **(Fig. 25-2)**.

Ascending colon is usually *fixed posteriorly* but can be mobile with a mesentery in 11–35% of individuals. In such situation, caecum will also be mobile along with ascending colon; it may lead into caecal volvulus along with ascending colon. Often there will be an abnormal

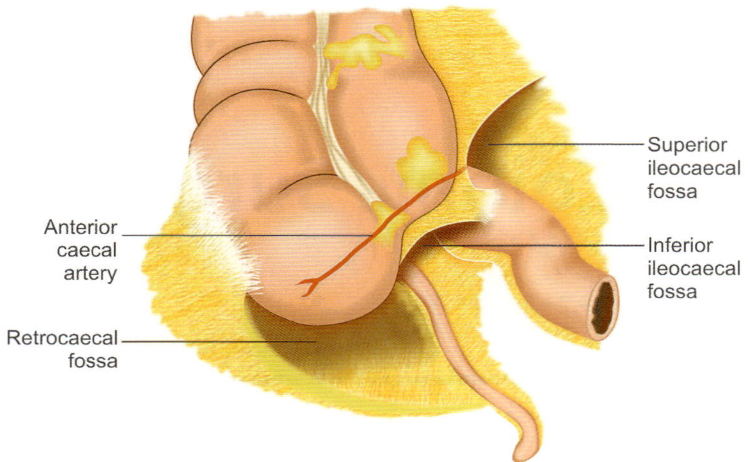

Fig. 25-2: Fossae in relation to caecum.

connective tissue band running across the ascending colon called as *Jackson's veil*; it may often be vascularised. From the right sided posterior abdominal wall it extends downwards and inwards getting attached to the anterior longitudinal ligament of ascending colon; often this veil may extend into caecum also. Ascending colon is 12 cm in length extending from caecum to hepatic flexure up to the inferior surface of the right lobe of liver. Behind it is related to iliacus, iliolumbar ligament, quadratus lumborum, transversus abdominis, lateral cutaneous nerve of thigh, ilioinguinal and iliohypogastric nerves, iliolumbar vessels, 4th lumbar artery and right kidney **(Fig. 25-3)**.

Right colic (hepatic) flexure: Ascending colon forms right colic/ hepatic flexure; hepatic flexure bends forwards, downwards and left to continue as transverse colon. Hepatic flexure is related to lower part of the right kidney and inferior surface of the right lobe of the liver.

Transverse colon is 50 cm in length extending from right flexure to left flexure. It hangs in the middle downwards like a suspension. It is suspended by transverse mesocolon, which is attached to anterior border of the pancreas and so creates wide range of mobility. In front it is related to greater omentum; behind it is related to 2nd part of the duodenum, head of the pancreas. Transverse mesocolon is double fold of peritoneum, which begins from the anterior border of the pancreas; middle colic artery runs in it. Middle colic artery may get damaged during gastrectomy during division of the greater omentum due to adhesions.

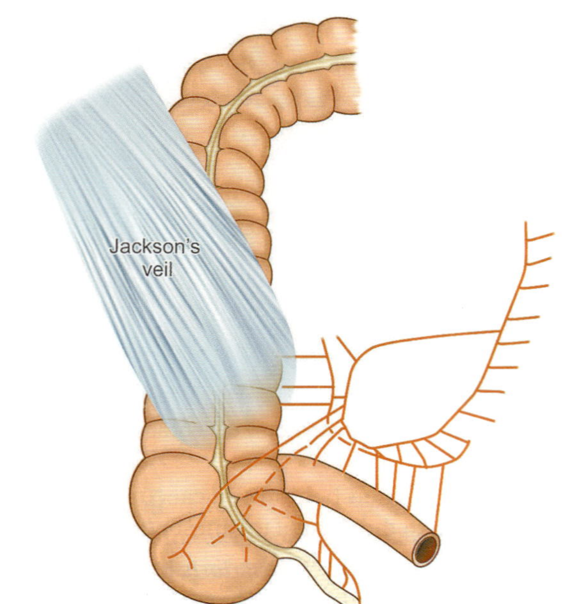

Fig. 25-3: Jackson veil/membrane extending from lateral abdominal wall on the anterior surface of the ascending colon.

Left colic (splenic) flexure: It extends from the junction of the transverse colon to descending colon; it bends backwards and downwards towards descending colon. It is related behind to left kidney and diaphragm below to anterior end of the spleen. *Phrenocolic ligament* extends as peritoneal fold from the splenic flexure to the 11th rib at midaxillary line; it also supports the spleen forming its bed. It forms the upper limit of the left paracolic gutter. Splenocolic ligament is located between spleen and splenic flexure **(Figs. 25-4A and B)**.

Descending colon is 25 cm long and extends from the left colic flexure to the sigmoid colon, vertically running up to iliac crest and medially on the iliopsoas muscle; in the pelvic brim it continues as sigmoid colon. Descending colon is retroperitoneal; it is rare to have a mesocolon. Behind it is related to transverse abdominis, quadratus lumborum, iliopsoas, iliohypogastric, ilioinguinal, lateral cutaneous, femoral and genitofemoral nerves, iliac branches of the iliolumbar vessels and testicular and external iliac vessels.

Sigmoid (pelvic) colon: It is about 35 cm in length extending from pelvic brim to 3rd piece of sacrum to continue as rectum. It is suspended with sigmoid mesocolon. Iliac part of the sigmoid is

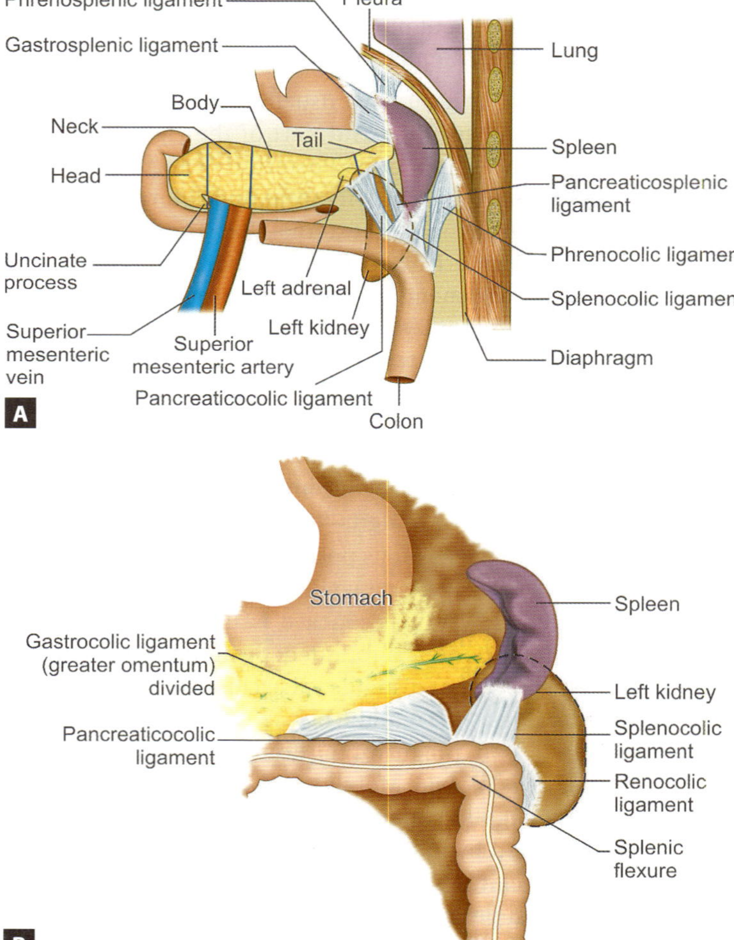

Figs. 25-4A and B: Splenic ligaments and relations of the splenic flexure of the colon. These relations are important in left sided colectomy.

fixed one; pelvic part is mobile one with sigmoid mesentery. Left ureter passes through the sigmoid colon through intersigmoid recess. Summit of the sigmoid is towards right iliac fossa. Pelvic mesocolon is inverted 'V' shaped; it has got two limbs—left limb is attached to brim of the left side pelvis; right limb is attached from apex to 3rd piece of the sacrum. Pelvic mesocolon carries superior rectal vessels; its apex is related to left ureter **(Figs. 25-5A to C)**.

Rectosigmoid junction is actually not a precise point as it is variable; it is marked by a distinct flexure. If the lesion is below the promontory it is called as rectal; rectosigmoid is 15 cm above the anal verge on sigmoidoscopy.

Colon does not have mucosal villi; its longitudinal muscularis externa has three discrete bands (taeniae). Appendices epiploicae are fat appendages attached to the surface of the colon; it is the site of infarction, torsion and site for diverticulae formation. While removing these appendages they should not be pulled out to avoid injury to the vessel underneath.

Blood Supply

Arterial Supply

Ileocolic, right colic, and middle colic arteries which are branches of superior mesenteric artery supply the colon from caecum to splenic flexure. Left colic, sigmoid, superior rectal arteries which are branches of inferior mesenteric artery supply the descending and sigmoid colon. The anastomotic arcade formed between the branches of superior and inferior mesenteric arteries is called '*arc of Riolan*.'

Ileocolic, right colic, middle colic (branches of superior mesenteric artery) and left colic artery and sigmoid branches supply the colon. Marginal artery connects branches of superior mesenteric and inferior mesenteric arteries. Marginal artery may be absent in 2% of individuals. Right colic artery may be absent in 12%; middle colic in 4% cases. Right (8%) and middle colic arteries (6%) or both (0.5%) may be often multiple. Atherosclerosis of the inferior mesenteric artery makes marginal artery poorer and unsuitable for colonic conduit. There is no marginal vein on the right side colon and it is said that anastomotic leak in 25% of right sided colonic conduit substitute is due to venous congestion rather than arterial.

Superior mesenteric artery (SMA) (artery of midgut) arises from the front of the abdominal aorta behind the body of pancreas at L1 vertebral level 1 cm below the coeliac trunk; it runs in front of the uncinate process crossing the 3rd part of the duodenum entering the mesentery to run in between its two layers. It ends at right iliac fossa by anastomosing with branch of ileocolic artery. Posteriorly above the root of the mesentery it is related to aorta, left renal vein, uncinate process and 3rd part of the duodenum; in the root of the mesentery it crosses the IVC, right ureter, right psoas muscle. SMV is on its right side; it is surrounded by superior mesenteric plexus of nerves. *Towards right side* it gives inferior pancreaticoduodenal, middle colic, right colic and ileocolic arterial branches. Middle colic artery arises just below the pancreas running downwards and forwards in the transverse mesocolon; its right branch communicates with right colic artery and its left branch with left colic artery. Right colic artery arises from SMA or as a common trunk with either middle colic or ileocolic arteries. It runs towards the upper part of the ascending colon; its descending branch anastomose with ileocolic artery and its ascending branch with middle colic artery. Ileocolic artery arises from SMA running downwards and towards right dividing into superior branch which anastomose with right colic artery and inferior branch which anastomose with terminal branch of the SMA. Inferior branch gives ascending colic branch, anterior and posterior caecal branches, appendicular artery and an ileal branch (terminal part of the ileum). Jejunal and ileal branches of SMA arise from its left side (fifteen in number) runs between two layers of the mesentery supplying the jejunum and ileum except terminal part of the ileum which is supplied by the ileal branch of the ileocolic artery. Jejunal vasa recta are longer and less numerous; ileal vasa recta are shorter and more in number.

The marginal artery of the colon, also known as the *marginal artery of Drummond* (Sir David Drummond (1852–1932) an English physician), is an anastomotic branch connects the IMA and SMA. It runs in the mesentery close to the bowel as part of the vascular arcade that connects the SMA and IMA. This artery is almost always present and its absence should be considered a variant.

The arc of Riolan (Riolan's arcade, Haller's anastomosis, 1803), also known as the 'meandering mesenteric artery' or central anastomotic mesenteric artery, is another inconstant vascular arcade present in the colonic mesentery that connects the proximal middle colic artery with a branch of the left colic artery. This artery is found low in the mesentery, near the root. Rarely, it can arise from SMA **(Figs. 25-6A to C)**.

Inferior mesenteric artery (artery of hindgut) (IMA) supplies colorectoanal region from left 1/3rd of the transverse colon to anal canal above the dentate line. IMA arises from front of the aorta 4 cm above the bifurcation of the aorta behind the 3rd part of the duodenum at L3 vertebral level. It descends downwards and left crossing the common iliac artery medial to the left ureter;

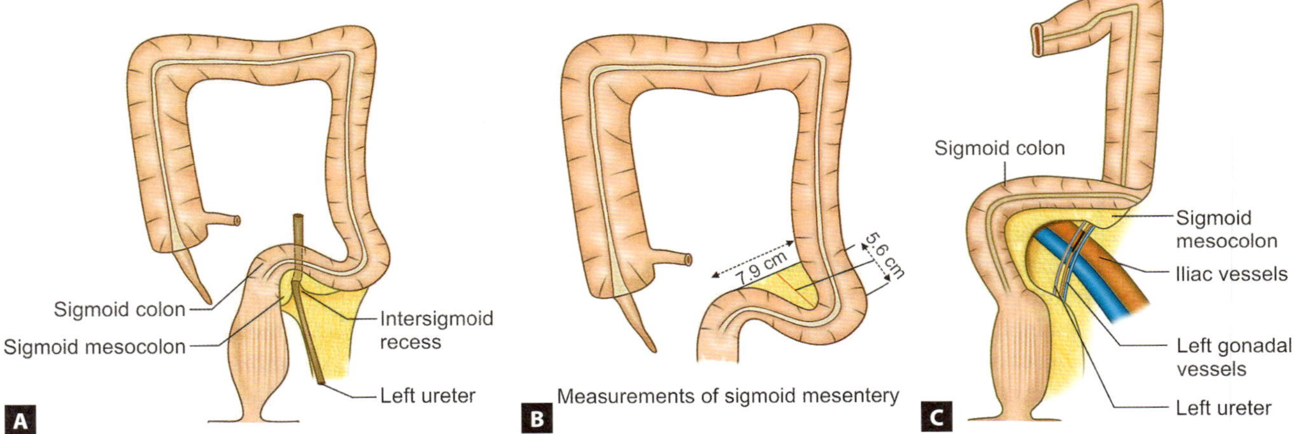

Figs. 25-5A to C: Relations and features of the sigmoid colon.

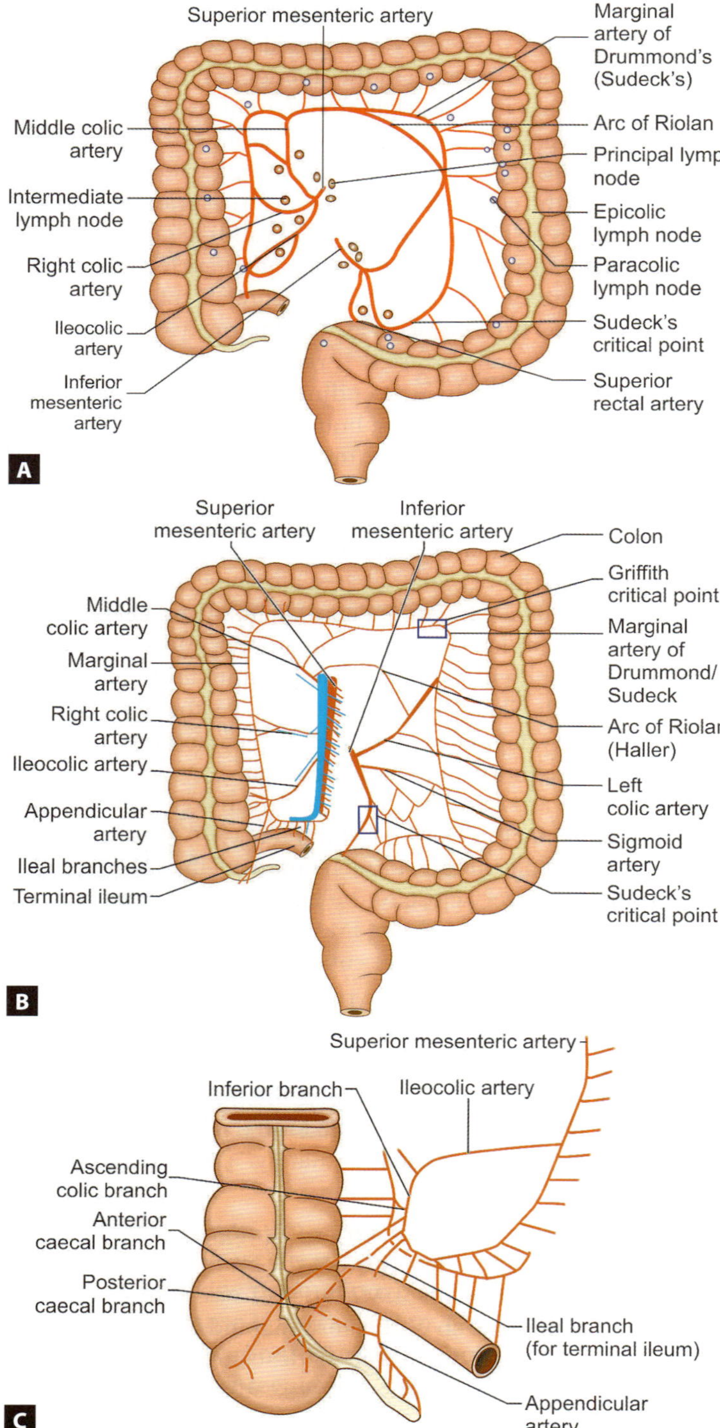

Figs. 25-6A to C: Blood supply and lymphatics of the colon.

in the sigmoid mesocolon it continues as superior rectal artery. *Left colic artery* is the 1st branch of IMA, runs upwards and left ends by dividing into ascending and descending branch. The ascending branch enters the transverse mesocolon and anastomoses with branch of middle colic artery. Descending branch anastomoses with 1st sigmoid artery. Left colic artery may be absent in 6% of cases. Sigmoid branches are 2-4 in number forms lowermost part of the marginal artery. Lowermost branch anastomose with superior rectal artery. *Sudeck's critical point* at the rectosigmoid junction is described as the point of origin of the last sigmoid arterial branch, originating from the inferior mesenteric artery (IMA). The Sudeck's critical point refers to a specific location in the arterial supply of the rectosigmoid junction, namely the origin of the last sigmoid arterial branch from the IMA. This arterial branch usually forms an anastomosis with a branch of the superior rectal artery. The anastomosis is small and often only singular. Sudeck's point has particular relevance in colorectal surgery and also forms a site of watershed susceptible to ischaemia. Superior rectal artery is the continuation of the IMA beyond the root of the sigmoid mesocolon. Opposite 3rd sacral vertebra it divides into right and left branches; each pierces the muscular coat of the rectum to supply rectum and anal canal communicating with middle and inferior rectal arteries. Right branch divides into anterior and posterior branches. Often a branch from proximal part of the left colic artery joins a branch from proximal middle colic artery to form arc of Riolan. IMA can be ligated and blood supply can be maintained through marginal artery (via SMA and through branches from internal iliac arteries). Marginal artery is weaker and less consistent in the splenic flexure and often absent in splenic flexure level and this point in splenic flexure is called as *Griffith critical point*.

Venous Drainage

Venous drainage occurs into superior mesenteric vein (which joins the splenic vein to form the portal vein) and inferior mesenteric vein (drains into the splenic vein). Venous drainage is similar to arterial supply. Marginal vein is often absent on the right side; but on left side marginal vein will be always present. So venous congestion can occur in right sided colon after surgery which may lead into venous infarction.

LYMPHATIC DRAINAGE

Mucosa contains no lymph channels, so mucosal cancers rarely metastasize. Nodes are *epicolic* (located in the colonic wall), *paracolic* (located along the inner margin), *intermediate* (located near the mesenteric vessels), *and principal* (located near main mesenteric vessels). Nodes situated along the main blood vessels like SMA, middle colic, right colic, ileocolic, IMA, left colic, sigmoid, superior rectal are called as proximal nodes; nodes along the next level branches are called as intermediate nodes, nodes in the colonic wall and its inner margin are called as distal nodes.

NERVE SUPPLY

Colonic motility is under control of autonomic nervous system; parasympathetic via vagi and pelvic nerves, sympathetic via superior and inferior mesenteric ganglia. The effect of meal on colonic activity is termed as *gastrocolic reflex*.

PRINCIPLES IN COLONIC SURGERY

Colonoscopy is essential in all colonic diseases prior to surgical intervention unless it is a surgical emergency. Proper preoperative staging using CT scan of abdomen and chest, endosonography is needed for staging. Carcinoembryonic antigen (CEA) is of no use for diagnosis; however, it is done to get a base line level so as to be utilised during follow up for comparison.

Preoperative preparation (of the bowel)

Principle behind bowel preparation: Colon contains large amount of bacteria up to 10^9/mL of faeces. Commonest anaerobe is bacteroides; commonest aerobe is *E. coli*; *Pseudomonas, Enterococcus, Proteus, Klebsiella, Streptococcus* are other organisms. Bowel preparation is done to clear this bacterial load to reduce postoperative complications.

Methods used are: *Mechanical bowel preparation* using PEG or sodium phosphate. *Polyethylene glycol (PEG)* is a non-absorbed sodium sulphate solution, 2–3 litres of which is asked to drink by the patient along with plenty of additional fluids. It cleans the bowel by passing loose stool for 10–15 times in 12 hours. It acts by its hygroscopic action. *Side effects* are—nausea, vomiting, and abdominal cramps. Antiemetics are often needed. It is ideal in renal failure, ascites, cirrhosis, CCF. *Sodium phosphate* is an alternative to PEG as smaller volume is sufficient to take. But it causes electrolyte imbalance. Its efficacy is similar to PEG. But patient compliance and cost is better acceptable. It can cause hyponatraemia, hypokalaemia, hypocalcaemia and hypophosphataemia in case of renal dysfunction. In such patients, it is contraindicated.

Other methods: (A) *Total gut irrigation* daily using 200 mL of *oral mannitol* or through nasogastric tube for 3 days prior to surgery; (B) *Bowel wash* daily for 3 days prior to surgery using 2 litres of normal saline (not water as it will cause water intoxication); it cleans the entire large bowel; (C) Senna, castor oil, bisacodyl; (D) Repeated enemas. *PEG or sodium phosphate has taken over all this methods. Contraindications* for mechanical bowel preparation: Complete bowel obstruction and perforation.

Antibiotics parenteral and as bowel antiseptics, oral neomycin (gentamycin, streptomycins were used in olden days) 1 gram, *erythromycin* 1 gram, is used 3 days prior to surgery. Alternatively *ciprofloxacin and metronidazole* are used. IV fluids should be given in addition to these patients to maintain hydration adequately. *IV antibiotics* given *4 hours before* making incision, reduces the incidence of sepsis (no clear evidence). Usually cephalosporins are given. ***Controversies***—There is doubt about the advantages of preoperative mechanical bowel preparation even though it is practiced universally. Oral antibiotics are used to reduce the bacterial load in the colon are also controversial. However, preoperative single dose parenteral antibiotic improves the result and reduces the sepsis.

Turnball no touch technique with ligation of pedicle at its origin prior to mobilising the colon and tumour reduces the chances of tumour spread. Avoiding breaching of the colonic wall, negative proximal, distal and radial margins are absolute need. Intraoperative frozen section biopsy of resected margin should be taken. Lymphovascular clearance is a must in colectomies for carcinomas.

Controversies still exist about the duration of nasogastric tube and beginning of oral feeding. Proponents of late oral feeding after 7 days believe that colonic stomal tensile strength and ability to withstand disruptive force takes 7 days and so oral feeding started after 7 days. Initially oral liquid then gradually solid food is started. Proponents of early feeding believe once bowel sounds is heard and patient has passed flatus without abdominal distension, feeding can be started; it is also believed by them that gradual feeding from oral liquid to solid is not necessary.

In colectomy for benign diseases initially colon is mobilised by opening the peritoneum along the paracolic gutter, and then vessels are ligated close to the bowel wall at its inner margin. There is no need to ligate vessels at its origin and no need to do lymphovascular clearance.

In *colonic perforation*—resection, creation of proximal stoma, closure of distal colon or creation of mucus fistula is better. Diversion may be loop ileostomy if perforation is in the right colon or proximal (right sided) colostomy if perforation is in left colon.

In colonic obstruction as general condition of the patient will not be good it is better to do resection and diversion.

Intestinal decompression can be done by doing a colostomy at the proximal site. On table colonic lavage as antegrade irrigation cleans the colon mechanically facilitating the one stage resection and primary anastomosis without diversion.

Meticulous anastomotic technique is important to avoid anastomotic dehiscence. Pulsatile arterial blood flow at the cut edge of the mesentery adjacent to the cut edge of the bowel is the deciding factor along with bleeding from cut edge of the bowel and pink, soft and pliable bowel are other deciding factors. Haematoma in the bowel wall, haematoma in the mesentery may reduce the blood supply. Single layer interrupted sutures using 3-0 silk is adequate. At every 3–5 mm distance sutures should be placed. Posterior layer knots are kept inside; anterior layer knots are placed outside. Two layers can be done with inner full thickness continuous or interrupted 3-0 vicryl sutures; outer interrupted seromuscular silk sutures. *Submucosa is strongest* layer and so bites should be taken through it during seromuscular sutures.

Different methods of anastomosis are used. ***Open method*** is commonly advocated. It can be single layer interrupted anastomosis or two layered anastomosis. ***Single layer*** has the advantages as it is easier, it maintains blood supply at the cut edges and prevents necrosis of the cut edges. Single layer bites can be *simple seromucosal full thickness sutures* or *mattress full thickness seromucosal* or *simple serosubmucosal sutures (mucosal bite is not taken here)* depending on the surgeons convenience and need of the patient. Whenever ***two layer anastomosis*** is done, inner continuous or interrupted full thickness sutures with outer seromuscular interrupted silk sutures are used. Usually 3-0 suture material is sufficient. Cut ends should be made of equal size by Cheatle's cut; occlusion clamps should be in place; initially bites are taken from mesenteric corner, antimesenteric corner and later bites are taken on either side. All suture bites should be ideally taken first and knots are tied later. Knots are placed inside in posterior layer and outside in anterior layer **(Figs. 25-7 to 25-9)**.

In closed method crushing clamps are placed on each side of the bowel; *serosubmucosal interrupted bites* are taken posteriorly; once all posterior bites are taken knots are tied outside. Then anterior serosubmucosal bites are taken and knots are tied outside. Once all knots are tied then only crushing clamps are released. With thumb and finger crushed inner parts of the cut ends of the bowel are separated properly (which are inside the lumen) and surgeon should confirm that lumen is made patent. Closed method prevents contamination; it is not commonly practiced. Still there are surgeons who advocate this method.

At least 1 cm of the bowel cuff is cleared of the fat, mesentery and epiploic appendices. Leak commonly occurs on the mesenteric side of the stoma. Mesenteric defect should be closed using interrupted or continuous sutures by absorbable (vicryl) or non-absorbable (silk) sutures. Tension free anastomosis should be achieved. Flexures whenever needed should be adequately mobilised to achieve free mobility of the stoma. Contamination should be avoided by using occlusion clamps, irrigation, and decompression. Fluid collection like blood, serous fluid should be avoided. Possible distal obstruction should be identified. It should be corrected otherwise it will cause anastomotic dehiscence. Patient who had radiotherapy earlier or if patient who was on steroids for long time needs special attention as stomal dehiscence and leak is very common in them. Omental wrap may be used around the anastomotic stoma.

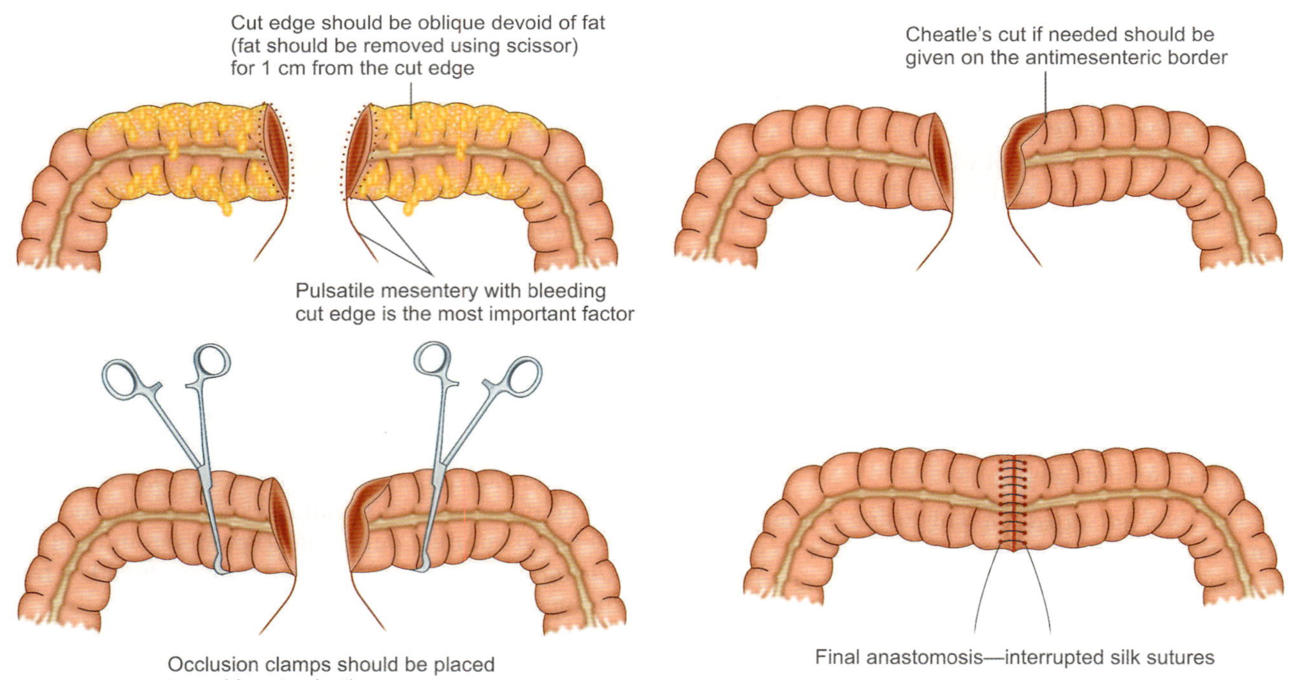

Fig. 25-7: Technique of colonic anastomosis.

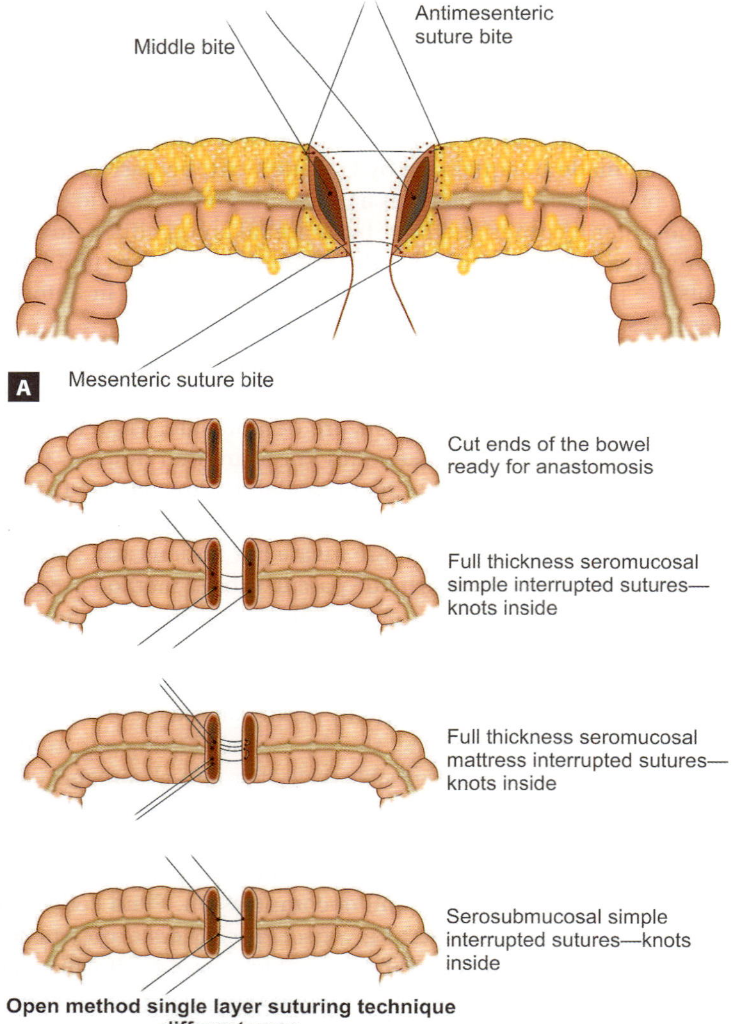

Figs. 25-8A and B: Suturing of the colon—different methods.

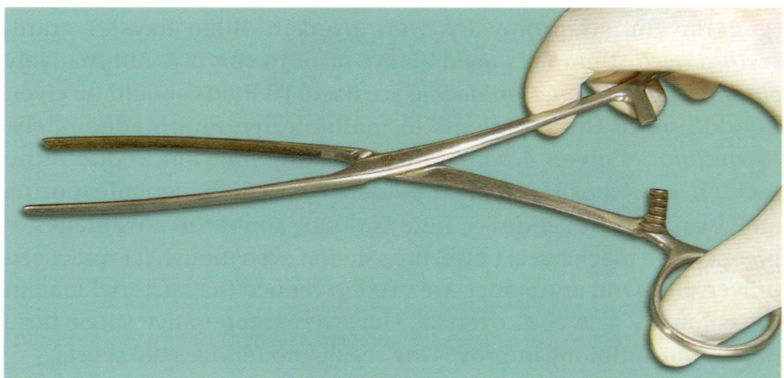

Fig. 25-9: Doyen's occlusion clamp is used during anastomosis as it is least traumatic.

Stapling is commonly used in colorectal surgery ***(Fig. 25-10)***

Stoma (colostomy/enterostomy) when planned should be sited properly. End ileostomy should protrude 1.5 cm from the abdominal wall; end colostomy should protrude 1.0 cm from abdominal wall. Stoma care should be meticulously followed. Stoma closure in temporary stomas should be done only after 3 months but not earlier; adequate time is taken to achieve stability of stoma and develop proper nutritional and biochemical optimum in the body. In loop ileostomy, site should be 10 cm proximal to the ileocaecal valve so that closure will be easier later. Nowadays end ileostomy is also commonly used as temporary one as it is easier to construct and easier to close at a later period. In permanent ileostomy Kock's continent type is often done with a nipple valve which facilitates collection of ileal excretions. It needs insertion of a tube into the continent pouch at regular intervals by patient himself to evacuate the contents. Kock's continent avoids usage of the stoma appliances. But problem herein is it needs re-surgery in up to 30% cases and complications are common. Permanent end ileostomy is needed in severe Crohn's disease where pouch is contraindicated or in ulcerative colitis wherein pouch has failed.

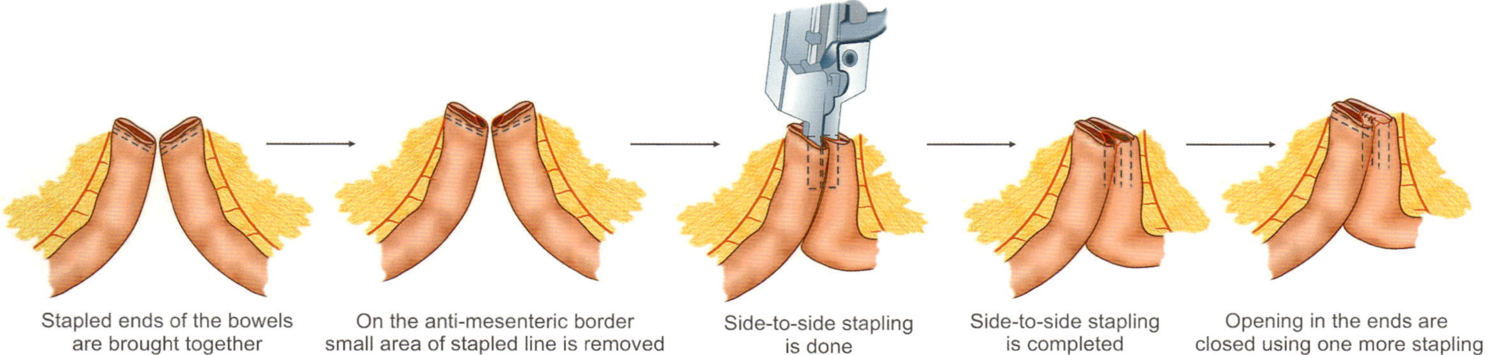

Fig. 25-10: Stapling is also used for colonic anastomosis. For anterior resection circular stapler is used.

Ureter is very important structure which should be safeguarded on both sides. Stenting prior to surgery may be needed if obstruction is suspected or observed in imaging. On right side duodenum, SMV are also important structures to be taken care of.

Bowel wall oedema may trouble proper approximation. Interrupted sutures, stapler usage are helpful. Otherwise diversion should be done instead of forcing the sutures.

Laparoscopic colectomy has become popular and safer on both right and left. In left colectomy circular stapler makes anastomosis easier and precise.

CAECOPEXY

It is rarely done nowadays. It is used whenever caecum and ascending colon is mobile with higher chances of precipitating volvulus. It is done by fixing the caecum and ascending colon to the lateral abdominal wall. Bites should be taken from the taeniae of the caecum **(Fig. 25-11)**.

CAECOSTOMY

Caecostomy is often done in acute colonic conditions as diversion procedure after surgery distally like perforation closure and resection. It is useful in pseudo-obstruction. But it is not as popular as colostomy because it may not function adequately, may get displaced or blocked. But it is technically easier and usually done by doing appendicectomy and passing Malecot's tube through appendicular stump. Removal is easier without any surgical intervention. Foley's catheter no. 30 F can be used. Purse string suture is placed around the tube by taking seromuscular bites with 3-0 vicryl or silk suture. It is also fixed by 2–3 interrupted sutures taken between seromuscular part of the caecum very close to the tube and parietal peritoneum (abdominal wall).

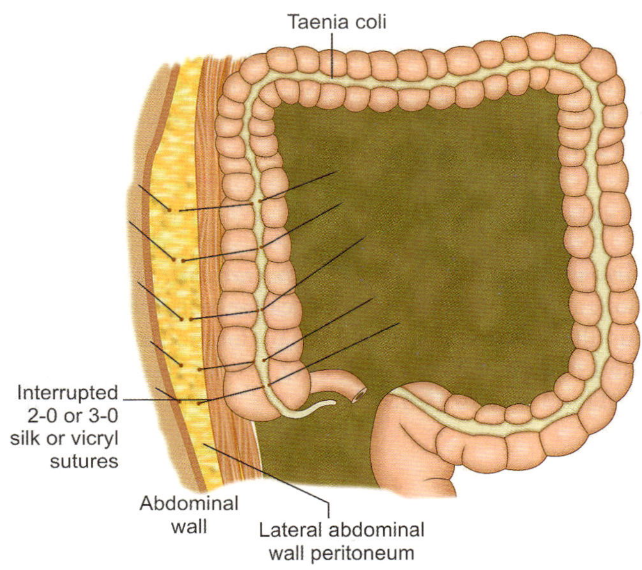

Fig. 25-11: Caecopexy technique.

It is often done along with other procedure during laparotomy. When only caecostomy is planned it is done through a oblique incision in right iliac fossa above the groin crease similar to Mc Burney's incision. Distended caecum is identified; an occlusion clamp is placed across the caecum; appendix removed with a purse string suture on the taeniae circumferentially. Appendix stump is not ligated; instead suction apparatus passed into that to suck the content to prevent spillage. No. 30 Foley's catheter is passed onto the caecal caecum; purse string suture is ligated. Second purse string suture is placed. Appendicectomy should be performed even if caecostomy is done on the anterior part of the caecum through taenia.

Tip of the tube is directed toward hepatic flexure. Non-functioning, blockage, slippage, leak are the complications **(Figs. 25-12A to D)**.

COLOSTOMY

It is an artificial opening made in the colon to the exterior (skin) to divert faeces and flatus.

Types

1. ***Temporary:*** Is done in conditions wherein diversion is required to facilitate healing distally in the rectum or distal colon. And this is closed once the purpose is over. Site of temporary colostomy is usually right hypochondrium and left iliac fossa.
2. ***Permanent*** colostomy is always *end/terminal colostomy* placed in left iliac fossa, 6 cm above and medial to the anterior superior iliac spine.

Colostomy Can be

Diversion colostomy: It is done when there is breach in bowel wall, trauma, destruction, sphincter injuries, Crohn's, carcinoma rectosigmoid. It is usually brought out as an end colostomy with a mucus fistula or with a Hartmann's resection. It can be at sigmoid, descending and transverse colon. ***Decompression colostomy:*** It is done for obstructive lesions in rectosigmoid, toxic megacolon. Types—(1) *Blow hole* procedure is done as a single or multiple small stomas onto the skin to decompress colon in acutely ill patients with massively dilated or impending perforation of colon. Problems are—

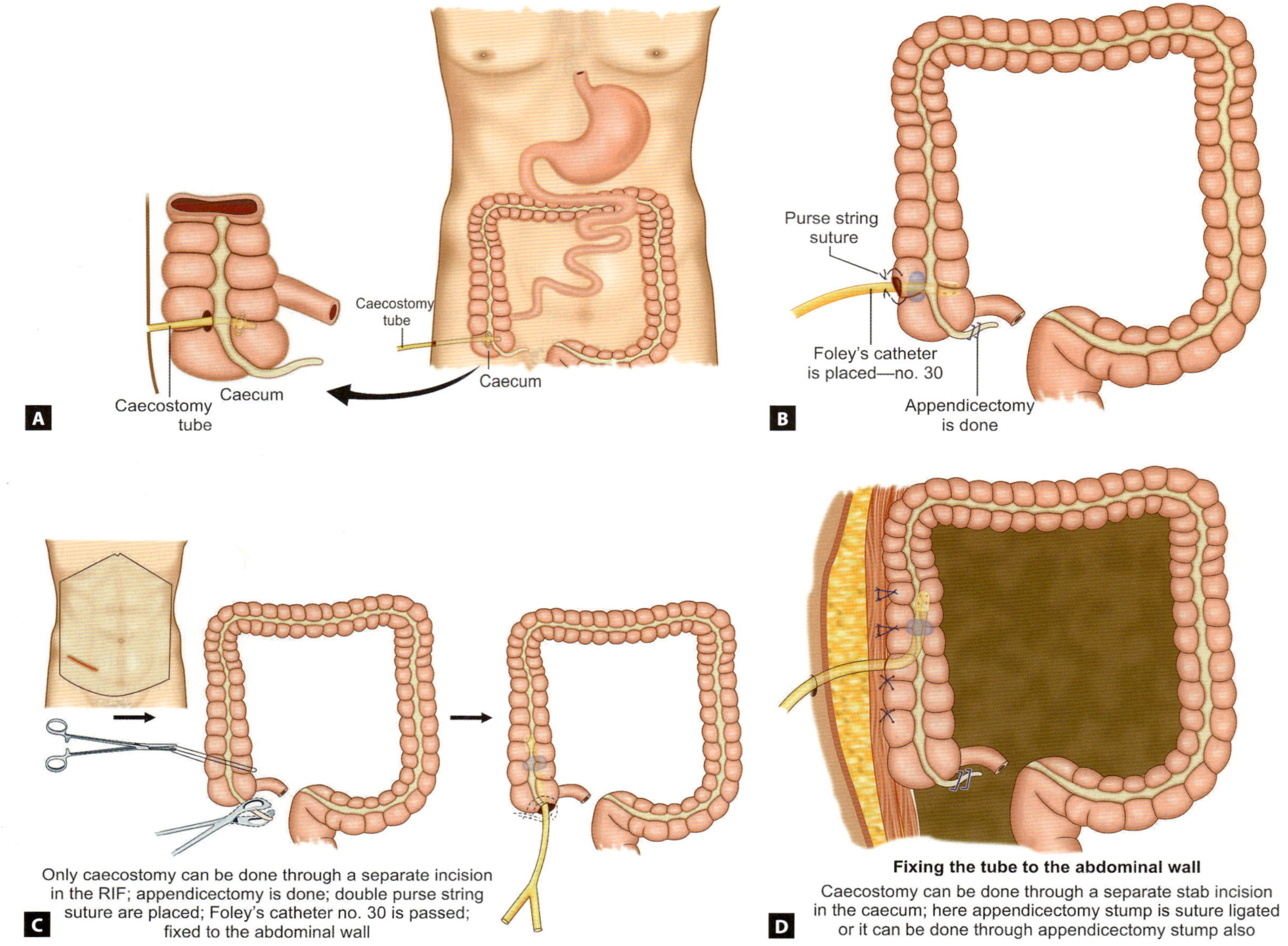

Figs. 25-12A to D: Caecostomy technique.

remaining possible ischaemic parts of the colon may not get identified thus risking perforation; peristomal skin complications and mucosal prolapse is also common. (2) *Tube caecostomy*—It is technically easier without much complications; but tube getting blocked limits its use regularly. (3) *Loop transverse colostomy*—It serves as decompressing and diverting long stoma without getting blocked. It is done only in mobile colon. *Irrigation colostomy:* It avoids the need of any appliance wear; reduces the passage of uncontrolled gas with less leak of stools. But it is time consuming with chance of water intoxication due to excess water absorption during irrigation.

Colostomy also can be

Loop colostomy *or double barrelled colostomy or* ***Devine's divided double-barrel colostomy*** (wherein there is a gap of skin between the two openings of colostomy which prevents spillage into the distal loop).

Loop colostomy is done temporarily to divert the stool. It is presently done to defunction distal anastomosis or in high fistulas or perianal traumas. It can be done at sigmoid colon at the junction of the sigmoid and descending colon as descending colon is fixed it, prevents colostomy prolapse. It can also be done more proximally at transverse colon in right hypochondrium. It is easier to construct. But prolapse is much more with colostomy than ileostomy; marginal artery may get damaged causing problematic eventual closure. Double barrel colostomy was done in olden days in sigmoid volvulus as Paul Mikulicz operation wherein a spur was created between two limbs at antimesenteric border.

Indications

Temporary: Congenital megacolon. ***Permanent:*** Abdominoperineal resection; anorectal malformations; carcinoma anal canal; sigmoid volvulus after Hartmann's operation; perforation of left sided colon; left sided colonic growth; high anal fistula; trauma to left sided growth **(Figs. 25-13 to 25-15)**.

Technique

Loop colostomy

It is ideally done under general anaesthesia; but can be done under spinal or local anaesthesia. It is done along with laparotomy for

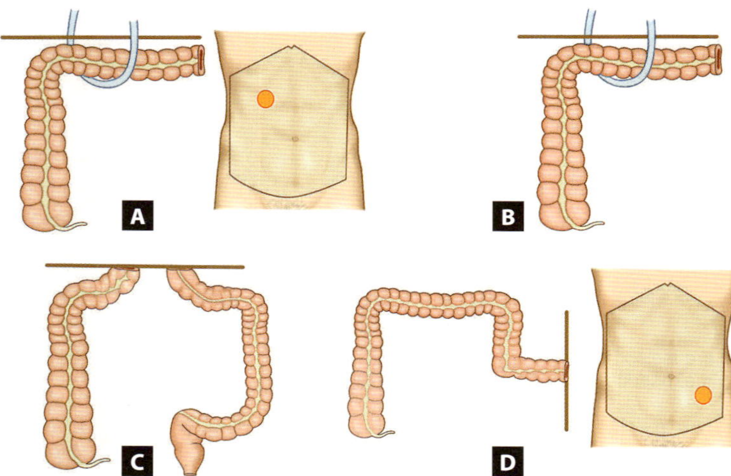

Figs. 25-13A to D: Types of colostomy. (A) Temporary colostomy; (B) Loop colostomy; (C) Devine's double barrel colostomy; (D) Permanent colostomy.

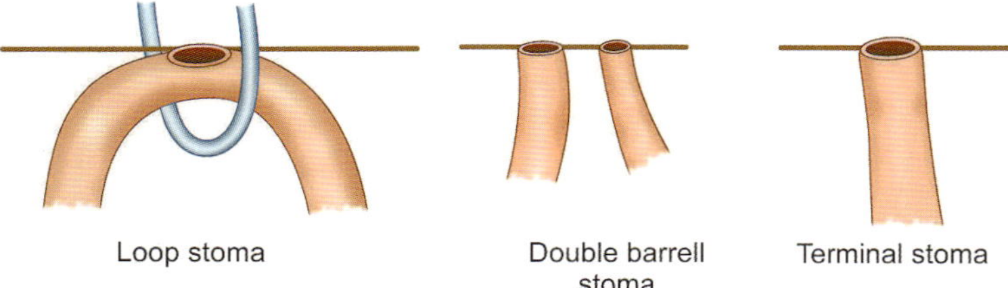

Fig. 25-14: Different types of stomas used in colostomy.

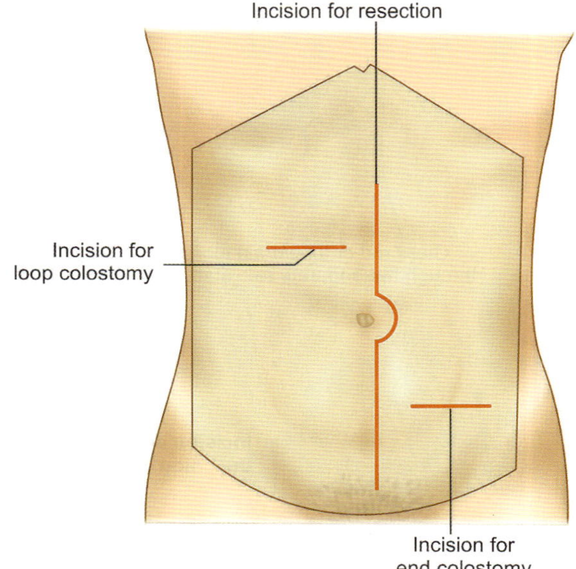

Fig. 25-15: Midline incision is used for resection. Incision in the right hypochondrium is used for loop colostomy (temporary). Permanent end colostomy is done after abdominoperineal resection (APR); here colostomy is sited at left iliac fossa.

definitive procedure or only loop colostomy at time and definitive procedure is done at a later period **(Fig. 25-16)**.

Incision is in the right hypochondrium midway between umbilicus and right costal margin, horizontally placed of about 6 cm in length, over the right rectus muscle with its right end ends just lateral to the lateral margin of right rectus abdominis muscle. Skin, two layers of superficial fascia and anterior rectus sheath is incised in the line of the skin incision. Rectus muscle is split vertically or horizontally cut; posterior rectus sheath and peritoneum are opened. Transverse colon is pulled out; omentum is detached from the colon for sufficient length—6 cm. Transverse mesocolon very close to the colonic wall is opened (window is created) in avascular plane and glass rod or stiff silastic tube/drain tube of 18 French size is passed across (which is usually removed in 8-10 days). Glass rod prevents retraction keeping colocutaneous suture line intact. But it is not mandatory to place a rod like this always; it is useful in obese patients. Glass rod often is brought out on either side by a separate stab incision which facilitated proper placement of sutures between colonic edge and skin. Colon is traditionally opened longitudinally along the taenia extending to both limbs of the loop. It is also practiced to open the colon horizontally which causes less damage to blood vessels. Both ways are accepted. After opening it is often a practice to place few interrupted 2-0 vicryl sutures between rectus sheath and seromuscular part of the colon away from the cut edge site. Usually 6 such sutures are placed. But it is again not mandatory to place such sutures in temporary colostomy. Interrupted sutures are placed between skin, subcutaneous and full thickness colonic cut edge. Many people use only subcuticular part of the skin for suturing instead of entire skin. Colostomy is ready for function. Stoma appliance is placed. Stoma should protrude outward at least 1-3 cm beyond skin margin **(Fig. 25-17)**.

Prasad end loop colostomy is often done along with laparotomy resection. Colostomy site is transected using stapler; proximal part is brought out through already created colostomy opening and is matured by releasing the stapler line; distal stapled colon is brought out adjacent to proximal loop. Proximal cut edge is sutured to skin using interrupted skin sutures. Distal loop stapled line is removed; it is partly sutured to skin; its inner part which is adjacent to proximal loop is anastomosed to it as side to side to create a modified loop colostomy.

End or Terminal Colostomy

End or terminal colostomy is done after abdominoperineal resection. It is permanent one. End colostomy site should be marked properly and a circular disc of skin is removed. Many do skin excision by holding the skin to be excised with a toothed forceps or Allis forceps and an elliptical-shaped skin is excised but it is actually inadequate but accepted. Similarly same sized superficial fascia and rectus sheath is excised at corresponding level. Rectus muscle is split and peritoneum is incised. Two fingers should be passed through the wound without any difficulties. End of the cut colon is brought out by passing a Babcock's forceps inside through the opening for about 5 cm outside. If possible when colon is intraperitoneal lateral space between mesocolon and abdominal wall is closed using interrupted silk sutures. It prevents herniation. Otherwise colon end itself can be made extraperitoneal and brought out. One should ensure that there is no tension and good blood supply at the end of the colon. Few interrupted vicryl sutures may be placed between rectus sheath and seromuscular colon 1 cm proximal to the colon end. Interrupted skin sutures are placed between colonic full thickness edge and skin with subcutaneous fat. Many people take bites from seromuscular part of the colon avoiding the mucosa but it is practically not necessary. Even fixing to the rectus sheath is not mandatory even though commonly practiced.

When stapler is used for resection of the colon, stapler end is brought out and then later stapler line is excised. Other option is maturation is done at a later period postoperatively. But nowadays preferred one is doing maturation in the operation table only after closure of the main laparotomy wound.

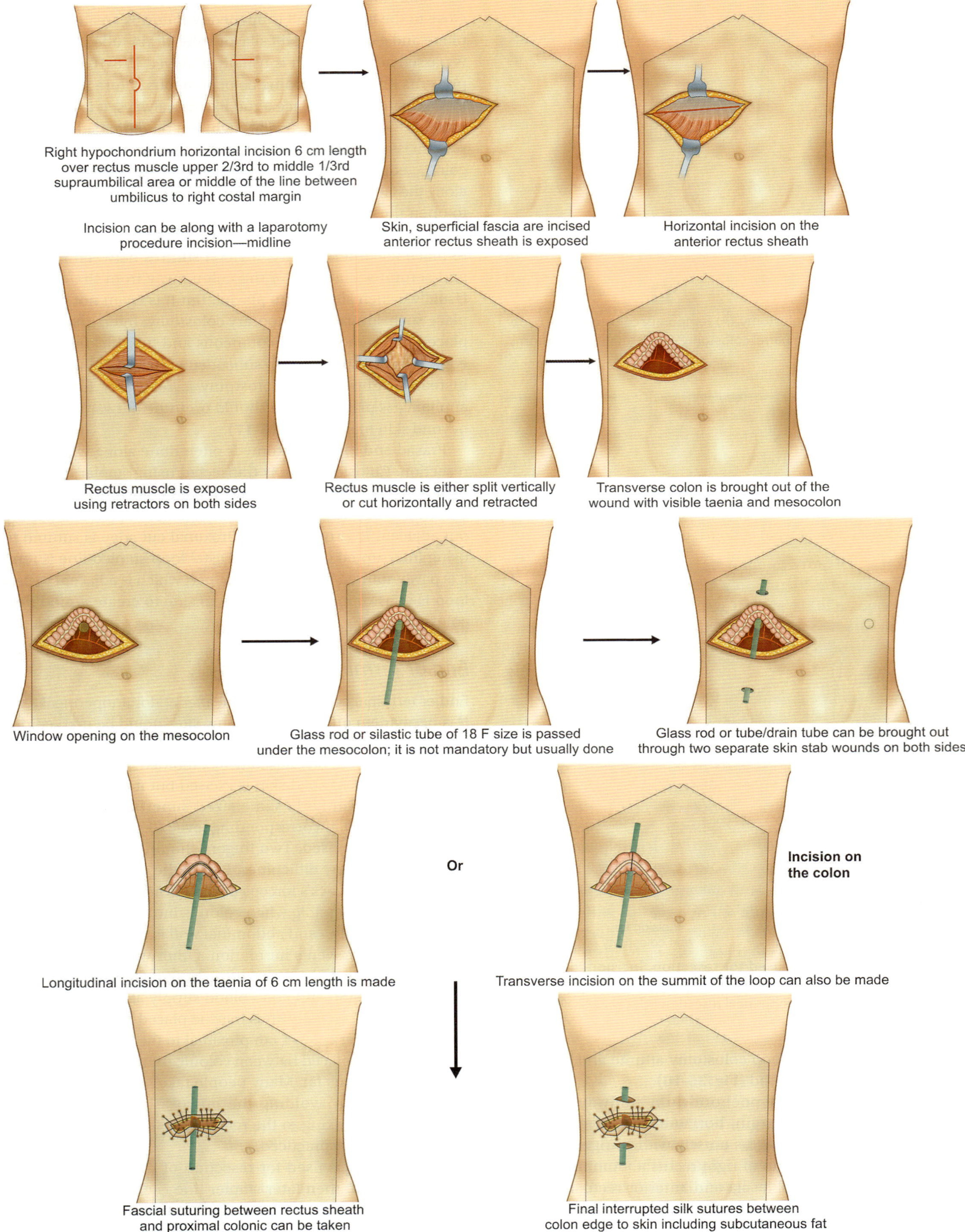

Fig. 25-16: Technique of loop colostomy.

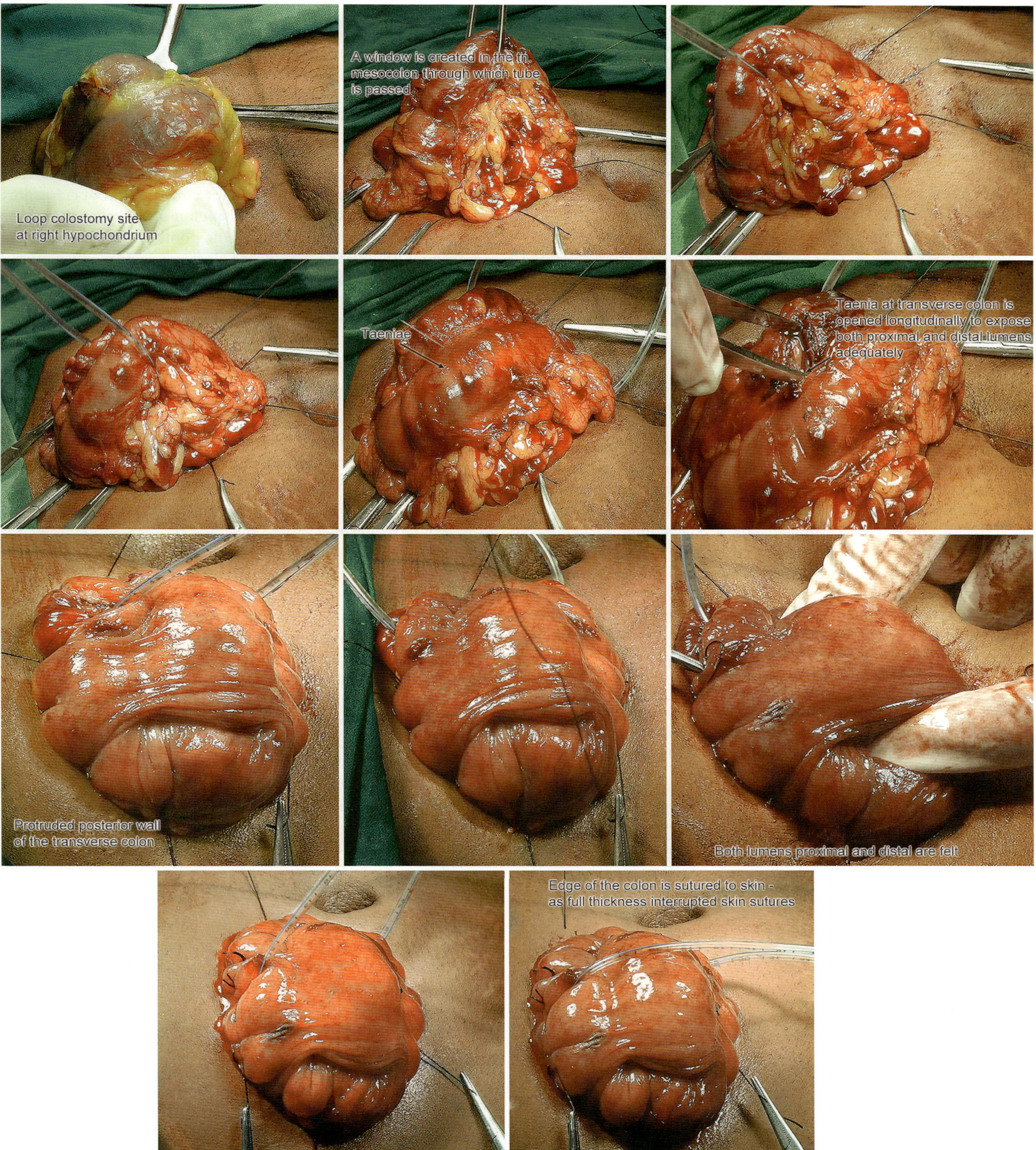

Fig. 25-17: Loop colostomy is usually done in right hypochondrium. It is a temporary colostomy.

Complications of Colostomy

Prolapse of mucosa (prolapse of distal loop mucosa is common)—commonest complication; retraction; necrosis; stenosis; herniation; bleeding; diarrhoea; enteritis; skin excoriation. Necrosis of stoma can be just mucosal or full thickness.

Mucosal necrosis is treated conservatively. Full thickness necrosis needs reexploration and creation of new stoma.

Colostomy prolapse is more common in loop type than in end type. It is initially treated conservatively; if troublesome then conversion into end colostomy and mucus fistula is safer. Mucus fistula is created at a separate opening.

Parastomal hernia is common in end colostomy. It is herniation of intestine on the side of bowel stoma—ileostomy/colostomy/other stomas. Incidence is 8%. *Classification (Devlin's)*: (1) Subcutaneous—intestine herniates along the side of stoma to reach subcutaneous plane—commonest. (2) Interstitial—along the side of stoma intestine herniates into intermuscular plane. (3) Intrastomal—bowel herniates between emerging and everted parts of the stoma. (4) Parastomal—herniation occurs between the layers of the prolapsed stoma. Parastomal hernia can cause obstruction and strangulation. *Features:* Pain, features of obstruction, stomal malfunction, swelling which is tender, toxicity. If it is distressing it should be treated. Local repair with or without mesh can be done; otherwise closure of the stomal site with hernial repair using a mesh and redoing the colostomy at different location is the only choice. Mesh may be placed intraperitoneally or extra-peritoneally. Rectus sheath which is closed often is supported with a local large Leslie skin flap.

Infection (enteritis/colitis), colostomy separation, skin excoriation, social problems, appliance problems are the ones which are often difficult to manage **(Fig. 25-18)**.

Colostomy Care

It is similar to stoma care. Initially stoma bag should be transparent as content is liquid stool but later it can be opaque. Regular consultation with stoma therapist; care of the skin; training for managing colostomy, its care to prevent leak, odour, and discomfort. Educating the patient regarding the proper usage of colostomy bags and proper care of the colostomy is very essential.

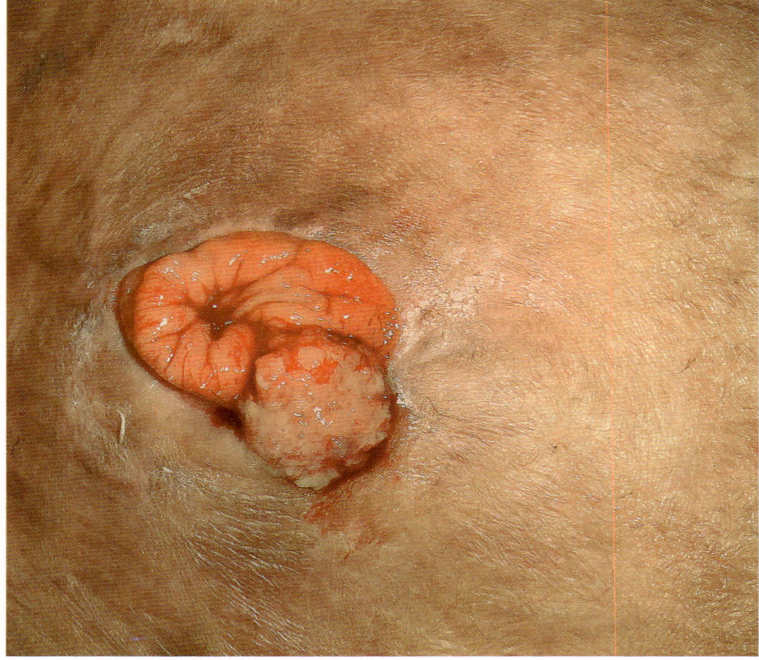

Fig. 25-18: Colostomy site recurrence of the carcinoma who has earlier undergone abdominoperineal resection.

CLOSURE OF COLOSTOMY

Criteria for temporary colostomy closure:

Integrity of distal colon should be normal and adequate; anorectal sphincter should be normal. Cause for construction of colostomy is cured completely without any suspicion of recurrence of same disease distally. When temporary colostomy is done, it is closed usually after 3 months. Closure of colostomy is done after proper bowel preparation, ideally under general anaesthesia. Colonoscopy is a must just prior to colostomy closure to confirm that distal colon is normal and without any obstruction and devoid of any disease.

Types of Colostomy Closure

Two types of closure are present: Extraperitoneal and intraperitoneal type. *Now intraperitoneal closure is done.*

Earlier extraperitoneal closure was done in loop colostomy by placing a spur in between and closing the antimesenteric part of the colon. It prevents the peritoneal contamination. But inadequate closure, leak, adhesions are the problems.

Intraperitoneal closure: Commonly advocated technique now. It is done by placing series of 6-8 silk sutures around the skin margin to give traction while dissecting, separating and mobilising the colon using circumferential incision over the margin with 2 mm skin edge. Incision is deepened to enter the peritoneum and the colostomy stoma is pulled out. Adequate mobilisation is essential to prevent tension over the anastomotic site. Part adjacent to the skin is resected and anastomosed using silk/vicryl. Two layer anastomosis using interrupted sutures is usually practiced. If there is an unhealthy edge then it is better to mobilise the hepatic flexure completely and do a small colonic segment resection and anastomosis. Sutured bowel is placed into the peritoneal cavity. Drain is placed into the peritoneal cavity. Abdomen is closed in layers **(Fig. 25-19)**.

Proper postoperative care is important. Patient should perform anal sphincter exercises to prevent sphincter atrophy and to maintain sphincter tone **(Fig. 25-20)**.

Complications of Colostomy Closure

Breakdown of anastomotic site and faecal fistula is the commonest complication; but it usually subsides unless there is distal obstruction. Distal anastomotic abscess formation, wound infection, wound dehiscence and later incisional hernia can develop.

TREATMENT FOR DIVERTICULAR DISEASE OF SIGMOID/COLON

Medical Treatment

High fibre diet; antibiotics; bulk purgatives; avoid constipation; regular follow-up of the progress of disease and onset of complications.

Abscess can be drained by CT guided aspiration or percutaneous drainage tube. *Guided aspiration* of the abscess is sufficient if abscess is small. Proper antibiotics are needed.

In acute stages, conservative treatment like bowel rest, anti-spasmodics, antibiotics are advised **(Fig. 25-21)**.

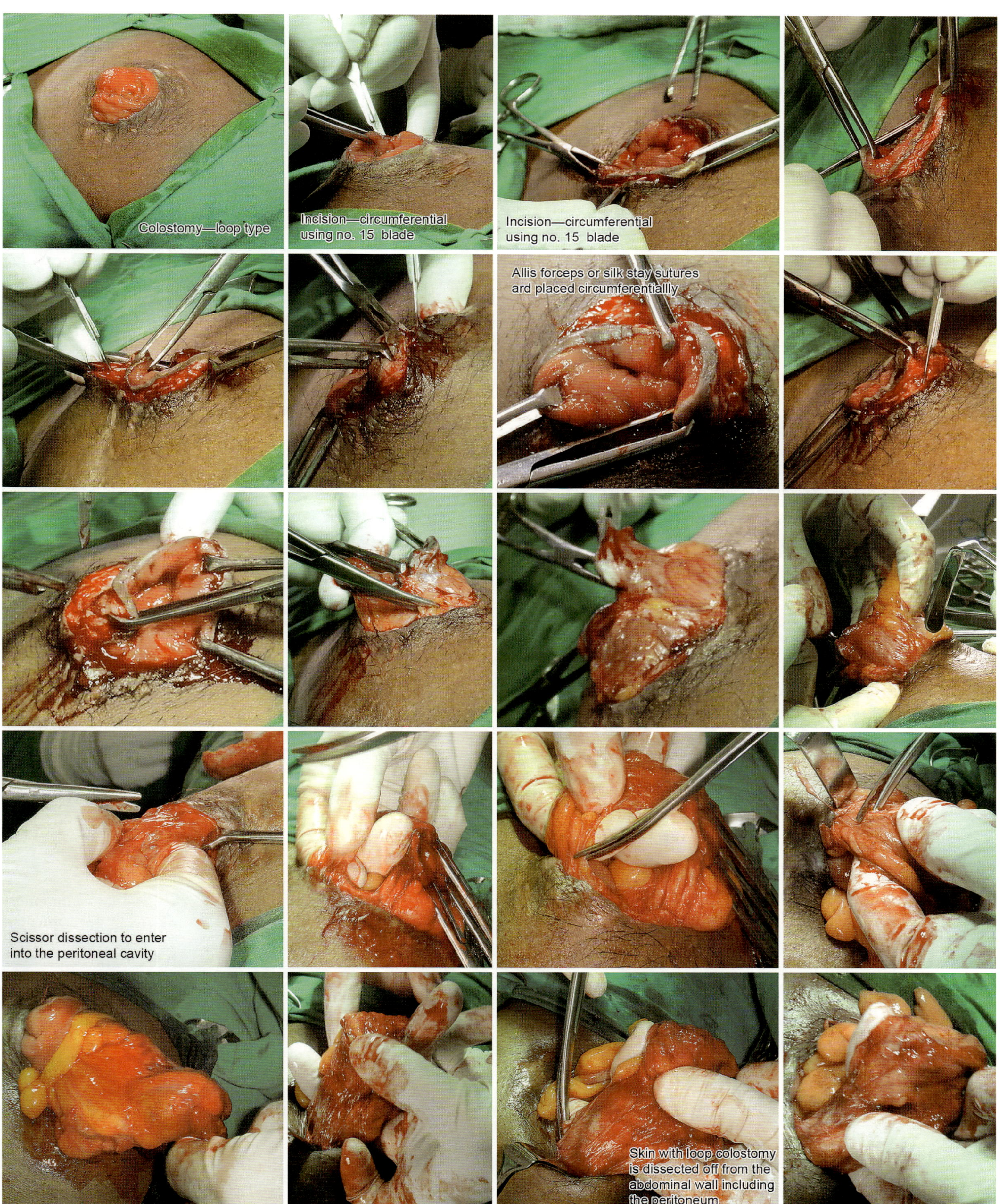
Colostomy—loop type
Incision—circumferential using no. 15 blade
Incision—circumferential using no. 15 blade
Allis forceps or silk stay sutures ard placed circumferentiallly
Scissor dissection to enter into the peritoneal cavity
Skin with loop colostomy is dissected off from the abdominal wall including the peritoneum

Figs. 25-19(1)

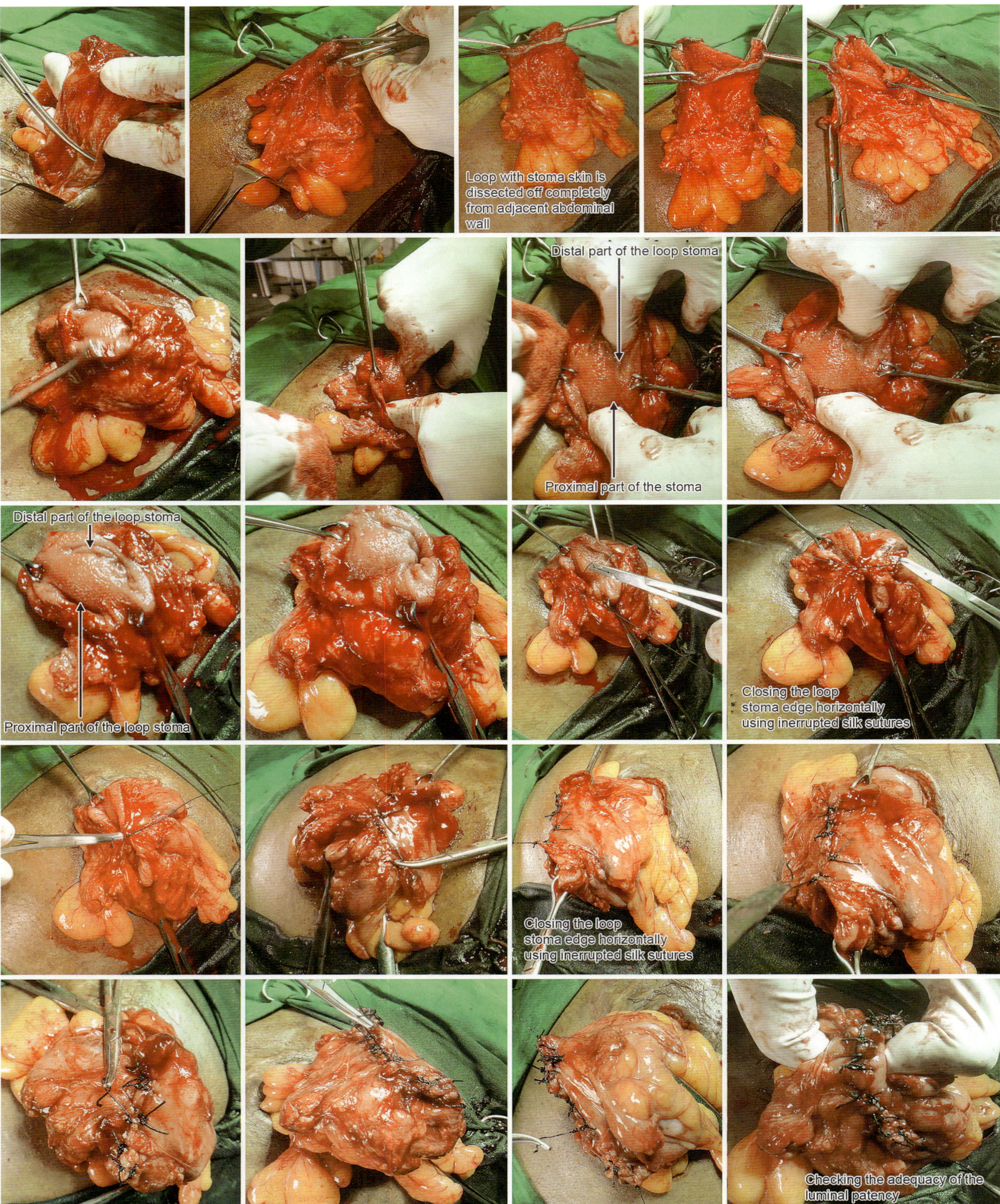
Loop with stoma skin is dissected off completely from adjacent abdominal wall
Distal part of the loop stoma
Proximal part of the stoma
Distal part of the loop stoma
Proximal part of the loop stoma
Closing the loop stoma edge horizontally using interrupted silk sutures
Closing the loop stoma edge horizontally using interrupted silk sutures
Checking the adequacy of the luminal patency

Figs. 25-19(2)

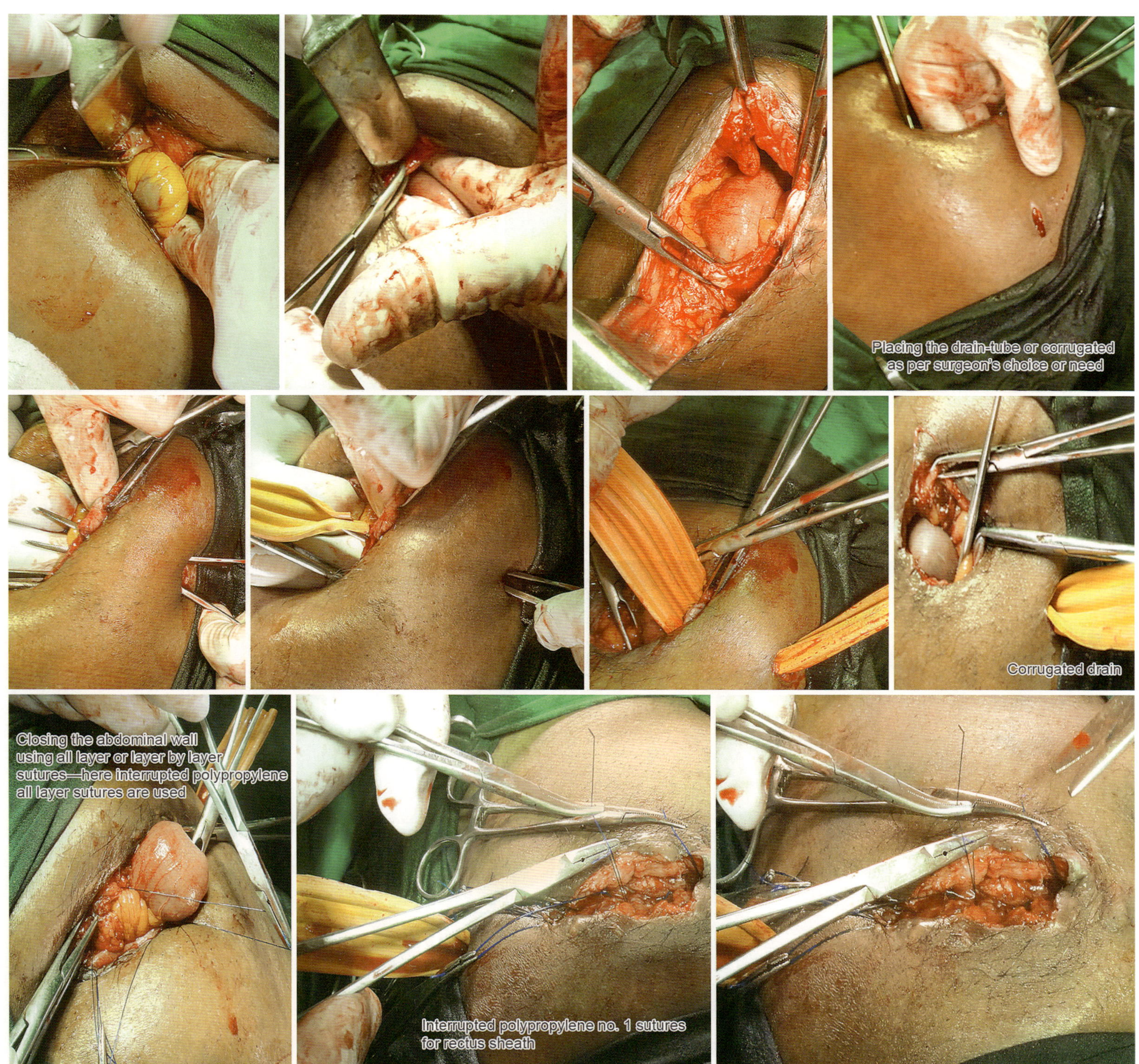

Figs. 25-19(3)

Figs. 25-19(1 to 3): Closure of loop colostomy—intraperitoneal type. After cleaning and draping stay sutures are placed circumferentially (alternatively Allis forceps can be placed); using no. 15 blade or cautery or both circumferential incision is made over the skin close to the colostomy margin. Incision is deepened across the abdominal wall layers to reach the peritoneal cavity. Scissor can be used for dissection. Bipolar cautery is used to achieve haemostasis. Colon proximally and distally is mobilised along with complete separation of the colostomy loop. Loop margin is trimmed using sharp scissor; bleeding from the cut edge ensures the viability which is most important in colostomy closure. Antimesenteric border of the trimmed colostomy loop stoma is approximated using 3-0 interrupted silk sutures. Two layer interrupted suturing can be done—inner vicryl and outer silk. Sutures ideally should be at 5 mm intervals. Stapler closure also can be used as an alternative effective method. Once closed properly patency of the lumen should be checked using thumb and index finger. Tube or corrugated drain can be placed depending on the surgeon's choice. Peritoneum is closed using vicryl. Abdominal wall is closed using interrupted polypropylene (non-absorbable) 1-0 sutures. All layers—as single layer closure can be done using interrupted sutures. Skin can be closed using stapler or non-absorbable monofilament interrupted mattress sutures.

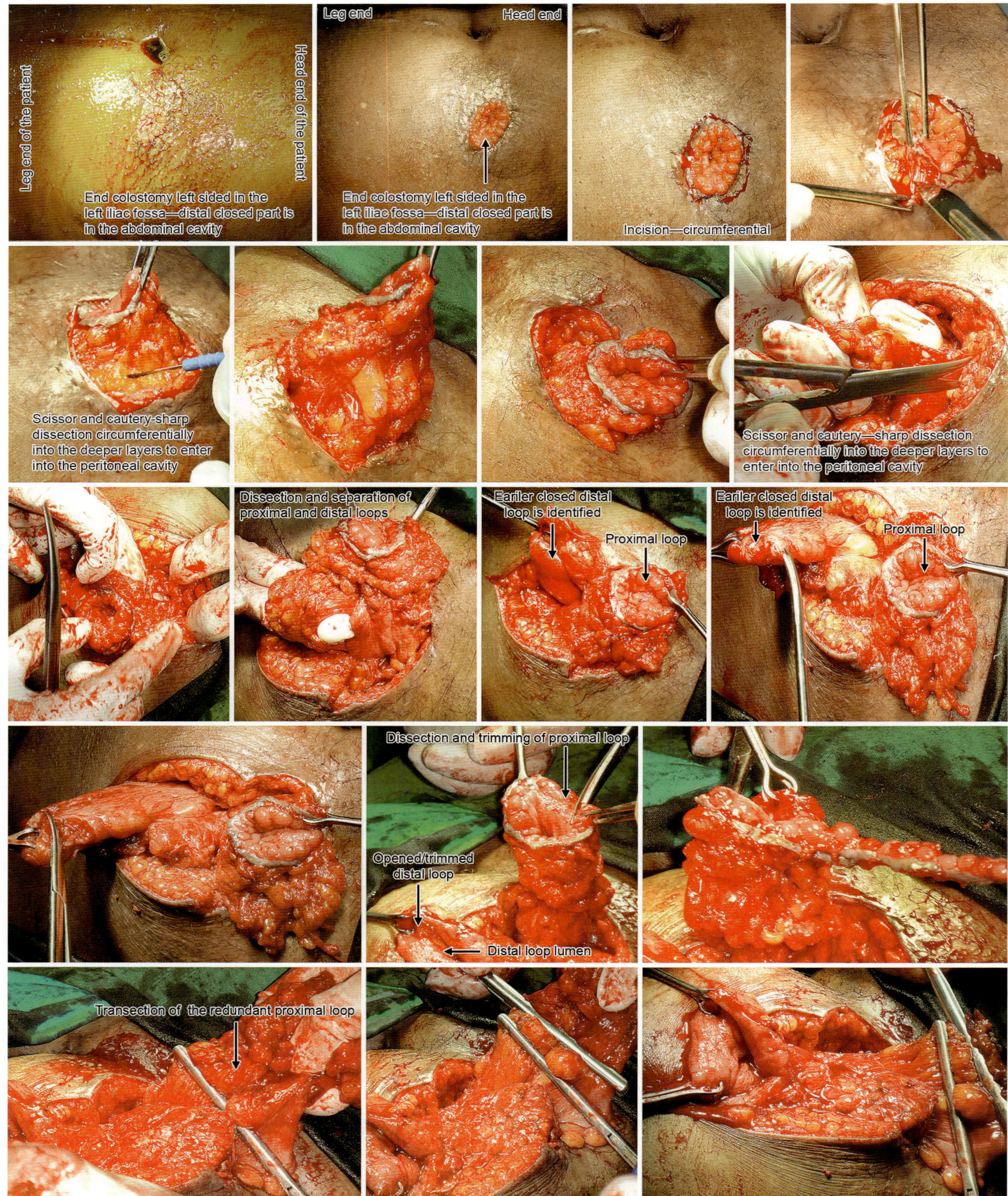
Leg end of the patient
Head end of the patient
End colostomy left sided in the left iliac fossa—distal closed part is in the abdominal cavity
Leg end
Head end
End colostomy left sided in the left iliac fossa—distal closed part is in the abdominal cavity
Incision—circumferential
Scissor and cautery-sharp dissection circumferentially into the deeper layers to enter into the peritoneal cavity
Scissor and cautery—sharp dissection circumferentially into the deeper layers to enter into the peritoneal cavity
Dissection and separation of proximal and distal loops
Eariler closed distal loop is identified
Proximal loop
Eariler closed distal loop is identified
Proximal loop
Dissection and trimming of proximal loop
Opened/trimmed distal loop
Distal loop lumen
Transection of the redundant proximal loop

Figs. 25-20(1)

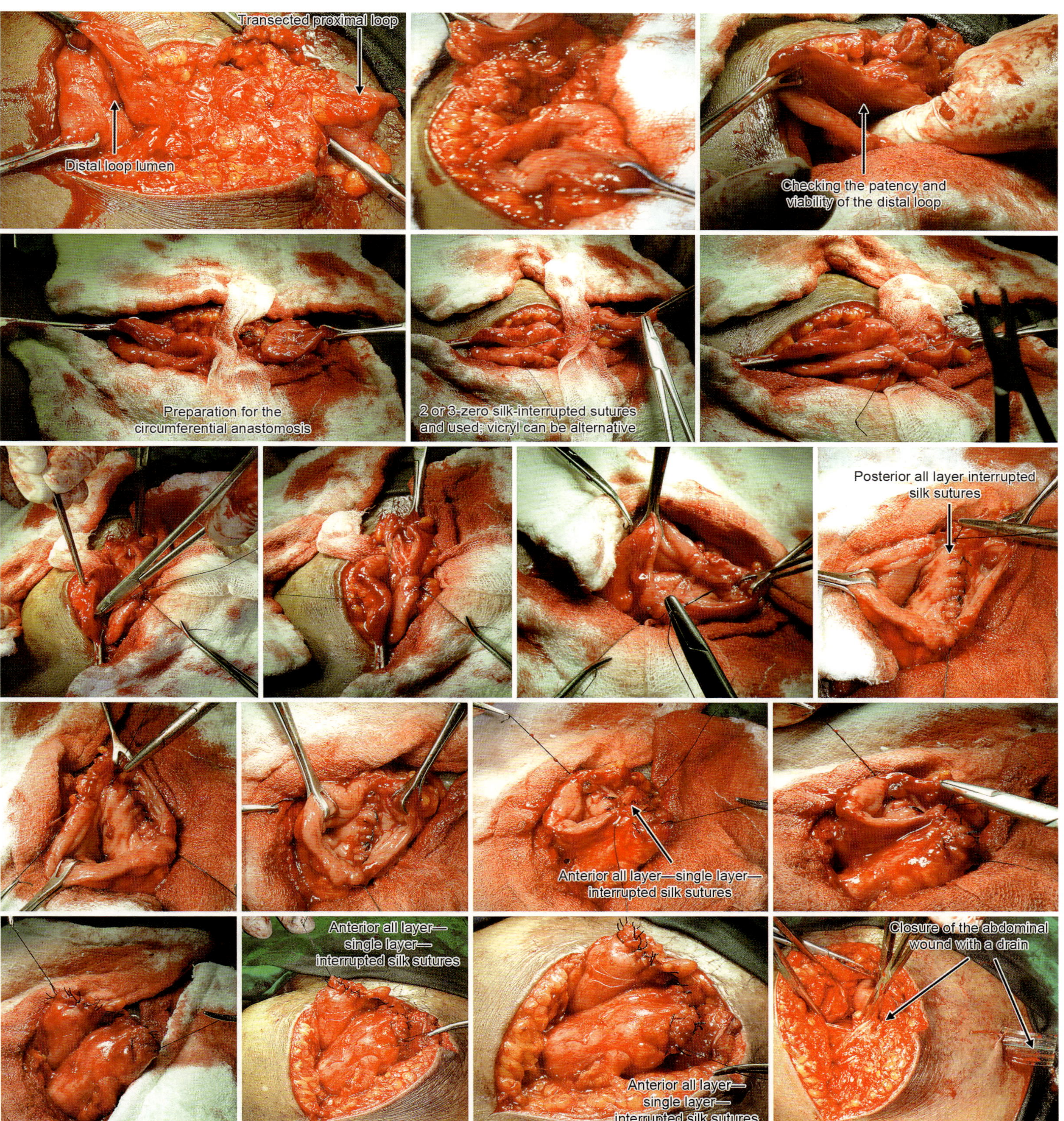

Figs. 25-20(2)

Figs. 25-20(1 and 2): Alternatively colostomy can be closed circumferentially all around. It is done if posterior bridge/part of the loop colostomy does not look viable or not healthy or if end colostomy done with distal part is closed and placed intraperitoneally. End colostomy is dissected circumferentially using sharp and cautery dissection; blind proximal end of the distal loop is identified, dissected adequately for significant length; proximal loop also mobilised properly to achieve tension free anastomosis. End of the dissected stoma is trimmed by excising the skin part on its edge; distal component is transected to enter into its lumen; proper bleeding is essential from cut edges of both parts. End-to-end anastomosis is done using interrupted single layered 3-0 silk sutures or inner vicryl and outer silk two layered interrupted sutures. Anastomosis should be tension free and viable. Abdominal wound is closed after placing a drain using interrupted monofilament sutures.

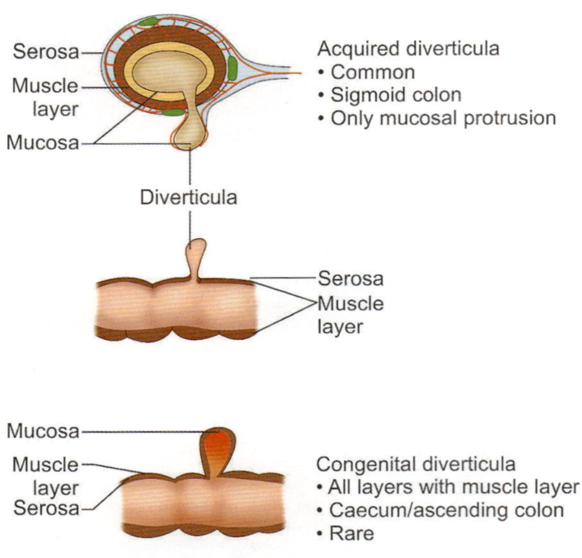

Fig. 25-21: Colonic diverticula—diagram.

Indications for Surgery

Recurrent diverticulitis; diverticulitis with complications.

Surgery required is—*resection of sigmoid colon and anastomosis (colorectal). Laparoscopic sigmoid resection can also be done* **(Fig. 25-22)**.

If colon is loaded with faecal matter, initially a transverse colostomy is done. Followed by resection and anastomosis; later colostomy closure is done as a staged procedure **(Fig. 25-23)**.

In case of perforation, proximal colostomy and exteriorisation of the affected bowel with later resection and anastomosis is done as it has high mortality **(Fig. 25-24)**.

Occasionally, Hartmann's procedure (combination of sigmoidectomy, end colostomy and closure of rectal stump) is better and life saving **(Fig. 25-25)**.

Fistulas are treated by resection of the diseased bowel and closure of the fistula along with diversion procedures like colostomy, cystostomy, ureterostomy.

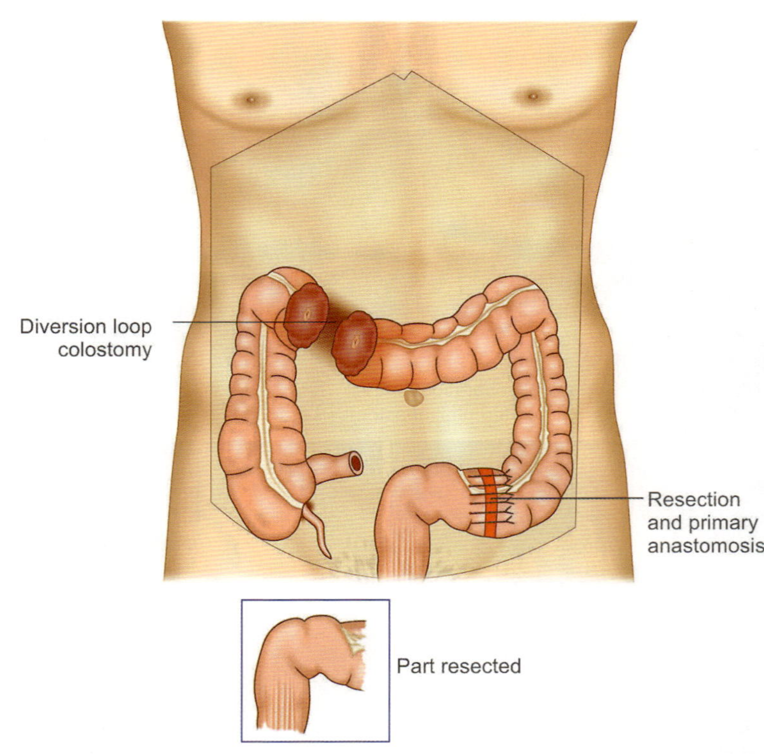

Fig. 25-23: Resection of sigmoid colon for sigmoid diverticula with primary anastomosis and defunctioning diversion colostomy.

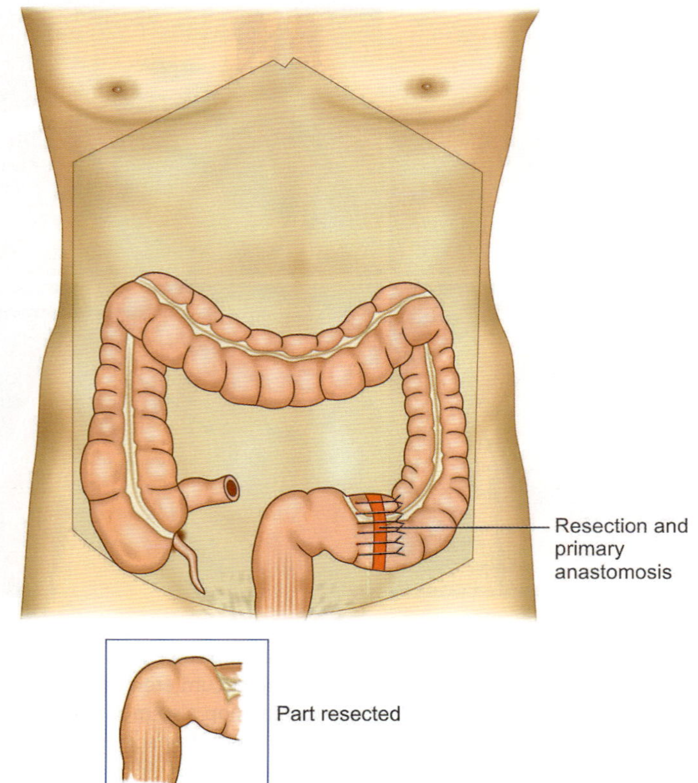

Fig. 25-22: Resection and primary anastomosis can be done in sigmoid diverticula after proper bowel preparation electively.

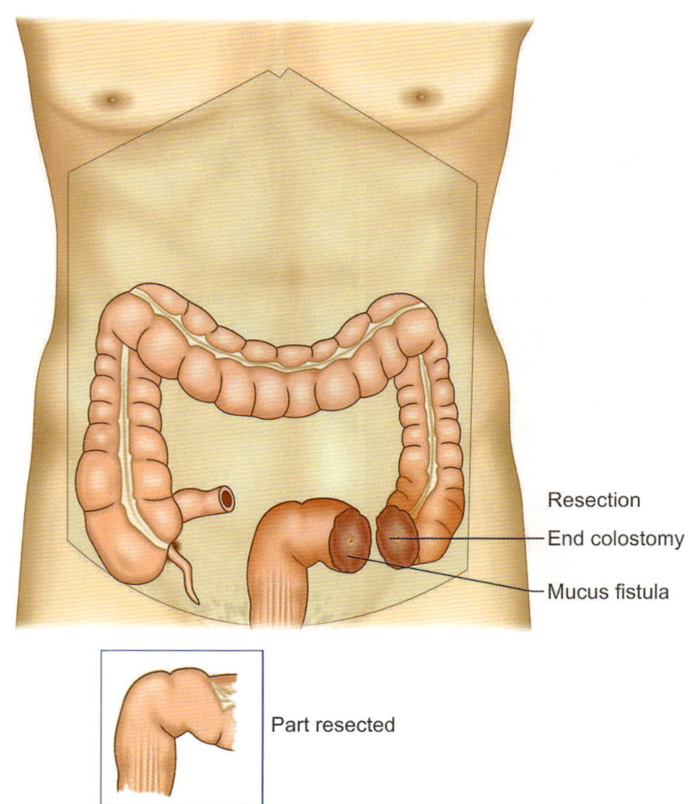

Fig. 25-24: Resection and formation of end colostomy and mucus fistula for acute sigmoid diverticulitis.

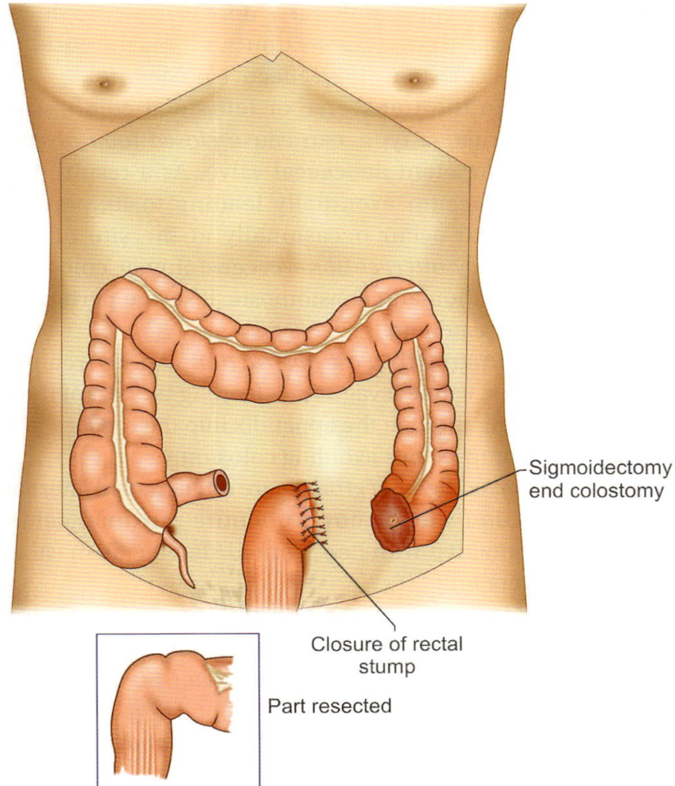

Fig. 25-25: Hartmann's operation for acute diverticulitis with sepsis/perforation/peritonitis. Here, after resection proximal colon is exteriorised as end colostomy. Distal rectal stump is closed.

In certain cases of diverticulosis, a longitudinal incision through the taenia and muscular layer without opening the mucosa is sufficient (like Heller's/Ramstedt's myotomy)—*Reilly's sigmoid myotomy.*

Note: It is basically **a benign condition**, therefore the prognosis is good. High fibre diet is advised. Complications like *perforation, fistulas are dangerous and life-threatening.* Right sided diverticulum in the caecum and ascending colon is usually solitary and congenital.

Myotomy

- Heller's myotomy—achalasia cardia
- Ramstedt's myotomy—congenital pyloric stenosis
- Reilly's myotomy—diverticulosis

TREATMENT FOR ULCERATIVE COLITIS

General: Correction of anaemia; fluid and electrolyte supplementation; nutrition (high protein, carbohydrate, vitamin, but low fat diet), TPN; sedatives and tranquillisers; psychological counselling.

Drugs: In active disease, drugs are used to *induce remission.* Later drugs are also given for *maintenance* of remission and to prevent relapses. Salazopyrine/sulphasalazine splits into 5 amino-salicylic acid and sulphapyridine in colon. It is used as *first line therapy.* Its dose is 2–4 g/day. It is mainly used to induce remission. It suppresses PGE1 and PGE2 thereby reducing the inflammation, inhibits proteolytic enzymes and also causes immunosuppression. 5 ASA is the most active ingredient. Side effects are skin rashes, bone marrow suppression, folic acid deficiency, haemolysis in glucose-6-phosphate dehydrogenase deficiency patients, temporary fertility problems in men. 5 ASA (Mesalamine) is also used in active disease as *first line therapy.* It is used with an azo bond to prevent its absorption in small bowel. Its induction of remission is same as sulphasalazine. Idiosyncrasy and temporary infertility is not present in mesalamine. Its *oral* dose is 2–4 g/day. It is also used as *retention enema* which is better than steroid enema in left sided ulcerative colitis/proctitis. But mesalamine enema (4 g in 100 mL saline) is costly. Enema is combined with oral mesalamine or oral steroid in acute cases. Mesalamine 500 mg *suppository* is also used in BID dose. Daily oral (1.6 gm) and topical 4 g enema, twice weekly is often used for maintenance therapy. Headache, dyspepsia and myocarditis are the complications. Steroids are used in cases where salazopyrine fail to induce remission. It is a drug for *refractory cases.* Oral prednisolone 60 mg/day tapering in 4 weeks is the dose. Intravenous hydrocortisone 100 mg 8th hourly is used in acute cases. 100 mg hydrocortisone enema/40 mg methylprednisolone enema (steroid retention enema) are used for 2 weeks in acute active diseases. Most patients with moderate to severe disease need steroid therapy. *Budesonide* a newer steroid hydrocortisone analogue is equally effective with lesser side effects and less adrenal suppression. Immunomodulators are used often to induce remission and for maintenance. Azathioprine and 6-mercaptopurine are used. They act at DNA level (purine ribonucleotide) and inhibit lymphocyte function (of T cells). But this action is slow. Cyclosporin is used in refractory, fulminant severe ulcerative colitis as a reserve drug. Dose is 4 mg/kg/day IV. Mebeverine HCl and Tegaserod (6 mg) are the other drugs used in ulcerative colitis. Other measures are using sucralfate, short chain fatty acids, probiotics, anti-diarrhoeal drugs (diphenoxylate, loperamide, codeine), avoiding milk products, fibre, fruits. Anti-tumour necrosis factor alpha—*Infliximab* is also used selectively (in some studies). It is given intravenously at interval of 6 weeks. It shows 70% remission in ulcerative colitis. Newer drugs with a targeted delivery into the colon is used nowadays. *For example* Olsalazine (azobond); Balsalazine (4 aminobenzoyl carrier).

Indications for Surgery—30% Cases

Intractability—commonest indication; toxic dilatation; perforation; haemorrhage; risk of malignant transformation, dysplasia (DALM); onset at early age; chronic invalidism; progressive disease with stricture, abscess, fistulae; steroid dependency, persistent active disease; malignancy; severe extraintestinal manifestations; growth retardation in children.

Toxic megacolon: It is 1.5% in incidence; common in transverse colon; colon more than 6.5 cm in diametre in transverse colon and more than 10 cm in caecum is likely to be toxic; colon is like wet blotting paper; commonly seen in ulcerative colitis; can occur in bacterial colitis, pseudomembranous colitis, fulminant amoebic colitis; may be precipitated by antidiarrhoeal drugs. It is treated by—IV fluids, blood transfusion, antibiotics, steroids; it can be life threatening; plain X-ray abdomen is very useful; emergency surgery, colectomy, colostomy/ileostomy may be required. In olden days *blow hole procedure* was advocated for toxic megacolon, may be still useful in severe cases. Skin level transverse colostomy, sigmoid colostomy and a loop ileostomy is done to decompress entire small and large bowel. After many months (6–8 months) once patient recovers from acute illness, total proctocolectomy with ileal pouch anal anastomosis is done.

Surgeries

Total proctocolectomy with ileo-anal anastomosis with pouches as reservoir ("J', 'S', or "W' pouches). It is called as *restorative proctocolectomy with ileal pouch anal anastomosis (IPAA)*. It is *ideal curative procedure* for ulcerative colitis. Anal sphincter complex is preserved. An 30 cm ileal pouch is created either hand sewn or with stapler. Created ileal pouch reservoir is anastomosed just above the anal canal using end-to-end stapler. Diametre of the pouch should be twice the diametre of the ileum. Obstruction (25%), diarrhoea, *pouchitis (25%)*, leak, sepsis, incontinence are the complications.

Total proctocolectomy with ileostomy (permanent, continent Kock's ileostomy, with one way valve is done). It is used at present only *in revision surgery* when needed after restorative proctocolectomy.

Total proctocolectomy with end non-continent ileostomy was the earliest operation done for ulcerative colitis. It is now *reserved only* for ulcerative colitis complicated with carcinoma of rectum. *Ileostomy site* should be marked in standing and sitting position. Stoma should be within the right rectus abdominis muscle at the summit of infraumbilical fat, away from midline incision, bony prominences and umbilicus.

Total colectomy with ileorectal anastomosis can be done. Proper follow up at regular intervals by sigmoidoscopic evaluation should be done as rectum is also diseased and vulnerable for complications. It is *not commonly* practiced now.

Total colectomy with rectal mucosectomy and anastomosis above the dentate line on posterior aspect is also occasionally used.

TREATMENT CONCEPT IN CARCINOMA COLON

Mainly Surgical

Right Sided Early Growth

Right radical hemicolectomy with ileotransverse anastomosis is done. Structures removed are terminal 6–15 cm of ileum, caecum and appendix, ascending colon, 1/3rd of transverse colon, lymph nodes (epicolic, paracolic, intermediate, principal).

In inoperable right sided growth, *ileotransverse anastomosis* is done as a by-pass procedure.

In transverse colon and hepatic flexure growth—*an extended right hemicolectomy* is the procedure done for transverse colon growth which includes division of right colic, middle colic arteries at their origin, with removal of terminal 6 cm ileum, ascending and transverse colon; anastomosing terminal ileum and proximal part of the descending colon—*ileocolic*. Alternatively, in mid transverse colon growth only transverse colon with both flexures can be removed; anastomosing cut ends of ascending and descending colon—*colocolic*.

Left Sided Early Growth

Left radical hemicolectomy is done, where in left ½ of transverse colon and descending colon is removed along with lymph nodes.

Left sided stenosing type of growth can present with acute intestinal obstruction, in which case initially colostomy is done. Later, after 3–6 weeks, following proper preparation, required formal procedure is done, followed by colostomy closure after 8 weeks (*3-stage operation*). Presently, it is done only in critically ill patient; otherwise it is proved that it is not necessary to do 3-stage procedures; instead primary resection and anastomosis with a proximal diversion colostomy is an effective procedure.

Often growth in the transverse or left sided colon, which is stenosing or obstructive type, can cause *closed loop obstruction* because of the competent ileocaecal valve. As a result, pressure increases in the caecum eventually leading to its perforation. Perforation can also occur occasionally at the site of tumour. They need *emergency intervention*—caecostomy or colostomy, or ileostomy with resection and anastomosis. If severe peritonitis sets in, it may be life-threatening.

Left sided colon growth *with obstruction* can be treated with resection of tumour, saline lavage and cleaning the rest of the colon by passing a catheter through the appendix into the caecum followed by primary anastomosis thus avoiding colostomy.

Severely *obstructed sigmoid growths* are often treated alternatively by tumour resection with removal of entire proximal colon and continuity is maintained with ileo sigmoid/ileo rectal anastomosis. It also avoids diversion.

During exploration, presence of any synchronous growths has to be looked for. Now, it is found that carcinoma colon can be *associated with tuberculosis or lymphoma colon*. So this association is also looked for.

In acute left sided growths, *transanal self-expanding metal stents* can be used instead of defunctioning colostomy.

Turnball's 'No touch technique': Here the vessels are ligated at its origin, at the beginning, in order to prevent the tumour spread—due to tumour handling. This medial to lateral oncological approach could be ideal in carcinomas. In laparoscopic colectomies, this medial to lateral approach is better as colon is fixed laterally making medial dissection easier.

Abdominal total colectomy with ileorectal anastomosis is done if there are multiple primary tumours or in HNPCC. Significant chronic diarrhoea is the problem due to defective water absorption.

In Liver Secondaries

In solitary liver secondary, segmental hepatic resection is useful.

In case of multiple secondaries confined to one lobe of the liver, hemihepatectomy can be tried.

Metastasectomy—it is done in one secondary/one lobe secondaries/less than 3 metastases in both lobes/without any extrahepatic spread.

A 'Second Look Operation'

It is most often helpful in carcinoma of colon, to resect the residual or recurrent tumours (*Owen Wangensteen's Second look surgery). Relaparotomy is done after a stipulated period at regular intervals once colectomy is done for carcinoma.*

Synchronous Growths

If there are synchronous growths or growth with other area having multiple potential polyps, then total *colectomy with colorectal* anastomosis is done.

Recurrent Tumour

Recurrent tumour should be treated by re-exploration and resection with adjuvant chemotherapy of different regime.

Laparoscopic Approach

Laparoscopic evaluation and resection is becoming popular. Laparoscopic assisted colonic resection is also done [*Hand assisted laparoscopic surgery (HALS)*].

Note

- Caecum and ascending colon—right radical hemicolectomy (terminal ileum to mid-transverse colon); hepatic flexure and transverse colon—extended right radical hemicolectomy (terminal ileum to proximal descending colon); splenic flexure extended left radical hemicolectomy (hepatic flexure to rectosigmoid); descending colon and sigmoid—left radical hemicolectomy (splenic flexure to rectosigmoid).
- Minimum 5 cm margin clearance at colonic side/sides is needed; 6 cm terminal ileum clearance is sufficient in case of right sided growth.
- Duodenum, ureter, IVC, superior mesenteric vein should be taken care of during dissection in right hemicolectomy; spleen, stomach, tail of the pancreas should be taken care of in left hemicolectomy.
- It is ideal to mobilise both flexures adequately in all colonic surgeries to reduce the anastomotic tension.
- Bleeding at edges of anastomotic site should be adequate; in emergency obstructive situation, better to do temporary covering colostomy or ileostomy to prevent anastomotic leak whenever necessary.
- On table and postoperative hypoxia and hypotension should be prevented to minimise anastomotic leak.
- Preoperative mechanical bowel preparation is important in elective colonic resection using polyethylene glycol/mannitol, oral bowel antiseptics like neomycin and metronidazole.
- Infiltration into adjacent local structures is not a contraindication for surgical resection.
- At least 12 nodes should be examined during histology after resection.
- Blood transfusion before or during surgery for colonic cancer may alter the immunological aspect of the colonic cancer and may increase the recurrence rate and so may alter the prognosis. It is presently not very well-proved. Reason thought is—Blood transfusion raises the level of suppressor T cells leading into immunosuppression. So autologous blood transfusion is better when needed.
- Proper preoperative bowel preparation by mannitol/polyethylene glycol/hypertonic saline/bowel wash/bowel antiseptics (neomycin or gentamycin or streptomycin and metronidazole orally).
- Antibiotic prophylaxis; DVT prophylaxis by crepe bandage or stockings bandage, heparin or low molecular weight heparin; pulmonary function tests and pulmonary exercise preoperatively as well as postoperatively; urinary catheterisation, nasogastric tube placement—are always needed.
- Postoperative proper care with fluid, electrolyte, drain care, early mobilisation, monitoring.
- Complications of surgery are leak (faecal fistula), bleeding, infection like intraperitoneal/pelvic abscess, respiratory problems, DVT, wound infection, burst abdomen.

RESECTION OF THE COLON

Colonic resection is of the common surgeries that surgeons will come across. It may be for benign diseases, acute conditions like obstruction, volvulus or perforation or diseases like severe ulcerative colitis, polyps of different type and cause, carcinoma at different levels. Technically even though colon resection is easier than biliopancreatic surgeries, to achieve an optimum result with least complications proper preoperative, operative and postoperative care should be undertaken.

Principles

Prior evaluation of the disease, extent, type of resection needed, and comorbid status should be evaluated by imaging, colonoscopy, biochemical and nutritional assessment, cardiac and respiratory evaluation. CT imaging is essential.

Need for diversion in obstruction and other acute conditions should be thought of. Diversion may be colostomy or ileostomy depending on the location of the pathology. Stoma appliances, stoma care should be planned.

Tumour may be closer to ureter or invading it; such situation warrants for ureteric stenting prior to surgery. Stent may be removed within 3 months.

Bowel preparation is routinely done with methods which surgeons are familiar. Bowel antiseptics, perioperative antibiotics are used. Nasogastric tube and urinary catheterisation is needed.

Epidural with General Anaesthesia is Commonly Used

Different types of colectomies are performed depending on the need; these terminologies are used based on the extent of the colon resected. In benign conditions vascular ligations are done very close to the colonic wall and conventional colectomies are done with colon being mobilised first from paracolic gutter inwards then vessel ligation followed by anastomosis. In carcinomas, resection begins with vascular ligation at its origin to achieve lymphovascular clearance. Ligation of the branch vessels at its origin, then followed by colon mobilisation from paracolic gutter to complete the resection—is termed as *radical resection* of the colon. Usually in *conventional colectomies* done for benign conditions colonic mobilisation is done first; whereas in radical colectomies done for malignancies lymphovascular ligation is done first at the origin of the branch vessels. But one should remember that radical colectomies can be achieved through conventional approach after colon is mobilised, vessels ligated at its origin to clear nodes. Ligation of vessels at its origin is not done in colectomies for benign diseases.

Different types of colectomies are shown in the diagram—they are—ileocaecal resection; segmental ascending colon resection; right hemicolectomy; extended right hemicolectomy, transverse colectomy, left sided hemicolectomy; extended left sided hemicolectomy; sigmoid colectomy; subtotal colectomy; total colectomy; total proctocolectomy **(Figs. 25-26 to 25-31)**.

RIGHT COLECTOMY

Conventional Right Hemicolectomy

Lengthy midline incision is used. Proper exploration is done - gall bladder, liver, pancreas, remaining parts of the bowel, pelvis, nodes should be assessed. Usually conventional right hemicolectomy is done for benign lesions. So lymph node clearance is not needed. But it is very well accepted that conventional colectomy can be used for malignancies but vessels should be ligated at its origin and lymphovascular clearance should be adequate and also gentle dissection and handling of the colon and tumour is needed. Self retaining retractor is placed. Surgeon can stand either on right side or on left side. Many prefer to stand on left side. Caecum, terminal ileum and ascending colon are gently retracted anteromedially. Posterolateral peritoneum (*Toldt's line*) gets stretched and is incised using cautery or scissor. As plane is natural and avascular gentle finger dissection using index finger will create a space underneath the peritoneum up to the hepatic flexure and peritoneum is incised to expose the psoas major muscle. If surgeon is holding the bowel assistant can incise the peritoneum or the otherwise. Ureter, gonadal vessels are identified and safeguarded. Duodenum is identified near hepatic flexure which is dissected and left in the retroperitoneum.

Posteriorly Gerota's fascia with kidney will be separated; Gerota's fascia is separated by dividing renocolic ligament. Gerota's fascia should not be opened. Junction of the ascending colon and hepatic flexure is adherent to the gallbladder and should be released using scissor and finger dissection (division of *hepatocolic ligament*). Greater omentum is ligated and divided to achieve further mobilisation. In benign lesions omentum can be divided close to the colon at avascular plane. While mobilising hepatic flexure and right half of the transverse colon, mesocolon is related to SMV, middle colic vessels. Veins are friable here, so gentle and careful dissection under vision is needed to avoid unnecessary troublesome bleeding. If bleeding occurs it is better to keep a mop for a while and the bleeder is identified and caught with a haemostat and transfixation ligation is done using 3-0 vicryl or polypropylene. Firm pressure for few minutes controls most of the bleeding here. SMV is identified and care should be taken not to injure it. Peritoneum incision on the mesentery of the terminal 15 cm ileum is completed and that part of the ileum is also mobilised.

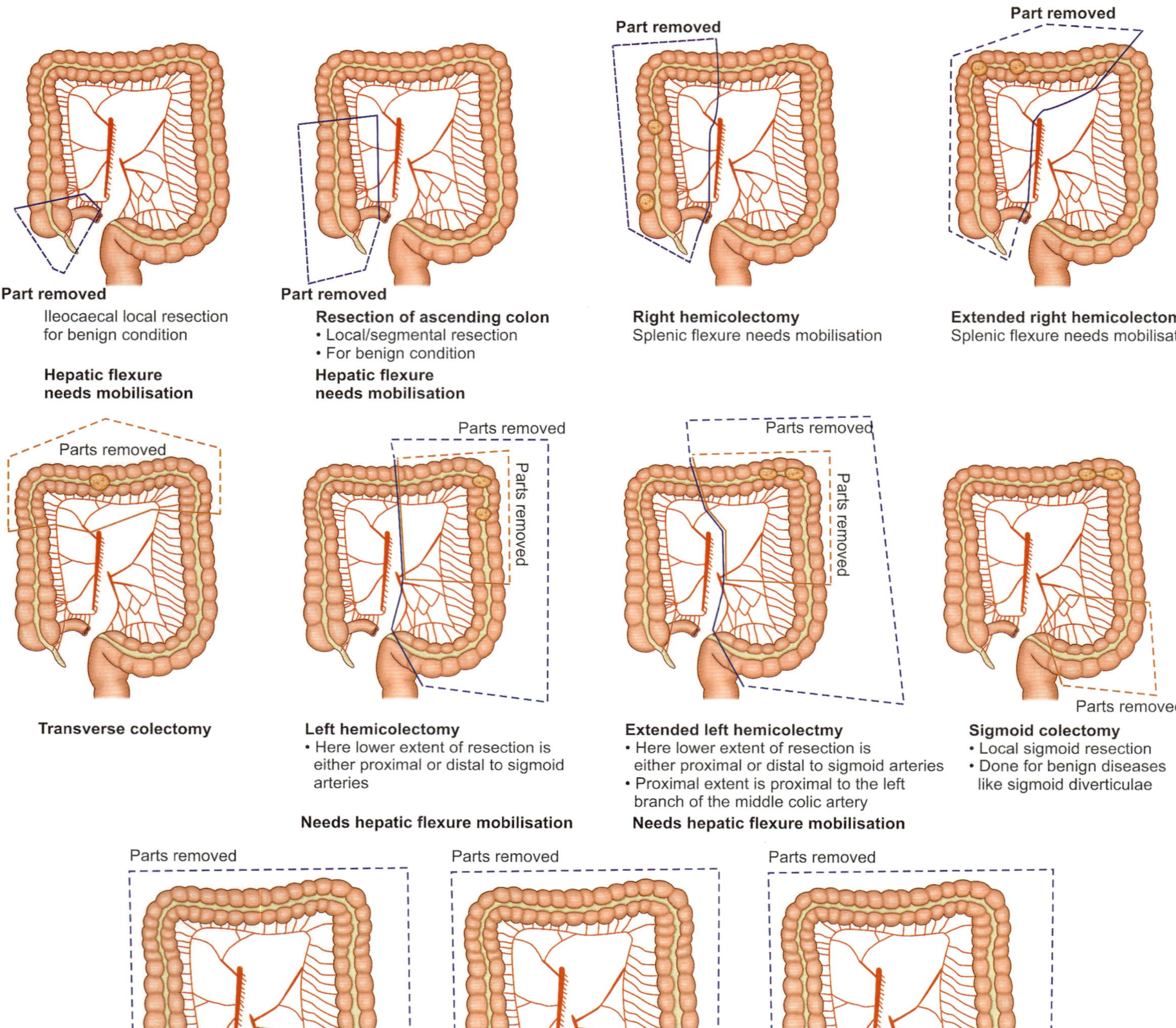

Fig. 25-26: Different types of colectomies with extents of resection.

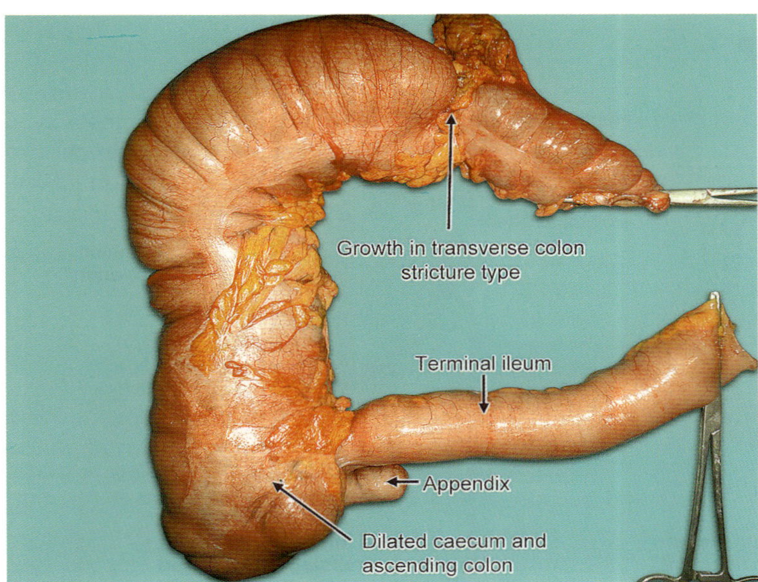

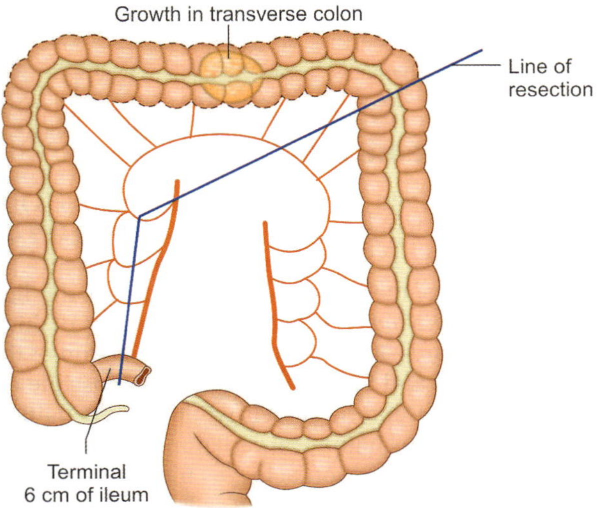

Fig. 25-27: Extended right hemicolectomy.

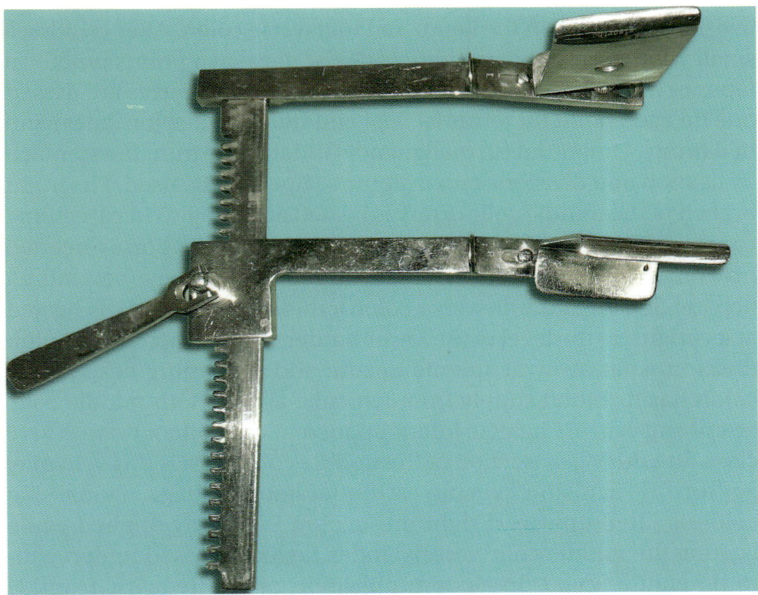

Fig. 25-28: Finochette retractor gives good exposure of the field keeping assistant's hands free for assisting.

Occlusion clamps are placed at the line of resection. Clamps are placed on the ileum obliquely; clamps should not extend onto the mesentery (only bowel part should be clamped). Another occlusion clamp is placed on the right 1/3rd to ½ of the transverse colon. Once right colon unit is completely mobilised, vessels are ligated. In benign diseases vessels are ligated very close to the bowel without intervening the main branch vessels. Often there will be fat in the mesentery which obviates the proper ligation; it is better to take short width of the mesentery of 1 cm for ligation; proximal double ligation or transfixation is needed and is safer. Vessels are identified through transillumination. In malignancy main vessels are ligated at its origin. Prior to ligation of the vessels one should confirm that ureter, gonadal vessels, duodenum are kept away from the site of resection. Once mesenteric ligation is done within the area between the occlusion clamps; crushing or Kocher's clamps are applied on the specimen side. Ileum is cut using no. 15 blade from inside mesenteric point to outside antimesenteric part; similarly colon is cut between clamps to retrieve the specimen. Occlusion clamps should be placed oblique outwards to maintain the blood supply of the colon at its antimesenteric part. In practice occlusion clamps are placed 10 mm from the cut edges of the ileum and transverse colon; but ideally clamps should be placed 10 cm from the cut edges even though it is not practiced by most of the surgeons. Bleeding from the cut edge should be confirmed as well as pulsatile mesenteric edge. Fat should be removed from the colon for 1 cm from the cut edges to prevent fat interposition during anastomosis. For anastomosis, single layer interrupted full thickness 3-0 silk sutures or two layered interrupted full thickness vicryl sutures and outer interrupted seromuscular 3-0 silk sutures can be used. Cheatle's cut may be needed on the antimesenteric border of the ileum. Mesenteric rent is closed using continuous or interrupted 3-0 vicryl or silk sutures.

Conventional right hemicolectomy

Midline laparotomy
↓
Exploration
↓
Mobilisation of the colon from paracolic gutter through avascular plane of *Toldt*
↓
Safeguarding the ureter, gonadal vessels
↓
Ascending colon and hepatic flexure is released from gall bladder by dividing hepatocolic ligament
↓
Mobilisation from the duodenum and Gerota's fascia
↓
Greater omentum is separated by ligation and division
↓
Care should be taken about SMV and its branches and bleeding
↓
Ligation of the vessels close to the colon in case of benign conditions; ligation of their branches at their origin from middle colic vessels to ileocolic vessels in case of malignancy to clear nodes
↓
Division of the terminal ileum and transverse colon between clamps
↓
Constructing a safe ileocolic anastomosis
↓
Closure of the mesenteric defect
↓
Suction tube drain and closure of the abdomen

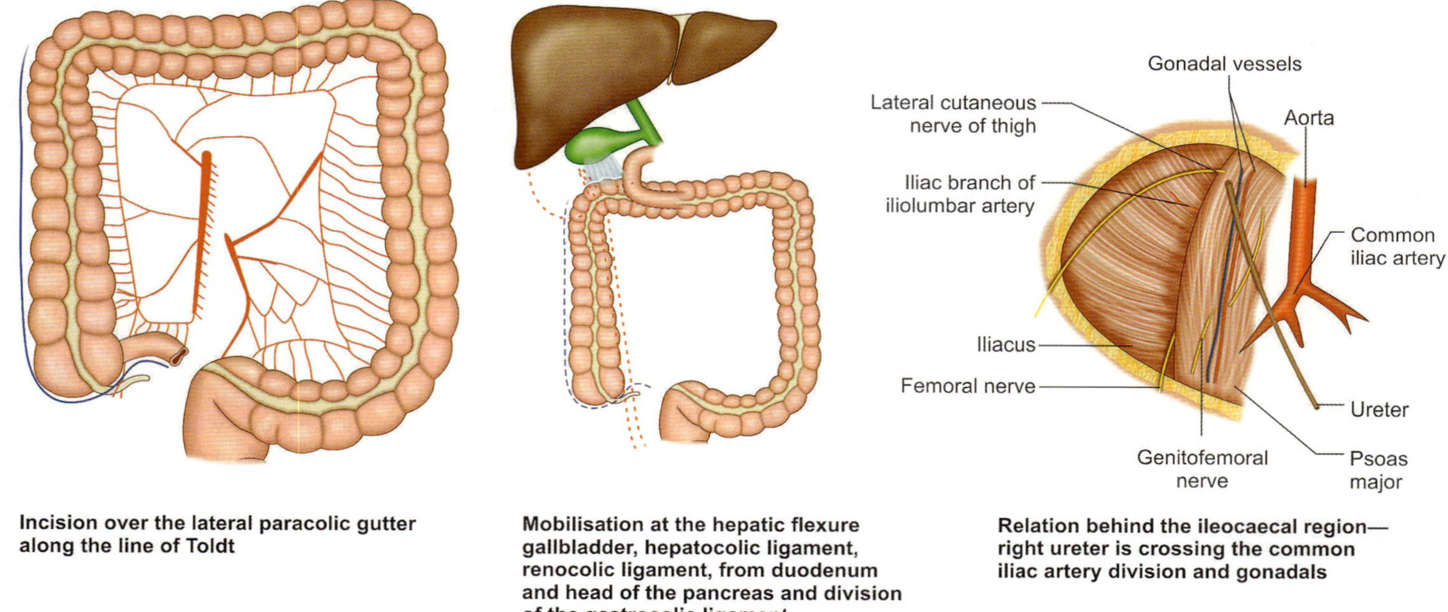

Fig. 25-29: Relations, structures which will come across while doing right hemicolectomy.

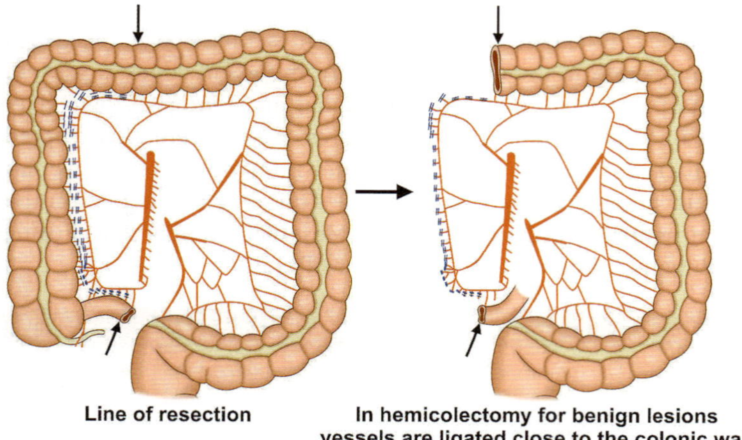

Fig. 25-30: In benign lesions, while doing hemicolectomy lateral to medial (conventional) approach is used with ligating the vessels close to the colonic wall without any lymphovascular clearance.

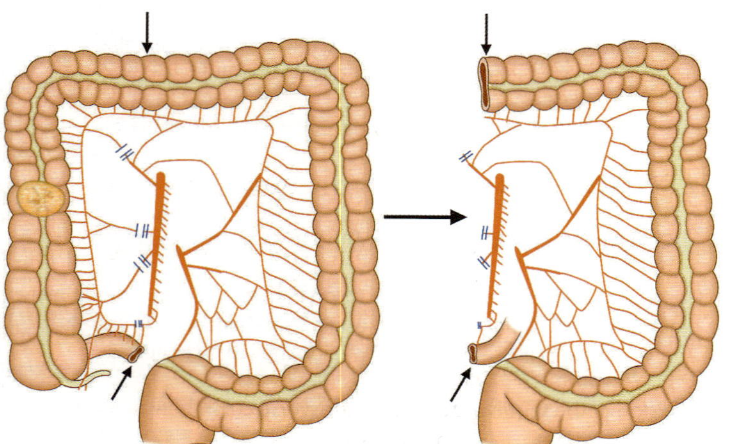

Fig. 25-31: In malignancy, medial to lateral approach (oncological) is used with proper lymphovascular clearance. Here vessels are ligated at their origin.

Radical Right Hemicolectomy

It is done commonly from medial to lateral with vessels ligated at its origin to clear the lymphovascular area. It clears the drainage lymph nodes properly in carcinomas. It also prevents spillage, avoids manipulation of the tumour area prior to vascular ligation—based on '*Turnball's no touch technique*'. Advantages of this medial to lateral technique are—it facilitates the early ligation of the main branches of the SMA and SMV and so prevents possible eventual trauma of superior mesenteric vessels while mobilising the colon; field will be clean and so anatomical variations are better identified. Early lymphovascular dissection achieves more precise dissection and clearance. Even though it is oncologically not very much proved, technically it is more precise. But surgeon should remember that radical hemicolectomy can also be done through conventional approach wherein after complete mobilisation of the colon, vessels are ligated at its origin to clear lymphovascular area.

Through transillumination vascular arcade is studied; site of division is decided in the ileum and transverse colon. After creating a small window at the mesenteric sides of these two points umbilical tapes or fine infant feeding tubes or two wet roller gauzes are passed one on each point (at terminal ileal and transverse colon sides) and tied firmly. Omentum (in malignancy) is detached from the stomach by ligation and divisions or harmonic scalpel can be used. First right branch of the middle colic artery is ligated at its origin (in carcinoma caecum and ascending colon); usually double ligation is needed proximally. In extended right radical hemicolectomy (carcinoma hepatic flexure and transverse colon), middle colic artery is ligated at its origin (at the level of the lower border of the pancreas) as colon division is far away at splenic flexure and remaining descending colon has its blood supply from left colic artery. Both middle colic artery and vein are ligated; inferior pancreaticoduodenal vein is very close and during dissection of the middle colic vessels this vein may get torn by avulsion causing torrential haemorrhage. Transverse colon is lifted upwards; right mesocolon is already opened while ligating the middle colic vessels; index finger is passed underneath to do gentle finger dissection; pulsation of the ileocolic trunk is felt. It is dissected from surrounding areolar tissue; ileocolic vein is also located adjacent to the artery which should not be injured.

SMA pulsation is also felt and is identified. SMA pulsation should not be mistaken for ileocolic arterial pulsation. Ileocolic artery and vein are individually ligated doubly using silk 1 cm distal to the SMA. Ileocolic vessels are divided. Ileal mesentery is divided for 10-15 cm (length of ileum removed depends on the location of the primary tumour). It is divided between ligatures.

Now right paracolic gutter is incised at avascular plane of Toldt from terminal ileum to hepatic flexure level using blunt finger and sharp scissor dissection. Ureter, gonadal vessels, Gerota's fascia, duodenum is dissected using bipolar cautery and sharp scissor dissection. Blunt dissection here may injure these structures or can cause bleeding. Gerota's fascia is separated by dividing renocolic ligament. Omentum is separated from the greater curvature of the stomach (partial omentectomy) up to the level of transection of the transverse colon. Ureter is easily identified by its tubular shining nature with good peristalsis. Ureter crosses common iliac artery where bifurcates into external and internal iliac arteries. Reflected peritoneum may be having attached ureter and so should be inspected and felt carefully in the peritoneum.

Ileum and colon is divided similarly like mentioned earlier in conventional method above. Anastomosis is done. Stapler transection can be done at both ends; later completion with side-to-side stapler anastomosis **(Fig. 25-32)**.

Radical right hemicolectomy—medial to lateral vessel first hemicolectomy (Turnball no touch method)

Midline incision, exploration, self-retaining retractor
↓
Umbilical tape or fine infant feeding tube or wet roller gauze is tied around the ileum and transverse colon at their line of resection
↓
Transverse colon is lifted up
↓
Middle colic vessels are identified
↓
In right radical hemicolectomy, right branch of the middle colic vessel at its origin is ligated (in caecal and ascending colon growth). Origin of the middle colic vessels at the lower border of the pancreas is dissected and double ligated in hepatic flexure and right side transverse colon growth (extended). Double ligation should be ligated.
↓
Right colic vessels are ligated (may be absent also)
↓
Larger ileocolic artery is identified, dissected and doubly ligated (should not get confused for SMA)
↓
Terminal ileal vessels (terminal 10–15 cm) are ligated
↓
Now colonic mobilisation is done along the paracolic gutter through the line of *Toldt*
↓
Ureter, gonadal vessels, duodenum, Gerota's fascia are identified and dissected away from right colon
↓
Ascending colon and hepatic flexure is mobilised by separating from gall-bladder, duodenum and by cutting the renocolic ligament using scissor and gentle finger dissection; partial omentectomy is done by dividing the omentum adjacent to greater curvature of the stomach
↓
Once complete mobilisation is over; specimen is divided between clamps on both sides. Fat at the colonic cut edges is freed for 1 cm
↓
End to end hand sewn or side to side stapler ileocolic anastomosis is done
↓
Mesenteric defect is closed; suction tube drain is placed; abdomen is closed in layers

Stapler anastomosis can be done as side to side. Few stapler area in the antimesenteric borders of each ends which are brought together are removed just sufficient enough to pass the arms of the stapler. Arms are passed through this across the antimesenteric border and stapler is fired to create the anastomosis as side to side. Now stapled ends of the each part are having a defect at the antimesenteric border which is closed by another linear stapling device.

Postoperative Care

Nasogastric tube is removed once bowel sounds appears; patient passes flatus; no distension in the abdomen. Drain is removed in 5 days. Oral fluid started in 3–5 days. Antibiotics are given. Fluid and electrolyte management is done judiciously.

Complications

Infection, subphrenic and pelvic abscess formation can occur. It is identified by CT imaging; initially can be treated with antibiotics conservatively but if persists or progress then US/CT guided pigtail catheter drainage or occasionally open drainage is done.

Anastomotic disruption is a dangerous complication. It causes leak from drain site or main abdominal wound. If it is a significant leak then re-exploration and re-anastomosis are done; commonly re-anastomosis is difficult due to friable inflamed oedematous bowel; ileostomy for diversion is best in such situation. If leak is less and patient is passing stool per anally then conservative treatment settles the leak. TPN, antibiotics, control of sepsis and observation, repeated imaging is the needed management.

Abdominal dehiscence is not uncommon; it needs resuturing of the rectus sheath, control of infection.

Injury to right ureter, duodenum can occur. Duodenal injury is sutured if it is small otherwise duodenostomy through a T tube should be done. Ureter injury when identified on table is sutured using interrupted 3-0 vicryl sutures. J stent should be placed in the ureter which is removed in 6–12 weeks.

LEFT COLECTOMY

Left hemicolectomy is done for both benign and malignant diseases. Principles are almost similar as right hemicolectomy. But no touch technique is difficult to apply to left-sided colectomy. Marginal artery should be retained in all these patients especially in malignancies to maintain the blood supply retained to colon and anastomotic site. Left branch of the middle colic artery when retained is adequate enough to maintain the blood supply. Inferior mesenteric artery is ligated and divided at its origin from the aorta and inferior mesenteric vein is divided at lower border of the pancreas. Even if most of the sigmoid colon needs resection, blood supply of the anastomotic site can be achieved from middle rectal and inferior rectal arteries along with marginal artery. In benign diseases vessels are not ligated at their origin but close to the colonic wall as lymphovascular clearance is not needed.

In no touch technique, inferior mesenteric vessels are ligated first with lymphovascular clearance (for carcinoma left side colon) then left colon mobilisation is done. In benign diseases first mobilisation of the left colon is done then vessels are ligated close the colonic wall.

Splenic injury can occur while mobilising the splenic flexure; alternatively spleen may get infiltrated by the splenic flexure growth which needs splenectomy. Gonadal vessels can be ligated if needed; but left ureter should be taken care of.

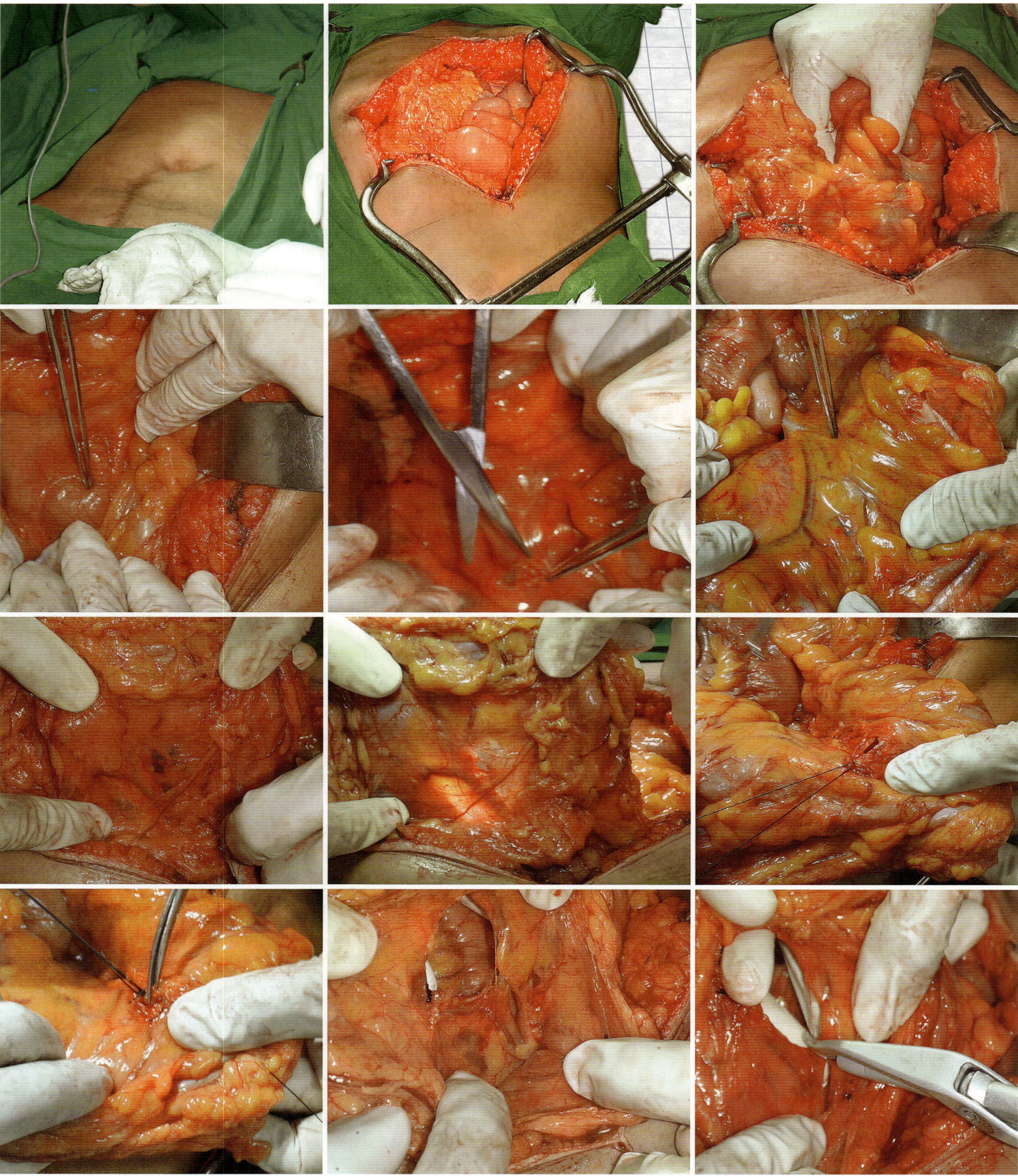

Figs. 25-32(1)

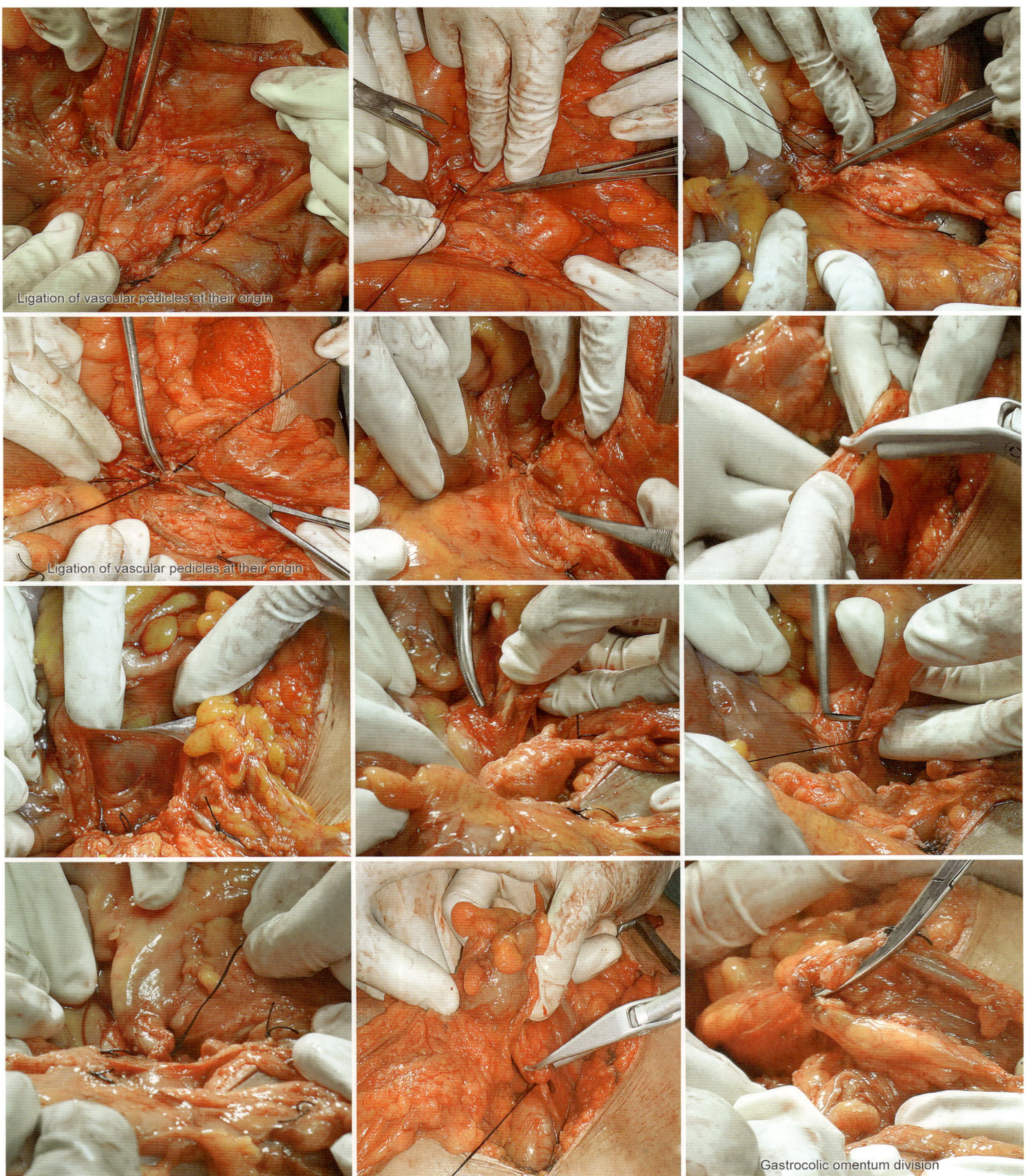
Ligation of vascular pedicles at their origin
Ligation of vascular pedicles at their origin
Gastrocolic omentum division

Figs. 25-32(2)

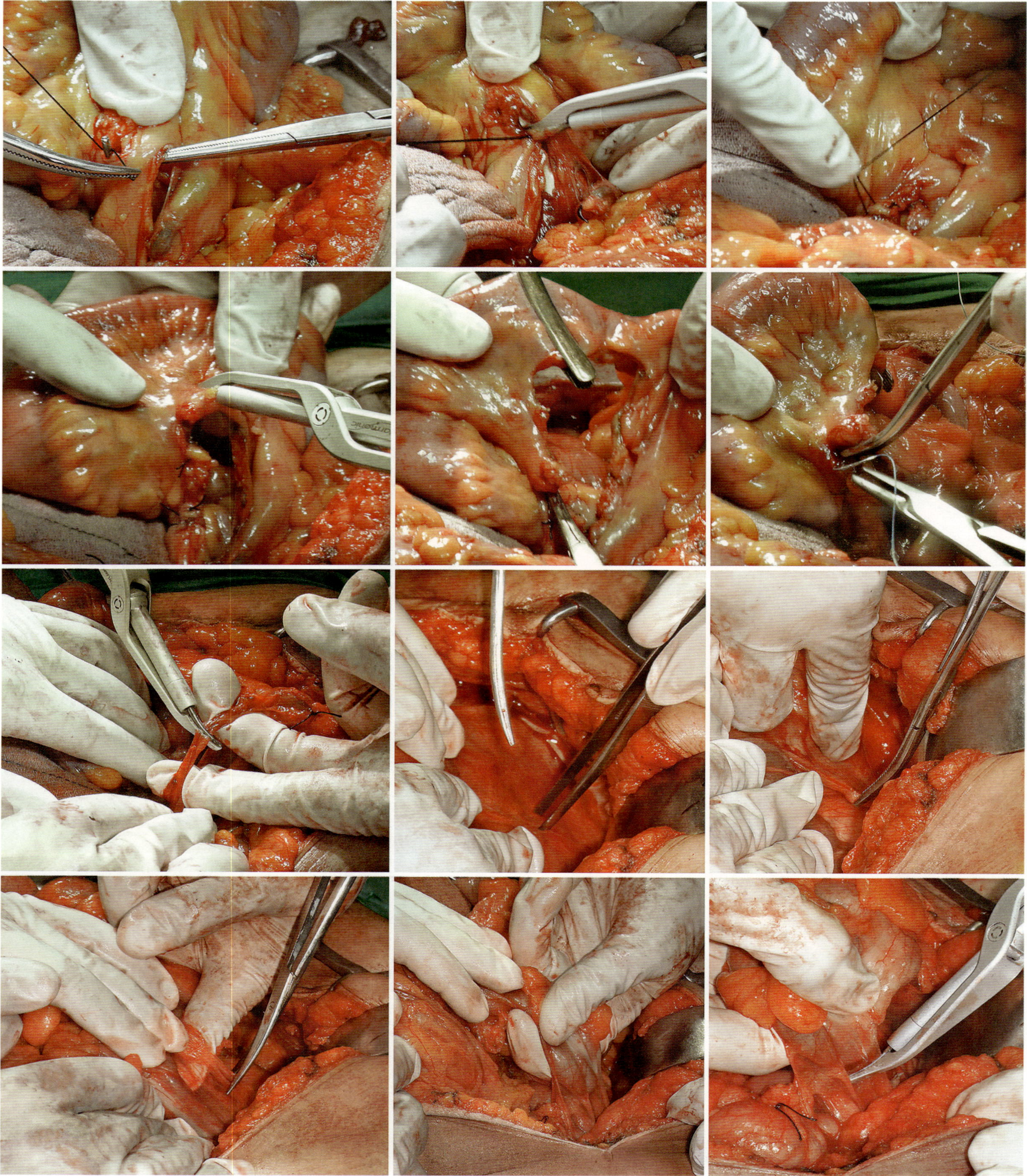

Figs. 25-32(3)

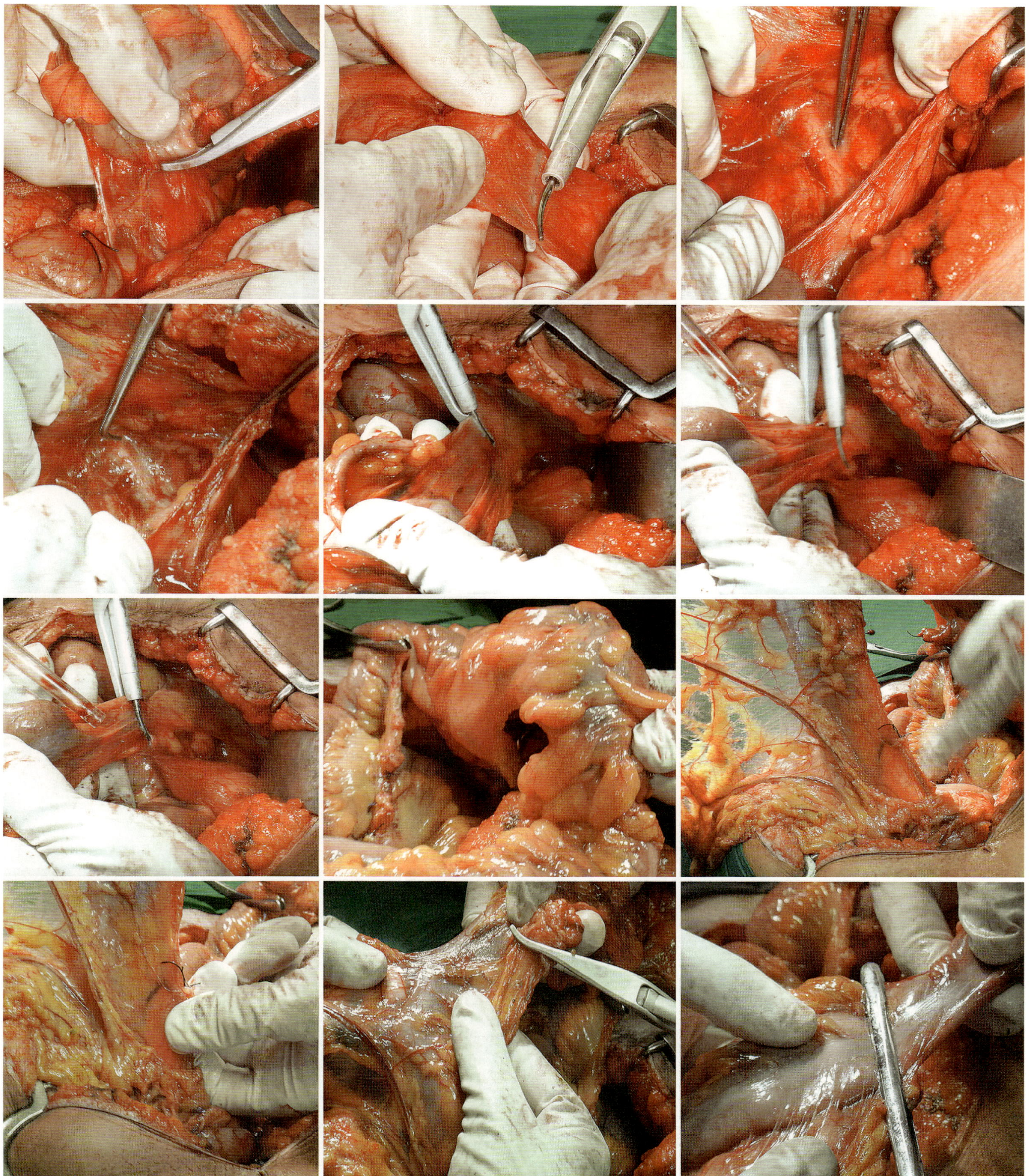

Figs. 25-32(4)

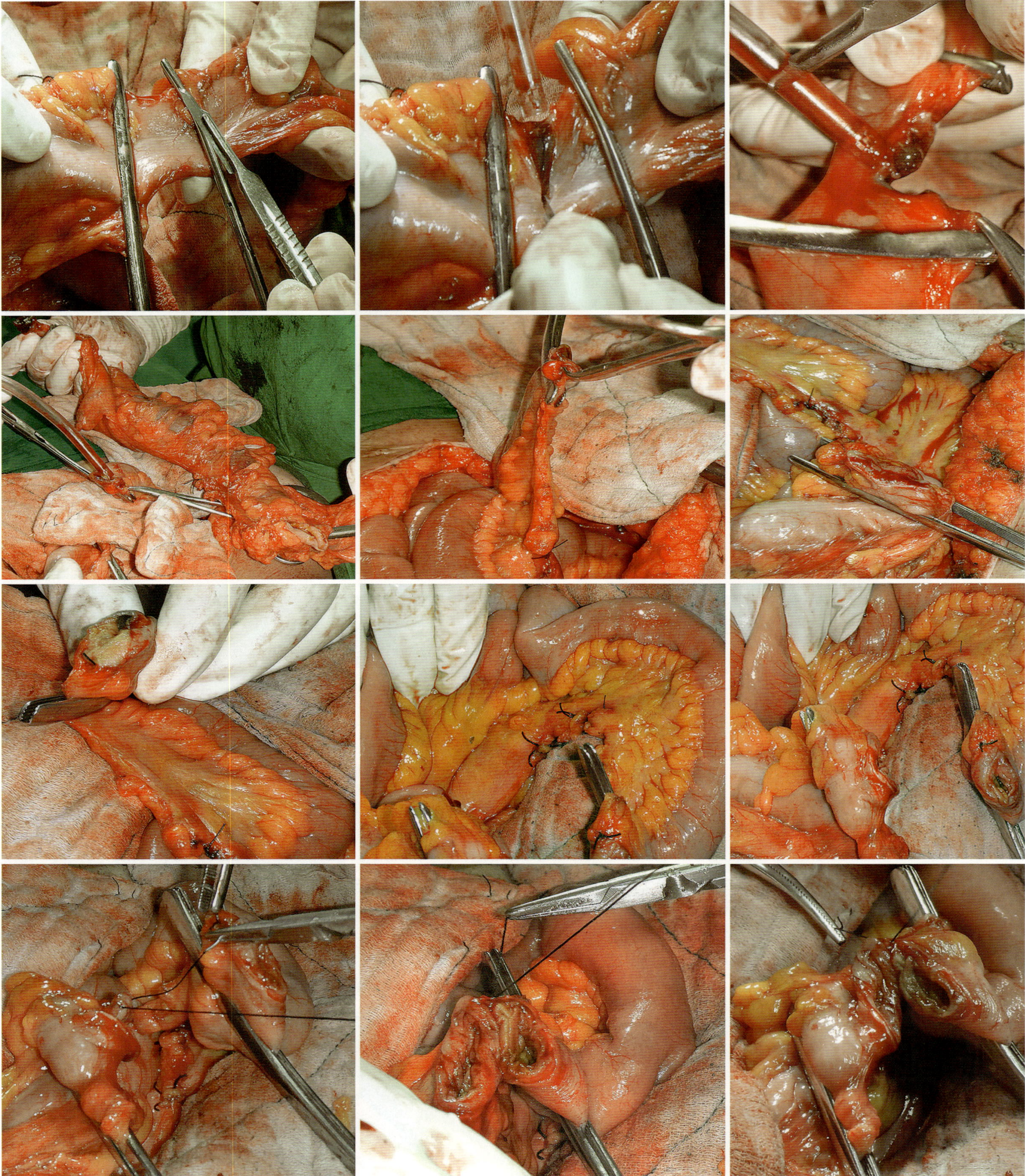

Figs. 25-32(5)

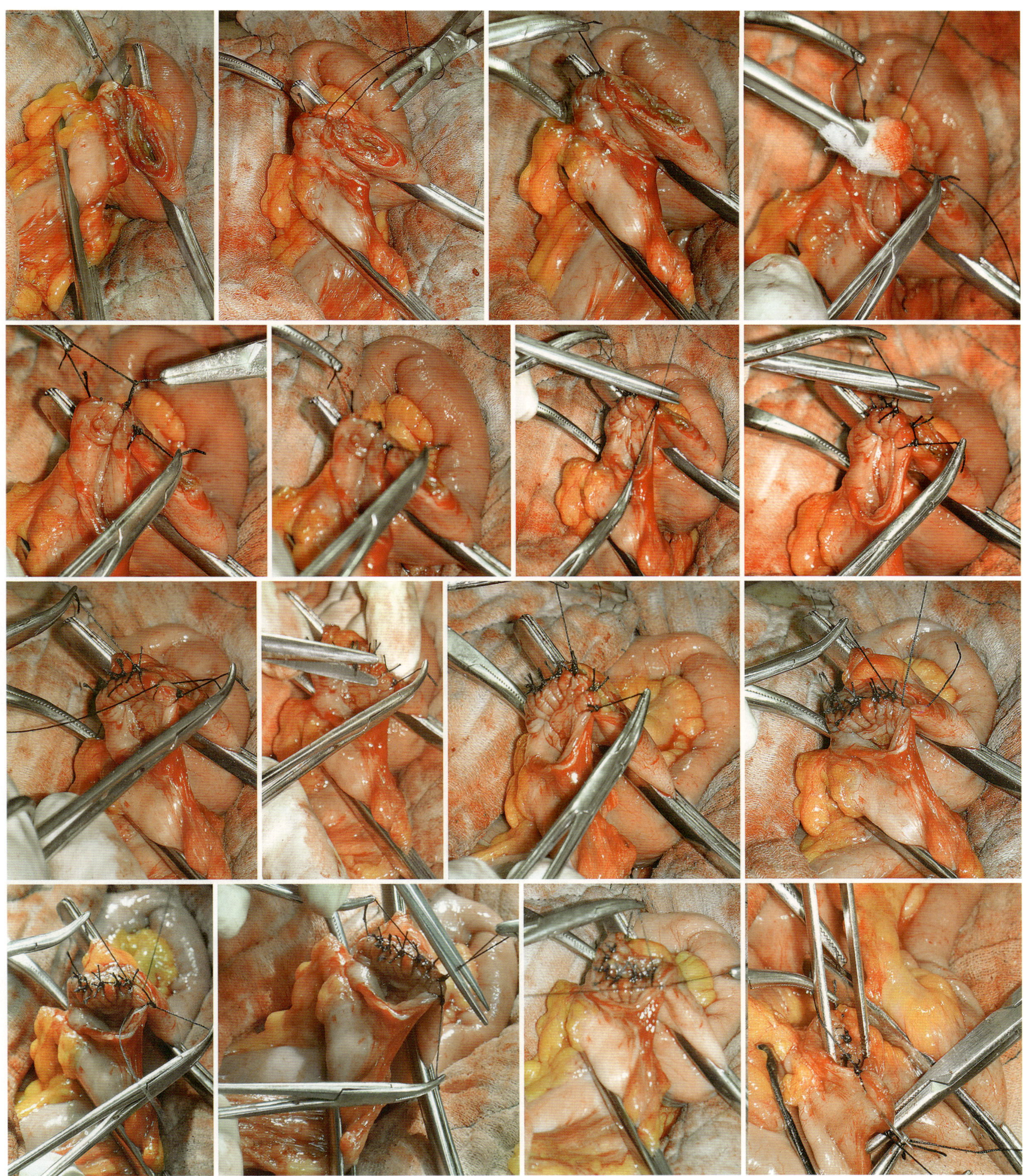

Figs. 25-32(6)

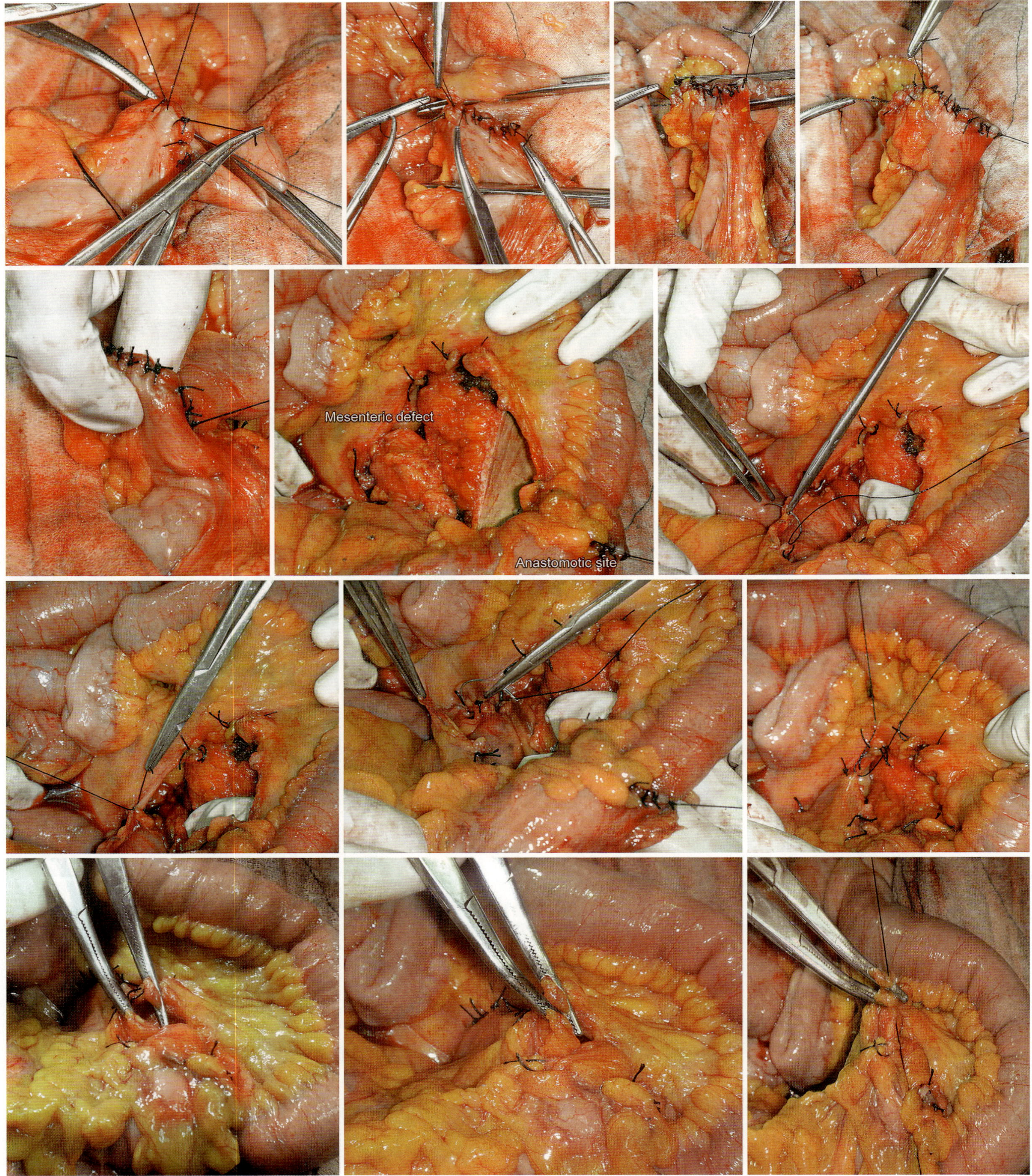

Figs. 25-32(7)

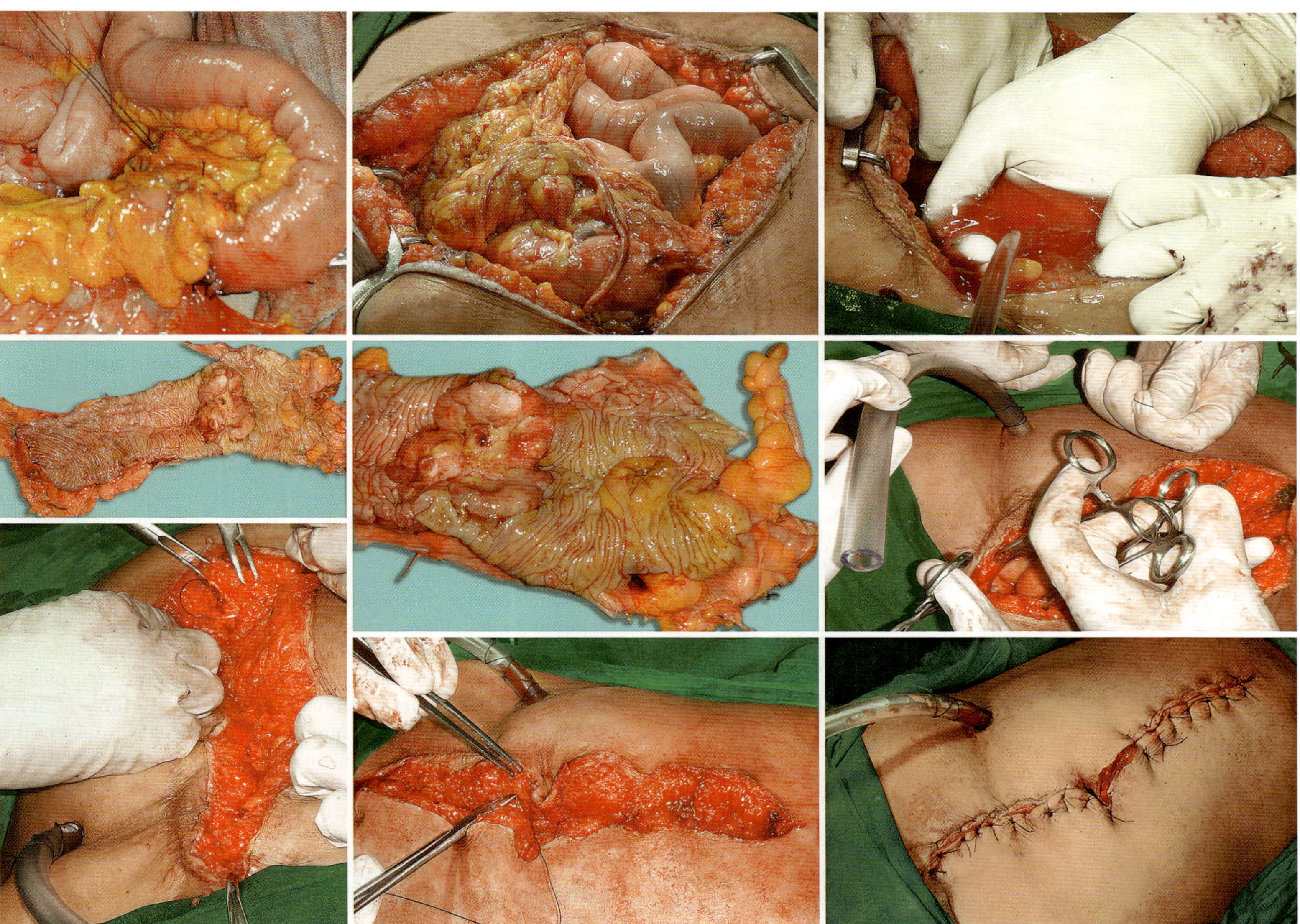

Figs. 25-32(8)

Figs. 25-32(1 to 8): Right radical hemicolectomy with lymphovascular clearance with medial to lateral approach. Vessels are ligated near their origin.

Technique

Epidural and general anaesthesia are given. Nasogastric tube and urinary catheter are passed. After cleaning and draping lengthy midline incision is made. Head down position is better. In sigmoid resection, when EEA stapler is used then low lithotomy position is better. Self retaining retractor like Finochette is used. Surgeon usually stands on the left side.

Sigmoid and descending colon is held towards right using a mop; peritoneum on the paracolic gutter is incised adjacent to sigmoid; left ureter and left gonadals are identified and safeguarded; incision is extended proximally towards splenic flexure; greater omentum attached to that part of the transverse colon close to the splenic flexure is divided between ligatures. Undue traction and blunt dissection should be avoided which may cause troublesome oozing. *Renocolic ligament* between capsule of left kidney and posterior part of the mesocolon is divided. *Lienocolic (splenocolic) ligament* is divided; *pancreaticocolic ligament* is divided to free the splenic flexure downwards. Appendices epiploicae of transverse colon may come across during dissection which when divided may cause bleeding; it needs proper ligation. While mobilising the splenic flexure adequate exposure is essential; undue traction on the colon may cause the avulsion on the omentum and bleeding; recognising the right plane and dissecting along that is needed; sharp scissor dissection with careful bipolar cautery fulguration is ideal rather than blunt dissection in splenic flexure mobilisation.

Duodenum, 3rd and 4th part will be visualised here. Mesocolon on the medial aspect is incised from splenic flexure downwards towards the sacral promontory level. Inferior mesenteric artery is identified emerging from the aorta; its origin is visualised; 1–2 cm distal to its origin artery is double ligated and divided. This allows safe preservation of the hypogastric nerve plexus which are in front of the aorta. Preaortic areolar tissue with lymph nodes is swept medially to clear all lymphovascular tissues. Preaortic sympathetic plexus should not be injured to prevent development of sexual dysfunction. Inferior mesenteric vein is identified which runs upwards behind the duodenojejunal junction behind the pancreas to join splenic vein **(Fig. 25-33)**.

Rest of the mesocolon is divided down towards the sigmoid colon; here marginal artery is divided to complete the mesocolon and vascular dissection and mobilisation. If dissection is carried out downwards up to the rectosigmoid junction; proximal rectum

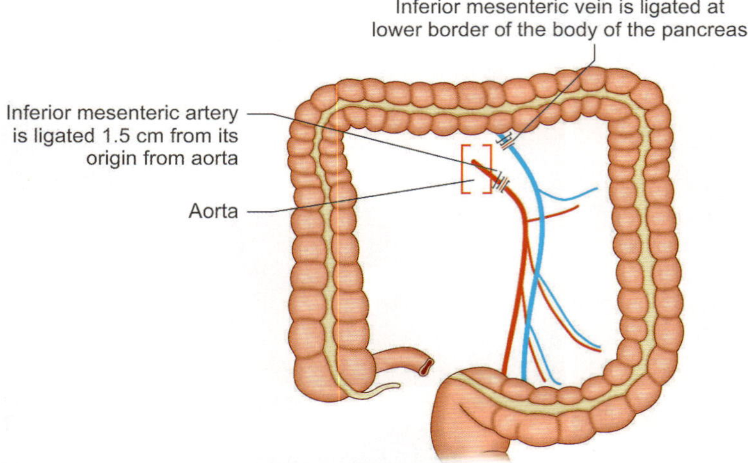

Fig. 25-33: Ligation of inferior mesenteric vessels in radical left colectomy.

which is covered by peritoneum is dissected for 3 cm above the sacral promontory by ligating and dividing the vascular pararectal tissues. Autonomic nerve plexus lying on the posterior pelvic brim is preserved. Fat around the rectum for 1 cm should be cleared meticulously to achieve optimum anastomosis. Occlusion clamp is applied to the transverse colon proximal to the mobilised splenic flexure; crushing clamp is applied towards specimen side and divided in between using cautery or ideally no. 15 blade. Proximal cut edge should bleed adequately for safe anastomosis. Distally proximal to the mobilised and dissected proximal rectum another curved crushing/Kocher's clamp is applied (towards specimen side); usually clamp is not placed on the rectal stump side; however a soft occlusion clamp can be used if necessity arises. Bleeders in cut edge of the rectum are ligated using fine 4-0 vicryl or bipolar cauterisation is done. Fat should be cleared from the cut both ends for 1 cm; bleeding cut edge should be confirmed. Proximal cut end of the transverse colon easily reaches the rectal stump at sacral promontory level. If tension is present then the hepatic flexure should be mobilised to make transverse colon tension free.

While anastomosing, the cut edges of transverse mesocolon should come towards the right side of the rectum. Usually two layered anastomosis is done; but single layer interrupted silk sutures are sufficient. Surgeon should stand on the left side while doing anastomosis. Initially two posterior seromuscular 3-zero silk sutures are placed on the medial and lateral aspects; knots are not tied now and these sutures act as marker/stay sutures to identify the medial and lateral edges of the rectal end. Then remaining 4–6 seromuscular sutures are placed at 5 mm gap; once all sutures are placed they are tied; leaving medial and lateral tied stay sutures long remaining sutures are cut. 2nd posterior full thickness interrupted 3-zero vicryl sutures are placed at 5 mm gap; once all sutures are placed they are tied together. 3rd layer anterior full thickness interrupted 3-zero vicryl sutures are placed and tied together. Lastly anterior seromuscular interrupted 3-zero silk sutures are placed. Site is checked for tension free anastomosis with adequate lumen inside **(Fig. 25-34)**.

Many use continuous 3-zero vicryl sutures for 2nd and 3rd layer. It is also practiced that if apposing area can be rotated for 180° then anterior layer seromuscular sutures are placed first; rotated fully to visualise the posterior layer through which anterior full thickness, posterior full thickness and posterior seromuscular sutures are placed and colon is derotated back to its original position. *End to end (EEA)* stapler can be used to achieve proper anastomosis. *Linear stapling device* can be used to transect at transverse colon level as well as rectal level.

It is often used to pass a wide Foley's catheter (no. 22 F) per anally and gently to negotiate across the anastomotic site to keep it there for 48 hours. After insertion of the Foley's catheter before negotiating across, anastomotic field is filled with normal saline and air is pushed across the Foley's catheter to check air bubbles in the field; if air bubbles are present then few more interrupted silk sutures may be placed at the site of the leak. Again even though it is not mandatory many do anal sphincter dilatation presuming that it will prevent distal obstruction and so reducing the chances of anastomotic leak. Tube drain is placed in the pelvis. Abdomen is closed in layers.

Postoperative Care

Nasogastric tube is removed in 72 hours; oral liquid is started. Drain is removed in 7 days. Skin sutures are removed in 10 days.

Complications

Intraoperative—injury to left ureter; spleen, haemorrhage—adequate exposure and careful dissection will prevent this.

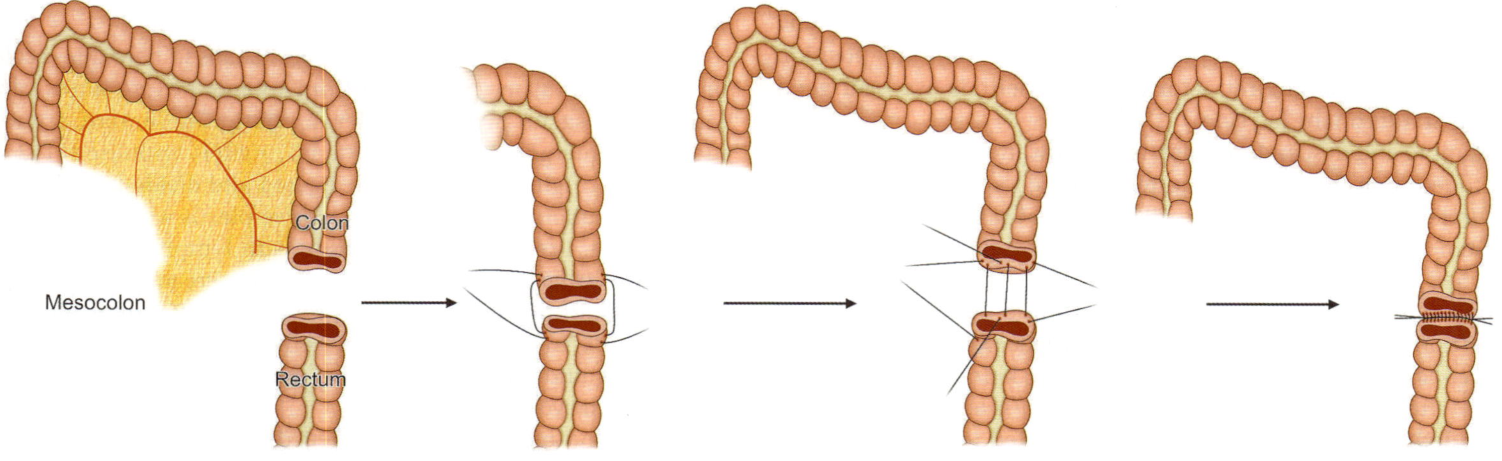

Fig. 25-34: Placing seromuscular sutures in colorectal anastomosis.

Postoperative—anastomotic leak can occur; it is usually partial leak and subsides gradually. If significant high fistula persists then covering diversion proximal colostomy or ileostomy should be done. Often peritonitis may develop in such situation, anastomotic site is detached and proximal colonic part of anastomosis is brought out as colostomy; distal rectal stump is closed (Hartmann's) which is sutured to sacral promontory by 2-3 silk sutures to prevent it from getting retracted; once patient recovers from sepsis, only after 3 months resurgery should be done to maintain the continuity. Pelvic abscess, left sided subphrenic abscess are other complications which can occur.

LAPAROSCOPIC COLECTOMY

Laparoscopy for colectomy right or left is now well-accepted approach. There is lack of tactile sensation; dissection in more than one quadrant needs the camera to be changed in different ports during dissection. Contamination, bleeding, spillage of the content, port site recurrence, conversion, long time, cost are different problems. Still colectomy either totally laparoscopic or hand assisted are accepted universally. Principles and technique are same as open surgery. Identification and localisation of the pathology, mobilisation of the needed part of the colon, devascularisation, restoration of the bowel continuity are essential steps of the colectomy. Different ports of different sizes, specialised instruments like bowel grasper and endostaplers are needed. Endostapler needs 12 mm port.

Different types of laparoscopic colectomies are practiced. In dissection facilitated laparoscopic colectomy, mobilisation of the colon is done through laparoscopy; and then through a small laparotomy incision, resection and anastomosis is done. In resection facilitated laparoscopic colectomy, dissection and resection is done through laparoscopy; specimen retrieval and anastomosis is done extracorporeally. In near total laparoscopic colectomy, dissection, resection and anastomosis is performed through laparoscopy; specimen retrieval and anvil of the circular stapler is passed through a small incision. In totally laparoscopic colectomy, dissection, resection, retrieval of the specimen and anastomosis are done through laparoscopy only; it is technically very demanding and time consuming.

Indications: Colonic malignancy, colonic tuberculosis, ileocolic Crohn's disease; diverticulitis, polyps which cannot be removed through the colonoscopy.

Contraindications: Faecal peritonitis, cirrhosis of liver, large abdominal aneurysm, pregnancy, cardiopulmonary problems, previous abdominal surgeries, blood dyscrasias.

Laparoscopic Right Hemicolectomy

Conventional lateral to medial approach and oncological medial to lateral approach are the two approaches. Former one is used in benign lesions and technically easier; latter one is used in malignancy wherein first vascular control is obtained prior to mobilisation. Nasogastric tube and urinary catheterisation are done. Under general anaesthesia, in supine position, cleaning and draping are done. Monitor is kept on the right side; surgeon stands on the left side; cameraman on the left of the surgeon; then scrub nurse.

Port positions: 10 mm umbilical port is created as open method (or closed Veress needle method can be used) which is used as right hand working port initially then later as camera port; suprapubic 10 mm port is used as camera port for mobilisation and later is used for retraction; left hand 5 mm working port is on the right iliac fossa; 10 mm epigastric port initially is used for retraction during hepatic flexure mobilisation and later as right hand working port **(Fig. 25-35)**.

Medial to lateral oncological approach: Here during initial dissection of lymphovascular tissue, lateral peritoneal attachment of the ascending colon, which is yet to be divided acts as a natural retractor facilitating the vascular dissection easily. Camera telescope is passed through the suprapubic 10 mm port; terminal ileum is held upwards; peritoneum is opened behind the terminal ileum and caecum; retroperitoneal tunneling is created; right ureter and right gonadal vessel are identified in this avascular plane; cranial dissection is done in front of the right ureter and right gonadal vessel till 2nd part of the duodenum is visualised; Gerota's fascia is seen during this dissection which is not opened. Duodenum, head of the pancreas and IVC is visualised. Stretching of the mesentery facilitates the identification of the ileocolic and right colic vessels from below upwards. Ileo colic vessels are dissected close to their origin to SMV and SMA; fat and lymphatics are cleared off from its surface; ileocolic artery and vein are individually clipped or ligated and divided. Right colic vessels are also divided; often right colic vessels may be absent. Mesentery is divided using harmonic scalpel. Mesentery division continues on the transverse mesocolon until the right branch of the middle colic vessels are identified which are individually clipped and divided. Patient's position is changed to head-up position (reverse Trendelenburg). Right flexure of the colon is retracted downwards and medially; now umbilical port is used as camera port; epigastric port is used for right hand working. Lesser sac is entered by dividing the greater omentum between transverse colon and stomach. Dissection continues laterally by dividing the peritoneum between duodenum and pancreas and transverse colon. Hepatocolic ligament is divided to release the hepatic flexure. Middle colic vessels can be ligated at this juncture as proximal as towards its origin. This completes the devascularisation of the entire right colon; mesentery of the terminal ileum is divided using harmonic scalpel. At the end lateral attachment of the colon is divided using harmonic scalpel to complete the dissection and devascularisation. Intracorporeal resection is done using endo stapler; specimen is retrieved through a small subumbilical incision and anastomosis is done extracorporeally. Alternatively after dissection and mobilisation, mobilised part is exteriorised through a small subumbilical incision; resection is done; anastomosis is done using hand sewn or lineal stapler.

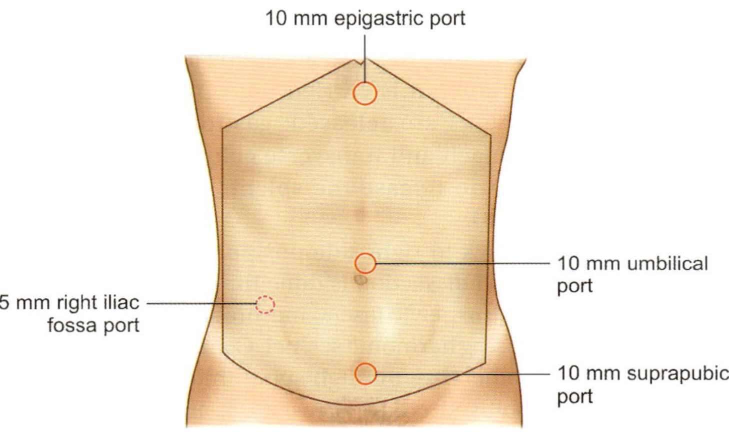

Fig. 25-35: Ports used for right laparoscopic colectomy.

Lateral to medial approach: It is conventional one wherein lateral peritoneal attachment (along the white line of Toldt) of caecum and ascending colon is incised and colon is mobilised; similarly hepatic flexure and transverse colon is mobilised using harmonic scalpel. Right ureter, vas deferens, gonadal vessels and duodenum are identified. Gastrocolic ligament is divided. Subumbilical midline incision is done for 5 cm; mobilised colon is brought out; ileocolic, right colic and middle colic vessels are ligated and divided extracorporeally; in benign conditions vessels are ligated close to the colonic wall as there is no need to divide branch vessels at their origin. Resection and anastomosis is done extracorporeally; mesenteric defect is closed; anastomotic parts is placed back into the peritoneal cavity; minilaparotomy is closed in layers; again pneumoperitoneum is created; peritoneal cavity and anastomotic site is inspected; port area are closed in layers.

Laparoscopic Left Hemicolectomy

Patient is placed in supine with semilithotomy position with thighs placed semiflexed and hips flexed to only limited 15°. Rotating table is a must to tilt the table as needed. Nasogastric tube insertion and urinary catheterisation is done. Monitor is placed on the left foot side. Wide area cleaning and draping is done; camera port (10 mm) is placed in supraumbilical position or right of the midline; 10 mm right hand working port is in the right iliac fossa; 5 mm left hand working port is in the right lumbar region; 10 mm colon retracting port is in the left lumbar area. Additional trocars may be added depending on need. Surgeon initially stands on the right side but changes the position to between legs for dissection of the splenic flexure and transverse colon on the left side. Head down with left upwards is the usual table tilt done to make small bowel to fall away from the pelvis.

Peritoneal cavity is explored including liver for initial assessment. Sacral promontory is identified; over the medial aspect of the mesosigmoid an incision is made; through the left lumbar midclavicular port sigmoid is grasped and retracted laterally. Avascular plane is reached by deepening the plane. Plane in front of the ureter, gonadal vessels and inferior mesenteric vessels is dissected carefully. Ureter is safeguarded. Inferior mesenteric vessels are dissected and, ligated and divided individually using silk (intracorporeal sutures). Dissection in this plane is continued upwards towards the splenic flexure. Gerota's fascia is visualised and kept undisturbed.

Now sigmoid colon is gently retracted medially and lateral colonic peritoneal attachment is incised along the white line of Toldt. Surgeon should stand in between legs incision; monitor is shifted towards head end; table may be tilted according to need. Dissection over the lateral peritoneum is carried out upwards. Renocolic, splenocolic attachments are released; gastrocolic omentum is divided between stomach and transverse colon. Pancreaticocolic ligament is dissected to release the splenic flexure adequately downwards **(Fig. 25-36)**.

Surgeon returns back to right side position; monitor is shifted back to foot end. Rectal dissection is done through avascular plane between the layers of the pelvic fascia; mesorectum is divided up to the line of resection using harmonic scalpel. Colon can be transected using endostapler; otherwise through subumbilical incision colon is exteriorised; mobilised colon is resected; and end to end or stapler anastomosis is done. Sterile barrier (plastic) should be used while retrieving the specimen to avoid port site complications. Alternatively after resection using stapler; anvil of the EEA stapler is sutured to proximal end using nonabsorbable purse string suture; both ends are dropped into the peritoneal cavity. EEA stapler is gently negotiated per anally towards peritoneal cavity; its sharp point is made to perforate away from stapler line; it is connected to the anvil already present in the peritoneal cavity along with the proximal cut end of the bowel with purse string and locked. Stapler is fired to complete the anastomosis. Device is removed; doughnut is observed.

Complications and Problems with Laparoscopic Colectomy

Difficulty in dissection and mobilisation; injury to vital structures; multiquadrant dissection; problems related to laparoscopy itself; inability to feel the tumour; problems with the retrieval of the specimen; port site problems; increased operating time; anaesthesia complications; availability of the instruments; cost are different problems.

Complications specific to technique are—anastomotic leak; abscess formation (pelvic/subphrenic); anastomotic stenosis. In such situation proximal diversion or colostomy with mucus fistula formation or Hartmann's procedure may be required. Inadequate clearance in case of tumours, port site recurrences are other complications.

Laparoscopic Subtotal/Total Colectomy

It is demanding technique as it needs mobilisation of the colon in different quadrants as well as in pelvis. Tilting table is a must as position has to be changed depending on the site of mobilisation. With steep head-down (Trendelenburg) position (similar like for left colectomy) after placing adequate proper ports dissection begins at rectosigmoid. Dissection here is same as for left colectomy mentioned above. Inferior mesenteric vessel ligation; splenic flexure mobilisation remains the same. Transverse colon mobilisation is carried out as continuation of the splenic flexure mobilisation; gastrocolic omentum is divided using harmonic scalpel; transverse mesocolon is dissected to identify the middle colic artery which is ligated and divided. SMA should be identified and safeguarded without injuring it.

Right colon mobilisation is done with surgeon standing on the left side similar to right colectomy. It is done from medial to lateral approach. Retroperitoneal tunneling is created; right ureter, gonadals are identified; plane in front is dissected upwards; ileocolic vessels are ligated; then right colic artery. Once vascular divisions are complete, lateral peritoneal attachment is incised and divided along the Toldt's line. Terminal ileal vessels are divided using harmonic scalpel.

Rectum is further mobilised depending on the level of resection; injury to sympathetic nerves should be avoided to prevent sexual dysfunction. Injury to sacral plexus vessels will cause torrential haemorrhage; it is difficult to cauterise them as they retract into the sacral foramina.

Rectosigmoid is divided using lineal stapler; minilaparotomy is done with a Pfannenstiel incision; protective plastic sheath is placed across the edge of the laparotomy; specimen is brought out; proximal part (terminal ileum) is transected. Ileo rectal continuity is achieved by intracorporeal suturing or if rectal end can be brought out to the wound it can be done using hand sewn technique; otherwise circular EEA stapler can be used to achieve continuity. Lower level resection decides the procedure as either subtotal or total colectomy.

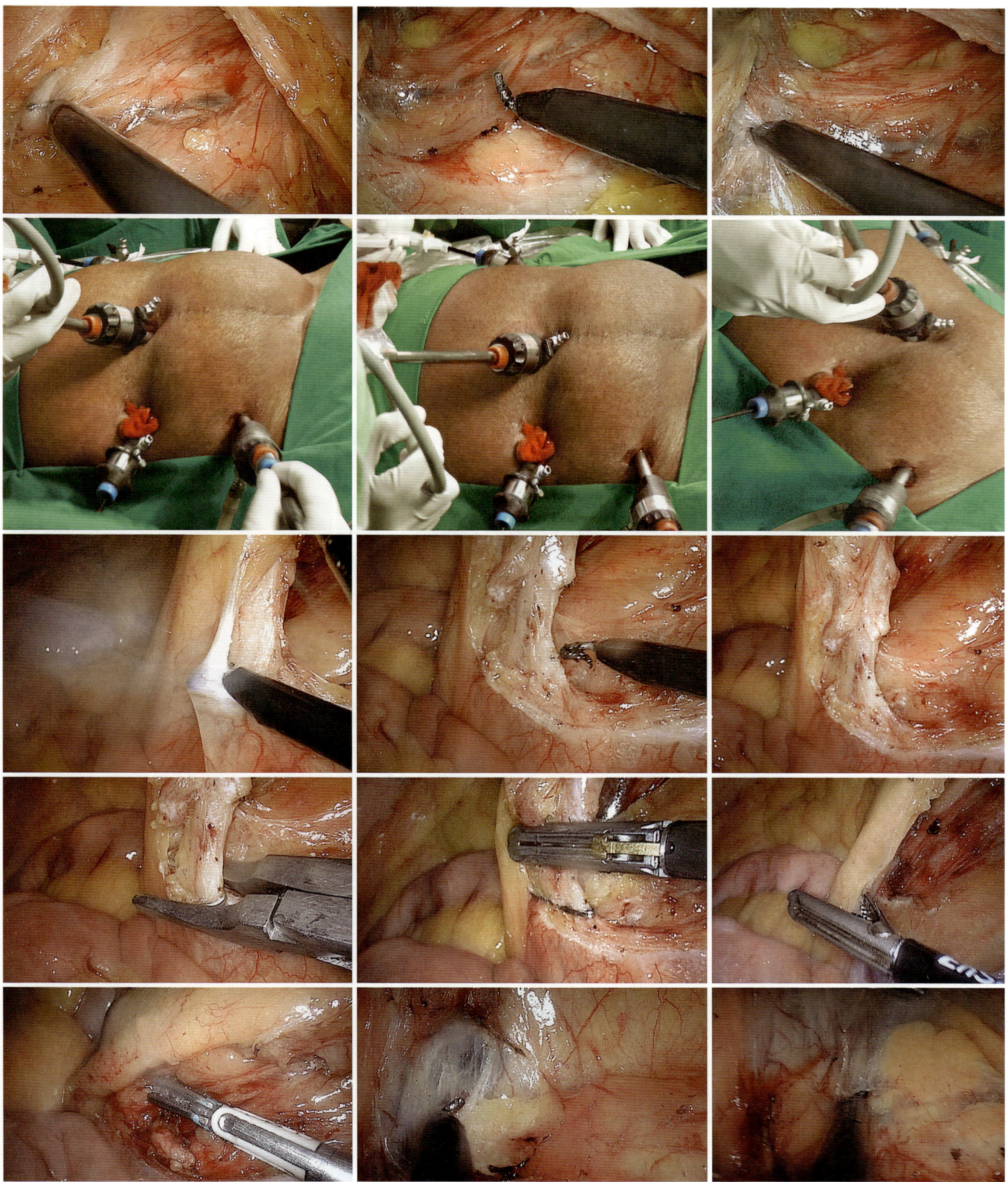

Figs. 25-36(1)

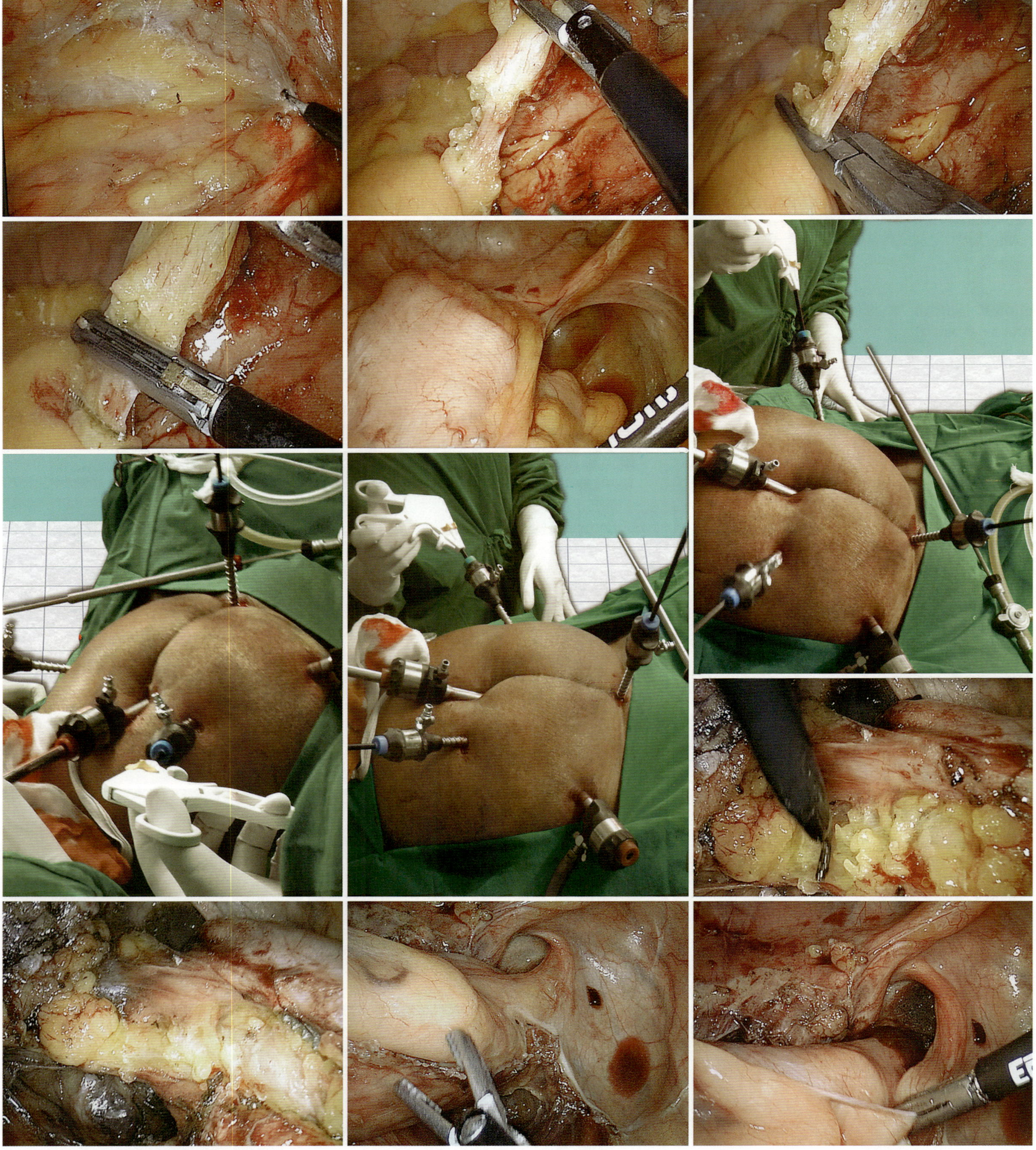

Figs. 25-36(2)

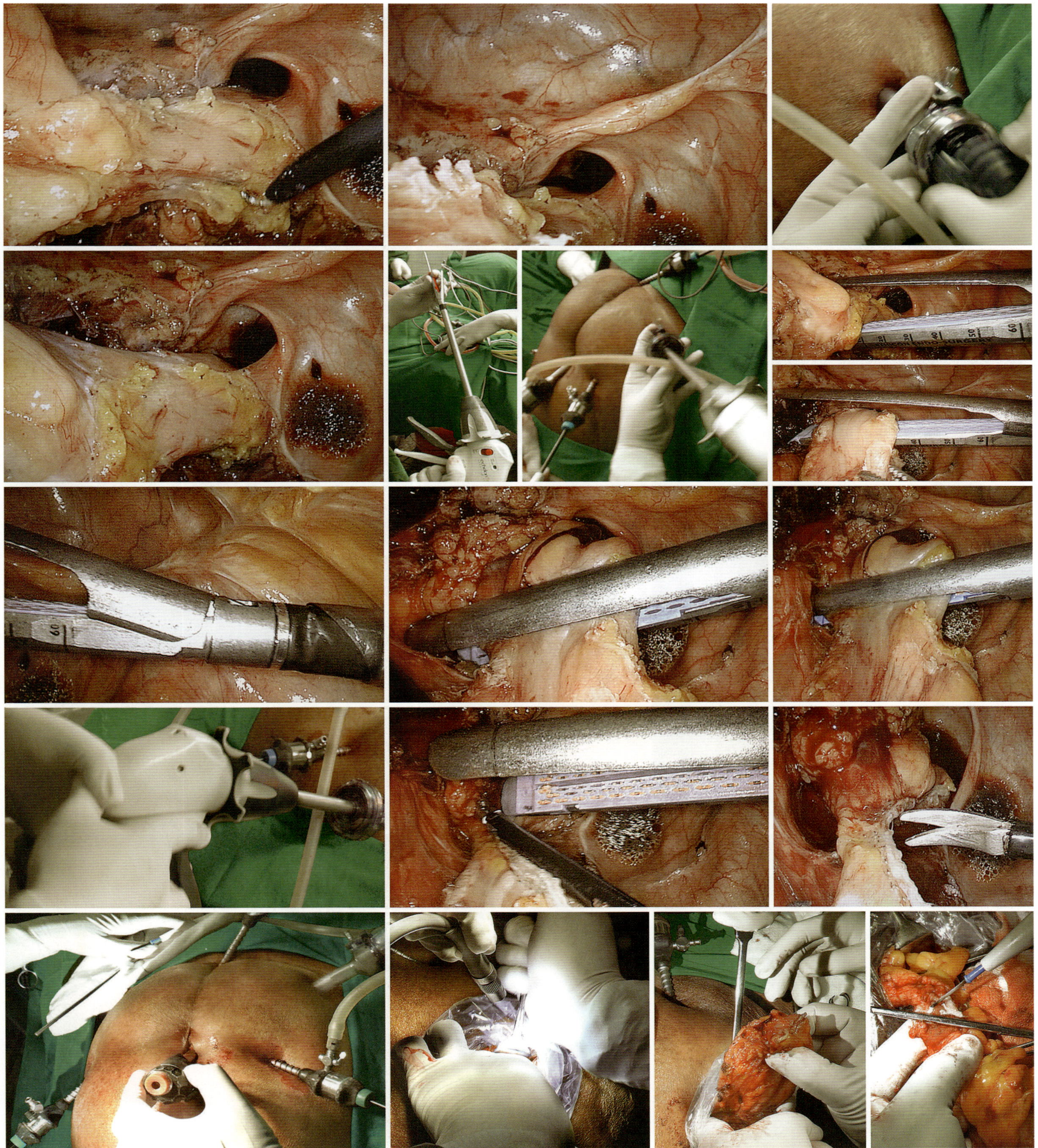

Figs. 25-36(3)

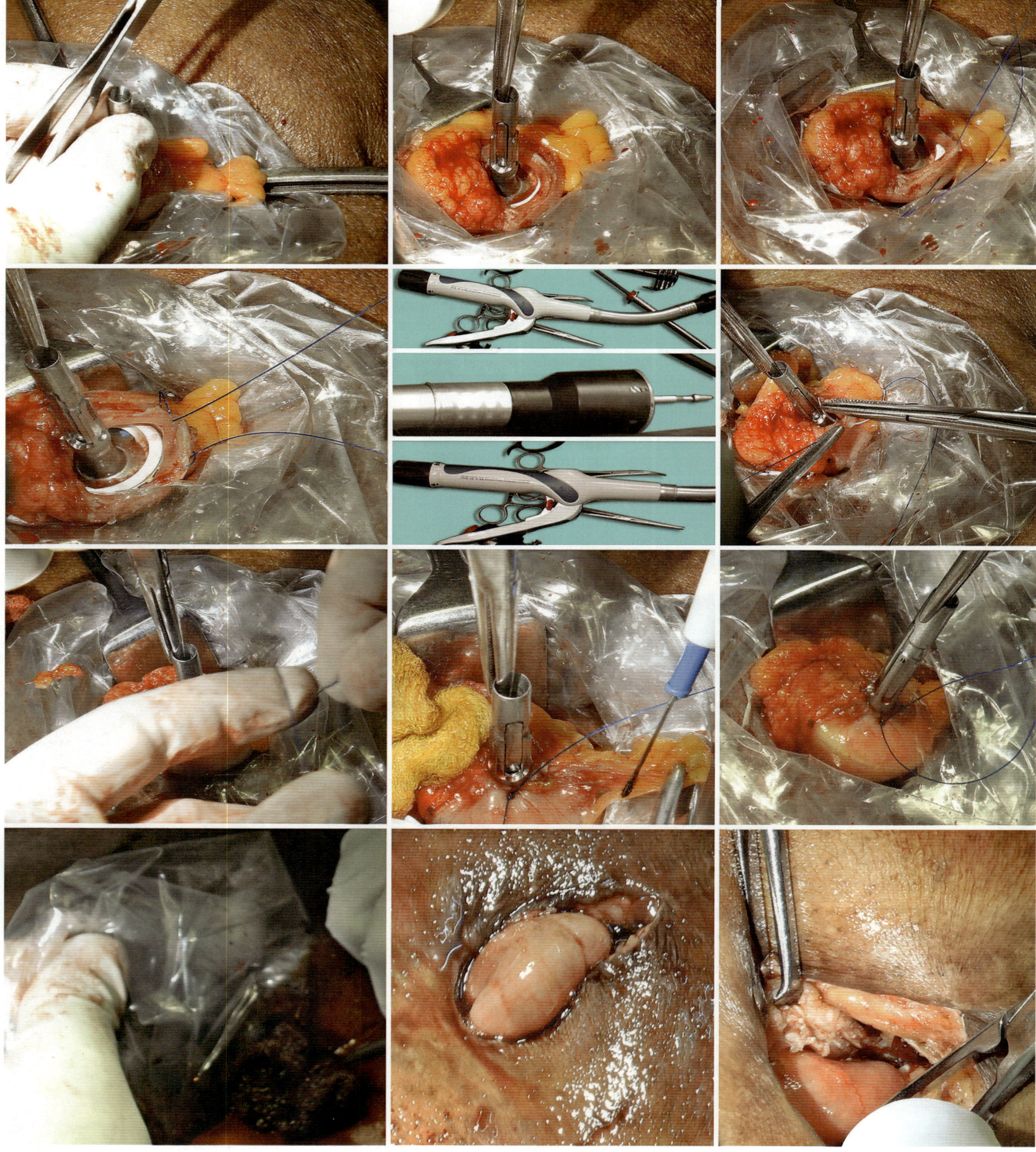

Figs. 25-36(4)

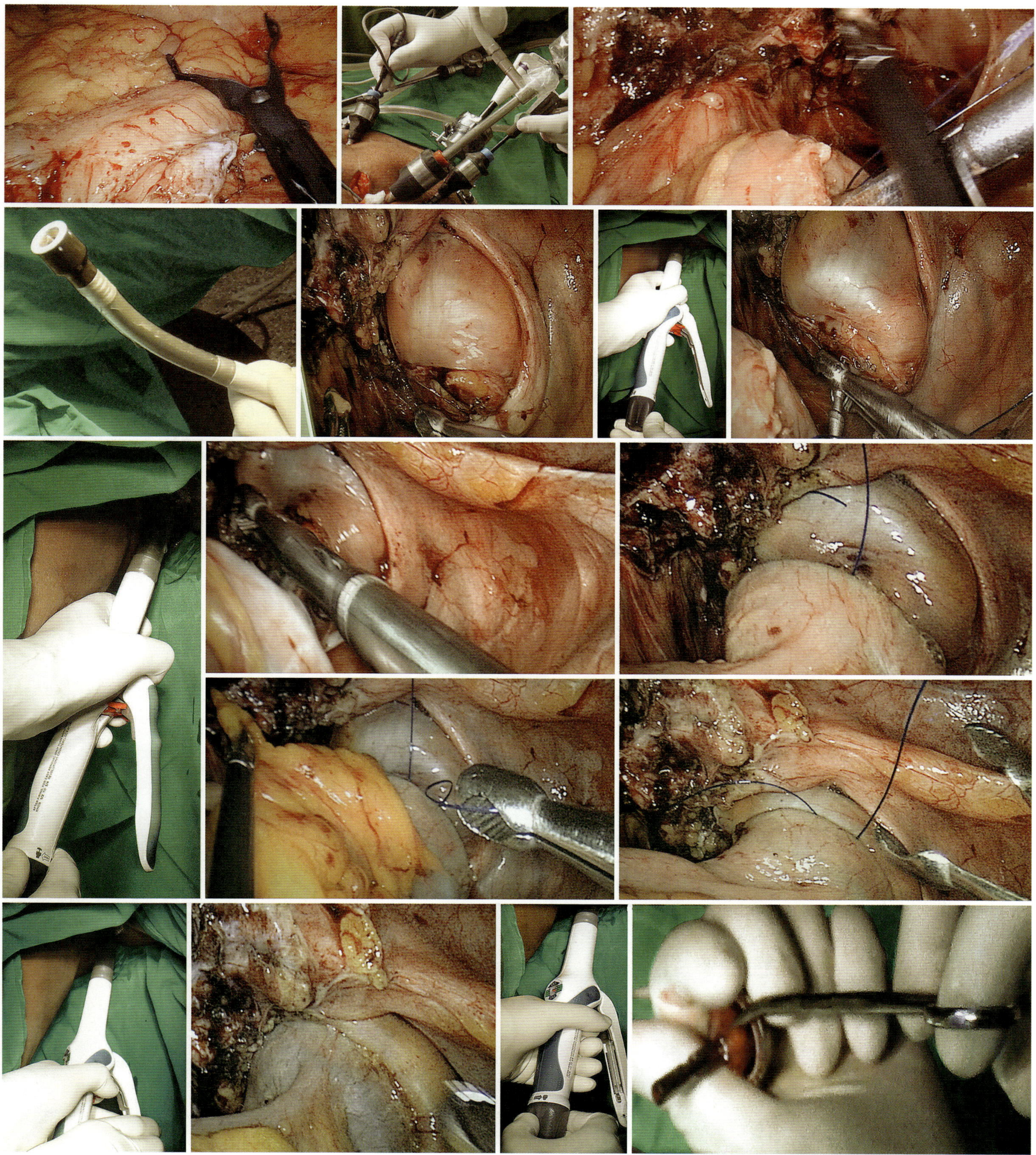

Figs. 25-36(5)

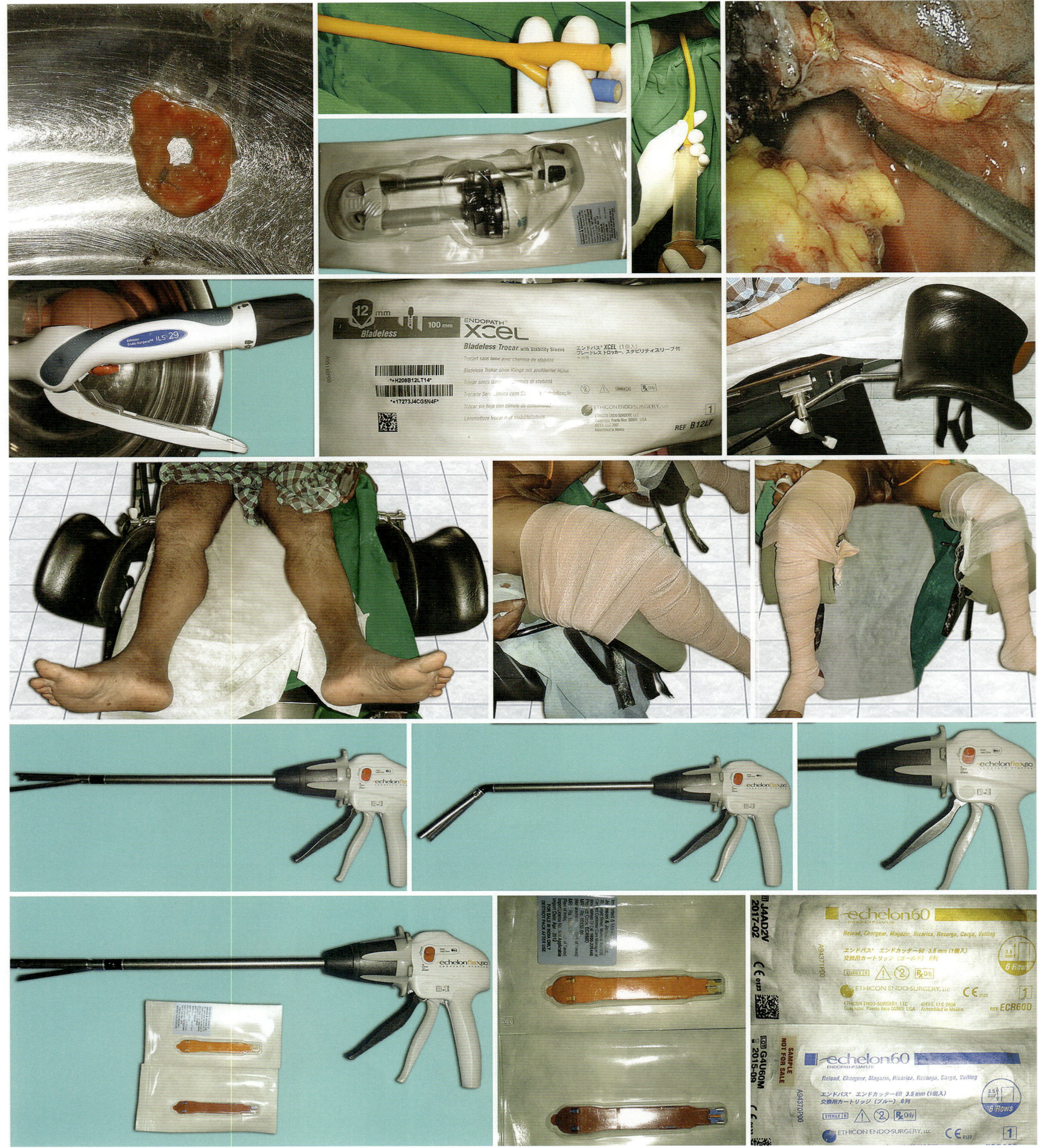

Figs. 25-36(6)

Figs. 25-36(1 to 6): Laparoscopic left colectomy. Note the angulated stapler used for transection. it needs 12 mm port. Note the patient position; port positions; steps; specimen retrieval; barrier plastic to the subumbilical minilaparotomy; anvil; placing purse string suture; circular stapler; firing the stapler; and other steps of dissection. Dissection here is done from medial to lateral. Main vessels (left colic) are clipped and divided using harmonic.

LOCALLY ADVANCED TUMOUR (INOPERABLE)

It is managed by colonoscopic decoring and stenting as a palliation. But it needs repetitive procedure. Alternatively bypass can be done either as ileo transverse anastomosis in case of hepatic *flexure* growth or colocolic anastomosis between transverse colon and descending colon in case of the left side advanced growth near or at splenic flexure **(Fig. 25-37)**.

Bowel proximal and distal are brought together confirming that there is no tension; if tension is there bowel mobilisation may be needed. Antimesenteric border of the ileum of 6 cm and antimesenteric border of the colon are incised at taenia at corresponding parts after placing occlusion clamps. Interrupted two layer anastomosis is done with inner full thickness and outer seromuscular sutures using 3-zero silk. Greater omentum may be wrapped around; clamps are removed. Usually drain is not required for bypass procedures unless there is contamination **(Fig. 25-38)**.

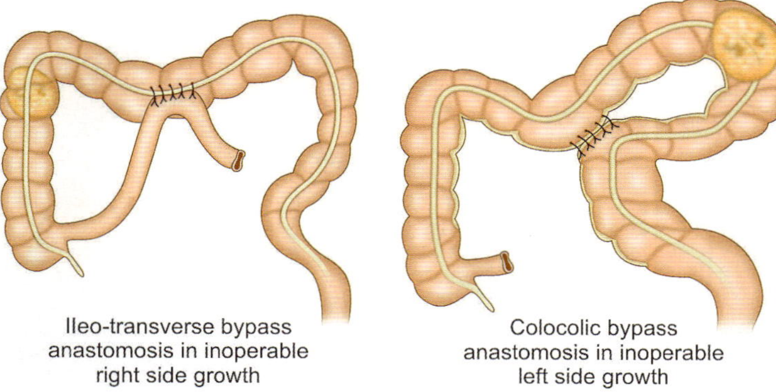

Fig. 25-37: Bypass colonic procedures in advanced malignancies.

SURGICAL MANAGEMENT IN LARGE BOWEL OBSTRUCTION

Large bowel obstruction faces problems with sepsis, dehydration, contamination during surgery, electrolyte imbalance and nutritional deficiency.

Presently resection and primary anastomosis is done as a possibility. However, surgeon should finally decide about the factors like patient's general condition to obtain optimum recovery. Decision should be individualised rather than generalised. If needed after resection and anastomosis for right sided obstruction, covering loop ileostomy should be done which is closed after 3 months.

In left sided obstruction commonly due to growth, resection and anastomosis with right side diversion colostomy is the choice. It is often preferable to do on table colonic lavage to reduce the contamination and sepsis. It is done by passing a catheter through appendicectomy opening or a separate ileal stab opening which is secured by a purse string suture. Left sided growth/obstruction is identified; colon is transected between clamps above the obstruction; proximal end of the bowel is directed outside the surgical field to empty the content or connected to a lengthy tube (Savaage's decompressor). Warm normal saline is run through the proximal catheter distally across the colon towards distal end to empty; around 10 litres of fluid is needed to clean the bowel adequately **(Fig. 25-39)**.

Treatment of Sigmoid Volvulus

Initial treatment—nasogastric tube aspiration; IV fluids; catheterisation; antibiotics; *a flatus tube or sigmoidoscope* is passed in operation theatre (proper care is taken otherwise it leads to perforation). If it derotates, patient will pass flatus and faeces; and distension reduces **(Fig. 25-40)**.

If derotation does not occur, laparotomy through midline incision should be done. Dilated sigmoid colon is derotated manually and checked for viability. If viable, it can be fixed to the lateral wall of abdomen or pelvis—***Sigmoidopexy***.

If sigmoid colon is gangrenous, it is resected and proximal cut end is brought out as colostomy and distal end is brought out as mucus fistula, from the rectum *(Paul-Mikulicz operation)*. Later after 6 weeks, continuity is maintained after proper preparation.

Resection of the gangrenous sigmoid done; proximal cut is brought out as end colostomy: distal end closed—*Hartmann's operation*. Later in 6-12 weeks colorectal anastomosis is maintained.

Primary resection and anastomosis is not advisable because of the contamination and anastomotic leak.

Mortality in sigmoid volvulus is due to *perforation, peritonitis and septicaemia* **(Fig. 25-41)**.

TREATMENT FOR HIRSCHSPRUNG'S DISEASE

Initially, colostomy is done either transverse or transitional, so to have normal bowel function, and nutritional supplementation. Once the child attains 10 kg of weight, definitive procedure is done, i.e. (a) Excision of aganglionic segment (spasmodic segment); (b) Maintenance of continuity by doing coloanal anastomosis; (c) Closure of colostomy later.

Common procedures done are:

Modified Duhamel operation: Resection of upper part of the rectum and a part of colon; anastomosis of colon to posterior part of the lower rectum and crushing the spurs to create the rectal pouch. It is *technically easier and a retro-rectal pull through*. New pouch is created by anterior part of the aganglionic rectum and by ganglionic proximal pulled down colon. Biopsy should be taken from proximal pulled down colon to look for evidence of ganglions. Pulled down proximal colon is sutured to full thickness posterior anal canal just above the dentate line. Spur between these two segments is crushed by Kocher's forceps or specialised instrument to create a single pouch **(Fig. 25-42)**.

Soave's mucosectomy and pull through operation: Through laparotomy approach rectum is mobilised deeply into the pelvis; circular myotomy is made on the rectal wall; submucosal plane is created up to the dentate line; denuded mucosa is excised; normal colon is brought down through this tube and coloanal anastomosis is done. In original Soave's technique, after telescoping the normal proximal colon through the rectal tube outside anus it is made to protrude outside for few cms which is not sutured and left like that to allow distal part to slough off to achieve continuity naturally.

Total proctocolectomy with ileo-anal anastomosis in case of total colonic Hirschsprung's disease.

Swenson's operation: Through abdomino-anal approach, aganglionic segment of the rectum is mobilised including proximal normal bowel.

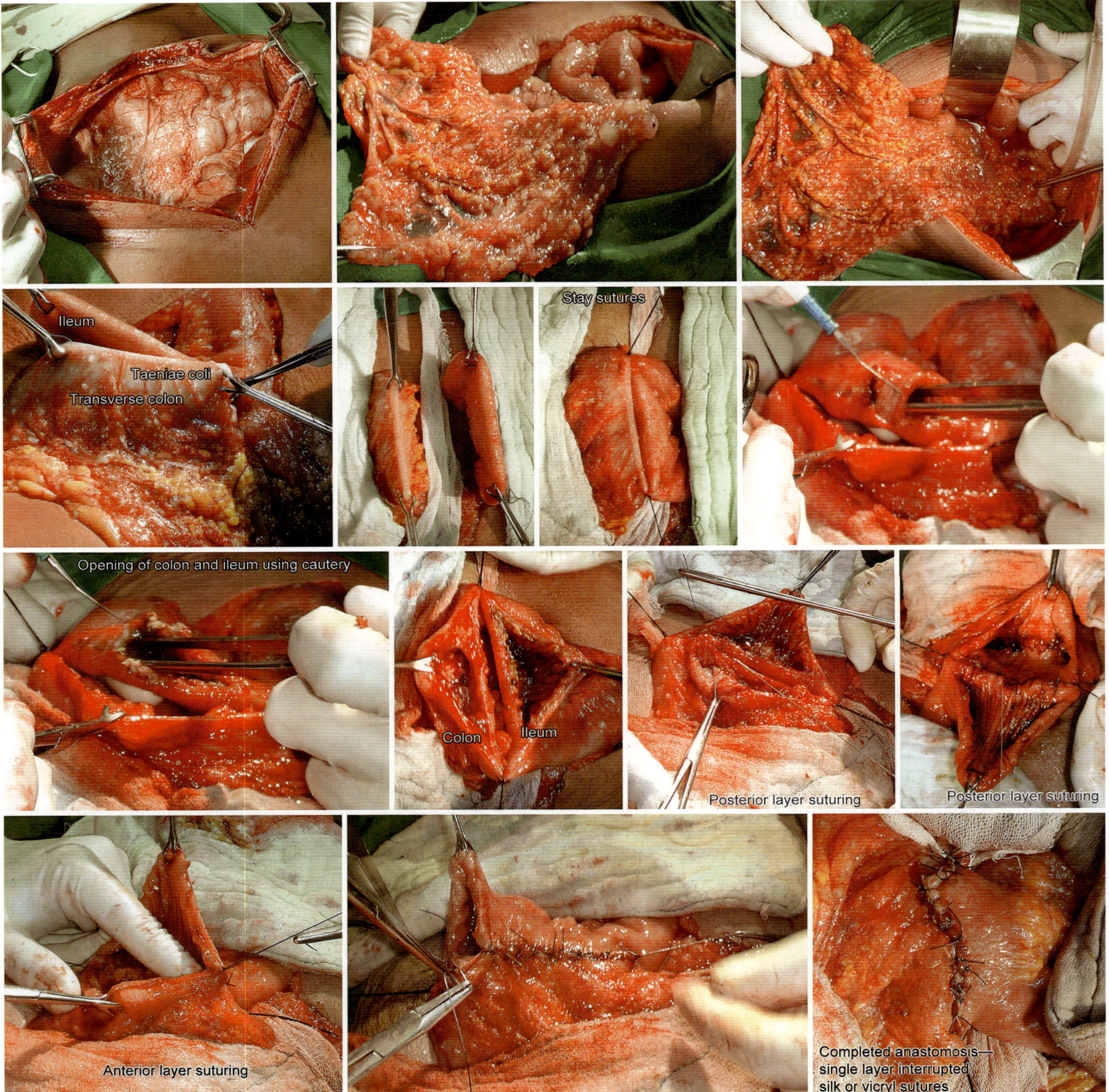

Fig. 25-38: Ileotransverse anastomosis is done in a patient with obstruction at ileocaecal region. It is done here as patient had abdominal tuberculosis involving peritoneum and omentum; hence resection is not done but less aggressive bypass was done. Single layer interrupted sutures are placed—silk suture material.

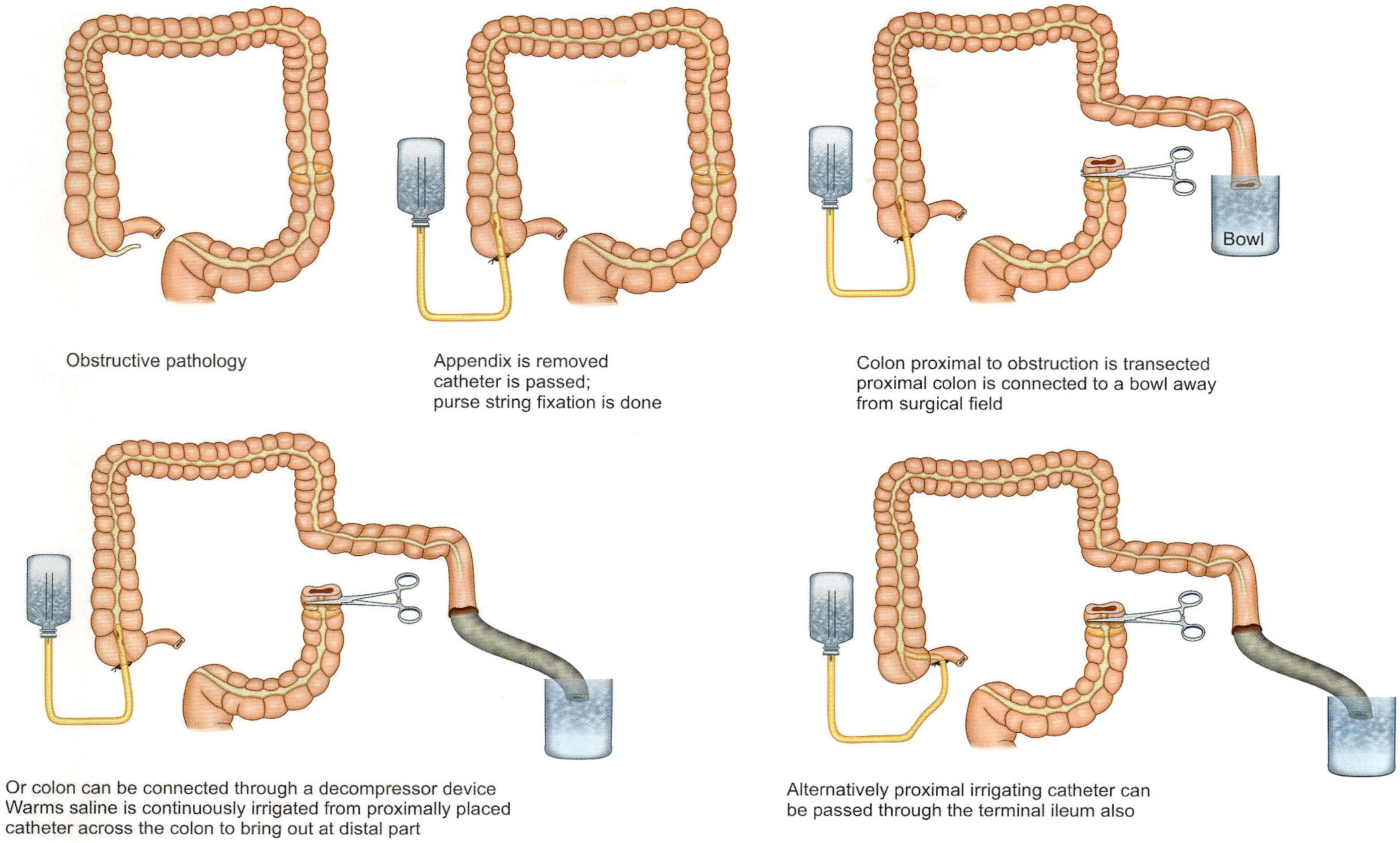

Bowl
Obstructive pathology
Appendix is removed
catheter is passed;
purse string fixation is done
Colon proximal to obstruction is transected
proximal colon is connected to a bowl away
from surgical field
Or colon can be connected through a decompressor device
Warms saline is continuously irrigated from proximally placed
catheter across the colon to bring out at distal part
Alternatively proximal irrigating catheter can
be passed through the terminal ileum also

Fig. 25-39: Technique of colonic decompression.

Band
Long sigmoid
colon
Long
mesentery
Narrow root

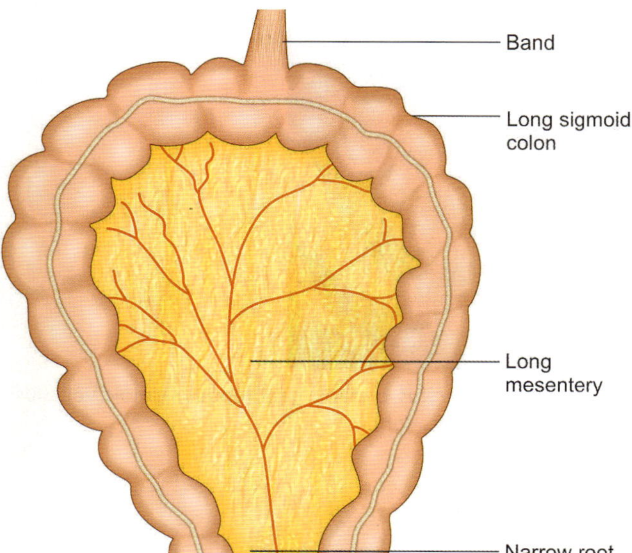

Fig. 25-40: Precipitating factors for sigmoid volvulus.

Rectum above the pathological level is transected; lower segment is everted through the anus; normal proximal colon is brought out through the everted rectum; everted diseased rectum is resected just above the dentate line, anastomosis is done between brought out colon and cut end of the rectum just above the dentate line. Anastomotic site is repositioned back by gentle push.

Anorectal myectomy is found to be very useful for ultrashort segment and short-segment Hirschsprung's disease. Mucosa is incised horizontally 1 cm proximal to mucocutaneous junction. A strip of muscularis with part of internal sphincter is excised with both muscle layers of the rectum for about 6–10 cm length. Mucosa is sutured back. Complications are abscess formation and failure.

Complications of Surgeries

Severe colitis often distressing; faecal fistula due to disruption of the anastomotic site; stenosis at anastomotic site; stunted growth of the child due to deficiencies.

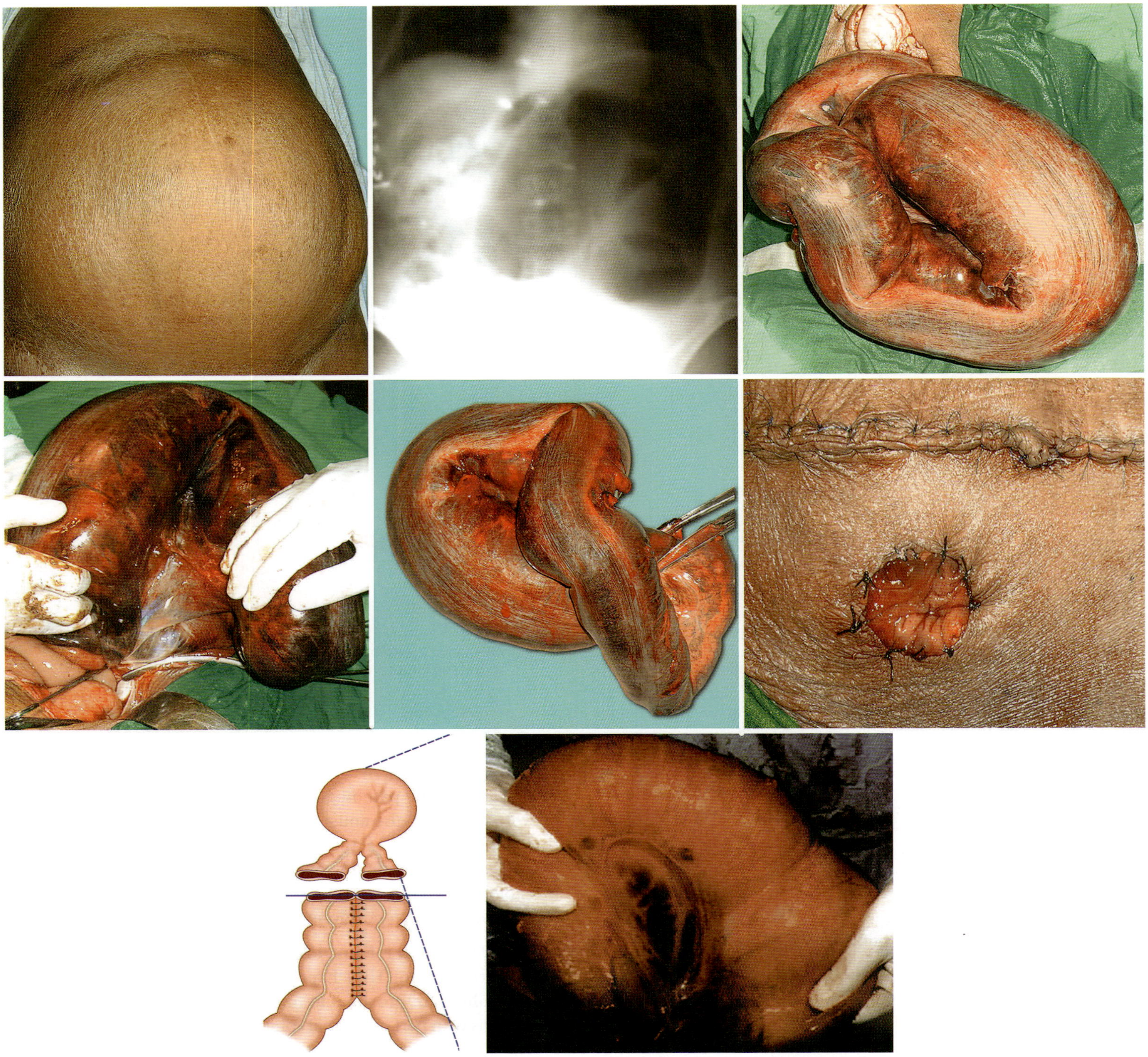

Fig. 25-41: Sigmoid volvulus: Note distended tympanic abdomen; X-ray showing typical sigmoid volvulus; on table gangrenous sigmoid volvulus; underwent resection with colostomy and mucus fistula (exteriorisation).

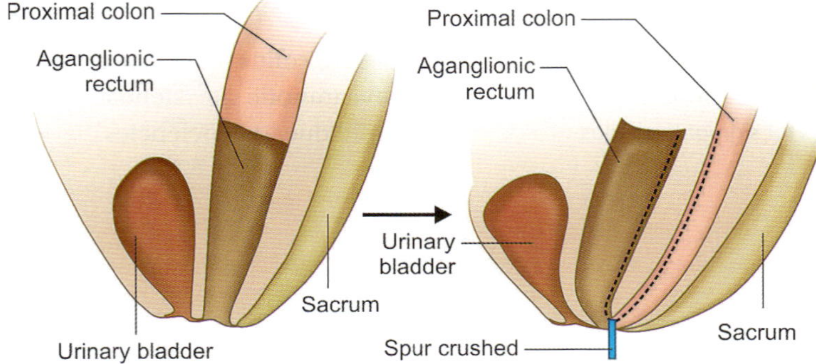

Fig. 25-42: Modified Duhamel operation. Normal colon is brought behind the aganglionic rectum and anastomosed just above the dentate line.

26

CHAPTER

Anorectal Surgeries

SURGICAL ANATOMY

Rectum

Rectum is connecting part between sigmoid colon above and anal canal. It is a misnomer as it is not straight; it has got curvatures anteroposteriorly and side to side. It is located in the posterior part of the lesser pelvis in front of the three sacral pieces and coccyx. It begins at 3rd sacral vertebra and ends at anorectal ring 2 cm in front and below the tip of coccyx at the apex of the prostate in males. It is 12 cm in length; proximally it has got same diameter as sigmoid colon; below it dilates to form rectal ampulla. Initially, it runs backwards and downwards then it runs forwards and downwards. In the sacrum and coccyx, it is concave in front; it bends backwards at the anorectal junction. It has got three lateral curves—upper lateral with convex towards right; middle lateral with convex towards left; lower lateral with convex towards right **(Fig. 26-1)**.

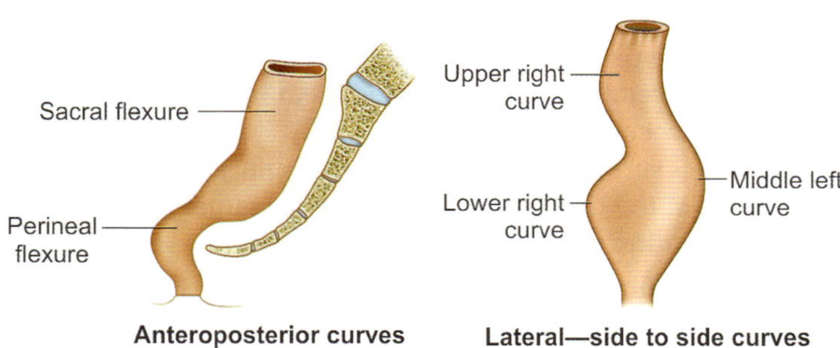

Fig. 26-1: Curvatures of the rectum.

The three cardinal features of large intestine (*sacculation, appendices epiploicae and taeniae*) are *absent* in the rectum.

Rectosigmoid junction implies a segment of bowel comprising the last seven centimeter of sigmoid colon and upper five centimeter of rectum. On sigmoidoscopic examination, it is taken as a point 15 cm from the anal verge. Taeniae of the sigmoid blends for about 8 cm to become longitudinal muscle coat of the rectum.

Relations of the Rectum

Upper 1/3rd is covered with peritoneum in front and sides; middle 1/3rd is covered by the peritoneum only in front; lower 1/3rd is not related to peritoneum but is dilated to form ampulla. Lower 1/3rd lies below the rectovesical pouch in males (pouch is 7.5 cm from the anus); below the rectouterine pouch (5.5 cm from the anus) in females. Anterior aspect of upper 2/3rd in males is related to rectovesical pouch, intestines and sigmoid colon; in females rectouterine pouch, intestines, sigmoid and anterior aspect of lower 1/3rd is related to base of the urinary bladder, ends of the ureters, seminal vesicles, vas deferens and prostate in males; lower part of the vagina in females **(Fig. 26-2)**.

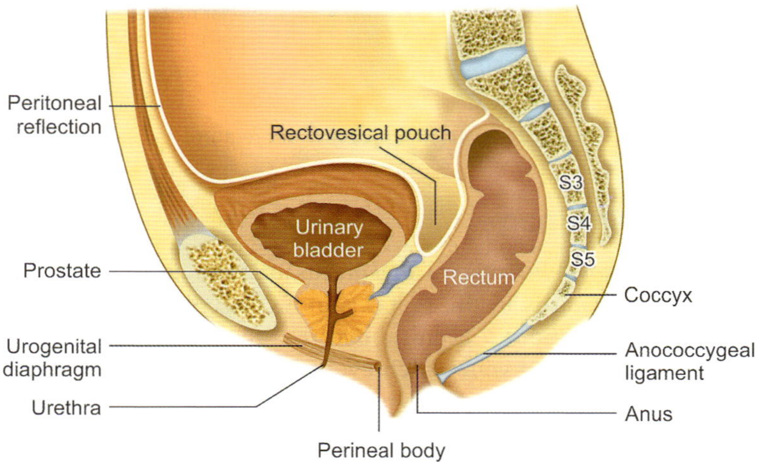

Fig. 26-2: Relations of the rectum.

Posteriorly rectum is related to lower three sacral pieces and coccyx, anococcygeal ligament, pyriformis muscle, coccygeus and levator ani, median sacral, superior rectal and lower lateral sacral vessels, sympathetic chain and ganglion impar, anterior primary rami of S3,4,5 and coccyx 1 nerves, pelvic splanchnic nerves, lymph nodes, lymphatics and fat.

Upper rectum contains 3 folds—left superior (12 cm from anal verge); right middle (10 cm from anal verge); left inferior (7 cm from the anal verge). These folds are called as valves of Houston.

Arterial Supply of the Rectum

Superior rectal artery, terminal branch of inferior mesenteric artery is the main artery of the rectum. It runs medial to left ureter at pelvic brim; opposite 3rd sacral vertebra it divides into right and left branches. Each branch divides into smaller branches to pierce the muscle wall of the rectum to run in the anal columns up to anal valves to form anastomoses.

Middle rectal artery arises from anterior division of the internal iliac artery runs in the lateral ligament supplies muscles of the lower rectum.

Median sacral artery arises from the back of the lower most part of the aorta descending in the median plane supplying the posterior part of the anorectum **(Fig. 26-3)**.

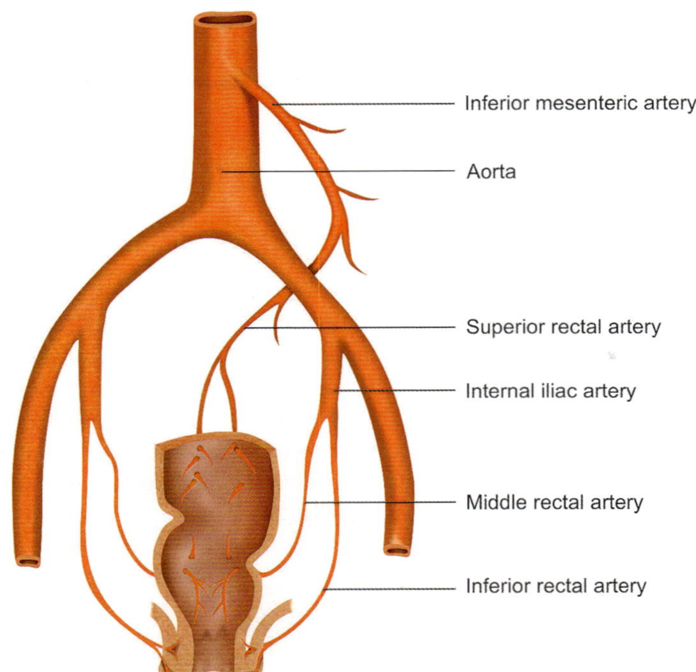

Fig. 26-3: Arterial supply of anorectum.

Venous Drainage

Superior rectal vein: Internal anal plexus forms about six tributaries which run upwards in the rectal submucosa; pierces the rectal muscular coat about 7.5 cm above the anus; join together to form superior rectal vein which eventually continues as inferior mesenteric vein.

Middle rectal veins drain from muscle coat of the rectum to end in internal iliac vein.

Submucous venous plexus drains into the venous plexus around the rectum, which communicates with the venous plexus in the base of the broad ligament in female and vesical plexus in male.

Lymphatic Drainage

Upper half of rectum along the superior rectal vessels drain into the inferior mesenteric nodes; and the lower half of the rectum drain along the middle rectal vessels into the internal iliac nodes.

Nerve Supply

Superior rectal, inferior mesenteric and inferior hypogastric plexus supply both sympathetic (L1,2) and parasympathetic (S2,3,4) components. Sympathetic nerve is vasoconstrictor, inhibits the rectal muscle, and constricts the internal sphincter. Parasympathetic nerve contracts the rectal muscle but inhibits the internal sphincter.

Supports of Rectum

Pelvic floor: It is formed by levator ani muscles.

Fascia of Waldeyer: It is the condensation of pelvic fascia behind rectum, contains superior rectal vessels and lymphatics. It attaches the lower part of the rectal ampulla to the sacrum. It is strong thick layer of parietal pelvic fascia adherent to sacrum and coccyx. Below it fuses with the rectum at anorectal junction. It is seen as a thick white fascial layer above the anococcygeal ligament. This Waldeyer fascia has to be divided to gain access to the retrorectal space; inadvertent dissection posterior to this fascia will injure sacral veins causing torrential haemorrhage.

Lateral ligaments of rectum: It is the condensation of pelvic fascia, attaches rectum to the posterolateral wall of lesser pelvis. They enclose the middle rectal vessels and branches of the pelvic plexus. It is also called as rectal stalk, is a dense fibrous tissue running from the 3rd piece of sacrum to the rectal wall. It contains nervi erigentes. These ligaments have to be divided during abdominoperineal resection.

Denonvilliers' fascia: It is the fascial condensation which separates rectum from prostate and seminal vesicles in males and vagina in females. It is densely adherent visceral pelvic fascia in front of extraperitoneal portion of the rectum extending above from upper peritoneal reflection below to urogenital diaphragm; laterally it continues with lateral ligaments. This fascia remains adherent to the posterior aspect of the prostate gland.

ANAL CANAL

Anal canal is 3.8 cm long extending from the anorectal ring to the anus directed downwards and backwards; it is situated below the level of pelvic brim; lying in the perineal anal triangle between right and left ischiorectal fossae. These fossae facilitate expansion of the anal canal during defaecation. Anal canal is surrounded by inner involuntary and outer voluntary sphincters. They keep the anal canal closed as an anteroposterior slit.

Anorectal junction is the junction where rectal ampulla narrows and pierces the pelvic diaphragm. It corresponds to the apex of the prostate. Anorectal junction is located 2 cm in front and just below the tip of the coccyx.

The anus is surface opening of the anal canal situated 4 cm below and in front of the tip of the coccyx. This has radial folds of the skin with pigmentation containing apocrine glands.

Relations: Anteriorly, it is related to perineal body; in males, membranous urethra and bulb of penis; in females, lower end of the vagina. Posteriorly, it is related to the anococcygeal ligament and coccyx. Laterally, it is related to the ischiorectal fossae. Sphincter muscles are around the anal canal.

Spaces Related to the Anal Canal

Ischiorectal fossa (pyramidal shape 5 cm depth and 2 cm width) lies between anal skin and levator ani. Right and left communicates with each other. Laterally, it is related to fascia covering obturator internus and ischial tuberosity; medially to levator ani and external sphincter; posteriorly sacrotuberous ligament and gluteus maximus; anteriorly urogenital diaphragm; below, the floor by skin. Above, it is related to lunate fascia and pudendal neurovascular bundle in pudendal canal (*Alcock's canal*). There is no deep fascia under the skin in ischiorectal fossa. *Fascia lunata* (semilunar shaped hence the name) covers fascia on the levator ani medially, covers fascia on the obturator internus laterally (pudendal canal is located between obturator fascia and fascia lunata transmitting internal pudendal vessels and nerves); in front it fuses with urogenital diaphragm; above fascia is arched as tegmentum creating suprategmental space above **(Fig. 26-4)**.

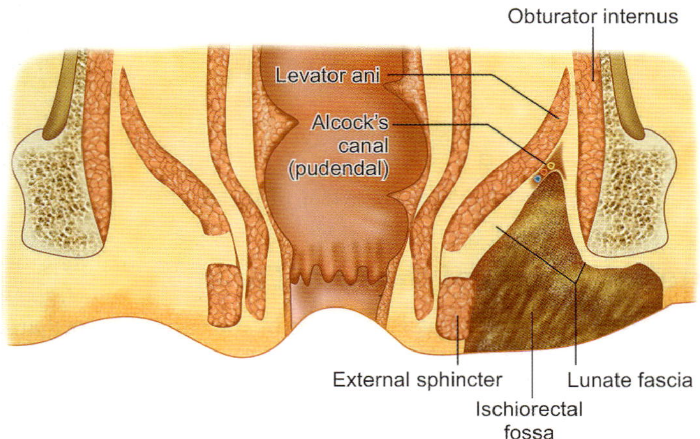

Fig. 26-4: Surgical anatomy of ischiorectal fossa.

The perianal space surrounds the anal canal below the white line. It contains subcutaneous external sphincter, external rectal venous plexus and the terminal branches of the inferior rectal vessels and nerves. Pus here spreads to white line or perianal skin but not into the ischiorectal space.

Submucous space lies above the white line between mucous membrane and internal sphincter, which contains internal venous plexus and lymphatics. Abscess here (submucous abscess) is not visible from outside; on rectal examination, it is felt as boggy tender swelling. It needs drainage under general anaesthesia.

Parts of the Anal Canal

Interior of the anal canal is divided into three parts **(Fig. 26-5)**.

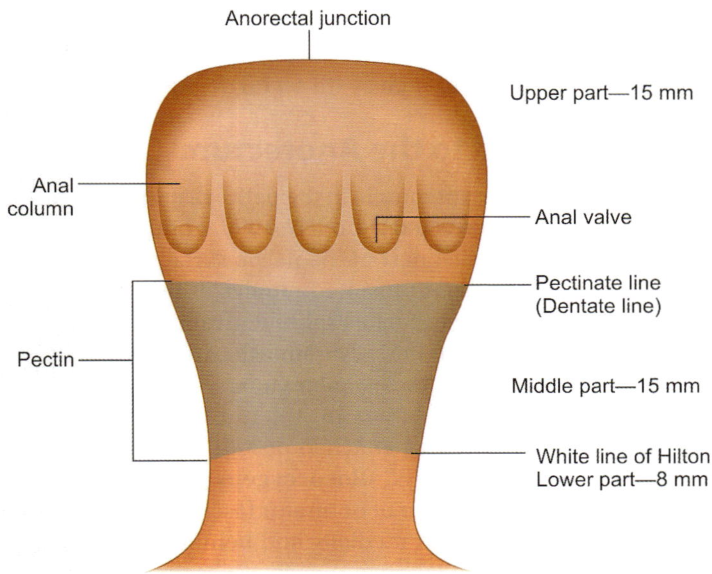

Fig. 26-5: Parts of the anal canal.

Upper part is 15 mm in length; lined by mucous membrane; endodermal origin. 6–10 vertical folds here are called as *anal columns of Morgagni*; lower ends of these columns joint together by transverse folds called as *anal valves*; depression above each valve is called as *anal sinus/anal crypt*. Anal glands about 5–10 in number opens into the anal crypts. Transverse line along the anal valves all around is called as *pectinate/dentate* line. Epithelial projections of the anal valve are called as anal papillae. Dentate line is situated opposite the middle of the internal sphincter.

Middle part of the anal canal is called as pectin or transition zone; is 15 mm in length; dense submucosal venous plexus makes it appear bluish; mucosa in this part is less mobile. Lower portion of middle part is whitish and is called as white line of Hilton, which defines the gap between subcutaneous part of the external sphincter and lower border of the internal anal sphincter. Middle part is thin, pale, glossy and is lined by stratified squamous epithelium without sweat glands.

Lower part of the anal canal is 8 mm in length and is lined by sweat and sebaceous glands like a true skin.

In normal situation anorectal angle is 90°; during defecation it becomes 120°. Miligan Morgan started the concept of *anatomical anal canal and surgical anal canal.* The anatomical anal canal is between anal verge and dentate line. Surgical anal canal is between anal margin and anorectal ring. Anal canal is 1.5 to 2.5 cm in front; 2–3 cm laterally; 3–4 cm behind. In 1975, Thomson described *anal cushions* as submucosa inside the anal canal as discontinuous series of cushions; usually three—right anterior, right posterior and left lateral (3, 7, 11 O'clock positions). They are hemispherical, deep purple protruding masses towards anal canal. These anal cushions contain loose areolar tissue, elastic muscle fibre, anorectal vascular plexus with superimposing vertical mucosal folds of Morgagni. These cushions are anchored to their normal position by ligament of Treitz which are muscle fibres originated from the conjoined longitudinal muscle. *These cushions have got two components: Vascular and non-vascular. Non-vascular are*—(1) Connective tissue between sinusoids; (2) Ligament of Treitz (this ligament has got anal submucosal muscle which fixes the cushions to internal sphincter and mucosal suspensory ligament which fixes the sinusoids to conjoined longitudinal muscle; (3) Sphincter like part in arteriole reducing the more arterial inflow which may be flat or absent in haemorrhoids; (4) Small calibre terminal arterioles. *Vascular one:* are haemorrhoidal arterial system which contains arterioles and venules without capillaries with arteriovenous network leading into hollow sinusoidal spaces in anal cushions. Three anal cushions are normal; often accessory anal cushion is present posteriorly. These sinusoids in anal cushions are called as corpus cavernosum recti. Anal cushions facilitate anal closure; maintains 20% resting anal pressure; protects sphincter while defecating.

Muscles of the Anal Canal

Internal anal sphincter is formed by thickened circular smooth muscle which is involuntary; extends and surrounds proximal 3 cm of the anal canal; below it ends at white line of Hilton. It is controlled by autonomic nervous system. Internal sphincter is light chicken meat coloured, firm structure which is well exposed during haemorrhoidectomy; its lower fibres are divided during sphincterotomy for fissure in ano. Under anaesthesia when anus is stretched, lower end of the internal sphincter is at a lower level than the lower end of the external sphincter **(Fig. 26-6)**.

External anal sphincter is striated voluntary muscle which surrounds the entire length of the anal canal and has three parts—deep, superficial and subcutaneous. *Subcutaneous part* is below the level of the internal sphincter; it is flat band of 15 mm size, which does

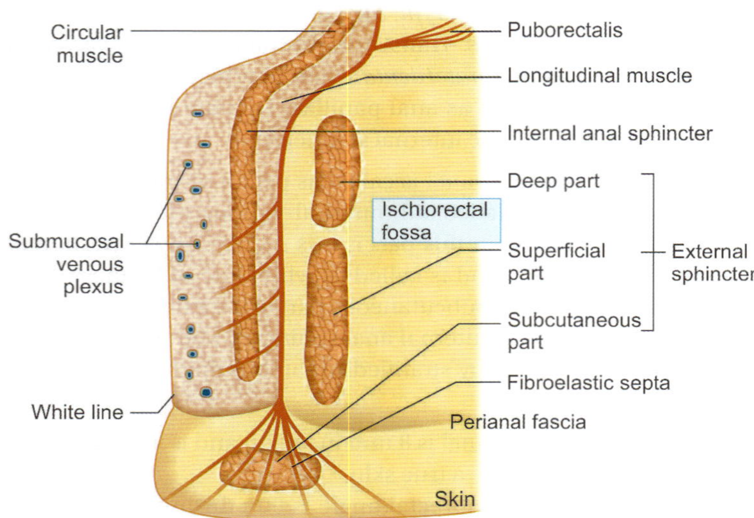

Fig. 26-6: Sphincters of the anal canal.

not have bony attachments. *Elliptical superficial part* arises from terminal coccygeal segment and anococcygeal ligament or raphe which after surrounding the lower part of the internal sphincter gets inserted into the perineal body. *Deep part* also does not have bony attachment; it surrounds the upper part of the internal sphincter to fuse with puborectalis above. External sphincter is supplied by the inferior rectal nerve and branch of the 4th sacral nerve **(Fig. 26-7)**.

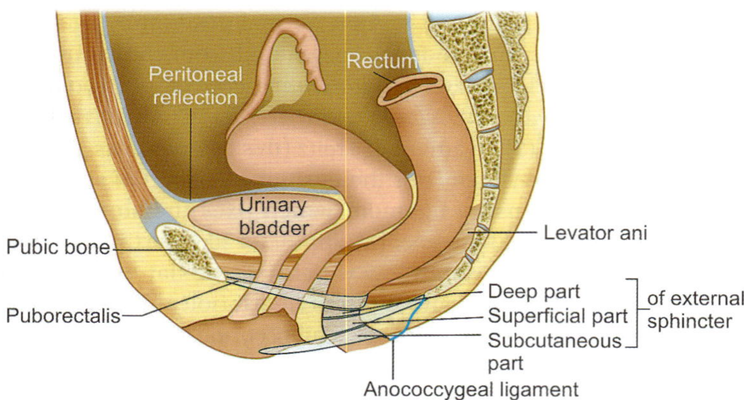

Fig. 26-7: External sphincter and puborectalis muscle. Deep part of the external sphincter fuses with the puborectalis above.

Conjoint longitudinal muscle coat is formed at the anorectal junction by the fusion of the puborectalis and longitudinal muscle coat of the rectum lying between external and internal sphincters. Below it forms fibroelastic band, which at the level of white line divides into many fibroelastic septa piercing the subcutaneous part of the external sphincter getting attached to the skin around anus. Lateral most septum is perianal fascia; anal intermuscular septum is most medial one.

Anorectal muscular ring is formed at the anorectal junction by the fusion of the puborectalis, deep external sphincter and internal sphincter. Ring is less prominent anteriorly as puborectalis fibres are absent anteriorly. Anorectal ring is palpable on digital examination of the rectum.

Puborectalis, deep and superficial parts of the external anal sphincter forms the triple *loop of Shafiq* which is important for incontinence. Sphincter mechanism consists of external and internal sphincters, anal cushions and puborectalis **(Fig. 26-8)**.

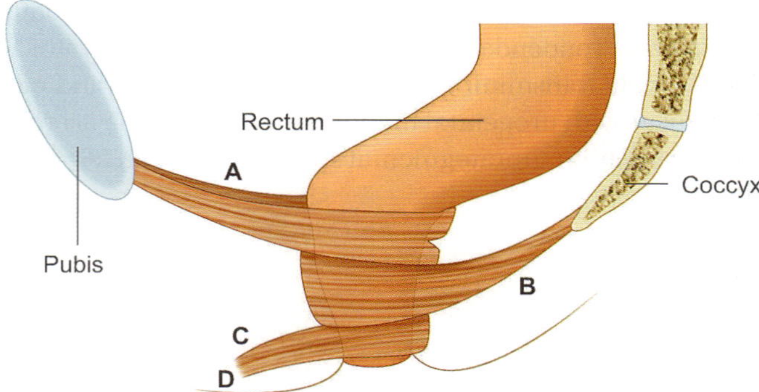

Fig. 26-8: Triple loop of Shafiq.

Arterial Supply of the Anal Canal

Part above the pectinate line is supplied by the superior rectal artery; part below is supplied by the inferior rectal artery.

Venous Drainage of Anal Canal

Internal rectal/haemorrhoidal venous plexus lies in the submucosa of the anal canal draining into the superior rectal vein and so inferior mesenteric vein; communicates freely with external venous plexus which drains into the middle (to internal iliac vein) and inferior rectal (to internal pudendal vein) veins—creating a porta systemic communication.

Lymphatic Drainage of Anal Canal

Lymphatics above the dentate line drains into internal iliac nodes; below the line drains into medial group of superficial inguinal nodes.

Nerve Supply of Anal Canal

Above the dentate line sympathetic by inferior hypogastric plexus L1,2 and parasympathetic by pelvic splanchnic nerve, S2,3,4; below the dentate line somatic inferior rectal nerve S2,3,4.

Internal sphincter contracts by sympathetic action; relaxes by parasympathetic action. External sphincter is supplied by the inferior rectal nerve and branch of 4th sacral nerve.

Muscles Related to the Anorectum

Levator ani: It is important muscle in the pelvic diaphragm. It has got two parts. **Pubococcygeus part**—*Anterior fibres* of the puborectalis originates from the medial part of the pelvic surface of the body of the pubis which surrounds prostate in males as levator prostatae; in females surrounds the vagina as sphincter vaginae. *Middle fibres* arise from the lateral part of the pelvic surface of the body of pubis as puborectalis which encroache the anorectum. The *posterior fibres* of the pubococcygeus originate from the anterior half of the white line of the obturator fascia getting attached posteriorly to anococcygeal ligament and tip of the coccyx. **Iliococcygeus part** arises from the posterior half of the white line of obturator fascia and pelvic surface of the ischial spine; inserted medially and behind to anococcygeal ligament and side of the last two pieces of coccyx. Levator ani is supplied by a branch from 4th sacral nerve and a branch from inferior rectal nerve or perineal division of the pudendal nerve **(Figs. 26-9 and 26-10)**.

Coccygeus: It is triangular in shape which is partly muscle and partly tendinous; originates from pelvic surface of the ischial spine and sacrospinous ligament to insert into the side of the coccyx and 5th sacral vertebra. Coccygeus is supplied by a branch from 4th and 5th sacral nerves.

Pyriformis muscle: It originates from pelvic surface of 2nd, 3rd, 4th pieces of the sacrum, upper margin of the greater sciatic notch, adjoining sacroiliac joint and sacrotuberous ligament; inserted into the apex of the greater trochanter of the femur. It is supplied by ventral S1, 2 rami.

Obturator internus: It originates from pelvic surface of the obturator membrane, body of the ischium, ischial tuberosity, ischiopubic rami, ilium below the pelvic brim; it is inserted into the medial surface of the greater trochanter of the femur after passing through the lesser sciatic foramen running laterally. It is supplied by nerve to obturator internus—L5, S1, 2.

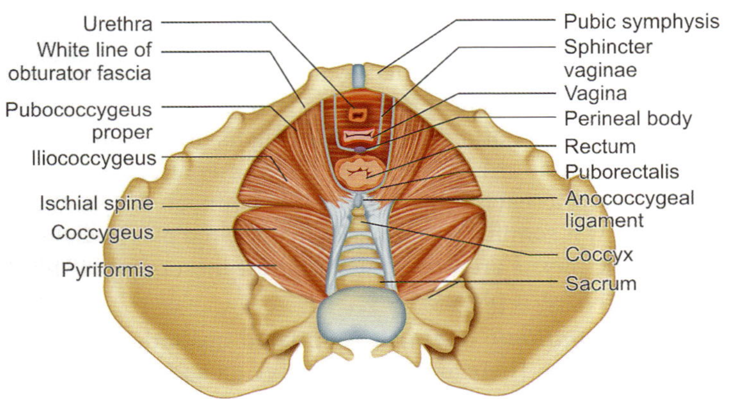

Fig. 26-9: Levator ani muscle.

Vessels of the Pelvis

Internal iliac artery (IIA) begins as smaller terminal branch of common iliac artery which is 3.75 cm in length. IIA in foetus transmits blood to the placenta through the umbilical artery. CIA → IIA → umbilical artery → placenta in foetus. After birth, only proximal part of the umbilical artery persists as 1st part of the superior vesical artery; remaining part of the umbilical artery obliterates as medial umbilical ligament. IIA begins in front of the sacroiliac joint at the level of disc between L5 and sacrum. It runs medial to psoas major downwards and backwards ending at the upper margin of the greater sciatic notch by dividing into *anterior and posterior divisions.* IIA is related in front to ureter, ovary and Fallopian tube in females; behind to internal iliac vein, lumbosacral trunk and sacroiliac joint; laterally to external iliac vein and obturator nerve; medially to peritoneum and small tributaries of IIV. IIA supplies all pelvic organs except those supplied by the superior rectal, ovarian and median sacral arteries; the perineum; greater part of the gluteal region; iliac fossa. *Branches* of anterior division are—superior vesical; obturator; middle rectal; inferior vesical; inferior gluteal (largest branch of anterior division) and internal pudendal. (In females, inferior vesical artery is replaced by vaginal artery; also uterine artery as an additional branch). *Posterior division branches are*—iliolumbar, two lateral sacral, superior gluteal arteries (runs above the 1st sacral nerve and enters the gluteal region by passing through the greater sciatic foramen above the pyriformis). Inferior gluteal and internal pudendal are terminal branches; in males there are six branches; in females seven branches (uterine artery is extra). Artery of vas arises from superior vesical artery **(Fig. 26-11)**.

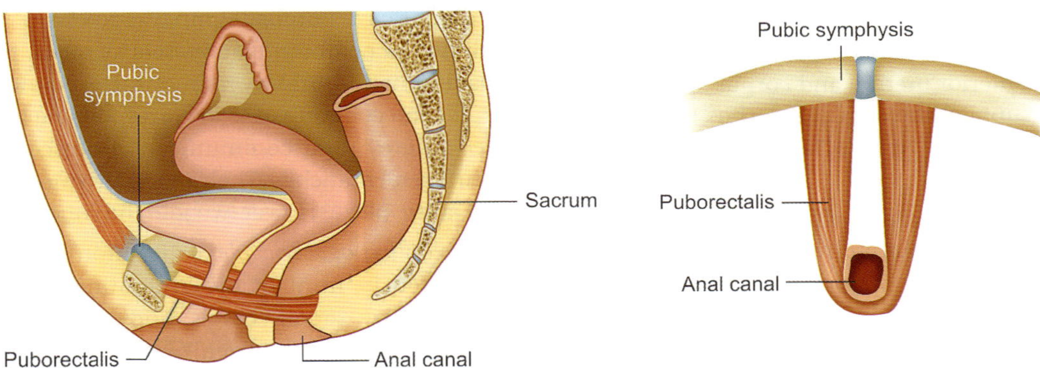

Fig. 26-10: Puborectalis sling.

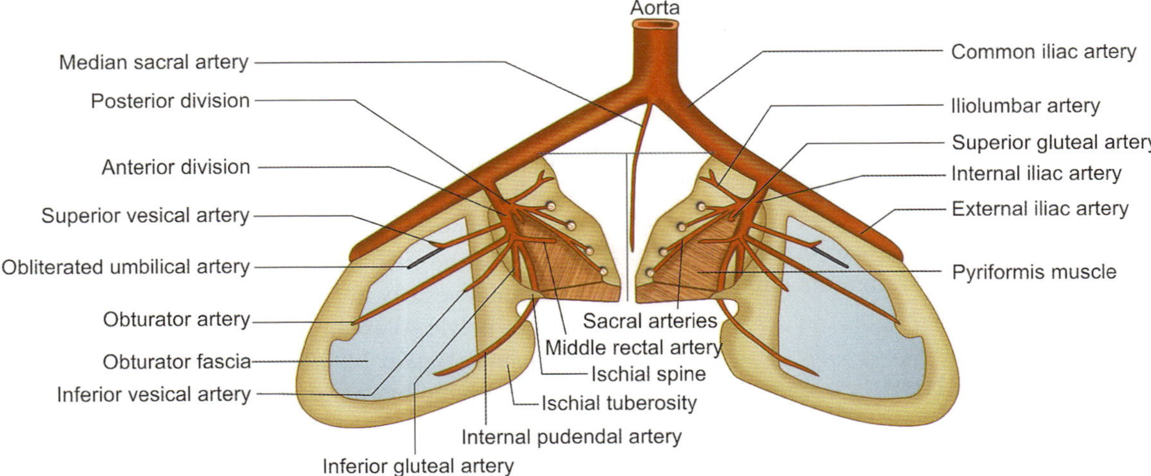

Fig. 26-11: Internal iliac artery and its branches in the pelvis.

Obturator artery runs in obturator fascia in between obturator vein (below) and nerve (above) enters the obturator foramen. It passes through the obturator foramen. It is crossed by ureter and vas deferens. It gives iliac, vesical branches and a pubic branch, which communicates with pubic branch of the inferior epigastric artery and with pubic branch of opposite side obturator artery.

Middle rectal artery originates with the inferior vesical artery; it supplies prostate, seminal vesicle and a little to muscle of the rectum; it may be absent in females.

Inferior gluteal artery is the largest branch of IIA running downwards in front of the sacral plexus and pyriformis and runs between pyriformis and coccygeus to enter lower part of the greater sciatic foramen to reach gluteal region. It gives muscular, fascial and vesical branches in the pelvis.

Internal pudendal artery is the main artery of the perineum and external genitalia. It is the smaller terminal branch of the anterior division of the IIA. In the pelvis, it runs on the pyriformis, sacral plexus, inferior gluteal artery enters the gluteal region by passing through the greater sciatic foramen; it runs for a short course in gluteal region; again through lesser sciatic foramen and then enters the pudendal canal. In the canal it is related to dorsal nerve and perineal nerve; gives inferior rectal artery posteriorly and perineal artery anteriorly; artery enters the deep perineal space as artery of penis or artery of clitoris. Artery of the penis divides just behind the arcuate pubic ligament as deep and dorsal arteries of the penis. Branches of the internal pudendal arteries are—*inferior rectal artery* that supplies skin and muscles of the anal region. Perineal artery pierces the base of the perineal membrane to reach the superficial perineal space dividing into transverse perineal and posterior scrotal arteries. Artery of the penis runs in the deep perineal space gives artery of the bulb (supplies the bulb of penis and posterior urethra); urethral artery (supplies anterior urethra and corpus spongiosum); deep artery of the penis supplies the crus and corpus cavernosum; dorsal artery of the penis supplies the skin, fascia of the body of the penis and glans.

Internal iliac vein lies posteromedial to the IIA joins the external iliac vein to form common iliac vein, in front of the lower part of the pelvic brim.

Lymph Nodes of the Pelvis

Internal iliac nodes receive lymphatics from all pelvic organs, deeper parts of the perineum, muscles of the buttock and back of thigh; efferents enter the common iliac nodes. Sacral and obturator nodes drain to these nodes.

External iliac nodes receive lymphatics from inguinal nodes of infraumbilical deeper parts of the abdominal wall, membranous urethra, prostate, base of the urinary bladder, cervix of the uterus, part of the vagina. Inferior epigastric nodes and circumflex iliac nodes drain to these nodes.

Common iliac nodes are 4–6 in number receive lymphatics from external and internal iliac nodes; their efferents enter the lateral aortic nodes.

Nerves Related to Anorectum

During dissection of the rectum, hypogastric nerves should be retained. So proper anatomical knowledge of nervous system in the pelvis is essential for a surgeon.

Autonomic Nervous System of Abdomen

Sympathetic nerves are derived from coeliac plexus formed by splanchnic from thorax supplies all abdominal organs and gonads; the lumbar sympathetic trunk has got somatic branches to lower abdominal wall and lower limb; visceral branches supply pelvic organs. Coeliac ganglion is the largest ganglion in the body situated one on each side of the coeliac trunk. Coeliac/solar plexus is located in relation to coeliac ganglion on the aorta around coeliac trunk and root of superior mesenteric artery (SMA). Coeliac plexus extends above to crura of diaphragm; overlapped by inferior vena cava (IVC) and pancreas. Its preganglionic fibres come from greater and lesser splanchnic nerves; preganglionic vagal fibres from right vagus mainly. Its branches are—plexuses of phrenic, hepatic, left gastric, suprarenal, renal, testicular/ovarian. Superior mesenteric plexus contains superior mesenteric ganglion. Abdominal aortic plexus is intermesenteric plexus formed by coeliac plexus and fibres from 1st and 2nd lumbar splanchnic nerves. Plexus is situated on the sides and in front of the aorta, between the origins of the superior and inferior mesenteric arteries with 6–12 intermesenteric nerves which are connected to each other. Above it is connected with coeliac plexus; below it continues as superior hypogastric plexus. Branches of this aortic plexus are—testicular, inferior mesenteric, iliac and superior hypogastric plexus.

Lumbar sympathetic chain: It is situated on both sides of the body of vertebrae. There are four ganglia as 1st and 2nd are usually fused together. It runs downwards closely related to psoas major and lumbar vessels; on right side it is covered by IVC; on left side by lateral aortic nodes. First ganglion is very closely related to crus of diaphragm. Lumbar sympathetic chain continuous below and behind the common iliac vessels as sacral part of the sympathetic chain. Anterior primary rami of corresponding lumbar nerves send white rami communicans to corresponding ganglion. Lumbar nerves receive grey rami communicans from corresponding ganglia as their lateral branches. Their upper two medial branches join coeliac and aortic plexus; lower two join the superior hypogastric plexus.

Superior hypogastric plexus is often called as presacral nerve; is located in front of the abdominal aorta, left common iliac vein, median sacral vessels, body of 5th lumbar vertebra, sacral promontory, and between two common iliac arteries. Plexus is located more towards left side. It commonly has multiple fibres. Plexus is formed by descending fibres of aortic plexus and 3rd and 4th lumbar splanchnic nerves. Above it gives branches to ureter, testis/ovary, and common iliac plexus branch; below it divides into right and left hypogastric nerves which on reaching the pelvis form inferior hypogastric plexus **(Fig. 26-12)**.

Inferior hypogastric plexuses are two—right and left. It is located in the pelvis extraperitoneally; lying on the side of rectum, seminal vesicle, prostate, posterior part of the urinary bladder in males; in females it lies on side of rectum, cervix and fornix and posterior part of the urinary bladder. In males, adjacent to prostate and seminal vesicle, in front of the Denonvilliers' fascia nervi erigentes from pelvic splanchnic nerves join sympathetic branches to form a *neurovascular bundle of Walsh*. Inferior hypogastric plexus gives sympathetic and parasympathetic branches.

Parasympathetic nerves are derived from vagus, which joins coeliac ganglion; pelvic splanchnic nerves join inferior hypogastric plexus. Pelvic splanchnic nerves (nervi erigentes) are sacral outflow of parasympathetic system. Nerves arise from ventral rami of S2,3,4. They pass through the sacral foramina and join the inferior hypogastric plexus to supply the pelvis; few fibres run upwards along with hypogastric nerves to join superior hypogastric plexus.

Pelvic sympathetic chain runs medially over the body of the sacrum along the medial margins of the foramina, one on each side, two chains join in front of the coccyx as ganglion impar.

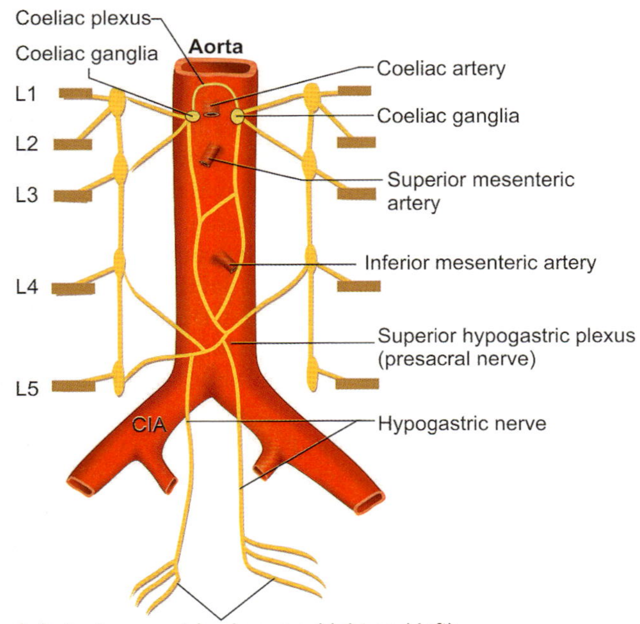

Fig. 26-12: Autonomic nervous system of the posterior abdominal wall and pelvis.

PRINCIPLES IN ANORECTAL SURGERIES

Lithotomy position is essential in most of the anorectal surgeries. Low lithotomy with legs at low position is better **(Fig. 26-13)**.

Entire abdomen, perineum should be cleaned and separately draped. Nasogastric tube and urinary catheterisation is needed in rectal surgeries and in selected anal surgeries. Head low position (reverse Trendelenburg/Fowler's) is also useful to keep small bowel upwards out of surgical field in the pelvis. Anatomical dissection in the rectum is difficult as it is a narrow compact area. Injury to sphincters will lead into incontinence. Buttocks should be abducted properly to facilitate the perineal dissection in abdominoperineal resection and also in anterior resection to negotiate the circular stapler across the anal canal.

Invasion of the tumor into the presacral nerves and prostate makes rectal cancer inoperable. Adherence to sacrum due to desmoplastic reaction is common and is not a contraindication for resection. In some patients with local invasion initial neoadjuvant chemotherapy or chemoradiation and later resection (APR) can be done probably after 3 cycles of chemotherapy.

Anastomotic leak can occur in rectal anastomosis. There is no serosa in the lower rectum and so barrier is not clear.

Nerves in the posterior plane may get injured which will cause impotence. Safeguarding the nerve is very important. Preaortic sympathetic nerves of the superior hypogastric plexus contribute to inferior pelvic hypogastric plexus; this plexus at sacral promontory forms two hypogastric nerves often each with many strands descends in the posterolateral wall of the pelvis close to IIA (hypogastric artery); injury to this will cause failure of ejaculation in males.

In carcinoma, achieving clearance circumferentially (CRM, circumferential resected margin) is important. Total mesorectal excision is ideal (TME) but technically it is demanding.

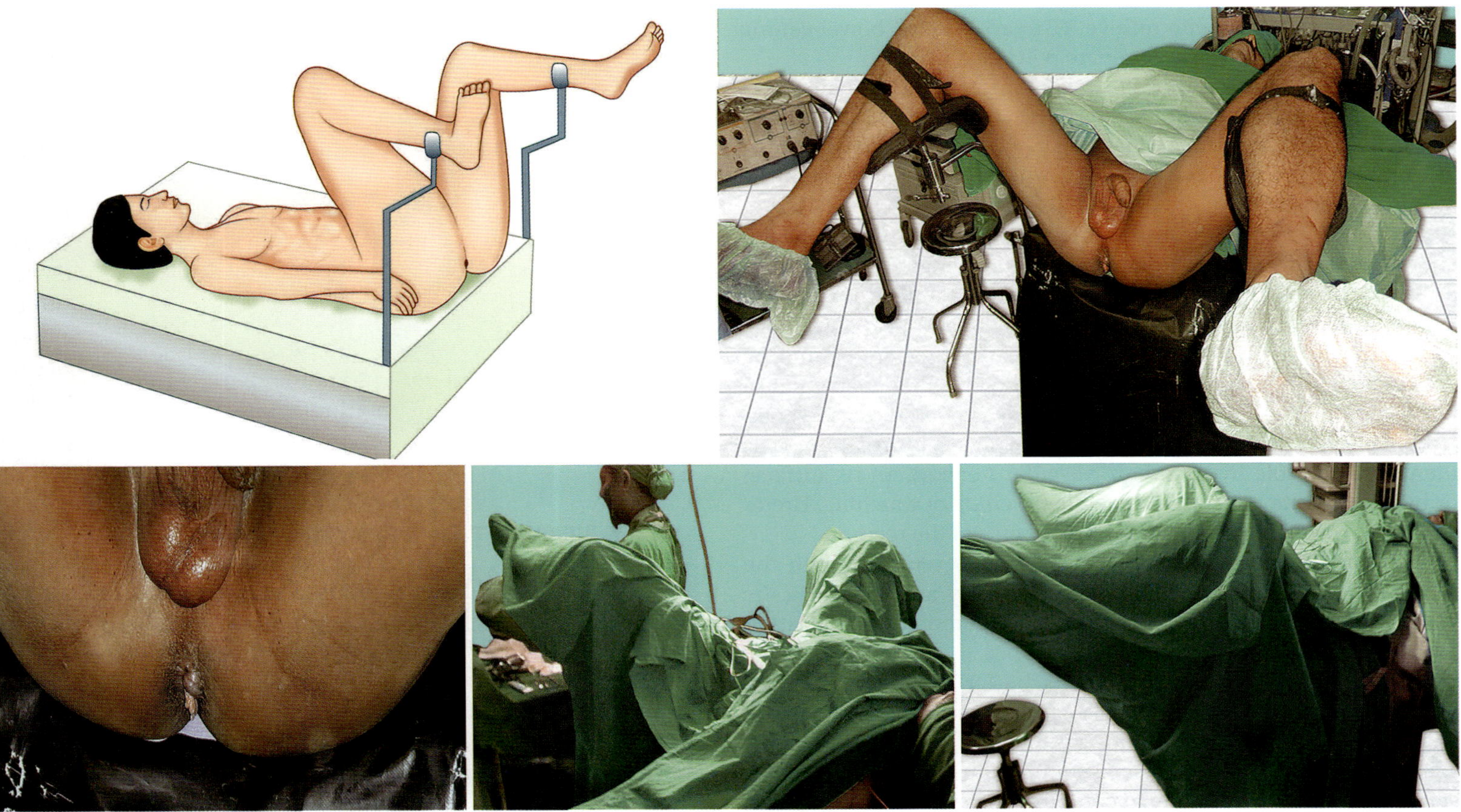

Fig. 26-13: Lithotomy position is commonly used for anorectal surgeries. Prone jackknife position is also used often.

Disparity between diameter of rectal ampulla (6 cm) and colon needs correction. Otherwise anastomotic dehiscence can occur. Side to end anastomosis between the colon and rectum will correct this problem. Tension free anastomosis is very important. Mobilisation of the splenic flexure is a must in all rectal cancer surgeries.

Oozing in the presacral space during dissection is common; it is often difficult to reach the instruments into deep pelvis for control of haemorrhage and dissection especially in open approach. Laparoscopic approach facilitates the instruments into the place and visual dissection. Haematoma is common in this space which will lead into sepsis, disruption of the anastomosis. It is better to place a suction drain in the presacral space. Dissection in presacral space very close to the periosteum will injure the veins draining through the sacral foramina which get retracted into the foramina. It is impossible to control such haemorrhage. Packing or placing surgicel on the presacral foramina or placing thumbtack on the foramina (Nivatvongs and Fang, 1986) or bone wax are the only options. If nothing helps then pack/mop kept in place firmly controls the bleeding almost always. Presacral bleeding can be avoided by doing sharp dissection rather than blunt dissection. Laparoscopic dissection is very helpful for presacral dissection. Dissection should be in front of the endopelvic fascia, which covers the presacral veins. If presacral dissection is bloodless then it means it is in proper plane.

Most of the bleeding in rectal surgeries are venous and careful bipolar cautery fulguration controls the bleeding often also with suture ligation.

Waldeyer fascia in the lower part behind the rectum is strong and tough and it should be dissected with sharp scissor or harmonic scalpel or using cautery. Care should be taken not to injure the rectal wall during this dissection.

Peritoneum in the pelvic floor after colorectal anastomosis should not be sutured as it will create a dead space around the anastomotic site. But it may be sutured after APR. Whether to sutured it or not is a debate in patients who receive RT to avoid small bowel getting radiation enteritis and so adherent to pelvis.

Adequate blood supply is an absolute need in colorectal anastomosis. Inadequate blood supply means inadequate healing of the anastomotic site. It is better to ligate vessel after the branching of the left colic artery instead of ligating the inferior mesenteric artery at its origin.

Both ureters should be identified and safeguarded in rectal surgeries. It is important to have a fair knowledge of the surgical anatomy of the ureter, rectum and pelvis while doing rectal surgeries. Blind surgeries, surgeries without anatomical knowledge in the anorectum will lead into complications. There cannot be presumption in surgical dissection and technique. Proper anatomical knowledge and safe dissection is an absolute need in rectal surgeries. Ureter crosses the common iliac artery at its bifurcation; it is identified on table by its colour, vascular network on its surface, or by eliciting the peristalsis by gentle pinching or touching. Ureter should be traced beyond the lateral ligaments of the rectum.

For most of the rectal cancers, sigmoid is removed with the rectal specimen and continuity is achieved by anastomosing the descending colon to the rectal stump after complete mobilisation of the splenic flexure.

Stapled (circular) anastomosis is better in low resections. In resection suturing anastomosis can be done 10 cm above the anal verge. Below that level suturing is difficult. Angulated stapler is used to divide and close the rectal stump from above; then circular stapler is passed from below to complete the stapled anastomosis. This avoids the difficult purse string suturing of the rectal stump.

Difficult low anastomosis should be complemented with proximal diversion colostomy of transverse colon at right hypochondrium.

Anastomotic site is often passed with a tube 28–30 French Foley's catheter across and can be kept in place for 4–5 days. Through this, air can be injected on table to observe the possible air bubble in a saline filled anastomotic site to identify the leak (leak test). Leak test is commonly done in anterior resection even though many surgeons do not keep catheter in place for long time (4–5 days). In olden days, it is practice to do sphincter dilatation in presumption of preventing distal obstruction and fair anastomotic take up. It is not proved as such and so is not mandatory.

In anorectal surgeries like for fissure in ano, haemorrhoids, Sitz bath is given. Patient sits in a warm water bowl dipping the anal canal region for 25–30 minutes two to three times a day; it reduces the oedema, promotes the healing and relieves the pain significantly. Local heat increases blood flow to the area, promoting healing. A plastic tub that can be fit over the toilet commode to which few centimetres depth warm water is added. Small quantities of eusol, povidone iodine or salt can be added to that. Delayed wound healing is common after excision of anal papilloma or similar lesions. Stricture is also common due to wound contraction and fibrosis **(Fig. 26-14)**.

Sphincter injury, stricture in anorectal surgery is common which should be avoided by careful dissection at anatomical plane.

All patients with colorectal surgery needs deep venous thrombosis (DVT) prophylaxis using low molecular weight heparin. Stoma therapist should give advice in relation to stoma care prior to surgery if patient needs colostomy or ileostomy.

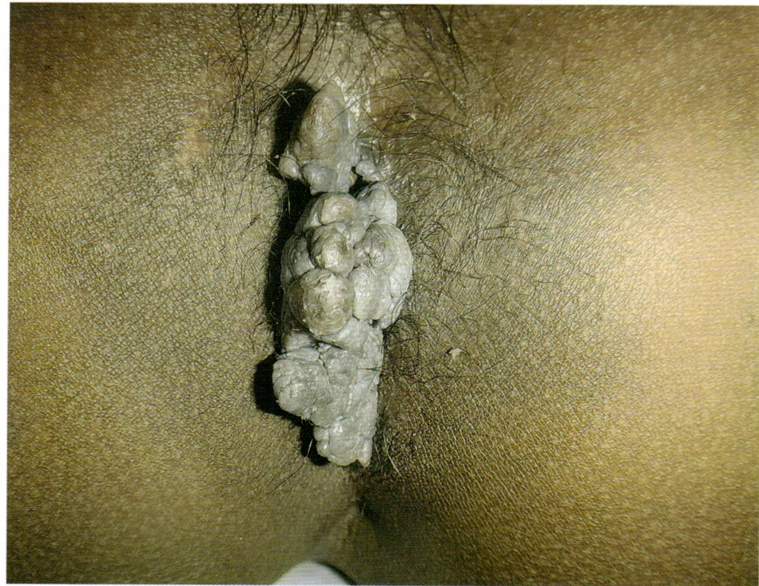

Fig. 26-14: Anal papilloma.

TREATMENT PLAN FOR CARCINOMA RECTUM

Surgical Principles

Surgery is the main method of treatment. Preoperative chemoradiotherapy is often used if growth is invading into adjacent tissues (T4). Adjuvant chemotherapy and radiotherapy is a must. Genetic, morphologic, biologic features of rectal cancers are similar to colonic cancers. But *anatomical factors* make it more complex than colonic cancers, like its location deep in the pelvis, relation to important structures like ureters, bladder, genital, autonomic nerves and anal sphincters. So surgical approach is very difficult. *Avascular endopelvic fascial plane (holy plane of Heald)* is important during dissection to avoid injury laterally to autonomic nerves (will cause impotence in men and bladder dysfunction in both sexes); more medial dissection leads into incomplete clearance and high local recurrence. *Abdomino-perineal resection (APR)* is the gold standard. But if tumour is well-differentiated and if there is adequate margin above the anal canal, a sphincter saving *anterior resection (AR)* can be done. *Low anterior resection (LAR)* is possible if EEA stapler is used for anastomosis. But anterior resection should not be done by compromising the adequacy of tumour clearance. Tumour clearance is still the priority in rectal cancer as it decides the eventual outcome. *Total mesorectal excision (TME) should be the goal* in all procedures as mesorectum contains nodes and lymphatics, clearance of which gives better result. It is a *sharp dissection* (not blunt) in avascular areolar plane between fascia of rectum which encroach the mesorectum and parietal pelvic wall fascia. Mesorectum should not be breached. Absolute haemostasis, *preservation of autonomic nerves* and dissection under vision are the essential principles. Both layers of membranous anterior Denonvilliers' fascia should be dissected off the prostate and seminal vesicles in male to have proper clearance. In TME for middle and lower rectum, entire mesorectum should be removed. For upper rectal tumours, TME is done 5–6 cm below the lower margin of the tumour. *TME improves the quality of life in relation to impotence, retrograde ejaculation and urinary incontinence. These complications are around 50% or more in APR whereas in TME it is less than 20%.* Recommended *distal rectal margin clearance is 5 cm*, however, 1–2 cm distal margin is an *acceptable* clearance. *Circumferential resected margin—CRM* (*radial margin, >2 mm*) is more important than proximal and distal margin. A 5-cm clearance of mesorectum from the primary tumour is essential as tumour implants can occur only for up to 4 cm from primary tumour margin.

Principles to be followed—Adequate lymphatic and vascular clearance; en bloc resection of primary tumour; no/less touch technique; avoiding spillage; adequate radical surgery. *Ultra low anterior resection or intersphincteric* resection can be considered in low rectal tumours. After resection (on table) *irrigation of rectal bed* with cetrimide or hypertonic solution like distilled water is often practiced as they are tumouricidal. Selection of the procedure, AR or APR is decided by proper staging using TRUS and MRI. Neoadjuvant chemotherapy or neoadjuvant chemoradiotherapy is often used in T3 lesions, which also may avoid APR; and AR may be sufficient. Local wide excision approaches are often used when tumour is <4 cm; <40% circumference involved.

T1 N0/T2 N0 tumour: *transanal approach* is used in small tumours that is 3–5 cm above the dentate line but within 10 cm from the anal verge; *transcoccygeal Kraske's approach* is used for posterior wall rectal tumours (dangerous posterior faecal fistula can occur). *Transanal endoscopic microsurgery* (Buess) using operating microscope and videoscope can also be done. This *endosurgical device* is 4 cm in diameter, specialised sealed proctoscope with ports for CO_2 insufflation, water irrigation, and suction and for monitoring intrarectal pressure. CO_2 insufflation distends the rectum and local excision is done with proper positioning of the device.

In females, partial vaginectomy with or without hysterectomy and bilateral oophorectomy may be needed in T4 lesions to achieve surgical resection. Removal of uterus and ovaries prevents patient from developing possible associated cancers of these organs. Carcinoma rectum also spreads to ovaries commonly, which can be prevented by oophorectomy. Often resection of liver secondaries can be undertaken in selected patients when one lobe is involved or solitary secondaries are present.

Laparoscopic APR/AR is becoming popular. *Features are:* Dissection will be more meticulous. Less blood loss, less postoperative pain; early bowel function; clearance is same as open method in relation to primary tumour and nodes.

Short hospital stay, mortality and morbidity are similar to open method. Chances of port site recurrence are 0.5–2% (Earlier it was higher; now it has reduced due to proper technique, careful handling of the specimen, specimen isolation prior to extraction, trocar site irrigation with cytotoxic agents and povidone iodine).

For carcinoma rectum presenting with obstruction, an initial proximal colostomy is done. Neoadjuvant chemoradiation is given. Patient is reassessed for operability. Then APR is done with permanent colostomy.

Incidence *of local recurrent rectal cancer* is 30%. About 80% of local recurrence occur within 2 years of surgery. Common site of recurrence is in the pelvic wall. It also can occur at distal anastomotic margin. Intractable pelvic pain, urinary symptoms, sepsis, bleeding, perineal sinus, swelling and induration, bowel disturbances are the features. It is evaluated by CEA, biopsy, CT abdomen, MRI of pelvis and PET scan. It is often difficult to manage **(Figs. 26-15 and 26-16)**.

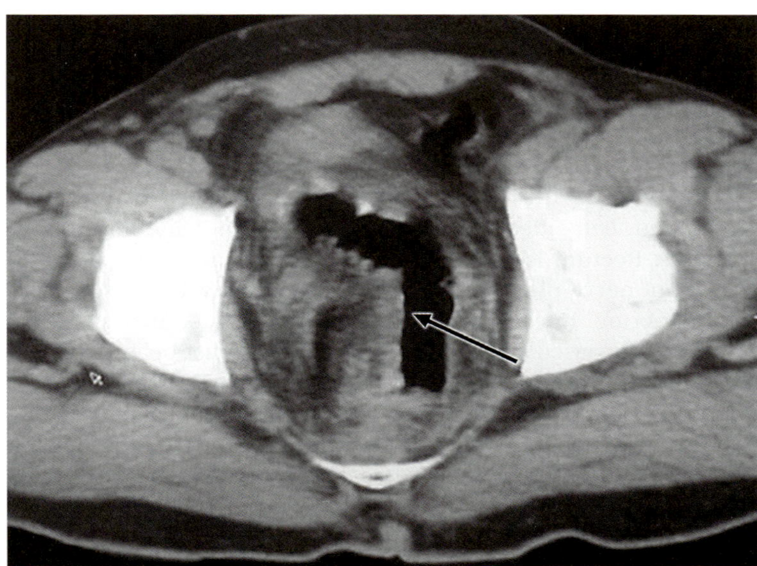

Fig. 26-15: CT scan showing extent of carcinoma rectum. CT is useful to assess nodal status.

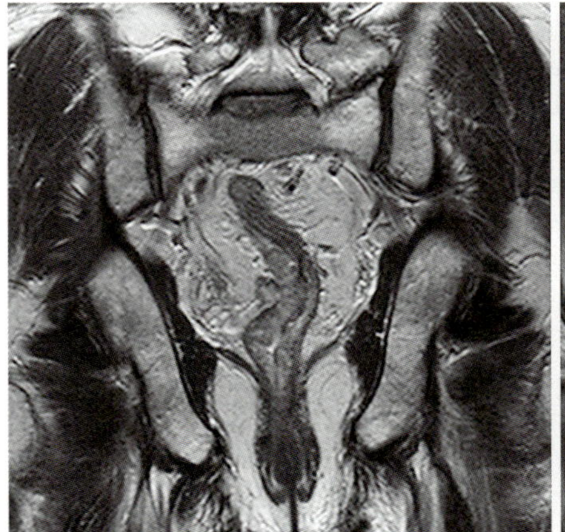

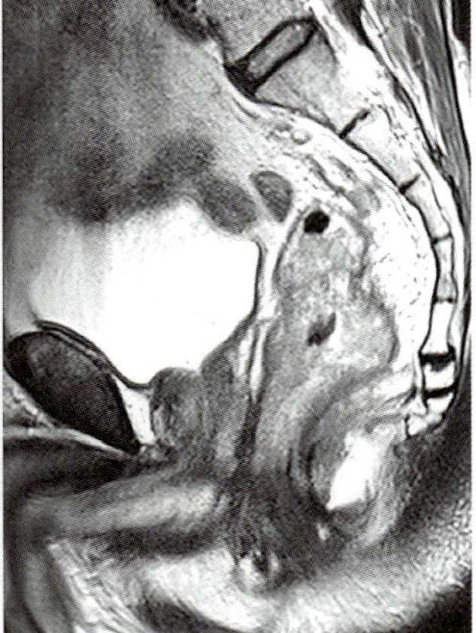

Fig. 26-16: MRI of rectum is useful to assess local infiltration.

Incidence of recurrence will come down to 5% in proper TME. Palliative chemoradiation, end colostomy, ureteral stenting are the palliation. RT controls pain and bleeding. Extensive radical surgery like removal of tumour with pelvic structures can be undertaken with diversions but with a high mortality rate and failure rate.

Proper *preoperative bowel preparation* is a must in all rectal cancers, which reduces the postoperative problems like sepsis, leak and increases the early chance of recovery. Bowel preparation by polyethylene glycol; electrolytes *orally*; bowel wash *per anally*; bowel antiseptics like neomycin 1 g tid previous day/erythromycin 1 g tid/metronidazole tid *orally*. Systemic antibiotics like cefazolin, metronidazole, gentamicin; prophylactic heparin or low molecular weight heparin; Foley's catheterisation and nasogastric tube—are other preparations. Preoperative adequate hydration using IV fluids; blood grouping and crossmatching and required bottles of blood should be reserved if needed to transfuse during the procedure.

Different Surgeries for Carcinoma Rectum

1. **Abdominoperineal resection** (AP resection) (APR) wherein sigmoid, descending colon and upper rectum is mobilised per abdominally. Anal canal with perianal and perirectal tissues are dissected per anally. Retained colon is brought out as *end colostomy* in *left iliac fossa*.

Abdominoperineal resection—types
Miles—abdomen first, perineum later
Gabriel—perineum first, abdomen later
Lloyd-Davies—synchronised (together), (combined)

   APR is done through lower midline incision in lithotomy position. Left-sided colon and entire rectum is mobilised from above. Rectum is mobilised posteriorly in avascular plane in front of nerve plane (hypogastric nerve) between mesorectum and sacrum. Inferior mesenteric artery is ligated high proximal (as lymphovascular ligation) at its origin or just beyond its first branch. Colon is transected and proximal cut end is fashioned for end colostomy in *left iliac fossa*. Through perineum, a purse string suture is placed around anal margin. Circumferential incision is placed around the anus. Dissection is deepened using scissor and cautery into the perineal body, coccyx, ischial tuberosity, ischiorectal fossa. First posterior and lateral dissections are undertaken until it reaches above. Lastly, anterior dissection is done to reach above and specimen is removed through perineal wound. Perineal wound is closed in layers often with a drain. Abdomen drain is placed. Colostomy is created by suturing skin to mucosa using silk. Colostomy done in left iliac fossa after APR. Colostomy care is important.

   Complications of APR: Bleeding; infection of perineal wound; complications of colostomy like prolapse, stenosis, and infection; injury to urinary system, ureter, impotence, urinary incontinence. Operative mortality is less than 2%. *APR is the treatment of choice when mesorectum is involved or when it is poorly differentiated tumour or when nodes are involved.* It gives adequate clearance.

   Sphincter saving APR with coloanal anastomosis: It is done in operable distal rectal tumour in young individual wherein within oncological principle anal sphincter need not be sacrificed but adequate oncological tumour clearance can be achieved. Here a permanent colostomy stoma is avoided. Approach is both abdominal and perineal. Initial dissection of rectal mobilisation is done from above; dissection of rectal mucosa from the anal sphincter at the level of dentate line and complete dissection of distal rectum is done through anal canal. Entire rectosigmoid is removed retaining only the anal sphincter. Colonic J pouch or coloplasty reservoir is created in the mobilised descending colon; coloanal anastomosis is done per anally using hand sutures under direct visualisation.

   APR with neosphincter reconstruction is also occasionally sought; but technically difficult with complications.

   Perineal colostomy is done with gracilis muscle wrap which is made to produce sphincter like muscle twitch using an implanted pacemaker.

2. **Anterior resection** (Abdominal radical restorative operation) is done in growths located in the mid and upper part of the rectum, which is well-differentiated, small-sized and with a clear adequate length for anastomosis after resection. *Anterior resection* is also called as *anterior proctosigmoidectomy* through *abdominal* approach wherein rectum *above* the peritoneal *reflection* is resected with colorectal anastomosis. *Low anterior resection (LAR)* is resection of rectum *below the peritoneal reflection* along with the sigmoid colon (as sigmoid should be removed due its precarious blood supply after dissection), with total mesorectal excision (TME) *through abdominal approach* (laparotomy) followed by *colorectal anastomosis* using *circular* stapler device (EEA stapler). Stoma should be inspected using proctoscope for integrity and when in doubt a covering temporary proximal colostomy should be done. LAR often leads to frequent small bowel movements causing more frequent stools called as *low anterior resection syndrome (LAR syndrome)/clustering*. It can be avoided by creating reservoir either by doing *colonic J pouch* or by doing *coloplasty* 6 cm from proximal divided end of colon (longitudinal colotomy between taeniae of 10 cm which is sutured horizontally).

   Criteria for anterior resection (Low anterior resection, LAR) are: Upper and middle third rectal growth; growth above the peritoneal reflection; well-differentiated tumour; <4 cm size tumour; in females, growth 7 cm above the anal verge; T1 N0/T2 N0 tumour; tumour without lymphatic or venous spread.

   Advantages: It avoids permanent colostomy; sphincter is retained and so patient's acceptance is high **(Fig. 26-17)**.

   Disadvantages: Uncertainty of clearance which is very important in cancer surgeries and so chances of local recurrence is high; anastomotic leak, infection; stenosis.

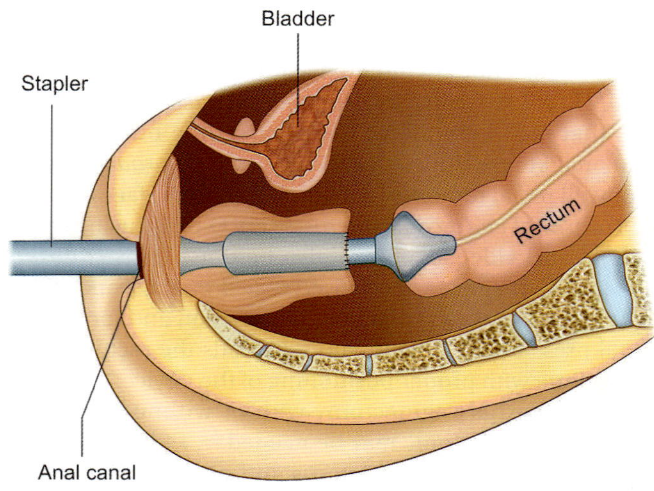

Fig. 26-17: Anterior resection for carcinoma upper rectum using stapler device.

3. **Hartmann's operation (Henri Hartmann, 1923)** is an excellent palliative procedure:
   It is done in elderly people who are not fit for major surgery like AP resection and also in locally advanced tumours. It is also done often in sigmoid diverticula with complications like abscess formation and sepsis. Here rectal growth is resected along with sigmoid colon and cut end of the rectum (rectal stump) is closed completely. Proximal colon is brought out as *end colostomy*. It is done as an emergency procedure wherein it is unsafe to perform a primary anastomosis and also due to insufficient length of the distal retained rectum it is also difficult to do mucus fistula. Midline laparotomy is done; sigmoid is mobilised similarly; ureter is safeguarded; vessels are ligated below the level of the left colic artery branch. Mesentery of sigmoid is divided. Distal dissection of the rectum is done just below the level of the peritoneal reflection. Rectum is resected using TA 55 linear stapler. Sigmoid is resected at its junction with descending colon; specimen is removed. Descending colon is mobilised to get adequate length for colostomy; extraperitoneal tunneling of the descending colon is not necessary as it is only temporary end colostomy. Drain is kept in the pelvis after thorough warm saline wash. Abdomen is closed. Complications are—burst abdomen; sepsis (pelvic abscess); rectal stump leakage; complications related to colostomy; haemorrhage; severe colitis; intestinal obstruction. As it is an emergency procedure got high mortality of 10–20%. Restoration of the continuity is done only after 3–6 months for benign conditions **(Figs. 26-18A to C)**.

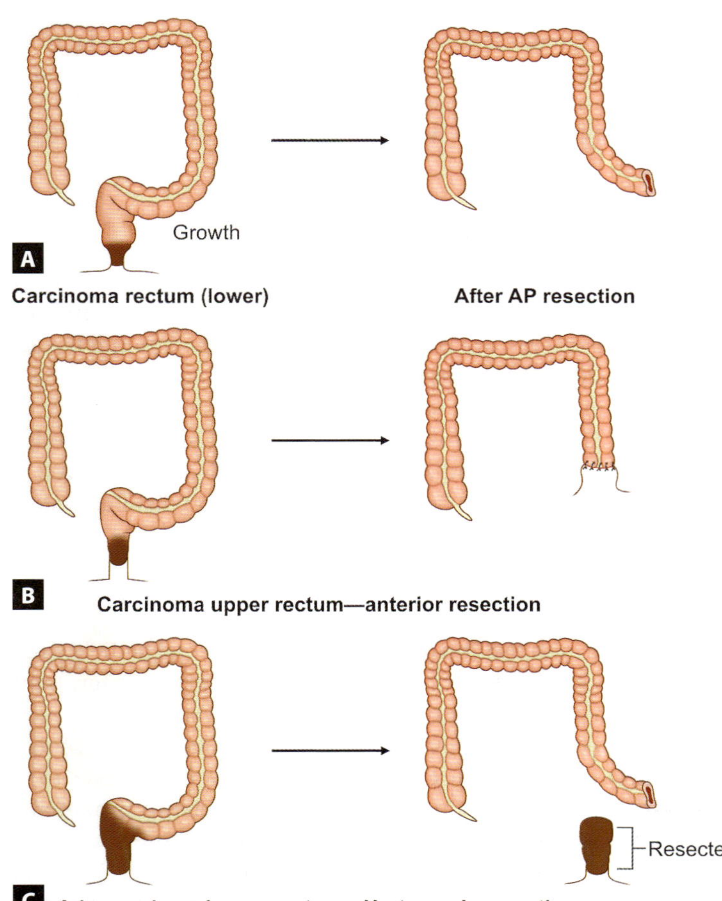

Figs. 26-18A to C: Surgeries for carcinoma rectum: (A) AP resection; (B) Anterior resection; (C) Hartmann's resection.

4. **Pelvic evisceration (Brunschwig's operation):** It is removal of rectum with the tumour along with all the lymph nodes, urinary bladder, fat, fascia, uterus, vagina, with colostomy and urinary diversion. It is neither favourable nor popular.
5. **Palliative colostomy** is done in advanced unresectable growth which presents with intestinal obstruction.

ANTERIOR RESECTION/ABDOMINAL RADICAL RESTORATIVE OPERATION/ ANTERIOR PROCTOSIGMOIDECTOMY (OPEN METHOD)

It is called as anterior resection as dissection is done from above in front through laparotomy. It is done in rectal carcinoma wherein tumour is above, 6–14 cm from the anal verge; i.e. middle and upper thirds of the rectum. Anterior resection is done as sphincter saving procedure otherwise patient might have undergone abdominoperineal resection with a permanent end colostomy.

Presently anterior resection of the rectum has widened definition than the earlier one due to availability of the modern laparoscopic set up. Anterior resection may be ***high*** (anastomosis above the peritoneal reflection); ***low*** (anastomosis below the peritoneal reflection; ***ultra-low*** (anastomosis within 2 cm of the dentate line with sphincter preservation). *Coloanal anastomosis as sphincter saving procedure* is done by anastomosing the colon to the dentate line or below it. Ultralow and coloanal types need laparoscopy for dissection and stapler for anastomosis. ***Low anterior resection (LAR)*** is commonly advocated either by open or through laparoscopy.

Preoperative evaluation and preparations are same—colonoscopy and biopsy; CEA; CT abdomen and pelvis to check nodal status and secondaries in liver; MRI pelvis to identify local infiltration; EUS is also very useful. Bowel preparation is done as similar for colonic diseases (please read in previous Chapter 25).

Technique

Position

Patient is kept in modified lithotomy position with steep head down at 40°. Surgeon stands on left side. One assistant stands on right side; another in between legs of the patient.

Incision

Lengthy midline incision is placed; abdominal cavity is explored for secondaries; self-retaining retractor is placed.

Sigmoid Dissection

Small bowel is pushed upwards and kept away from the pelvis. Distal sigmoid may be occluded using a tape. Sigmoid colon is retracted medially. Peritoneum on the left lateral paracolic gutter is exposed; held between two haemostats and incised using scissor. Adhesions in this lower part are common which are released carefully. Peritoneal incision on the lateral paracolic gutter is extended towards the splenic flexure. Left ureter, left gonadal vessels are identified. Left ureter is dissected carefully and plastic loop is passed around it. Ureter is dissected carefully downwards using scissor and bipolar cautery down into the pelvis. Left hypogastric nerve in front of the internal iliac artery is identified and safeguarded. Sigmoid colon is retracted medially;

incision is made on the right side of the sigmoid mesocolon. Dissection is done from bifurcation of the aorta downwards into the pelvis. Right ureter is also identified as it crosses the bifurcation of the common iliac artery in front of it. Right hypogastric nerve is identified now. Incision is made on the rectovesical or rectouterine pouch to mobilise the rectum from front. This also can be done at later period during rectal mobilisation.

Vascular Ligation

Colon is mobilised and held upwards and left with traction. Gonadal vein is separated. Inferior mesenteric artery originating from the front of the aorta is identified; fat and lymphatics (lymphovascular bundle) are swept towards the specimen colorectum; inferior mesenteric artery is divided 1.5 cm from its origin; it is also ligated and divided after it gives off left colic branch to maintain the adequate blood supply in the eventual anastomotic site which is essential. Preaortic sympathetic nerve should be retained.

Presacral Dissection

Sigmoid is retracted upwards and towards left to identify a tissue band between posterior aspect of the rectum. It should be divided using cautery as it contains branches of the middle sacral artery. Loose avascular areolar tissues on both sides of this band are identified. Dissection is continued in this avascular holy plane *(avascular plane of Heald)* using scissor; blunt dissection as it is tempted for will open the posterior endopelvic fascia to expose presacral veins which if injured cause torrential haemorrhage. Slow gentle meticulous sharp dissection is better. Posterior presacral dissection is done down into the pelvis up to the coccyx. Ureter and hypogastric nerves are visualised again for safety. Laterally lateral ligaments are identified by stretching the rectum towards opposite side. Lateral ligament is dissected and divided using cautery with right angle forceps underneath. Once both lateral ligaments are divided, tough Waldeyer's fascia is seen extending from the coccyx to the posterior rectal wall which is divided with sharp dissection. If difficulty is anticipated in dissection of ureter then by imaging study prior stenting of the ureter is ideal. If on table ureter is injured then it can be closed primarily with 4-zero vicryl interrupted sutures with a J stent inside or by ureteric reimplantation into the bladder or ureteroureterostomy to opposite ureter. If hypogastric nerve is infiltrated by tumour one nerve can be sacrificed.

Anterior Dissection of the Rectum

Anteriorly peritoneum in rectovesical/rectouterine fold is incised. Dissection is carried out downwards behind the prostate and seminal vesicles along the Denonvilliers' fascia. Initially sharp dissection, then blunt and sharp dissection helps to separate this fascia and rectum from prostate and seminal vesicle. Rectal wall and tumour should not be breached to avoid tumour spillage and contamination of the field. Dissection in woman is between the uterus and rectum and posterior wall of the vagina and rectum. Bilateral salpingo-oophorectomy is often done by few surgeons in anticipation of spread of tumour from rectum to ovaries. It is not mandatory.

In low and ultralow anterior resection, Waldeyer fascia should be divided completely; Denonvilliers' fascia in front should be dissected adequately beyond the apex of the prostate up to the urethra; laterally beyond the lateral ligaments down to the puborectalis, pubococcygeus proper and iliococcygeus (parts of levator ani). Dissection should not go beyond the puborectalis. All fat and lymphatics should be cleared up to this point. Distal tumour clearance in such patients will be only 1 cm which is oncologically sufficient.

In females, anterior dissection is done between vagina and rectal wall and Denonovilier's fascia is less developed in females; posterior to cervix and posterior fornix this fascia is vascular due to venous plexus. Cuff of the vagina may require to be excised to include with the specimen. Often, if tumour is infiltrating the cervix hysterectomy is done along with the procedure like in APR.

Nervi erigentes curves anteriorly from sacral foramina to converge and join the presacral nerves and form *neurovascular bundle of Walsh* at 2 and 10 o'clock positions in the Denonvilliers' fascia just behind the lateral edges of the seminal vesicles. This bundle controls both potency and bladder function. If seminal vesicles are involved by tumour infiltration in rare occasion, only then are also excised along with the specimen; in such situation, it is difficult to preserve nerves in Denonsvillier's fascia.

Extended anterior resection may be advocated. It means removal of the involved internal iliac nodes and lateral pelvic wall. Plane of dissection here is lateral to the anterior division of internal iliac vessels; so these vessels are ligated at their origin/joining.

Haemostasis

Presacral haemostasis is a must. It is usually venous bleeding which stops by pressure. Presacral venous tear may be torrential; it is controlled by gel foam, surgicel, bone wax, pressure, titanium thumbtack—titanium preloaded haemorrhage occlude pin with applicator, muscle fragment welding (rectus abdominis muscle piece is harvested and placed on the bleeding vein in the foramina and held with forceps and high coagulation current is passed to the muscle through the forceps), silastic tissue expander tamponade. Occasionally, need may arise to pack the presacral area with mops which are removed in 48 hours once control of haemorrhage is obtained.

Splenic Flexure Mobilisation

Adequate mobilisation of the splenic flexure is done to avoid tension at anastomotic site. Renocolic, splenocolic, pancreaticocolic and gastrocolic ligaments are divided to mobilise the splenic flexure; mobilisation should be done under vision and so adequate exposure through lengthy incision is ideal always. Colon is divided above the sigmoid level using an occlusion clamp; bleeding from the cut edges should be ensured; fat and appendices epiploicae are cleared off for 1 cm from the cut edge. Colonic wash with warm distilled water is also often used; it will be beneficial.

Division of the Rectum

After complete mobilisation of the rectum, mesorectal pedicle which runs on the posterior aspect of the rectal wall containing few blood vessels is ligated securely distal to the line of division. Distal rectal stump is dissected to remove all fat and perirectal tissues so as to expose the longitudinal muscles. Rectum is divided 3 cm distal to the rectal tumour after applying curved crushing clamp proximal to the line of division. Distally soft curved occlusion clamp may or may not be needed; often even if clamp is applied it tends to slip. Distal rectal stump is irrigated with ½ to 1 litre of sterile warm water or warm dilute povidone iodine solution. There should be adequate bleeding from the cut edge of the rectum. Specimen is retrieved.

Specimen and lymph nodes should be marked. Line of resection distally taken as 3 cm is sufficient; even 1–3 cm is adequate enough as it is proved that microscopic mural spread beyond the palpable lower edge of the tumour is very rare.

In low and ultralow anterior resection (open method), resection at lower end of the tumour on the rectal stump is difficult. Strong right angle clamp is placed 1–2 cm distal to the tumour after thorough irrigation of the rectum per anally using warm distilled water. Small incision is made distal to the clamp on the anterior surface of the rectum; polypropylene 1-zero continuous suture bites are taken from the distal cut edge with 5 mm gap with 5 mm thickness; sequentially rectum is cut part by part and suturing is continued as *whip stitch* until entire rectum is transected beyond the clamp to retrieve the specimen. Frozen section biopsy from distal end should be done ideally. One should remember that it is not possible to take circumferential stitches around the stump after transection of the rectum in open method. Stapler should be used for anastomosis. J pouch may be done if surgeon is well versed with technique in ultralow resections.

Anastomosis

It is achieved usually as end to end two layer or one layer anastomosis. 3-zero or 2-zero silk or vicryl is used. In single layer anastomosis interrupted silk sutures are used. In two layer, outer silk and inner vicryl or silk interrupted sutures are used. Full thickness horizontal mattress sutures also can be placed. If there is discrepancy between colonic end and rectal stump (rectal ampulla is wider often 6 cm or more) then side to end anastomosis can be done to correct the discrepancy (Baker). Circular stapling anastomosis can also be done. Rectal stump can be transected using linear stapler and also the proximal colonic resection site. Anvil is passed to the proximal colonic end and fixed using polypropylene purse string sutures; circular stapler is passed per anally across the distal rectal stump; if linear stapler is not used then circular stapling end is fixed to rectal stump using similar purse string sutures. Anvil is connected to the circular stapler and is fired. Stapler with anvil is removed with completion of the colorectal anastomosis. Doughnut should be observed for adequacy. Fat should be cleared for 1.5 cm in both ends prior to stapler anastomosis as fat interposition can cause disruption and leak. Blood vessels adjacent to bowel wall near cut edge should be ligated or fulgurated properly otherwise after stapling troublesome bleeding can occur.

Closure

Pelvic peritoneum should not be closed. Large Foley's catheter is passed per anally towards the anastomotic site; pelvis is filled with warm distilled water; air is infused through the Foley's catheter to check the leak from the anastomotic site by seeing the air bubbles; if present additional silk sutures may be needed. Suction tube drain is placed into the pelvis and abdomen is closed in layers. Usually covering proximal colostomy is not needed as bowel is already been prepared as an elective surgery. If there is lot of contamination in the field or if it is very low anterior resection, then diversion colostomy should be done.

Postoperative Care

Nasogastric tube is removed in 5 days; drain is removed in 5–7 days. Foley's catheter from the urinary bladder is removed in 7 days. Oral fluid is started in 5 days. Observation for leak, sepsis, should be done.

Complications

Injury to ureter: If it occurs it should be sutured on table using 4-zero vicryl interrupted sutures with a J stent within. Ureteric reimplantation to the urinary bladder or ureteroureterostomy are other options.

Haemorrhage from pelvic presacral veins can be dangerous; surgicel, bone wax, packing are the options. Blood transfusions are required.

Pelvis abscess formation or pelvic infection or pelvic irritation is common. Fever with chills, lower abdomen pain, tenesmus, tenderness on gentle rectal examination, raised total count are the features. US may show abscess. CT is confirmative. CT guided percutaneous drainage, posterior colpotomy and drainage may be needed. If still persists then open drainage with diversion colostomy is needed. As already there is an anastomotic site per rectal drainage is impossible.

Sexual dysfunction in males if nerves in the pelvis are injured. Use of excessive monopolar cautery in posterior dissection may cause nerve injury; so judicious use of monopolar cautery or use of bipolar cautery or harmonic scalpel (open, focus) is better.

Bladder dysfunction is common in males which is usually mild and subsides gradually.

Anastomotic leak due to disruption can occur. It needs diversion proximal colostomy.

Stenosis at anastomotic site is not uncommon. Sigmoidoscopy confirms it. It should be differentiated from recurrence and so needs biopsy in suspected cases. Dilatation is sufficient usually; occasionally resurgery is required.

Abdominal wound infection, wound dehiscence and incisional hernia also can occur.

ABDOMINOPERINEAL RESECTION

Abdominoperineal resection (APR) is based on the concept that lymphatics spread from the rectum occur upwards, laterally and downwards and so entire field is removed. In 1908, *West Ernest Miles* did first APR. Presently APR is done if LAR (low anterior resection) is not possible or in invasive rectal cancers **(Fig. 26-19)**.

Abdominal Part

Initial evaluation, abdominal phase of surgery are same as in anterior resection described above. Urinary catheter, nasogastric tube, steep head down low wide lithotomy position under epidural/general anaesthesia—are the preliminary steps. Incision is midline with umbilical curve towards left/colostomy site is in left iliac fossa **(Fig. 26-20)**.

Extent of resection is up to the sigmoid colon above and below to the level of the left colic artery level. Peritoneum in the left paracolic gutter is incised and extended proximally across the sigmoid mesentery; below it is extended into the pelvis; left ureter is identified. Peritoneum on the right side is incised and sigmoid is retracted towards left; upward it is dissected up to the sacral promontory and aortic bifurcation. Right ureter is identified and preserved. Inferior mesenteric vessels are ligated and divided. IMA is ligated after the origin of the left colic artery. Sigmoid mesentery is dissected up to

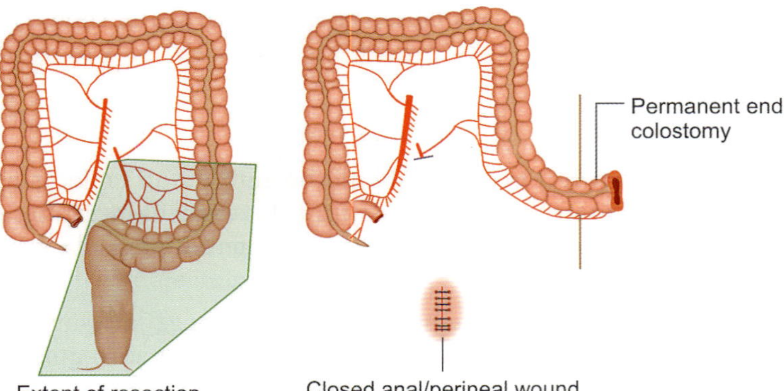

Fig. 26-19: Extent of resection and citation of colostomy in APR.

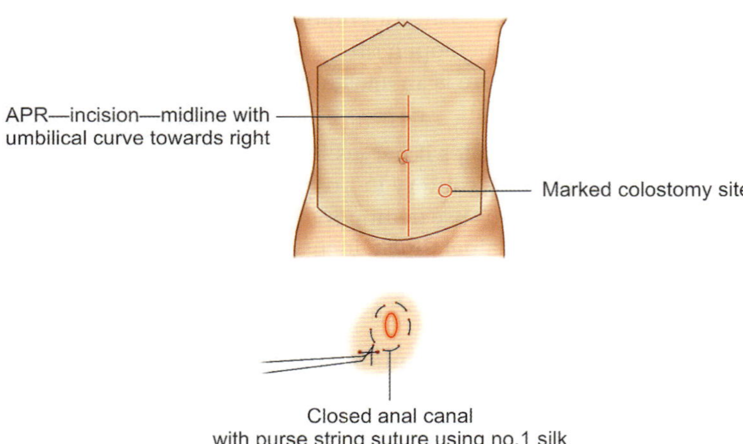

Fig. 26-20: Midline incision with umbilical curve towards right side; colostomy site should be marked. Anal canal should be closed using no. 1 silk with purse string suture.

the colon margin. Presacral dissection is done in similar fashion like low anterior resection. Lateral ligaments are divided. Anterior dissection is done by incising the rectovesical peritoneal fold. It is extended downwards behind the prostate and seminal vesicle up to the membranous urethra in males and posterior fornix in females. In females, vaginal cuff may be removed; or hysterectomy can be done if needed. Further, dissection is done to complete the division of the entire lateral ligaments downwards which will facilitate the mobility of entire rectal tube. Levator ani muscle on both sides should be visualised to complete the abdominal part. Colon is resected after deciding the line of resection. Distal part is tied with an umbilical tape or roller gauze if stapler transection is not done. Proximal part is left for colostomy with an occlusion clamp.

Perineal Part of the Surgery

Purse string suture is placed using no. 1 silk suture using cutting needle around the anus so as to close the aperture. Elliptical incision is made beginning 3 cm in front of the anus extending posteriorly towards the coccyx. Incised skin is held with Allis' forceps with purse string silk suture; dissection is carried out in the posterior plane in front of the coccyx. Coccyx can be excised if needed. Inferior haemorrhoidal arteries are identified, ligated and divided. Anococcygeal ligament is visualised and divided using cautery or scissor. Waldeyer's dense condensed fascia extending between the lower rectum and the lower presacral and precoccygeal region is divided using cautery. Often this fascia is divided from above through abdominal approach. Levator ani muscle is divided on either side to reach the abdominal pelvic area after incising the peritoneum there. Lateral dissection is done upwards by giving traction on the specimen towards the opposite side.

Lastly, anterior perineal dissection is done; lower edge of the transverse peronei muscle is identified; plane below it is dissected which is a natural plane separating rectum and urinary system. Incision on the anterior aspect is deepened to reach the apex of the prostate. Plane behind the prostate is dissected; rectourethralis muscle is transected to reach the peritoneal cavity behind the urinary bladder. As dissection is completed, all around specimen is removed. In females, dissection between vagina and rectum is done; if tumour is closer then cuff of the vagina adjacent to tumour is also removed. If vaginal cuff is not removed then during dissection blood supply to vagina should be retained otherwise it will cause perineovaginal fistula which may persist for long time.

Closure of the perineal wound—all bleeders are cauterised. Wound is washed with warm distilled water and warm saline. Two suction drains one on each side is placed; deeper vicryl sutures are placed. In case wound is contaminated with faecal matter thorough wash is given; deeper vicryl sutures are placed and external wound is kept open. This wound is dressed regularly and allowed to granulate and heal on its own.

Many surgeons use prone jackknife position for perineal surgery, which is said to be better, but not popular. Here once abdominal part is entirely completed with closure and creation of colostomy, patient's position is changed to prone position for perineal part of the dissection **(Fig. 26-21)**.

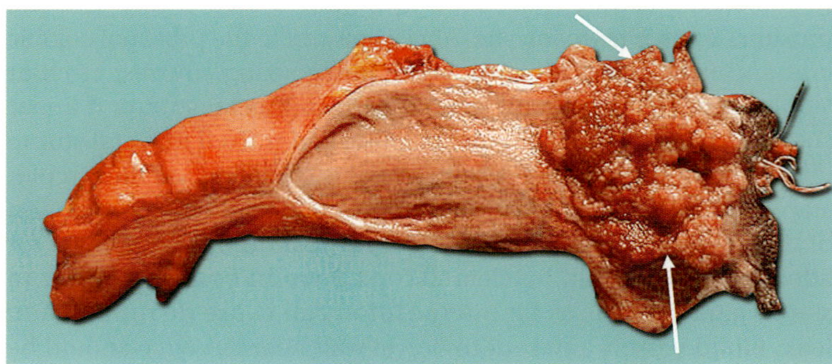

Fig. 26-21: Specimen of carcinoma rectum after APR.

Creation of Colostomy

Colostomy is created as end one in the left iliac fossa on the rectus muscle. A circular piece of skin is excised. Anterior rectus sheath is excised; muscle is split; peritoneum is opened to bring the end of the colon outwards. It can be brought out extraperitoneally to prevent herniation. Seromuscular suture bites are taken from the colon 5 cm proximal to cut margin which is also passed through the peritoneum and rectus sheath; interrupted vicryl sutures are placed. After closure of the abdominal wound, maturation of the colostomy is done by trimming the end if there is stapler line and suturing the full thickness edge of the colon to the skin using interrupted silk sutures.

Closure

Pelvic peritoneum is irrigated. Pelvic peritoneum can be closed in APR if it is amenable for closure. Usually, there is no need to place the drain into the peritoneal cavity. If pelvic cavity is not sutured and kept open (can be kept open without suturing also) then abdominal drain may be needed. Omentum is brought out lateral to the colostomy part of the colon towards the pelvis to fill the free space. It also absorbs fluid, prevents sepsis and supports urinary bladder. Alternatively if omentum is not adequate then absorbable mesh of large size can be sutured to posterior and lateral abdominal wall without injuring the ureters. In females uterus if not removed will fall retroverted and fill the pelvic cavity. Few surgeons do the caecal mobilisation so as to allow it to drop into the pelvic cavity to fill the space. Abdomen is closed in layers. Pelvis is already drained from below.

Colostomy care: Immediate care is given by doing irrigation daily with 1 L warm saline to the proximal colon through colostomy. It is to distend the proximal colon so as to produce reflex peristalsis to empty the entire colon; so patient should feel colicky pain after saline infusion. Infusion is done through a tube, which should be gentle otherwise perforation may occur.

Postoperative Care

Nasogastric tube can be removed in 24 hours. Usually, colostomy starts functioning early. Oral feeding can be started in 48 hours. Perineal drain is removed in 7 days. Urinary catheter is removed in 7–10 days.

Colostomy bag is placed and colostomy care should be given. Colostomy site should be observed for mucosal necrosis; hence, initially transparent bags are used to visualise the mucosa easily. Perineal suture is removed in 14 days. *Sitz bath* to the perineal wound helps in faster healing of the wound.

Complications

Bleeding during abdominal dissection due to tear of presacral vein or dissection; bleeding from perineal wound can occur from inferior haemorrhoidal vessels and branches of the internal iliac vessels.

Injury to ureter during abdominal and presacral dissection can occur. Urethral injury can occur while dissecting the rectum in front either from above or from below.

Small bowel adhesions can occur onto the pelvic suture line; or herniation of the small bowel across the pelvis leading into *intestinal obstruction* can occur. Colostomy in such situation will not function. Contrast CT is useful to confirm the obstruction. Initially it is treated conservatively; if patient is not responding then laparotomy may be needed.

Infection—wound infection, pelvic infection, septicaemia and urinary infection can develop after abdominoperineal resection **(Fig. 26-22)**.

Bladder dysfunction is very common due to lack of pelvic support to urinary bladder. *Sexual impotence* is common after APR due to nerve damage (>50%).

Colostomy complications can develop—necrosis, retraction, prolapse, parastomal hernia.

Problems in healing of the perineal wound—wound may partially heal forming a chronic sinus. Wound healing may be delayed often. Persistent discharging sinus can occur; it will last for years often; it needs exploration of the sinus, excision of the sinus with coccyx; once it granulates split skin graft is placed on the raw area.

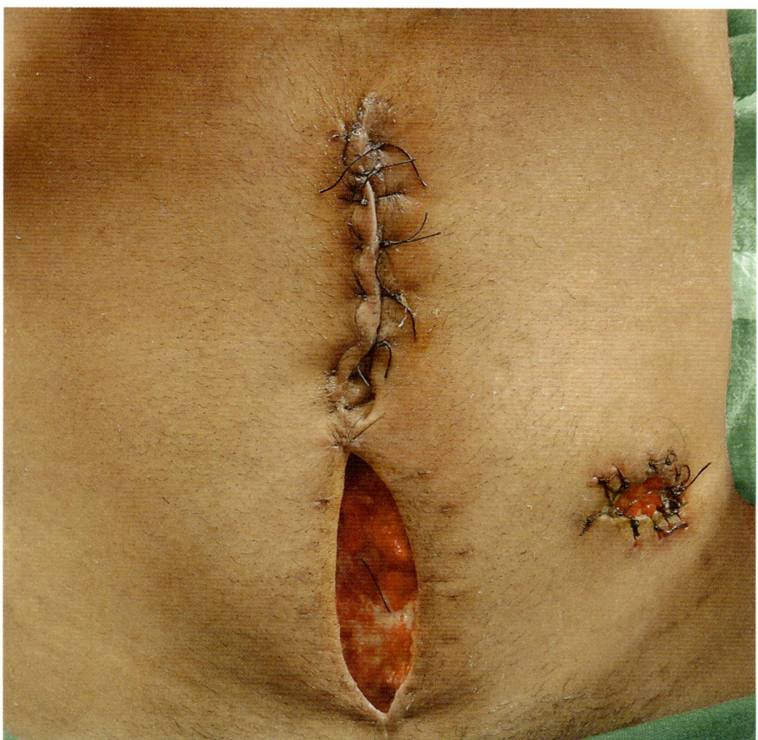

Fig. 26-22: Wound infection after APR.

LAPAROSCOPIC ABDOMINOPERINEAL RESECTION

First laparoscopic APR was done by Sackier in 1991. Laparoscopic abdominoperineal resection with formation of the colostomy is commonly done. Here abdominal part dissection is easier under direct vision; perineal dissection is same as in open procedure. It is technically easier compared to laparoscopic anterior resection as anastomosis is not done **(Fig. 26-23)**.

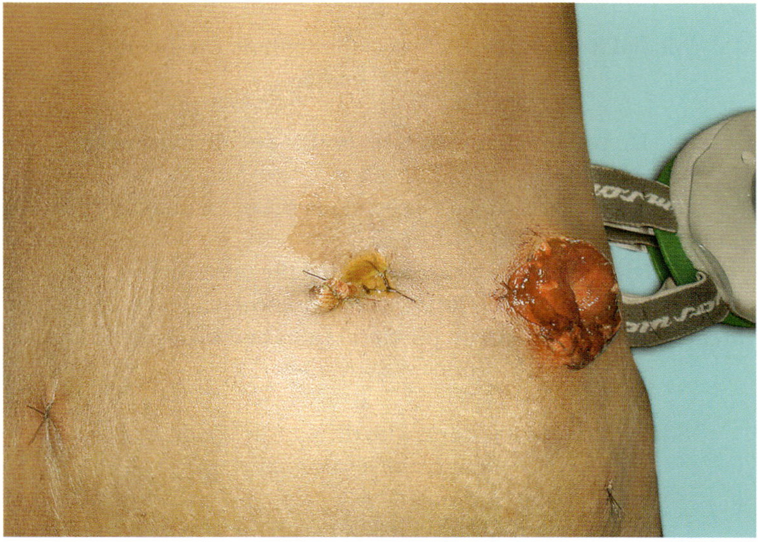

Fig. 26-23: Laparoscopic APR. Colostomy is in left iliac fossa.

Present indication for laparoscopic APR—tumours within one cm of the anal verge; invasive rectal cancers.

Contraindications—perforated or obstructed tumours; severe obesity; previous pelvic surgeries. Tumours invading the bladder, pelvic wall, uterus needs open approach.

Patient position, trocar placements are same as described in laparoscopic low anterior resection. But here dissection is done much more distally beyond the levator ani posteriorly and up to proximal urethra beyond the apex of prostate anteriorly.

Laparoscopic USG is better to confirm the operability and to rule out any possible metastases in liver, nodes and retroperitoneum.

Abdominal part of the technique is same as laparoscopic anterior resection. Perineal part is same as perineal part of the open APR.

Steps in Laparoscopic APR

Proper positioning—lithotomy with steep head down; proper port placement

↓

Release of adhesions; in women elevation of uterus towards abdominal wall using silk sutures

↓

Holding the sigmoid up and left

↓

Opening the mesocolon adjacent to sacral promontory and dissecting upwards

↓

Identification of left ureter and gonadal vessels; dissection should not be too anterior and too posterior

↓

Ligation of inferior mesenteric artery after dissection beyond the origin of the left colic artery.

↓

Division of IMA is done using ligatures, endovascular stapler, clipping, ligasure.

↓

Division of the inferior mesenteric vein at the lower border of the pancreas.

↓

Splenic flexure mobilisation is not necessary but paracolic gutter along the line of Toldt needs to be incised.

↓

Medial to lateral dissection of the sigmoid mesocolon up to the colon margin.

↓

Ureter, gonadal vessels on both sides are preserved.

↓

Posterior presacral dissection along the avascular holy plane of the Heald which is identified by loose areolar tissue; in front endopelvic fascia is present enveloping the mesorectum; behind presacral pelvic (parietal) fascia will be present which should not be breached to avoid injury to presacral veins and hypogastric nerves (one on each side).

↓

Sharp dissection is done with division of Waldeyer fascia to identify the levator ani.

↓

Lateral ligaments are divided between mesorectum and the autonomic nerves using harmonic scalpel; mesorectum should not be breached and autonomic nerves should not be injured.

↓

Mobilisation in front between the anterior rectal wall mesorectum and prostate and seminal vesicles along and in front of the Denonvilliers' fascia beyond the prostate apex to urethra up to the pelvic floor; in females anterior dissection is done between vagina and rectal wall and Denonvilier's fascia is less developed in females; posterior to cervix and posterior fornix this fascia is vascular due to venous plexus. Cuff of the vagina may be required to be excised to include with the specimen. Often, if tumour is infiltrating the cervix hysterectomy is done along with APR (like in open). Nervi erigentes curves anteriorly from sacral foramina to converge and join the presacral nerves and form *neurovascular bundle of Walsh* at 2 and 10 o'clock positions in the Denonvilliers' fascia just behind the lateral edges of the seminal vesicles. This bundle controls both potency and bladder function.

↓

Sigmoid is divided along the proposed line of resection using linear stapler.

↓

Perineal procedure—elliptical skin incision; dissection in front of coccyx; division of anococcygeal ligament; division of levator ani on both sides; division of superficial transverse muscles in front; then puborectalis and rectourethralis muscles.

↓

Retrieval of specimen through perineal wound.

↓

Suction tube drains are placed on both sides of the perineal wound; levator on both sides are approximated using vicryl in front of the coccyx; skin is closed using interrupted sutures.

↓

Pneumoperitoneum is recreated; proximal cut end of the colon is observed to rule out any twist and kept ready for colostomy; pelvic floor is visualised for any bleeding; omentum is brought into the pelvic cavity which minimises the fluid collection and so sepsis; it supports the urinary bladder in front in males so as to reduce residual urine; it prevents the small bowel adhesions also.

↓

Creation of the terminal permanent colostomy.

LAPAROSCOPIC LOW ANTERIOR RESECTION (LAR)

Indication: Rectosigmoid and rectal growth 4 cm proximal to the dentate line. In LAR, resection is done 2 cm above the dentate line. Presently high, low, ultralow anterior resections can be done through laparoscopy with expertise.

Advantages: Magnification, better visualisation, better dissection, preservation of the nerves, easier dissection through the avascular holy plane of Heald; better haemostasis, faster recovery.

Problems: Learning curve, need for modern equipment and cost, time consuming, inability to feel the tumour.

Preparation: Colonoscopic confirmation with biopsy is done. CT abdomen and pelvis is done to see nodal status, liver secondaries and local invasion. Carcinoembryonic antigen (CEA) estimation is done as a base line level for later follow up. Patient is prepared using polyethylene glycol or sodium phytate solutions 12 hours prior to surgery. Oral aminoglycoside and metronidazole may be given as bowel antiseptic.

Anaesthesia: General anaesthesia is used. Perineal scrub cleaning is done properly.

Position: Low lithotomy position with steep head down like for laparoscopic hysterectomy to make small bowel to settle in proximal abdomen. Cleaning and draping is done. Left side of the patient is raised to allow small bowel to fall out of the pelvis.

Surgeon stands on right side. Camera surgeon stands on left side of the surgeon; scrub nurse in between legs; first assistant on the left side of the patient near left shoulder to hold the colon using bowel grasper. Monitor is placed on the left side near foot end.

A 10-mm umbilical port is used for 30° telescope. *5 mm port is placed in midclavicular line on right side.* 10 mm port is placed at right iliac fossa 2.5 cm medial and above the anterior superior iliac spine. This port later requires to be converted to 12 mm port to pass *articulating endostapler* to staple the low rectum. Additional 5 mm port is later required in midline just above the symphysis while mobilising the splenic flexure.

After pneumoperitoneum, with assistant holding and pulling sigmoid upwards and towards left (through left upper 5 mm port); surgeon does dissection through two working ports—right 5 mm upper port and right 10 mm lower port; medial side of the mesocolon is incised from below upwards from left rectovesical/rectovaginal peritoneal reflection extending proximally across the sacral promontory upwards towards inferior mesenteric artery (IMA) origin. Left ureter and left gonadal vessels are identified and dissected off the posterior peritoneum. Sympathetic nerve at the level of the sacral promontory is preserved. IMA near its origin (usually after it gives left colic branch in case of carcinoma rectum) is clipped/ligated and divided using ligaseal or harmonic scalpel. Dissection further towards left visualises Gerota's fascia covering the left kidney. Colour of Gerota's fascia is more deep yellow than the surrounding fat. Incision is further extended upwards towards the duodenojejunal flexure. Inferior mesenteric vein is identified close to the ascending branch of left colic artery at the lower border of the pancreas which is double clipped and divided. Accessory left colic artery when present should be preserved carefully.

Now it is better if surgeon shifts his position in between legs of the patient to do mobilisation of the splenic flexure of the colon. Right lower and suprapubic ports are used for splenic flexure mobilisation. Dissection begins at the left paracolic gutter extending upwards towards splenic flexure; renocolic, splenocolic, gastrocolic and pancreaticocolic ligaments are incised. Splenic flexure is mobilised from left kidney, spleen and pancreas. It can be done from left side towards right or from middle level of transverse colon by dividing gastrocolic omentum towards left using harmonic scalpel.

Once splenic flexure is mobilised, surgeon again shifts his position towards right with working ports on right upper and lower area.

A 30° camera is placed on the right 10 mm port to visualise the pelvis for pelvic dissection. Plane of dissection is in a potential space between parietal and viscera pelvic fascia, which is avascular. Incised peritoneum on the sacral promontory is extended downwards on the right side of the rectum towards pelvis. Superior hypogastric plexus and two hypogastric nerves are identified and preserved. Peritoneum is incised on the left side and in front like U on the rectovesical or rectouterine fold. Dissection is continued in this *avascular holy plane of Heald* down towards the levator in front of the parietal pelvic fascia to clear the mesorectum. Levators are clearly seen now; midline raphe and Waldeyer fascia, which is strong and condensed is divided using harmonic scalpel. Mesorectum should be removed up to the levator ani.

Lateral mobilisation is done by dividing the lateral ligaments on both sides close to the rectum. It contains middle rectal vessels. Medial part of the autonomic plexus and branches passes through the lateral ligament. These nerves should be preserved.

Anterior mobilisation is done along the Denonvilliers' fascia behind the prostatic capsule up to the apex of the prostate. Mesorectum also should be cleared.

At the end circumferential dissection is done to achieve fully mobilised rectal tube. Fat and fascia of the rectal tube is removed to achieve complete denudation and muscularisation. This is essential step prior to stapler application. Cautery should not be used as it may injure the rectal wall; sharp dissection should be done; mucosa should not be breached. Rectal examination and proctoscopy can be done to assess the completion of the mobilisation.

Using *roticulating stapler* rectum is transected. Per anally warm distilled water wash is given to the rectum. This needs conversion of 10 mm port into 12 mm port (of suprapubic port). If this is not available then small Pfannenstiel incision (5 cm), made through which conventional linear stapler is used to divide the rectum. Tumour distal margin is felt for clearance. Bowel is brought out of the wound and specimen is removed after placing a sterile plastic sheath in the abdominal wound to prevent contamination and tumour spillage on the abdominal wound **(Fig. 26-24)**.

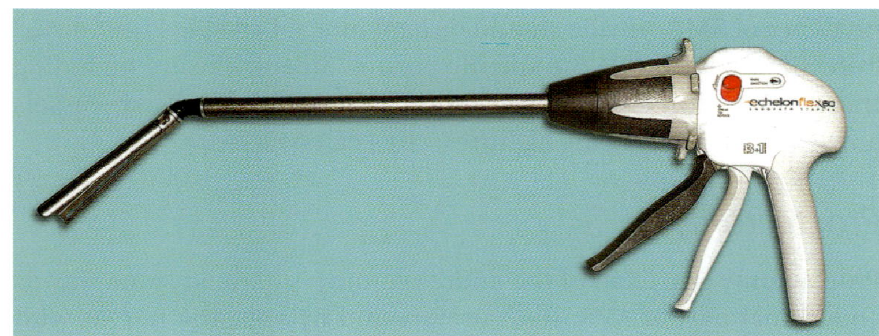

Fig. 26-24: Roticulating stapler is used to transect the rectum.

Transected proximal colon is prepared for anvil of the circular cartridge placement. After positioning the anvil, using 2-zero polypropylene purse string suture is placed around it through the cut edge of the colon. Colon with anvil is dropped into the peritoneum carefully without allowing the rotation. Circular stapler cartridge is passed through the anus carefully gently towards rectal stump and is perforated just adjacent to the stapler line in the middle; cartridge is locked to the anvil using two instruments. While locking the instrument care should be taken not to interpose other structures. It is done by counter clockwise movement of the shaft of the stapler. Stapler is fired through circular anastomosis. One minute after firing stapler is released by clockwise movement with careful rotation.

Pelvis is filled with warm distilled water and Foley's catheter is passed per anally; air is infused to check the air bubble leak in the pelvis. After completion, tension in the anastomotic site is assessed. Tube drain is placed through one of the 10 mm ports. Diversion colostomy is done if needed.

TOTAL PROCTOCOLECTOMY WITH ILEOANAL POUCH

It is removal of entire colon and rectum with creation of ileal distal pouch and doing ileoanal anastomosis.

Indications

Ulcerative colitis; indeterminate colitis; familial adenomatous polyposis, multiple sessile polyps, synchronous multicentric carcinomas.

Contraindications

Crohn's disease is a contraindication as terminal ileum is involved now or may get involved later after anastomosis leading into failure of the treatment.

Preoperative Preparation

Preoperative planning is essential. Colonoscopy, biopsy, marking of stoma, mechanical bowel preparation, nasogastric tube and urethral catheter placement and rectal washes with normal saline is done.

Total Colectomy

Lithotomy with head down position and lengthy midline incision is used under general anaesthesia. Mobilisation is same as combinations of right and left colectomies with proctectomy. Right paracolic gutter is incised and right colon is mobilised from lateral to medial approach unless malignancy is confirmed or suspected wherein dissection is done from medial to lateral. Right ureter, gonadals, duodenum, SMA, SMV are carefully preserved after dissection. *Vessels are ligated either close to colon wall*. Once ileocolic artery is ligated terminal ileum is supplied by jejunal branches of SMA; arcade should be kept intact. Left side is mobilised from sigmoid towards the splenic flexure. Splenic flexure including transverse colon is mobilised fully. Sigmoid is mobilised; vessels are ligated securely using ligatures; clips can be used.

Proctectomy

Proctectomy (Excision of the entire rectum) is done in same way as abdominal part of APR. Both ureters and hypogastric nerves with autonomic plexus are retained carefully. Presacral dissection is done in avascular holy plane of Heald which is identified by loose areolar tissue. One should not open posterior presacral fascia to avoid injury to presacral veins and nervi erigentes. Waldeyer fascia is divided. Lateral dissection is done by dividing the lateral ligaments; autonomic nerve plexus are close to it; one should avoid injuring it. Anterior dissection is done behind the Denonvilliers' fascial plane; behind prostate and seminal vesicles. Neurovascular bundle of Walsh is at 2 and 10 o'clock positions. Posterior dissection is done up to levator ani muscles. Entire rectal tube is mobilised. Distal small length of the mucosa if retained needs anorectal mucosectomy prior to doing hand sewn ileoanal anastomosis. Distal rectum is transected. Entire colorectum is removed after transecting the ileum very close to the caecum between soft occlusion clamps retaining its blood supply.

Mobilisation of the Small Bowel for Adequate Length

Small bowel mesentery is mobilised up to the 3rd part of the duodenum and inferior border of the pancreas. If still mobilisation is needed, then all peritoneal tissues are cleared from right of the superior mesenteric vessels. Using transillumination, superior mesenteric vessels and arcade should be identified for preservation. Small tiny 1 cm transverse incisions are made carefully on the peritoneum overlying the superior mesenteric vessels and also Kocherisation of the duodenum will also be helpful.

Construction of Ileal Pouch

Different pouches are used. J, S, W, H are different types. S pouch is easier to reach to the anal canal (more than 3–4 cm better than J pouch). J pouch is easier to construct. Possibility of tension free pouch should be confirmed prior to construction of the pouch. Pouch plan is done; proposed apex is held with Babcock's forceps which is pushed down towards the anal canal; finger is placed in the anal canal to feel the tip of Babcock easily without tension confirming that pouch is tension free. A point in the ileum 20 cm from the cut end if able to be brought down 6 cm beyond the pubic symphysis, it is said that tension free pouch is possible. Pouch is created either by hand sewn or by stapler. Interrupted or continuous inner full thickness vicryl sutures and outer seromuscular interrupted silk sutures are used to create the pouch after doing enterotomy on the antimesenteric border. Stapler can be used to create pouch. 15 cm each limb (total of 30 cm of terminal ileum) J pouch is created. Pouch should be checked for leak proof by infusing saline into the pouch. Apex of the pouch is opened; saline filled syringe is passed through this enterotomy and pushed to check for leak. Syringe is removed. Anvil of the circular stapler is passed into the pouch through the enterotomy and purse string suture is placed using 2-zero polypropylene sutures **(Fig. 26-25)**.

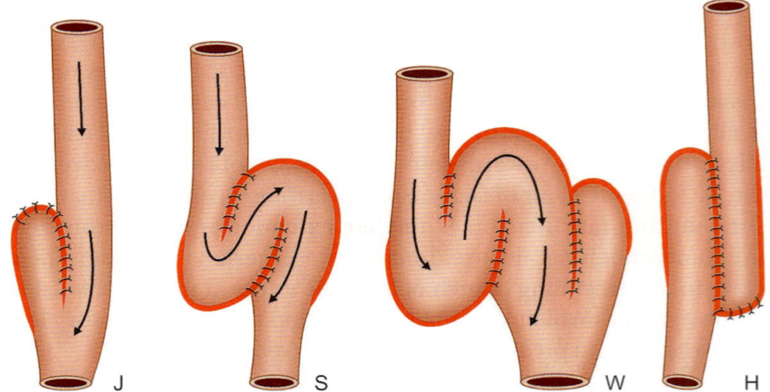

Fig. 26-25: Different pouches are used—J, S, W, H.

Ileal Pouch Anal Anastomosis

When stapler is used, anastomosis is achieved at anorectal ring at the top of the anal column; here anal sensory epithelium is retained and anastomosis is tension free as it is higher level than hand sewn. Stapled anastomosis at further lower level is not possible as it will damage the internal sphincter. Stapled type is easy to do with less infective complications and better function. But there is potential risk of malignant transformation in transitional zone (4–5%). So, whenever biopsy report shows dysplasia then mucosectomy with hand sewn anastomosis should be done. Cartridge is passed into the anal canal; rectal stump is already stapled during transection; cartridge is punctured through rectal stump and is locked with anvil of the pouch; stapler is fired to achieve the anastomosis. Stapler is removed; doughnut is checked. Sphincter should not be included in the stapler; posterior vaginal wall should not be included to avoid formation of pouch-vaginal fistula. Apex of the J pouch or end of the S pouch is used.

When *mucosectomy* is needed in patients with dysplasia, rectum is transected just above the levator ani; mucosa is stripped off the muscular layer of the rectum from dentate line up to the anorectal ring/levator ani. Ferguson anal retractor is needed for this purpose. 10–20 mL of 1 in 2,00,000 units of adrenaline solution is used to raise the mucosa from the muscle layer. Every parts of the mucosa should be removed carefully and gently. Frozen section biopsy of the excised mucosa is a must to rule out carcinoma and Crohn's disease. Cautery is used to control bleeding.

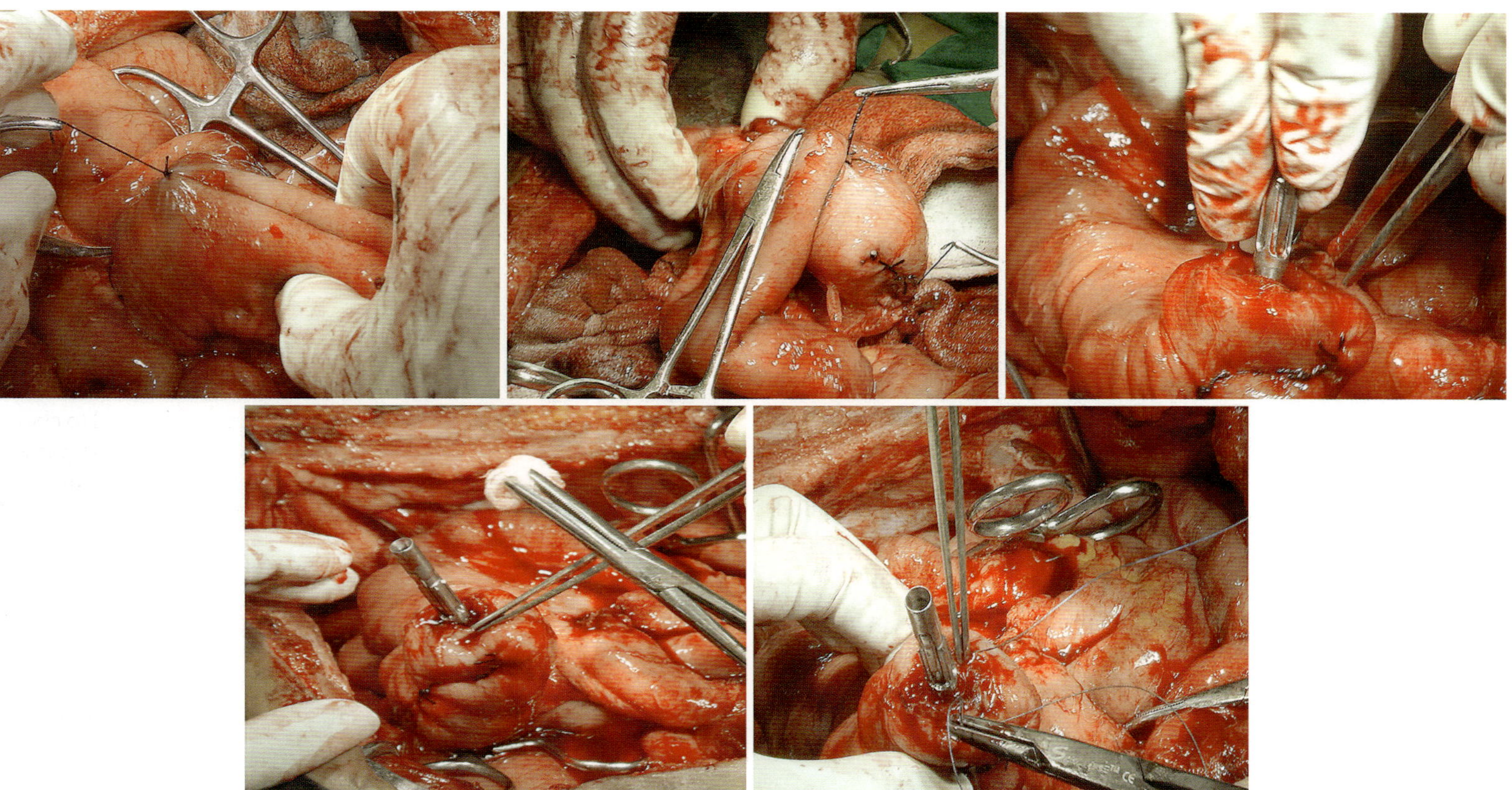

Fig. 26-26: Construction of ileal pouch and placing anvil in the pouch.

CUSA can be used to do mucosectomy. Mucosectomy is better achieved in prone Jackknife position. Sullivan and Garnjobst in 1982 started to do mucosectomy prior to abdominal procedure in prone position. Mucosectomy is done from dentate line upwards for 4–6 cm in a tubular fashion **(Fig. 26-26)**.

Pouch is brought down towards anal canal and is anastomosed to anal canal. Hand sewn anastomosis is technically difficult and demanding. Ileal pouch end is brought down into the anus after mucosectomy. Bivalved Park's retractor is of great help for this. Two Gelpi retractors one at right angles to each other are also very useful. 4-zero vicryl interrupted sutures are taken. Bites should be taken from few fibres of underlying internal sphincter muscle.

Covering Diversion Loop Ileostomy

Covering diversion loop ileostomy is done 20 cm proximal to the pouch which should not have any tension. Routinely diversion should be done as usually patients are on high dose of steroid, malnourished, toxic, anaemic. In selected patients restorative proctocolectomy with ileal pouch anal anastomosis is done without any diversion ileostomy. Transanal pouch (32 French) catheter is placed often for 5 days.

Postoperative Care

Ileostomy created is usually of high output that drains about 1 to 2 litres of liquid causing severe dehydration and electrolyte imbalance. One should avoid hot weather, exercise, high fibre diet; plenty of oral fluids should be taken. Loperamide orally is useful to reduce the pouch output. If patient is on steroids; it should be tapered gradually under observation. Antibiotics, correction of nutrition and anaemia are needed depending on the individual patients.

Complications

Usual complications are anastomotic leak, stricture, recurrent pain, diarrhoea, perianal ulceration, perianal infection, pelvic abscess formation, irritable pouch syndrome.

Pouchitis is a specified complication in ileal pouch surgeries. In pouchitis patient presents with acute diarrhoea, urgency, rectal bleed, suprapubic pain. *Pouchitis disease activity index* is often used to assess the severity of the pouchitis—by features, endoscopy and biopsy. Local steroid, mesalamine are useful. If persists then pouch excision and permanent ileostomy should be done.

Cuffitis, cuff abscess if inadequate mucosectomy is done.

Technical complications like injury to ureter, bleeding, impotence, sepsis, intestinal obstruction can occur.

Faecal incontinence is another distressing problem.

TREATMENT FOR RECTAL PROLAPSE

Treatment for Partial Prolapse

In children the nutrition of the child is improved and digital repositioning is tried. *Correction of constipation* is important **(Fig. 26-27)**.

Submucosal injections of 10 mL of 5% phenol in almond oil or ethanolamine oleate is given into the apex of the prolapse under general anaesthesia so as to create an aseptic inflammation leading to tethering of mucosa to the underlying muscular coat. Injection can also be given at the base or both at the apex and base. Alternatively, 30 mL of tetracycline or oxytetracycline or hypertonic saline injection can also be used. Initial injection is supported by *Thiersch wiring* using (temporary) chromic catgut until adhesion occurs between the mucosa and muscular layer (in 3 weeks). In adults,

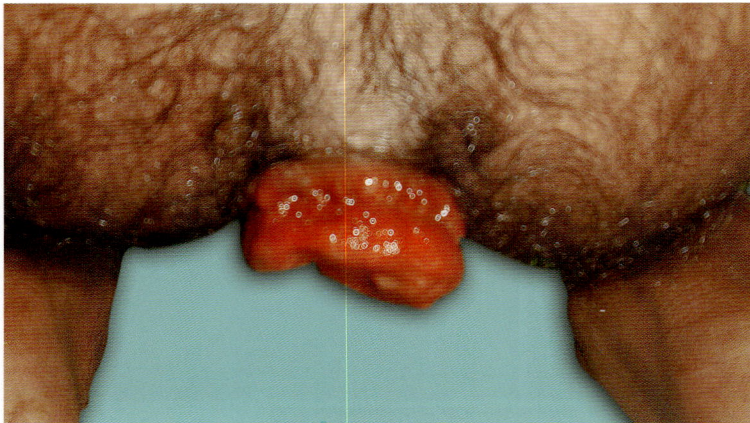

Fig. 26-27: Partial rectal prolapse.

injection therapy is tried for partial prolapse, results are not as good as in children.

Thiersch wiring alone is tried with good success rate in children.

Goodsall's operation is excision of the prolapsed mucosa at its base, usually in three positions. Stapled transanal rectal resection surgery *(STARR)* is also often used **(Fig. 26-28)**.

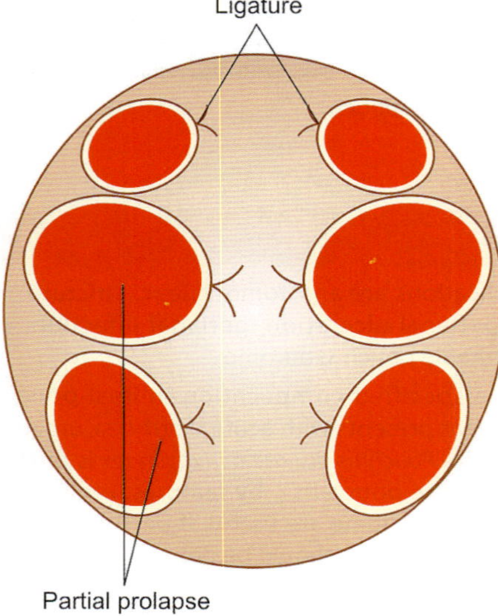

Fig. 26-28: Goodsall's ligature for partial prolapse. Prolapsed mucosa is ligated at different positions using non-absorbable suture material often with double needled. Usually, it is done for one side in three portions.

Treatment for Complete Prolapse

Principles

Surgery is done to *control* the prolapse; to *restore* continence; to *prevent* constipation **(Fig. 26-29)**.

In young males, abdominal repair should be avoided as it injures pelvic nerves leading to sexual impotency. So perineal approach is better.

Rectopexy is fixing the rectum to sacrum by sutures or mesh after complete mobilisation of the rectum. Laparoscopic rectopexy using polypropylene mesh and sutures gives good result and has become very popular.

Delorme's operation is better option in young individual with complete prolapse. In elderly perineal proctectomy with anterior and posterior reefing of the sphincter muscle is the accepted method now. It is similar to Altemeier technique (It is perineal rectosigmoidectomy). Here entire prolapsed rectum and redundant sigmoid is resected through perineum prior to reefing of the sphincter. Anal encircling surgeries using synthetic wires/mesh/suture materials are limited to extremely ill patients and elderly who will not withstand perineal proctectomy. *Choice of procedure* depends on age, sex, operative risk, pelvic floor defect, degree of incontinence, history of constipation.

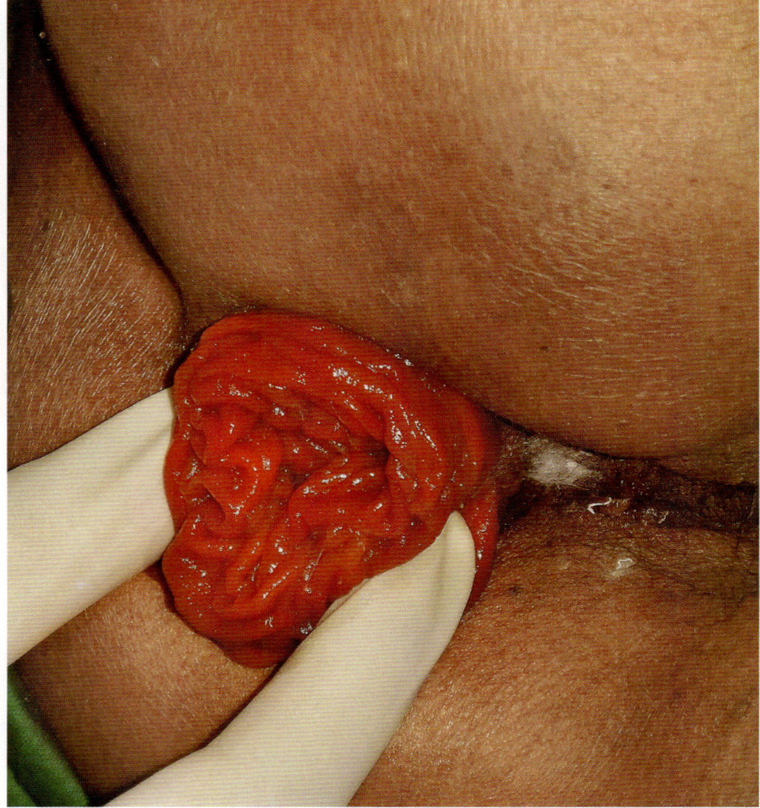

Fig. 26-29: Complete rectal prolapse.

Colonoscopy, defaecating proctography, bowel preparation, nasogastric tube, urinary catheterisation and perioperative antibiotics are needed in preoperative preparation.

Procedures for repair of rectal prolapse

Perineal operations	*Abdominal operations: Open/laparoscopic*
• Mucosal sleeve resection (Delorme) • Perineal rectosigmoidectomy (Altemeier) • Posterior fixation of the rectum of Lockhart-Mummery • Wyatt operation • Mickulicz Miles perineal transanal rectosigmoidectomy/amputation of prolapse • Anal encircling (Thiersch)	• Suture rectopexy–Goligher, Lahaut, Devadhar, Rosoe Graham • Prosthetic or mesh rectopexy— Anterior/posterior—Ripstein, Well's • Resection rectopexy—Muir's • Anterior resection • Lahaut's operation

Surgery—Types

Abdominal Procedures

Laparoscopic Rectopexy

It is ideal and good approach to fix the rectum to sacrum. *Laparoscopic posterior mesh rectopexy* ***(LPMR)*** is the procedure done. Prior colonoscopy and bowel preparation is needed using exelyte or Peglec. Head down, low lithotomy position is needed. Ports placement is same as for anterior resection or APR. 10 mm umbilical camera port; 10 mm right lower pararectus right hand working port; 5 mm left lower pararectus left hand working port; 5 mm left lumbar port for traction to the sigmoid colon; another extra 5 mm suprapubic port in female patients to fix the uterus **(Fig. 26-30)**.

Sigmoid colon is held with left sided port. Surgeon does dissection from right side. Peritoneum on the right of the rectum is opened from sacral promontory downwards to reach avascular holy plane of Heald which is identified by typical presence of loose areolar tissue. Care should be taken to avoid injury to autonomic nerves, ureters. Dissection is extended down as posterior mobilisation into the pelvis with adequate mobilisation of the rectum. Lateral peritoneal reflection on left side is incised and is dissected to connect on both sides of the mesorectum. Left ureter is preserved. Presacral mobilisation is done below up to levator ani muscle. Lateral ligaments are either divided or left alone. It is divided usually in elderly; it is preserved in young individuals unless there is a need to correct undue redundancy of the rectum. *Anterior mobilisation* is also important. Anterior mobilisation along the Denonvilliers' fascia is done 5 cm below the peritoneal reflection. 15 × 10 cm polypropylene mesh is placed in the presacral space deep to rectum, which is fixed to presacral fascia along the sacrum and sacral promontory. Mesh is also sutured to rectal wall on both sides using interrupted polypropylene sutures to create a mesh wrap around the mobilised rectum. Only partial wrapping of mesh is done. This partial wrap corrects the prolapse completely without incontinence and constipation. Partial wrap may be ½ or 2/3rd or 3/4th one. Peritoneum is closed using vicryl to extraperitonealise the mesh. Many advocate laparoscopic mobilisation and fixation of mobilised rectum to sacral promontory using polypropylene sutures without mesh.

Laparoscopic sigmoid resection and rectopexy (Laparoscopic resection rectopexy, LRR) is done when there is rectal prolapse with constipation, with excess redundant sigmoid colon with kinking. Here complete resection of the sigmoid colon is done with colorectal stapled anastomosis. Suture rectoplexy is done by suturing the rectal wall to the mesorectum and the presacral fascia below the level of the sacral promontory. Usually three interrupted sutures are placed. Often fixation between lateral ligaments and sacral promontory is also done. Sigmoidoscopy is done to check the anastomosis. In LRR mesh should not be used as field may be contaminated during resection.

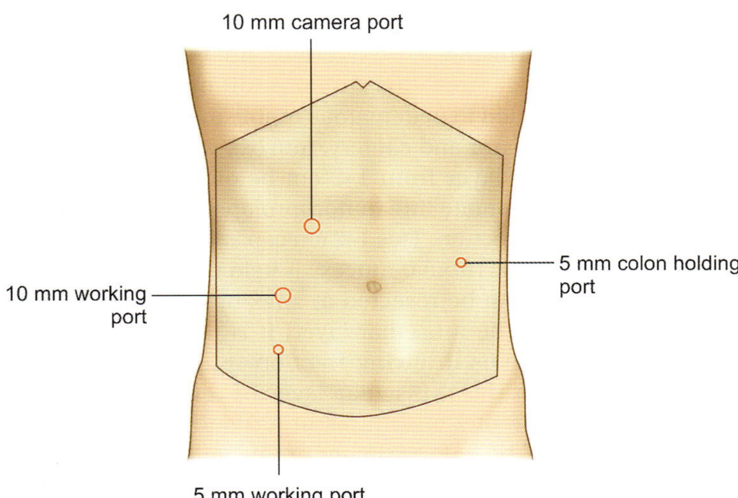

Fig. 26-30: Ports placement for laparoscopic rectal prolapse.

Well's (Britain, 1959) Operation

Polyvinyl alcohol sponge is wrapped around the mobilised rectum posteriorly (from behind) and is fixed to sacrum. Infection, fistula formation is high. Polypropylene mesh is used as a modification now instead of polyvinyl sponge; wrapping is only partially done to reduce the incidence of constipation. But this Ivalon sponge is not approved by USA FDA. Teflon (poly carbon fluoride) and polypropylene mesh are commonly used now. Patient under general or epidural anaesthesia is placed in supine head down position. After midline laparotomy, small bowel is pushed and packed upwards. Peritoneum on both sides of the rectosigmoid is incised 5 cm above the pelvic brim one after the other. Both ureters are identified and protected. At the sacral promontory posterior peritoneum is incised; avascular presacral holy plane of Heald is identified by the presence of loose areolar tissue. Dissection is done in this plane. Anteriorly mesorectum should not be disturbed and posteriorly presacral fascia should not be breached to avoid injuring the presacral veins and nerves. Dissection is done using cautery and scissor up to the coccyx. Tougher Waldeyer fascia behind the lower rectum and coccyx is also divided. Anterior dissection is done carefully up to distal part of the seminal vesicles. Care should be taken not to injure the neurovascular bundle of Walsh at 2 and 10 o'clock positions. Lateral ligament if needed should be divided to avoid the redundancy. Full mobilisation is essential to avoid redundancy and so recurrence. Proper haemostasis is achieved. Ivalon sponge 22 × 10 cm size × 3 mm thickness is used, which is fixed to presacral fascia using three interrupted 2-zero polypropylene sutures posteriorly. All three sutures are taken first then sutures are moved deep down into the pelvis to tie knots. 3/4th circumference of the rectum is encircled by the sponge and is fixed on both sides to the rectal wall using three interrupted 3-zero polypropylene sutures. Pelvic peritoneum is closed using continuous vicryl sutures to extraperitonealise the sponge. Now polypropylene mesh (6 × 4) is used **(Fig. 26-31)**.

Ripstein Operation (Charles Benjamin Ripstein, Canada, 1965)

After mobilisation of the rectum, 5 cm width Teflon mesh sling is passed around the rectum from front to fix it behind to fascia 5 cm below and in front of the sacral promontory. Sling is also fixed in front and laterally to rectum. As anterior fixation is dangerous, this procedure is not advocated now **(Fig. 26-32)**.

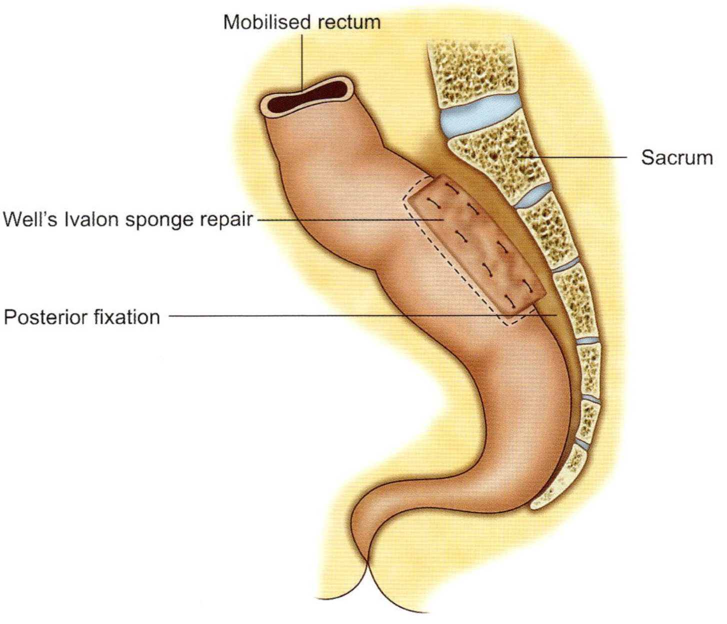

Fig. 26-31: Well's Ivalon sponge repair—posterior repair.

Suture Rectopexy

Rectum is mobilised fully; rectum is secured to sacral fascia or bone using interrupted non-absorbable sutures. It is simple, easy to undertake with high success rate; but causes evacuation disturbances, constipation and obstruction **(Fig. 26-33)**.

Goligher's Operation

Rectum is entirely mobilised up to anorectal ring and its posterior muscular layer is fixed to presacral fascia using interrupted polypropylene sutures.

Devadhar Rectal Plication

Through abdominal approach, junction between thick lower part and thin upper part of the intussusception is identified. A purse string suture using silk is placed in front and laterally; further 3–4 interrupted submucosal Lembert sutures are placed to create reverse intussusception.

Lahaut's Operation

Rectosigmoid is mobilised fully; mobilised loop of rectosigmoid is passed in front through posterior rectus sheath behind the rectus muscle; extraperitonealisation is done to pull the rectus forward to prevent descent.

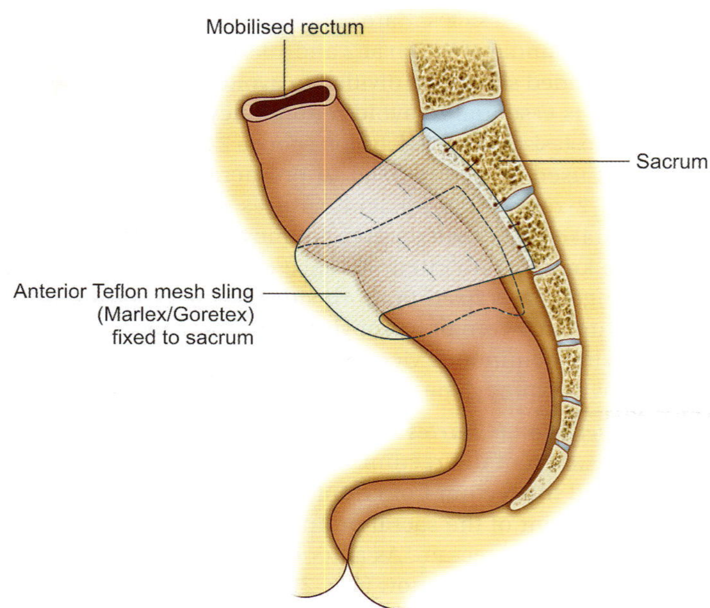

Fig. 26-32: Ripstein repair—anterior repair.

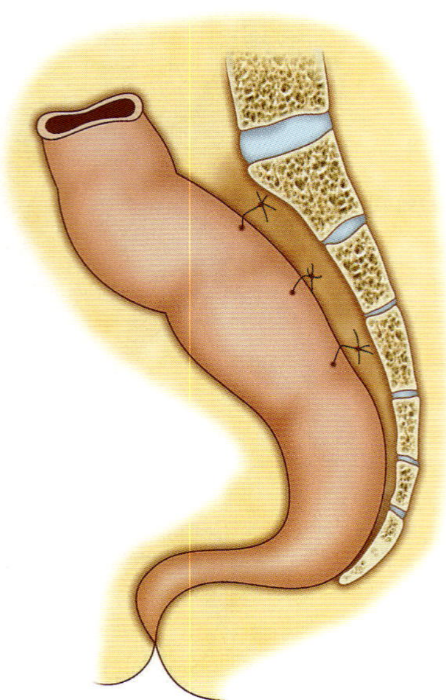

Fig. 26-33: Suture rectopexy.

Rosoe Graham Operation

After mobilisation of the rectum, levator muscles are exposed and sutured in front of the rectum along with removal of pouch of Douglas.

Dumphy Operation

It is done through combined abdominoperineal approach with perineal rectosigmoidectomy. Both procedures control prolapse well but not incontinence.

Muir Low Anterior Resection

In a redundant rectosigmoid with prolapse, rectosigmoid resection is done; excision of redundant pouch of Douglas is done; rectum is fixed to sacrum behind.

Nigro Teflon Halter Operation

It is suspension of the rectum through intra-abdominal sling approach from pubis around the mobilised rectum using 4 × 20 cm mesh sling middle part of the mesh is sutured to rectal wall using interrupted sutures. Pubic rami are dissected in space of Retzius. Each end of the mesh is sutured to pubic ramus on each side to suspend the rectum.

Orr (1947) Fascia Lata Sling Suspension

Fascia lata sling is taken from lateral part of the thigh; it is sutured to the wall of rectum and sacrum with interrupted sutures on both sides after complete mobilisation of the rectum. Nylon is used by many instead of fascia lata for similar suspension.

Complications of Abdominal Procedures

Intraoperative: Presacral bleeding, nerve plexus injury, injury to ureter.

Postoperative: Intestinal obstruction, adhesions, faecal impaction, fistula formation, mesh erosion, recurrence, stricture formation. Constipation rate is more if lateral ligaments are divided; if slings are placed anteriorly also along with posterior slings. Pelvic abscess is common especially in Well's operation which can be prevented by proper bowel preparation prior to surgery. Once abscess forms, Ivalon sponge or mesh has to be removed. Preoperative antibiotics are used to prevent this complication.

Perineal Procedures

Delorme's operation (Mucosal sleeve resection and rectal muscle plication, Edmond Delorme, French surgeon, 1900)

After prior bowel preparation, under spinal anaesthesia, in lithotomy position, completely prolapsed rectum is held with Babcock's forceps. 1 in 2,00,000 adrenaline solution is injected into the submucosal plane of the rectum to cause haemostasis. Rectum is pulled down to create complete prolapse and held using Babcock's forceps at the apex. A circumferential incision is made 1–2 cm away from dentate line; often additional longitudinal incisions may be needed in oedematous friable mucosa. Dissection is done with sharp scissor and cautery; mucosa is stripped off from the deeper muscular layer from 1–2 cm below the anal margin (1–2 cm proximal to dentate line in non-prolapsed position) to the apex of the prolapsed rectum. This 1–2 cm gap is needed to preserve the anorectal sensation. Tubular mucosa is held down with traction; this stripped sleeve can be resected at apex now or later placing plication sutures on the muscular layer; it is better to keep if it is not friable as it helps in giving traction to the rectum while placing plication sutures. Muscular layer of rectum is plicated using absorbable vicryl 2-zero interrupted sutures all around; approximately 12–15 plication stitches are needed. These sutures are tied after finishing the passage of all sutures. Cut end of the mucosa of the apex is sutured to anal margin using interrupted vicryl sutures. It is technically easier **(Fig. 26-34)**.

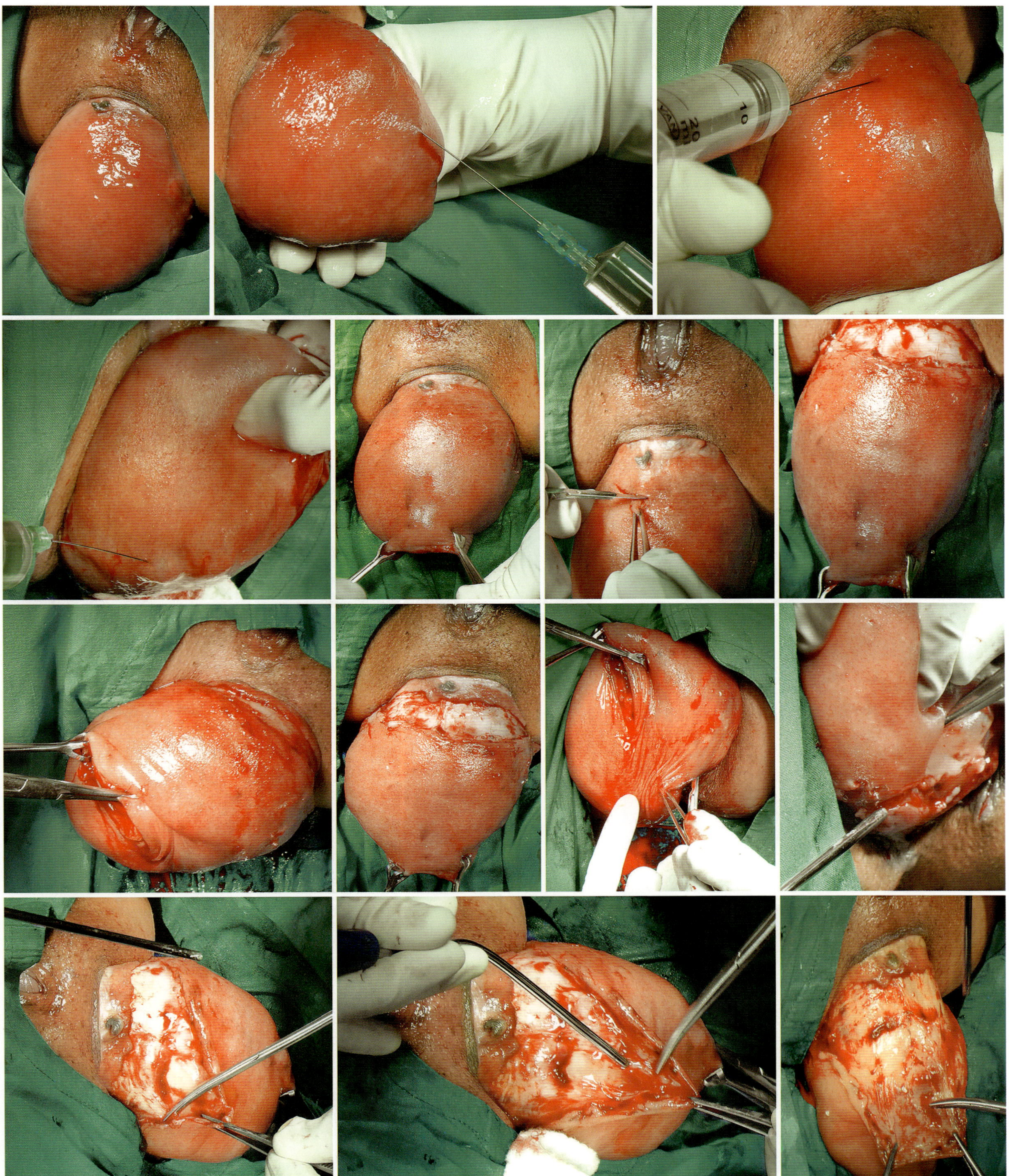

Figs. 26-34(1)

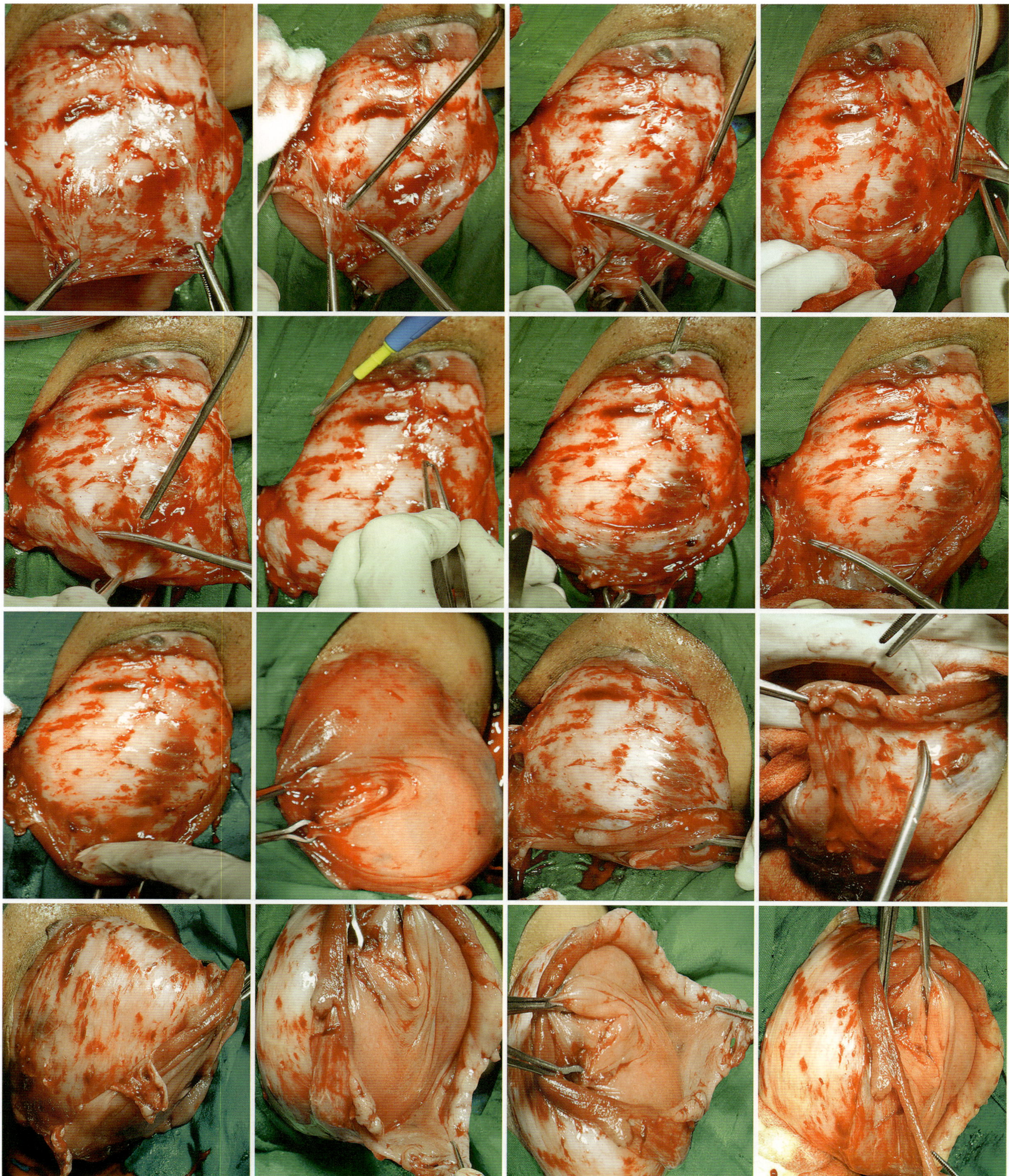

Figs. 26-34(2)

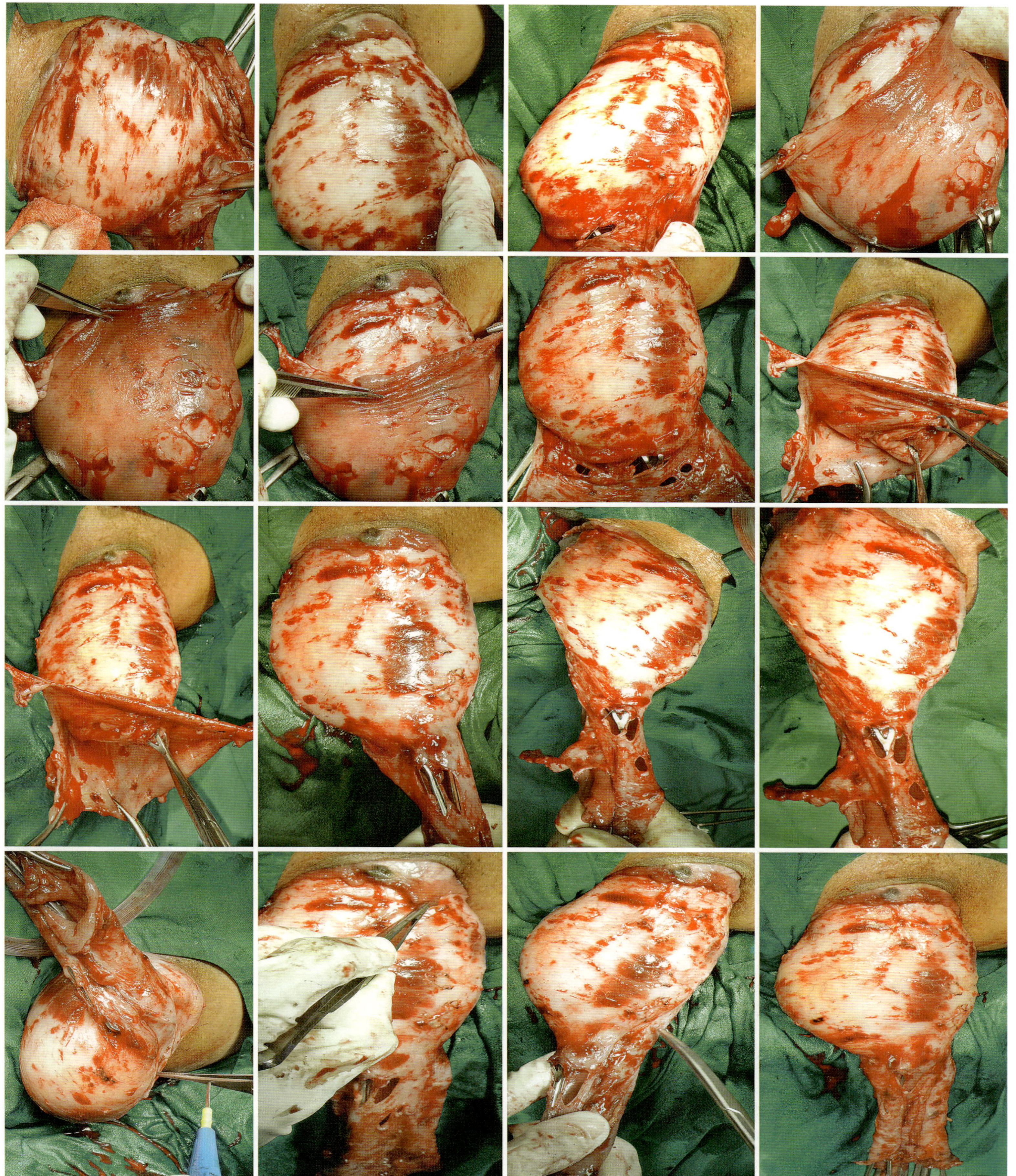

Figs. 26-34(3)

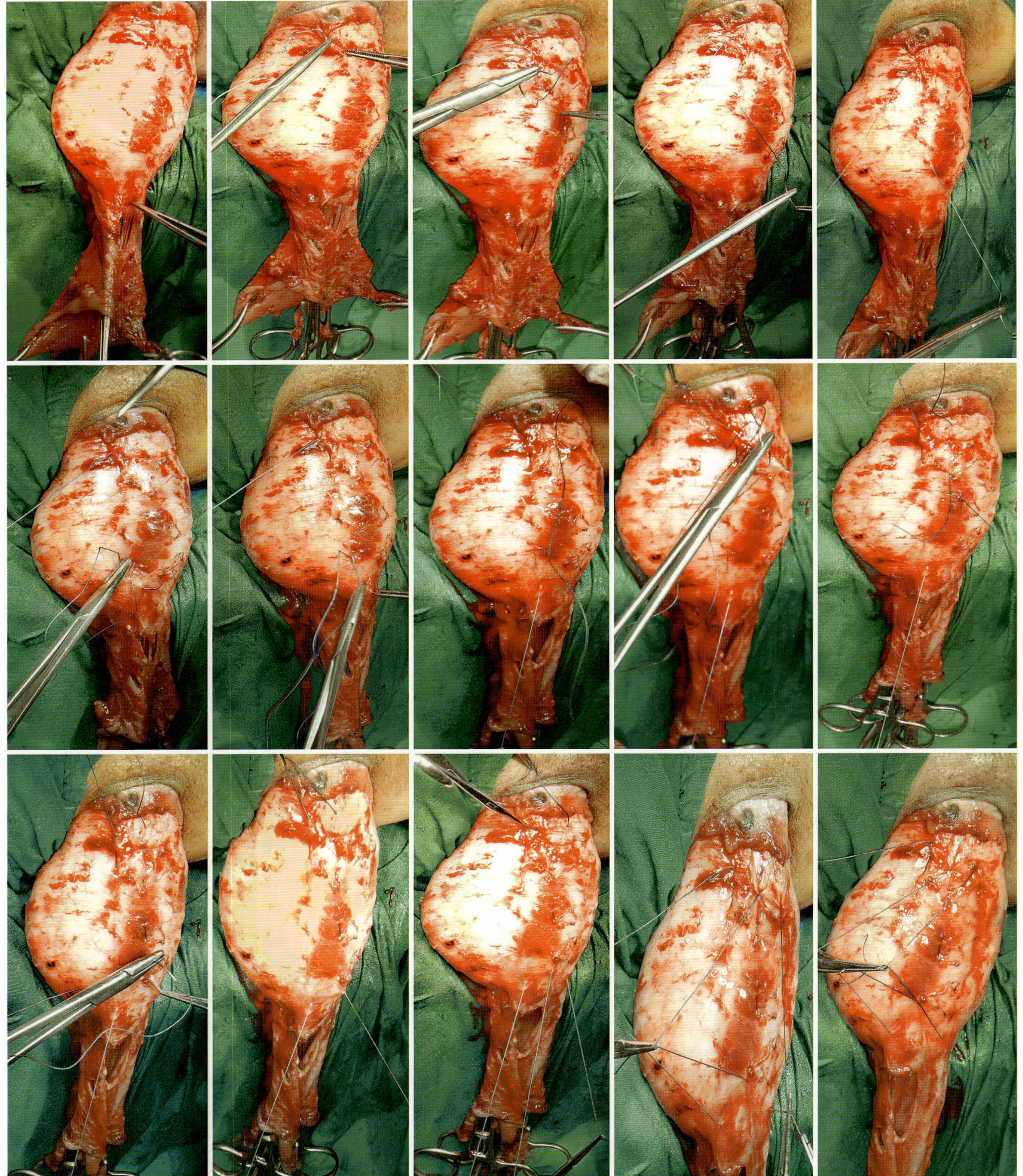

Figs. 26-34(4)

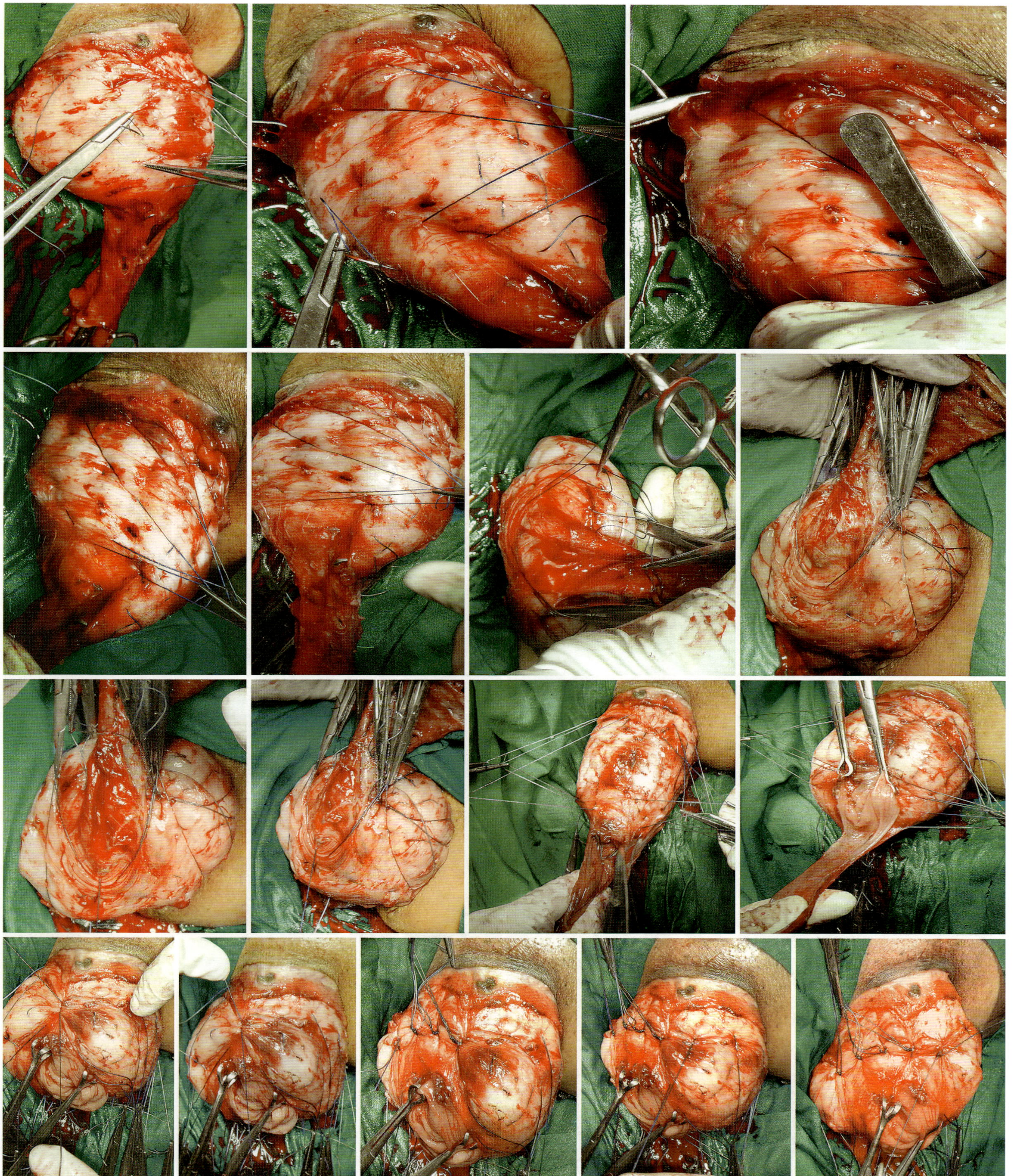

Figs. 26-34(5)

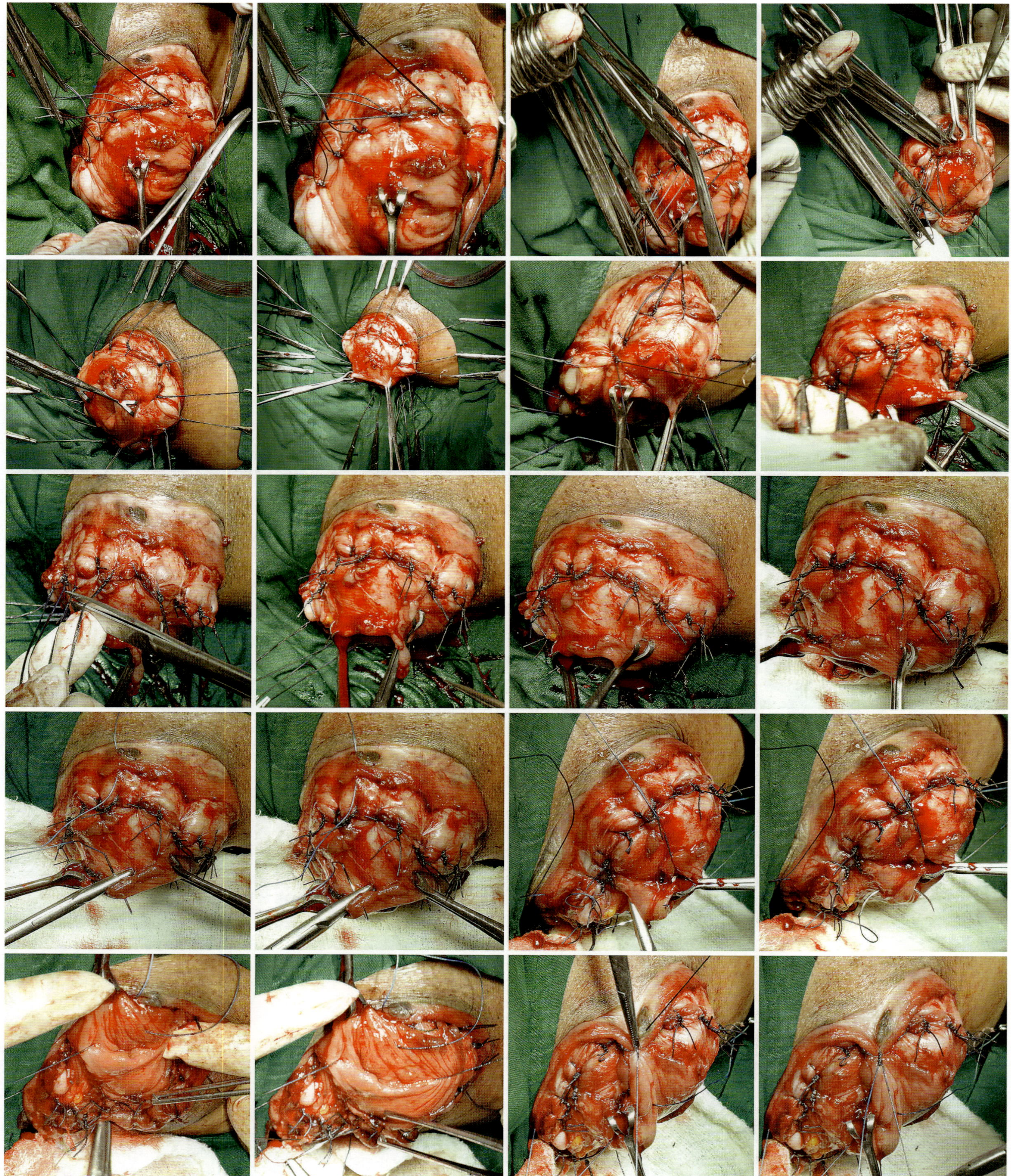

Figs. 26-34(6)

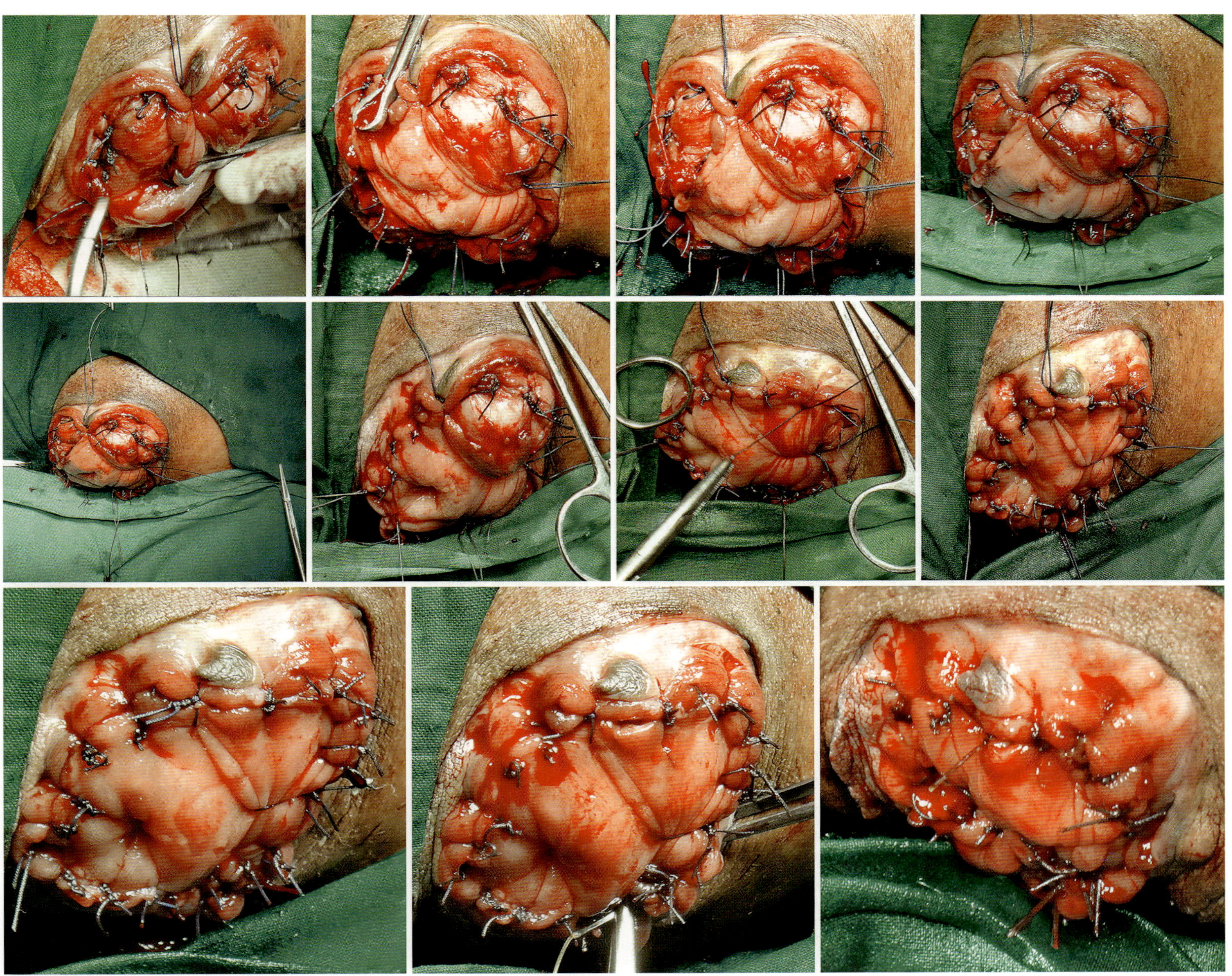

Figs. 26-34(7)

Figs. 26-34(1 to 7): Delorme's procedure for rectal prolapse.

Complications: It causes alteration in rectoanal inhibitory reflex, complete loss of rectal reservoir function, incontinence may persist and recurrence chance is high. Abscess in plicated segment can occur. Occasionally stricture can develop.

Perineal Posterior Fixation of the Rectum of Lockhart-Mummery

Retrorectal space is dissected through perineal approach and posterior rectal wall is sutured to sacrum and coccyx, additionally placing a retrorectal gauze pack to stimulate adhesions.

Wyatt Operation

Through perineal post-anal approach, dissected retrorectal space is placed with a Marlex/mersilene mesh which is sutured high to the sacral promontory and rectal wall laterally.

Mickulicz Miles Perineal Transanal Rectosigmoidectomy/ Amputation of Prolapse

Prolapsed rectum is excised and sigmoid is sutured to the anal margin.

Altemeier's Perineal Rectosigmoidectomy (1952)

After rectosigmoidectomy, colonic anastomosis and pelvic floor is supported by suturing puborectalis muscle in front of the rectum using non-absorbable sutures.

Rectum is fully prolapsed and held with Babcock's forceps. 1:2,00,000 adrenaline is injected to the submucosal plane. Circumferential incision is made 1.5 cm away from the dentate line; first on the posterior surface then on the anterior surface. All the layers of the rectal wall is incised to its full thickness.

Perirectal fat is identified between two outer and inner rectal tubes. Inner rectal wall is not incised. Mesorectum between two tubes is identified. Mesorectum is carefully ligated using two ligatures proximally sequentially at proximal level. Peritoneal cul de sac of sliding hernia is identified and opened. Bowel contents inside peritoneal cavity is pushed upwards; further ligation, division and mobilisation of the mesorectum and mesosigmoid is done. Hernial sac is closed with absorbable vicryl sutures. Levator ani is sutured posteriorly using 2–3 interrupted 2-zero polypropylene sutures to achieve levatorplasty; often anterior levatorplasty is also done. Sigmoid on its anterior part is cut and is sutured to the anal canal above the level of pectinate line to preserve columns of Morgagni; preservation of columns of Morgagni retains the fine anal continence and reduces the chances of anal stricture formation after surgery. Once anterior part of sigmoid colon is cut and sutured (using 3-zero vicryl) only then posterior part of the sigmoid colon is cut and sutured to anal canal. This avoids retraction of the cut part of the sigmoid colon proximally. Anastomosis can also be done using circular stapler.

Complications are—bleeding, anastomotic dehiscence, sepsis, anal stenosis, which may require regular dilatation.

Gant-Miwa Operation (1920, Japan)

Placement of 30–40 absorbable interrupted sutures incorporate the mucosa and submucosa from the apex of the prolapse 1 cm above the dentate line with each at 5 mm apart; with anal encirclement. It has got 15% recurrence rate.

Anal Encircling

In 1891, Thiersch did anal encircling using silver wire to provoke inflammatory fibrosis as well as to give mechanical support to the anal orifice—*Thiersch wiring*. It is done under local anaesthesia. Two small incisions are made at lateral parts or anterior and posterior parts of the anal canal. Submucosal tunnel is created using a curved haemostat. Silver wire is passed around deeper to these incisions and tied after placing the *index finger* into the anal canal. Wire can be removed after 12 months. Polypropylene, nylon are the other materials that can be used. Ribbon shaped prosthetic mesh also can be used. Procedure leads into partial closure and narrowing of the anal canal. *Temporary wiring* along with Goodsall's ligature or injection sclerotherapy using thick catgut are often advocated. *Complications:* Pain due to wire erosion, infection, faecal impaction, incarceration, rectal prolapse, recurrence (80%).

Supralevator high encirclement of anal orifice (of Notaras) is done above the level of levator muscles by placing Teflon or nylon ribbons through anterior and posterior incisions. It gives better support and will not cut through. *Thoralsksen* modified this by placing plastic/mersilene tape around the bowel high up.

Complications of rectal prolapse surgery

- Injury to hypogastric nerve causing impotence.
- Bladder dysfunction.
- Bleeding from presacral venous plexus.
- Injury to rectum and colon causing faecal fistula.
- Constipation after rectopexy is a known complication.
- Recurrence of prolapse.
- Incontinence persists in 50% of cases postoperatively.
- Infection—proctitis/pelvic abscess.

TREATMENT OF PILONIDAL SINUS

Pilonidal sinus may consists of primary and secondary sinuses. It is common in hairy people. Tuft of hairs in the track is common presentation **(Figs. 26-35 and 26-36)**.

In Acute Phase Initially

Drainage of the abscess is done and antibiotics are given; later definitive treatment is undertaken.

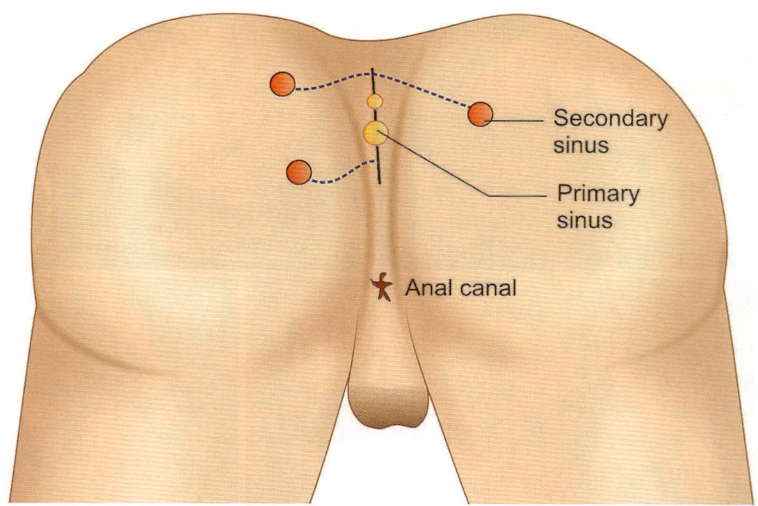

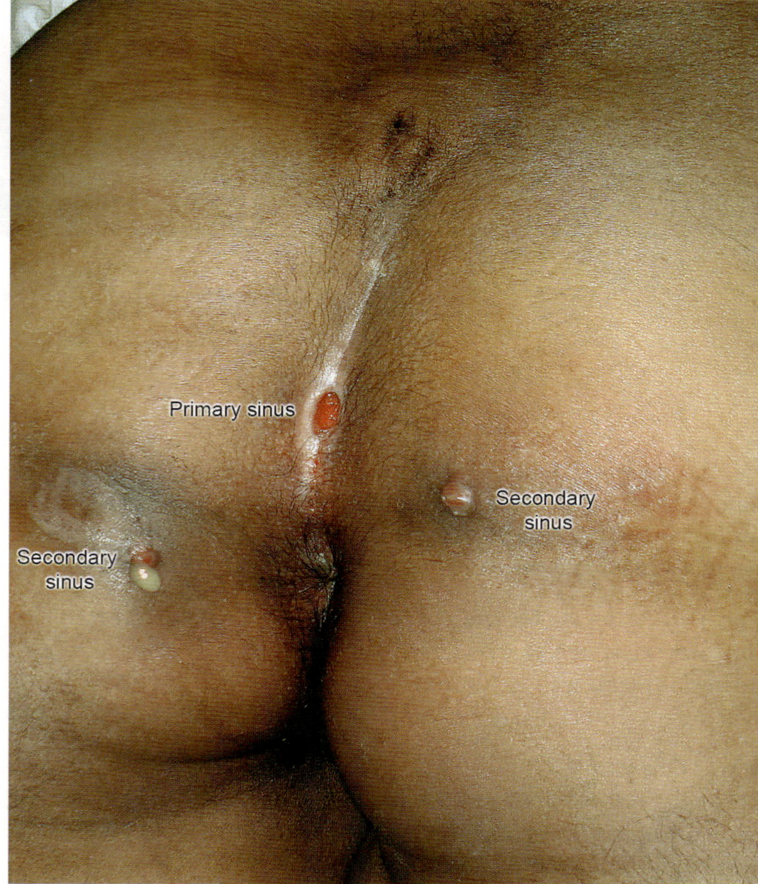

Fig. 26-35: Primary and secondary pilonidal sinus tracks.

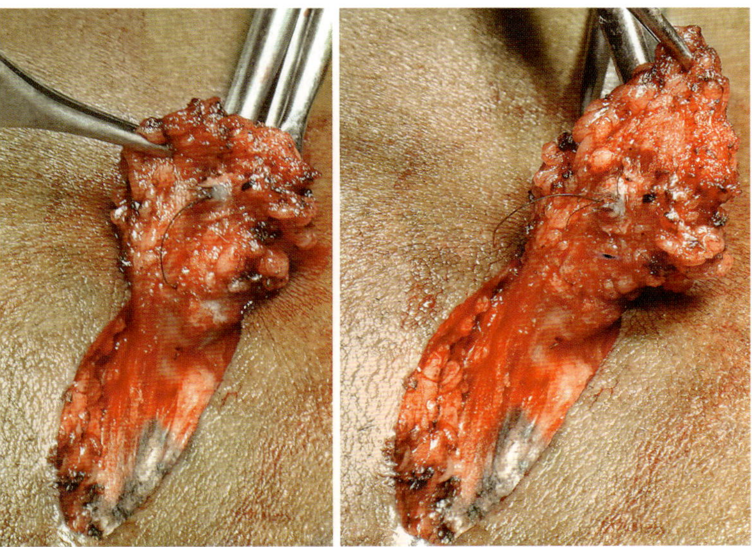

Fig. 26-36: Tuft of hairs in pilonidal sinus track.

Definitive Treatment

Excision

In prone position (*jackknife* position, i.e. prone with buttocks elevated) excision and primary closure is done under general anaesthesia or local anaesthesia. All sinus tracks, unhealthy granulation tissues with hairs are removed completely. Methylene blue is injected to demonstrate the multiple tracks properly. Excision and skin grafting—has got high recurrence rate **(Figs. 26-37 and 26-38)**.

Excision with Z Plasty

It shows good result. Excision with multiple Z plasty is said to be better but technically difficult **(Figs. 26-39 and 26-40)**.

Karydakis Excision

It is done through a semilateral incision and lateralised suturing of the wound away from the midline, gives good result. In prone position with buttocks strapped outwards, paramedian vertically elliptical incision of 5 cm length 2 cm from the midline is placed; edges of the ellipse should be symmetrical; elliptical skin, fat and deep fascia is excised. Medial part of the ellipse will cross the midline to include all midline primary sinuses. Medial flap of the incision is raised for 2 cm further towards midline and opposite side and all fat and deep fascia under the entire length of the medial flap is excised. Haemostasis is maintained. Suction drain is placed. Buttock straps should be released prior to wound closure. Pressure dressing is placed. Subcutaneous tissue and skin are closed. Sutured wound will lie away from newly formed midline **(Fig. 26-41)**.

Rhomboid Flap

Excision with closure using *Limberg (Rhomboid) buttock flap* (single or double rhomboid flaps)—good result. Under general or local anaesthesia, in prone position buttocks are strapped outwards to table using wide plaster. After cleaning and draping, rectangular (rhomboid) tissue of full thickness skin and subcutaneous fat is excised including the midline with its long axis in the midline. Angles of rhomboid should be 60° and 120°. Angles are adjusted meticulously as shown in the pictures; flaps are elevated, rotated and sutured using 3-zero polypropylene or polyethylene.

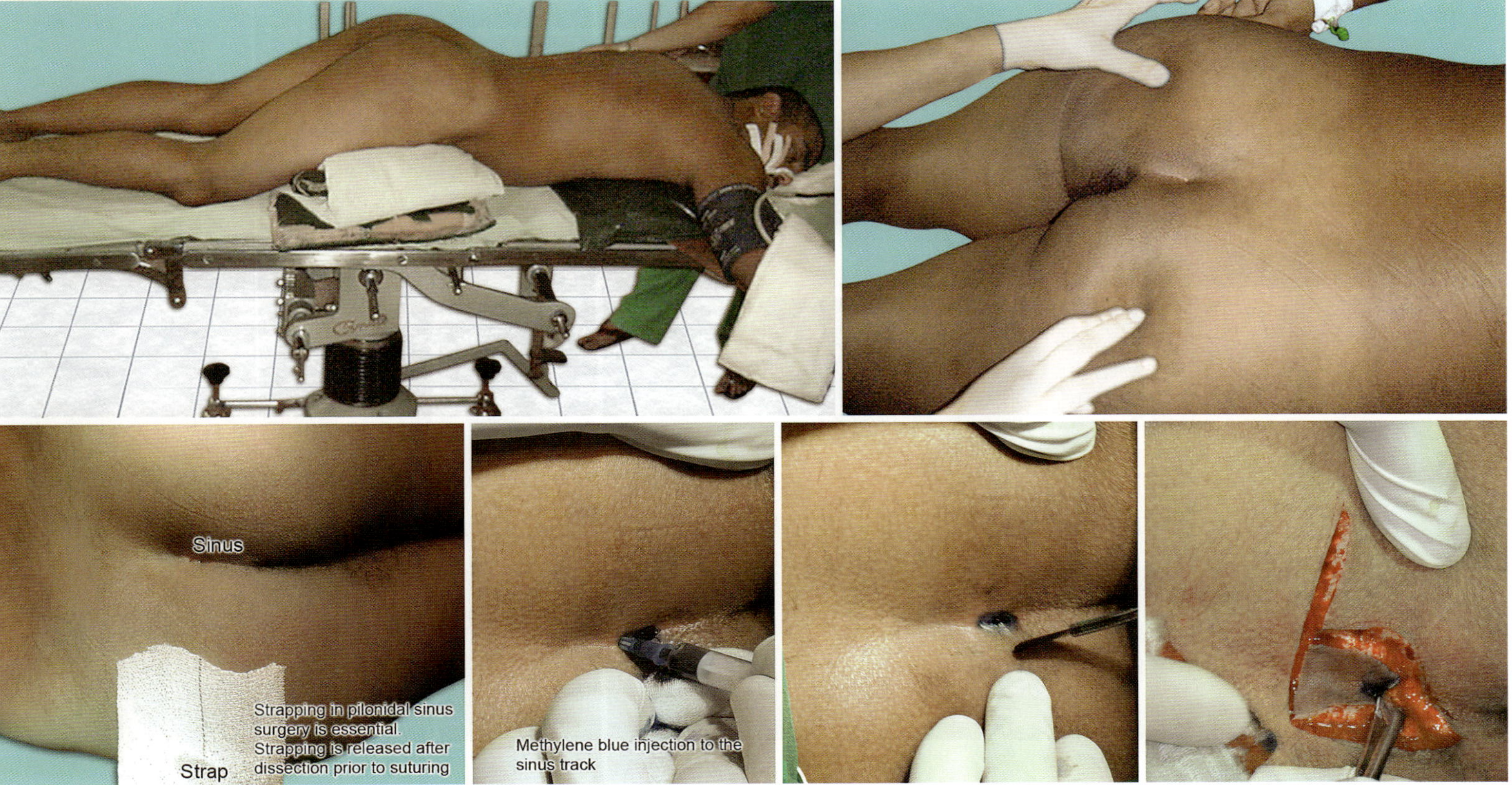

Fig. 26-37: Pilonidal sinus—operative jackknife position; making incision for the same.

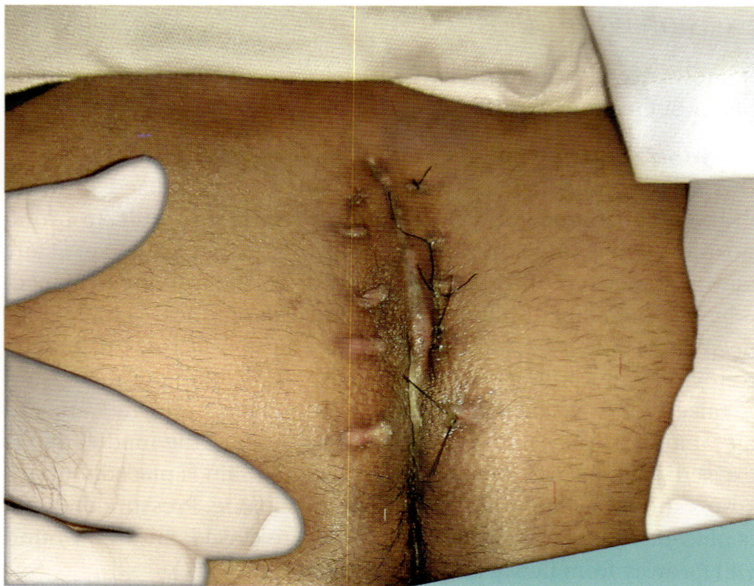

Fig. 26-38: Excision and primary suturing of the pilonidal sinus. It has got high recurrence rate as scar formed here is in the midline.

While elevating the flap monopolar cautery should be avoided or used only with care; bipolar cautery is better. No. 15 blade or fine scissor is always better to retain the blood supply of the flap. Suction drain is placed underneath. Buttock straps should be released before suturing. Subcutaneous absorbable sutures are placed. First sutures should be placed over the angles and then other sutures. Pressure dressing is placed **(Figs. 26-42 to 26-44)**.

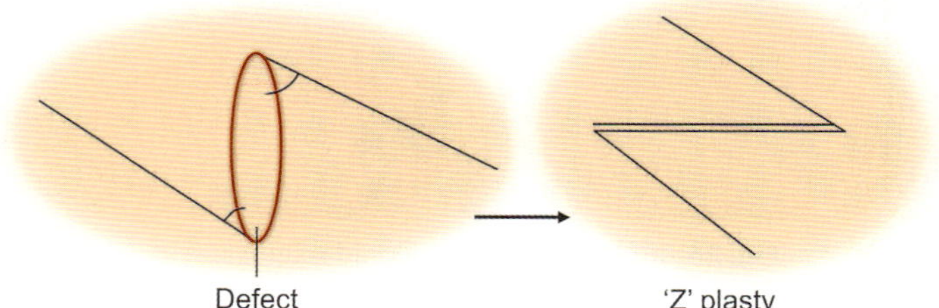

Fig. 26-39: Incision and mobilisation for Z plasty.

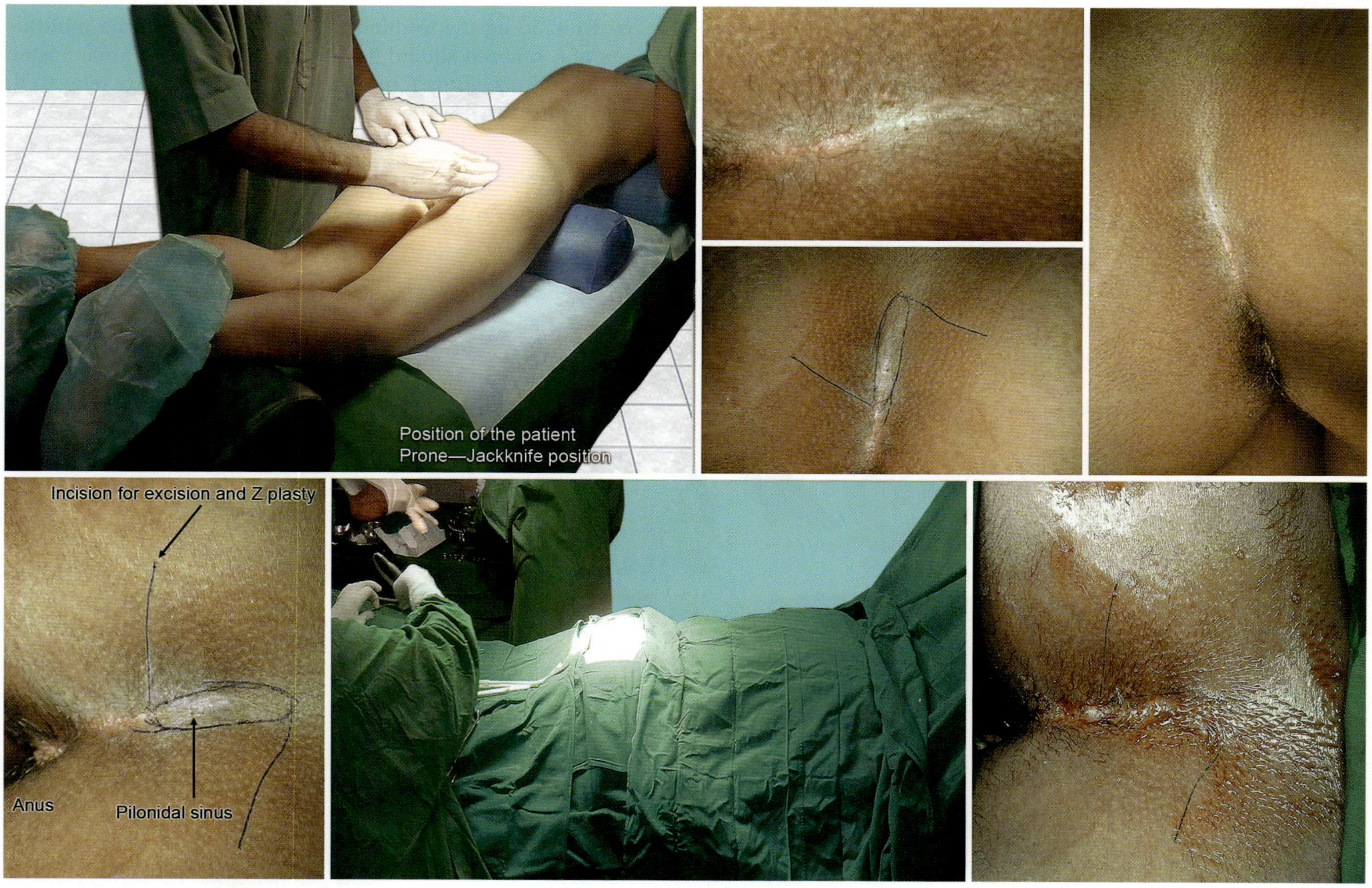

Position of the patient
Prone—Jackknife position

Incision for excision and Z plasty

Anus

Pilonidal sinus

Figs. 26-40(1)

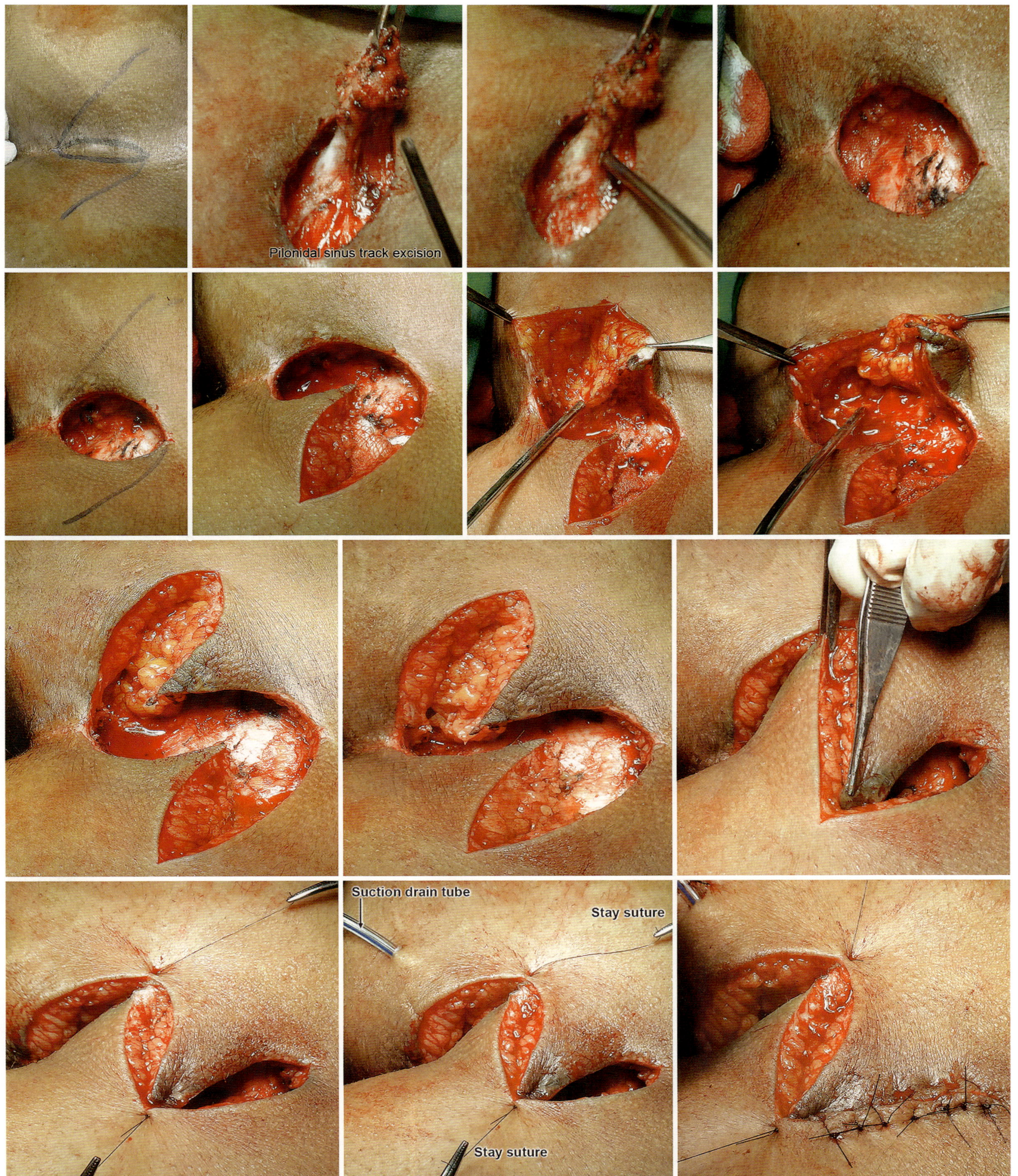
Pilonidal sinus track excision
Suction drain tube
Stay suture
Stay suture

Figs. 26-40(2)

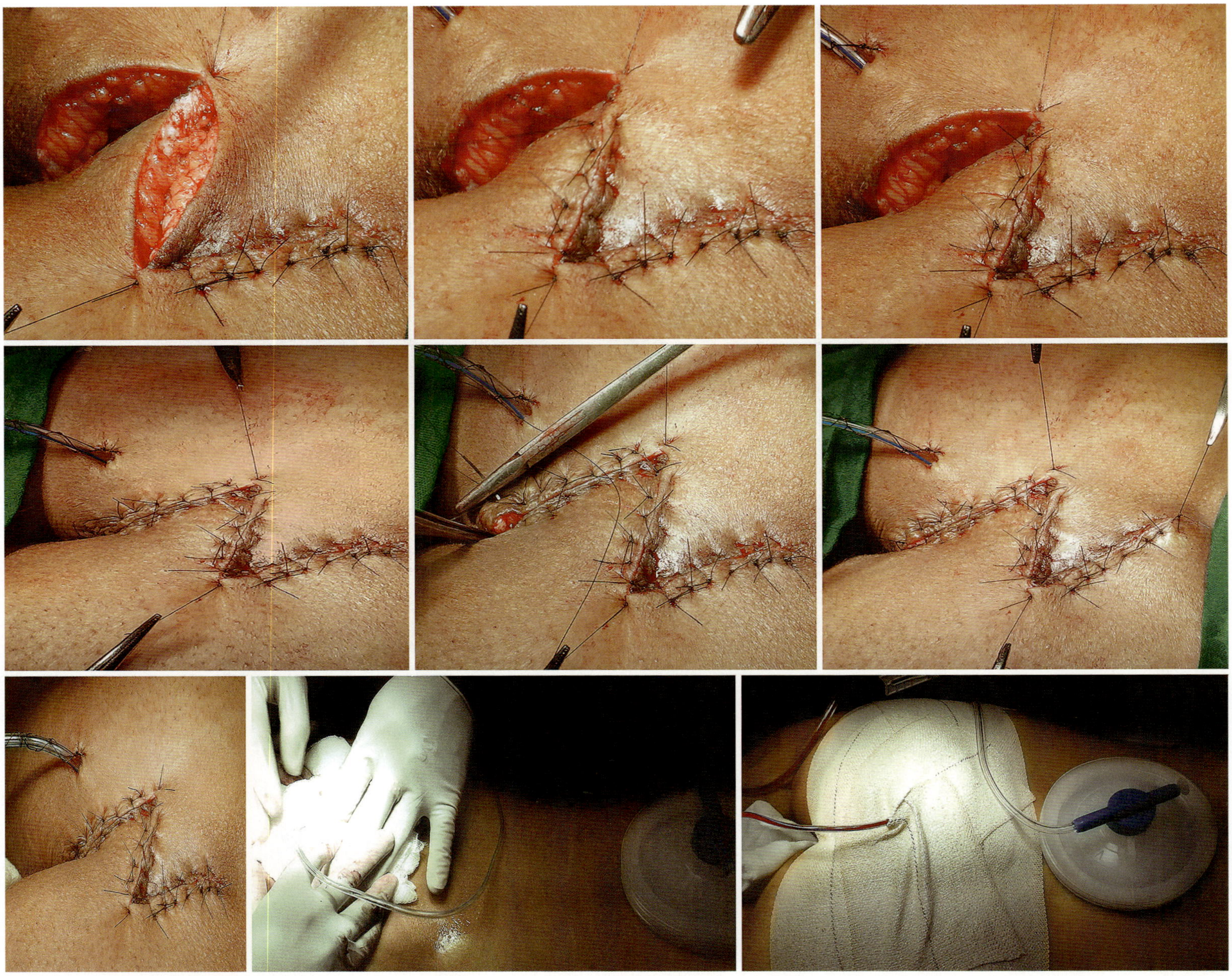

Figs. 26-40(3)

Figs. 26-40(1 to 3): Technique (Steps) in 'Z' plasty—done for pilonidal sinus. It gives good result. Multiple Z plasties are also used.

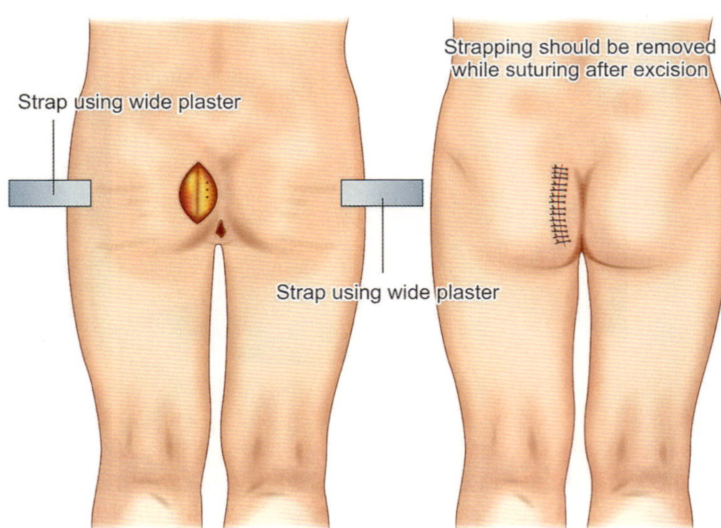

Fig. 26-41: Karydakis excision.

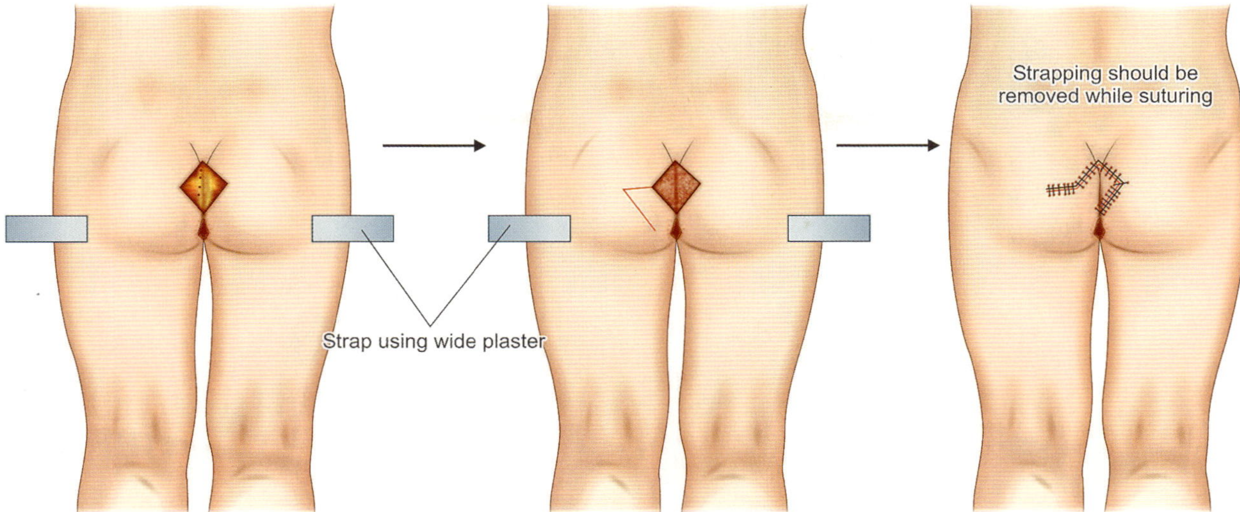

Fig. 26-42: Limberg-rhomboid flap used for pilonidal sinus.

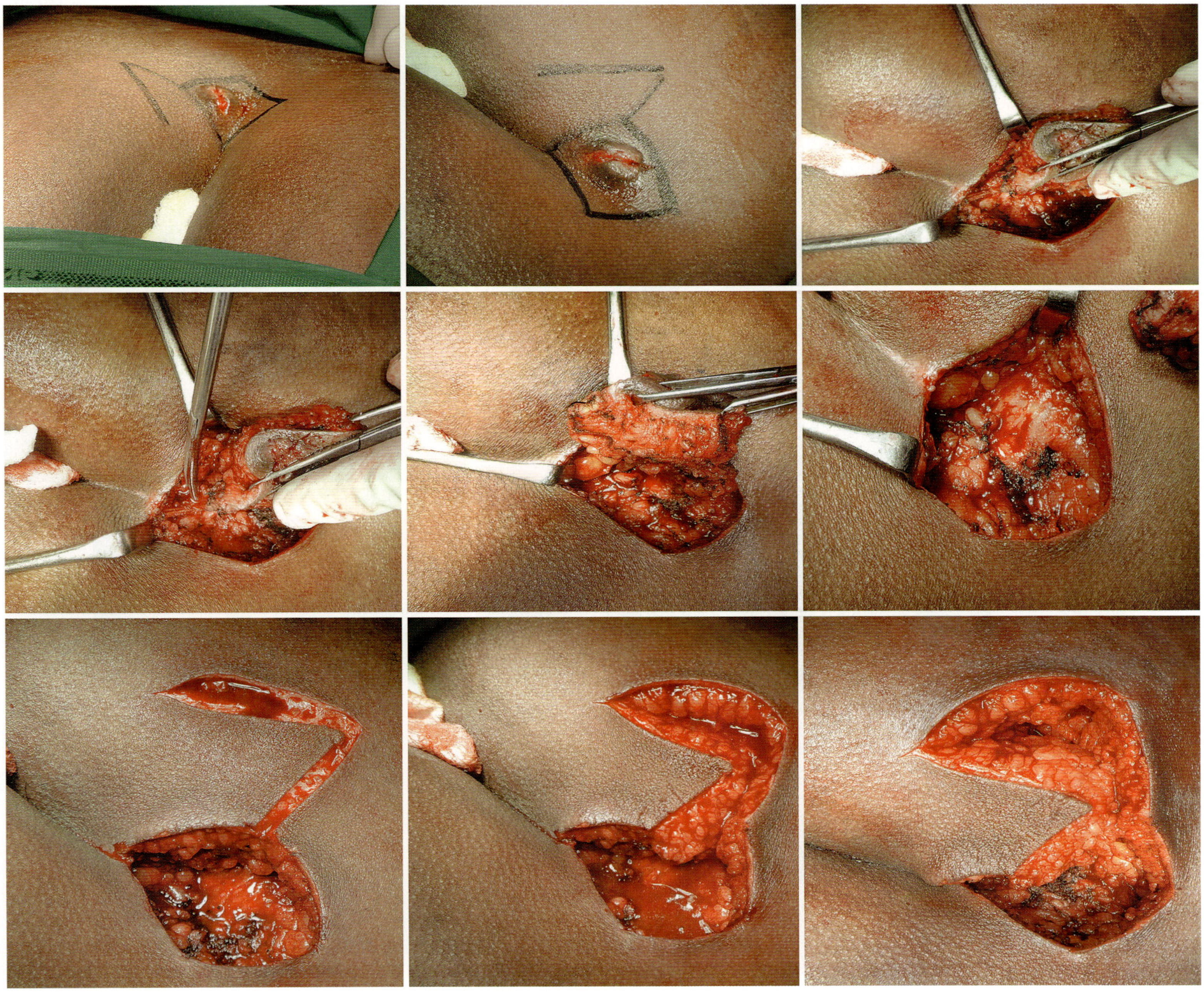

Figs. 26-43(1)

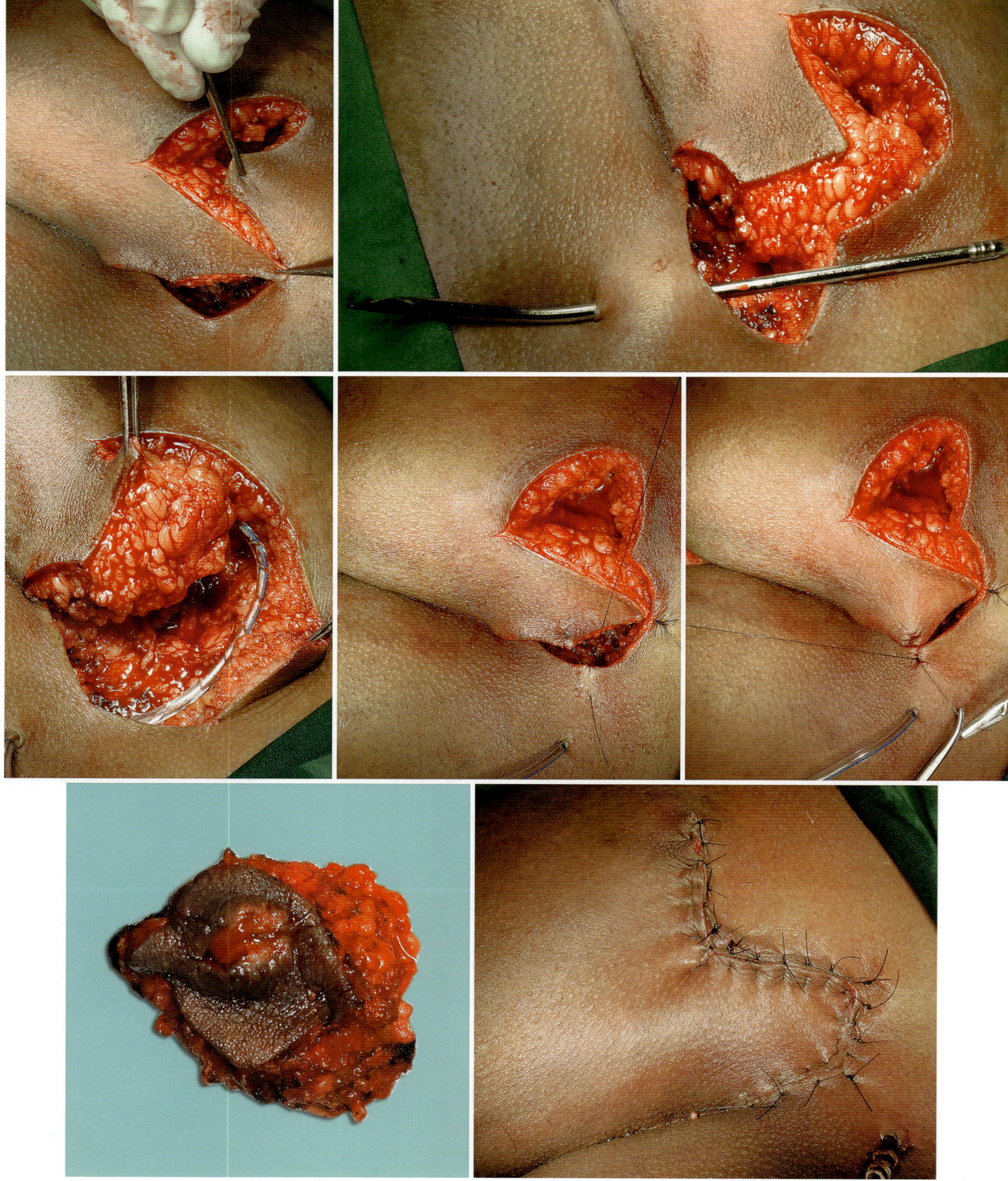

Figs. 26-43(2)

Figs. 26-43(1 and 2): Rhomboid flap for pilonidal sinus.

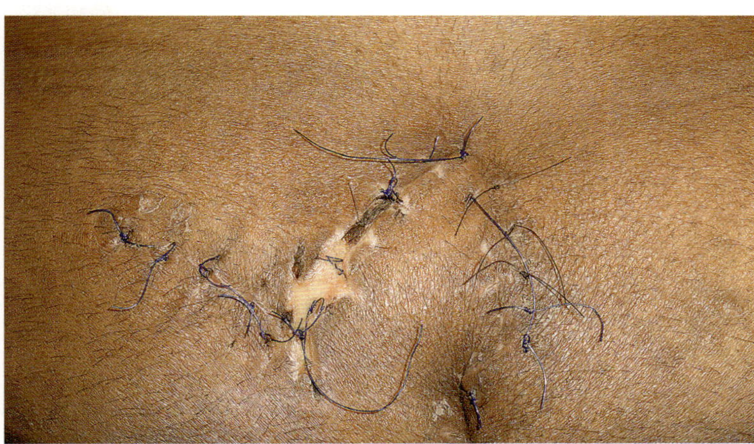

Fig. 26-44: Rhomboid flap after healing—scar will not be in midline.

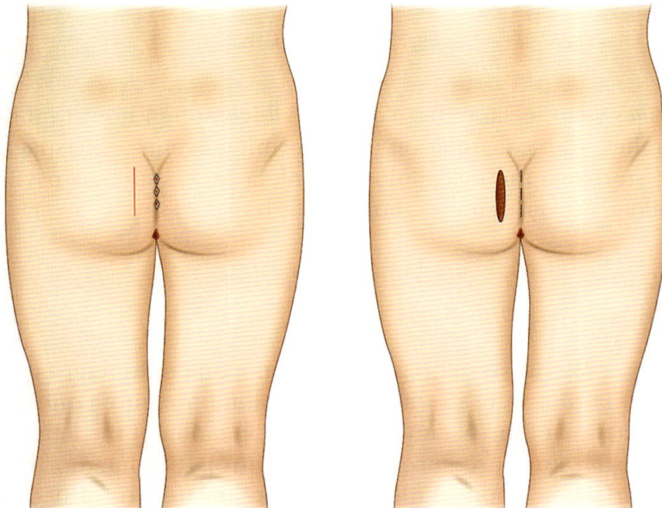

Fig. 26-45: Bascom technique.

Bascom Technique

It is the excision of the pilonidal sinus through lateral approach—is a good method. Through a lateral incision or multiple small lateral incisions 2–4 mm sized sinus is approached and pus is drained; hairs are removed with only minimal excision of sinus. Cavity walls are not excised. Lateral small wounds are either sutured or left open for spontaneous healing. Procedure is done under general/local anaesthesia in prone Jackknife position. After cleaning and draping, small pits in the midline primary site are approached through tiny 3 mm diamond incisions and skin is excised. A probe is passed through one of these opened pits to identify the side towards which sinus tracks. A vertical 3 cm incision is made in the paramedian area deep enough to reach the sinus cavity. All unhealthy tissues including track and hairs are removed. Thorough wash is given. Fibrofatty flap is rotated towards midline. In modified Bascom technique this rotation is not done. Tiny diamond midline wounds are closed with subcuticular non-absorbable sutures. Lateral wound is left open to granulate on its own **(Fig. 26-45)**.

V-Y Gluteal Advancement Flap

V-Y gluteal advancement flap is useful in recurrent and wide area involvement.

Lahey and Cattell's Method

Lahey and Cattell's relaxing skin incisions on one buttock is done to relieve tension on main wound sutures with later closure of secondary wounds by sutures or advancement.

Davies and Starr Buttock Skin Flap Rotation

Davies and Starr buttock skin flap rotation into the defect and secondary defect is closed at a later period.

After complete excision of entire sinus, wound is left open to granulate and heal by epithelialisation with regular dressings.

Buie's Marsupialisation

Buie's marsupialisation of the sinus track, 1944—after making incision on the sinus track, edge of the laid opened area is sutured to the skin edge all round using silk or vicryl. This reduces healing time and promotes healing.

Lord and Millar's Limited Excision

Lord and Millar's limited excision of primary track for 0.5 cm depth with removal of tuft of hairs, debris and unhealthy granulation tissue using tiny brush and nylon bristle.

Excision with Primary Suturing

Excision with primary suturing is done only when disease is confined to midline; but creating a midline scar increases the chances of recurrence as hairs can penetrate midline scar easily.

Excision of all Granulation Tissues

Excision of all granulation and unhealthy tissues from both primary and secondary sinuses with *deroofing* and allowing it granulate and heal by secondary intention. It is better than primary closure. Problem is healing takes 6–8 weeks and creates wide scar which can breakdown. Present principle is to avoid any midline scar in pilonidal sinus surgery.

Injection of Phenol to the Track

Injection of phenol to the track destroys the epithelium after removal of the tufted hairs. Phenol is allowed to be in contact with epithelium for 3 minutes to create a blanch in the track orifice.

Non-operative Treatment/Prevention of Recurrence after Surgery

Regular shaving of natal cleft to have meticulous hair control and proper perineal hygiene is essential. *Laser, depilatory cream, electrolysis* are other methods used.

Causes for High Recurrence Rate

Improper removal (technical); overlooking of existing diverticulum; entry of new tuft of hairs; breakage of scar. *Note:* Condition has got high recurrence rate (20%).

TREATMENT OF HAEMORRHOIDS

Parts of piles—pedicle (internal) and external component **(Fig. 26-46)**.

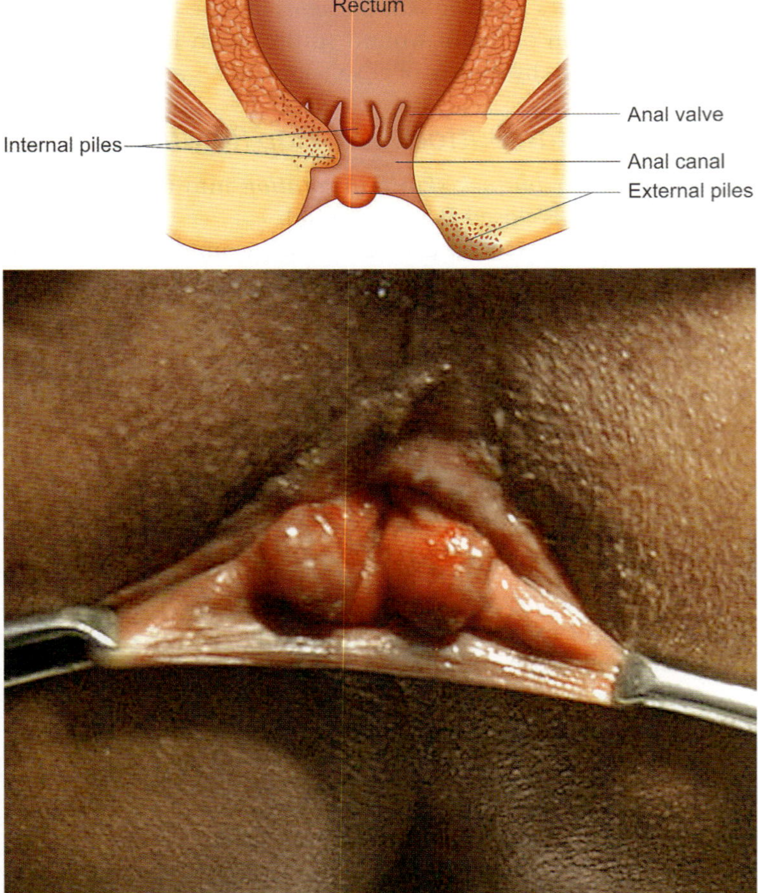

Fig. 26-46: Parts of piles—internal and external.

Preventive Therapeutic/Curative

Preventive	Parasurgical
Diet—more fibre/liquid Laxatives	♦ Sclerotherapy ♦ Banding ♦ Cryotherapy ♦ Infrared coagulation (IRC) ♦ Laser therapy ♦ Doppler-guided haemorrhoidal artery ligation (DGHAL)
Medical	*Surgical*
Local applications; Sitz bath, diet, laxatives, drugs—analgesics	♦ Open haemorrhoidectomy ♦ Closed haemorrhoidectomy ♦ Stapled haemorrhoidopexy ♦ Anal stretching—Recamier, Lord's

Non-operative

Sitz bath—means the patient has to sit in a wide tub containing warm water with the anal region dipped in water for 20 minutes, 2–3 times a day. This reduces the oedema, pain and promotes healing. Specialised toilet trays are available which can be placed over the commode on which patient can sit for Sitz bath **(Fig. 26-47)**.

Local applications to reduce pain, itching and oedema can be used. Antibiotics, laxatives, anti-inflammatory drugs are beneficial. Other different methods are—fibre diet 35 gram/day, plenty of water; *fibre alternatives* can be used to supplement a high-fibre diet; squatting position may reduce the incidence of piles; plenty of liquid intake; *laxatives* such as lactulose solution which soften bowel motions and relieve the constipation (bulk-forming agents, e.g. ispaghula husk, sterculia, methylcellulose); bulk laxatives such as psyllium mucilloid, Konsyl or polycarbophil may be necessary.

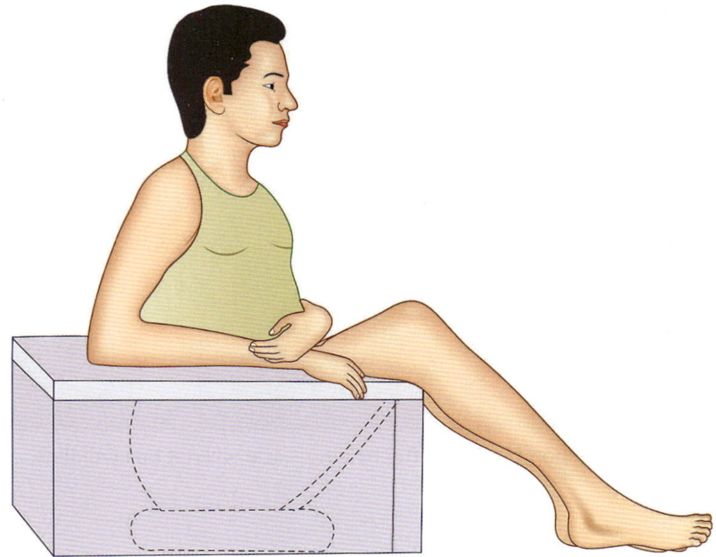

Fig. 26-47: Sitz bath.

In Case of Inflamed, Permanently Prolapsed, Oedematous Piles

Initially, manual stretching of the anal canal sphincter is tried. In 1968, Lord proposed that increased anal pressure contributes the formation of the haemorrhoids; so dilatation of the anal canal reduces the anal pressure thereby controls the haemorrhoids. A constriction to the outlet is present in 3rd and 4th degree haemorrhoids which is relieved by gentle firm stretching of the lower rectum and anal canal until constriction disappears. Eight fingers are passed as high as possible to achieve this. This prevents congestion of anal cushions and relaxes the anal sphincter, as a result of which the prolapsed piles gets reduced—*Lord's dilatation (8 fingers)*. Once oedema subsides, in 1–2 weeks, formal procedure is done. **Complications of anal dilatation—**incontinence—rectal—usually temporary; infection; haemorrhage/haematoma; prolapse rectum **(Fig. 26-48)**.

Note: Lord's dilatation is presently not accepted.

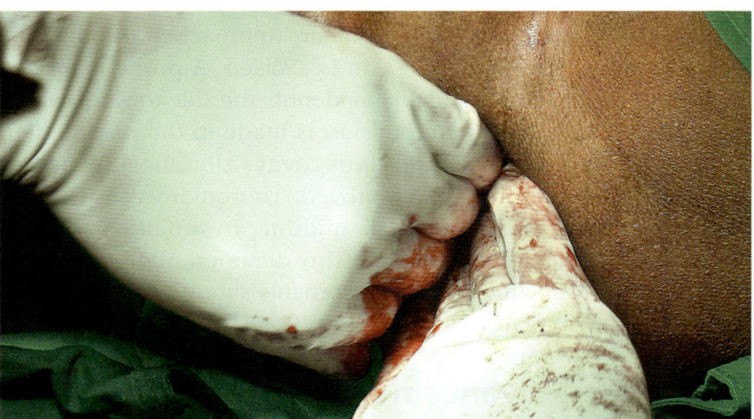

Fig. 26-48: Lord's dilatation—it is 8 finger dilatation of the anal canal; it may cause anal incontinence.

Injection—Sclerosant Therapy

It is done in first degree and early second degree piles (internal)—outpatient procedure. Using proctoscope and Gabriel syringe, 3–5 mL of 5% phenol in almond oil is injected into the submucosal plane just above the anorectal ring to the pedicle. All three piles can be injected separately—3–5 mL to each site in single sitting. Technique can be repeated after 6 weeks. This technique is not done in the presence of sepsis or prolapse. The drug causes fibrosis in the submucosal region (sclerosis leading to mucosal fixation on to deeper planes and occlusion of lakes) which in turn causes fixation of the anal cushions so that it do not prolapse, causes strengthening of the vessel wall and obliteration of the vessel lumen. It is quick and painless; gives 95% cure rate in first degree piles; done on OP basis. *Contraindications are*—thrombosed/prolapsed piles, presence of proctitis/fissure/fistula-in-ano, pregnancy and diabetes mellitus. Sclerotherapy has not gained popularity, oily solution is difficult to handle and inject. *Complications*—recurrence (15%), pain in the hypochondrium due to entry of drug into the portal system, tenesmus, mucosal sloughing/ulceration, submucosal abscess, anal canal pain, anal stricture.

Inadvertent deep injection can precipitate pelvic abscess, prostatitis, impotence, rectovaginal fistula **(Fig. 26-49)**.

Other sclerosants used are—Sodium tetradecyl sulphate (setrol); polidocanol 3%; aluminium potassium sulfate/tannic acid (Japan).

Rubber Band Ligation/Banding

It is done for second degree piles. It causes ischaemic necrosis and piles fall off. At one time only two piles can be banded. Repeat banding can be done only after 3 weeks. Band should be placed 2 cm above the dentate line. Usually 2 bands are used for pile mass to take care of breakage. Tissue sloughs off in 1–2 weeks leaving an ulcer which heals by scarring. Equipment is inexpensive, simple to perform; done without anaesthesia on OP basis; results are consistent, stops bleeding and tackles the prolapsing of anal cushion. Different Band ligators are available now. Barron's (1962), McGivney ligator, McGown one hand ligator, etc. **(Fig. 26-50)**.

It is contraindicated in fissure/fistula/proctitis.

Complications: If applied low into skin it causes severe pain; discomfort; secondary haemorrhage; ulceration; thrombosis; slippage; sepsis.

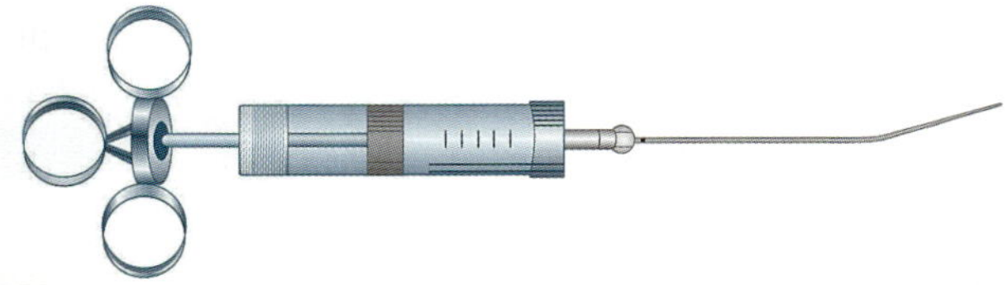

Fig. 26-49: Gabriel syringe—it is used for injection sclerotherapy for internal piles using 5% phenol in almond/olive oil (almond/vegetable oil acts as a vehicle which holds phenol for long period of action). It is a stainless steel syringe with two metallic finger brims near the proximal end. One more metallic finger brim is present on the proximal end of the piston to place thumb while injecting.

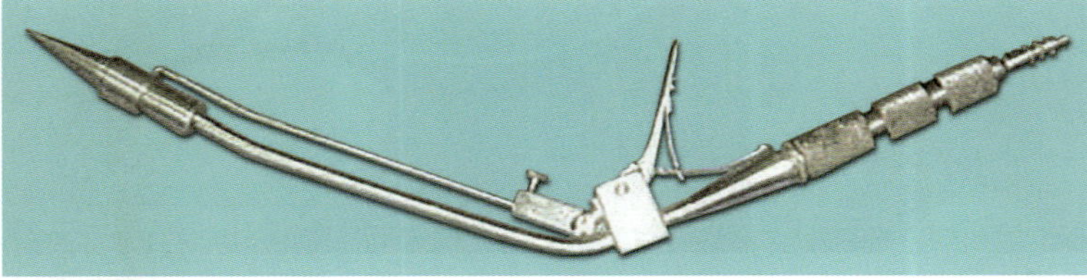

Fig. 26-50: Rubber band ligation instrument for first and early second degree piles.

Note:
Suction banding is used presently—Lurz Goltner suction ligator; O'Regan disposable suction banding system. Suction is used to suck the internal pile into the banding gun.

Cryosurgery

Using nitrous oxide (-98°) or liquid nitrogen (-196°), extreme cold temperature is used to coagulate and cause necrosis of piles which gets separated and falls off subsequently. It is relatively painless and can be done on OP basis. All masses can be tackled at one sitting. This is carried out with the help of a *cryoprobe.* Nitrous oxide is preferred since it produces adequate freezing. Nitrous oxide delivery system/cryoprobe does not require special rewarming circuit. Liquid nitrogen produces quick destruction and damage of sphincter muscle; also needs special rewarming circuit for its release and is costlier. Under lithotomy position, cryoprobe is applied in the longitudinal axis of internal pile above the dentate line; the pressure must be maintained above 700 lb continuously; rapid adhesion with freezing (white area formation on piles) occurs; traction and slight rotation in both directions is done to draw entire pile mass to come in contact with the probe; after entire tissue is frozen in 20–30 seconds, the probe is detached after warming (defrosting/thawing). Procedure is repeated on other pile masses **(Figs. 26-51 and 26-52)**.

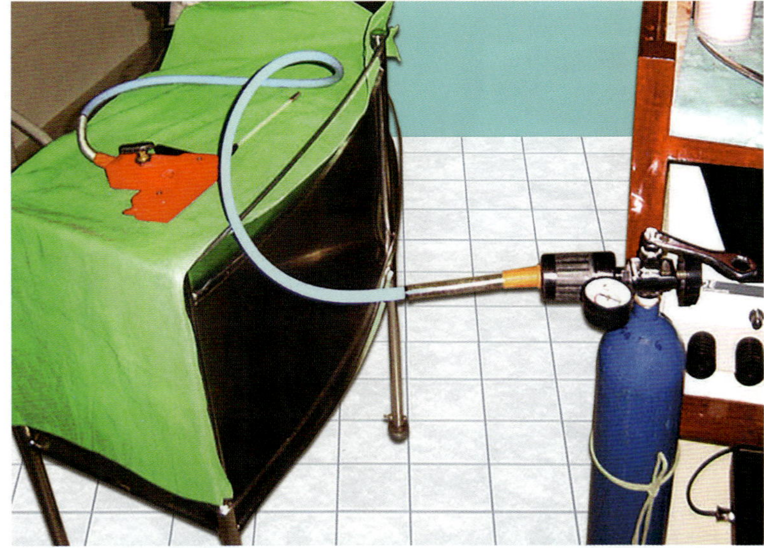

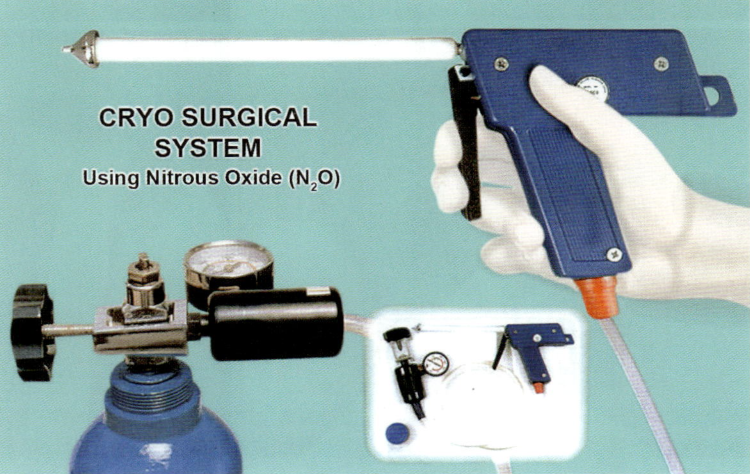

Fig. 26-51: Cryosurgery instrument set up for cryohaemorrhoidectomy.

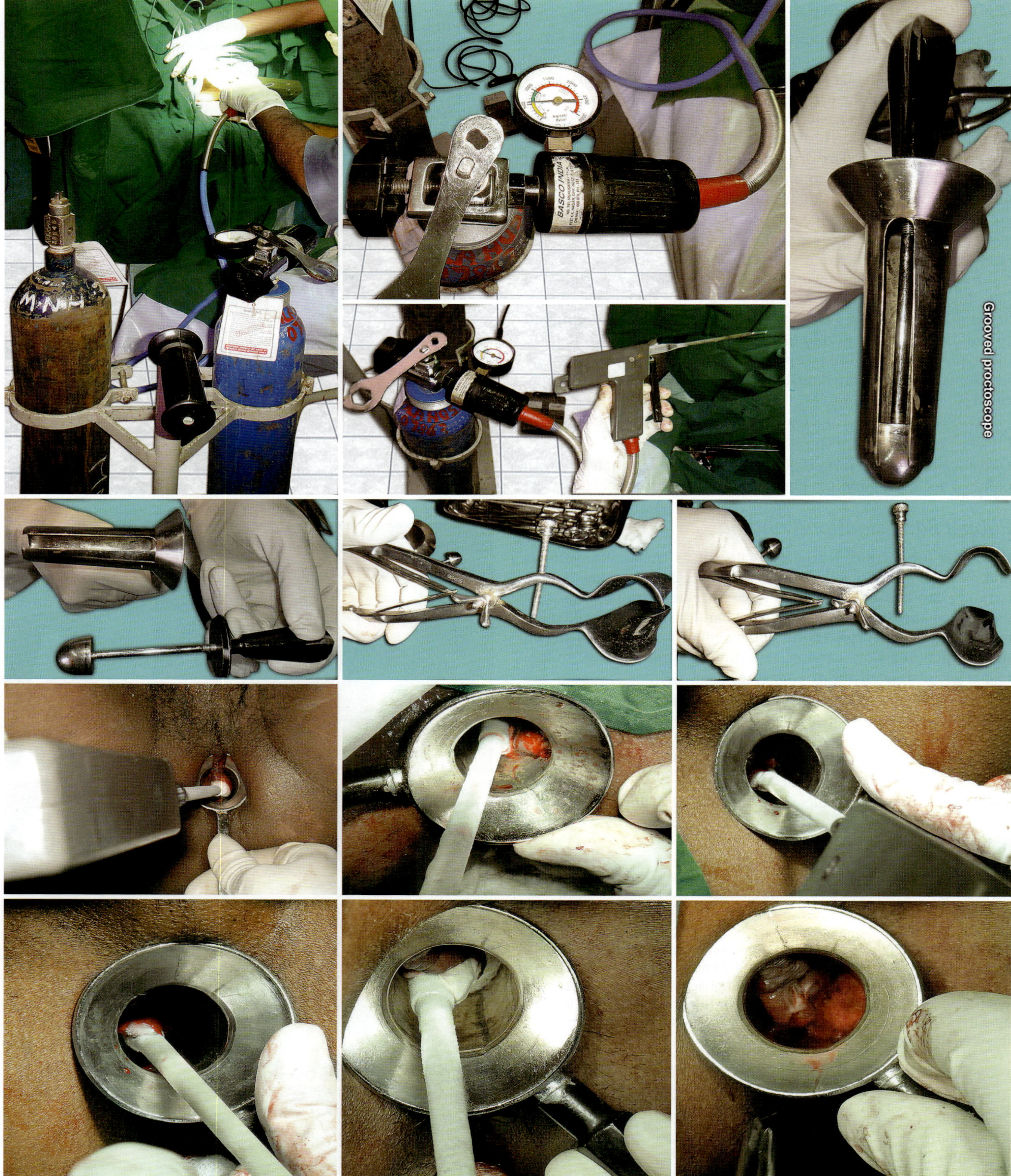

Fig. 26-52: Cryosurgery for piles.

Advantages: It is reasonably painless, simple, safe, can be done on OP basis, with less bleeding.

Disadvantages: It causes *profuse watery discharge*, itching, pain if skin is frozen; marked oedema of adjacent skin, incontinence occasionally.

Infrared Coagulation

Here heat is used to burn the piles so as to allow it to fall off. Pulses of infrared radiation are applied through a handheld applicator. The specific infrared wavelengths produce chemical changes that cause blood coagulation within the haemorrhoid itself, which causes the haemorrhoid to seal, shrivel, shrink or slough off. Source of infrared rays of 14 volt Wolfram halogen lamp with a gold plated reflector rays are transmitted from fibreoptic cable, which terminates in a probe or pistol for coagulation. In left lateral position, the probe is applied at the base of pedicle above the dentate line and bursts are given in clover leaf fashion. Timer is set at 2 secs giving a depth of 2 mm; total time taken is 2–5 minutes. It is done in first, second and third degree piles. It produces a discrete area of necrosis (coagulates tissue proteins and evaporates water from the cells), which heals to form a scar; reduces or eliminates blood flow through the haemorrhoid thereby shrinking it and mucosa becomes fixed to the underlying tissue. Often 3 or 4 sittings are needed at 1 month intervals. It does not cause non-contact coagulation; does not cause interference with electromagnetic devices such as pacemakers. It is *contraindicated* in external pile, proctitis. Long-term results are not good. Equipment is expensive; multiple sessions are needed **(Fig. 26-53)**.

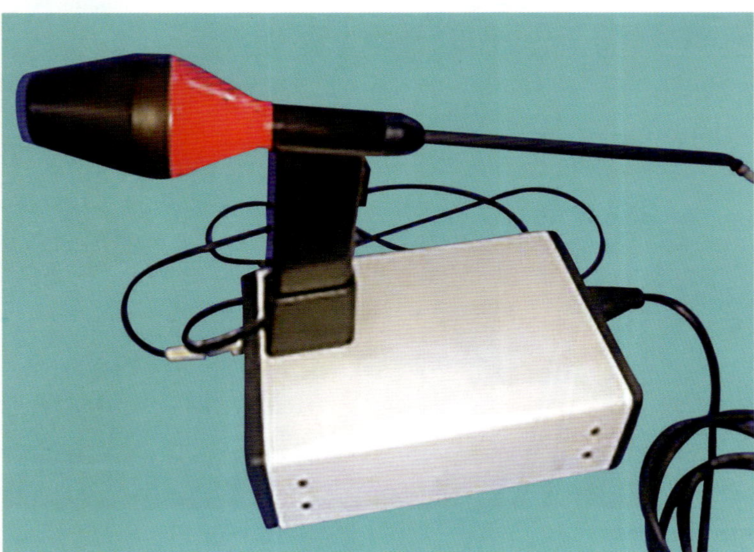

Fig. 26-53: Infrared coagulation device for piles.

Laser Therapy for Piles

It is used for third degree piles. Nd-YAG, diode and carbon dioxide lasers can be used but are expensive and tedious. The intense beam of light interacts with tissue and can be used to cut, coagulate or ablate the tissue, seal off nerves and tiny blood vessels. By sealing superficial nerve endings patients have minimum postoperative discomfort. Laser is used for dissecting and excising pile masses. It is done for internal haemorrhoids.

Advantages—less operative time; less intraoperative and post-operative bleed and pain; rapid healing; quick recovery; done under LA/SA; less complications; minimal pain, constipation and urinary retention.

Disadvantages—needs skill; sphincter should be taken care of; non-contact burning can occur; secondary haemorrhage can occur due to heat tissue destruction; and also injury to sphincter can occur **(Fig. 26-54)**.

Newer concepts in laser haemorrhoidoplasty: Now diode laser is used with different probe tip. Often it is combined with Doppler or Finger Guided Haemorrhoidal Artery Ligation (DGHAL/FGHAL) as hybrid procedure. Laser is haemostatic, less painful, bactericidal. It preserves the anal cushions physiology. Here diode laser energy is delivered into the haemorrhoidal mass allowing protein denaturation and fibrosis. Corpus cavernosum recti (CCR) vascular component of the anal cushions are addressed. Photocoagulation occurs due to protein denaturation which begins at 72.6°C till 132°C and photo vaporisation occurs when 1470 mm diode laser passes through pile mass with blood causing vaporisation of the water with shrinkage of tissues. Laser fibre here is conical with specialised curved probes through which fibre is passed through and makes fibre to protrude nearly 1 cm beyond. Total Joules used per pile mass should be within 200 Joules. At the point of entry 6 W, 1 second pulse; during activation 6–9 W, 3 seconds pulse. Point of entry of fibre is mucocutaneous junction. Half cut semilunar proctoscopy is used. Eye goggles should be worn. Red glow at the laser tip after entry is observed; it should not be more which means it is close to mucosa; and it should be very dim which means it is deep close to sphincter; both may get damaged if so. Tip should be in pile mass. Laser is activated slowly withdrawing from distal to proximal with rotation and fan-shaped movements. After withdrawal, ice packs are placed to prevent oedema formation for 10 minutes. Remaining pile masses and accessory pile mass is also dealt with similarly. FGDHL is added as hybrid procedure. Through cut proctoscopy, above the pile mass haemorrhoidal artery is felt and ligated using vicryl. Blaisdell or Farag's mucopexy can be added in bulky pile masses; it is done by taking three interrupted sutures through mucosa and submucosa above the dentate line to cause mucosal fixation.

Doppler-guided Haemorrhoidal Artery Ligation (DGHAL, Morinaga, 1995)

The DGHAL is an advanced instrument that works under Doppler-guided ultrasound. It is painless, 20-minute procedure that cures all degrees of haemorrhoids. It causes choking and blocking of the blood supply of piles. It is done using proctoscope with an incorporated Doppler probe (modified proctoscope with built in ultrasound transducer, light and special window echo sounder). This proctoscope is inserted and used to locate the haemorrhoidal arteries by an audible signal. Once located, a needle holder is inserted into the lumen of the proctoscope and the artery ligated with a 'figure of eight' absorbable suture into the submucosa. The procedure is repeated until no more Doppler signals are identified. It is the transanal dearterialisation technique.

Advantages: Anaesthesia is not needed; blood loss, pain, residual problems are minimal; done as day care surgery; early return for work; may be safe in diabetic, cardiac, old age patients, and in pregnancy. It is under trial and too early to confirm the efficacy.

Ultroid

It is monopolar, low voltage device having a generator unit, an attachable handle, single use sterile probes, a grounding pad,

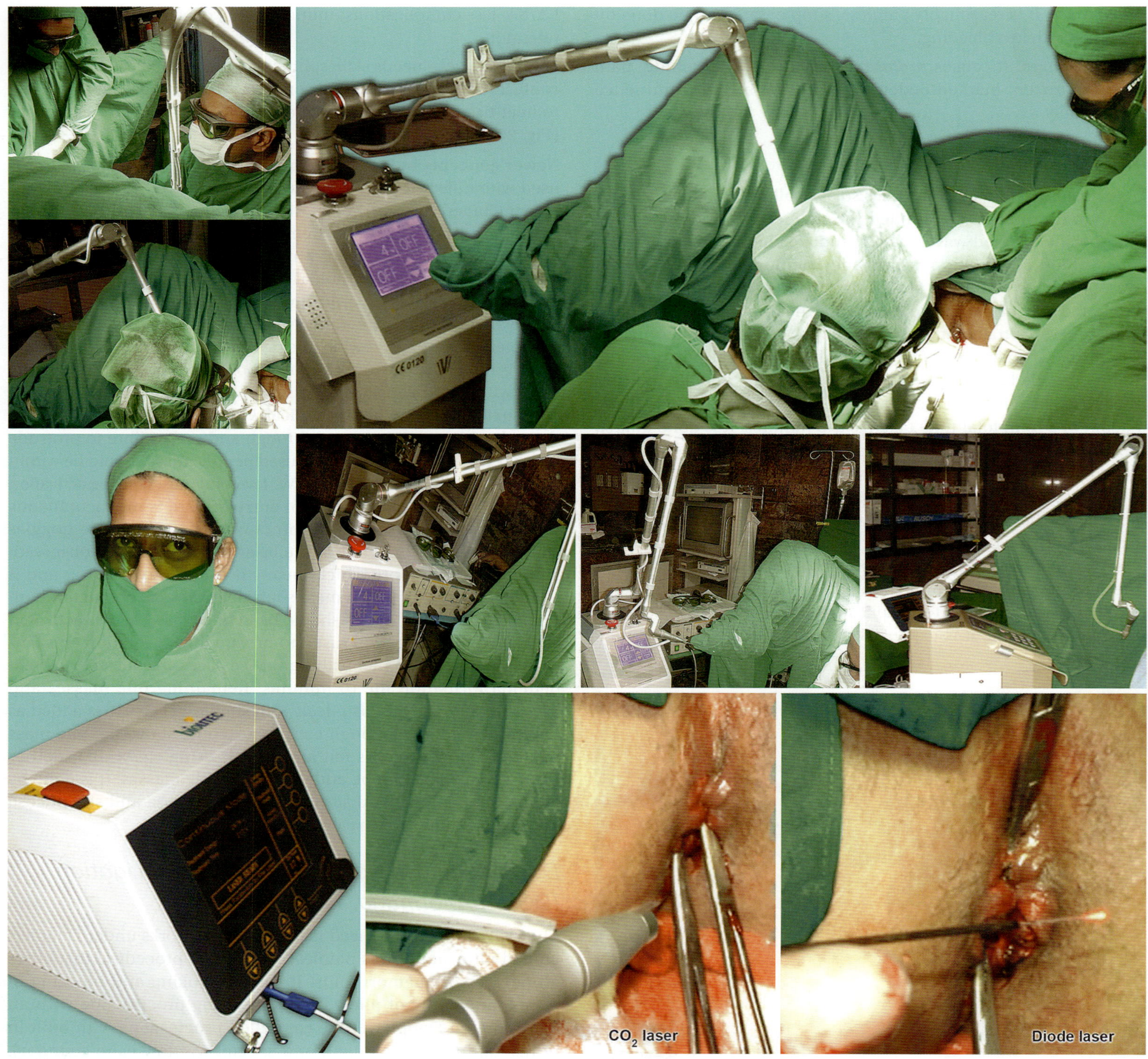

Fig. 26-54: Laser surgery for piles.

non-conductive anoscope. Device acts by production of sodium hydroxide at the negative electrode. Probe tip is placed at the apex of the pile mass above the dentate line and amperage of 6–16 mA is passed. Probe is kept in position for 10 minutes until sound ceases. Only one pile mass is treated during one sitting. Technique is not popular.

Stapled Haemorrhoidopexy (Antonio Longo, 1998)

It is circumferential excision of the mucosa and submucosa 4 cm above the dentate line using circular haemorrhoidal stapler passed per anally (MIPH—minimally invasive procedure for haemorrhoids; PPH—procedure for prolapse and haemorrhoids). It is not called as stapled haemorrhoidectomy as neither anal mucosa nor haemorrhoidal tissues are removed.

Advantages are—it is less painful; less blood loss; faster recovery; short hospital stay and equally efficacious. It is done only for prolapsed piles **(Fig. 26-55)**.

This procedure avoids wound in the sensitive perianal skin thereby reducing the postoperative pain. Under spinal or general anaesthesia, circular anal dilator is passed (CAD 33) into the anal canal; it is anchored to skin; circular purse string suture anoscope is passed into the anal canal. It can be rotated so the purse string suture can be placed 4 cm above dentate line on the rectal mucosa.

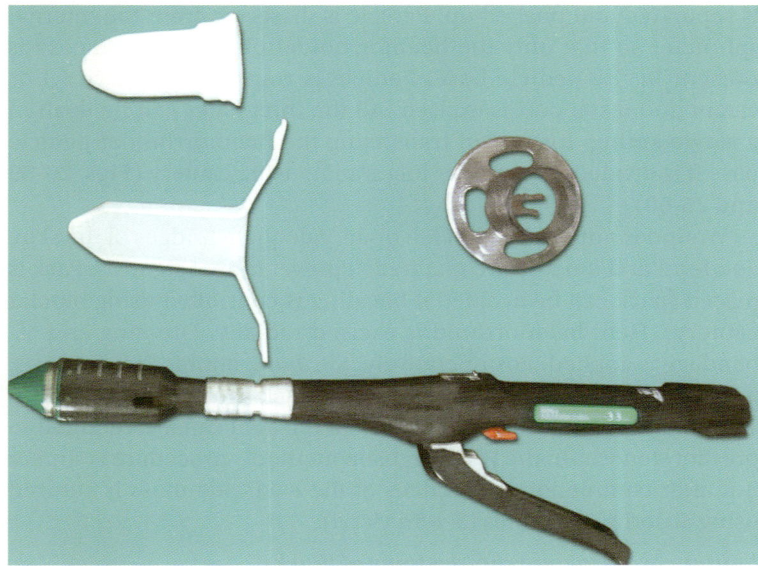

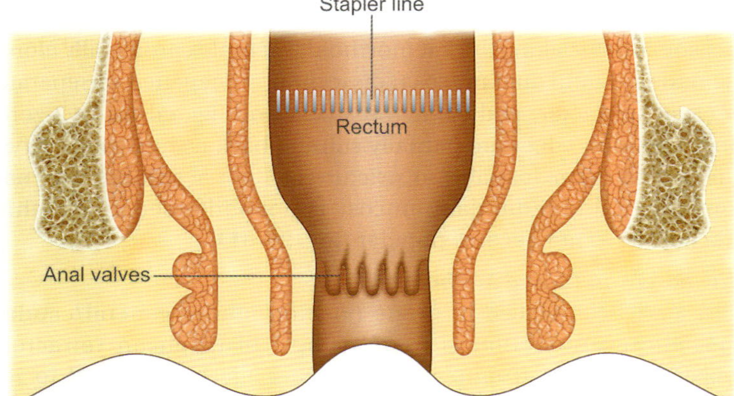

Fig. 26-55: Stapled haemorrhoidopexy. It is minimally invasive procedure for haemorrhoids. It is high mucosal rim excision including vascular pedicles using circular (single use) staplers. It is done for prolapsed piles.

Small bites which are close together are taken from mucosa and submucosa; muscle layer should not be included in the bites. There should not be any gaps or dog ears in the purse string suture. Fully opened stapler head is inserted into the anal canal and through the purse string beyond it; purse string is tied with one throw knot; two tiles of the suture are passed through the lateral channels in the head of the anvil with the suture threader. External knotting of the suture tails is done. Stapler is closed completely and fired with continuous downwards traction on the purse string suture. Using stapling gun, a unique circular stapler which reduces the degree of prolapsed piles by excising a circumferential strip of mucosa from the proximal anal canal. The strip of mucosa and submucosa is excised circumferentially above the dentate line. The veins leading to the haemorrhoids are thus incorporated in this excision. Activation of the gun also simultaneously recovers the cut mucosa and submucosa by stapling the edges together.

Disadvantages: Need for experience, as it is advanced surgical skill; costlier; may cause a full-thickness excision of the rectal wall; may injure the anal sphincter. *Improper purse string* can cause incomplete doughnut leading to severe haemorrhage.

Contraindication: Associated anorectal disease like fissure, fistula in ano; full thickness complete rectal prolapse; anal stenosis; gangrene and abscess, acute thrombosis.

Note:
Doughnut should be *sent for histology* for muscular layer; proper doughnut should not contain muscular layer.

Open Operative Methods: Still Gold Standard

Indications
Third degree piles; failure of non-operative methods; fibrosed piles.

Haemorrhoidectomy is the best treatment for haemorrhoids. The haemorrhoidectomy is performed using an open or closed technique. The open technique is commonly used in UK and is known as *Milligan-Morgan operation*. The *closed technique (Hill Ferguson)* is more popular in USA. Both involve ligation and excision of the haemorrhoid, but in the open technique the anal mucosa and skin are left open to heal by second intention, and in the close technique, the wound is sutured. Efficacy of surgery is 95% with 2–5% recurrence rate **(Figs. 26-56 and 26-57)**.

Methods

Ligation and excision of piles—commonly done procedures *(Milligan-Morgan) (Open method)*.

Under anaesthesia, in lithotomy position (Few advocate initially sphincter dilatation/stretching to reduce the postoperative pain.

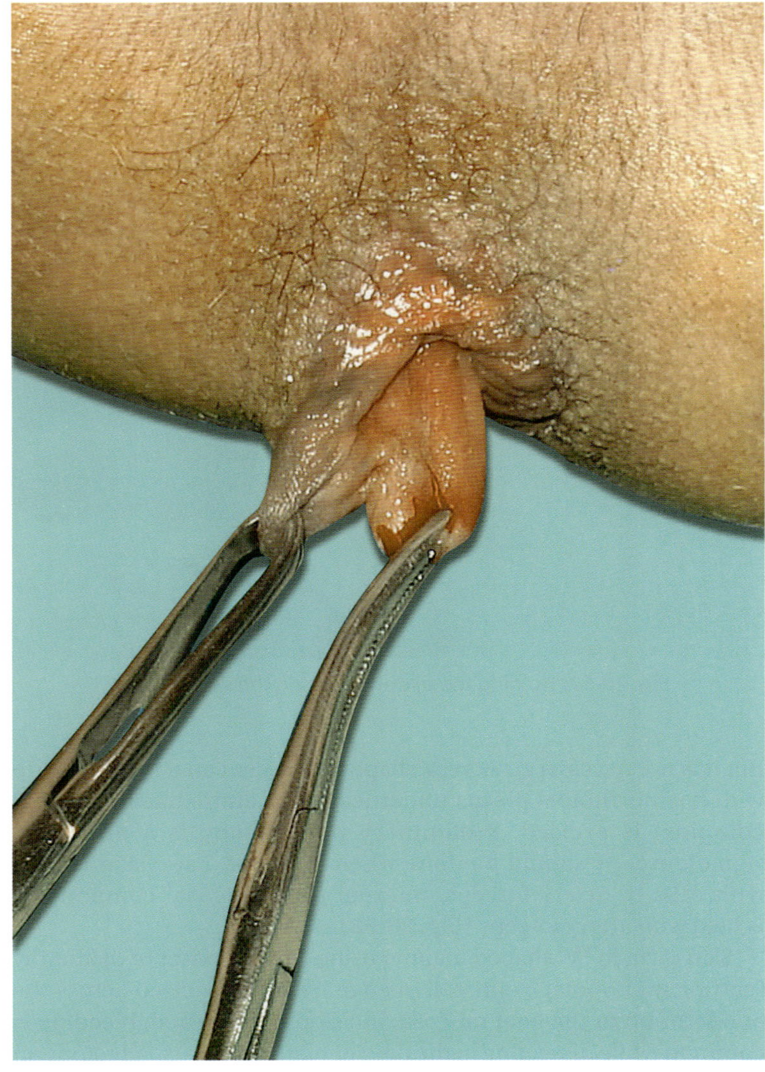

Fig. 26-56: Holding pile mass for haemorrhoidectomy.

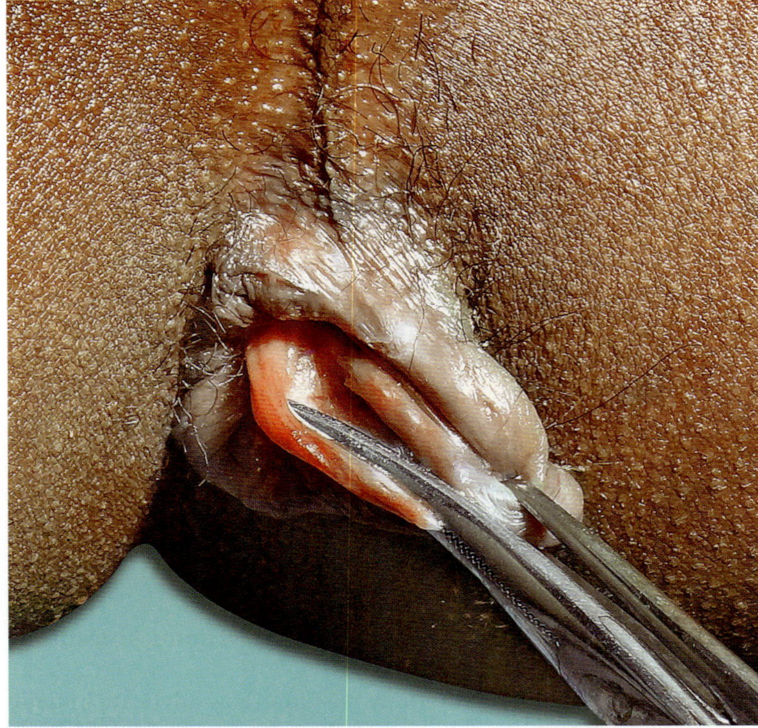

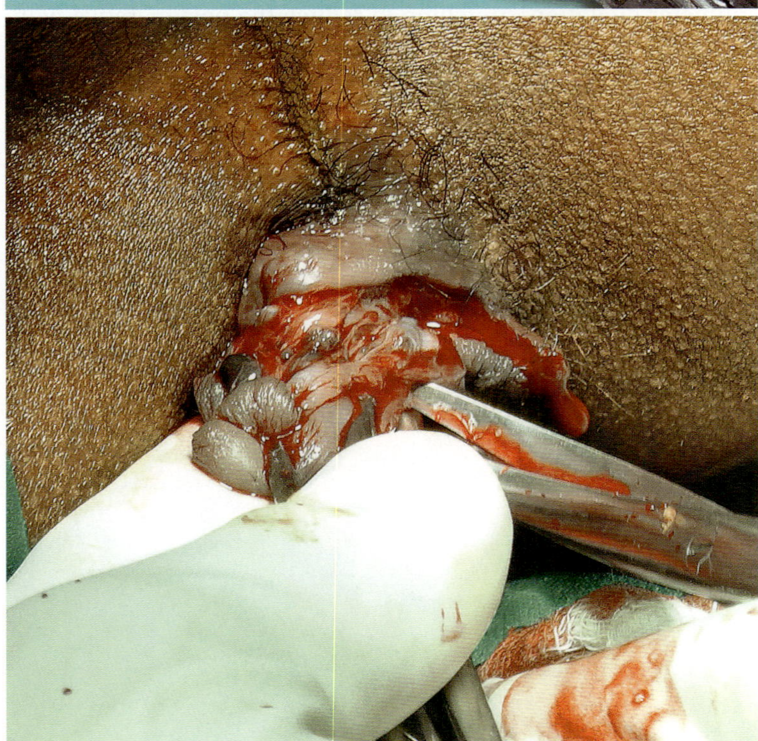

Fig. 26-57: Holding the pile and incising the skin—'V' cut.

But it is not necessary). Skin (V shaped), adjacent anal mucosal strip with haemorrhoidal plexus underneath (i.e. entire haemorrhoidal complex) is excised. Preliminary proctoscopy is a must and sigmoidoscopy should be done when in doubt. Later skin is held with Allis or artery forceps, internal pile (mucosal component) is held with artery forceps **(Fig. 26-58)**.

Skin is cut in "V' shaped manner using curved scissor or diathermy (cutting monopolar); entire skin edge has to be incised across the anoderm up to the anal mucosa; incision is deepened; bleeding is common while dissecting in the deeper plane which usually stops on its own but often may require bipolar cautery and internal sphincter is separated and pushed up. Pedicle is dissected from the internal sphincter so that only the haemorrhoidal plexus with mucosa is present in the pedicle base. Pedicle is transfixed with vicryl or catgut and distal part is excised. All the three piles can be dealt in a single sitting. Instead of transfixing the haemorrhoidal pedicle base it is divided after proper fulguration using cautery **(Figs. 26-59 and 26-60)**.

Wound is not sutured but left open. Adequate bridges of the skin, anoderm and mucosa are retained; it prevents anal stenosis. Pack is placed (pack can be avoided if bleeding is controlled using bipolar cautery). Here haemorrhoid is excised radially. Dressing and 'T' bandage is applied. Postoperatively, *Sitz bath*, antibiotics, laxatives, analgesics, local applications are given. Pack should be removed in 12 hours. Often few finger dilatation of the anal canal is required to prevent stenosis. In the Hill–Ferguson method—procedure is similar but after completion, skin edges of the each pile mass is sutured using absorbable sutures (3-zero vicryl).

Submucosal Haemorrhoidectomy of 'Parks'

Approach here is above the skin through submucosal plane. Radial incision is made along the haemorrhoidal complex proximally along the anoderm and anal mucosa; dissection is deepened to separate internal sphincter; pedicle is transfixed and ligated using 2-zero vicryl. Incision edges are partially sutured back using 3-zero vicryl. There is no tissue loss and so stricture will not occur; but external component and redundant mucosa is not addressed and so this procedure has not become popular **(Fig. 26-61)**.

Hill-Ferguson Closed Method

Here patient is placed in prone position, under general/caudal anaesthesia, retraction is done using Hill-Ferguson retractor. Incision is made around pile mass, pedicle is dissected to its proximal base; it is ligated with transfixation using 2-zero vicryl or silk; mucosa and anal skin is sutured using 3-zero vicryl/dexon after proper haemostasis using cautery.

Whitehead (Whitehead, England, 1882) Haemorrhoidectomy

Here mucosa is sutured to the anal canal above the pectinate line through a circumferential incision. It is technically difficult, causes mucosal ectropion (wet anus, Whitehead deformity). Procedure is rarely done now.

Management of Strangulated/Thrombosed/Gangrenous Piles

Here initially conservative treatment is done using warm water Sitz bath; antibiotics; elevation; bed rest; saline compression dressing; analgesics. This reduces the oedema and piles shrink. Later in 15–20 days haemorrhoidectomy is done. Doing haemorrhoidectomy immediately may precipitate portal pyaemia, bleeding and also increases risk of developing anal stricture **(Fig. 26-62)**.

Newer Methods

Using ultrasound or controlled electric energy (Harmonic scalpel or ligasure or laser), haemorrhoidectomy can be done with less postoperative pain. But tissue charring may precipitate secondary haemorrhage. Sentinel pile often requires excision under local anaesthesia **(Figs. 26-63 and 26-64)**.

Transanal suture mucopexy (Chivate, 2012): Chivate introduced transanal suture mucopexy in which ligation of mucosa, submucosa is done in two level circumferential locking sutures; one 4 cm

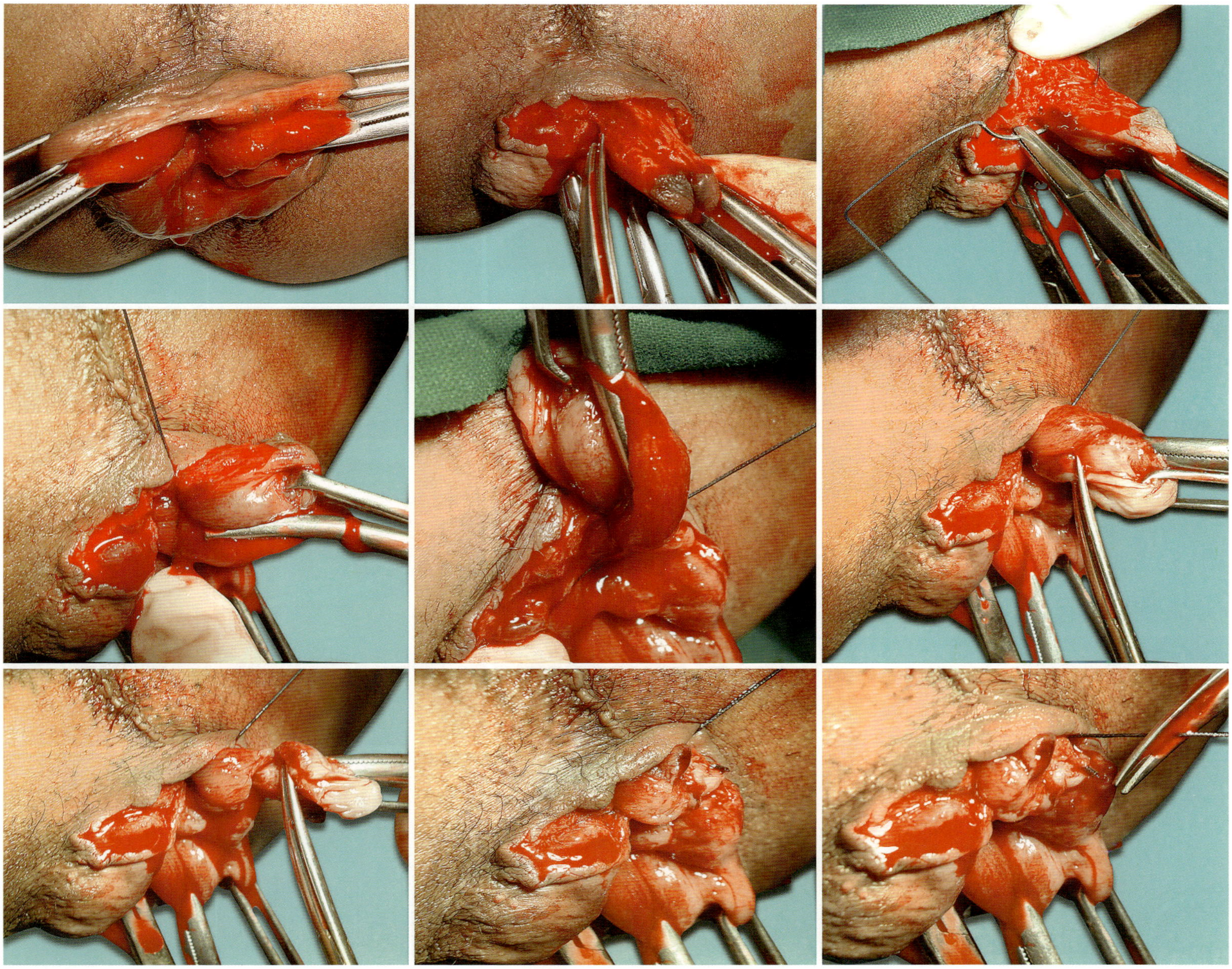

Fig. 26-58: Transfixation of the pile mass.

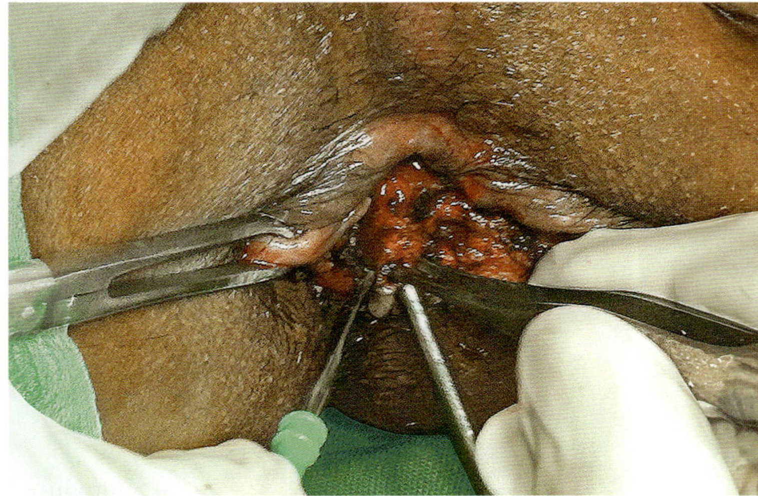
Fig. 26-59: Cautery can be used carefully for fulgurating pedicle and also to make skin incision.

proximal to dentate line, another circumferential suture line is done 2 cm proximal to dentate line using 2 zero vicryl/polyglactin suture. Postoperatively pain is less and less chances recurrence and incontinence. Concept here is—lowered anal cushions which is abnormal is restored to their original positions and ligation of blood flow to anal canal and cushions. It is effective in grades III and IV haemorrhoids. It is done in jackknife position or lithotomy position.

Postprocedure Complications

Pain—due to spasm, nerve irritation, muscle injury; retention of urine—commonest—50%.

Reactionary or secondary haemorrhage—secondary haemorrhage is more problematic as infected friable granulation tissues will bleed torrentially and it is not possible to cauterise or ligate the bed; blood transfusions is often required; antibiotics, inflating the balloon of a 30 French Foley's catheter inside the canal is tried.

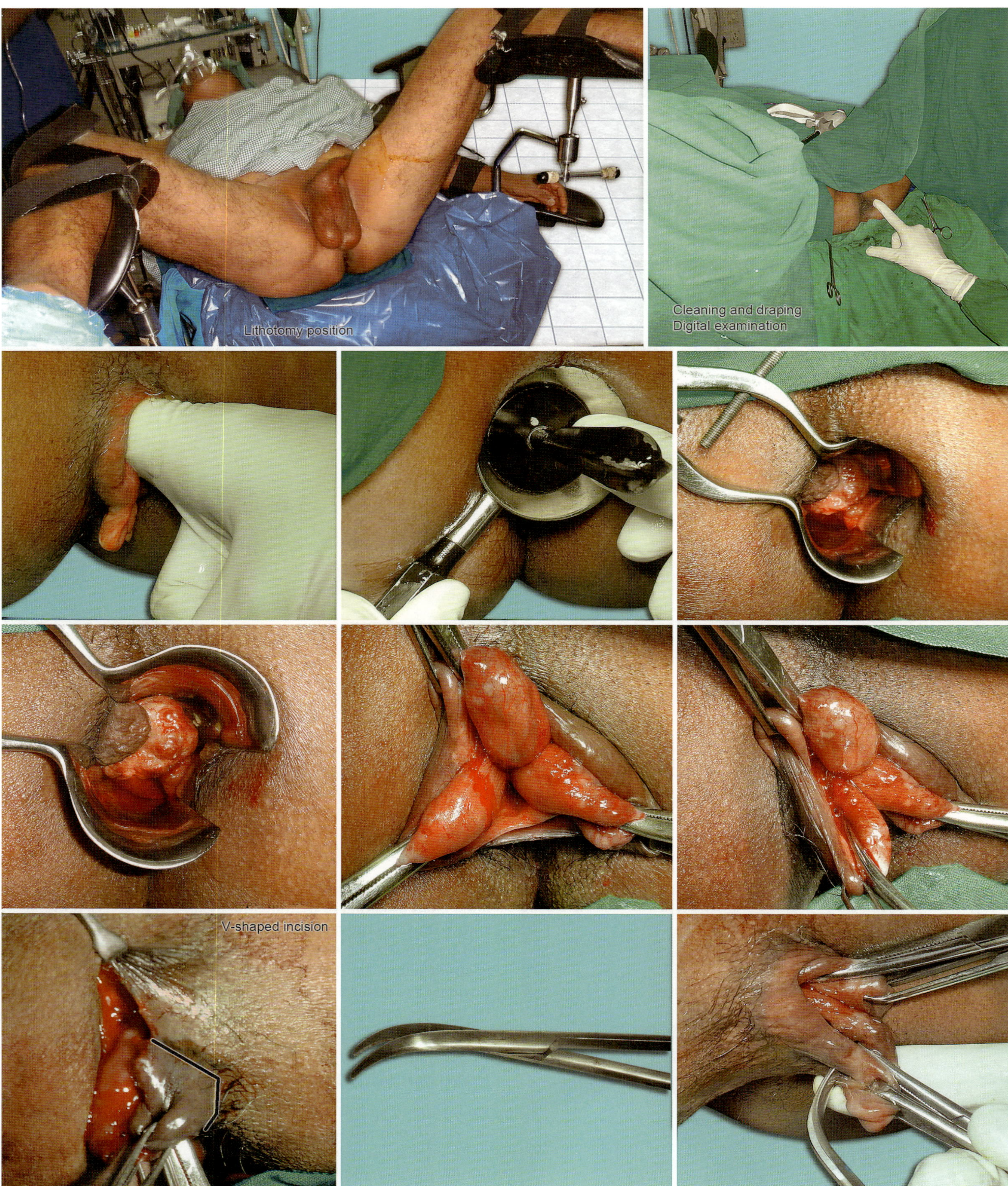
Lithotomy position
Cleaning and draping
Digital examination
V-shaped incision

Figs. 26-60(1)

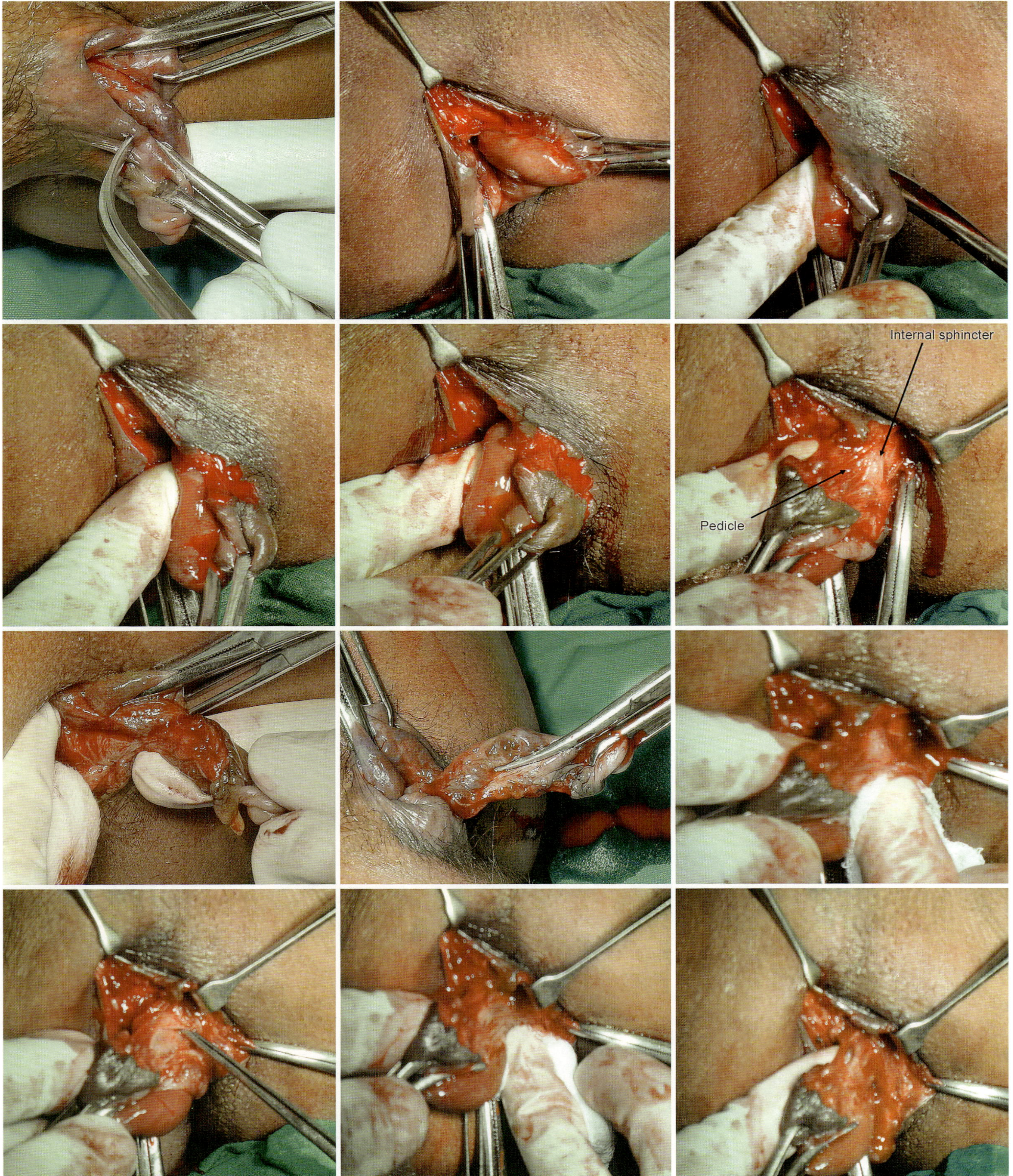

Figs. 26-60(2)

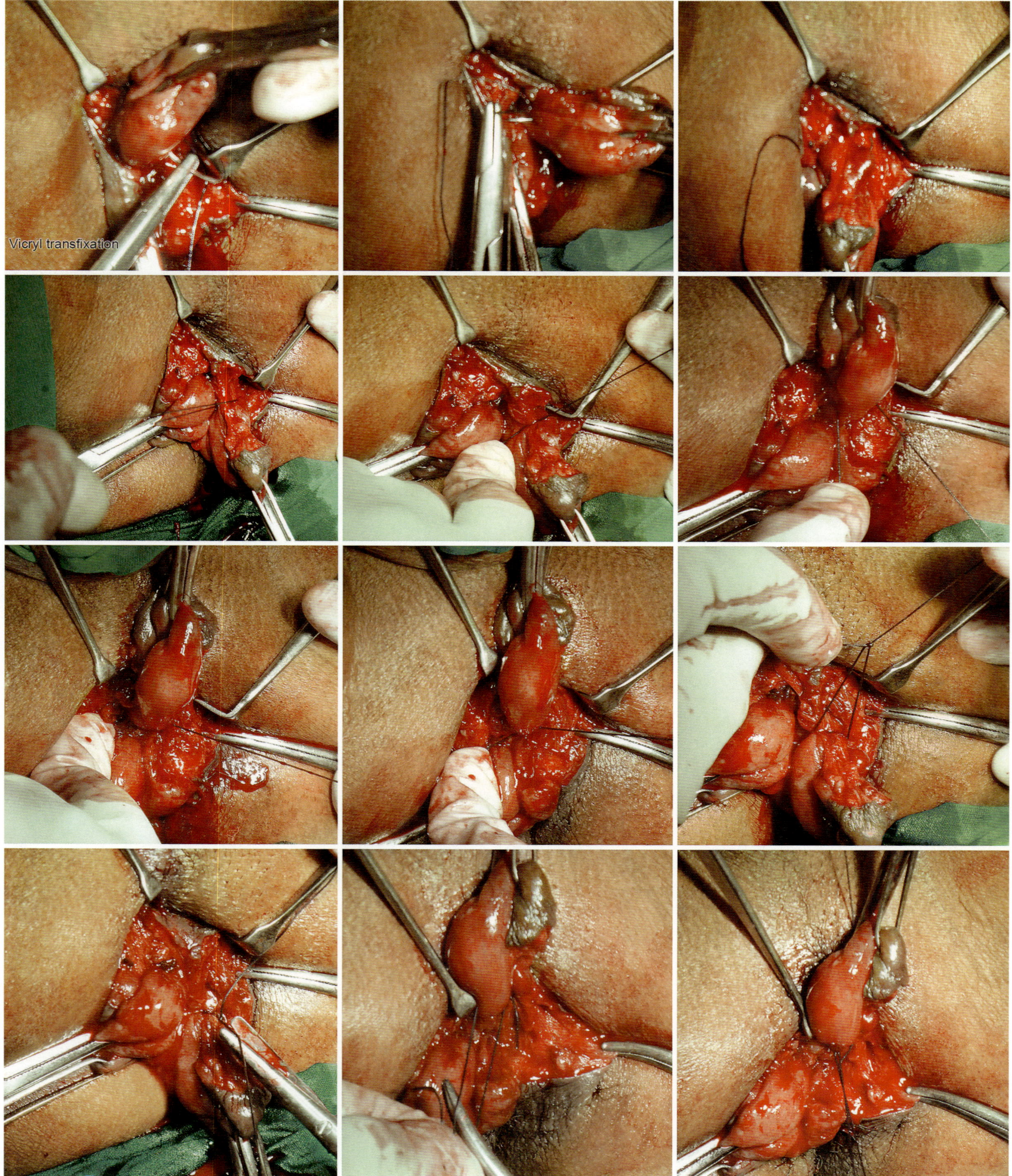

Figs. 26-60(3)

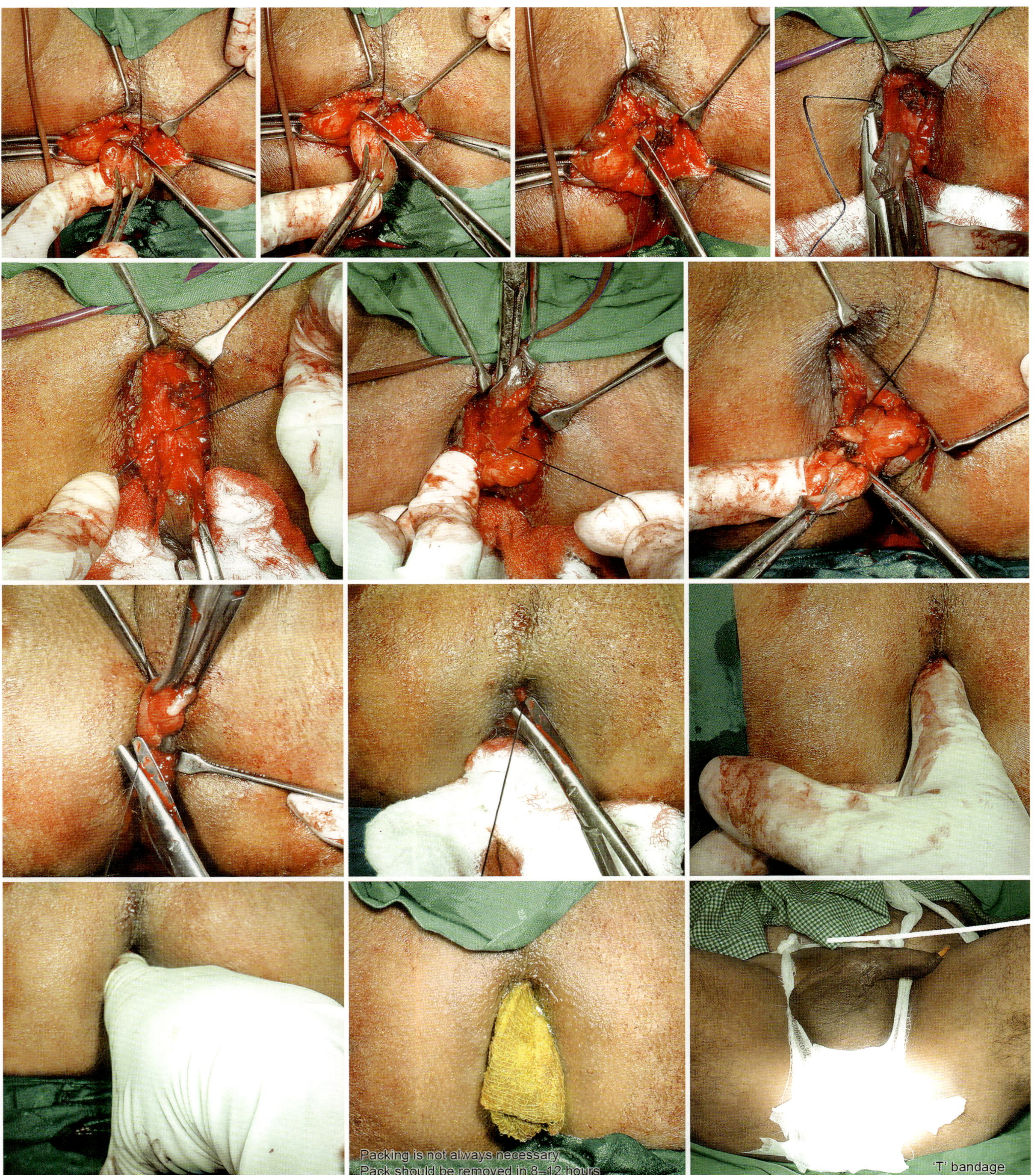

Figs. 26-60(4)

Figs. 26-60(1 to 4): During haemorrhoidectomy, skin part is held with Allis forceps; internal pedicle is held with artery forceps. A 'V' cut is placed over the outer skin up to mucocutaneous junction. Dissection is deepened to visualise the internal sphincter. Once pedicle is dissected, it is transfixed using vicryl suture material. Distal tissue is excised. Technique is repeated on other sites also.

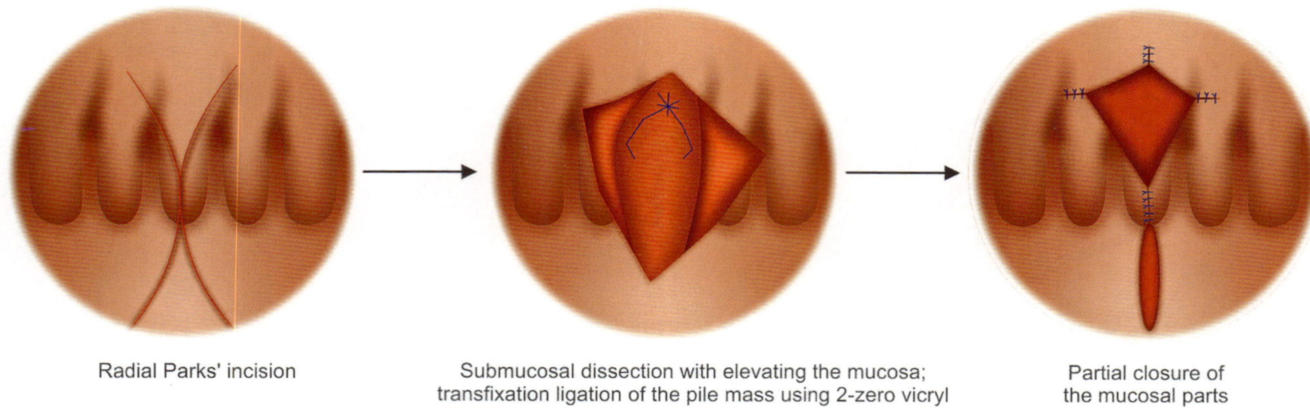

Fig. 26-61: Parks' submucosal haemorrhoidectomy.

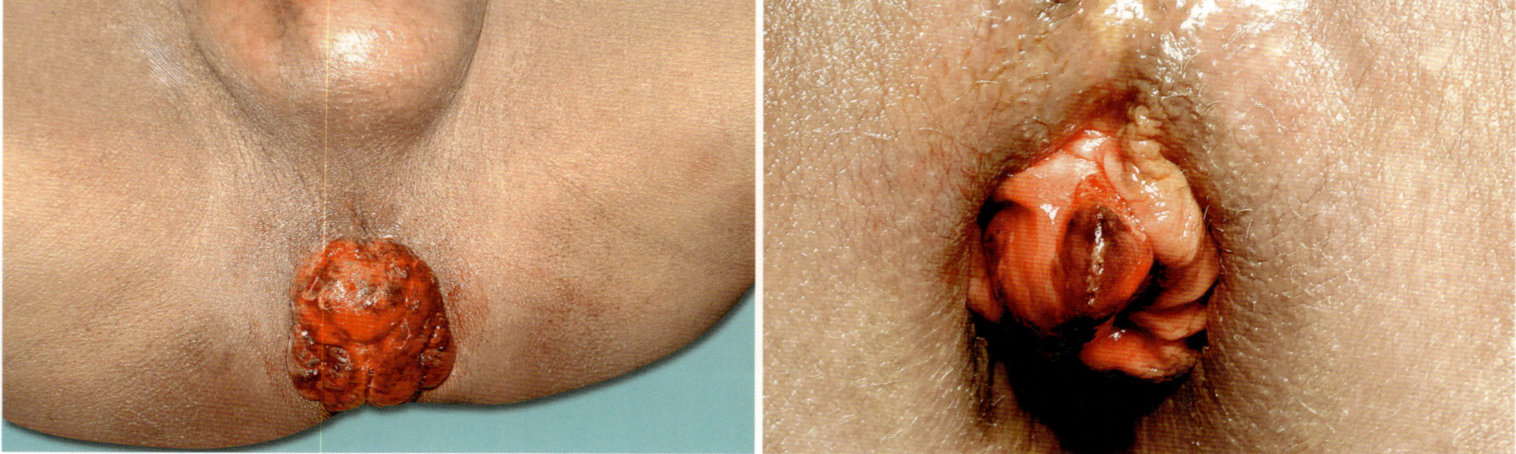

Fig. 26-62: Prolapsed thrombosed pile. It needs initial conservative treatment and later definitive treatment. Anal sphincter stretching may be useful.

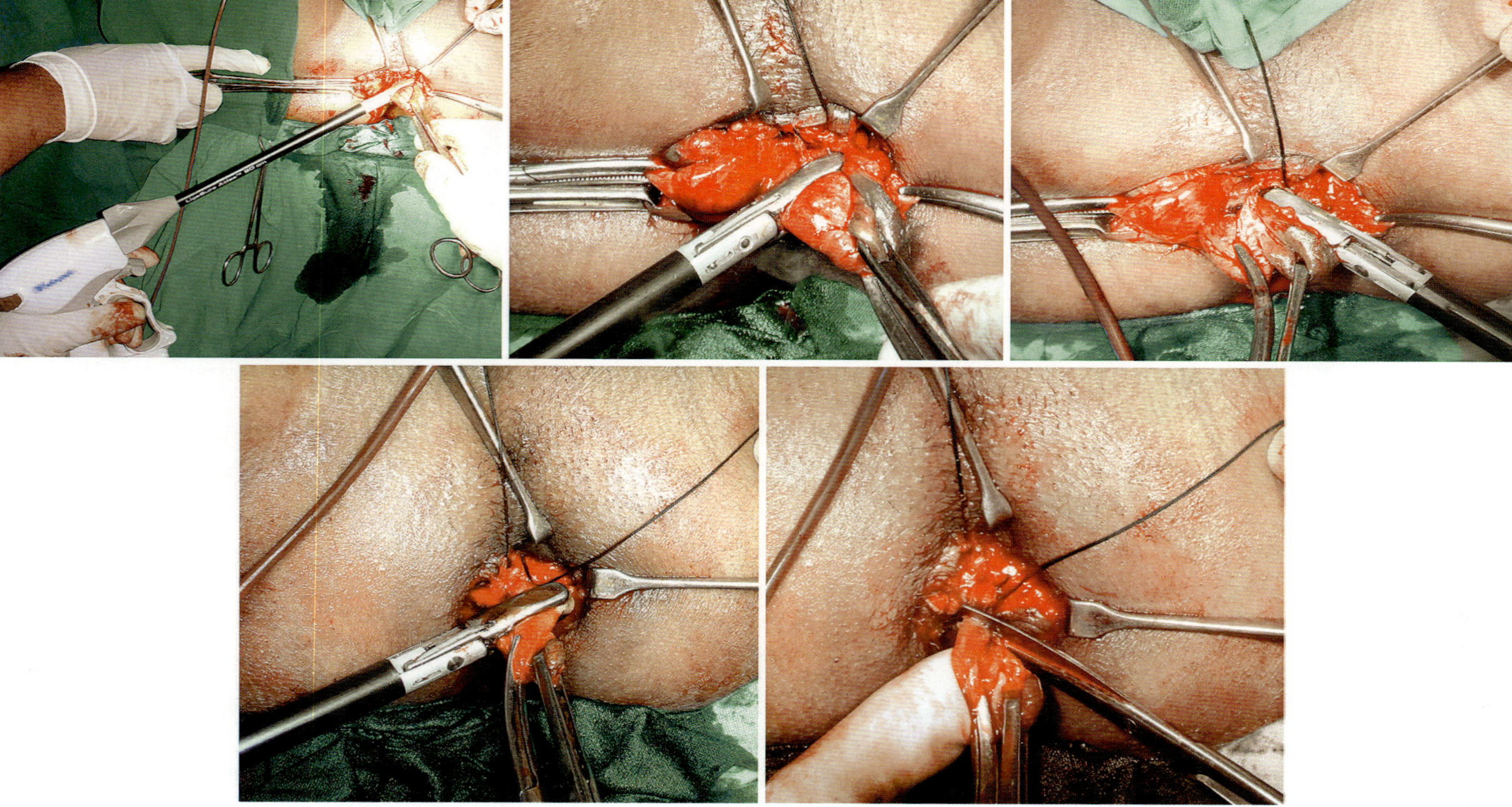

Fig. 26-63: Ligasure is often used in haemorrhoidectomy; it avoids suture ligation of the pedicle.

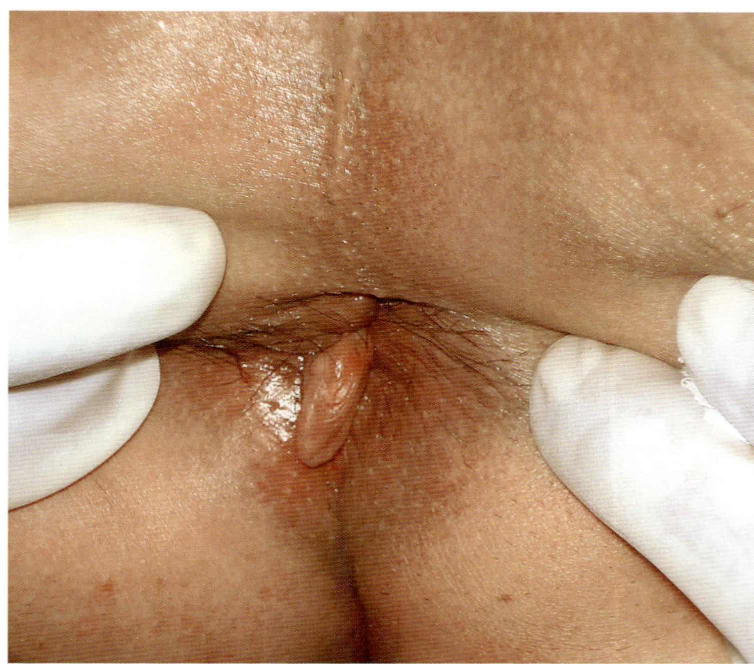

Fig. 26-64: Sentinel pile often requires excision under local anaesthesia.

Anal stricture is not uncommon; needs regular dilatation by patient himself; usually done two times a day for 6–8 weeks will stretch the anal canal correcting the stricture. Severe cases need stretching under general anaesthesia or anoplasty to rectify the problem **(Fig. 26-65)**.

Anal fissure due to breakdown of the anoderm.

Recurrence is not very high—2–5%.

Anal discharge for sometime which usually subsides in 2 weeks.

Incontinence for faeces or gas is common; but subsides in 4–6 weeks.

Ectropion (Whitehead deformity) of the anal mucosa; it commonly regresses once healing occurs as mucosa will be drawn upwards towards the muscle.

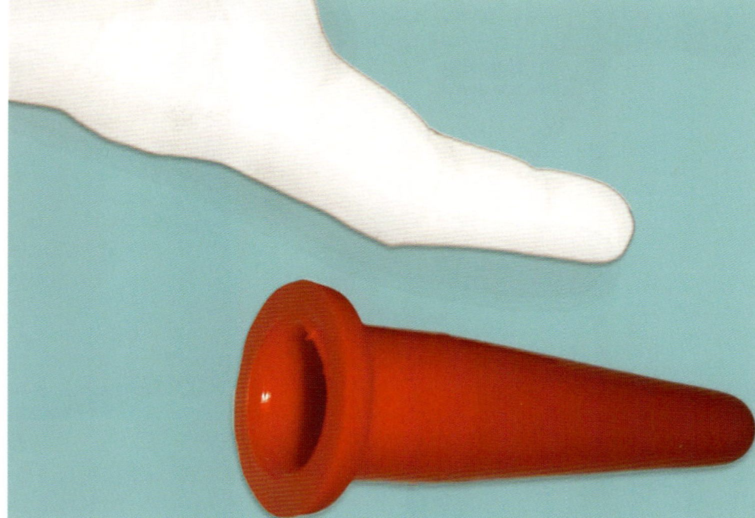

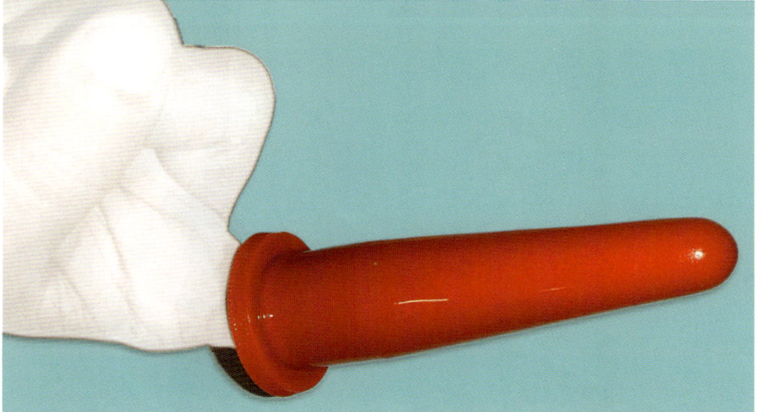

Fig. 26-65: Anal dilator. Many anorectal surgeries require regular anal dilatation postoperatively. Note how to hold the dilator to pass into the anus after applying lubricant.

TREATMENT OF ANAL FISSURE

General Measures for Anal Fissure

Adequate fluid intake (6–8 glasses of liquids); fibre rich diet (vegetables, fruits, brown rice); bulk forming agents (psyllium husk, bran); stool softeners (lactulose); local anaesthetic agents (lignocaine 5%); Sitz bath; avoid constipation; once recovers, regular anal dilatation **(Fig. 26-66)**.

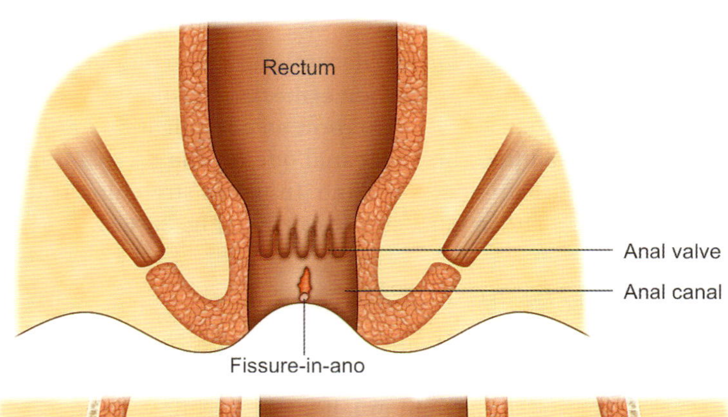

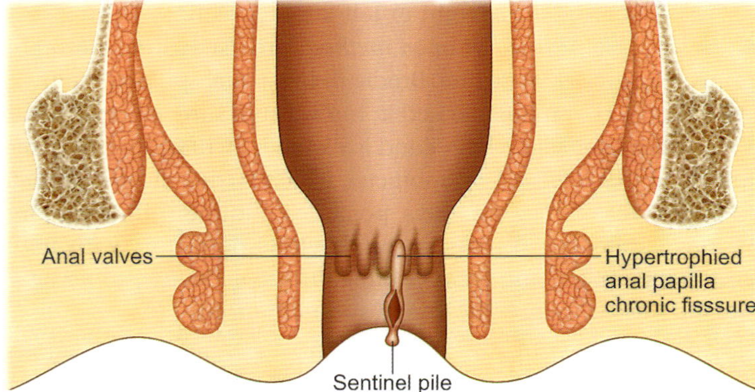

Fig. 26-66: Fissure-in-ano and its surgical anatomy.

In an Acute Case

Lord's Dilatation

It is done under general anaesthesia to relax the sphincter. It is the *manual dilatation* (Lord, 1968–1969) of the anus under general anaesthesia with relaxation using *four fingers of each hand* (*8 fingers*) to cause vigorous stretching of the anal canal to break the circular constricting band in the wall of the anorectum. It is found that it causes tear of levator ani reducing its tone and so it is not universally accepted even though it gives early pain relief; but incidence of symptomatic incontinence is surprisingly not very much. Later, use of laxatives, xylocaine surface anaesthetic application, and anal dilatation with finger can be carried out for certain period. Bed rest; 2% nifedepine ointment.

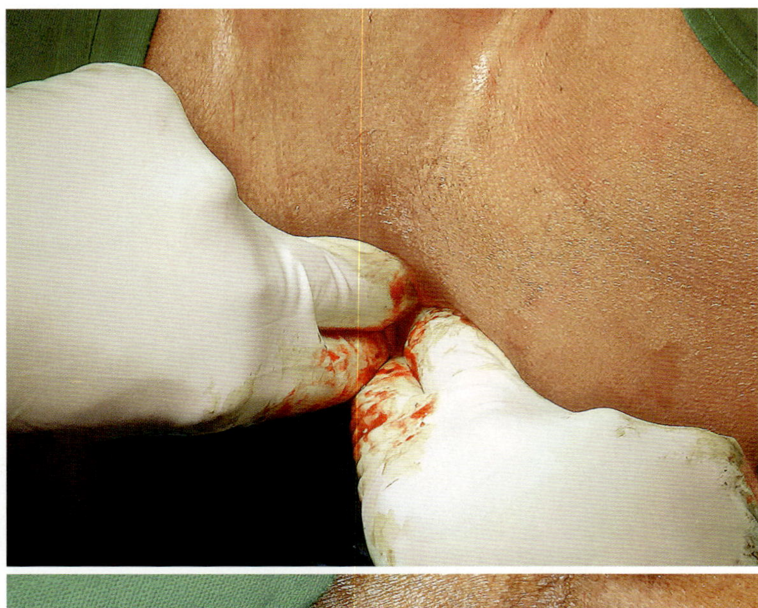

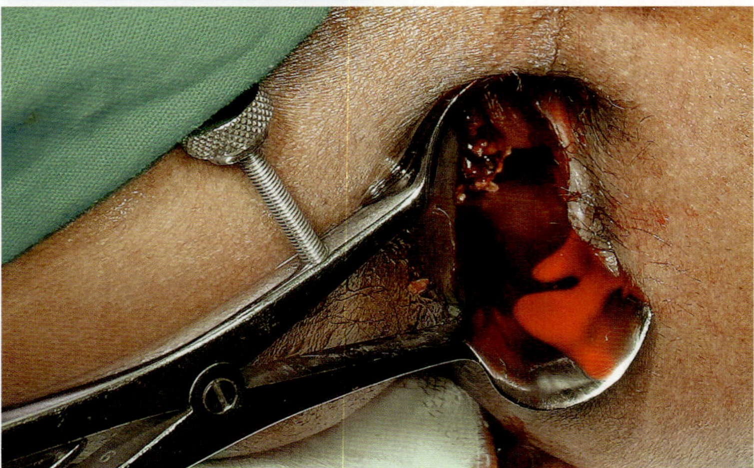

Fig. 26-67: Stretching of the anal canal is done using four fingers (two fingers of each hand). Instrument stretching can be done.

Stretching of the anal sphincter (Recamier, 1829) using *two fingers of each hand* (*4 fingers*) under anaesthesia is also an alternative one. It is better than Lord's dilatation as complications are less. Fingers are passed into the anal canal one by one up to 4 fingers; gradual persistent stretching is done. In males stretching is done anteroposteriorly and in females transversely **(Fig. 26-67)**.

For Chronic Fissure (Fig. 26-68)

Lateral anal sphincterotomy (Subcutaneous lateral internal sphincterotomy): Here internal sphincter is divided partially away from the fissure either in right or left lateral positions (also gives a good result). Here *closed or open methods* are used. Sphincterotomy is done below the dentate line. Brodie did first anal sphincterotomy in 1839. In 1863, Hilton popularised it; but was not sure which structure is torn. Miles later said pectin band is divided. In 1951, Eisenhammer understood that it is internal sphincter, which is truly divided partially in this procedure. In olden days, posterior midline sphincterotomy was in practice; but it was causing keyhole deformity with flatus incontinence (34%) and faecal soiling. In 1969, Eisenhammer again modified the technique into lateral sphincterotomy.

In *closed method* (Notaras, 1969), bivalved retractor is passed first to stretch the sphincter gently so as to make it taut which facilitated its cutting easier; no. 11 blade is inserted into the intersphincteric groove to pass upwards. Blade is moved medially to cut lower 1/3 or 1/2 of the internal sphincter. Cataract surgery knife (Beaver cataract blade, 25.5 × 2.2 mm) is better instrument (Notaras). Hook knife is also used. External sentinel pile and inner fibroepithelial polyp on the inner end is excised. Closed method is simple but effective method. It can very well be done under local anaesthesia with 1:2,00,000 adrenaline as office or day care surgery. Lateral, prone jackknife or lithotomy positions are used. Right lateral 9 o'clock position is the preferred site/point/area than left (In left side 3 o'clock position left haemorrhoidal vessels are located. So, chances of haematoma are more); but right hand surgeon finds difficult to give a

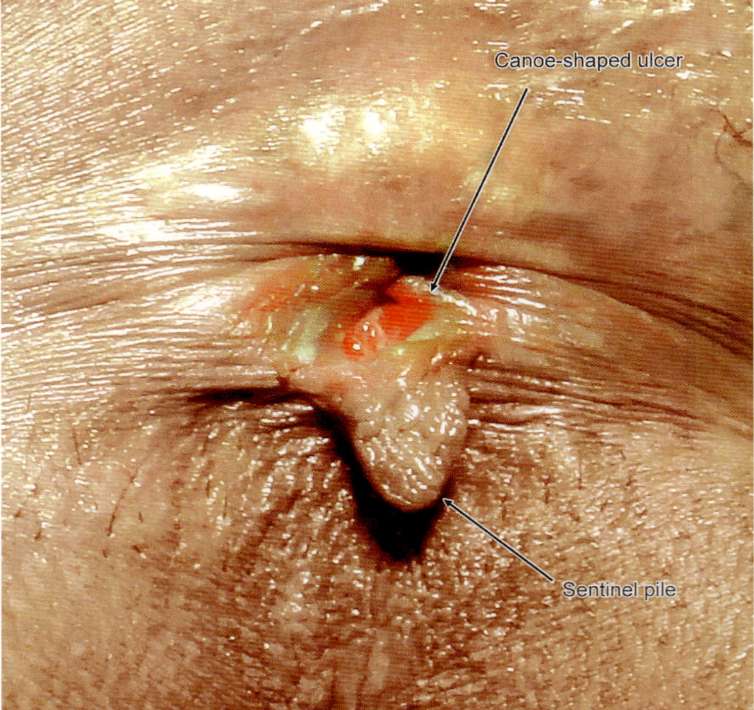

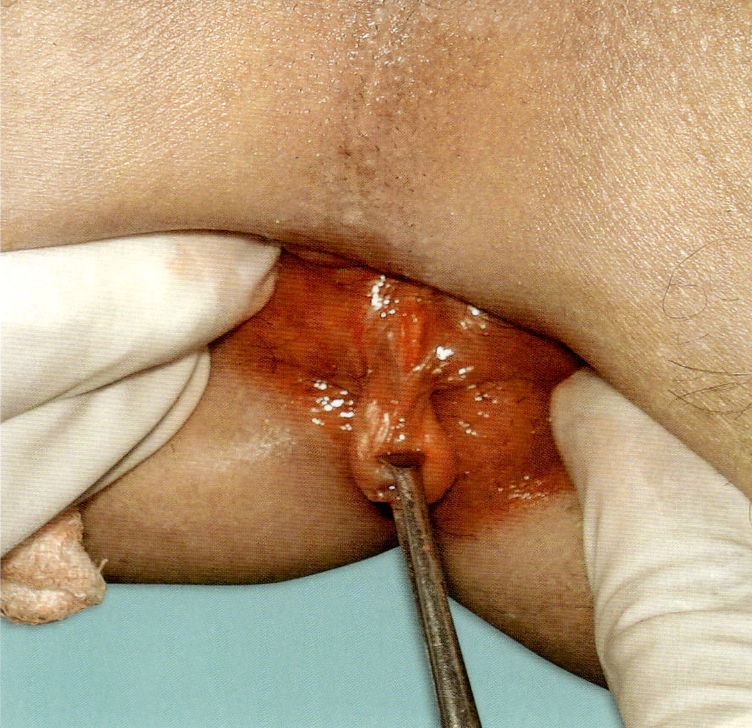

Fig. 26-68: Chronic fissure-in-ano and its parts.

backhand cut on the sphincter than left hand surgeon; so many right hand surgeons prefer to do from left side. Digital examination of the rectum is done; intersphincteric groove is identified; retractor can be placed gently if needed; after sphincterotomy residual sphincter fibres can be broken using finger. Reintroduction of blade should be avoided **(Fig. 26-69)**.

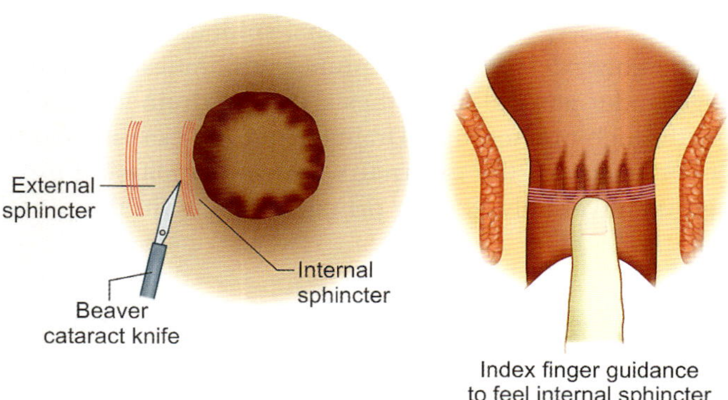

Fig. 26-69: Closed method of lateral sphincterotomy.

In *open method*, skin is incised laterally circumferentially for 2 cm at 9 o'clock position (radial incision also can be used); free edge of the internal sphincter is dissected external to anal verge. Hypertrophied band of lower part of internal sphincter (free lower edge) is dissected and divided. If wound has to be closed absorbable 4-zero vicryl should be used. Wound may be left open to allow it to granulate. Haematoma, ecchymosis, perianal abscess, bruising, fistula, incontinence are the complications of lateral sphincterotomy. Flatus incontinence is more common in women. Recurrence rate of sphincterotomy is 2–4%. Complications are little less in closed approach but recurrence rates are same in both.

Dorsal fissurectomy with sphincterotomy is done under anaesthesia. Specimen should be sent for biopsy to rule out carcinoma, tuberculosis, Crohn's disease, etc. Here, transverse lower fibres of internal sphincter are divided in the floor of the fissure. Keyhole deformity is a troublesome effect of fissurectomy. But for *chronic fibrotic anal fissure, fissurectomy has to be the treatment* along with sphincterotomy. Sphincterotomy can be done in the fissure floor after excision or lateral sphincterotomy can be added.

Topical nitroglycerine 0.2% can also be used to relax the sphincter. It causes severe headache. Botulinum toxin 25 units injected into the internal sphincter. It causes temporary denervation of the internal sphincter; reducing its tone, improving the blood supply and controlling ischaemia. It causes temporary incontinence for flatus (10%). Diltiazem (2%), and L arginine are the other agents that can be used. Regular anal dilatation is also important to prevent recurrence.

ANORECTAL ABSCESS

Most common causative organism is *E. coli (60%)*. Others are *Staphylococcus, Bacteroides, Streptococcus, B. proteus.* Commonly occurs due to infection of anal gland in perianal region. 95% of anorectal abscesses are due to infection of anal glands in relation to crypts—*cryptoglandular* disease. Common in diabetics and immunosuppressed **(Fig. 26-70)**.

Other Causes

Injury to anorectum; cutaneous infection (e.g. Boil); blood borne infections; many anorectal abscesses are associated with anal fistulas; fissure-in-ano; perianal haematoma; post-anorectal surgery; Crohn's disease; tuberculosis **(Fig. 26-71)**.

Differential diagnosis of anorectal abscess: Periurethral abscess; Bartholin abscess; tuberculous abscess.

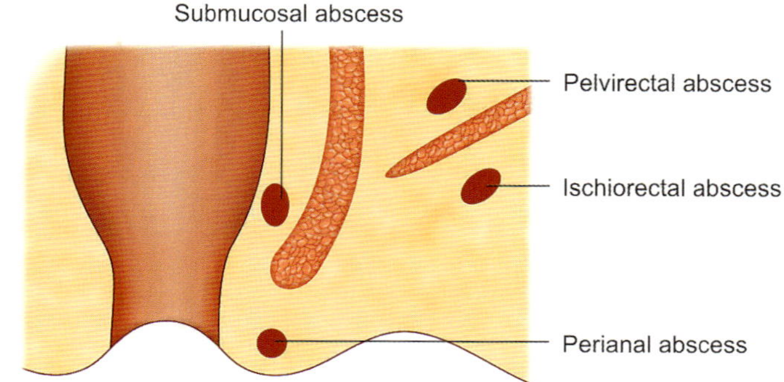

Fig. 26-70: Anatomy of anorectal abscess.

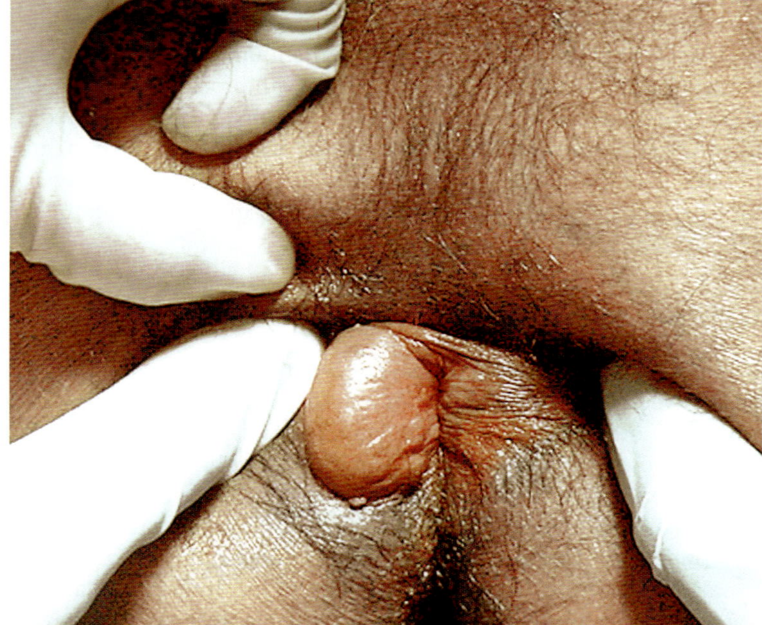

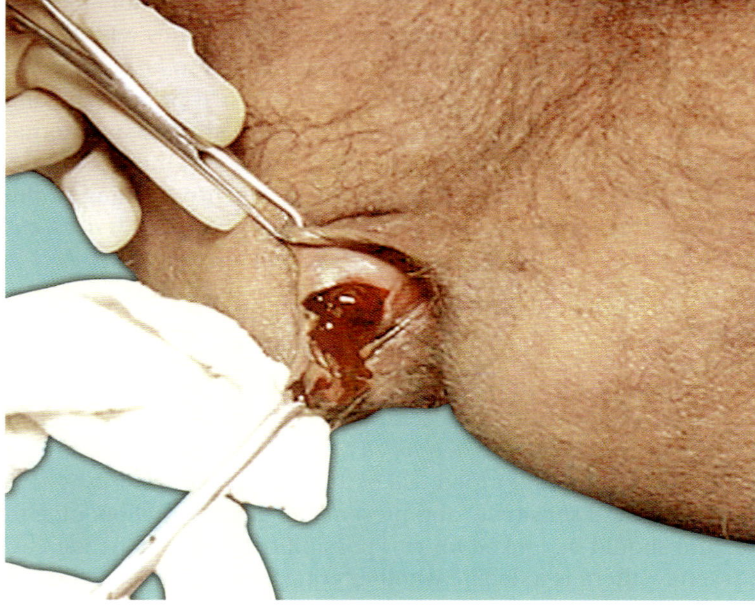

Fig. 26-71: Perianal haematoma and its drainage. It can be done under local anaesthesia.

Investigations

MRI is the *investigation* of *choice* for anorectal abscess; *perineal and anal US* is also very useful; investigations relevant to specific cause may be done; proctosigmoidoscopy is needed to identify secondary cause in anorectum.

Classification

1. Perianal.
2. Ischiorectal.
3. Submucous.
4. Pelvirectal.
5. *Fissure abscess* (in relation to fissure-in-ano).

Perianal Abscess (60%)

This usually results due to suppuration of anal gland or suppuration of thrombosed external pile or any infected perianal condition. It lies in the region of subcutaneous portion of external sphincter. After drainage under general anaesthesia, pus should be sent for culture. Patient should be re-examined in 2 weeks with proctosigmoidoscopy. If patient develops abscess later then patient should be warned of need of fistulotomy or fistulectomy which should be done at a later period. Anal fistula is not recognised at the time of drainage of the abscess; so fistulotomy is usually delayed until fistula manifests **(Fig. 26-72)**.

Ischiorectal Abscess (30%)

Ischiorectal fossa (pyramidal shape 5 cm depth and 2 cm width) lies between anal skin and levator ani. Right and left communicates with each other. Laterally, it is related to fascia covering obturator internus; medially to levator ani and external sphincter; posteriorly sacrotuberous ligament and gluteus maximus; anteriorly urogenital diaphragm; below, the floor by skin. Above, it is related to lunate fascia and pudendal neurovascular bundle in pudendal canal (Alcock's canal). Commonly, it is due to extension of low intermuscular anal abscess, laterally through external sphincter. But often it can be blood or lymphatic borne. Fat in the fossa is more prone for infection because it is least vascularised. Fossa communicates with that of opposite side through post-sphincteric space and so *horse-shoe like* abscess can occur. When swelling is pressed just prior to making incision, if pus exudes per anal canal it means there is an internal opening and patient is likely to develop a trans-sphincteric fistula. Abscess presents with tender, indurated, brawny swelling in the skin over the ischiorectal fossa with high fever. *Swelling is not well-localised and fluctuation is absent in ischiorectal abscess.*

Treatment

Under general anaesthesia in lithotomy position, through a cruciate incision a portion of skin is excised (de roofing) and pus is drained. Cruciate incision should be placed close to the anal verge, so that subsequent fistula if formed will be having short track. Pus is sent for culture and sensitivity and presence of any internal opening to rectum should be looked for (for possibility of an existing fistula). Presently, there is a debate whether cruciate incision is needed or not **(Figs. 26-73 and 26-74)**.

Submucous Abscess (5%)

It occurs above the dentate line, causing aching pain in the anorectum with significant perineal discomfort. On digital examination (P/R), tender, soft, smooth swelling in the lower rectum and anal canal is felt. It may be missed clinically as there is no obvious swelling externally. It is called as deep post-anal abscess if it originates from posterior crypt above the external sphincter in front of and below the coccyx. *Treatment* is proper antibiotics; incision and drainage under general anaesthesia can be drained with sinus forceps through proctoscope. Drainage of deep post-anal abscess requires division of the external sphincter by passing a probe through the invariably existing primary opening in the posterior midline (Hanley).

Intersphincteric Abscess (2%)

It begins in a cryptogland in the intersphincteric plane, which burrows cephalad to present as a mass in the lower rectum. Abscess differs from submucous abscess as it is not in the submucosa plane but it is in the intersphincteric plane. Features are anorectal pain which is exacerbated during defaecation; rectal examination reveals a tender mass. It requires admission and hospital treatment under general anaesthesia. Abscess wall should be marsupialised along with excision of the part of the internal sphincter with crypt. Abscess cavity is allowed to drain into the lumen.

Pelvirectal Abscess

It is situated between the upper surface of levator ani and pelvic peritoneum. It is almost like a pelvic abscess; develops secondary to appendicitis, salpingitis, diverticulitis, Crohn's. Ultrasonography of abdomen is done to rule out the above factors. Treated accordingly, after thorough investigations for diabetes, Crohn's and other conditions. Occasionally, it can develop as in continuity cephalad extension of a trans-sphincteric or retrosphincteric abscess. US abdomen and pelvis or CT scan is must. MRI may be needed if there is intersphincteric pathology. Usually, it is treated like a pelvic abscess drained under general anaesthesia either per rectally in males or per vaginally (posterior fornix) in females. Malecot or Foley's catheter is placed. External drainage is rarely done; it is done only in few occasions' like Crohn's disease with abscess where long-term drainage is needed. Through intersphincteric space after placing an incision close to the anal canal, abscess is reached and Malecot's catheter is placed.

Problems with anorectal abscess: Recurrent abscess formation; fistula formation is common. Other than this in diabetic patients anorectal abscess may cause necrotising fasciitis or Fournier's gangrene. Perianal abscess may be often associated with leukaemia, neutropenia (neutrophil count less than 500/mm^3).

FISTULA-IN-ANO

It is a track lined by granulation tissue which connects perianal skin superficially to anal canal; anorectum or rectum deeply. It usually occurs in a pre-existing anorectal abscess which rupture spontaneously **(Fig. 26-75)**.

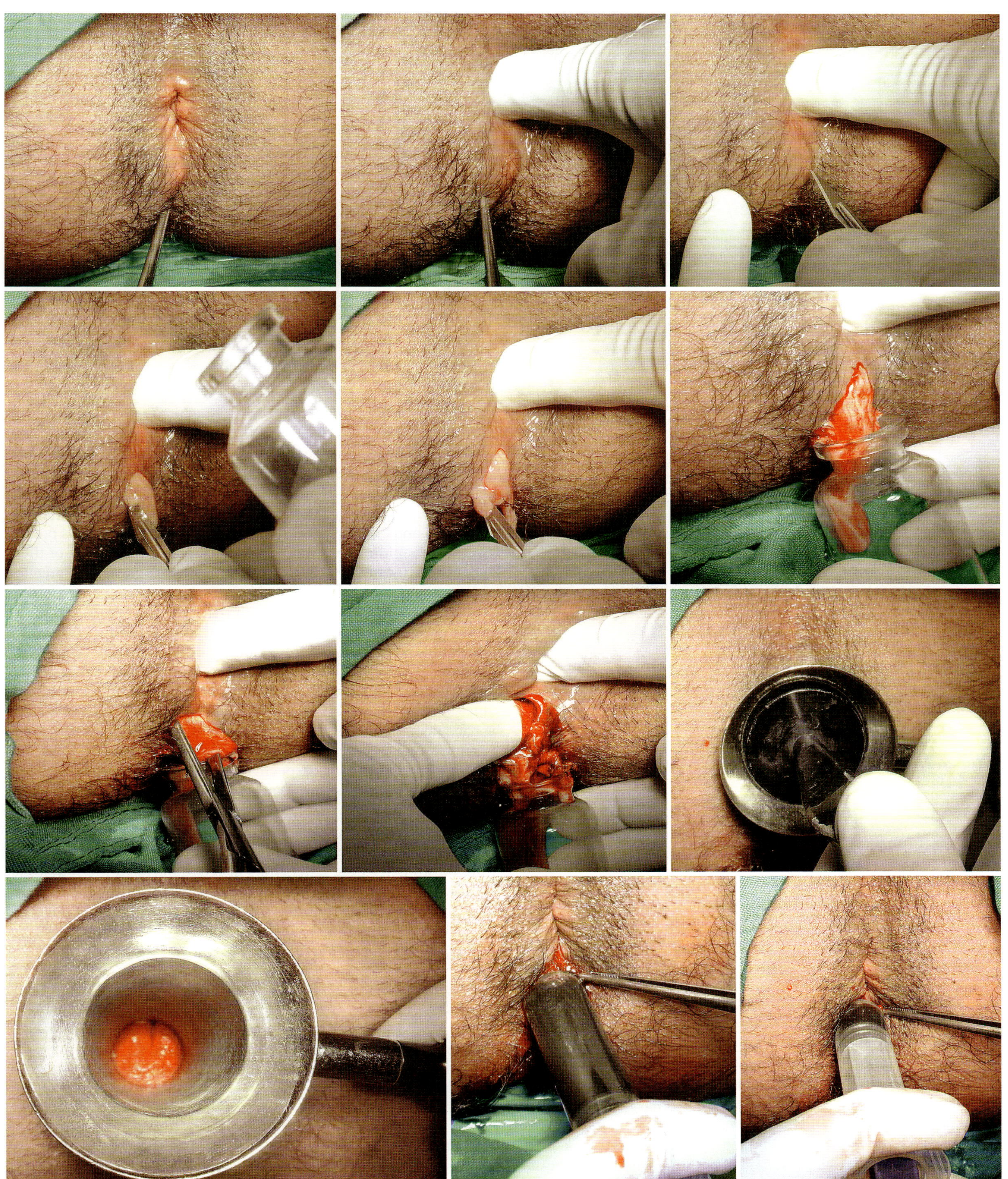

Figs. 26-72(1)

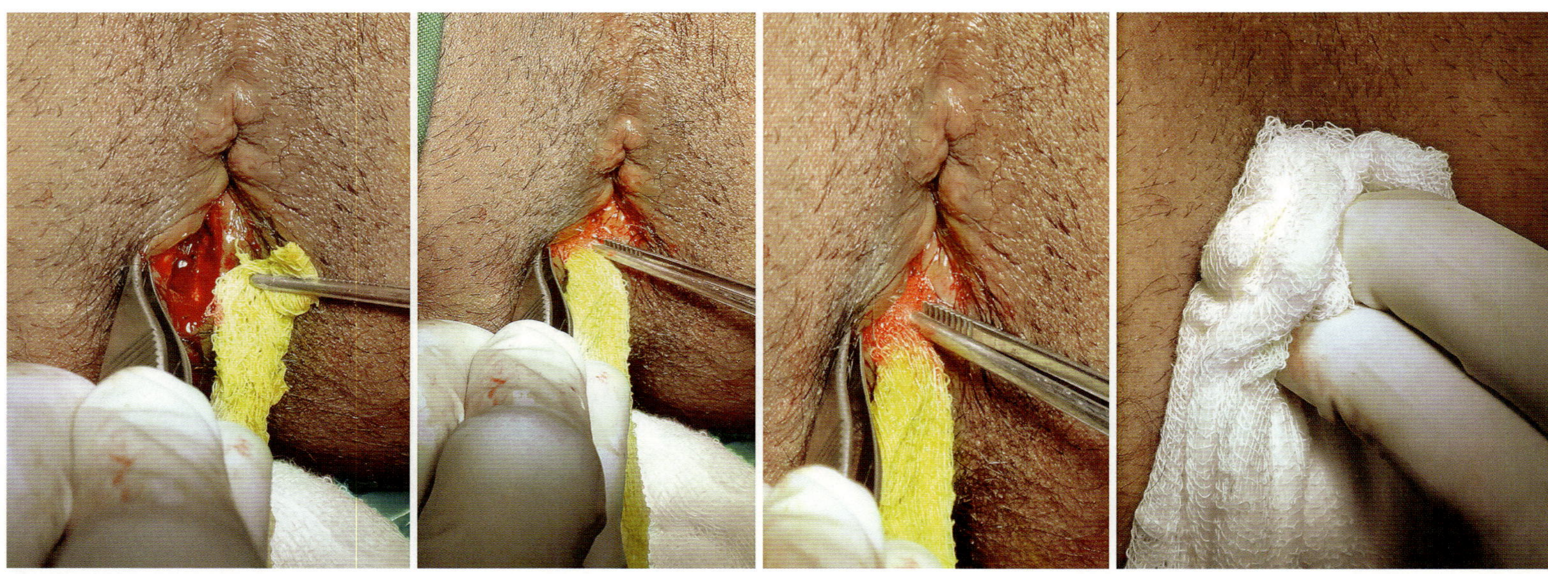

Figs. 26-72(2)

Figs. 26-72(1 and 2): Drainage of perianal abscess.

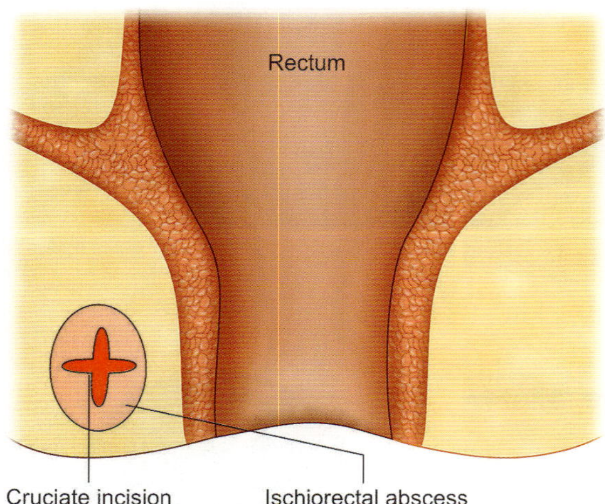

Fig. 26-73: Cruciate incision is used for drainage of ischiorectal abscess.

Types of Fistula-in-Ano

Cryptoglandular or Non-cryptoglandular

Non-cryptoglandular (other causes)—10%—tuberculosis, carcinoma, Crohn's disease, ulcerative colitis, lymphogranuloma venereum, hydradenitis suppurative, traumatic.

Cryptoglandular Hypothesis (90%)

The intersphincteric space is the surgical plane between the internal and external sphincters and is found between the longitudinal muscle and external sphincter, where it exists as a sheet of fat containing loose areolar tissue. The fat-filled ischioanal fossa lies lateral to the sphincter complex and is traversed by a network of fibroelastic connective tissue. Proximal half of the anal canal is characterised by longitudinal mucosal folds, the anal columns of Morgagni. The distal aspect of each column is linked to its neighbour by a small semilunar fold (the anal valves), which in turn, forms small pockets (the anal sinuses, or *crypts of Morgagni*). The distal undulating limit of these valves is the dentate (pectinate) line, which also marks the most distal aspect of the anal transitional zone, a histologic junction between anal squamous and rectal columnar epithelium. The dentate line lies 2 cm proximal to the anal verge and is important landmark in fistula-in-ano because the anal glands empty into the crypts that lie proximal to the valves. These glands secrete mucus to lubricate anus, and are the source of infection. These glands present in the subepithelium, internal sphincter, and two-thirds of these glands are located within the intersphincteric space. The infection of these intersphincteric glands initiates the fistula in ano, according to "*cryptoglandular hypothesis*".

These glandular infection leads into an intersphincteric abscess due to blockage of the draining duct by infected debris. This abscess may resolve by spontaneous drainage into the anal canal or may progress to an acute anorectal abscess. Treatment of this abscess is incision and drainage; but source of infection in the intersphincteric space persists, leading into development of a fistula-in-ano. Acute anorectal abscess and fistula-in-ano are believed to be acute and chronic manifestations, respectively of the same disease.

While most fistulas start as a *simple single primary tract*, recurrent infection eventually causes formation of *extensions (secondary tracts)*. Extensions may be intersphincteric, ischioanal, or supralevator (pararectal). The ischioanal fossa is the commonest site for an extension. Extensions also can occur in the horizontal plane known as "horseshoe" if there is ramification each side of the internal opening **(Fig. 26-76)**.

Classification (Figs. 26-77 to 26-79)

Standard (Milligan Morgan, 1934; Goligher 1975)	*Park's classification (1976)*
♦ Subcutaneous—commonest ♦ Low anal—common ♦ Submucous ♦ High anal ♦ Pelvirectal	♦ Intersphincteric—commonest (70%) ♦ Trans-sphincteric (25%) ♦ Supralevator/suprasphincteric (4%) ♦ Extrasphincteric (1%)

Fistula can be:

1. ***Low level fistulas:*** *These open into the anal canal below the internal ring.*
2. ***High level fistulas:*** *These open into the anal canal at or above the internal ring.*

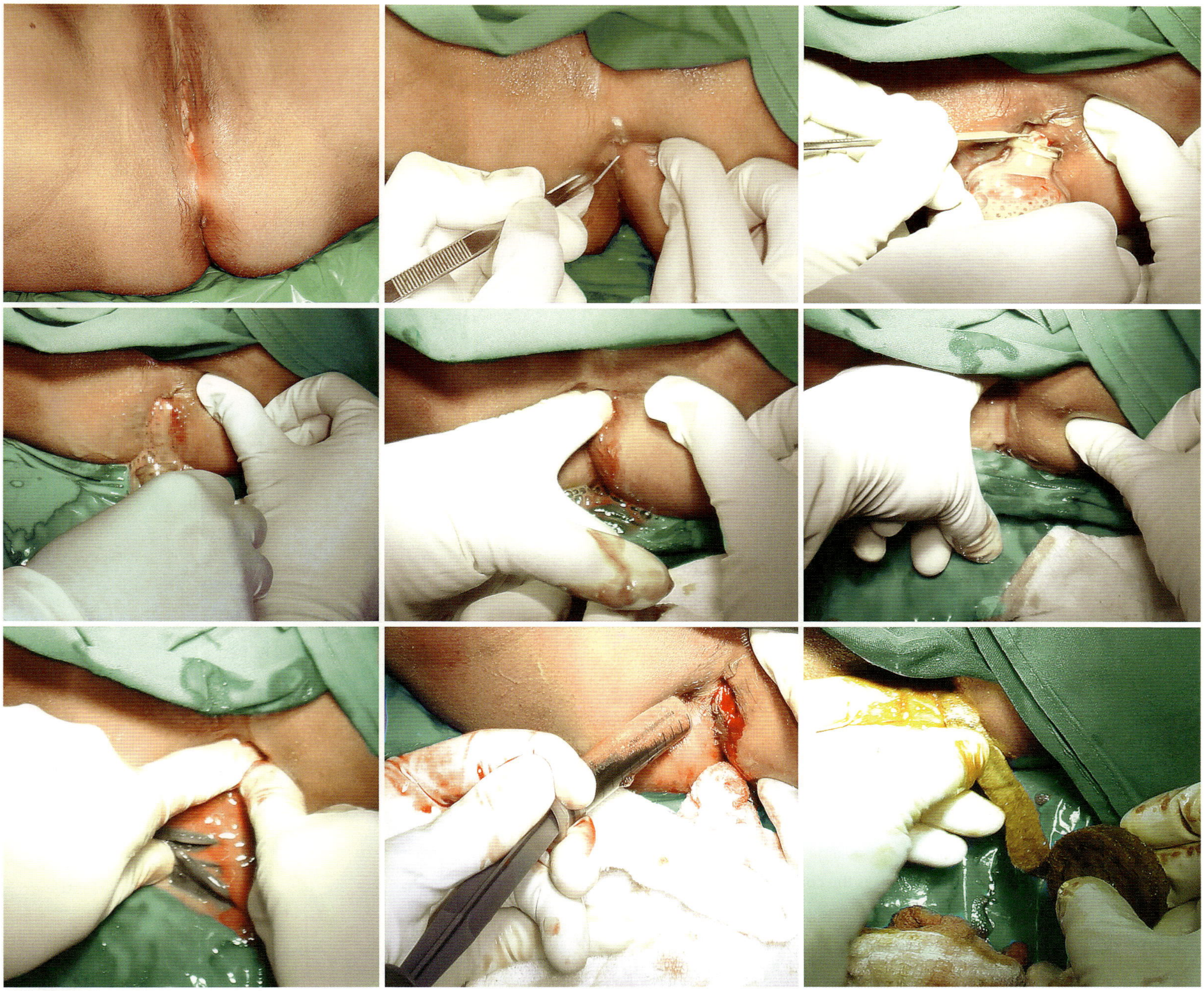

Fig. 26-74: Drainage of ischiorectal abscess. Cruciate incision can be used; but its need is a debate. Packing the cavity to drain is a must.

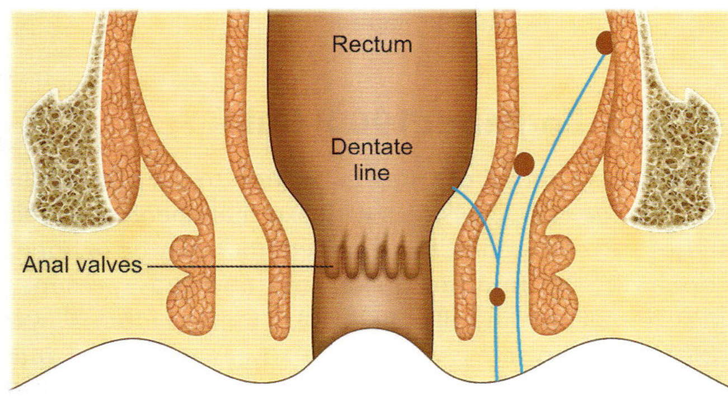

Fig. 26-75: Anatomy of fistula-in-ano.

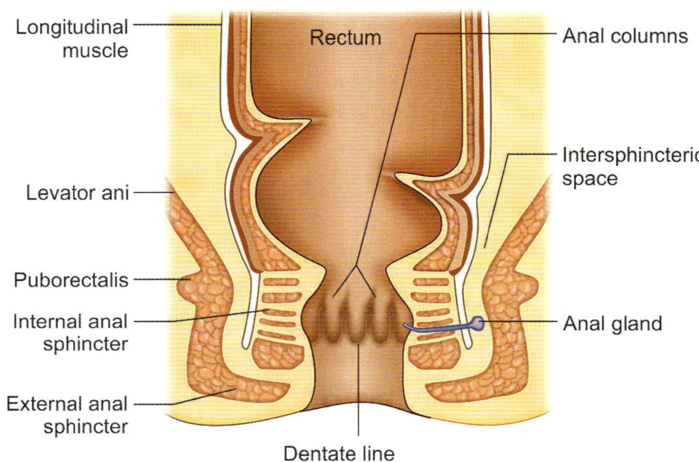

Fig. 26-76: Anatomy of anal glands (cryptoglands of Morgagni).

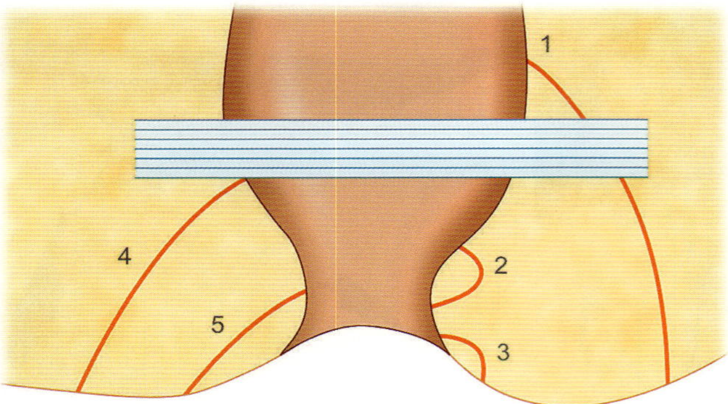

Fig. 26-77: Standard classification of fistula-in-ano.

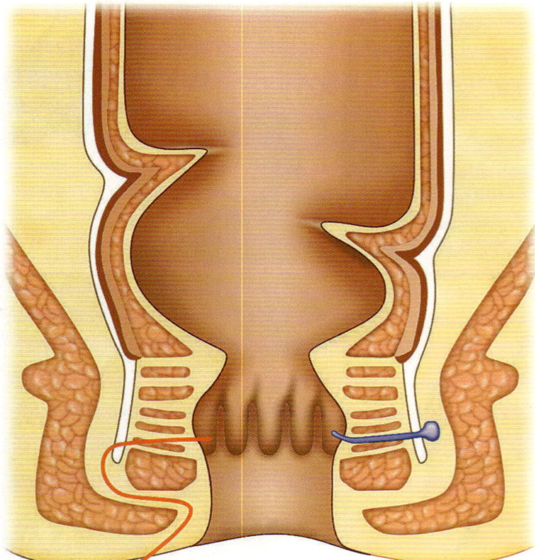

Fig. 26-78: Intersphincteric fistula is the commonest type.

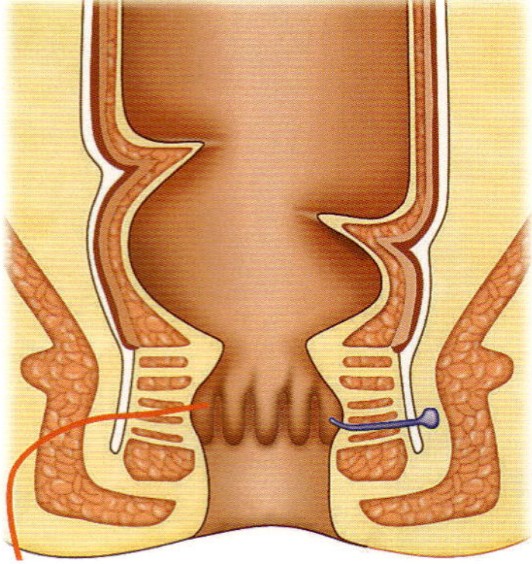
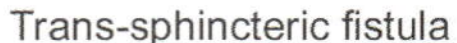

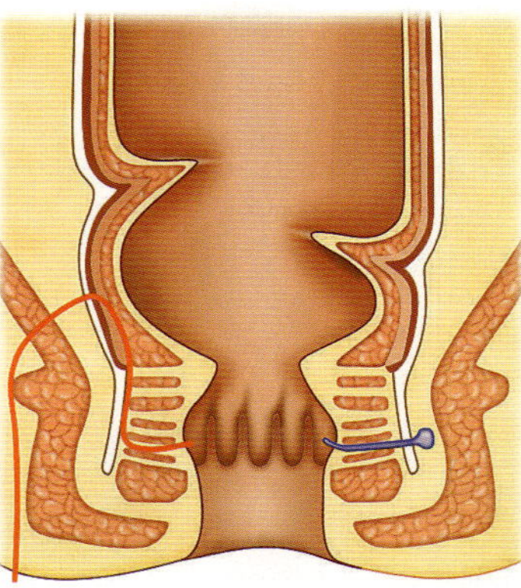

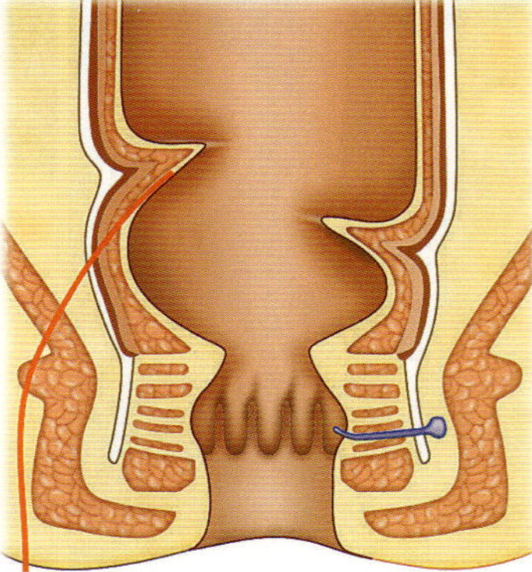

Fig. 26-79: Trans-sphincteric, supralevator, extrasphincteric types of fistulas.

Fistula can be

- *Simple fistula* without extensions.
- *Complex fistula* with extensions **(Figs. 26-80 and 26-81)**.

Fistula can be with

Single external opening.

Multiple external openings which are often seen in tuberculosis, ulcerative colitis, Crohn's disease, lymphogranuloma venereum (LGV), hidradenitis suppurativa, actinomycosis **(Figs. 26-82 and 26-83)**.

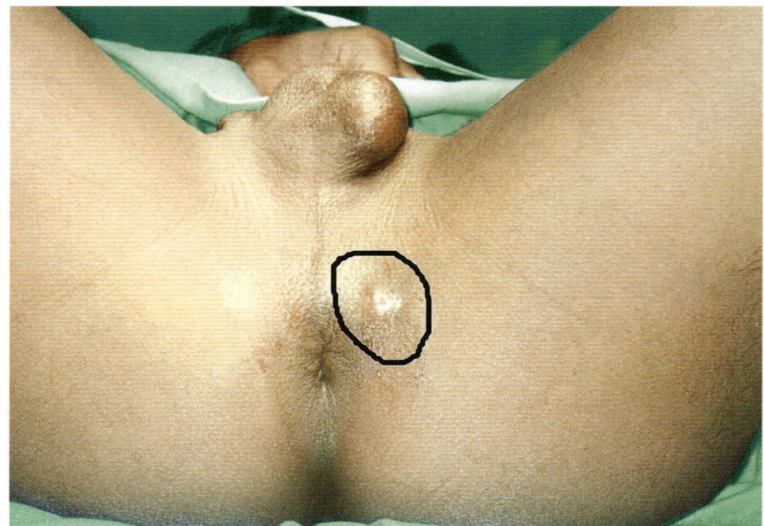

Fig. 26-80: Simple fistula-in-ano.

Low-level Fistulas

It has a prevalence of 0.01% and is common in young adult males (2:1, male to female). It presents with seropurulent discharge (65%), along with skin irritation and one or more external opening may be present with induration of the surrounding skin. Often it may heal superficially but pus may collect beneath forming an abscess, which again discharges through same or new opening.

Ischiorectal fossa on each side, most often communicates with each other behind the anus causing *horseshoe* fistula.

Goodsall's (England, 1900) Rule

Fistulas with an external opening in relation to the anterior half of the anus is of *direct type*. Fistulas with external openings in relation to posterior half of the anus, has a curved track may be of horseshoe type, opens in the midline posteriorly and may present with multiple external opening all connected to a single internal opening **(Fig. 26-84)**. *Per-rectal examination shows indurated internal opening usually in the midline posteriorly*. Most of the fistulas are on posterior half of anus.

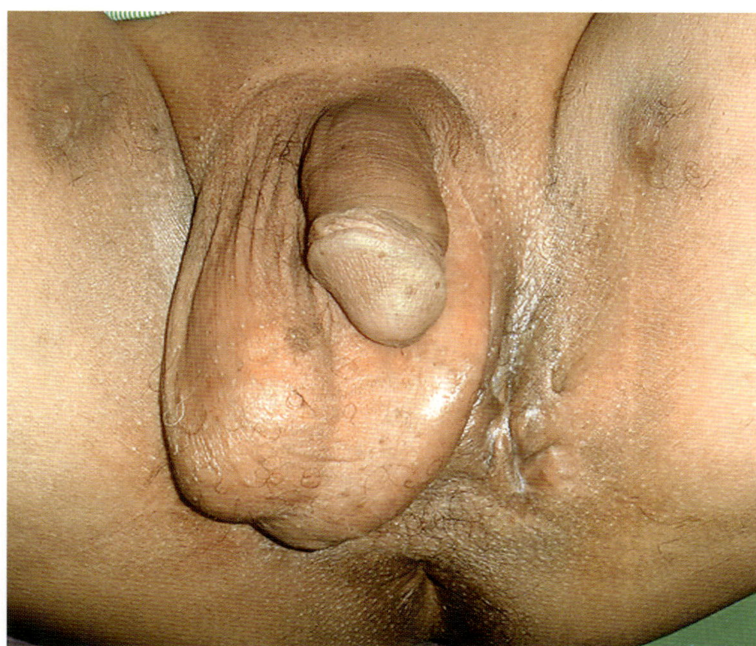

Fig. 26-81: Complex fistula-in-ano.

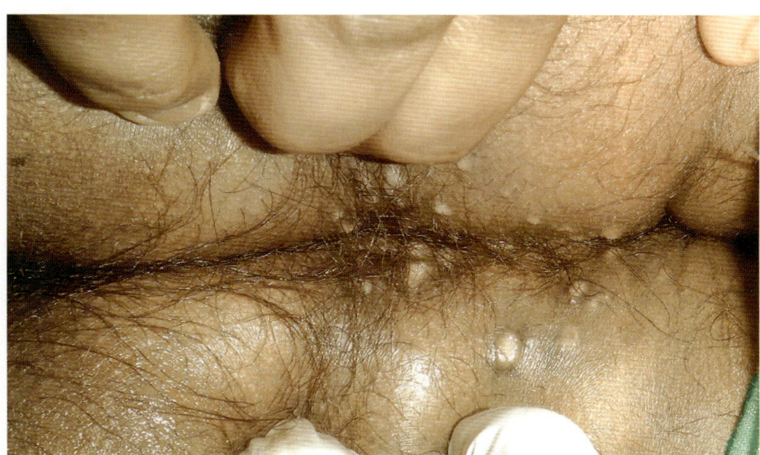

Fig. 26-82: Multiple fistula-in-ano.

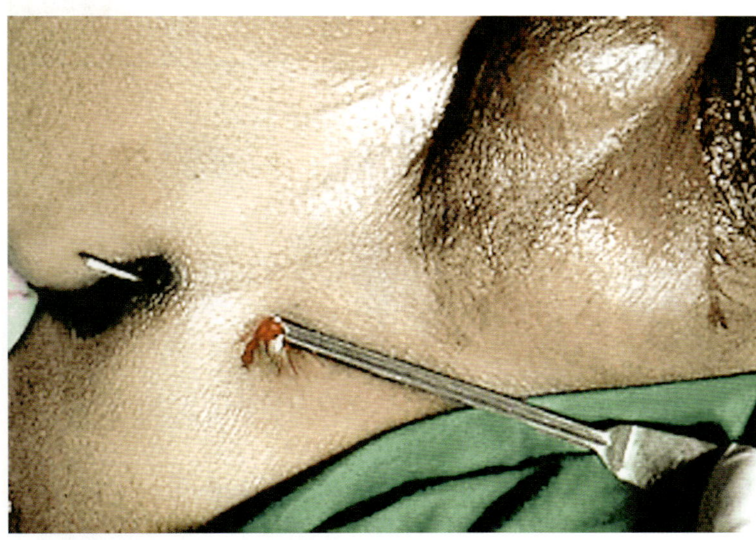

Fig. 26-83: Probing of fistula should be done in operation theatre prior to surgery.

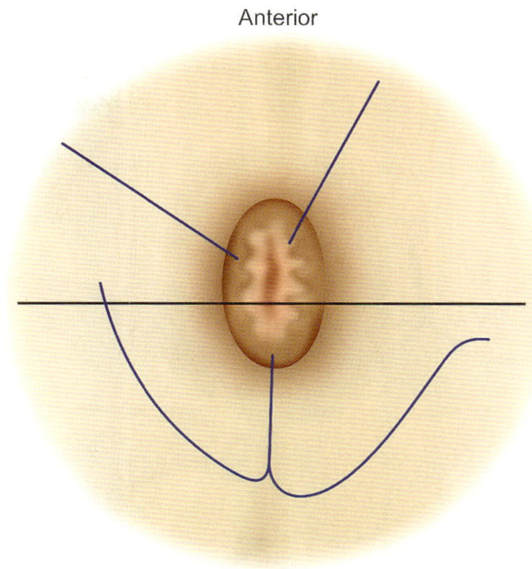

Fig. 26-84: Goodsall's rule.

Investigations

Chest X-ray, erythrocyte sedimentation rate (ESR) and barium enema X-ray; *if required fistulogram is done only under anaesthesia*. MRI/MR fistulogram ideal. Endorectal US (US perineum) is useful to assess deeper plane. Discharge study, methylene blue dye study, biopsy. Colonoscopy often is done when ulcerative colitis/ Crohn's is suspected. Specific blood tests if needed should be done **(Figs. 26-85 to 26-87)**.

Note: *Probing and fistulogram in the ward* before surgery using *Lipiodol* is not advisable as it may cause recrudescence of inflammation. It can be with adequate precaution in the operation theatre under general anaesthesia otherwise it can *create extensions*.

Differential diagnosis for fistula-in-ano: Urethral fistula in male; chronically infected Bartholin's gland; pilonidal sinus; hidradenitis suppurative; carcinoma; Crohn's disease; tuberculosis, ulcerative colitis.

Treatment of Fistula-in-Ano

Principles in management	*Procedures*
♦ Identify the cause—cryptoglandular or other ♦ Delineate exactly the fistula-in-ano by—MRI/EUS ♦ Identify relation of fistula to anal sphincter ♦ Drain all sites of infection ♦ Eradicate track and secondary extensions ♦ Preserve anal continence of function The *primary objectives* are to eradicate the tract and drain all associated sites of infection while simultaneously preserving anal continence.	♦ Laying open of fistula—fistulotomy with curetting ♦ Fistulectomy ♦ Gluing of fistula—not much useful ♦ Mucosal flap procedure ♦ Fistulectomy with primary repair ♦ Fistulectomy with primary repair with episiorectopexy ♦ Fistulectomy with secondary repair ♦ Anal fistula plug (AFP) repair ♦ LIFT technique (ligation of intersphincteric fistula track) ♦ Seton technique (Latin—seta—a bristle) ♦ Colostomy—lay open, fistulectomy, later closure of colostomy—for high type ♦ VAAFT procedure (video assisted anal fistula track ligation)

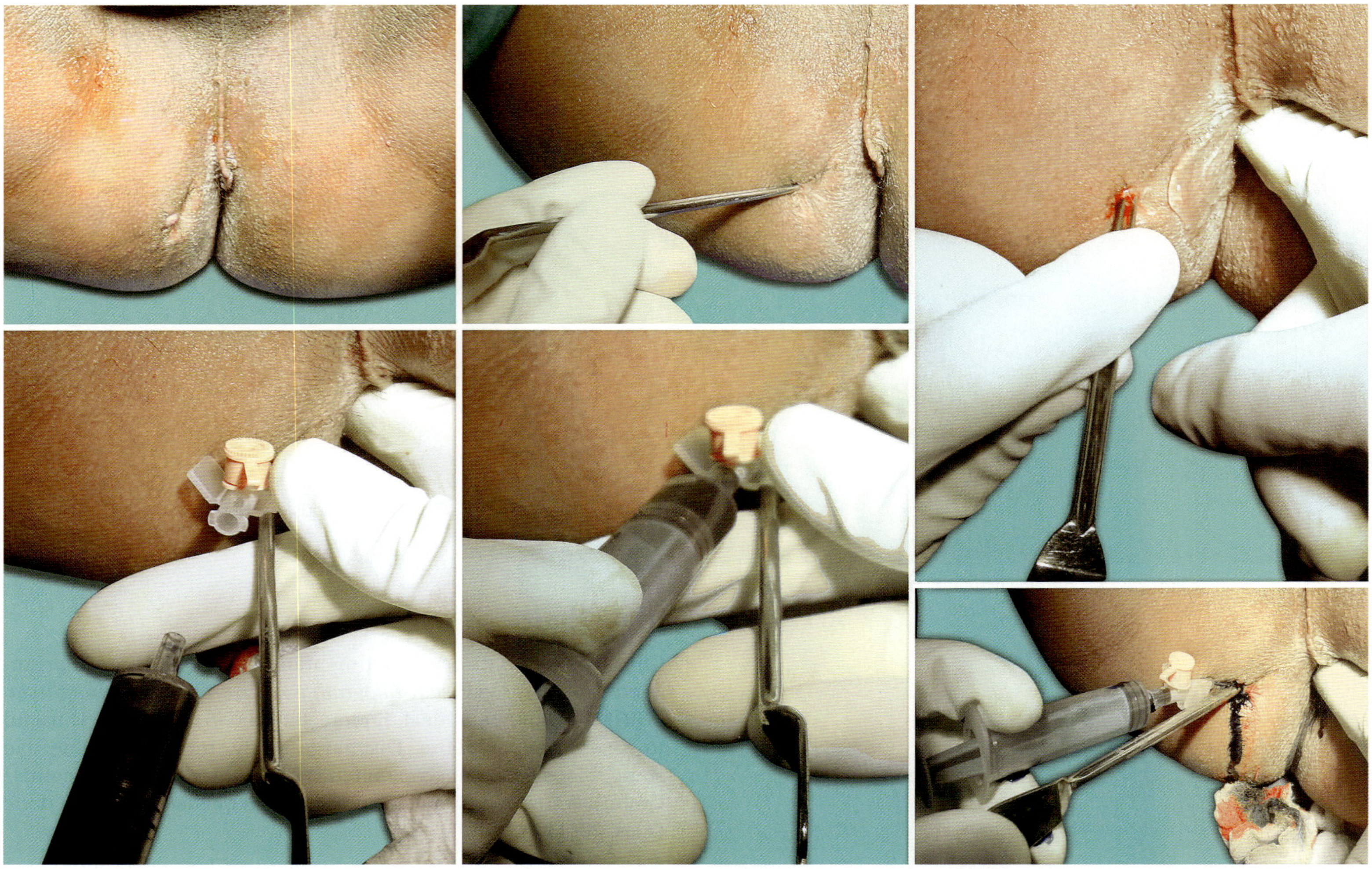

Fig. 26-85: Methylene blue injection study in fistula-in-ano. It is usually done on table prior to surgery to identify track.

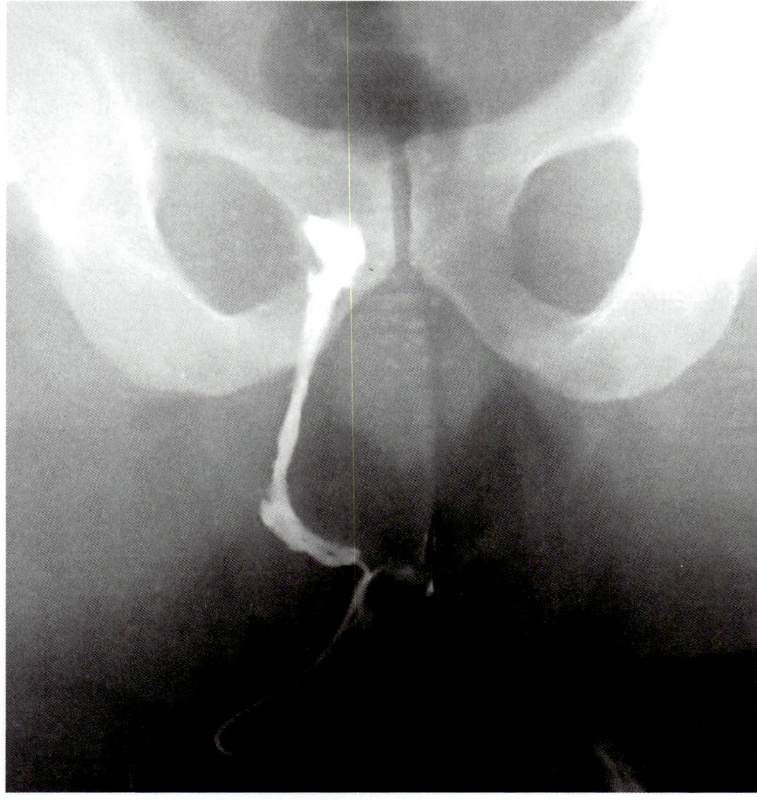

Fig. 26-86: Fistulogram for fistula-in-ano.

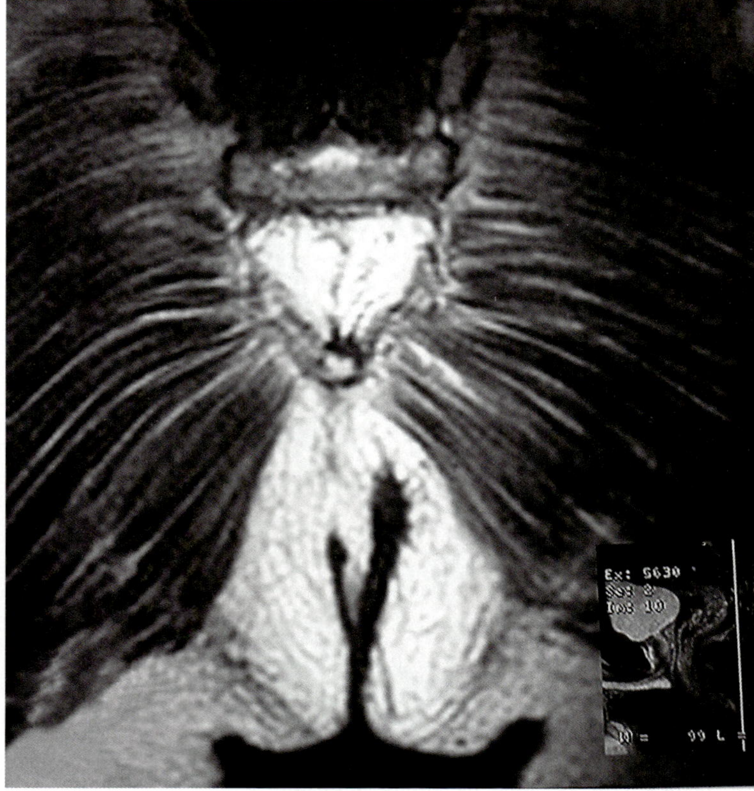

Fig. 26-87: Magnetic resonant fistulogram.

Principles in management

- Delineate exactly the fistula anatomy—MRI/EUS
- Identify the cause—cryptoglandular or other
- Methylene blue injection on table
- Fine ureteric catheter may be placed into the track
- Drain all sites of infection
- Eradicate track and secondary extensions
- Preserve anal continence function
- Fistula surgery should be done in a dry field
- Careful use of cautery is ideal

Evaluation of Fistula-in-Ano

Identification of pathological anatomy of the fistula-in-ano is crucial. Digital rectal examination *(DRE)* is important. Often examination under general anaesthesia may be helpful to assess especially in recurrent/anterior/multiple/complex fistulas.

MR fistulogram is ideal. It has got 100% specificity; 97% sensitivity. It is relatively precise, non-invasive. It detects the track, extent, sphincter complex relations, abscess formation, extensions, horse-shoe type, etc. anorectal endosonography (EUS) is also quiet useful; but extrasphincteric and suprasphincteric tracts are difficult to delineate. Fistulogram, CECT scan are other evaluator imaging methods.

Discharge for culture and sensitivity, discharge for AFB and cytology for specific causes should be done. Haematocrit, blood sugar, serum creatinine, ESR, CEA are other evaluation methods. Biopsy may be indicated in suspected malignancy, tuberculosis, Crohn's disease, ulcerative colitis. Colonoscopy should be done in such patients without fail.

Evaluation of incontinence: Incontinence for three components should be assessed—(1) Liquid; (2) Solid; (3) Flatus/gas. Causes may be—rectal or sphincter dysfunction OR neurological disorders. *Wexner's score* is used for incontinence assessment **(Table 26-1)**.

TABLE 26-1: Wexner's continence/incontinence score.

	Never	*Rarely*	*Sometimes*	*Usually*	*Always*
Solid	0	1	2	3	4
Liquid	0	1	2	3	4
Gas	0	1	2	3	4
Wears pad	0	1	2	3	4
Lifestyle alteration	0	1	2	3	4

Never—0
Rarely—<1/month
Sometimes—>1 per month; <1 per week
Usually—<1/day; >1 per week
Always—>1 per day

Total score 0—Perfect
Total score 20—Complete incontinence

One should remember that

- It is not easy to treat fistula
- Needs proper assessment and planning
- Right method to right type
- High, complex fistula—a risky one
- MR fistulogram with EUS may be ideal to delineate track
- Beware of high recurrence rate and specific causes

Fistulotomy

It is done in low anal fistula. It is technically easier. Methylene blue solution may be injected to the external opening. Track is identified. After passing the probe through the entire fistulous track, incision is made over the probe to cut and lay open the fistulous track. It is allowed to granulate and heal from the floor/surface. Technique is safe, easy and can be done on outpatient basis. Only outer part of the track is excised for histology purpose. External opening part is widened as skin part will heal more rapidly than mucosal part. Anal opening (only, not mucosal) is sutured to the internal sphincter for haemostasis as an optional technique. Dressing is done. Postoperative pain is very less. There is not much difference in outcome between fistulotomy and fistulectomy. Fistulotomy wound heals faster **(Figs. 26-88 and 26-89)**.

Advancement Flaps

They are used occasionally to get better result—mucosal flap procedure. Procedure is done per anally under spinal anaesthesia. Lithotomy position is used. Flap of mucosa with underlying internal sphincter with its blood supply is mobilised to cover the internal opening of the fistula properly and securely. Advancement can be done from above or from below. Problems are—it is technically demanding; flap failure; incontinence; it needs expertise to do.

Gluing of the Fistula Track

It is tried but success rate is not good. Fibrin glue is a multicomponent system containing mainly human plasma fibrinogen and thrombin. Once prepared, it is injected into the fistula track, which hardens in few minutes and fills the entire track. Success rate is 70%.

Anal Fistula Plug (AFP) Repair

Surgisis anal fistula plug (*porcine small intestine submucosa, SIS*) is used with 85% success rate in simple fistula. It contains naturally derived extracellular matrix which acts as scaffolding, ingrowth of tissue, remodelling **(Fig. 26-90)**.

LIFT Technique (Ligation of Intersphincteric Fistula Track):

It is high ligation of the fistula track with lateral approach. Here fistula tract is securely close to the internal sphincter, which probably avoids the reinfection of the intersphincteric space. Further resection of the intersphincteric tract and curettage of the remaining outer tract eliminates the diseased cryptoglandular tissue; distal tract when closed prevents its re-infection. Under anaesthesia in lithotomy position, methylene blue is injected into the track; fine ureteric catheter is passed gently through the fistula track from the external opening; intersphincteric space is reached through a 2-cm transverse incision in the intersphincteric groove adjacent to the fistula site. Fistula running across is identified and is clamped on the inner side with a haemostat; part of the fistula track in the groove is excised and sent for histology. Clamped fistula track on the inner side is suture ligated very close to the internal sphincter using 3-zero vicryl securely. External opening and the fistula track up to the intersphincteric space is gently curetted to clear all infected granulation tissue **(Fig. 26-91)**.

Track opening in the intersphincteric space towards the external sphincter is sutured using 3-zero vicryl. Dissected external sphincter and transverse incision in the intersphincteric groove is also sutured using interrupted 3-zero vicryl sutures. LIFT avoids incontinence

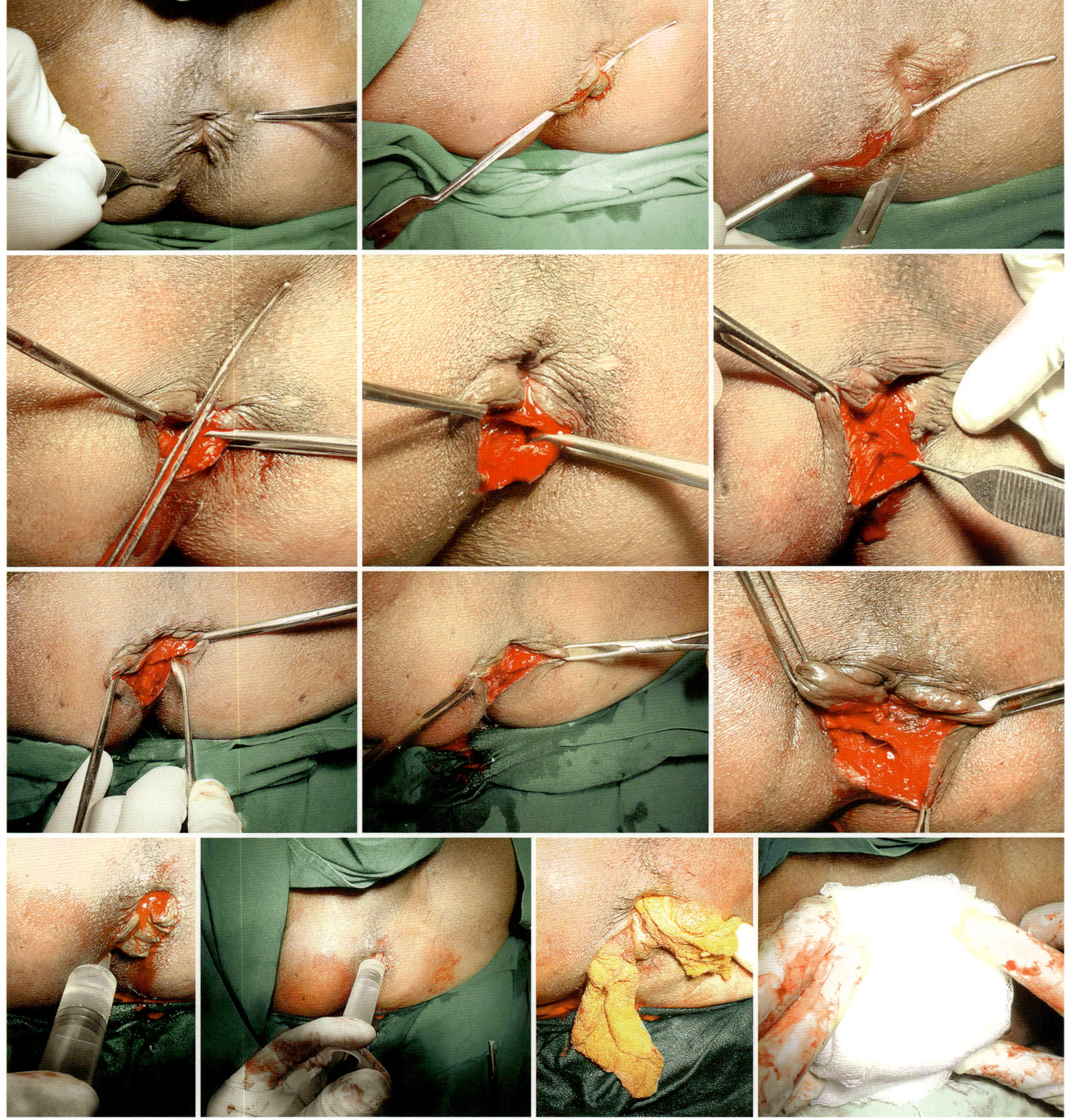

Fig. 26-88: Fistulotomy—laying open of the fistula track is the commonly done procedure.

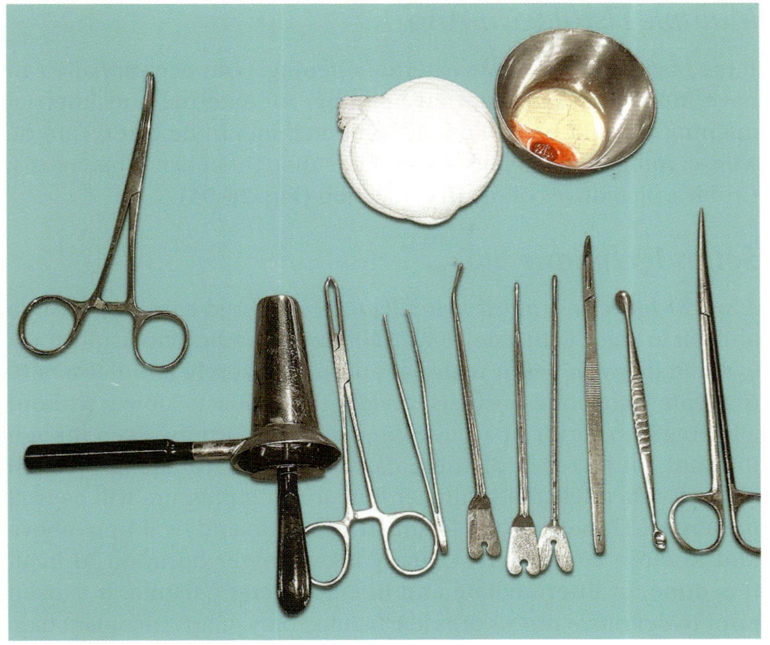

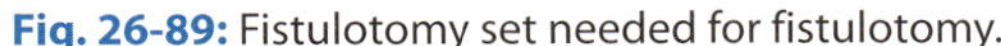

Fig. 26-89: Fistulotomy set needed for fistulotomy.

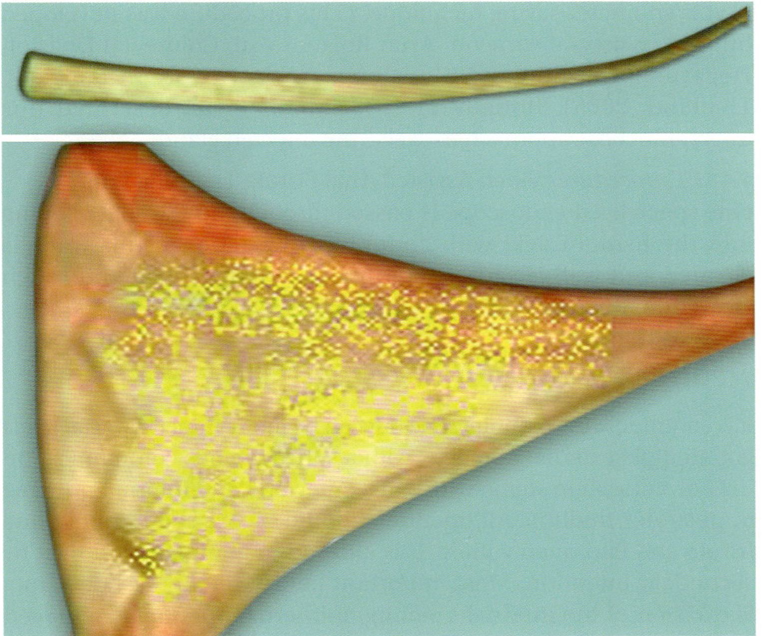

Fig. 26-90: Anal fistula plug.

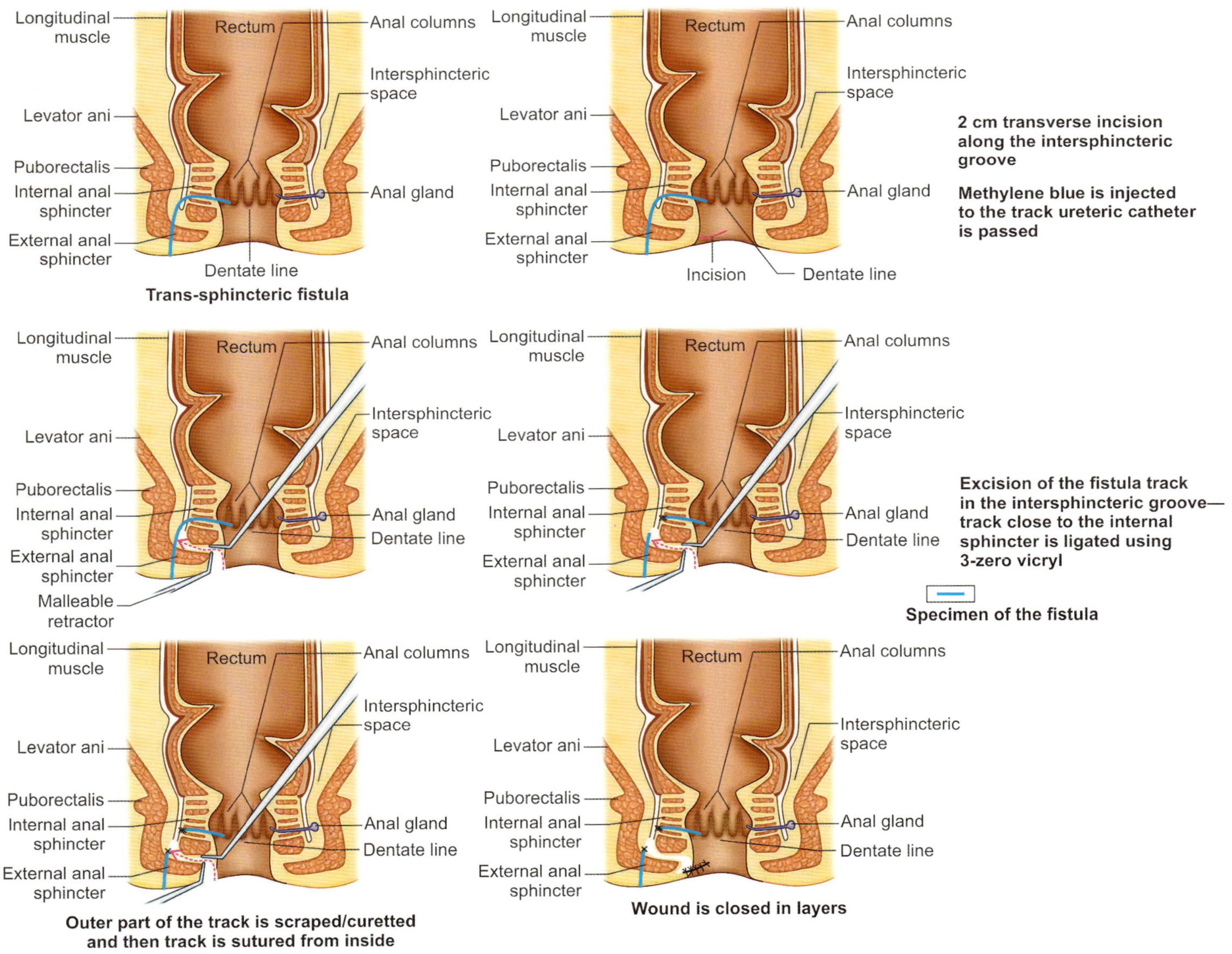

Longitudinal muscle
Rectum
Anal columns
Intersphincteric space
Levator ani
Puborectalis
Internal anal sphincter
Anal gland
External anal sphincter
Dentate line
Trans-sphincteric fistula

Longitudinal muscle
Rectum
Anal columns
Intersphincteric space
Levator ani
Puborectalis
Internal anal sphincter
Anal gland
External anal sphincter
Incision
Dentate line

2 cm transverse incision along the intersphincteric groove

Methylene blue is injected to the track ureteric catheter is passed

Longitudinal muscle
Rectum
Anal columns
Intersphincteric space
Levator ani
Puborectalis
Internal anal sphincter
Anal gland
Dentate line
External anal sphincter
Malleable retractor

Longitudinal muscle
Rectum
Anal columns
Intersphincteric space
Levator ani
Puborectalis
Internal anal sphincter
Anal gland
Dentate line
External anal sphincter

Excision of the fistula track in the intersphincteric groove—track close to the internal sphincter is ligated using 3-zero vicryl

Specimen of the fistula

Longitudinal muscle
Rectum
Anal columns
Intersphincteric space
Levator ani
Puborectalis
Internal anal sphincter
Anal gland
Dentate line
External anal sphincter
Outer part of the track is scraped/curetted and then track is sutured from inside

Longitudinal muscle
Rectum
Anal columns
Intersphincteric space
Levator ani
Puborectalis
Internal anal sphincter
Anal gland
Dentate line
External anal sphincter
Wound is closed in layers

Fig. 26-91: Ligation of intersphincteric fistula track (LIFT).

as it is sphincter saving technique. (This procedure was developed by Thai colorectal surgeon, Arun Rojanasakul, Colorectal Division Department of Surgery, Chulalongkorn University in Bangkok, Thailand, 2005). Initially in 1993, Matos et al. described this intersphincteric approach to excise the infected gland.

VAAFT procedure (Video Assisted Anal Fistula Track ligation): Fine specialised endoscope is passed through the external opening into the fistula track; with continuous irrigation fistula track is cleaned and wall is cauterised. Inner opening is ligated through vicryl from luminal side.

Treatment of Horseshoe Fistula

It is commonly trans-sphincteric but can be intersphincteric also. It has got multiple external openings with a subcutaneous communication in U or horseshoe shape with arms anteriorly and internal opening in posterior midline. All openings should be excised in horseshoe fistula and laid open widely. It is allowed to granulate and heal by secondary intention. Most important part in the horseshoe fistula is excision of the internal opening; if internal opening is removed then external openings will close (Hanley). It requires unfolding of the posterior midline to drain the deep post-anal space adequately. External openings and their tracks in such situation are individually approached, curetted and packed. Laid open deep post-anal space is also packed **(Fig. 26-92)**.

Fistulectomy

Under general or spinal anaesthesia, probe is passed through external opening up to the internal opening, which is felt as an induration. Fistula is opened along the probe using a knife. Fibrous track along with unhealthy granulation tissue and additional external openings are excised. Specimen is always sent for histopathology. *Fistulectomy for low level fistulas do not cause rectal incontinence.* Proper curetting of the infected anal gland area is essential. It is done in recurrent, chronic fibrotic fistulas **(Fig. 26-93)**.

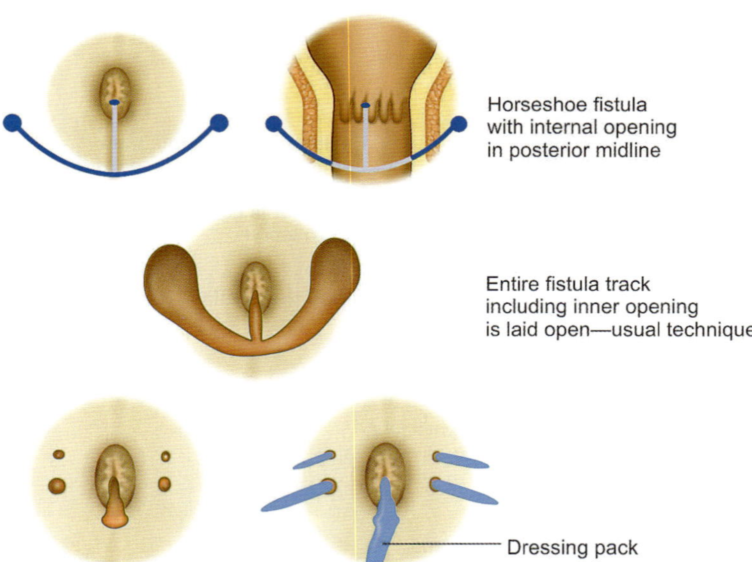

Fig. 26-92: Management of horseshoe fistula-in-ano. Both sides are laid open including the internal opening. When there are multiple external openings, they are individually curetted; internal opening is laid open properly.

Multiple Fistulae-in-Ano

It means usually multiple external openings; but occasionally can have more than one internal opening. All external and internal openings should be laid open. Sphincter should be taken care of. Non-cryptoglandular causes should be thought of like tuberculosis, Crohn's, ulcerative colitis, HIV infection **(Fig. 26-94)**.

Seton Technique

A silk or linen or braided nylon ligature is passed across the fistula and left in place with a tie. *Striated muscle* superficial to fistula track is encircled with Seton material and tied securely and left in situ to create ischaemic necrosis, dividing the muscle slowly without allowing it to spring apart avoiding gutter deformity. Even though internal sphincter is divided, causing adequate laying open of entire fistula track, the sphincter function and pressure will be well preserved. This allows the fistula to granulate and heal from above and to close completely. Usually takes longer duration to heal. It is done for intermediate and intersphincteric fistula. It is used prior to definitive procedures like fistulectomy or advancement flap.

Seton can be kept for 3 months. It can be regularly replaced by new silk or any material by rail road technique without anaesthesia **(Fig. 26-95)**.

Two types of setons are present. Loose setons are used mainly to drain for long period in recurrent/postoperative fistulas and due to specific causes like Crohn's. There is no tension in seton. Soft braided nylon is used.

Cutting setons are used when enclosed muscle is needed to cut (cheese wiring through ice effect). It is placed tight. It is used as a definitive treatment. It divides the sphincters slowly and track progressively becomes lower until seton falls out on its own. So, sphincter is divided part by part so that time is given for healing to the divided part prior to the next portion of the sphincter is divided. It is said to retain the sphincter function and so continence.

Other Methods

There are still many more methods for treating fistula. As recurrence rate is higher and is common disease, more and more procedures will evolutes–like laser, etc. Their real advantages over standard technique is not sure **(Fig. 26-96)**.

Fistula laser closure (FiLaC): The procedure is applied by the closure of the internal opening and then passing the laser fibre through the catheter into the tract and delivering energy with a wavelength of 1470 nm. Laser ablates the unhealthy granulation tissue and obliterates the tract. Radial fibre is used here.

Fistulectomy and primary sphincteroplasty (FIPS): Here fistulectomy with immediate sphincter repair is done. It avoids keyhole deformity; reduces faecal incontinence and recurrence.

Fistula clip closure: Closure of the internal fistula opening with a superelastic clip made of nitinol (over-the-scope clip - OTSC) – by German surgeon Ruediger Prosst.

Submucosal ligation of Fistula Tract (SLOFT) (Dr DU Pathak 2014): Here probe is passed through external opening; just at the entry to internal opening probe is kept and 2 zero polyglactin submucosal suture ligation of the internal opening is done; normal saline is infused through external opening to confirm the secure nature. Tract is fulgurated using cautery or laser. External opening is kept open for drainage.

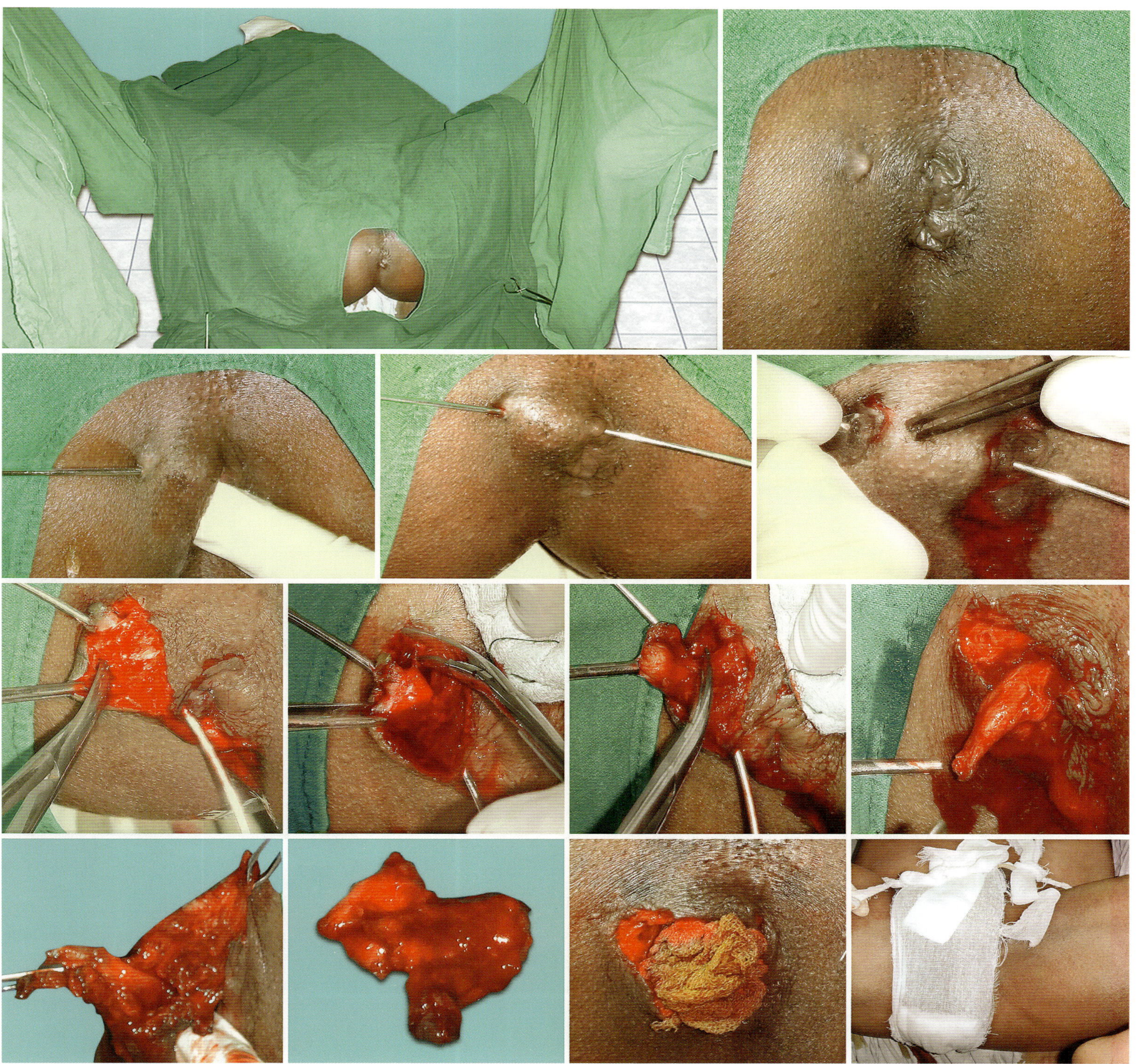

Fig. 26-93: Fistulectomy technique for fistula-in-ano. Entire track is removed and bed is curetted and left open; healing is slower in fistulectomy compared to fistulotomy.

VAAFT with LIFT (VA-LIFT): Video-assisted fulguration of fistula lining is done with intersphincteric fistula tract part ligation.

Subcutaneous incision of the fistula tract and internal sphincterotomy (SIFT–IS) (Rikisabura Sahara): It is a novel surgical procedure for transsphincteric anal fistula wherein fistula tract is incised through external opening and sphincterotomy is added from inside anoderm.

Other procedures: Distal laser and proximal SLOFT (DLPS); Distal coring with proximal fistulotomy with laser ablation (DCPF); Proximal superficial cauterisation, emptying regularly fistula tracts and curettage of tracts (PERFACT) procedure, transanal opening of intersphincteric space (TROPIS), and tunnel-like fistulectomy plus draining Seton combined with incision of internal opening of anal fistula (TFSIA).

Advanced regenerative medicine, such as tissue engineering and stem cell therapy, provide clinicians in colorectal surgery with novel and highly efficient techniques for treating perianal fistula in patients with underlying diseases such as Crohn's and other IBDs.

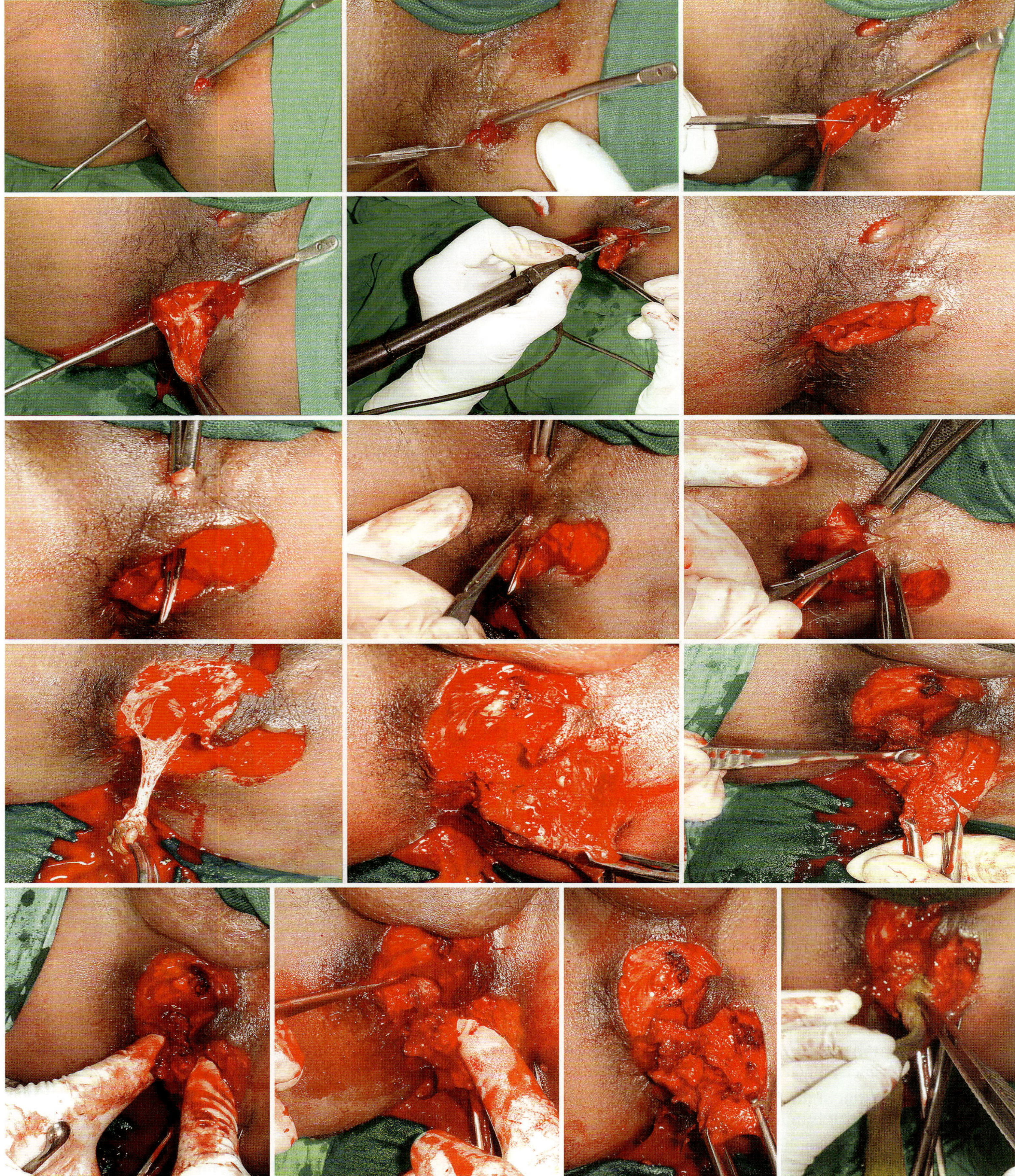

Fig. 26-94: In managing multiple fistulae, all external and internal openings including extensions should be laid open and curetted.

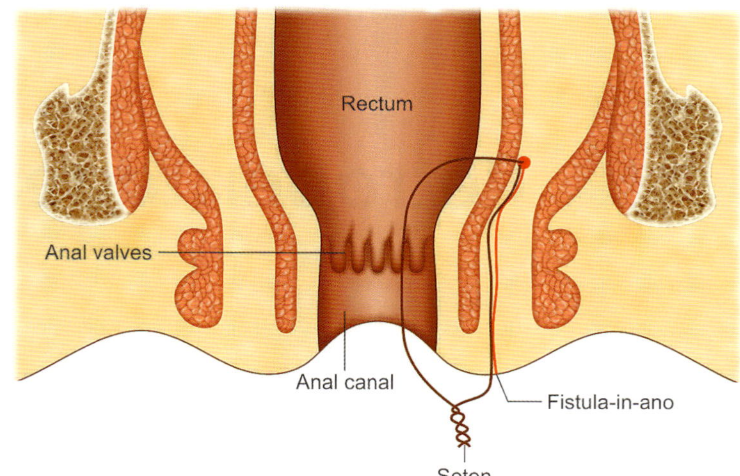

Fig. 26-95: Seton technique.

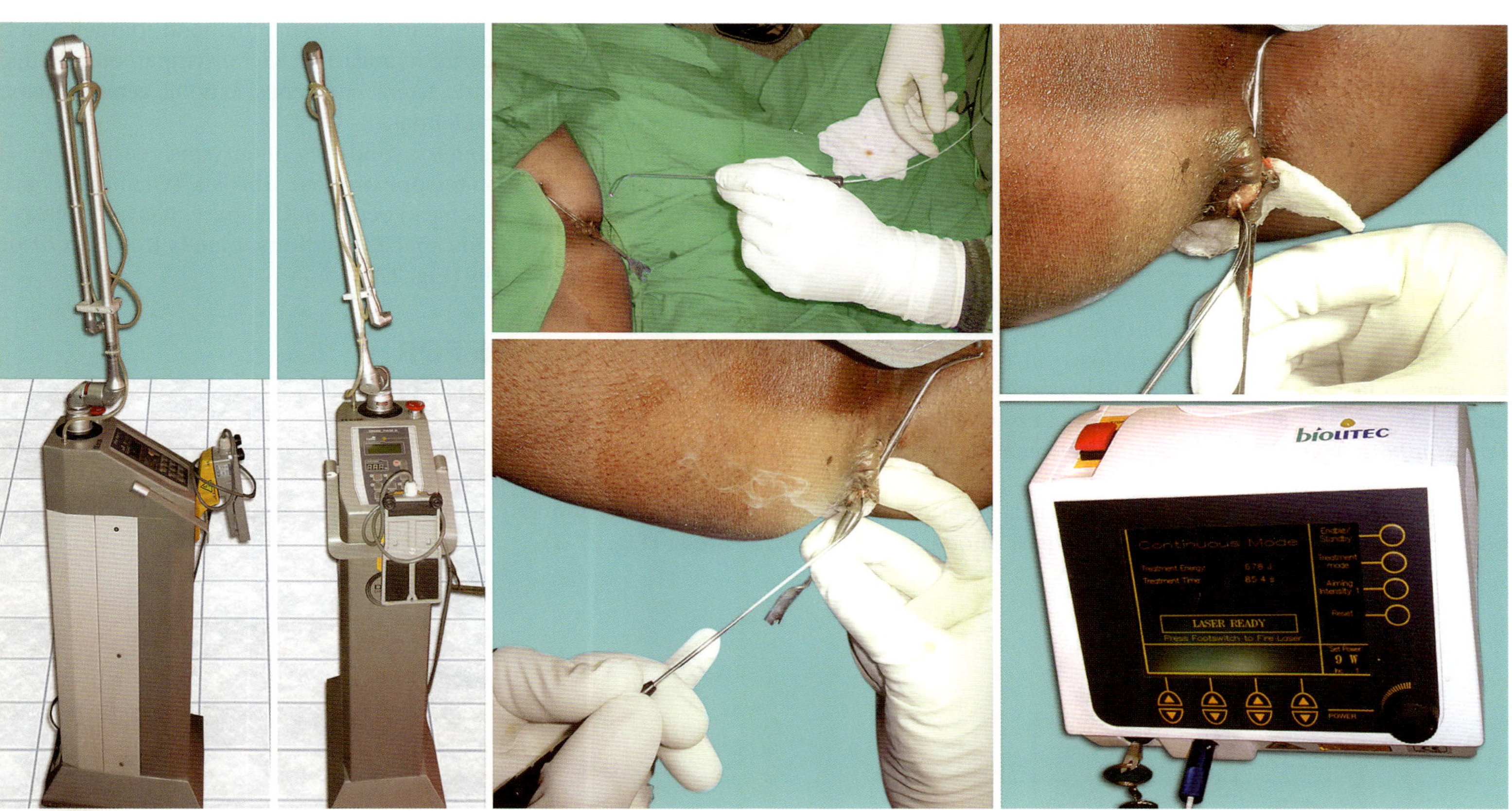

Fig. 26-96: Laser in fistula surgery. It controls bleeding well.

Postoperative Care

Sitz bath, antibiotics, analgesics, laxatives are given. Regular dressing is done. Wound usually granulates well and seals.

Complications

Fistula surgery is demanding and needs meticulous approach otherwise complications will occur. Incontinence for flatus and often faeces are the main complications. Infection, discharge, delayed healing, spread of infection are other complications.

27

CHAPTER

Retroperitoneal Surgeries

SURGICAL ANATOMY

This is the space between the peritoneal cavity and posterior abdominal wall. It is bounded anteriorly by posterior parietal peritoneum and contents of the peritoneal cavity; posteriorly by vertebral column, psoas, iliacus, quadratus lumborum muscles, and tendinous portion of transversus abdominis muscles; superiorly by diaphragm; inferiorly by pelvic levator muscles (by Ackerman). It is real potential space **(Fig. 27-1)**.

Three spaces are defined in the retroperitoneum. *Anterior paranephric space* is located between the parietal peritoneum and Gerota's fascia. *Middle perinephric space* is bounded in front by Gerota'a fascia and behind by Zuckerkandl's fascia; it contains kidney, adrenal, renal pelvis and proximal ureter and renal vessels. *Posterior paranephric space* is located between Zuckerkandl's fascia and transversalis fascia.

Retroperitoneum contains vessels (aorta, inferior vena cava, portal veins); kidney and ureters; pancreas, duodenum, parts of colon, rectosigmoid; lymphatics, cisterna chyli and thoracic duct; celiac, superior and inferior hypogastric, sacral sympathetic chains; ilioinguinal, iliohypogastric, lateral cutaneous, femoral, genitofemoral, obturator, sciatic and pudendal.

Retroperitoneal tumours, secondaries, aneurysms, retroperitoneal haematoma, abscess, retroperitoneal fibrosis (Ormond's) are different conditions which can occur in this space. It is an extensive space. Dissection in this space is tedious, bleeds from major or small vessels torrentially **(Fig. 27-2)**.

APPROACHES FOR RETROPERITONEUM

Transperitoneal lengthy midline incision is very useful approach for both sides of the retroperitoneum.

Loin incision extraperitoneally like approaches to kidney and ureter **(Fig. 27-3)**.

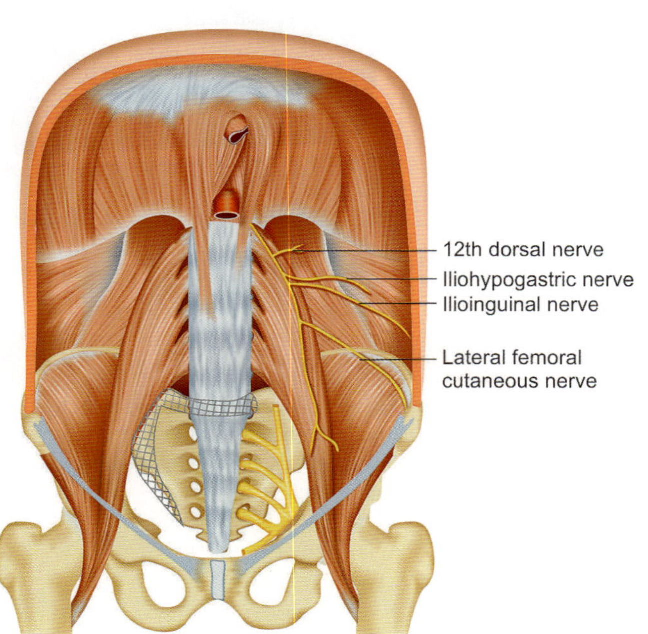

Fig. 27-1: Retroperitoneal anatomy.

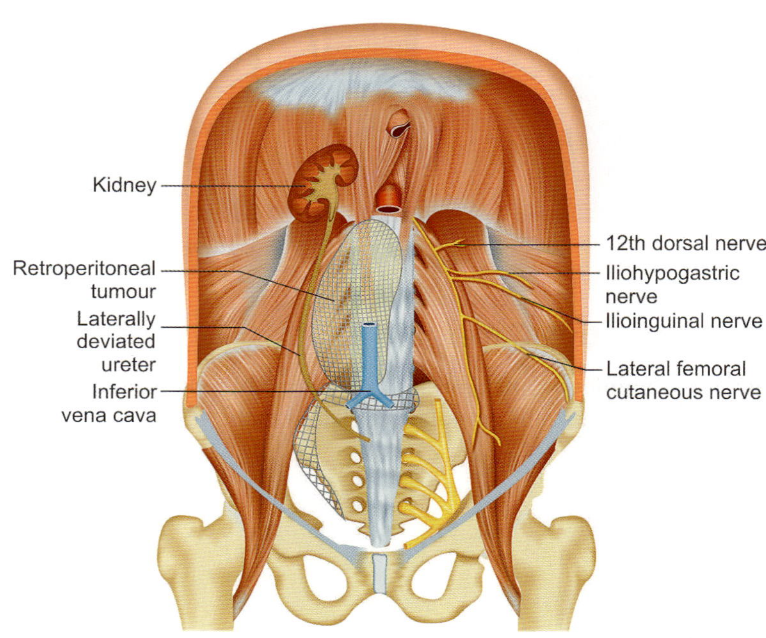

Fig. 27-2: Retroperitoneal tumour.

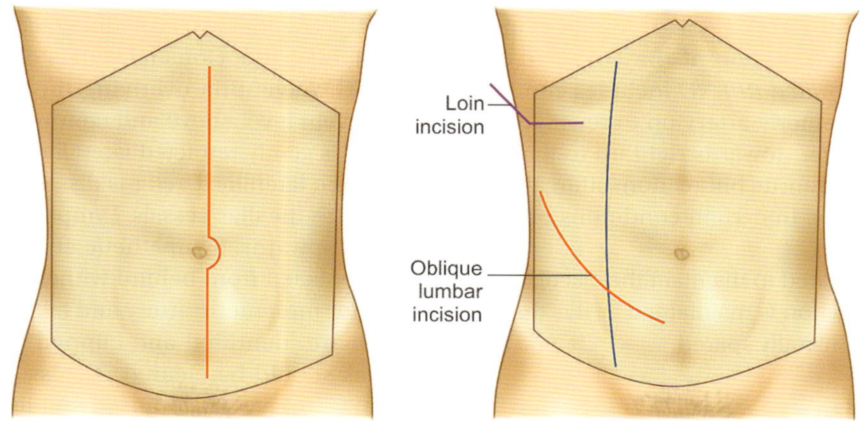

Fig. 27-3: Approaches for retroperitoneum—lengthy midline; oblique loin or loin incision in lateral position.

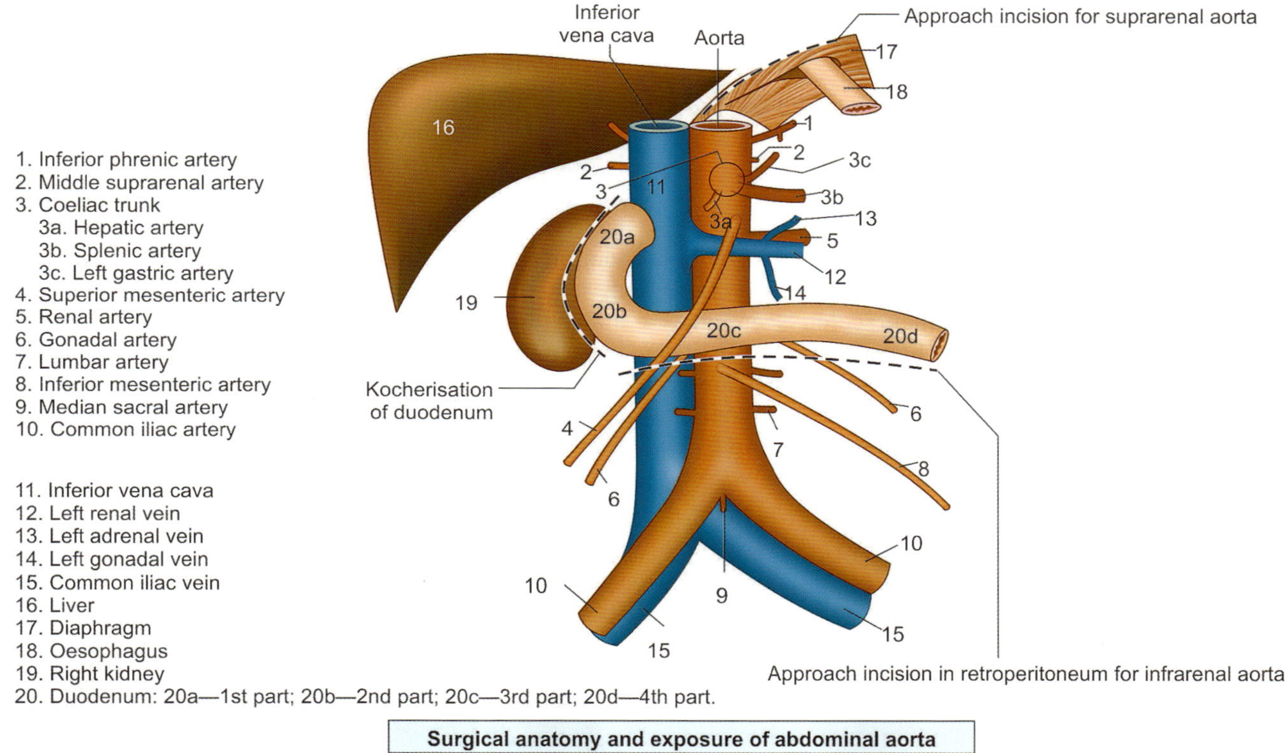

Fig. 27-4: Retroperitoneal approaches for aorta and lymph nodes.

Laparoscopic approach is very good to do retroperitoneal lymph node dissection.

Robotic assisted laparoscopic RPLND—is current trend.

Structures approached through retroperitoneum (other than kidneys and ureters) (Fig. 27-4) are:

- Aorta and its major branches.
- Retroperitoneal lymph nodes.
- Retroperitoneal tumour.
- Inferior vena cava and portal veins.
- Lumbar sympathetic chains.

RETROPERITONEAL LYMPH NODE DISSECTION (RPLND)

RPLND is often specifically commonly done for testicular and ovarian tumours. It is often also done in other malignancies like carcinoma cervix, endometrium, rectum, etc. Nonseminomatous germ cell tumour of stage I and IIa shows good benefit. RPLND is used for staging as well as for therapy.

Both open and laparoscopic approaches are used. Laparoscopic approach is better as magnification and dissection is better. Nerve sparing is better.

Right-sided RPLND includes complete dissection above the inferior mesenteric artery up to renal vessels; laterally up to both ureters; below along the bifurcation of the common iliac vessels on same side (right). *Left-sided RPLND* includes complete dissection above the inferior mesenteric artery up to renal vessels; laterally on left side up to left ureter; towards right up to the right margin of the IVC; below along the aortic bifurcation/bifurcation of common iliac vessels on same side. In certain conditions bilateral RPLND is also done.

Sympathetic nerve should be spared to maintain the ejaculation—nerve sparing RPLND. Erectile function is maintained as it is through parasympathetic fibres which are usually spared.

Preoperative Preparation

Patient should undergo complete metastatic work up RPLND is contraindicated as if there is evidence of blood spread or peritoneal spread. Peritoneal infection also temporarily preludes the surgery. Blood should be kept ready. Mechanical bowel preparation is needed. Nasogastric tube and Foley's catheter is passed.

Principles

Principles in RPLND are adequate exposure; meticulous dissection; haemostasis; use of bipolar cautery, proper retraction, safeguarding the bowel.

Technique

Right-sided RPLND: Right peritoneal fold (Toldt's line) is incised from hepatic flexure to medial umbilical ligament; colon is retracted medially by sharp dissection; colorenal and hepatorenal ligaments are divided by sharp dissection. Kocher's duodenal mobilisation is done. Great vessels are exposed. Right spermatic cord and internal inguinal ring are identified. Vas deferens crossing ureter and iliac vessels is dissected, clipped and transected. External, iliac vessels should be safeguarded. Gonadal vein is dissected up to its joining to IVC; gonadal artery is dissected up to a point where it crosses and joins aorta. Gonadal vein is clipped and divided at its joining to IVC. Adventitia overlying the IVC is dissected carefully from renal vein level above and common iliac vessels level below. Right ureter is gently retracted laterally and lymphatics are dissected and retracted laterally. Ureter is dissected distally up to the point where it crosses the iliac vessels. Lymphatics with nodes are dissected and swept upwards. Sympathetic chain is identified and lymph nodes are dissected from behind without injuring the sympathetic chain. Inferior mesenteric artery and left renal artery is identified. Lumbar veins are identified and clipped before division. Intercavoaortic nodes should be cleared. Accessory renal artery and retroaortic renal vein may get confused and ligated inadvertently; this should be avoided. IVC is retracted gently in front and tissues are dissected and brought towards specimen. Dissection up to the left ureter should be done in right RPLND **(Fig. 27-5)**.

Left-sided RPLND: Dissection here is above up to left renal vein; left ureter laterally; bifurcation of left common iliac veins below; right margin of IVC towards right side. Left paracolic gutter peritoneum is incised. Left colon is mobilised including splenic flexure by dividing left renocolic, phrenocolic, splenocolic, gastrocolic and pancreaticocolic ligaments; left renal vein is identified and dissected. Below up to the bifurcation of the common iliac vessels dissection is done. Colon, spleen above mobilised medially; left internal inguinal ring and left vas deferens is identified; left vas deferens is divided after clipping. Left gonadal vein is dissected up to its joining into the left renal vein. Aorta and left ureter is identified and dissected to clear para-aortic lymph nodes. Dissection from aorta above towards iliac vessels downwards along the origin of inferior mesenteric artery is carried out to clear all lymph nodes. Lymphatics along the intercavoaortic region from renal vein level to IMA level are cleared. IVC is dissected and retracted towards right to identify lumbar veins which are ligated and all tissues are swept towards left specimen side **(Fig. 27-6)**.

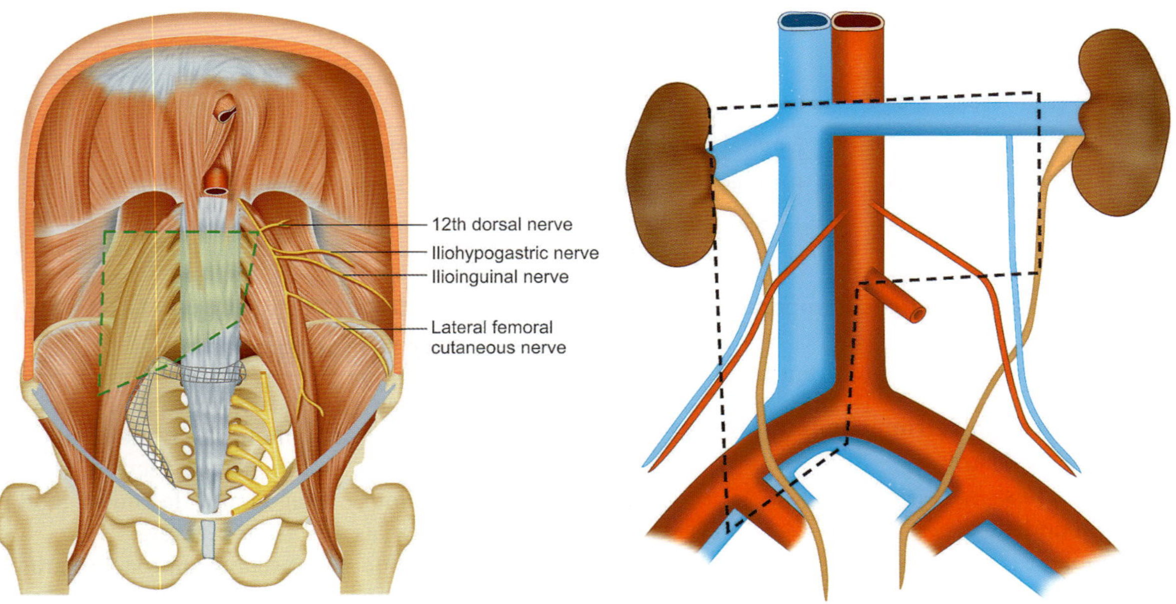

Fig. 27-5: Template for RPLND right side.

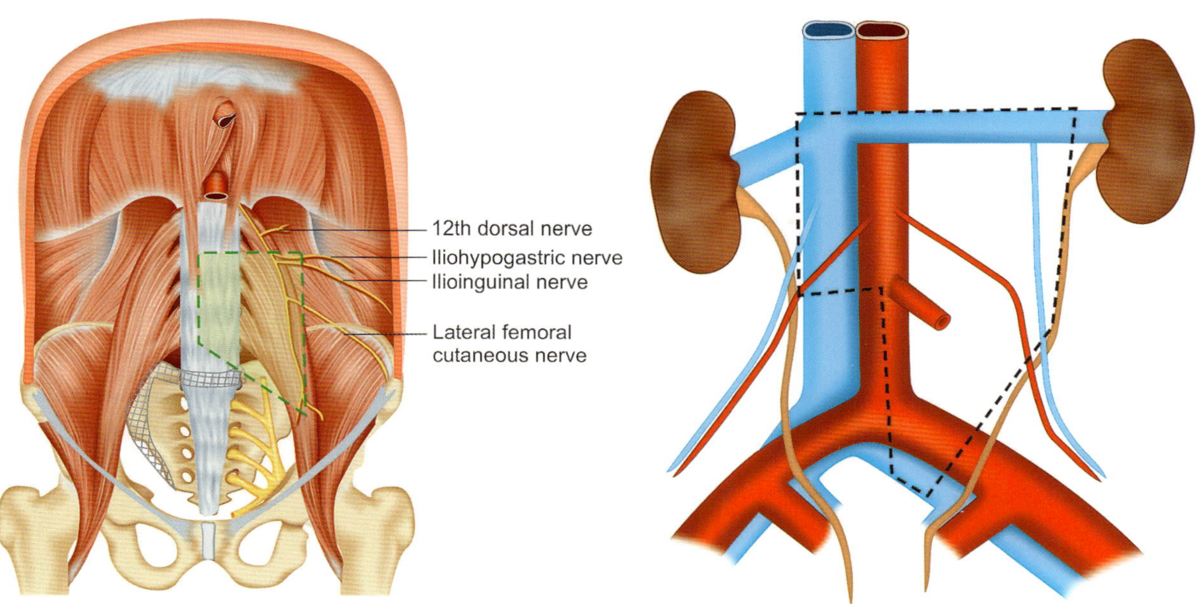

Fig. 27-6: Template for RPLND left side.

Complications

Haemorrhage occurs while dissecting and mobilising the IVC especially from its tributaries. Clipping the vessels is better way to prevent the haemorrhage.

Injury to ureter, stricture ureter (5%), and hydronephrosis due to surgical trauma can occur.

Lymphocele, chylous ascites due to lymphatic dissection is likely to develop often (3%).

Retrograde ejaculation due to sympathetic nerve damage can occur (5%). Nerve sparing surgery, avoiding monopolar cautery close to the sympathetic chain prevents this.

Contd...

Contd...

Paralytic ileus is common due to retroperitoneal dissection. If it persists long time one should suspect haematoma, pancreatitis, urinary extravasation.

Sepsis is not uncommon—retroperitoneal or intra-abdominal abscess formation can occur. It is diagnosed by CT scan, usually responds with higher generation antibiotics; may require guided catheter drainage; occasionally only needs open drainage.

28

CHAPTER

Urologic Surgeries

SURGICAL ANATOMY OF KIDNEY

They are a pair of excretory organs situated retroperitoneally, on the posterior abdominal wall; one on each side of vertebral column. Vertically, it extends from the upper border of T12 vertebra to the centre of the body of L3 vertebra. The right kidney is slightly lower than the left, left kidney is slightly nearer to the median plane. Each kidney is about 11 cm long, 6 cm broad, and 3 cm thick; 150 gram in weight; reddish brown in colour. Lateral border is convex. Medial border is concave with a hilum. Structures seen in the hilum are (from anterior to posterior)—(1) renal vein, (2) renal artery, (3) renal pelvis. Upper pole is related to suprarenal gland; lower pole lies 1 inch above the iliac crest. Capacity of renal pelvis is 10 mL. The angle between the 12th rib and the outer border of the sacrospinalis is the kidney/renal angle. Fetal kidney has got 12 lobules which fuse after birth to become smooth. Hepatorenal pouch (Morrison's kidney pouch) is a peritoneum lined deep recess, related to the upper pole of kidney. It is the lowest site when the body is in horizontal position, excluding the pelvis. Collection of extravasated fluid is likely to occur in this pouch following surgeries of the liver and biliary tract.

Kidney occupies lumbar, epigastric, hypochondriac, umbilical region. It extends vertically from upper border of 12th thoracic vertebrae to the centre of the body of 3rd lumbar vertebra. Right is lower than left; left is more medial than right. Upper pole is more medial than lower as long axis is directed downwards and laterally. Transpyloric plane passes through the upper part of the right renal hilum and lower part of the left renal hilum. Hilum lies opposite the lower border of the 1st lumbar spine; right hilum is lower **(Fig. 28-1)**.

Morris parallelogram is surface marking drawn from behind; two horizontal lines are drawn one at the level of the 11th thoracic spine, other at the level of 3rd lumbar spine; two vertical lines are drawn one 2.5 cm and other 9 cm from the midline. From front on the right side hilum lies 5 cm from the median plane below the transpyloric plane; and above on the left side medial to the tip of the 9th costal cartilage. Upper pole lies midway between xiphisternum and transpyloric plane 5 cm from midline; lower pole 7 cm from midline at umbilical plane on the right side and at subcostal plane (little above) on the left side. Lower pole is 2.5 cm above the iliac crest.

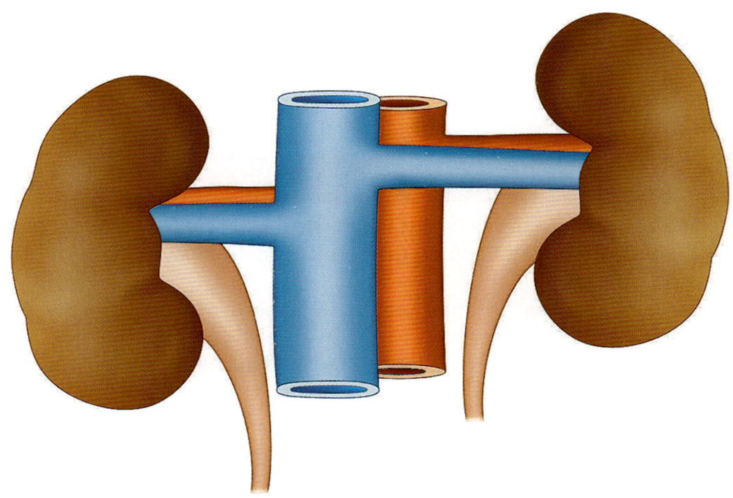

Fig. 28-1: Location of both kidneys and configuration. Right kidney is lower than left. Left renal vein is longer and runs in front of the aorta and behind the SMA.

Relations of Kidney

Posterior relations: Diaphragm, medial and lateral arcuate ligaments; psoas major muscle; quadratus lumborum; transversus abdominis; subcostal vessels; subcostal, iliohypogastric, and ilioinguinal nerves. Right kidney is related 12th rib; left one to 11th and 12th ribs **(Fig. 28-2)**.

Anterior relations: Right—Right adrenal gland; 2nd part of the duodenum; right flexure of the colon; small bowel; partly covered by peritoneum at hepatic and bowel parts. *Left*—Left adrenal gland; spleen; stomach; pancreas; splenic vessels; left colonic flexure; descending colon; jejunum. Gastric, splenic and jejunal surfaces are covered by peritoneum.

Capsules of Kidney

Proper fibrous capsule: It is fibrous membrane which can easily be stripped off from the organ. This is a thin membrane which closely invests the kidney and lines the renal pelvis.

Perirenal/perinephric fat is in the space of Gerota—it is the layer of fat outside the fibrous capsule.

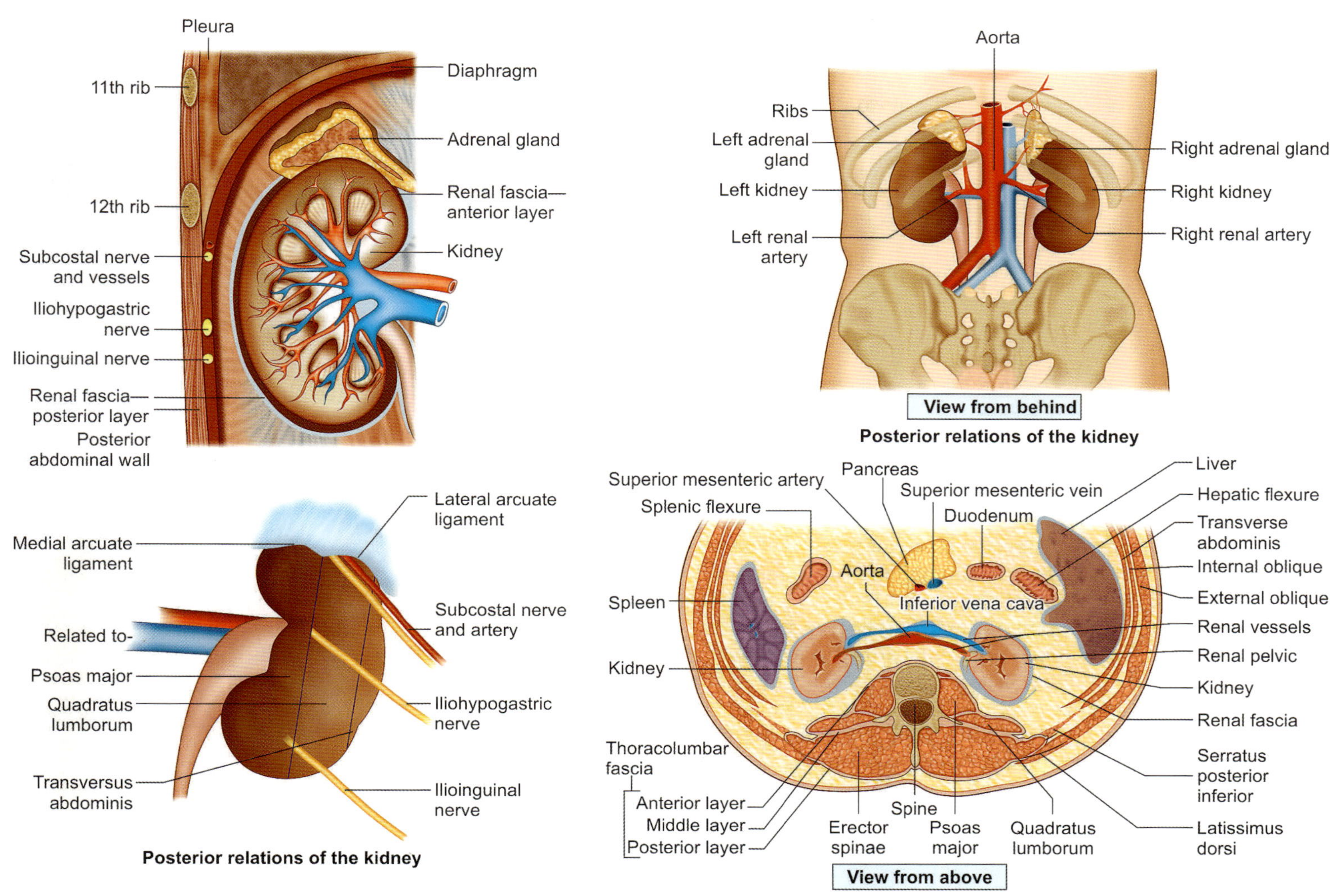

Fig. 28-2: Relations of kidney.

Renal fascia of Gerota: It is fibroareolar sheath which covers the kidney and perinephric fat. It has got anterior layer *(Fascia of Toldt)* and posterior layer *(Fascia of Zuckerkandl)*. Many trabeculae runs in this plane from fibrous capsule to the renal fascia. Above two layers of renal fascia encloses the adrenal gland as a separate compartment and fuse each other; continuing with fascia under the diaphragm. Below two layers are separate enclosing the ureter; anterior layer merges with the connective tissue of the iliac fossa; posterior layer blends with the fascia iliaca. Laterally two layers fuse to continue as fascia transversalis. Medially anterior layer passes in front of the renal vessels and merges with the connective tissue around the aorta and IVC. The posterior layer gets fused with the fascia covering the quadratus lumborum and psoas major; to the vertebra and intervertebral disc. Medially it forms a septum to get pierced by renal vessels preventing perirenal fluid to cross to opposite side.

Pararenal/paranephric body of fat is fat lies outside the renal fascia more on backside and lower pole filling paravertebral gutter to create a cushion for kidney.

Structure of Kidney

Gross

Coronal section shows outer brownish cortex, inner pale medulla, and renal sinus. Renal sinus is a space that extends into the kidney from hilum. It contains (1) branches of renal artery, (2) branches of renal vein, (3) renal pelvis.

The pelvis divides into 2–3 major calyces which in turn divide into 7–13 minor calyces.

Histology

Each kidney is composed of 1–3 millions of uriniferous tubules; each of which has a collecting part *(collecting tubules)* and secretory part *(nephron)*.

Blood Supply

Arterial Supply

It is from renal artery, which arises from the aorta at right angles, at the level of intervertebral discs between L1 and L2 vertebrae just below the level of the origin of the SMA. Right renal artery passes laterally behind the IVC and head of the pancreas to reach the right renal hilum. Left renal artery runs behind the left renal vein, splenic vein, body of the pancreas and duodenojejunal flexure. Each renal artery gives inferior adrenal artery and ureteral branches. About 95% of abdominal aortic aneurysm arises below the level of origin of renal artery **(Fig. 28-3)**.

The kidney is divided into anatomic segments based on blood supply. In the hilum, the main artery, divides into anterior and posterior divisions. The anterior division supplies the apical, upper, middle and lower segments; posterior segment is supplied by the posterior division. The knowledge of this is important in the

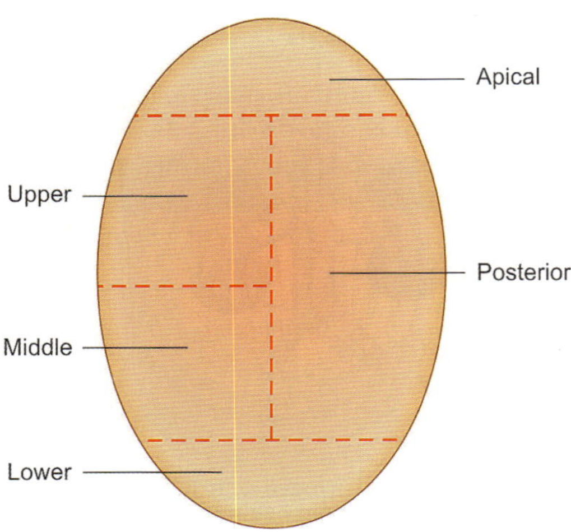

Fig. 28-3: Segments of kidney.

operation of anatrophic nephrolithotomy, where a functionally *avascular plane* (*Brodel*) between the posterior segment and the upper and middle segments exist on the posterior half of the kidney, about two-thirds of the way from the hilum to the lateral margin of the kidney. There is no collateral circulation between segments of the kidney but veins will communicate freely between segments.

Main renal artery → division → segmental artery → lobar artery to each pyramid → 2 interlobar arteries run on each side of the pyramid → 2 arcuate arteries interlobular arteries run radially to cortex → afferent arteriole to glomeruli and also branches to renal capsule which forms capsular plexus. Afferent glomerular arteriole → glomerulus → efferent glomerular arteriole → peritubular glomerular plexus. Renal medulla derives its blood supply from efferent arterioles. Free circulation in the cortex is glomerular; restricted circulation in the medulla bypasses cortical glomeruli which is more rapid **(Fig. 28-4)**.

Accessory renal artery (30%) may arise from aorta running parallel to renal artery entering the kidney either at poles or at hilum.

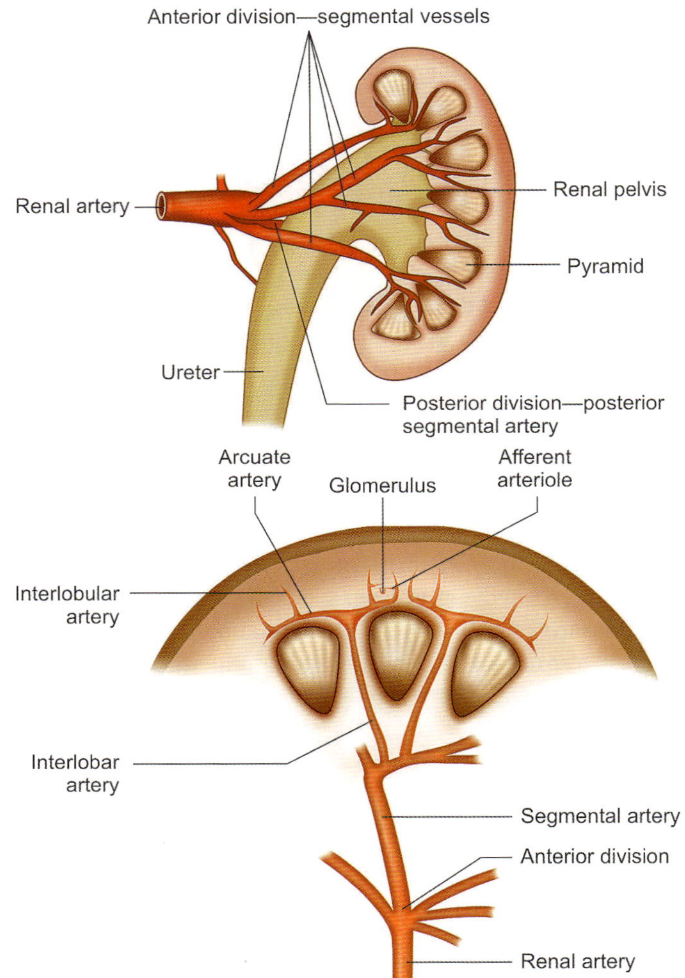

Fig. 28-4: Arterial segments and their distribution in the kidney.

Venous Drainage

Peritubular capillary plexus → interlobular veins → arcuate veins → interlobar veins → renal vein at renal sinus → join IVC just below the transpyloric plane. Left renal vein is longer than right one. Renal vein lies in front of the renal artery. Right renal vein lies behind the second part of the duodenum. Left renal vein crosses in front of the aorta lying behind the pancreas and splenic vein. Tributaries of left renal vein are left adrenal and left gonadal veins.

Nerve Supply

T10,11,12 through the lesser and lower splanchnic nerves.

Lymphatics

They are drained into para-aortic (lateral aortic) nodes. Perinephric fat is removed during nephrectomy (for malignancies), as intrarenal lymphatics freely communicates with the plexus in the perinephric fat.

SURGICAL ANATOMY OF THE URETER

Each ureter is 25–30 cm long. It begins within the renal sinus as a funnel-shaped dilatation called renal pelvis. It enters the bladder wall obliquely to open at the lateral angle of the trigone. It lies in the retroperitoneal space not attached to any fixed structures, so can be displaced or obstructed by retroperitoneal masses like tumours or aneurysms. Abdominal portion of ureter lies on the medial portion of psoas major muscle near the tips of transverse processes of lumbar vertebra (which is very well seen in IVP). The ureter enters the pelvis crossing the end of common iliac or beginning of external iliac artery. In females, uterine artery crosses the ureter from lateral to medial side, about 2 cm lateral to the cervix (this has to be remembered while ligating the uterine arteries in hysterectomy).

Ureter is marked by a line running downwards and medially from the tip of the 9th costal cartilage to the pubic tubercle; behind it is marked by a line running vertically downwards from the 2nd lumbar spine till the posterior superior iliac spine.

Ureter runs downwards and medially on the psoas major muscle and enters the pelvis by crossing the common iliac artery in front near its bifurcation. In the true pelvis ureter runs downwards, backwards and laterally along the anterior margin of the greater sciatic notch; opposite the ischial spine it runs forwards and medially to reach the base of the urinary bladder. It enters the bladder obliquely to open at trigone.

Normal sites of constrictions: (1) PUJ, (2) At the brim of lesser pelvis, (3) Along its passage through the bladder wall.

Abdominal Part of Ureter

Right Side

It is related to 3rd part of the duodenum; right colic, ileocolic, right gonadal vessels; root of the mesentery; terminal part of the ileum. Right ureter is related medially to IVC.

Left Side

Left ureter is related to gonadal artery (not gonadal vein but it is adjacent and medial to left ureter), left colic vessels, sigmoid colon, sigmoid mesocolon. Posteriorly, the ureter lies on psoas major, tips of transverse processes of lumbar vertebrae; genitofemoral nerve. Left ureter is related to left gonadal vein medially.

Pelvic Part of Ureter

Initial Part

Initially, it runs forward. Here, it is related behind to internal iliac artery, origin of its anterior trunk, internal iliac vein, lumbosacral trunk, sacroiliac joint. It is related laterally to superior vesical artery, obturator nerve, obturator artery and vein, inferior vesical vein, middle rectal artery, in females, it is posterior boundary of the ovarian fossa.

Later Part

Later, it runs forward. In males—vas deferens crosses the ureter above from lateral to medial side, the seminal vesicle lies below and behind the ureter, vesical veins surround its terminal part. In females, it lies in the lower medial part of the broad ligament of the uterus. Uterine artery lies initially above and in front, later it crosses the ureter from lateral to medial side "*water under the bridge*", ureter lies 2 cm lateral to the supravaginal portion of the cervix, then above the lateral fornix of the vagina and end lies in front of the vagina. Interureteric distance of the ureters inside the bladder is 5 cm in full bladder and 2.5 cm in empty bladder.

Arterial Supply

Upper segment of ureter receives blood supply from branches of renal, gonadal and adrenal arteries; the middle portion from the aorta and branches of arteries of posterior abdominal wall; the pelvic portion from the branches of internal iliac arteries. Vessels reach the abdominal portion of ureter on the medial side; whereas the pelvic portion receives on the lateral side (This has to be remembered while mobilising the ureter). The vessels form an anastomotic plexus in the adventitia of the ureter, which is found to be deficient in 10–15% of individuals leading to necrosis of cut ends of ureter following extensive mobilisation. Arteries divide into ascending and descending branches which first form a plexus on the surface of ureter.

Nerve Supply of Ureter

Sympathetic comes from T10-L1 segments and parasympathetic from S2-S4 nerves. It arises from renal, aortic and hypogastric plexuses.

ANATOMY OF URINARY BLADDER

It is a muscular reservoir of urine situated in the pelvis, posterior to the pubic bone from which it is separated by the retropubic space. The size, shape, position of bladder depends on the amount of urine it contains. In females, the peritoneum is reflected from the superior surface of the bladder onto the anterior wall of the uterus close to the junction of the body of uterus and cervix. In males, the peritoneum is reflected from the superior surface of the bladder over the superior surface of the ductus deferens and seminal vesicles. The neck of the bladder is the most fixed part, lies 3–4 cm behind the pubic symphysis. In males, it lies on the prostate and in females it rests on the anterior vaginal wall which is also supported by the levator ani muscle **(Fig. 28-5)**.

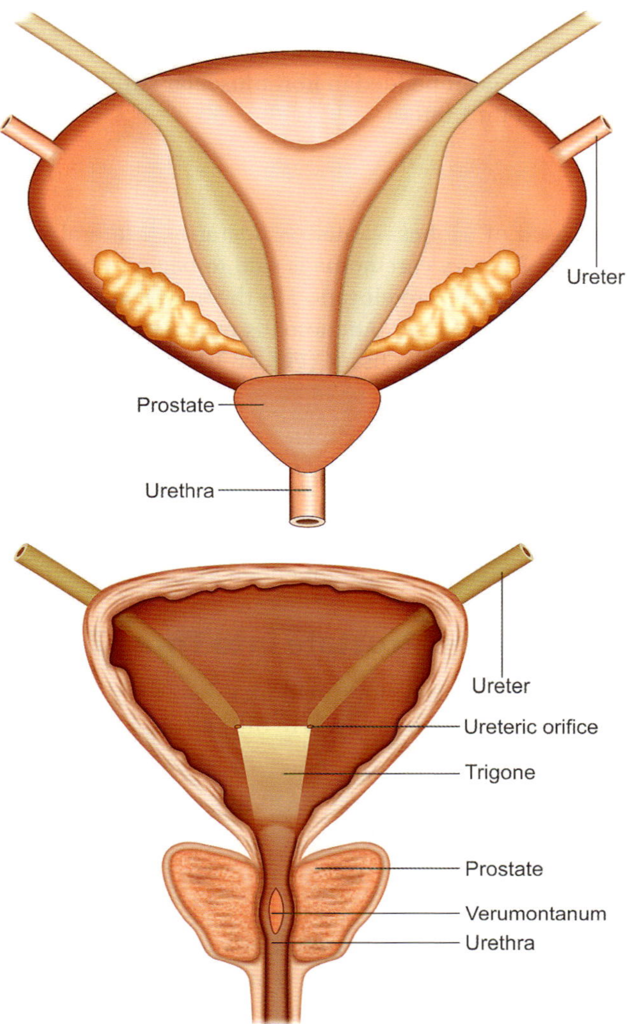

Fig. 28-5: Anatomy of urinary bladder—posterior aspect and interior part.

Structure of the Bladder

The bladder wall consists of interlacing fibres of smooth muscle. The urothelium consists of transitional epithelium which is loosely attached and easily separated from the bladder wall except over the *trigone*. *Trigone* is a triangular area over the lower part of the base of the bladder. The ureters open into the posterolateral angles of the trigone. The internal urethral orifice opens at the inferior angle of trigone.

Sphincters

Internal sphincter: Smooth muscle, situated at the neck of the bladder, micturition follows its relaxation. It is innervated by autonomic nervous system.

External sphincter: It consists of striated muscle, innervated by the perineal branch of pudendal nerve (S2,S3).

ANATOMY OF PROSTATE

It is an accessory gland of male reproductive system. It is composed of glandular tissue embedded in fibromuscular stroma. It surrounds the first 3 cm of the urethra.

Lobes

It is composed of 5 lobes—anterior, posterior, 2 lateral, 1 middle/median lobe. Primary carcinoma is said to begin in posterior lobe. Middle lobe produces an elevation in the lower part of the trigone of bladder *(uvula vesicae)*. Adenoma is more common here due to more amount of glandular tissue **(Fig. 28-6)**.

Capsules

1. *True capsule:* Formed by the condensation of the peripheral part of the gland; continues with the stroma of the gland.
2. *False capsule:* Derived from the pelvic fascia. On each side prostatic venous plexus are embedded in it.

McNeal Divided Prostate into Three Zones

1. *Peripheral zone*—prone for carcinoma.
2. *Periurethral transition zone* where BPH arises.
3. *Central zone.*

Note: Prostate carcinoma develops in prostatic gland proper; BPH develops in submucosal glands.

Blood Supply

Superior and inferior vesical arteries, branches of anterior division of internal iliac artery, obturator and inferior gluteal arteries supply the bladder. In females, uterine and vaginal arteries supply the bladder instead of inferior vesical artery.

Venous drainage is by the vesical plexus of veins, which drains into the internal iliac veins. These veins connect directly to veins of hip bones, the heads of femoral and vertebral bodies. This accounts for the site of occurrence of bony metastasis in carcinoma of the bladder and prostate.

ANATOMY OF URETHRA

Male Urethra

Male urethra is 20 cm long and is S-shaped. It extends from internal urethral orifice (neck of the bladder) to external urinary meatus (tip of penis).

Posterior urethra:
- Prostatic urethra.
- Membranous urethra.

Anterior urethra:
- Bulbar urethra.
- Penile urethra.

Prostatic urethra is 3 cm in length runs vertically downwards from internal urethral orifice through the anterior part of the prostate. It is widest part of the male urethra (mainly in its middle). It is most dilatable also. It joins membranous urethra. Its orifice is star-shaped; posterior mucosa contains median longitudinal mucosal ridge as urethral crest/verumontanum; in the middle of this crest an elevation called as colliculus seminalis is present. Prostatic utricle opens into the urethra into a slit like orifice on this elevation. Prostatic utricle is a blind sac of 6 mm length in the prostate directing upwards and behind between median and posterior lobes. Opening of ejaculatory ducts are present on both sides of this slit. Two vertical grooves one on each side of this crest are called as prostatic sinuses. Around 30 prostatic glands open into these sinuses.

Membranous urethra is 2 cm in length runs downwards and forward through the deep perineal space; pierces the perineal membrane about 2.5 cm below the pubic symphysis. It is the narrowest part of the urethra in males. It is surrounded by external urethral sphincter. Many urethral glands open into this urethra. *Cowper's bulbourethral glands* are located one on each side of this urethra. Their ducts travel down and open into the spongy part of the urethra after piercing the perineal membrane.

Penile/spongy urethra is 15 cm in length has got *proximal bulbar urethra* running forward and upward in the bulb of penis; later it bends downwards in front of the lower part of the pubic symphysis to run in the corpus spongiosum of penis. Diameter of penile urethra is 6 mm in diameter and is narrow in its beginning; beyond the membranous urethra it is dilated to form intrabulbar fossa which bulges into the floor on each side; terminal navicular fossa in the glans bulges into the roof on each side. External meatus is 6 mm sagittal slit bounded by tiny labium on each side. Ducts of Cowper's bulbourethral gland open into penile urethra one on each side. Plenty of urethral glands of Littre open into penile urethra with their openings facing forward. Many small lacunae of Morgagni open obliquely forwards; biggest lacuna on the roof of the navicular fossa is called as sinus of Guerin **(Fig. 28-7)**.

Internal urethral involuntary sphincter contains smooth muscles, elastic and collagen fibres which is supplied by sympathetic nerves (supply above the level of the ejaculatory duct).

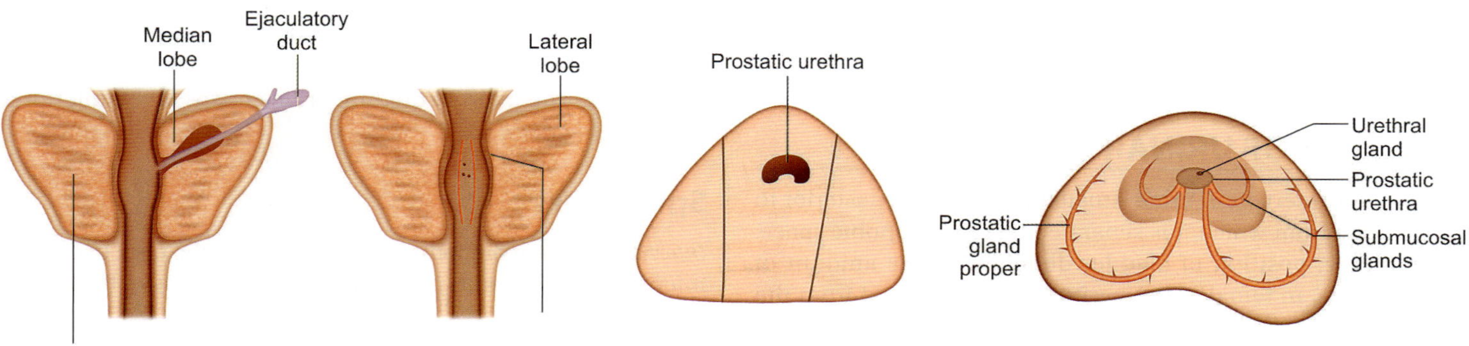

Fig. 28-6: Anatomy of prostate.

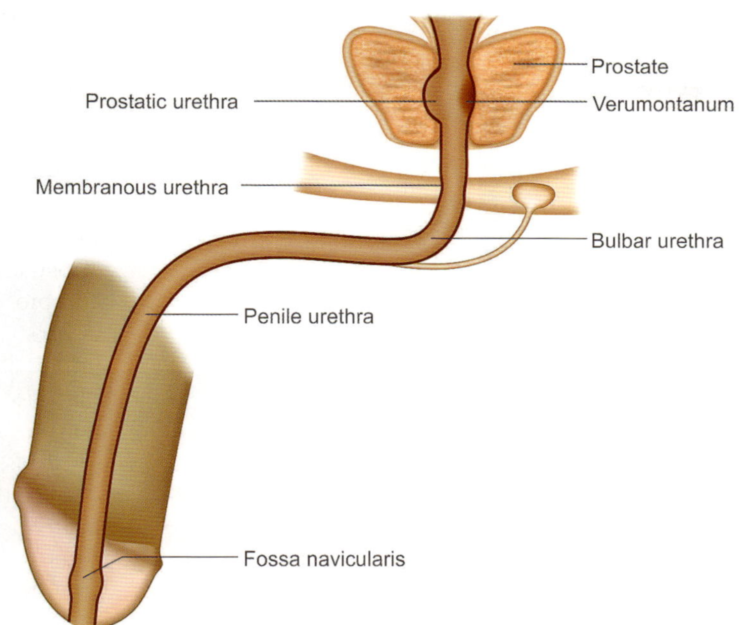

Fig. 28-7: Anatomy of male urethra.

External voluntary urethral sphincter controls the membranous urethra and is supplied by the perineal branch of the pudendal nerve (S2,3,4).

Female Urethra

Female urethra is 4 cm long and 6 mm in diameter. It corresponds to the prostatic urethra of male above the level of prostatic utricle. It starts at internal urethral orifice 5 cm behind the pubic symphysis runs downwards and forwards embedded in the anterior wall of the vagina crosses the urogenital diaphragm end at the external urethral orifice in the vestibule. Proximally, it is crescentic; middle, it is star-shaped; transverse distally. External meatus is sagittal. Paraurethral glands of Skene are collection of mucous glands on each side in the proximal part corresponds to prostate in males.

APPROACHES TO KIDNEY

Approaches may be posterior (loin) or anterior (per abdomen) or thoracoabdominal **(Figs. 28-8 to 28-10)**.

Loin approach is the standard approach. It is retroperitoneal approach. It is posterior subcostal with oblique lumbar incision. It is useful for pyeloplasty, nephrectomy for benign conditions like pyonephrosis with non-functioning kidney, tuberculous kidney, nephron sparing nephrectomies. Loin approach is in lateral position; with raised kidney bridge (or sand bags under the loin); with one knee flexed; large flat pillow between two legs; Mayo's table to keep instrument; arm is abducted and placed on an arm rest; with proper cotton padding to all pressure areas. Patient should be fixed to the table with tying belt and side supports. 12th rib excision is often required. 11th rib excision approach is done whenever 12th rib is rudimentary or absent.

Excision of along 11th rib along with the 12th to achieve extensive loin approach is called as *Nagamatsu approach* is used for large renal tumours.

Transperitoneal abdominal approach (anterior approach) is useful in renal malignancies.

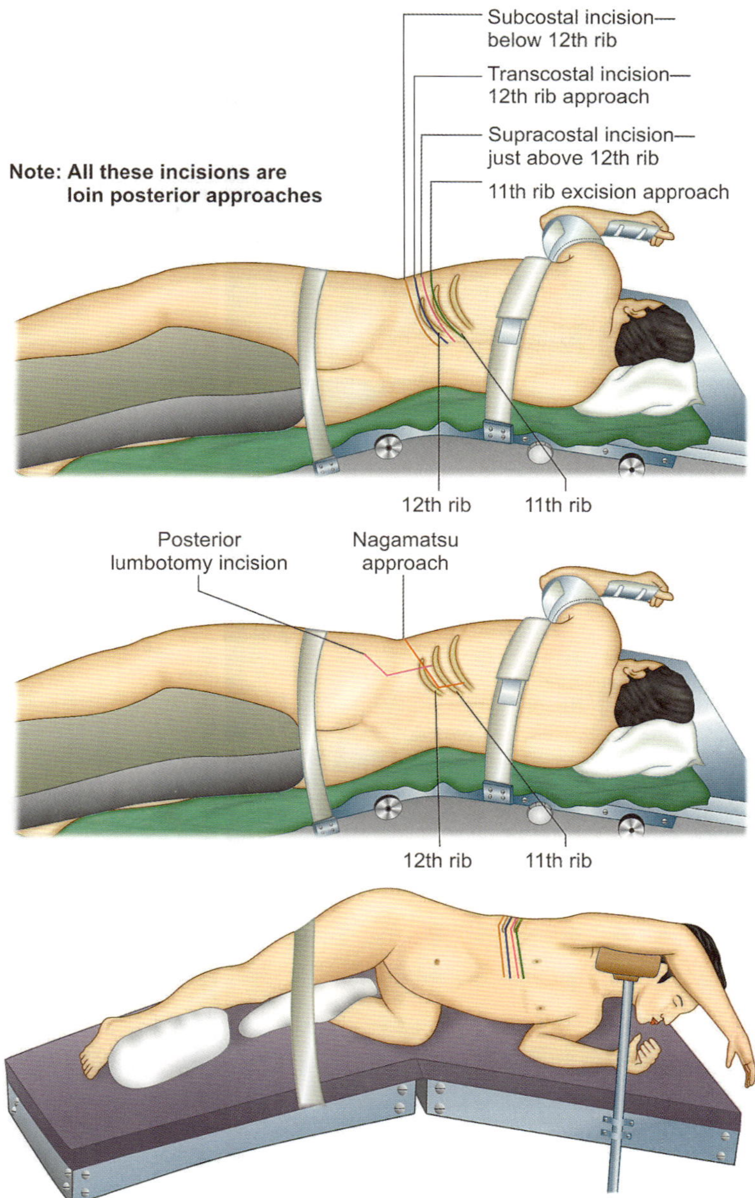

Fig. 28-8: Different approaches to kidney.

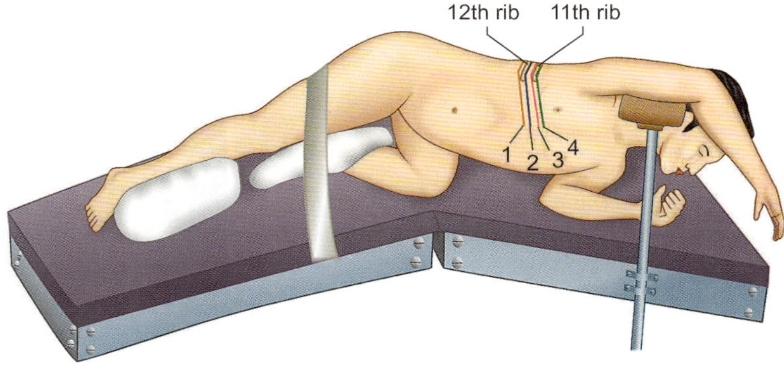

1. Subcostal approach—below the 12th rib
2. Transcostal approach—through 12th rib resection
3. Supracostal approach—just above the 12th rib
4. 11th rib excision approach

Note: All these incisions are loin posterior approaches

Fig. 28-9: Posterior loin approaches as viewed from front of the patient.

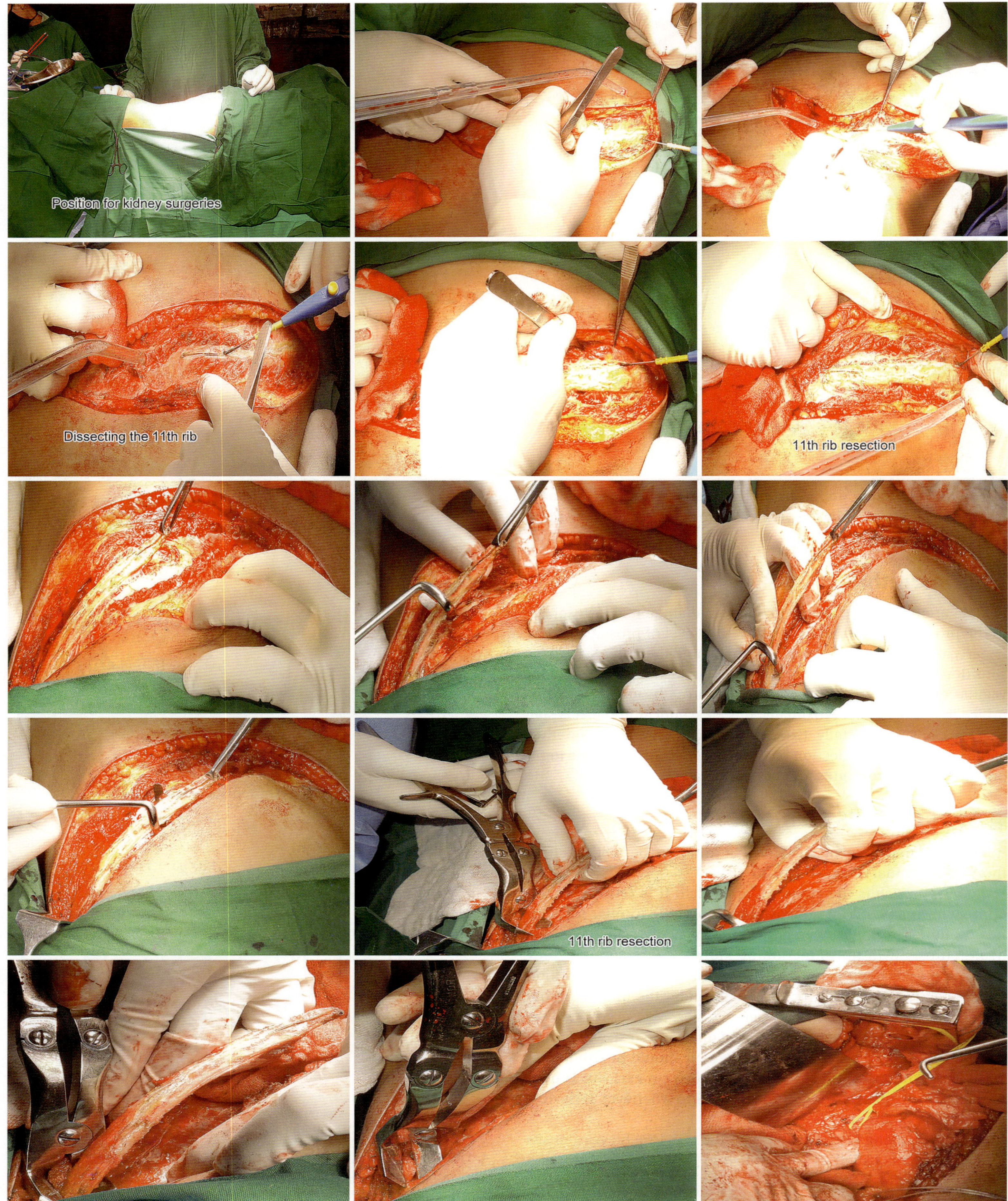
Position for kidney surgeries
Dissecting the 11th rib
11th rib resection
11th rib resection

Figs. 28-10(1)

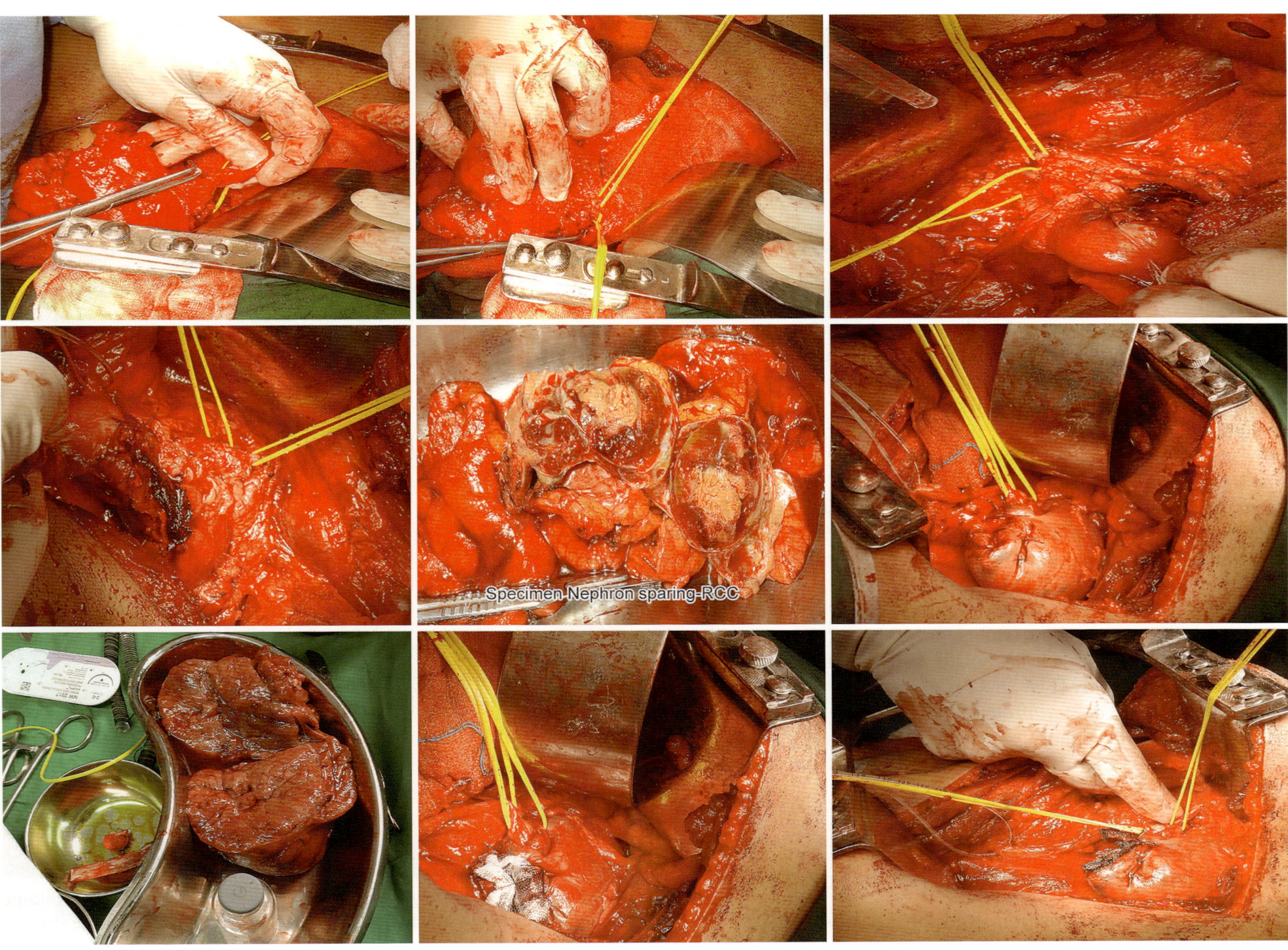

Figs. 28-10(2)

Figs. 28-10(1 and 2): Patient is positioned laterally (left lateral with right up for right sided kidney posterior loin incision. Mayo's table should be used to keep instruments safely. Cautery plate should be placed properly; both monopolar and bipolar (non-sticky) cauteries should be available. Pressure points should be supported with cotton cushion. Right hand is placed in arm rest. Intravenous cannula should be on to right hand; central line and arterial lines if needed should be placed for use. Blood pressure should be adequate; if there is drop in blood pressure adequate fluids should be given; only when blood pressure becomes optimum then kidney bridge should be raised; raised bridge may kink or cause angulation of the IVC leading to reduced cardiac input. Loin incision should be marked using marker pen; if rib resection is needed (in malignancy 11th rib resection is commonly done) rib should be marked. After making incision using no. 22 blade, incision is deepened using monopolar cautery. Subcostal nerves and vessels need to be cut after fulguration. Posteriorly incision is deepened on to the 11th rib; anteriorly external oblique, internal oblique muscles are cut along the line of the incision. 11th rib is dissected close to it using cautery; vessels at its lower part is ligated and cut or bipolar fulguration can also be done. Rib tip is held with Kocher's forceps and rib is separated off from its muscle and fascial attachments until posteriorly for adequate length up to the posterior end of the wound. Periosteal elevator and rib raspatory are used to elevate the rib properly and rib is transected using rib/bone cutter. In the upper part care should be taken not to open the pleura which are very close to the 11th rib. Anteriorly transverses abdominis muscle is split from behind forward; as in front muscle is adherent to peritoneum. Pleura is reflected carefully upwards posteriorly. Below blunt or peanut dissection is done along the psoas major muscle. Right sided colon along with peritoneum is dissected medially using finger dissection. IVC is identified as bluish structure; duodenum is identified and dissected medially and in front to get full length of the IVC under vision. Ureter is identified below and is slinged using infant feeding tube. It is dissected above to reach pelvis. Fatty and areolar attachments above the kidney towards the diaphragm are also dissected carefully; adrenals are identified at its superior pole as firm yellowish structure. Plane can be created above the adrenals or between the adrenal and superior pole of the kidney also. Finachutte retractor is applied to achieve proper exposure of the renal hilum for dissection. Kidney is held laterally to dissect the hilum. Using hydrodissection with a saline filled syringe plane is identified. Fascia covering the hilum is dissected using bipolar cautery and sharp dissection. Here blunt dissection should be avoided as it may tear small veins entering the renal vein causing bleeding and obscuring the field. It is better to ligate every fine tissue or cauterise using bipolar cautery which prevents bleeding, and allows clean surgical field for further anatomical dissection and also prevents lymph ooze postoperatively as lymphatics are also obliterated by this meticulous technique. Careful, meticulous dissection with patience with proper retraction is essential here. Renal vein is identified medially and dissected carefully to its adequate length and slinged using blue soft tape. It is often difficult to identify renal artery; it is felt posteriorly once kidney is brought medially. Once pulsation is felt it is dissected carefully for required length. Anomalies of both renal vessels are common; it should be always kept in mind while dissecting the hilum. All tissues should be dissected using bipolar cautery or fine ligatures and scissor without any hurry and hilum should be held with only its vessels and renal pelvis. It facilitates the easier application of vascular clamps to renal vessels as well as IVC whenever needed either in nephron sparing nephrectomy or radical nephrectomy.

Thoracoabdominal approach may be needed in large upper pole tumours. Patient is placed in supine position with two sandbags one under the shoulder and another under the buttock of the side of the surgery. Incision runs along the 10th or 9th rib extending from posterior axillary line to the midline and continuing downwards as midline incision. Hyperextension is provided by breaking the table. Posteriorly latissimus dorsi, serratus posterior inferior are incised using diathermy; 10th rib is resected (instead intercostal muscles may be cut above the rib); external oblique, internal oblique and rectus muscles are cut; costovertebral ligament behind and costal cartilage in front are cut. Pleura is identified and opened along the line of incision. Lung is retracted upwards; diaphragm is cut in the line of incision. Rectus sheath and peritoneum is opened up to the lower end of the incision. Large self-retaining retractors are used to retract wound edges to expose the field. While closing the wound, peritoneum is closed first; diaphragm is sutured using polypropylene or vicryl (no. 1); ribs are approximated using no. 1 polypropylene; pleura and intercostal muscles are sutured after placing a intercostal tube to the pleural cavity through the 6th intercostal space in the midaxillary line. Loin muscles are sutured – latissimus dorsi, serratus posterior inferior and external oblique are sutured. Other layers of the abdomen are closed. Skin is apposed using skin staplers **(Fig. 28-11)**.

Anterior supine paramedian vertical extraperitoneal approach is also popular for approaching while managing the benign conditions.

Laparoscopic approach is said to be ideal for many diseases including nephrectomy **(Fig. 28-12)**.

Retroperitoneoscopic approach is often used; but laparoscopic approach gives more space to work on it.

Posterior lumbotomy approach in prone position is no longer advocated.

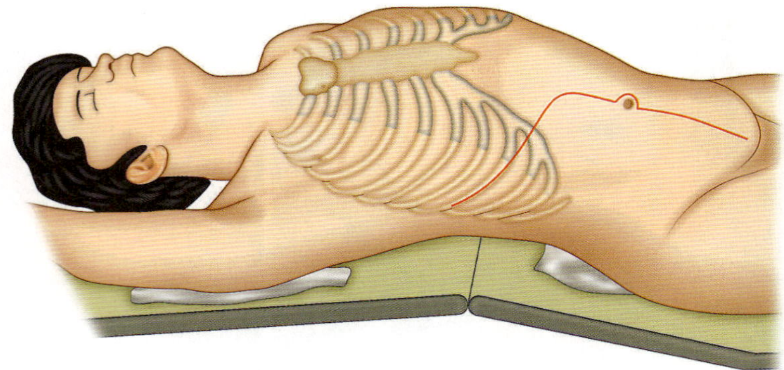

Fig. 28-11: Thoracoabdominal approach for kidney is done for large tumours.

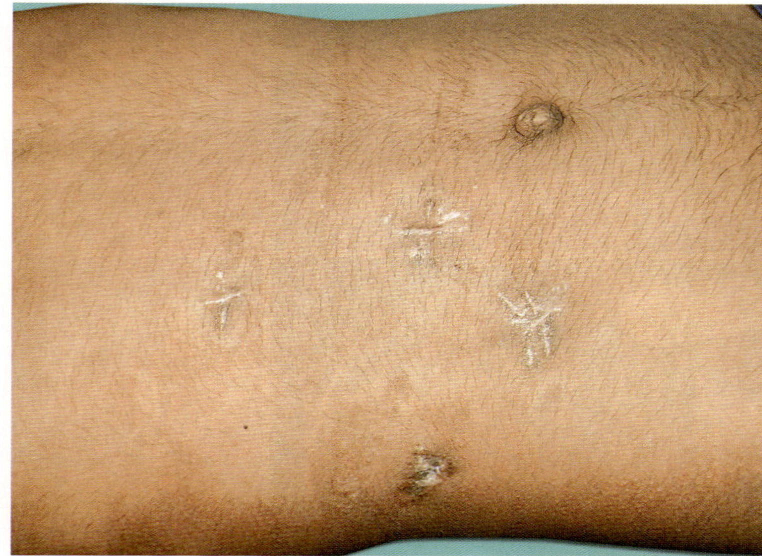

Fig. 28-12: Laparoscopy is very well accepted for most of the urologic surgeries; becoming standard also. But technique and principles are same as open method.

Loin Incision (Posterior Approach; Morris Incision, Sir Henry Morris London)

Loin position is usual position used for renal surgeries. It can be subcostal (classical Morris incision is subcostal type); transcostal (12th rib); supracostal (above the 12th rib in the intercostal space). Subcostal is used for the benign diseases and lower pole diseases. Transcostal, supracostal and 11th rib excision approach is for difficult cases and upper pole tumours.

Patient is placed in loin position. It is usually transcostal 12th rib excision loin approach. Full lateral position with kidney bridge raise (to break the table 40° to horizontal) with flexion of the knee of the leg which is on the theatre table is done (lower side leg—90°). Flat wide pillow should be kept between legs. Arm facing upwards is positioned towards head end with a support (cradle support). Patient is strapped firmly to table to prevent tilting or changing of the position during surgery. Back support is often needed. Mayo's table is placed on the leg side which facilitates to keep instruments safely after draping **(Fig. 28-13)**. Anaesthetist should observe blood pressure as it may drop after raising the kidney bridge by compression on the IVC.

After cleaning and draping, incision begins posteriorly behind the posterior axillary line in posterior subcostal line extending forward towards the outer margin of the rectus muscle. It usually marks angle of the 12th rib posteriorly to 15 cm beyond the tip of 12th rib. Rectus is usually not cut. Skin, subcutaneous tissue and superficial fascia are cut. Posteriorly latissimus dorsi, serratus posterior inferior and quadratus lumborum are cut; anteriorly external and internal oblique muscles are cut. Usually 12th or 11th rib is cut. Rib is identified. Incision is made over its periosteum. Periosteum is reflected using periosteal elevator and rib raspatory. Care should be taken to avoid injury to vessels underneath which often need proper ligation. Rib after mobilisation, is cut using bone cutter. Cut end is often smoothened using bone file. Pleura is very close to the rib which should not be opened. If opened pneumothorax develops; which is usually managed by placing vicryl sutures to pleura while anaesthetist keeps ventilating the lung with adequate expansion. Usually intercostal tube is not necessary. Postoperative check X-ray is needed for the evidence of pneumothorax. Transverse abdominis muscle is usually split from posterior to anterior. Peritoneum is adherent to the abdominal wall in front. So care should be taken not to tear on the anterior aspect. Peritoneum is swept forward to reach the Gerota's fascia **(Figs. 28-14 and 28-15)**.

Nagamatsu approach gives excellent exposure of the kidney and its pedicle. It is done in same lateral loin position. Incision extends initially vertically from above at its angle inferiorly to the angle of the 12th rib and then running obliquely forward along the 12th rib towards umbilicus just lateral to the rectus muscle. Periosteum of the both 11th and 12th ribs are removed and ribs are excised.

Note: In supracostal and transcostal approaches, diaphragmatic and pleural attachments are released; pleura is pushed upwards

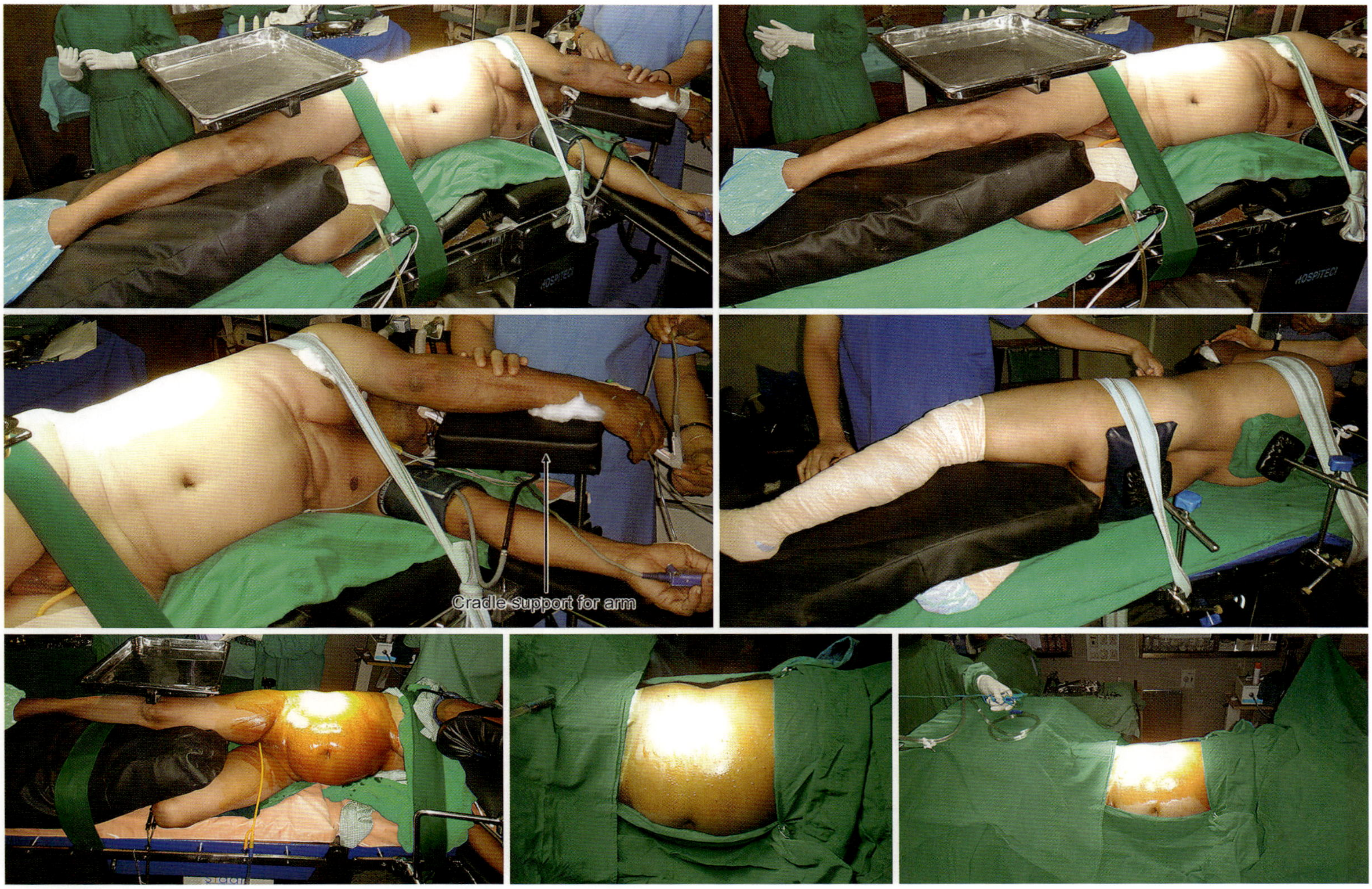

Fig. 28-13: Position of the patient for loin incision to approach kidney.

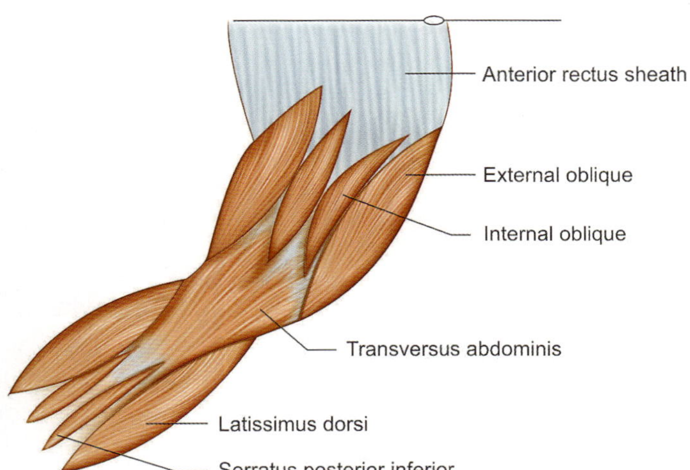

Fig. 28-14: Muscle and fascial layers which come across during posterior approach to kidney.

carefully without opening it. Costovertebral ligament should be divided. Iliohypogastric nerve should be mobilised below; subcostal nerve superiorly. Due to lateral position with raise of kidney bridge or breaking of the table venous return to heart decreases as due to IVC compression. One should inform anaesthetist while positioning the patient **(Fig. 28-16)**.

For many procedures of the kidney like nephron sparing nephrectomy, anatrophic pyelolithotomy ice packs are placed on the kidney surface for 20 minutes to increase the cold ischaemic time **(Fig. 28-17)**.

Closure of the Loin Wound

It is done in two layers. Transversus abdominis and internal oblique muscles are closed using continuous vicryl suture as inner layer. External oblique is closed using non-absorbable or delayed absorbable continuous suture as outer layer. Covering fascia should be included in the bite which is stronger than muscle itself. Drain when needed should be kept below the lower margin of the wound and on the anterior aspect in front of level of the anterior superior iliac spine; through a separate stab incision.

Incision can be extended into the thorax or into the peritoneal cavity as needed.

High 11th rib excision approach (both 12th and 11ribs are excised subperiosteally) is called as *Nagamatsu approach* which is used in approaching upper pole renal cell carcinoma (RCC).

Problems with Loin Incision

It is more painful, time consuming to open and close. Pleural and peritoneal opening is problematic in this approach. However, it is

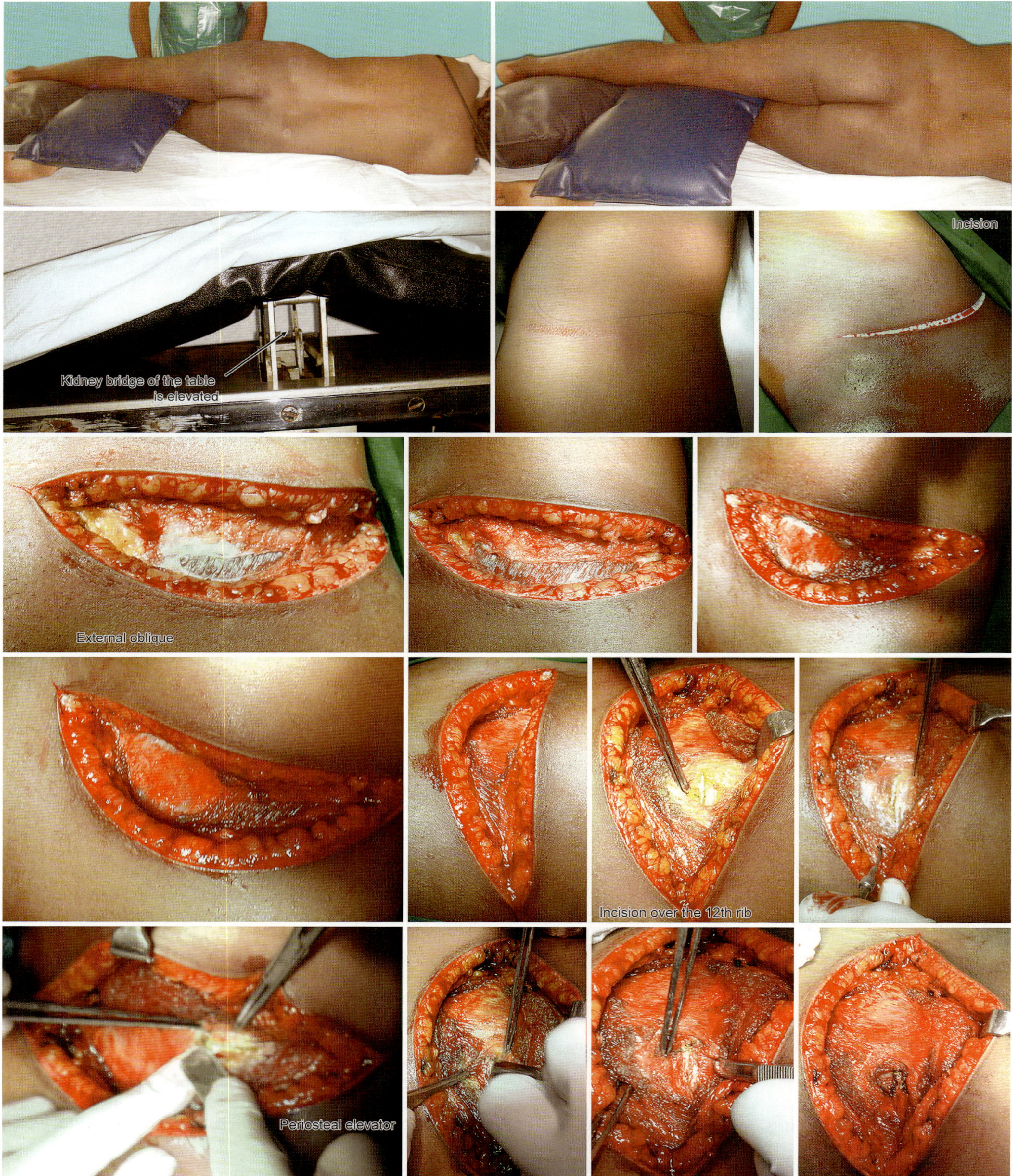
Kidney bridge of the table is elevated
Incision
External oblique
Incision over the 12th rib
Periosteal elevator

Figs. 28-15(1)

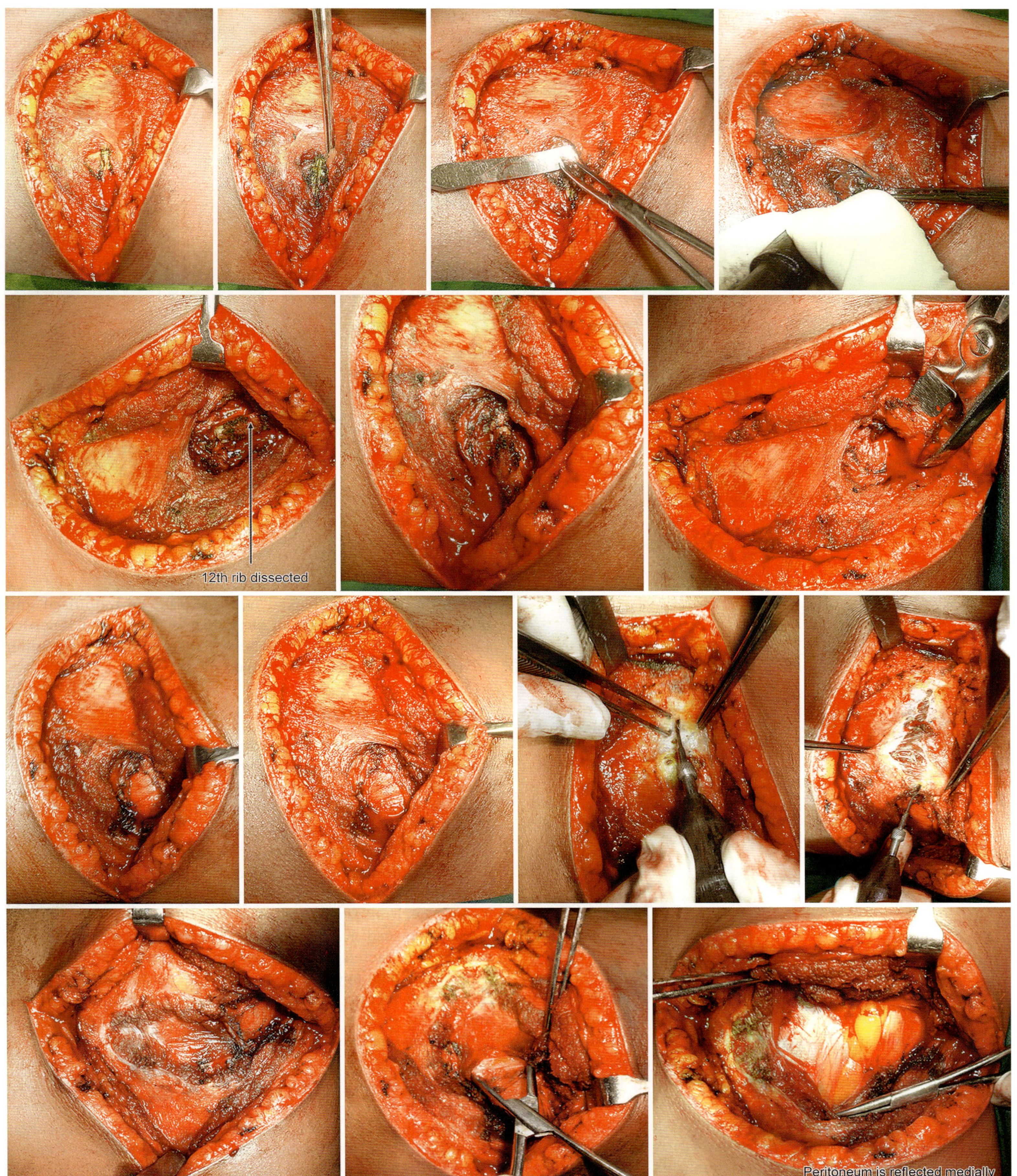

Figs. 28-15(2)

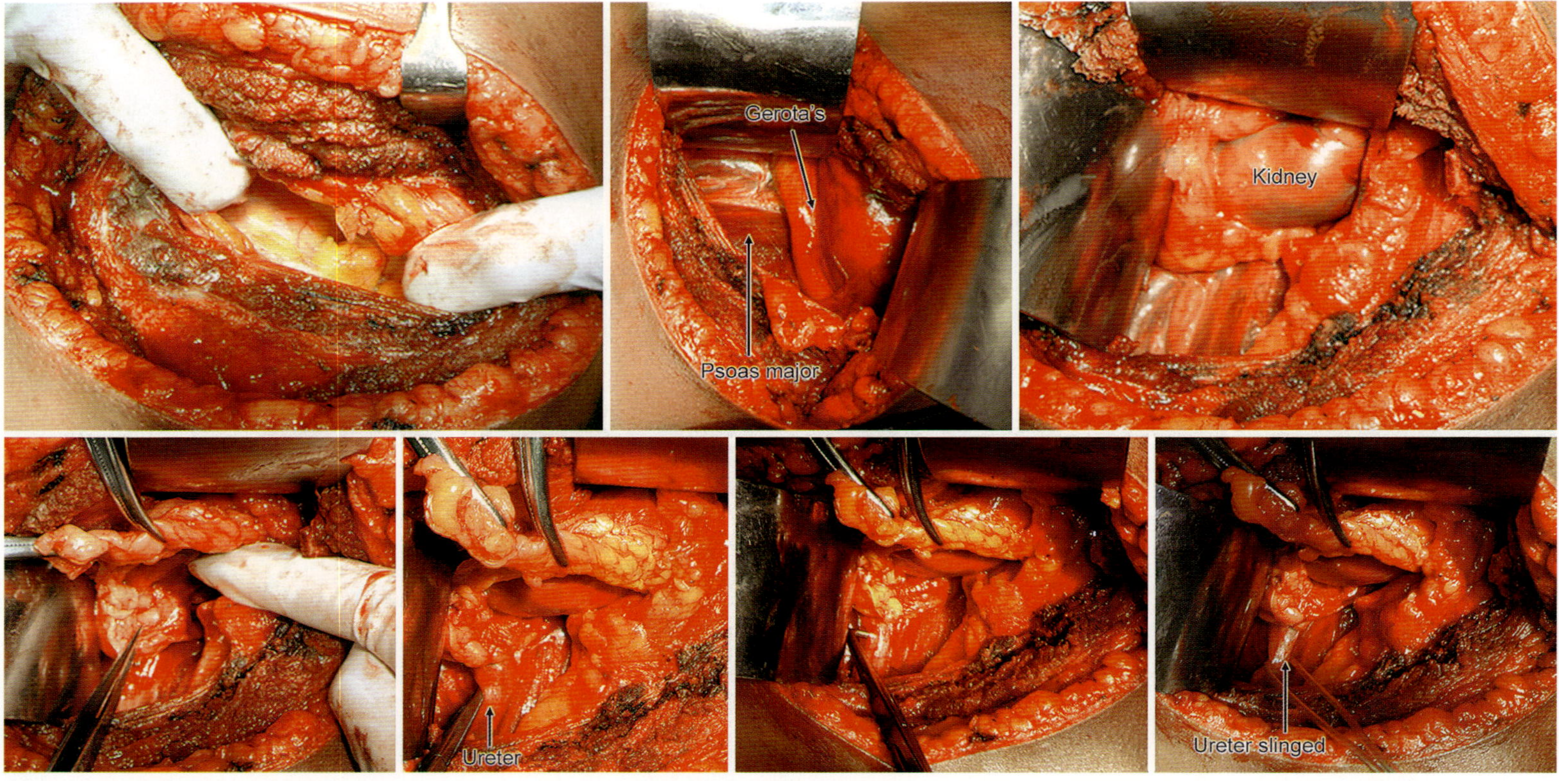

Figs. 28-15(3)

Figs. 28-15(1 to 3): Transcostal approach to kidney.

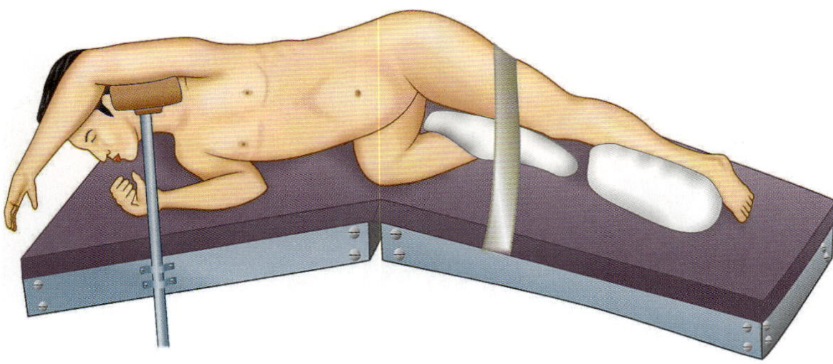

Fig. 28-16: Position of the patient usually used for loin approach for all common procedures including laparoscopic surgeries.

the most commonly used open approach for surgical intervention of the kidney.

Lumbotomy Incision (Gil-Vernet)

It is done in prone position for both sides; lateral position is possible for unilateral lumbotomy incision, two separate incisions can be placed on both sides in bilateral approach. It is used in bilateral partial nephrectomies, bilateral adrenalectomies. Unilateral lumbotomy incision can be placed in loin position; but it is more painful and retraction is difficult.

It is vertical posterior incision from 12 rib level to iliac crest. Incision is along the lateral border of the sacrospinalis. It extends from the upper border of 12th rib at lateral side of erector spinae downwards and forwards to the level of iliac crest for about 10 cm. It is deepened through latissimus dorsi, serratus posterior inferior, lumbosacral fascia, quadratus lumborum. Subcostal neurovascular bundle and 11th intercostal nerve should be mobilised and preserved. Gerota's fascia is visible; kidney is approached. If needed 12th rib or 12th and 11th ribs need to be excised to have better access. Pleura should not be injured.

Anterior Approaches

Anterior transperitoneal approach: It is done by lengthy midline or paramedian incision. Once laparotomy is done abdomen is explored; paracolic gutter is incised; colon is mobilised medially; Gerota's fascia is identified; ureter is identified by its location, peristalsis (elicited by tapping), feel, vascular pattern. Pelviureteric junction (PUJ) is identified; gonadal vessels are identified which crosses the ureter from front. IVC is identified and exposed for its full length while doing nephrectomy and vascular ligations.

Anterior extraperitoneal approach may be used: Here paramedian incision is placed; anterior rectus sheath is incised vertically; rectus muscle is retracted laterally; posterior rectus sheath is incised vertically without opening the peritoneum; peritoneum is reflected by finger dissection medially to reach the retroperitoneum renal area.

Thoracoabdominal approach is also anterior approach.

DISSECTION OF THE KIDNEY

It is always better to identify and dissect the vessels to have vascular control prior to dissecting the kidney. In benign diseases Gerota's fascia is opened to reach the kidney, pelvis and upper 1/3rd ureter. In malignancy, Gerota's fascia is not opened except in nephron sparing surgeries. It is always better to keep Satisnky vascular clamp ready in the theatre table during nephrectomy.

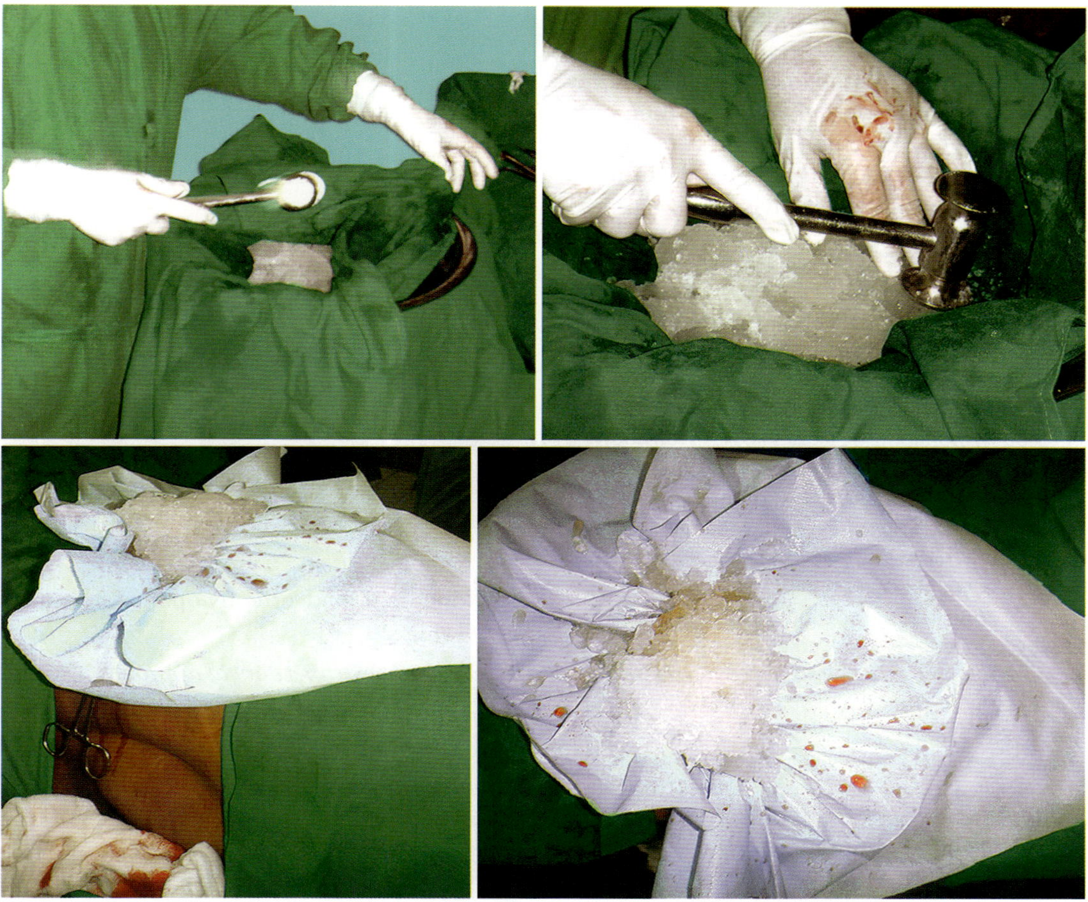

Fig. 28-17: Ice crystals placement on the kidney.

Right-sided Kidney Dissection

Right side faces challenges due to presence of the IVC, liver and right adrenal vein. Peritoneum is swept by blunt finger dissection medially; right colon will be located deeper to the peritoneum; after mobilisng it medially Gerota's will be exposed fully. Below ureter is identified by finger and cautery dissection. It is slinged using fine polythene tube or infant feeding tube. Gonadal vessels crossing the right ureter is identified. Right gonadal vein joins the IVC behind the duodenum; right gonadal artery and arises from aorta above the origin of the inferior mesenteric artery at the lateral margin of the aorta crosses the ureter. Ureter below crosses the junction of common iliac artery and its branches in front of it. IVC is dissected from common iliac vein junction to the level of duodenum. Duodenum is mobilised medially. Renal vessels are identified; right renal vein variations are common in its location, and branches. Sometimes double right renal veins may be present. Renal vein is carefully dissected using right angle instrument. It is not ligated but gently kept aside; right renal artery which is deeper and above is identified by its pulsation, isolated and doubly ligated using vicryl no. 1 or divided after transfixation. Aberrant renal artery is identified, dissected and ligated if present. Renal vein is double ligated using vicryl no. 1 and divided. Prior division between clamps followed by ligation should not be done because if clamp slips torrential haemorrhage can occur. It is always better to keep the Satinsky vascular clamp ready in case needed in torrential haemorrhage. Often tumour extends close to the IVC and it is difficult to dissect in such situation; right renal artery is identified between aorta and IVC, as after its origin, it runs behind the IVC to reach the right kidney and is ligated and divided at this juncture.

Tumour thrombus may extend across the renal vein into the IVC. If such thrombus is of short length in the IVC then after applying oblique Satinsky vascular clamps IVC is opened vertically to remove all tumour thrombus, and later venotomy in the IVC is sutured using 3-zero polypropylene continuous suture. If thrombus extends still more proximally extensively then veno cardiac bypass has to be done to achieve complete clearance of the tumour thrombus.

Often tear can occur in the IVC causing torrential haemorrhage (*Pack; Patience; Plan; Proceed* whenever there is bleed); tear should be occluded with thumb and Satinsky clamp should be applied obliquely and IVC is sutured with continuous 4-zero polypropylene sutures.

Left-sided Kidney Dissection

Approach is left loin posterior one. All layers are opened to reach the kidney. Peritoneum is usually not breached. Descending colon and splenic flexure is separated by dividing splenocolic ligament and mobilised fully medially to expose the entire left side Gerota's fascia and also left renal pedicle. This also requires dividing the lienorenal ligament. Renal pedicle is dissected; renal vein is in front of the renal artery. Renal vein is carefully dissected and kept aside. Often initially, there will be more than one tributaries of the renal vein, in such situation each is isolated and kept aside. By palpating with the finger for pulsation, left renal artery is identified, dissected and doubly ligated. Clips, haemoclips, vascular staplers can be used. Left adrenal vein joins the left renal vein vertically from above; it often needs ligation otherwise torrential haemorrhage can occur. Left inferior phrenic vein joins left adrenal vein which is also should be taken care off. Tail of the pancreas and splenic vein are very close to the upper part of the left kidney and its hilum; they are in front of the kidney. Care should be taken not to injure them which are separated by gentle finger dissection. Once left kidney is dissected fully medially with proper vascular control then only lateral dissection should be done in carcinoma kidney. In benign conditions like pyeloplasty pedicle dissection is not needed; Gerota's fascia is opened to reach the kidney and renal pelvis.

Different types of nephrectomies

Nephroureterectomy: It is done in transitional cell carcinoma of kidney pelvis wherein entire kidney with Gerota's fascia is removed along with entire length of the ureter up to the ureteric orifice.

Nephrectomy: It is done in benign conditions of kidney which is not functioning—non-functioning hydronephrotic kidney (DTPA scan shows function less than 20%).

Radical nephrectomy: It is removing the entire kidney, Gerota's fascia, fat, adrenal gland, lymph nodes, and entire ureter. Presently adrenal gland is removed only if it is invaded by RCC. Lymph node clearance is done only if imaging shows lymph nodes or on table lymph nodes are found.

Subcapsular nephrectomy: It is done in non-functioning benign/infective kidney like pyonephrosis wherein kidney is removed at subcapsular plane. As dissection outside capsule is impossible due to dense inflammatory adhesions; if attempted likely to injure the major vessels like IVC to land in disaster.

Heminephrectomy: it is done in duplex kidney wherein one part is totally separate from other anatomically and functionally even though they are covered by a single capsule. Non-functioning part is removed after pedicle dissection to identify the specific vessels of that particular part/moiety; those vessels are ligated securely. Dissection through the parenchyma after vascular ligation is very easy as plane is entirely avascular.

Nephron sparing nephrectomy: It is becoming more popular and acceptable method of treatment to surface RCC which is small and well localised wherein kidney is salvaged. Only diseased part with clearance margin is removed and frozen section biopsy is done to confirm the clearance.

Partial nephrectomy: It is removal of one of the poles of the kidney retaining the other pole. It is done when disease is limited to that particular pole only.

Donor nephrectomy: It is done in renal transplantation. Usually left kidney is used as left renal vein is longer.

APPROACHES TO URETER

Oblique Iliac Incision (Abbernethy's/Modified Gibson's)

It is used for *extraperitoneal approach* for ureteric stone, urinary bladder, lumbar sympathectomy. It is muscle cutting incision. It can be used for transperitoneal approach also.

Position is partial or complete lateral one depending on the side the surgery is needed. Incision is placed from mid-axillary line at the level of the umbilicus directing downwards and forwards towards pubic symphysis up to the lateral margin of the rectus muscle. Skin, subcutaneous fat, superficial fascia, external oblique muscle and aponeurosis below are incised layer by layer in the line of incision. Internal oblique and transverse abdominis muscles are also cut in the line of incision. Under transversalis fascia extraperitoneal fat and peritoneum is visualised. In extraperitoneal approach, peritoneum is swept forward from behind by blunt finger dissection. Psoas major muscle, genitofemoral nerve and inferior vena cava are identified. Ureter with its typical look and peristalsis (*vermiculations*) is also identified. Depending on the type of surgery further procedure is undertaken. Muscle is retracted using self-retaining retractor.

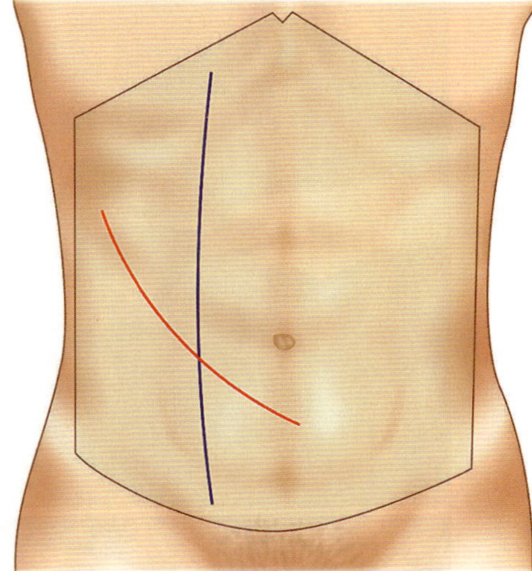

Fig. 28-18: Oblique iliac incision (Modified Gibson's).

Peritoneum if inadvertently opened, it can be sutured using 2 zero vicryl **(Fig. 28-18)**.

Paramedian extraperitoneal approach also can be used.

Transperitoneal approach is used when additional abdominal procedures are also warranted.

Laparoscopic and retroperitoneoscopic approaches are good other alternatives.

TREATMENT OF RENAL TUBERCULOSIS

Antitubercular therapy is started. INH, rifampicin, ethambutol and pyrazinamide. Duration of treatment is *one year* **(Fig. 28-19)**.

Surgeries

After 6–12 weeks of drug therapy, surgical treatment is planned. Kidney is exposed. Pyocalyx is drained. Cut edge of the capsule is sutured—*Hanley's renal cavernostomy.*

Hydronephrosis—*Anderson Hynes* operation or nephrostomy or stenting ("J" stent) of ureter is done.

Renal tuberculous abscess not resolving for 2 weeks should be drained.

Ureteral stricture—stenting/reimplantation of the ureter into the bladder/psoas hitch/Boari's flap/ileal conduit (*Koch's ileal conduit*).

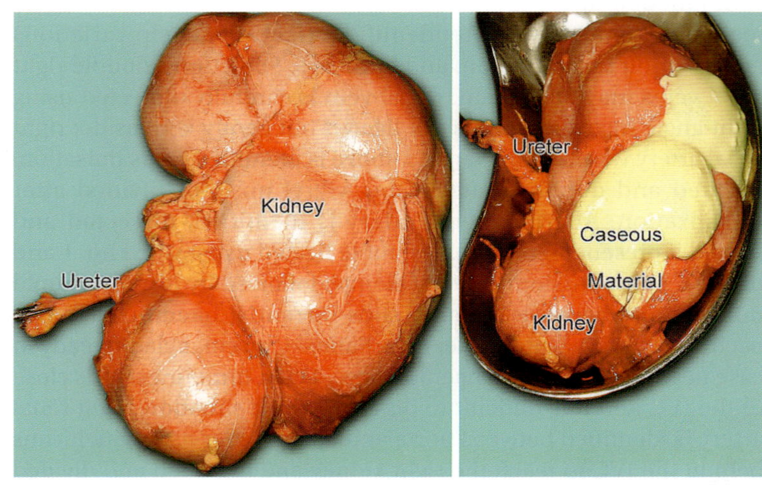

Fig. 28-19: Renal tuberculosis.

Thimble bladder—hydraulic dilatation/ileocystoplasty/caecocystoplasty/sigmoid colocystoplasty is done.

In unilateral lesion, with gross impairment of renal function—*nephroureterectomy* is done. Indications for nephroureterectomy are—non-functioning kidney; disease extensively involving the kidney; disease causing hypertension and severe obstruction; tuberculous pyonephrosis; coexisting renal cell carcinoma.

TREATMENT FOR HYDRONEPHROSIS

Always conservative surgeries which are aimed at conserving the kidneys are done. Nephrectomy is not done unless indicated **(Figs. 28-20 to 28-22)**.

The cause is treated: Stone, congenital anomaly, aberrant renal vessels, stricture urethra (dilatation, urethrotomy, urethroplasty); phimosis (circumcision); BPH (TURP); posterior urethral valve (cystoscopic fulguration of valve).

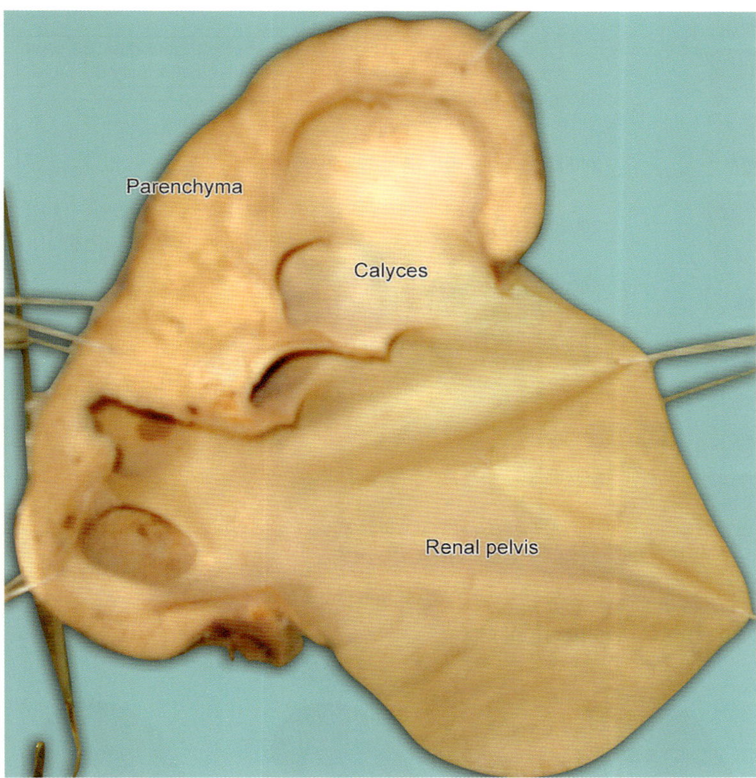

Fig. 28-20: Specimen of kidney showing hydronephrosis.

Pyeloplasty may be dismembered or non-dismembered; open or laparoscopic approach. In bilateral cases side which is functioning well should be operated first; after 6 weeks opposite side is operated.

Anderson-Hyne's Operation (Dismembered Pyeloplasty)

This procedure was first done in 1847 for retrocaval ureter. In congenital PUJ obstruction, the spasmodic segment and redundant pelvis are excised. A new pelvis is created and the cut end of pelvis is anastomosed to the ureter in the *dependent* position. Vascular, funnel shaped, dependent, tension free anastomosis should be done. Open approach is usually through loin in lateral position. Once peritoneum is pushed medially; colon is also pushed medially adequately. Ureter in the middle is identified; stent if present in the ureter will guide the identification easier; otherwise it can be identified by its look, peristalsis, location. Peristalsis can be elicited on it. Ureter is dissected and slinged. Proximally dissection is continued towards renal pelvis. PUJ with pelvis and lower pole kidney is identified and dissected properly. Small bleeders in the junction are cauterised using bipolar cautery. Stay sutures are placed one at the upper part of the pelvis laterally; another at lateral lower part of the pelvis medially; one more at the upper end of the ureter **(Fig. 28-23)**.

Pelvis which is redundant is excised within the stay suture area including the diseased PUJ. Specimen is sent for histology. Fish mouth cut is given to the ureter. Lower angle of the ureter is sutured to the lower angle of the cut end of the pelvis. J stent is passed across the ureter and pelvis. Further sutures either continuous or interrupted are placed using 3-zero vicryl sutures to complete the anastomosis. Further left open cut end of the renal pelvis is sutured. Anastomosis should be tension free, dependent. Adequate mobilisation of the lower ureter is often required. Tube drain is placed; wound is closed in layers. Drain is removed in 7 days; J stent is removed in 3–6 weeks **(Figs. 28-24 and 28-25)**.

Complications are—urine leak; infection; inadequate functioning of the kidney; stricture formation at anastomotic site **(Fig. 28-26)**.

Non-dismembered pyeloplasties: Here PUJ is not transected. Reconstruction is done without PUJ transection by different methods, e.g. Foley's Y-V plasty.

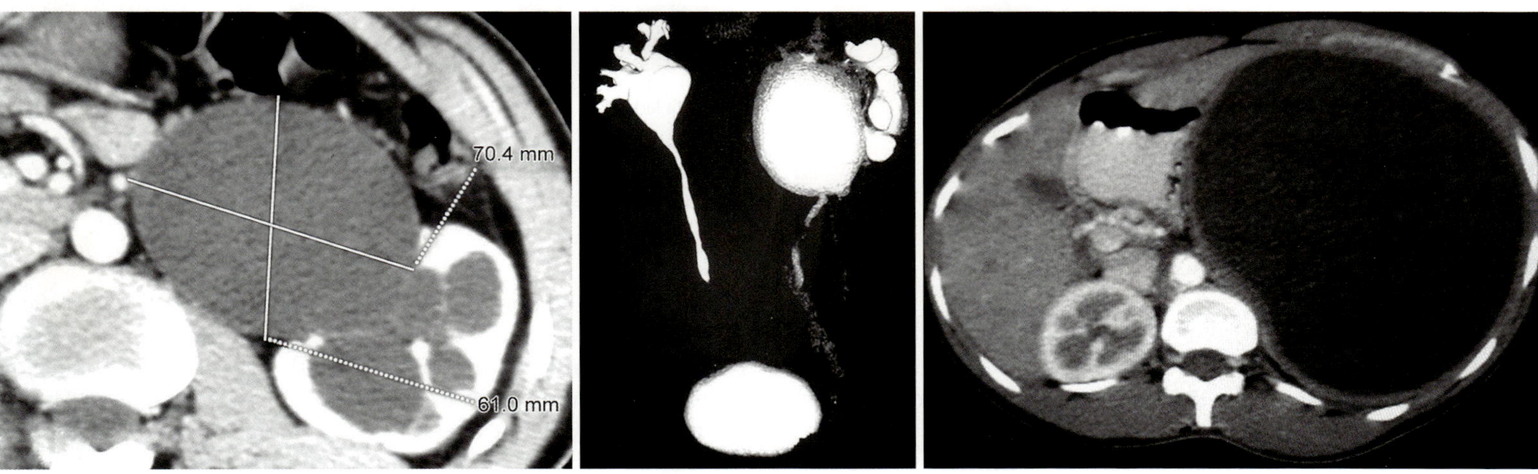

Fig. 28-21: CT scan showing unilateral and bilateral hydronephrosis in different patients.

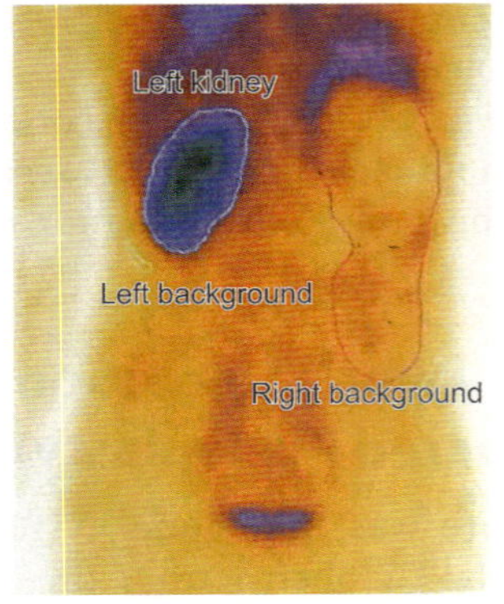

Summed function image

	Left kidney	Right kidney
Uptake % (2–3 min.)	61.95	38.15
Time to peak (min.)	2.88	18.88
Time to ½ (min.)	15.03	0.00
Peak count rate (C/min.)	21,044.00	21,690.18

Renogram analysis results

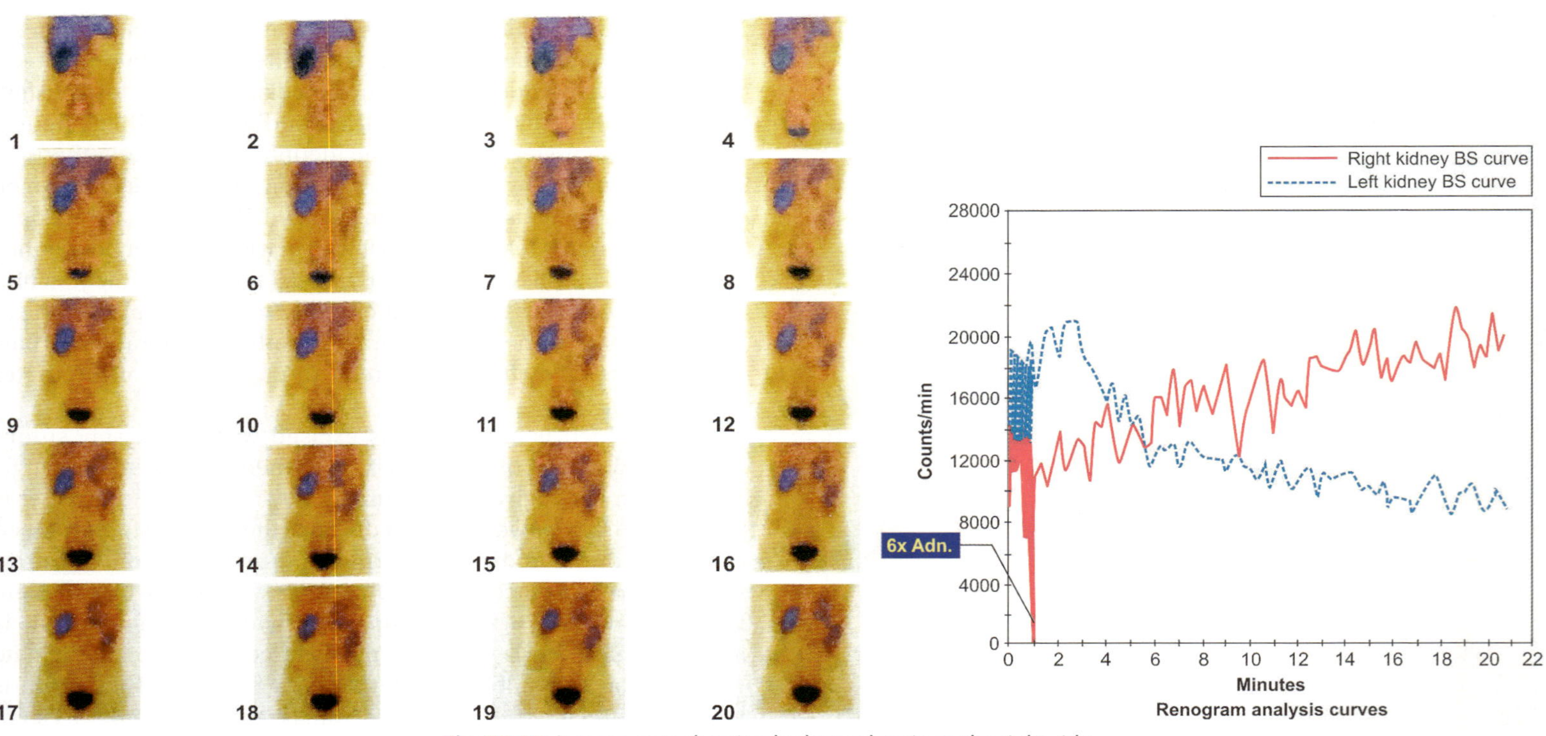

Fig. 28-22: Isotope scan showing hydronephrosis on the right side.

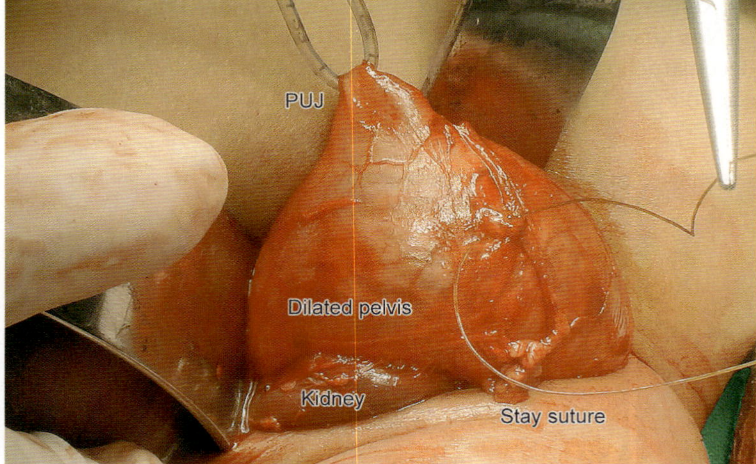

Fig. 28-23: Stay sutures placed for pyeloplasty.

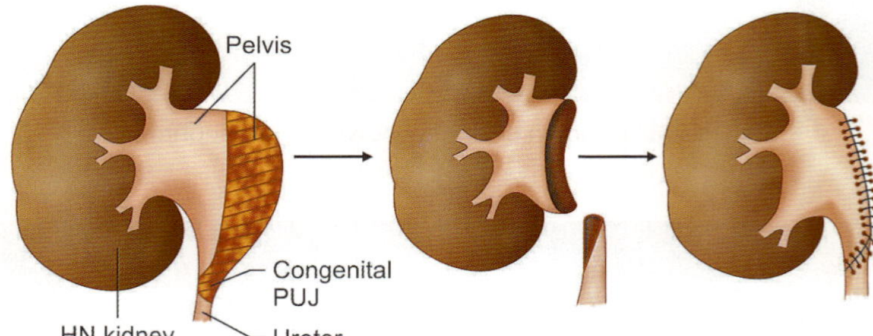

Fig. 28-24: Principles of Anderson-Hyne's operation. Excision of PUJ and redundant pelvis; anastomosis of the ureter with vascularised, tension free, funnel-shaped, dependent stoma.

Davis T-tube ureterostomy: Placement of T tube in the ureter by making longitudinal incision.

In bilateral HN, without renal failure, *kidney which is functioning better should be operated first.* Three months later, otherside kidney is dealt with. In bilateral HN with renal failure, *bilateral nephrostomy and haemodialysis* support is required initially. After 3–6 weeks IVU is done and the functions of both kidneys are looked for. If they function, then are treated accordingly by Anderson-Hyne's operation. *If kidneys are still not functioning (renal function <20% on isotope study) then nephrectomy and renal transplantation* is the only option left.

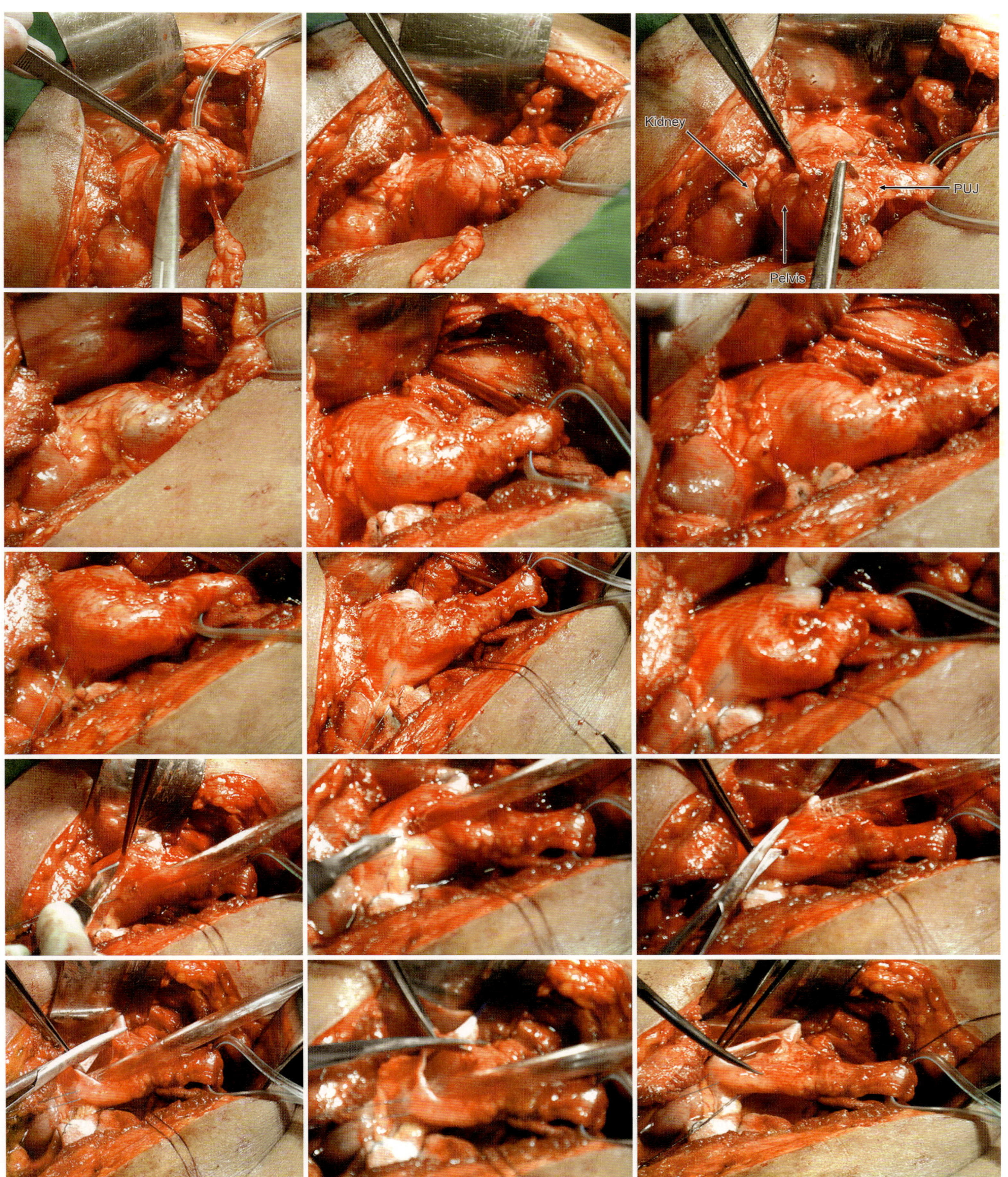

Figs. 28-25(1)

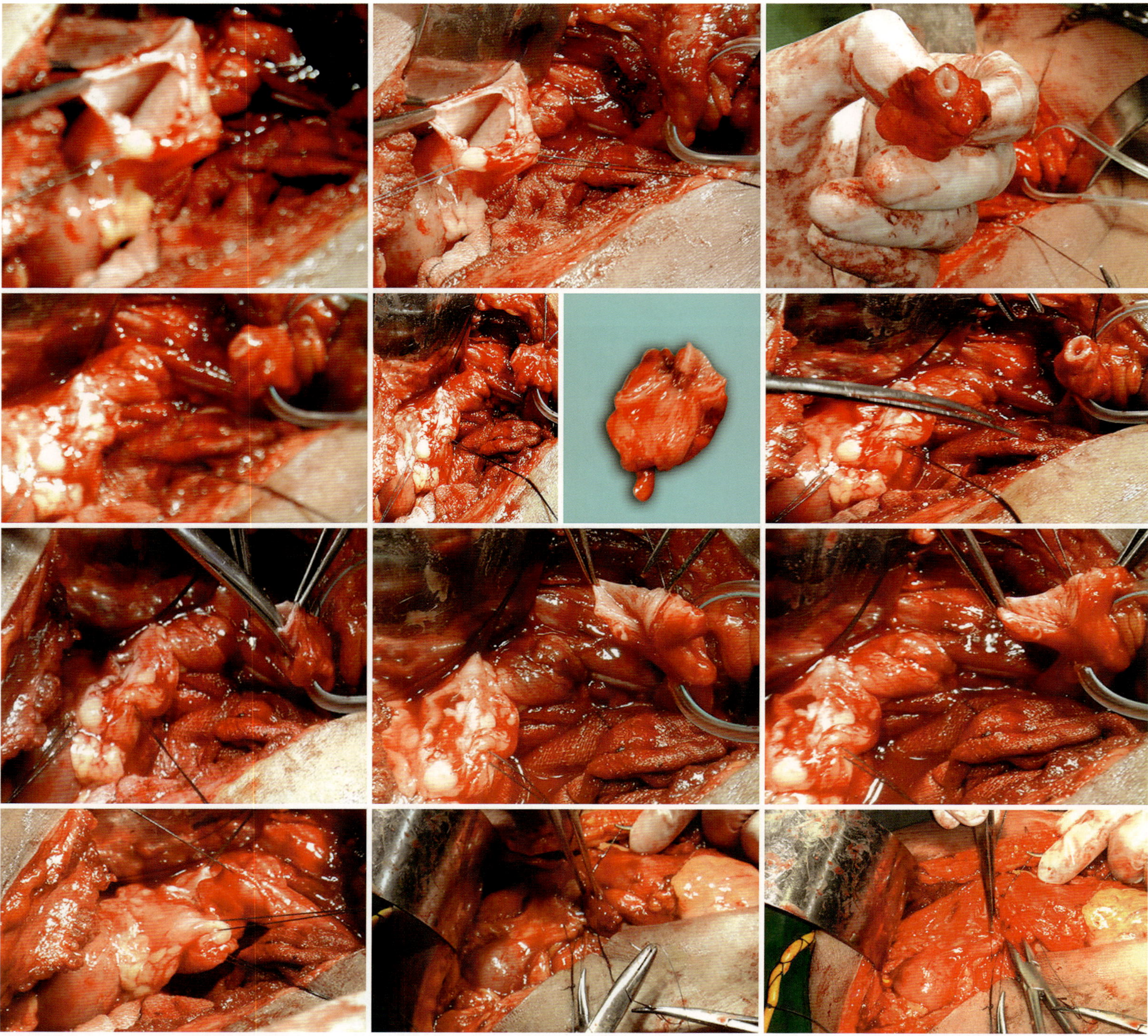

Figs. 28-25(2)

Figs. 28-25(1 and 2): Anderson-Hyne's operation—pyeloplasty in an adult.

Laparoscopic or *retroperitoneoscopic pyeloplasty* is becoming popular but is expensive and time consuming. It gives good result as well **(Fig. 28-27)**.

Endoscopic pyelolysis, even though technically easier results are not assured.

Aberrant renal artery or *vein* in the lower pole of kidney can compress the PUJ causing HN. Renal angiogram confirms the diagnosis. *Treatment of aberrant renal vessels*—If it is a vein it can be ligated safely. But if it is an artery, it exclusively supplies the lower pole of the kidney and so cannot be ligated. So kidney is mobilised; upper and lower poles are approximated together so that artery is made to slip away from the site of compression—*Hamilton Stewart operation*. Nowadays, this operation is not done. Vessels are dissected carefully and kept aside (preserved) and PUJ is transected and anastomosed in front of the vessels **(Fig. 28-28)**.

TREATMENT OF PYONEPHROSIS

After starting antibiotics, pus is immediately drained from the kidney through a loin incision and *nephrostomy* tube (Cabot's nephrostomy) (Malecot's catheter) is placed. If kidney is totally destroyed, *subcapsular nephrectomy* is done. This also prevents other kidney from getting infected through perirenal lymphatic connections. Approach is though loin. Adhesions are common.

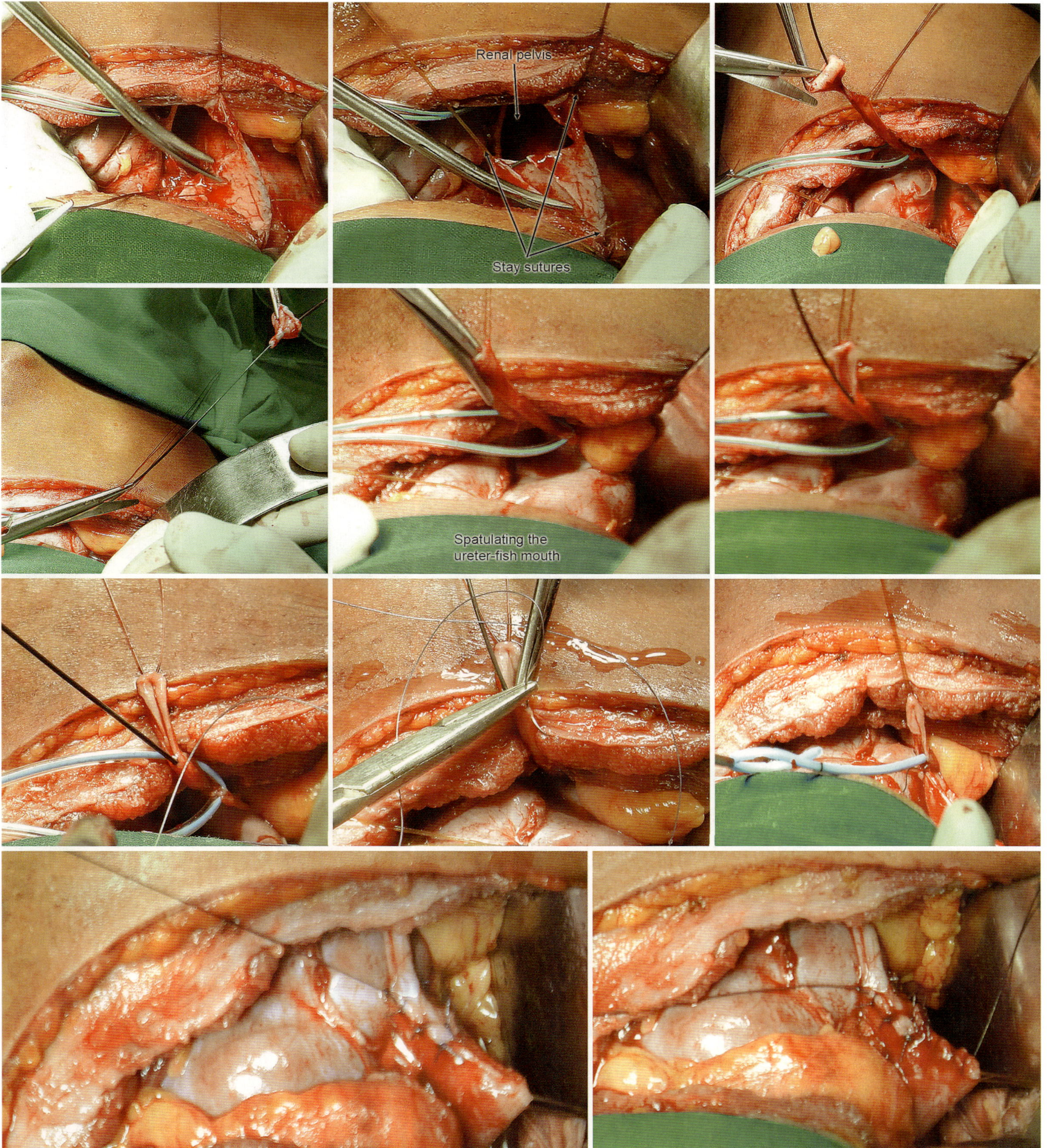

Fig. 28-26: Anderson-Hyne's operation—pyeloplasty in a child.

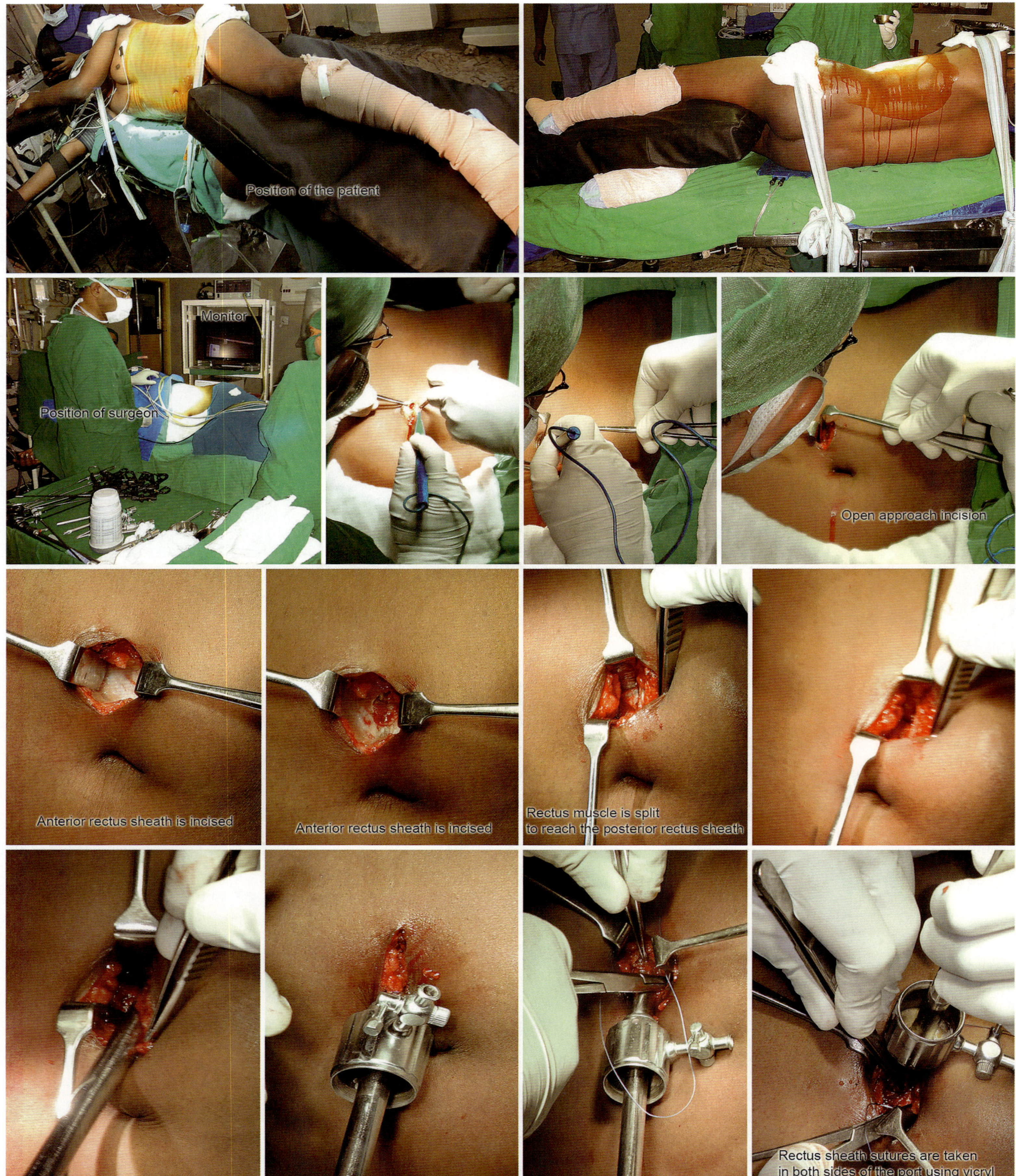
Position of the patient
Monitor
Position of surgeon
Open approach incision
Anterior rectus sheath is incised
Anterior rectus sheath is incised
Rectus muscle is split
to reach the posterior rectus sheath
Rectus sheath sutures are taken
in both sides of the port using vicryl

Figs. 28-27(1)

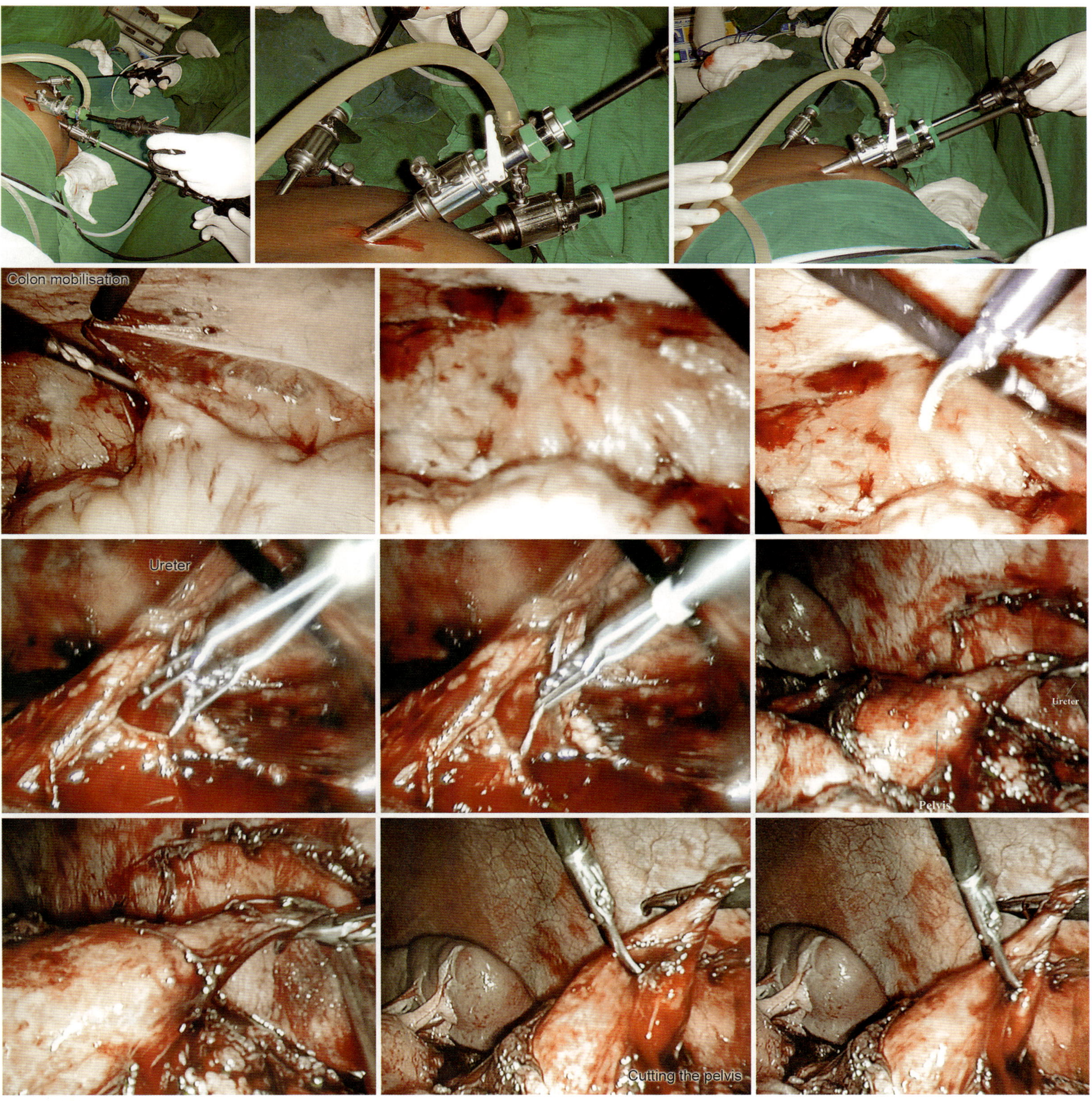
Colon mobilisation
Ureter
Ureter
Pelvis
Cutting the pelvis

Figs. 28-27(2)

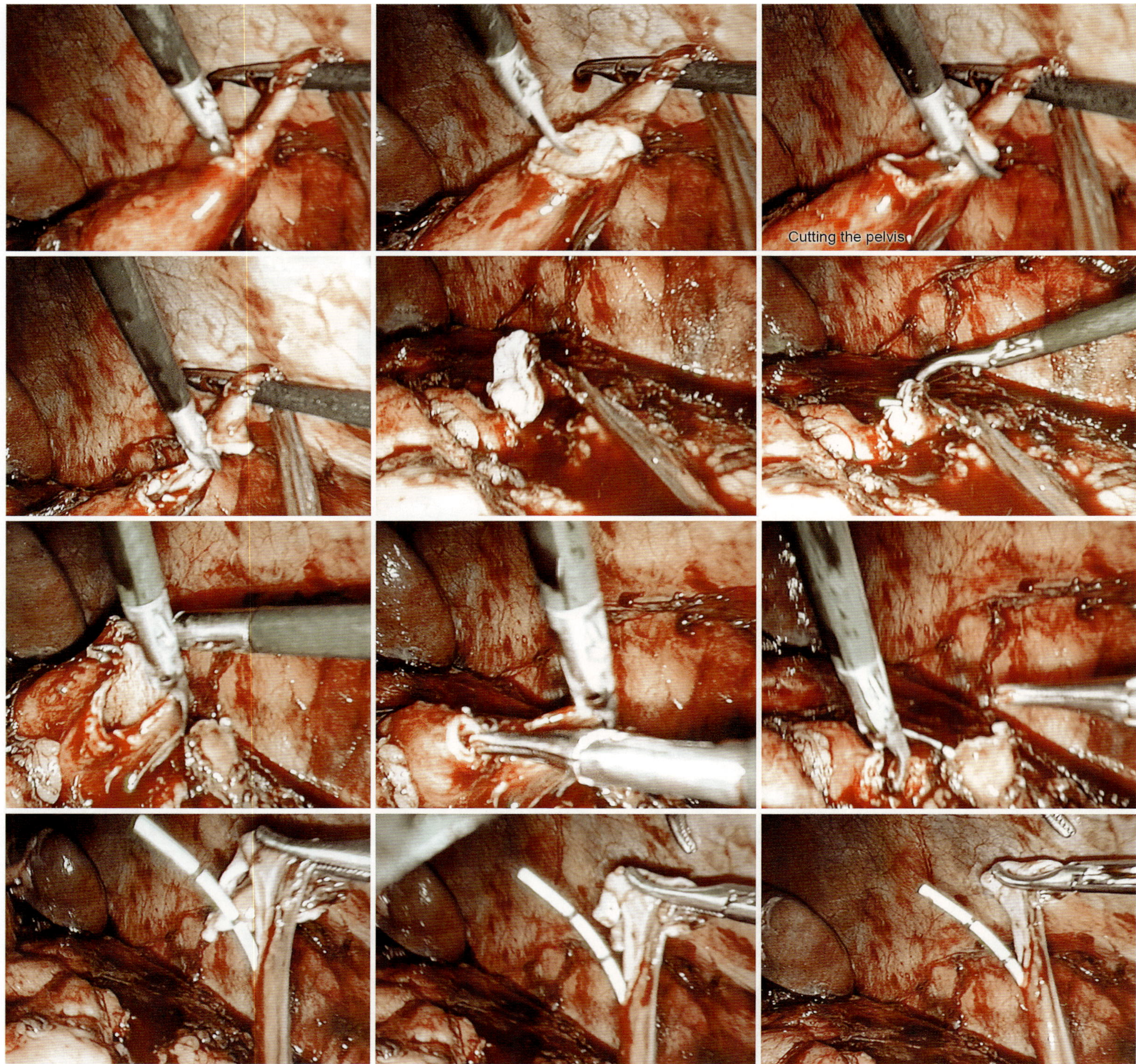

Figs. 28-27(3)

Figs. 28-27(1 to 3): Laparoscopic pyeloplasty is standard now. Initially cystoscopy is done to pass a ureteric catheter or J stent. Loin position (lateral) is used. Camera port is at the level of the umbilicus through the rectus muscle. Horizontal 1.5 cm incision is made; anterior rectus sheath is incised horizontally; rectus muscle is split; posterior rectus sheath and peritoneum is opened. 10 mm port is passed; two vicryl sutures on two diagonally opposite sides of posterior rectus sheath is taken and kept long for tying at the end of the procedure. Pneumoperitoneum is created. One 10 mm and another 5 mm ports on either side and laterally are passed under vision as working ports. Additional 5 mm working port can be added if need arises. Lateral paracolic gutter is incised along the Toldt's line; colon is mobilised fully medially from the Gerota's fascia; i.e. right side hepatic flexure and left side splenic flexure. Ureter is identified; gonadal vein is crossing the ureter on right side; on left side gonadal vein lies adjacent to ureter on its medial aspects without crossing it. Ureter is identified by its tubular nature, colour, peristalsis, vascular network. IVC is identified on the right side. Ureter is dissected upwards towards the renal pelvis which is mobilised all around. PUJ is identified and dissected. Renal pelvis is incised and cut in V-shaped manner. PUJ is also excised along with that. Spatulation of ureter (fish mouth) is done on its lateral side from its cut end using scissor. J stent is passed if not passed earlier; it is pushed towards the renal pelvis. Bite with 3-zero vicryl is taken from its apex of the spatulation from outside to inside then it is passed to the lower cut end of the pelvis from inside to outside. Knot is placed outside. One should not place knots inside in the urothelium anywhere. Continuous sutures are taken, first posterior layer is done between ureteric cut part and pelvis cut part; once posterior layer is finished knot is tied. Using new 3-zero vicryl anterior layer sutures are taken similarly. Proximal part of the renal pelvis is again separately sutured and closed. Secure dependent vascular funnel-shaped tension free anastomosis is achieved. Tube drain is placed; port sites are closed.

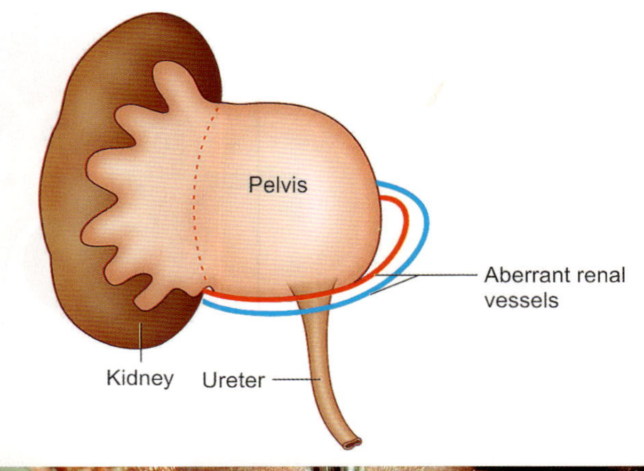

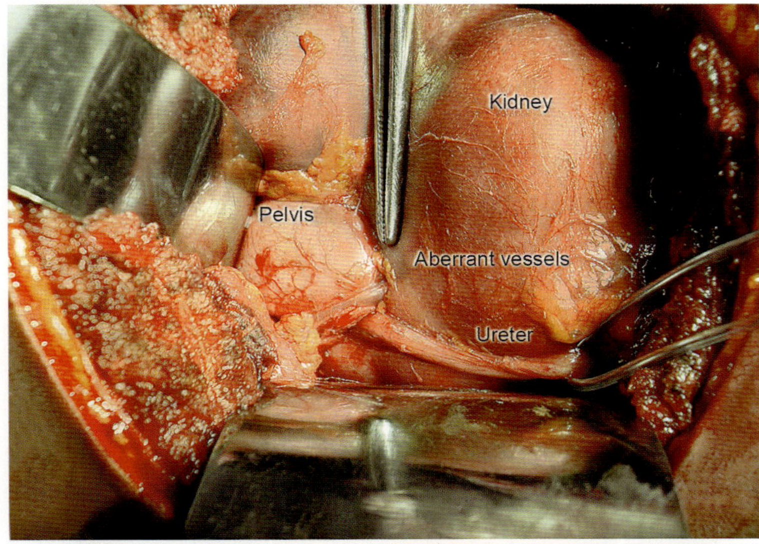

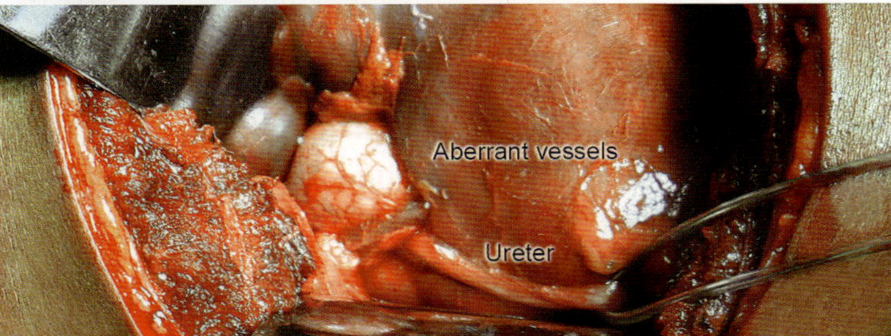

Fig. 28-28: Aberrant renal vessels.

It is often difficult to identify the major vessels and renal pedicle. Injury to renal vein, IVC is known to occur. Often mass clamping at the pedicle with transfixation ligatures using polypropylene sutures are better rather than individually identifying and ligation the vessels. If IVC tear is suspected the incision is extended, peritoneum is opened; duodenum and posterior abdominal wall is dissected to identify the IVC completely. Tear is identified with placement of vascular clamps. Tear is sutured. In bilateral pyonephrosis, *bilateral nephrostomy* is the only choice. *'J' stenting* is done often to keep the ureters patent.

NEPHROSTOMY

It is the method of draining the urine directly from the kidney across the loin outside by placing a tube of varying sizes. It is done in draining pus from kidney, urine on obstructed distal system, trauma. It also facilitates the further access to the renal collecting system to dissolve stones, to infuse drugs like chemotherapeutic agents, to irrigate renal collecting system; it also allows imaging of the distal system by antegrade radiography. Tumours blocking ureters, retroperitoneal fibrosis, and ureteral strictures need diversion either temporarily or permanently so that definitive procedures can be undertaken at a later period as elective surgery. It also gives antegrade access to flexible antegrade pyeloureteroscopy. In 1912, cystoscope is passed into the kidney percutaneously by Hampton Young in a massive hydronephrotic kidney. Willard Goodwin in 1955 did first Percutaneous nephrostomy. Percutaneous method is the current standard under image intensifier guidance **(Fig. 28-29)**.

Open method is the method used in olden days. Here under local or spinal anaesthesia, through an incision in the loin posteriorly kidney is reached by careful dissection across the muscle layers, renal and Gerota's fascia; through the convex surface of the kidney tube is passed across the renal parenchyma to reach the renal pelvis and calyces. Tube is fixed to the skin securely. Usually, small incision of 4 cm is made and insertion of tube can be confirmed by contrast X-ray—Cabot's nephrostomy. This procedure can also be done after open renal surgeries like for pyonephrosis, hydronephrosis, traumatic kidney if open intervention is done (in 20% of cases), distal blockage wherein other methods fail.

In open method, once renal pelvis is opened for removal of stone or correction of PUJ, tube which is having multiple openings on the central part is passed across the pelvis through the kidney parenchyma and both ends of the tube is brought out as drainage ends percutaneously outside so that tube stays like a 'C' with central part with openings (side holes). This facilitates drainage of the urine from both ends so that chances of blockage are less and also saline wash or irrigation can clear blockage if it happens. It also facilitates the replacement with a newer tube if needed using 'railroad' technique. But infection is the problem in there tubes—*Tresidder's nephrostomy*.

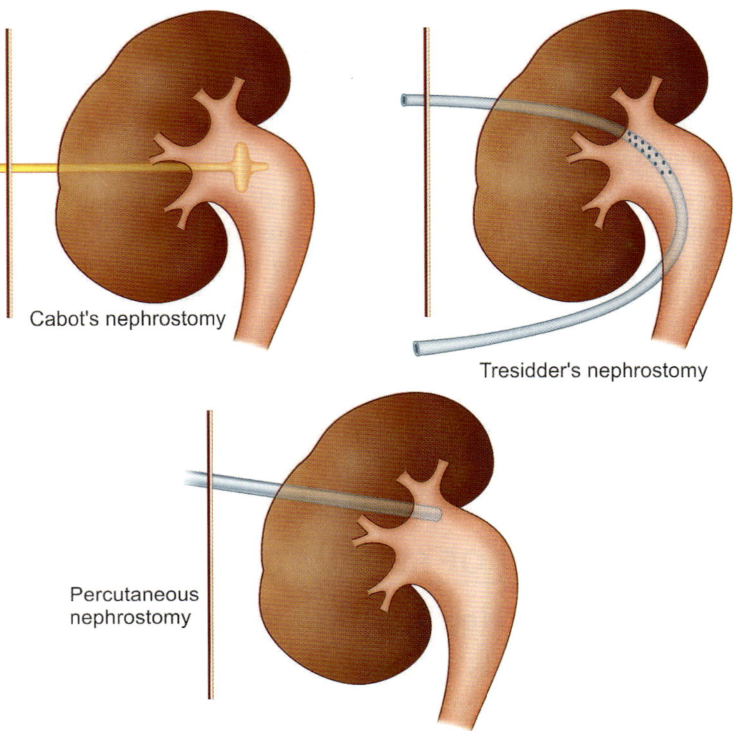

Fig. 28-29: Types of nephrostomies—Cabot's; Tresidder's; percutaneous. Percutaneous nephrostomy is the current standard.

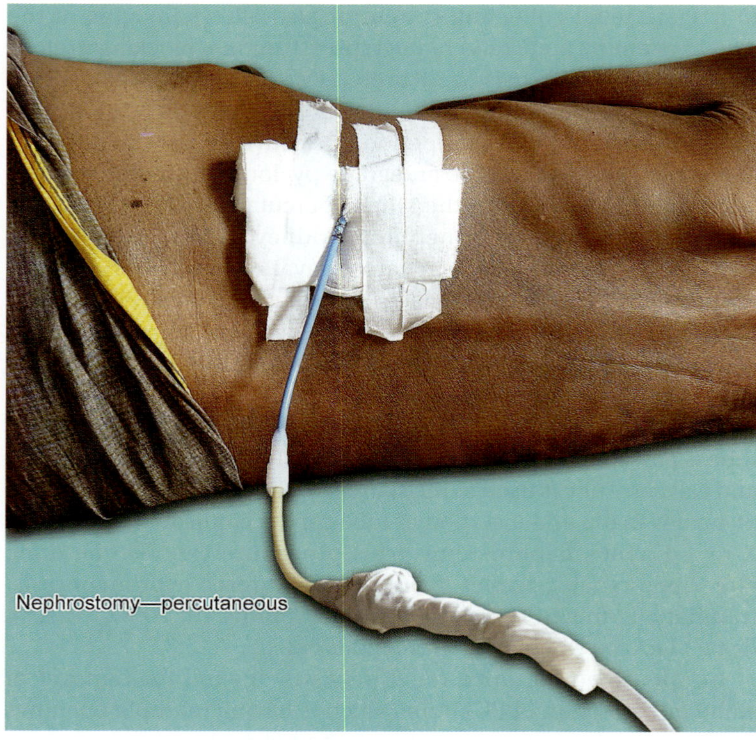

Fig. 28-30: Percutaneous nephrostomy.

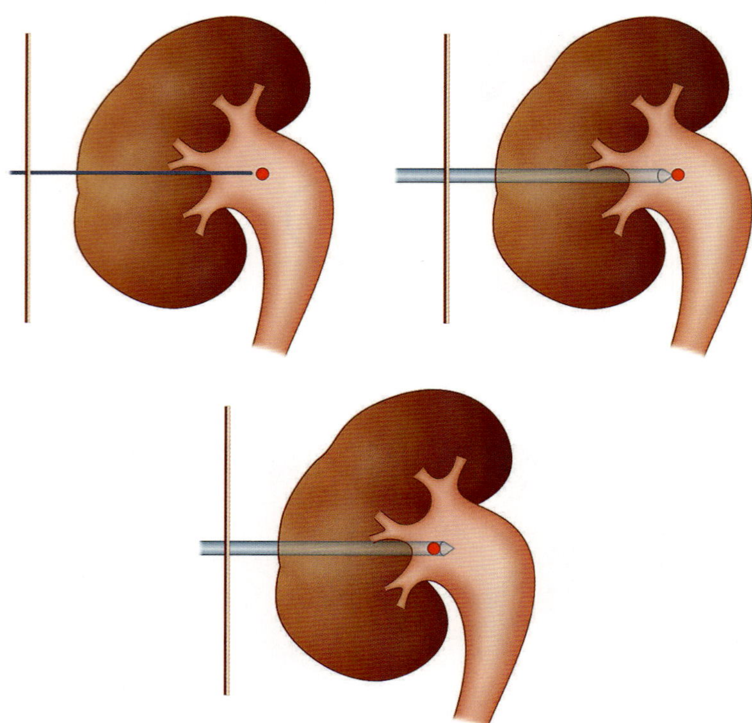

Fig. 28-31: PCNL—technique. It is commonly done procedure now for renal stone.

Percutaneous nephrostomy—is the standard presently. Under image guidance, needle is passed into the renal pelvis from behind across the loin through the kidney parenchyma; contrast dye is injected and position is confirmed by screening; guide wire is passed through percutaneous needle; needle is removed; serial dilators are passed through the guidewire into the renal pelvicalyceal system under guidance; once track is adequately dilated nephrostomy tube is passed into the system; it is confirmed again by injecting contrast agent with image guidance. Tube is secured to the skin. Bilateral percutaneous nephrostomy can also be done **(Fig. 28-30)**.

Contraindications for nephrostomy—bleeding diathesis; anticoagulant therapy.

Complications—bleeding from renal small vessels or may be from major vessels; usually stops by few transfusions; but if torrential bleeding occurs then exploration may be needed; consent for nephrectomy should be taken. Blockage of the tube, urosepsis, perirenal haematoma formation, severe pain and discomfort are other complications. Pneumothorax, haemothorax can occur by inadvertent pleural puncture. Organ injuries like of liver, spleen, colon, duodenum is also known to occur. Delayed haemorrhage is also known to occur. Failed access occurs in <5% cases. Reattempt after collecting system dilatation may be helpful.

TREATMENT OF RENAL STONES

Percutaneous Nephrolithotomy (PCNL)

Indications are—stones more than 2.5 cm in size; multiple stones; Stones not responding for ESWL.

Procedure: Initially cystoscopy is done and ureteric stent/catheter is placed and renal pelvicalyceal system is identified under C-arm guidance. Under the guidance of C-arm or U/S, needle puncture is made in the loin percutaneously. Through kidney, calyx and pelvis are approached. Guide wire is passed. Graduated dilators are passed and so track is widened. Then through that track, a nephroscope is passed. After fragmentation, stone is removed using different methods [Laser (Holmium), pneumatic, ultrasonic or electrohydraulic] **(Fig. 28-31)**.

Complications of PCNL: Haemorrhage; perforation of collecting duct causing extravasation of irrigation fluid; *injury to colon or pleura* while creating initial track for nephroscope.

Extracorporeal Shock Wave Lithotripsy (ESWL) (Fig. 28-32)

Piezo-Ceramic or *Electromagnetic* shock waves are passed to the stone through water bath or water cushion which acts as a media. Shocks are produced at 2/sec. 1000–4000 shocks are required for each stone. *Dornier Lithotripter* is used for fragmenting stones. Stone is located and observed through fluoroscope (C-arm) or ultrasound. Shock waves are triggered to create *compressive waves* over the stone, to fragment it. These fragments are flushed out later.

Advantages: No anaesthesia is required. Can be done as an OP procedure, less than 2.5 cm sized stones are well fragmented, hard stones, oxalate stones are better eliminated by ESWL, ESWL can be done repeatedly in different sittings, if it is not successful one can switch over to PCNL.

Complications: Renal haematoma; Severe haematuria; injury to adjacent structures; fragmented stone retains in the ureter.

Contraindications: Pregnancy; bleeding disorders; patients with abdominal aneurysms; sepsis and renal failure (Serum creatinine more than 3 mg%).

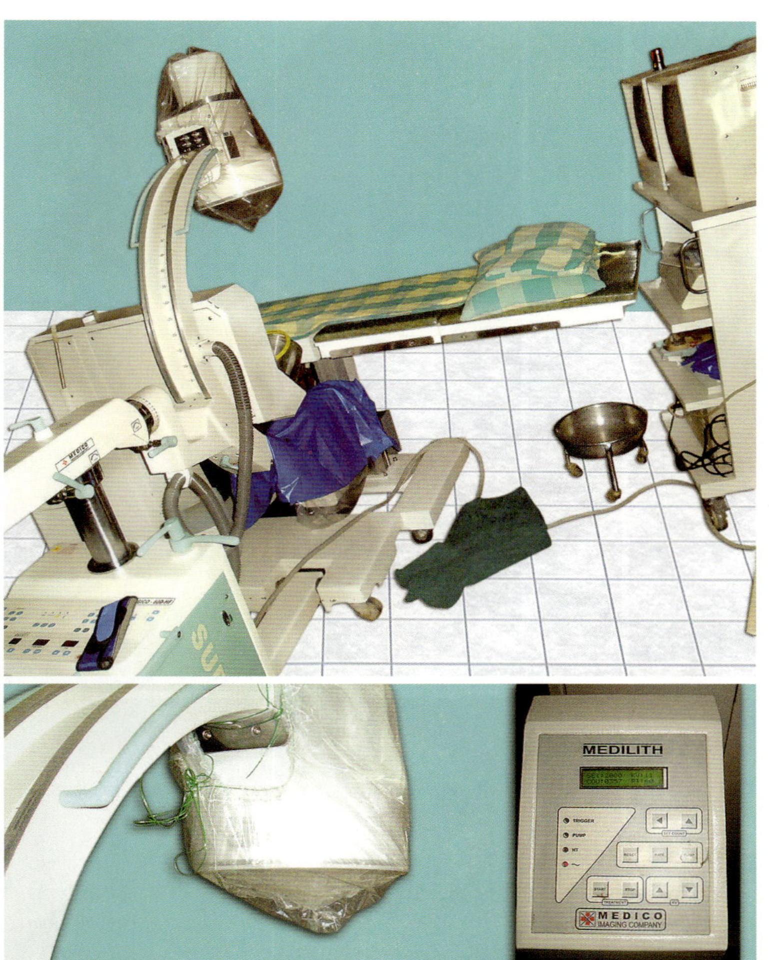

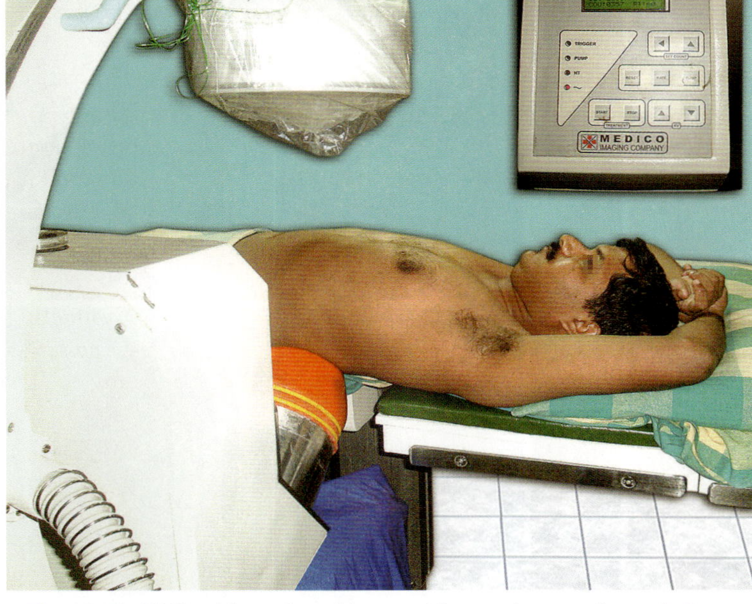

Fig. 28-32: ESWL table and machine used for renal stones. It needs C-arm to guide the exact point of stone to be fragmented.

Surgeries (Fig. 28-33)

Pyelolithotomy: It is suitable for stones in extrarenal pelvis. By loin (posterior subcostal) incision, kidney is approached. Renal pelvis is opened, the stone is removed and the pelvis is closed using 3 zero vicryl. A drain is placed and wound is closed **(Figs. 28-34 and 28-35)**.

Extended pyelolithotomy (Gil-Vernet): In case of intrarenal pelvis, incision is done on the hilum between the pelvis and kidney over the renal sinus, dissection is carried out so as to remove the stones from pelvis as well as calyces.

Nephrolithotomy: By placing incision just behind the most convex surface (Brodel's line), stone is removed.

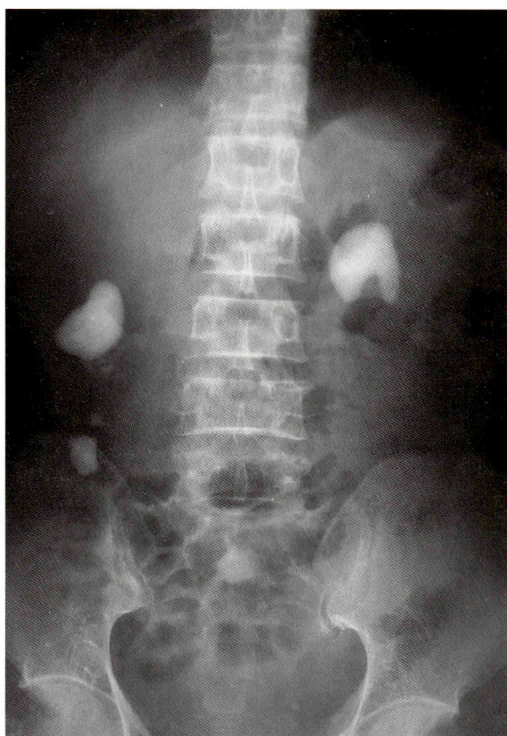

Fig. 28-33: Bilateral renal stones (large) with right ureteric stone.

Nephropyelolithotomy: By making incisions both over the kidney and pelvis, stone/stones are removed. It is often done in *staghorn calculus* **(Fig. 28-36)**.

Partial nephrectomy: Done when there are multiple stones occupying a pole, usually lower pole of the kidney or when there is damage to the calyx, if not removed may encourage further stone formation.

Bench surgery: Kidney is removed out temporarily, cooled by ice packs or inosine or liquid nitrogen. Stones are searched and removed completely. Later kidney is replaced in right iliac fossa.

Coagulum pyelolithotomy: Coagulum solution which contains fibrinogen is poured into the renal pelvis. It is activated so that it solidifies, meanwhile entangling the stones in renal pelvis. This entangled mass is removed en masse.

Anatrophic pyelolithotomy: After exposing the kidney, it is cooled with ice packs for 20 minutes and posterior branch of the renal artery is clamped temporarily using bull-dog clamp. The most avascular plane behind the Brodel's line is thus visualised properly. Kidney is opened through this line and stone/stones are removed (anatrophic means "to prevent atrophy") **(Fig. 28-37)**.

REMOVAL OF URETERIC STONE

Problems with ureteric stones—obstruction, hydronephrosis; infection, impaction, ureteric stricture **(Fig. 28-38)**.

Surgical Intervention for Ureteric Stones

Indications: Size of the stone more than 5 to 8 mm. IVU showing deterioration of function. Coexisting infection. If stone is impacted in the ureter with persistent symptoms **(Fig. 28-39)**.

Upper third stone: ESWL is used for stone in upper third ureter. The stone is pushed into the renal pelvis and then PCNL is done.

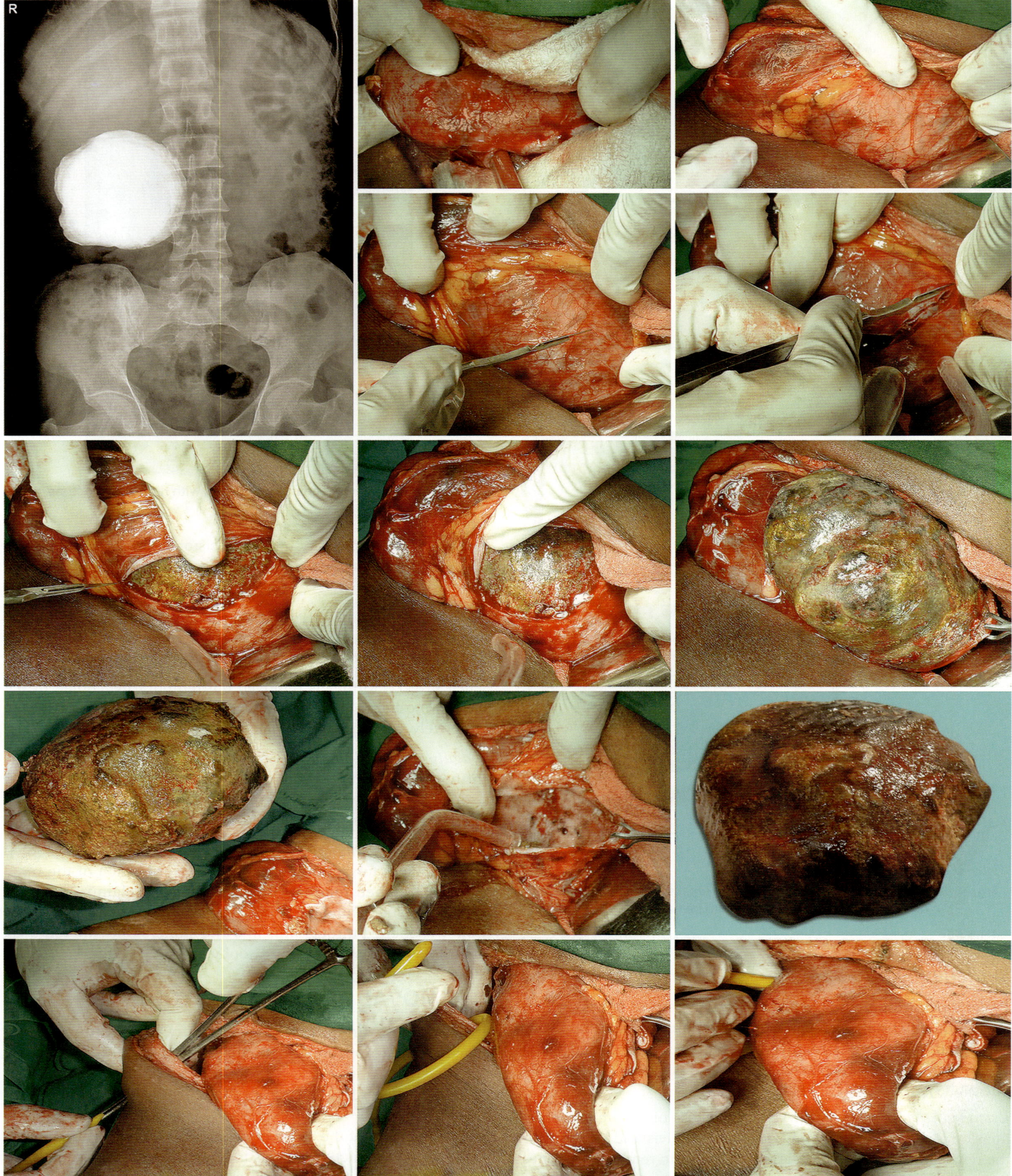

Figs. 28-34(1)

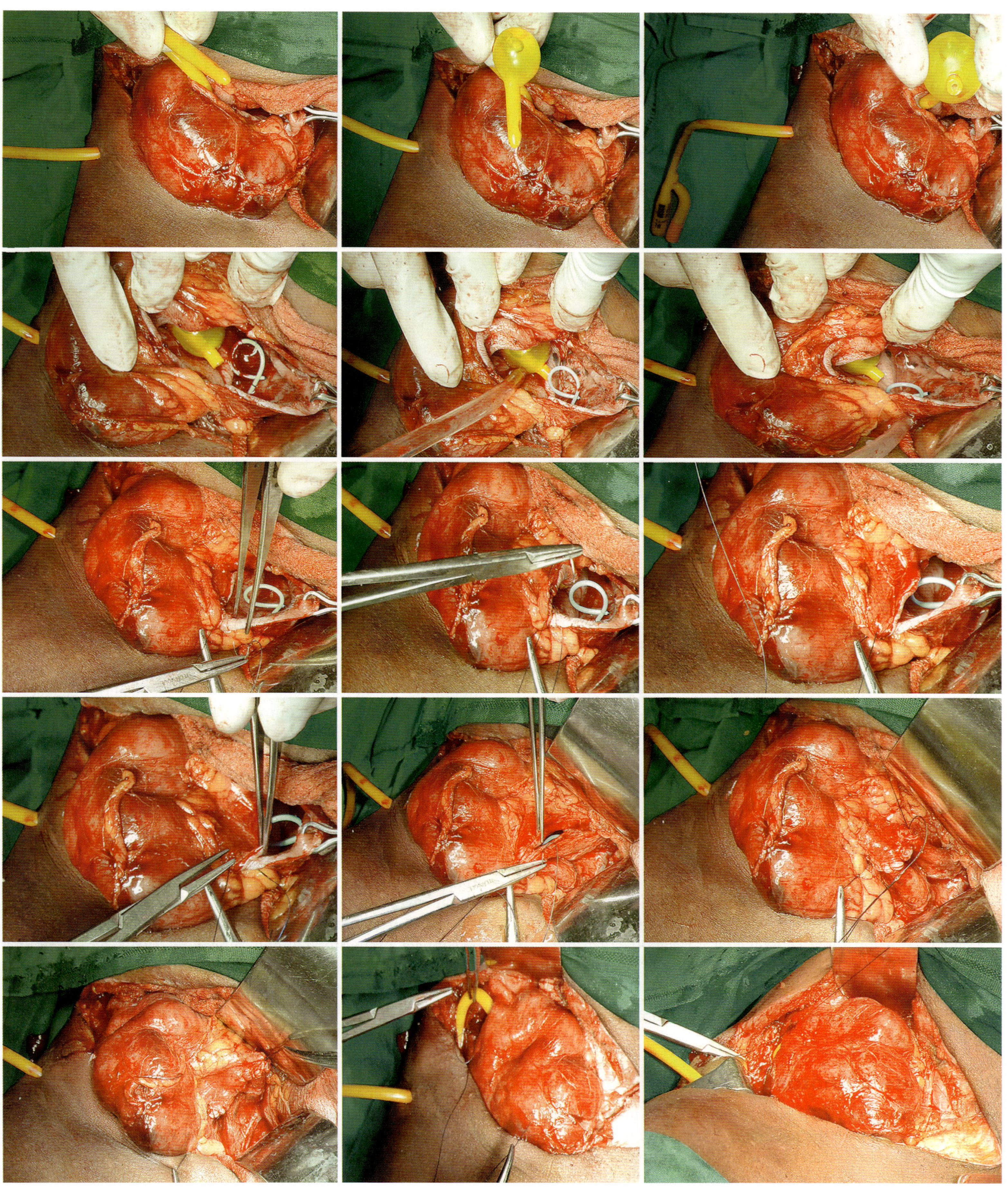

Figs. 28-34(2)

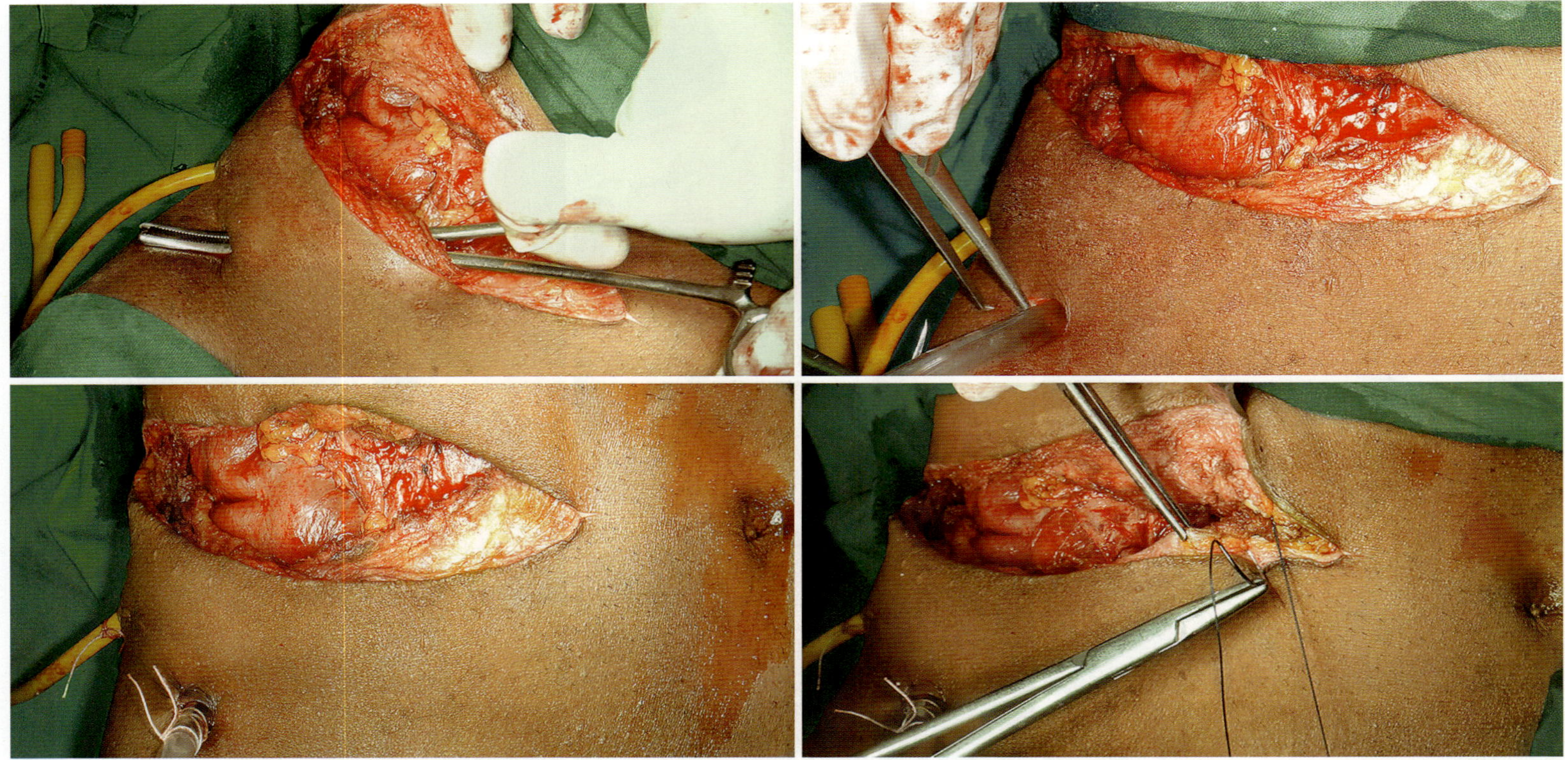

Figs. 28-34(3)

Figs. 28-34(1 to 3): Very large renal pelvic stone of more than 8 cm in size weighing 610 grams. It is one of the largest renal stone extracted.
Courtesy: Dr Ashok Pandit, MCh, Urologist, Mangala Hospital, Mangaluru, Karnataka, India.

Ureterorenoscopic stone removal (URS): Through ureteroscope, stone is visualised and often fragmented using pneumatic bombarder. It is then extracted by ureteroscope. Complications are perforation of ureter and extraperitoneal leakage of urine, bleeding. Open *ureterolithotomy is done* through loin incision **(Fig. 28-40)**.

Stone in middle third ureter: URS; open ureterolithotomy; laparoscopic stone removal.

Stone in lower third ureter: URS; *Dormia basketing* **(Fig. 28-41)**.

Indications for Dormia basketing: Stone in lower third ureter, stone below pelvic brim, stone less than 10 mm size, single stone, basket is passed into the proximal ureter beyond the stone and opened. The stone is then pulled out.

Complications of Dormia basket: Stone dislodgement, urethral injury, avulsion of ureter, stricture ureter, open ureterolithotomy.

Using cystoscope under general anaesthesia, *uretericmeatotomy* is done for stones impacted at the ureteric orifice. It is released by cutting the orifice at upper and lateral aspects.

Note: All ureteric stones can also be removed through laparoscopy or retroperitoneoscopy.

Open Ureterolithotomy

Nowadays, open approach is not commonly done; however surgeon should be familiar with the technique. On the day of surgery, plain X-ray KUB should be taken to confirm the location of the stone or ultrasound should be done. Large impacted stone which is not amenable to remove by any endourology technique is removed by open method. Oblique loin incision (*Modified Gibson's*) extending down towards the hypogastric region suprapubically—is used. It is an extraperitoneal approach. Skin, superficial fascia, external oblique, internal oblique are cut in the line of incision; transversus abdominis is split from behind forward as its posterior aspect not adherent to the peritoneum compared to anterior aspect; this avoids inadvertent opening of the peritoneum. Peritoneum is swept forward and medially by blunt finger dissection and this plane is avascular. Care should be taken not to enter behind the psoas major; if it happens plane will be lost and unnecessary troublesome bleeding can develop. Genitofemoral nerve is identified; ureter is identified by its peristalsis; it is dissected and sling is passed around it. Gently ureter is palpated towards the distal narrower part from proximal dilated part (due to impacted stone). Stone is palpated without giving room for its slippage; carefully ureter distally is also dissected and held with a tape/sling. Both slings held taut to prevent the slippage of the stone in both directions. Two 3-zero vicryl stay sutures are placed; stone is steadied between fingers; longitudinal incision is made directly on the stone from below upwards; grating sensation will be felt while making the incision; stone is retrieved; using fine polythene tube warm saline irrigation is flushed both proximally and distally to clear small particles of the stone. An infant feeding tube is passed distally to confirm that there is no obstruction. J stent is passed across the ureter which is removed after 6 weeks. Ureter incision is closed with 3-zero interrupted vicryl sutures taking bites only from the muscular layer. If wall of the ureter is oedematous and friable it is not necessary to suture the ureter; J stent placement is sufficient. Tube drain is placed into the cavity. Wound is closed in layers.

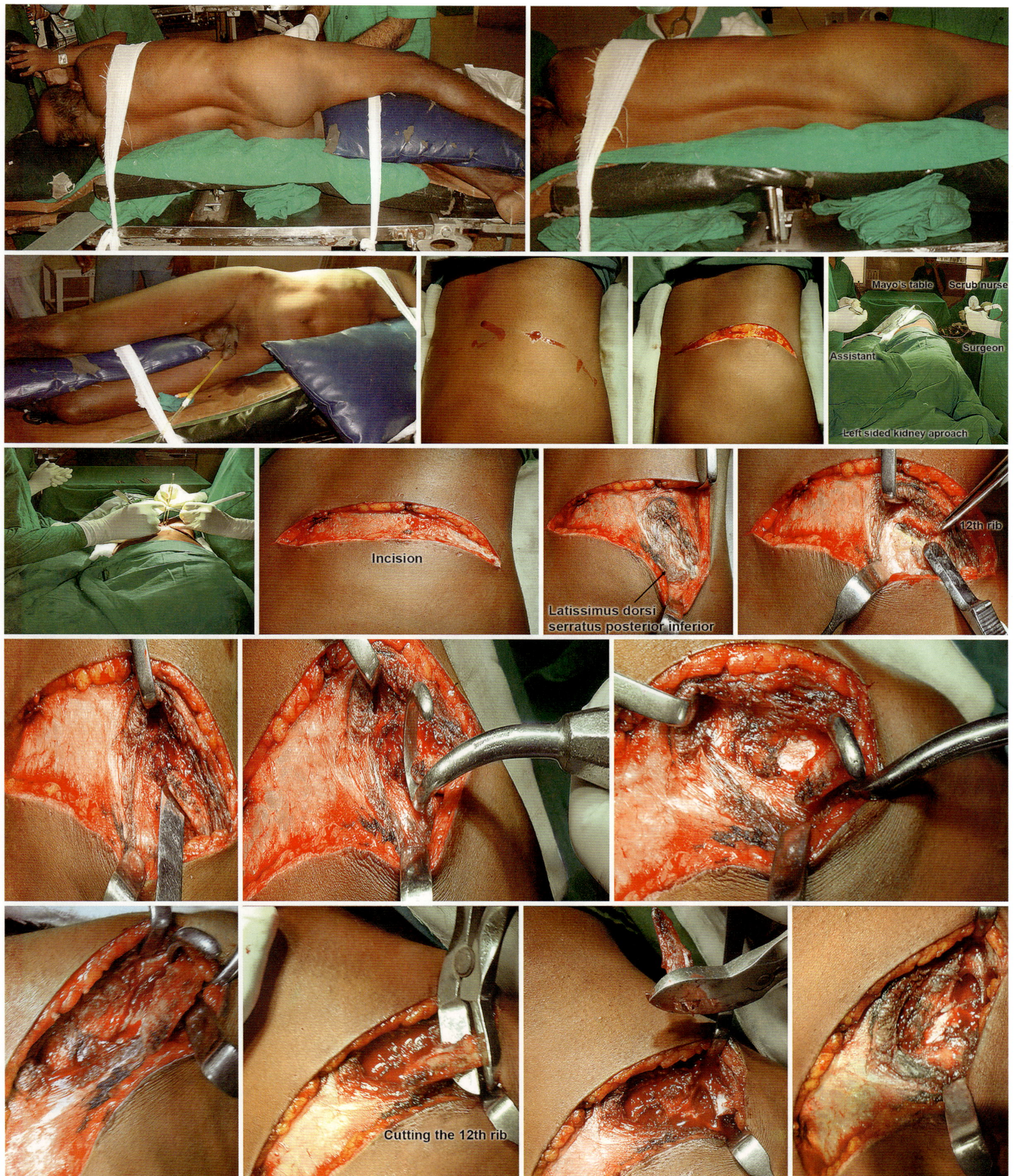
Mayo's table
Scrub nurse
Surgeon
Assistant
Left sided kidney aproach
Incision
12th rib
Latissimus dorsi
serratus posterior inferior
Cutting the 12th rib

Figs. 28-35(1)

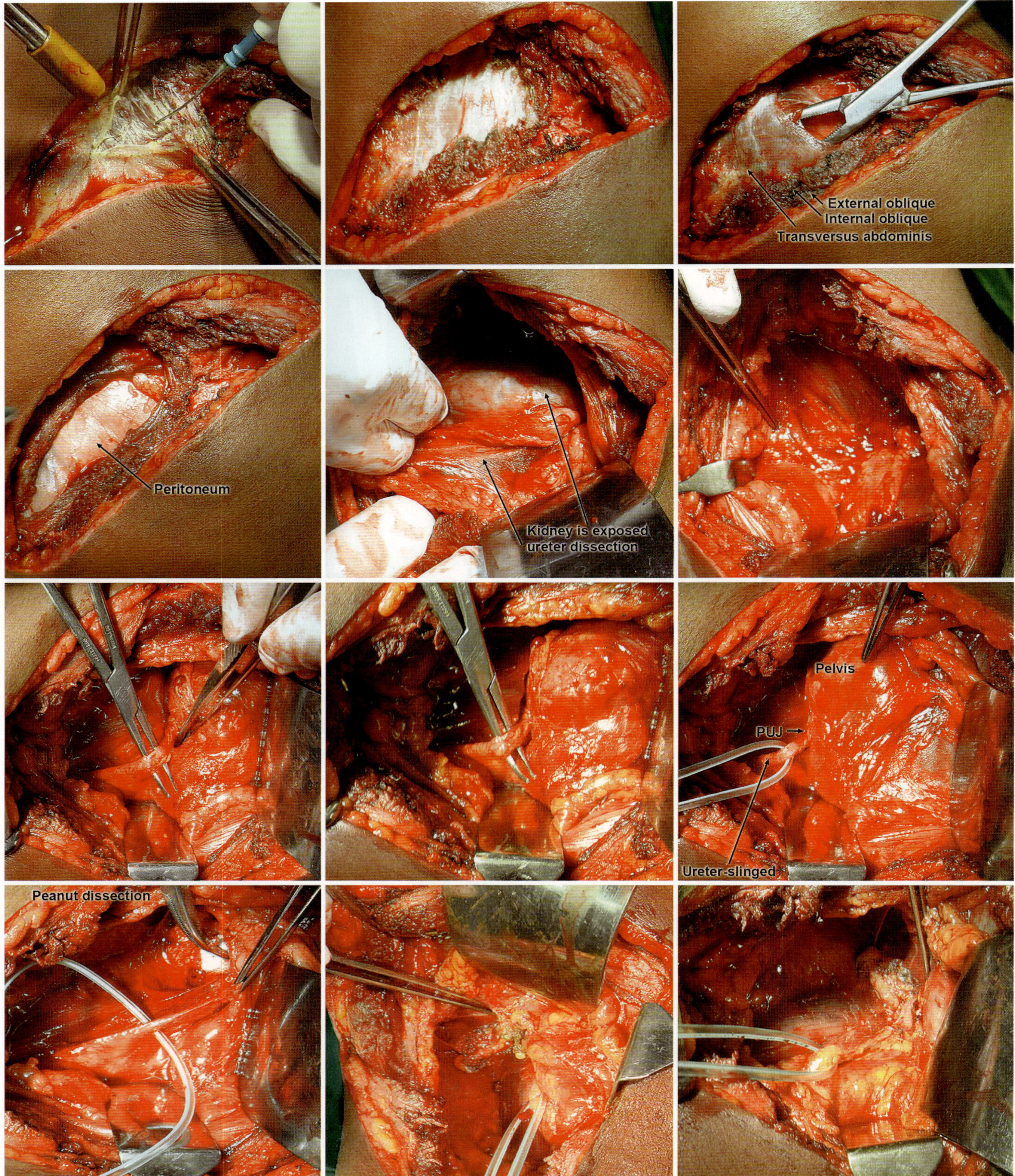
External oblique
Internal oblique
Transversus abdominis
Peritoneum
Kidney is exposed
ureter dissection
Pelvis
PUJ
Ureter-slinged
Peanut dissection

Figs. 28-35(2)

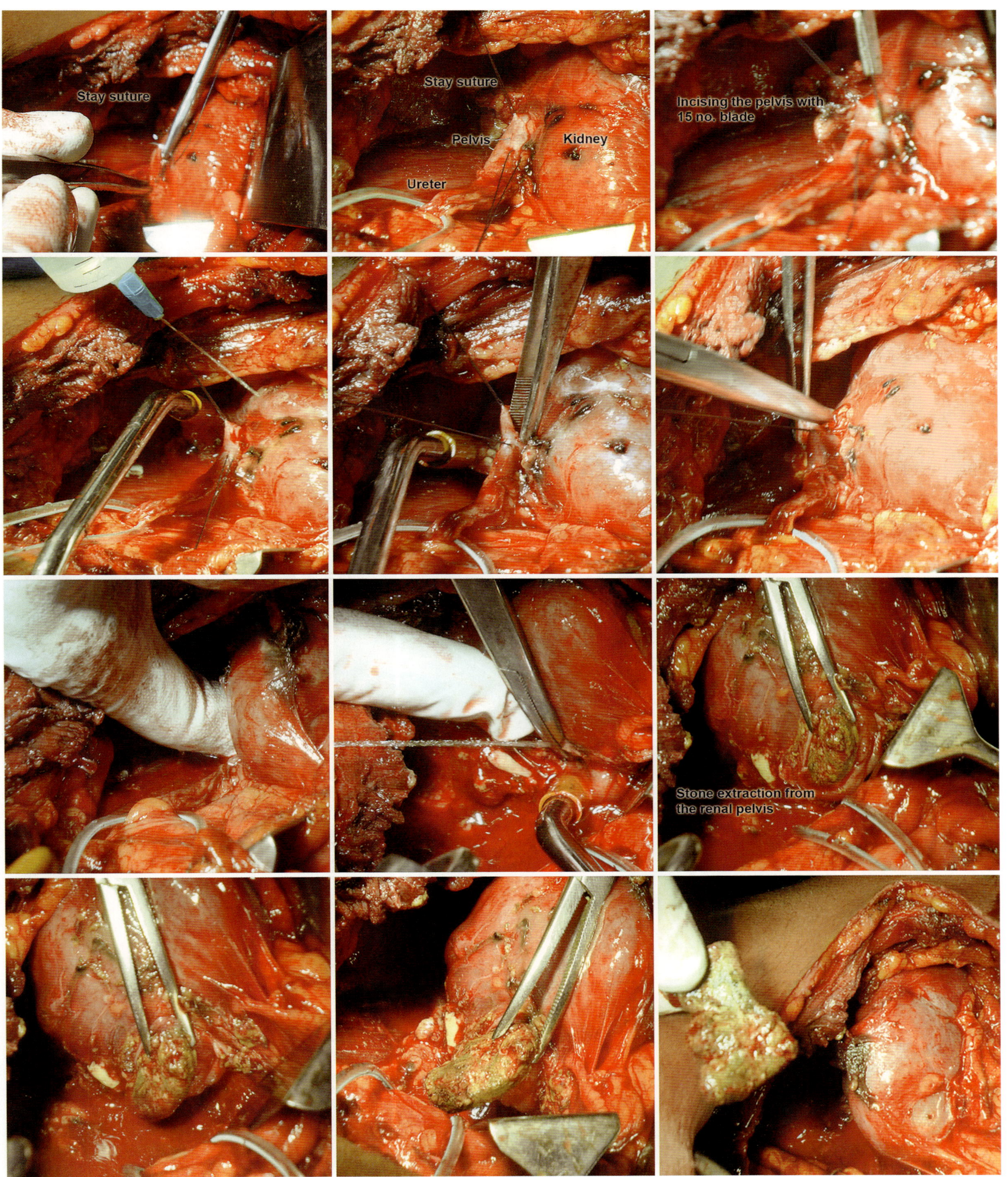
Stay suture
Stay suture
Pelvis
Kidney
Ureter
Incising the pelvis with
15 no. blade
Stone extraction from
the renal pelvis

Figs. 28-35(3)

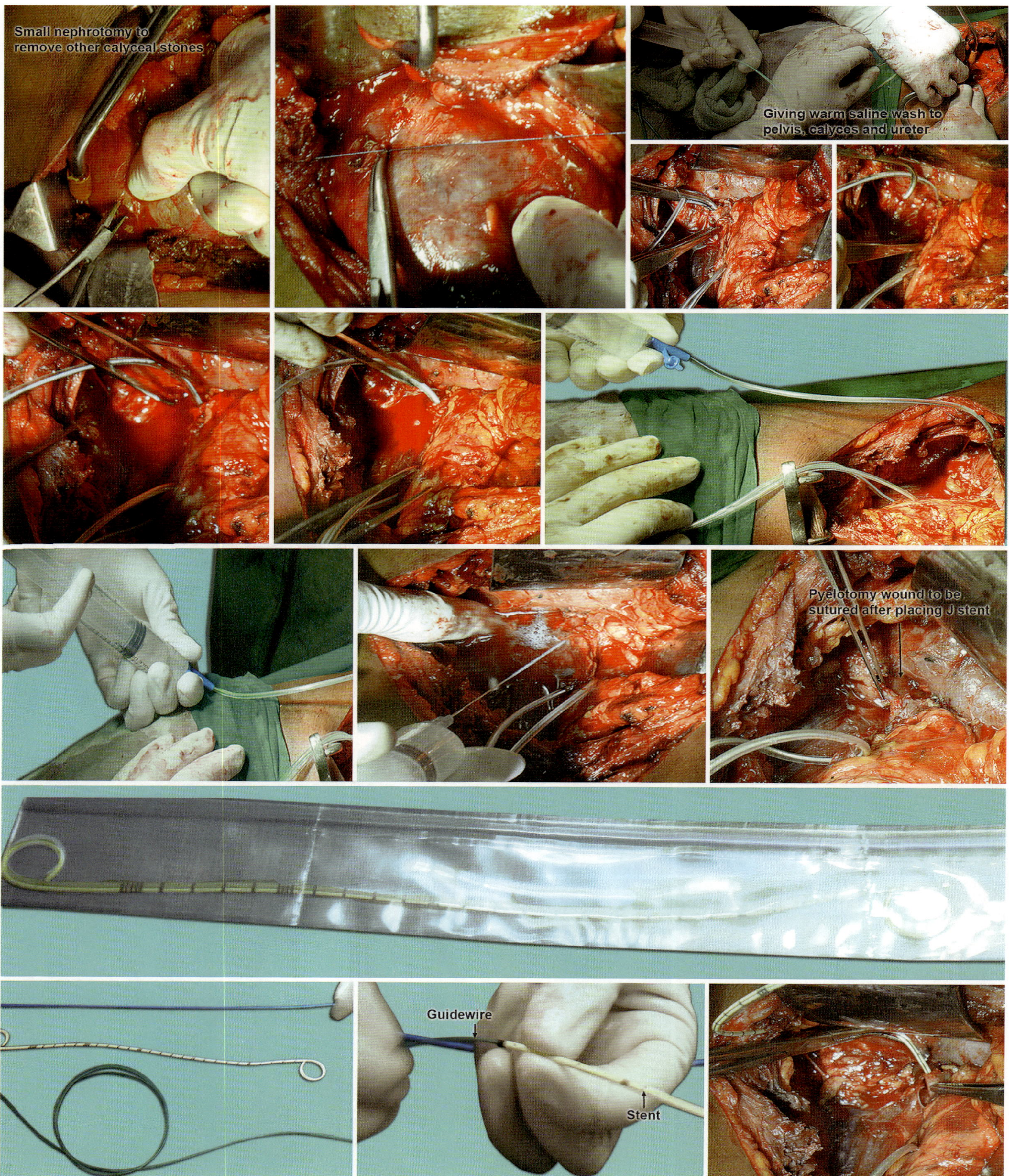
Small nephrotomy to remove other calyceal stones
Giving warm saline wash to pelvis, calyces and ureter
Pyelotomy wound to be sutured after placing J stent
Guidewire
Stent

Figs. 28-35(4)

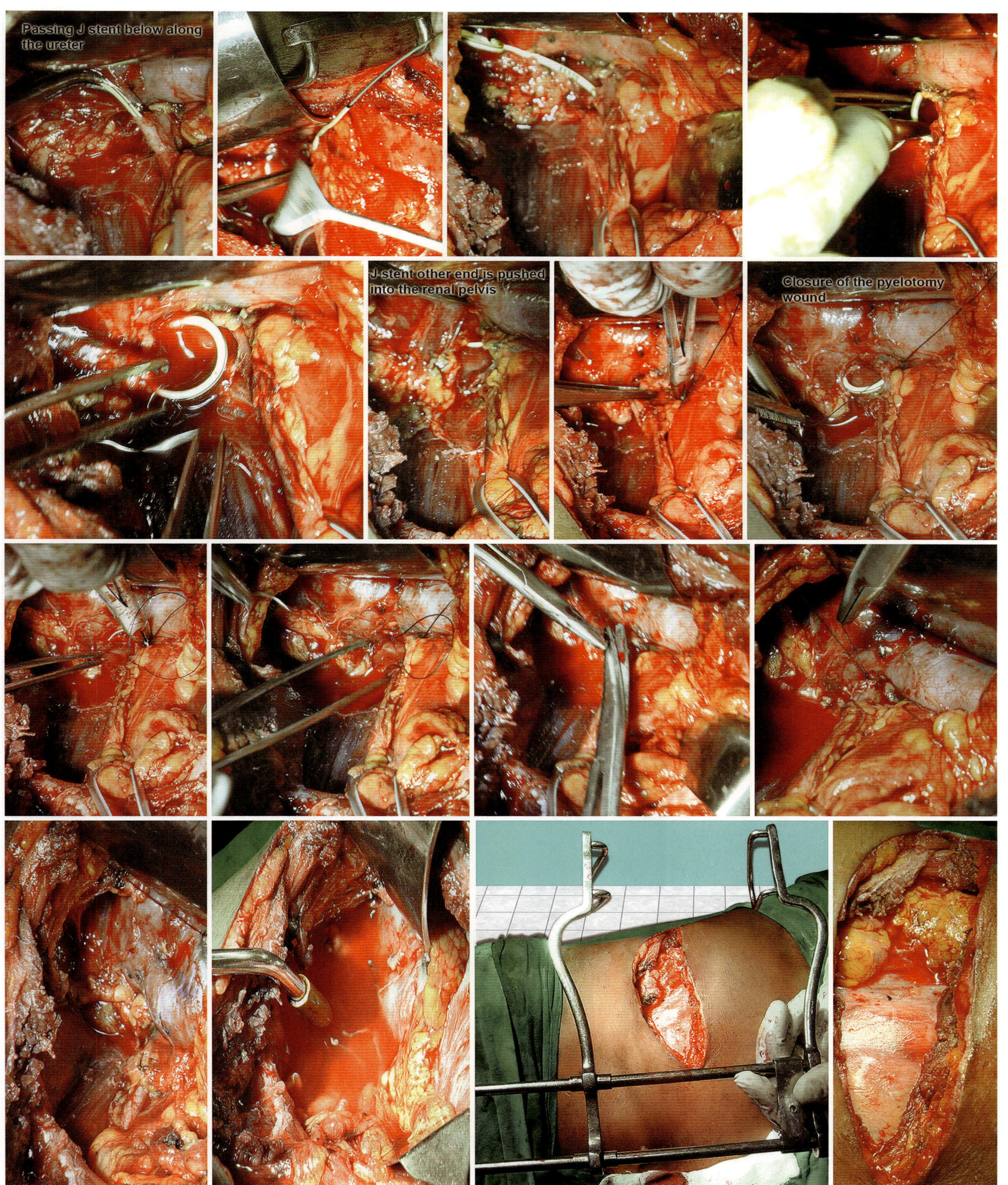
Passing J stent below along the ureter
J stent other end is pushed into the renal pelvis
Closure of the pyelotomy wound

Figs. 28-35(5)

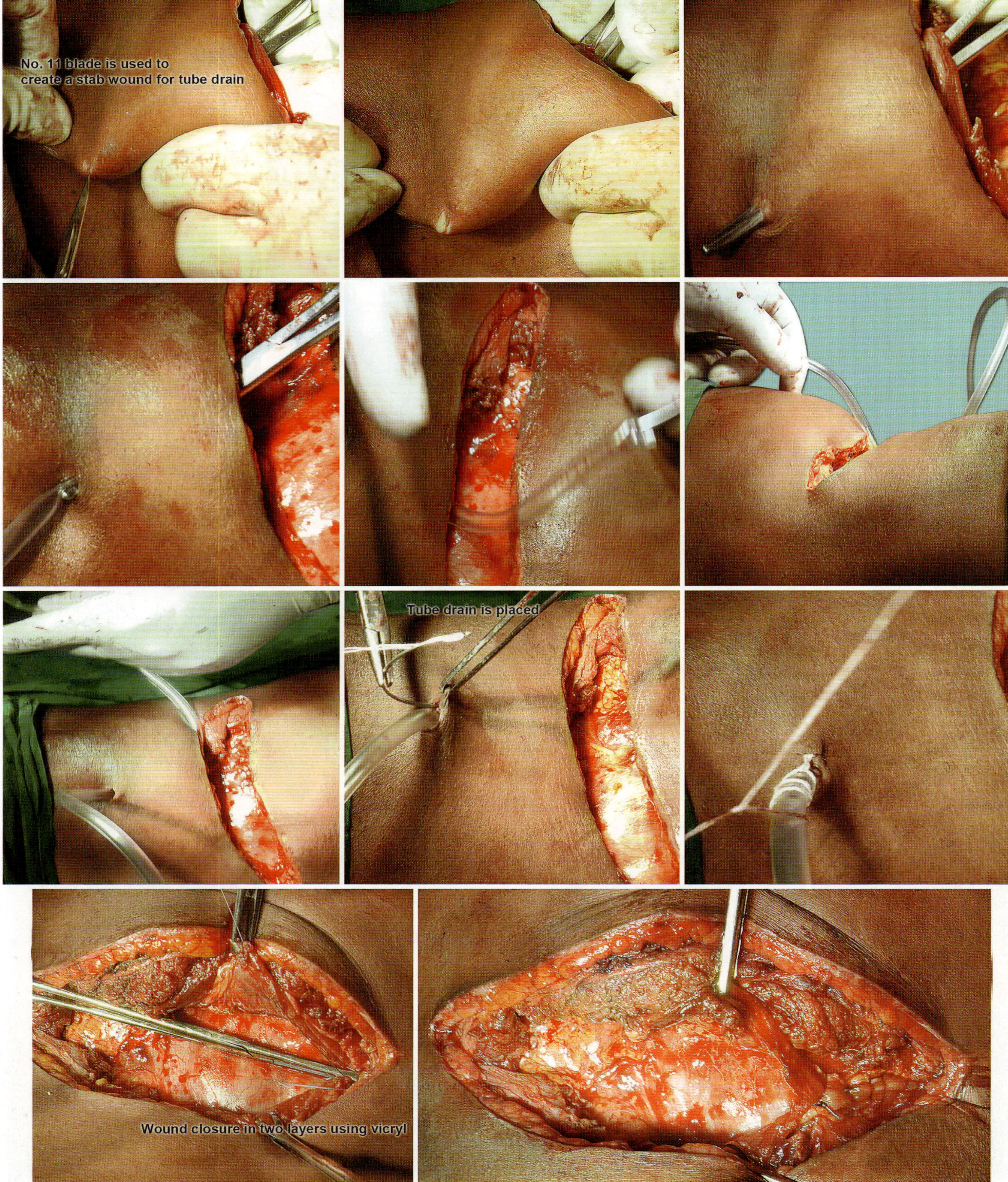

Figs. 28-35(6)

Figs. 28-35(1 to 6): Technique pyelolithotomy—open method. Now usually stones are removed through PCNL, ESWL or laparoscopic approach.

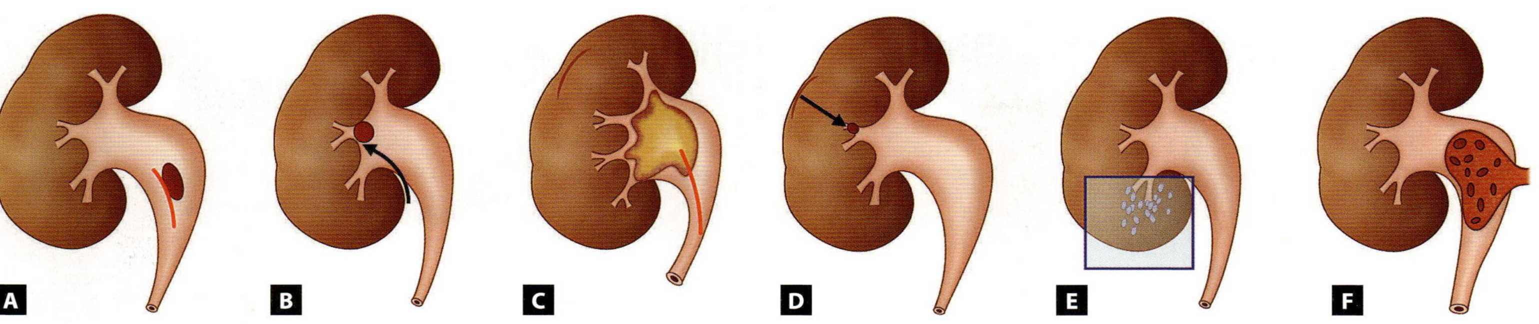

Figs. 28-36A to F: Surgeries for renal stones. (A) Pyelolithotomy; (B) Extended pyelolithotomy; (C) Nephropyelolithotomy; (D) Nephrolithotomy; (E) Partial nephrectomy; (F) Coagulum pyelolithotomy.

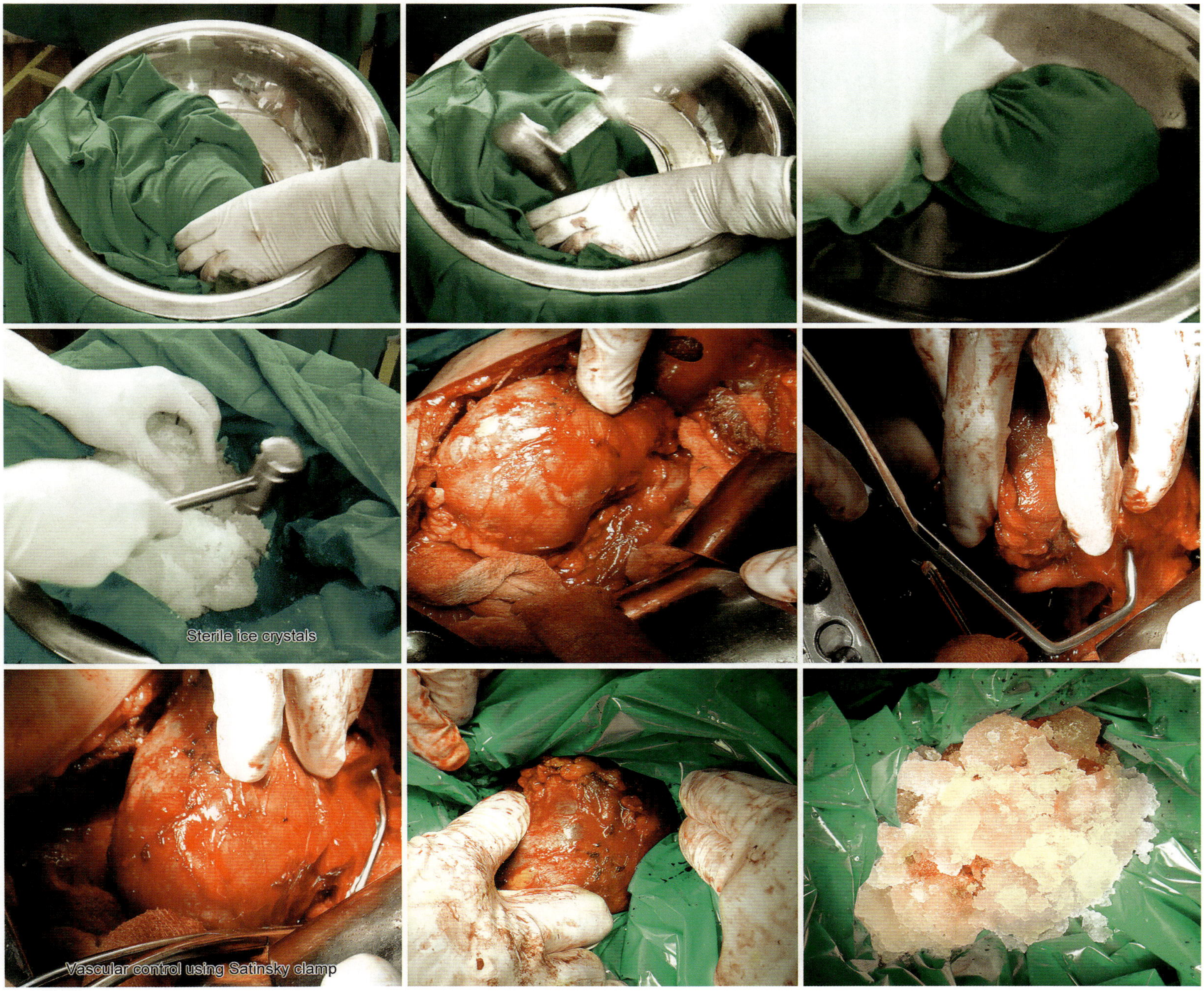

Sterile ice crystals

Vascular control using Satinsky clamp

Figs. 28-37(1)

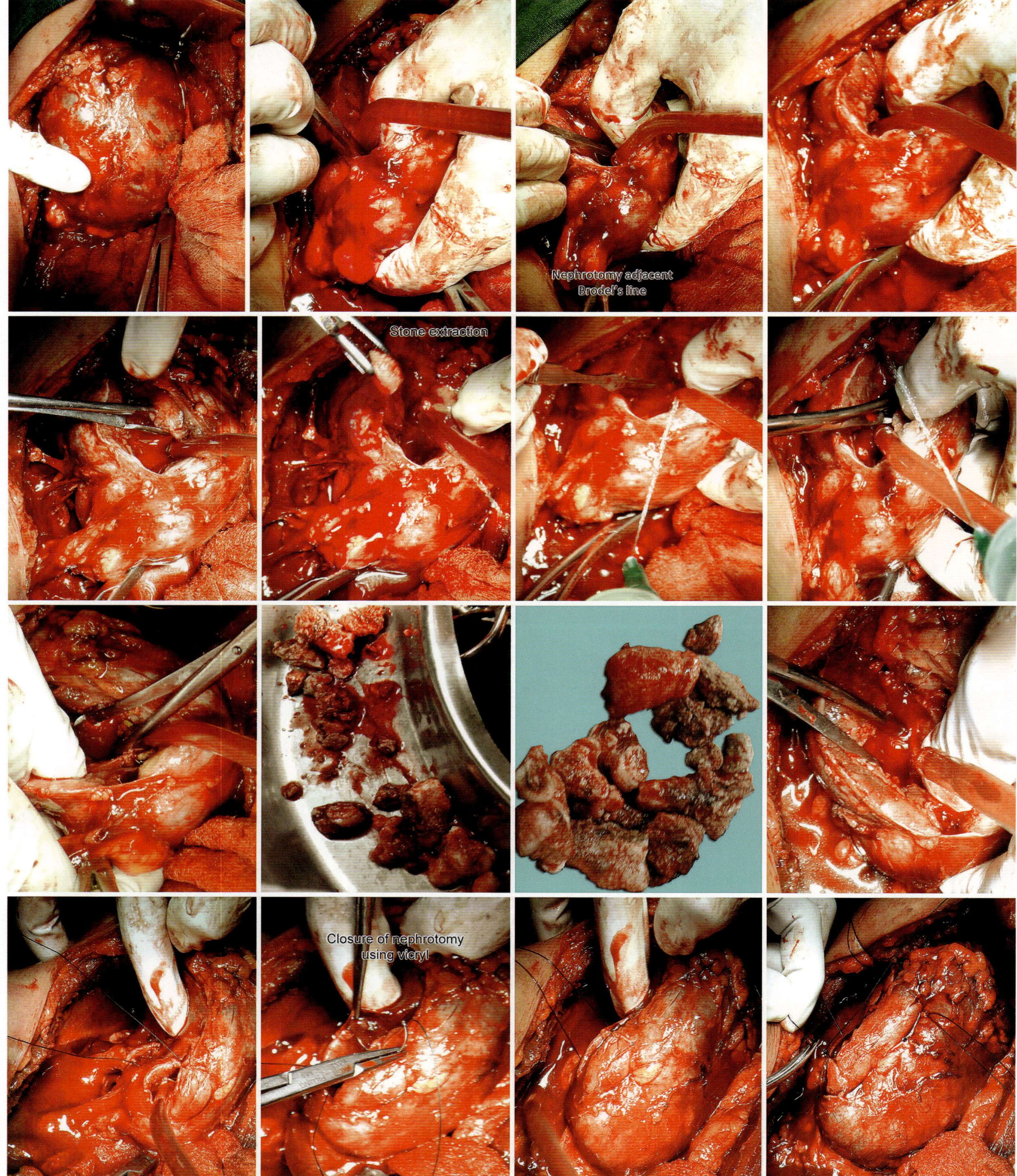
Nephrotomy adjacent
Brodel's line
Stone extraction
Closure of nephrotomy
using vicryl

Figs. 28-37(2)

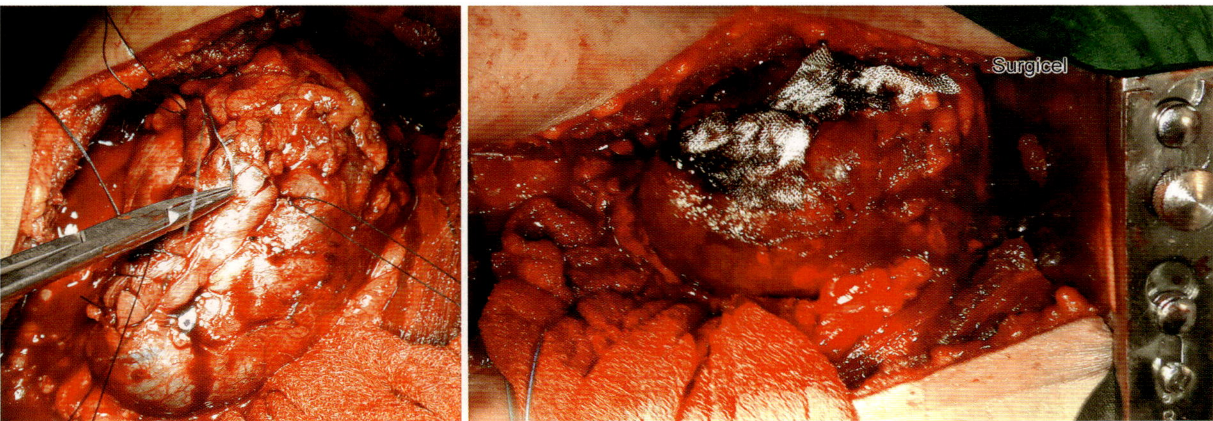

Figs. 28-37(3)

Figs. 28-37(1 to 3): Anatrophic nephropyelolithotomy. Vascular clamp is applied to the pedicle. Ice packs are kept over the kidney for 20 minutes; nephrotomy is done adjacent to Brodel's line to remove all stones. Nephrotomy wound is closed using vicryl. Nephrostomy (optional) and J stent (always) is kept in place. Vascular clamp is removed. Tube drain is placed; wound is closed in layers.

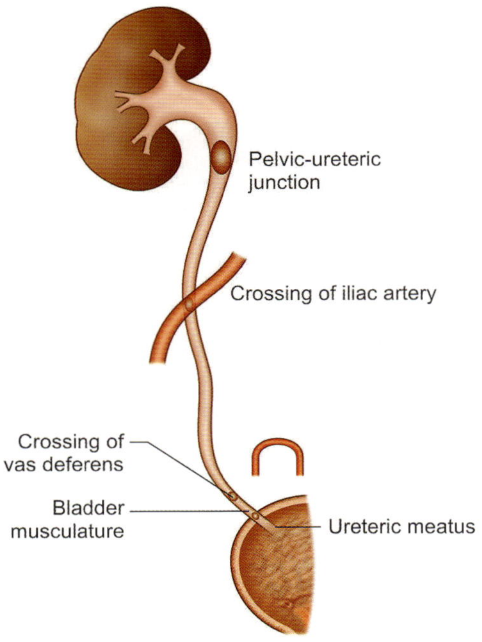

Fig. 28-38: Sites where a stone can get impacted in the ureter—narrow parts of the ureter.

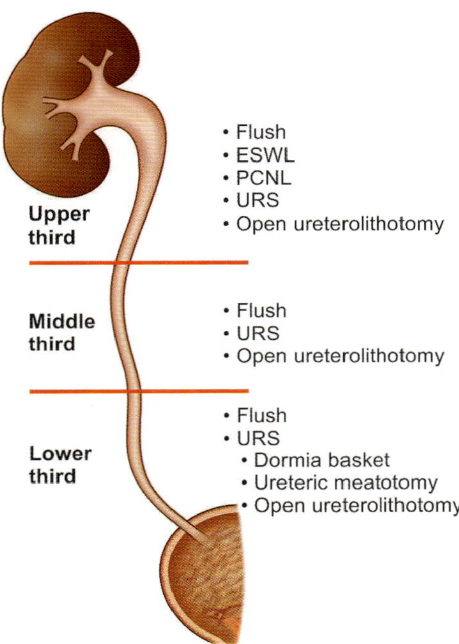

Fig. 28-39: Approaches for ureteric stones at different levels. (ESWL: extracorporeal shock wave lithotripsy; PCNL: percutaneous nephrolithotomy; URS: ureteroscopy)

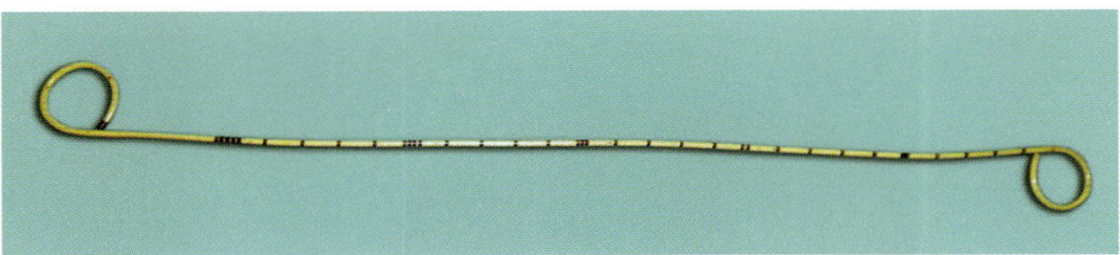

Fig. 28-40: J stent is commonly used for all urologic surgeries whether open or laparoscopic.

TREATMENT OF STAGHORN CALCULUS

Antibiotic is started. *Unilateral stone* is removed by *nephropyelolithotomy*. Multiple incisions are made over the Brodel's line (avascular plane) and assisted by pelvic incision. Stone is removed. Blood transfusion may be necessary as bleeding can occur. After that, nephrotomy and pyelotomy incisions are sutured with 3-zero vicryl **(Figs. 28-42A and B)**.

In *bilateral cases*, IVU is very essential. The kidney which is functioning better should be treated first. After 3 months, the other side kidney should be operated upon. If there are *bilateral staghorn calculi with pyonephrosis*, then initially bilateral nephrostomy is done using Malecot's catheter *(Cabot's nephrostomy)*. IVU is done later to see the renal function. If good function is present on both sides then both kidneys are operated one after the other in a gap of 3 months. They often need *haemodialysis*. Sometimes in case of severe infection *nephrectomy* is required. *Presently, PCNL is becoming a popular procedure for unilateral or bilateral staghorn calculi*. But when required, *conversion to open nephropyelolithotomy* should be considered **(Fig. 28-43)**.

Complications of staghorn calculus: Pyelonephritis, pyonephrosis, perinephric abscess, renal failure **(Fig. 28-44)**.

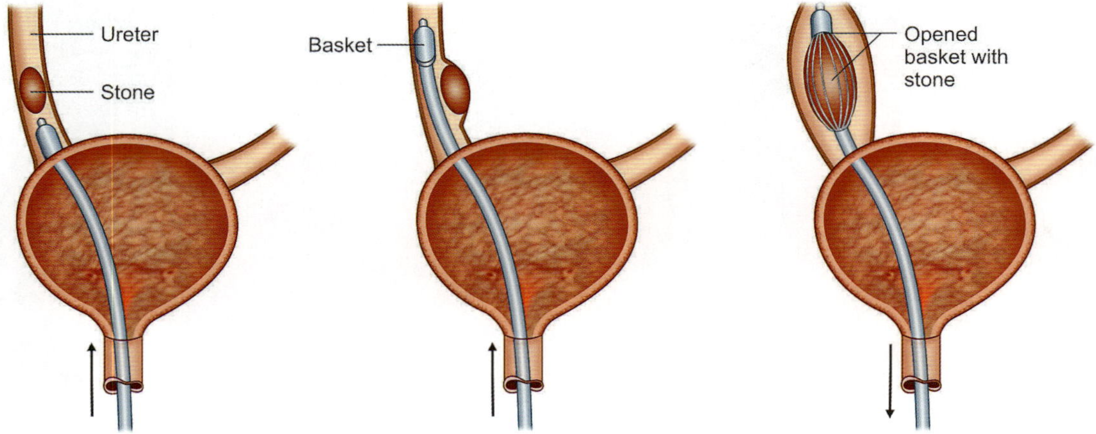

Fig. 28-41: Dormia basket is used to remove the stone in the lower ureter. Single stone less than 1 cm can be removed.

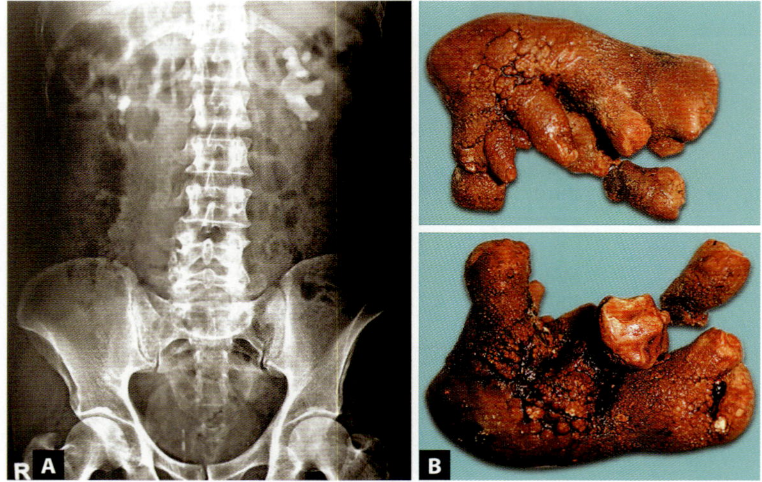

Figs. 28-42A and B: (A) X-ray showing staghorn calculus; (B) Large staghorn calculus removed from another patient.

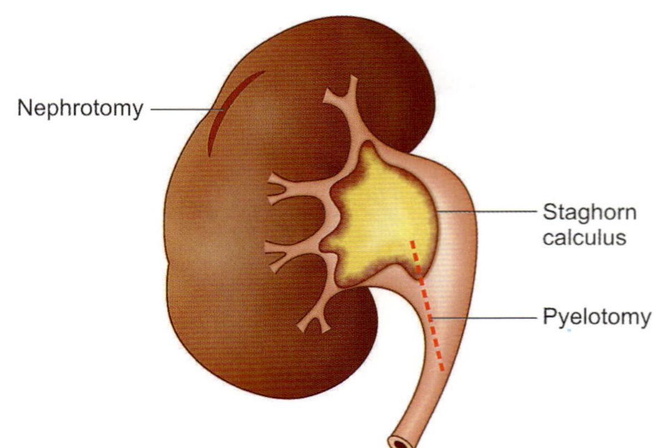

Fig. 28-43: Nephropyelolithotomy. *Note* the incisions placed.

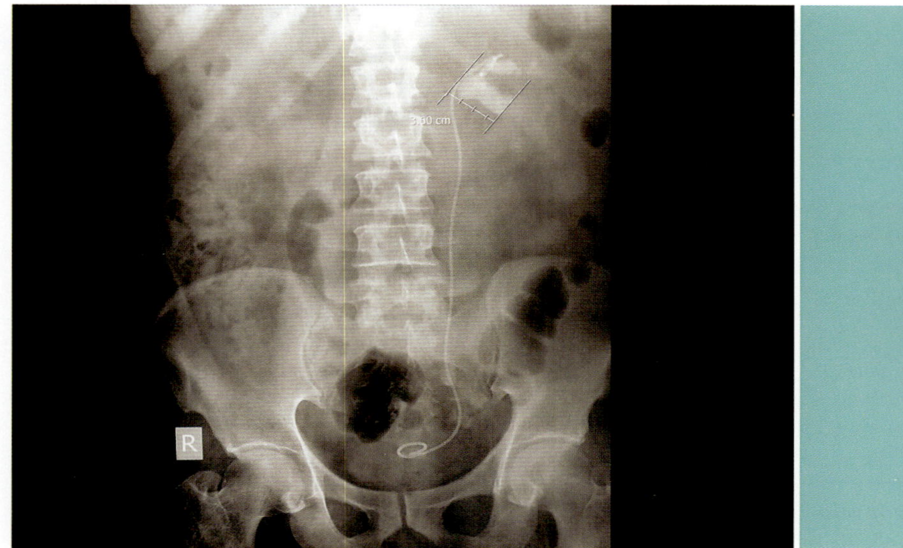

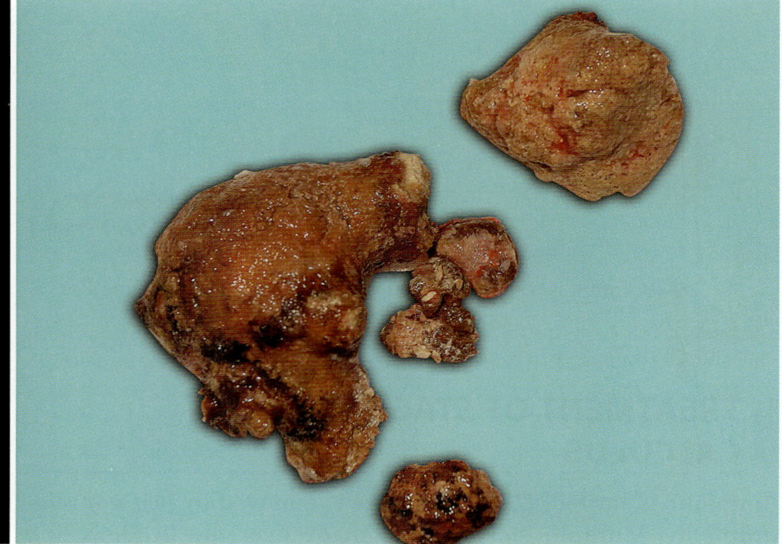

Fig. 28-44: X-ray and look of typical staghorn calculus—left sided. Open nephropyelolithotomy is done.

TREATMENT OF RENAL CELL CARCINOMA

Surgery is the treatment of choice. Initial CT imaging and proper evaluation is a must **(Figs. 28-45 and 28-46)**.

Radical nephroureterectomy: *Structures removed are* entire kidney along with tumour; perinephric tissue; ipsilateral adrenal gland (adrenal gland can be spared); proximal 2/3rd ureter/as low as possible; lymph nodes from crus of diaphragm to aorta bifurcation with renal hilar nodes. Transperitoneal approach is often used. Retroperitoneal/Nagamatsu (resection of 11th ribs) approach/ thoracoabdominal approach/posterior vertical are other approaches used. Patient will be in lateral position. After laparotomy, colon is mobilised medially. Vessels are identified and dissected and ligated securely (transfixation and three ligatures proximally using non-absorbable silk/polypropylene sutures). Preoperative renal artery embolisation can be done to decrease vascularity and to facilitate the removal of entire tumour. Renal artery which is posterior is dissected and clamped or ligated in continuity; then renal vein is ligated and divided; later ligated renal artery is divided. In case of IVC extension of tumour thrombus (8%), after applying an oblique vascular clamp, IVC is opened, tumour thrombus is removed and IVC is sutured. In supradiaphragmatic vena caval extension of thrombus, cardiopulmonary bypass is necessary. First renal vessels (artery and vein) should be ligated to prevent tumour dissemination and bleeding. Lymphadenectomy is not necessarily undertaken routinely; it is only done when imaging shows significant nodal enlargement or on table findings shows enlarged nodes **(Figs. 28-47 and 28-48)**.

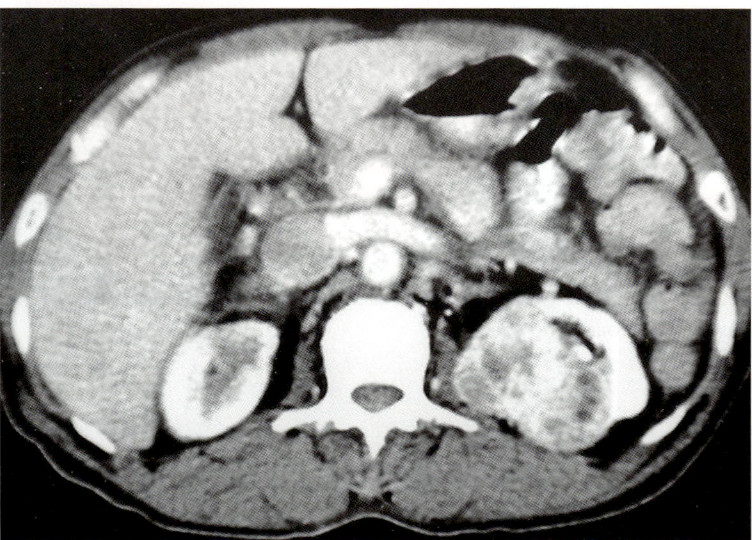

Fig. 28-45: CT scan of renal cell carcinoma.

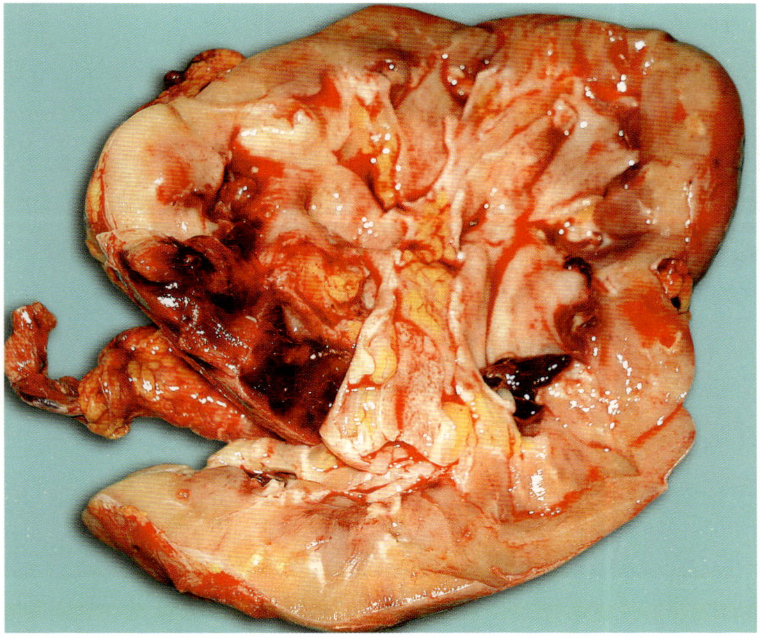

Fig. 28-46: Large upper pole renal cell carcinoma.

Even in large fixed tumour, palliative nephrectomy or debulking is advised as it may cause regression of secondaries **(Figs. 28-49 and 28-50)**.

Nephron sparing surgeries are done in bilateral RCC (bilateral partial nephrectomy). Renal artery is temporarily occluded using vascular clamps and kidney is cooled to have proper control of bleeding and adequate visualisation of the line of resection. Partially resected specimen is assessed by frozen section biopsy. Retained partial capsule is sutured after haemostasis. Renal arterial clamp is released. It is presently done for unilateral localised tumours also. After isolation of the renal artery with placing icepacks to control the ischaemic time, artery or its branch is clamped using vascular clamp. Icepacks are already in place. Tumour with clearance margin of 5 mm to 10 mm is excised; sent for immediate frozen section biopsy. Bleeding is controlled using continuous 3-zero vicryl sutures. Methylene blue is injected from below across the ureteric catheter; if renal excised wound stains blue that means there is disruption of the calyces and it should be sutured. Arterial clamp is released. Any bleeding points if present are sutured. Surgicel is placed on the raw area. Drain is placed. Loin wound is closed. Warm ischaemic time for kidney is 30 minutes; cold ischaemic time is up to 4 hours **(Figs. 28-51 to 28-53)**.

Partial nephrectomy (Carl Boye Semb, university of Oslo): It is done when disease is limited to one of the poles usually lower (T1a, T1b). Polar vessels are ligated and polar segment of the kidney is resected. Cut raw area is sutured with continuous 3-zero vicryl sutures. Tube drain is placed. Procedure is done through loin incision **(Figs. 28-54 and 28-55)**.

Complications

Intraoperative

Bleeding can occur from IVC, renal vein or branches. Vascular clamps should be used to control the bleeding. Vessel wall is sutured using continuous polypropylene 4-zero or 3-zero sutures.

Bowel injuries can occur especially to colon which is close to Gerota's fascia. If injury occurs then temporary colostomy or ileostomy is needed for 3 months after which it is closed. Sharp dissection injuries or cautery injuries can occur.

Injuries to liver, gallbladder, spleen (on left side) can occur during dissection due to avulsion. Pancreatic injury on left side can also occur. Injury to pleura, diaphragm are not uncommon **(Fig. 28-56)**.

Postoperative

Delayed bleeding, pseudoaneurysm formation, arteriovenous fistula can occur in nephron sparing nephrectomy. It is usually treated by therapeutic angioembolisation.

Infection, abscess formation, septicaemia can occur after any type of nephrectomy. Lymphocele can develop after lymphadenectomy.

Raised creatinine level in postoperative period in many nephrectomies.

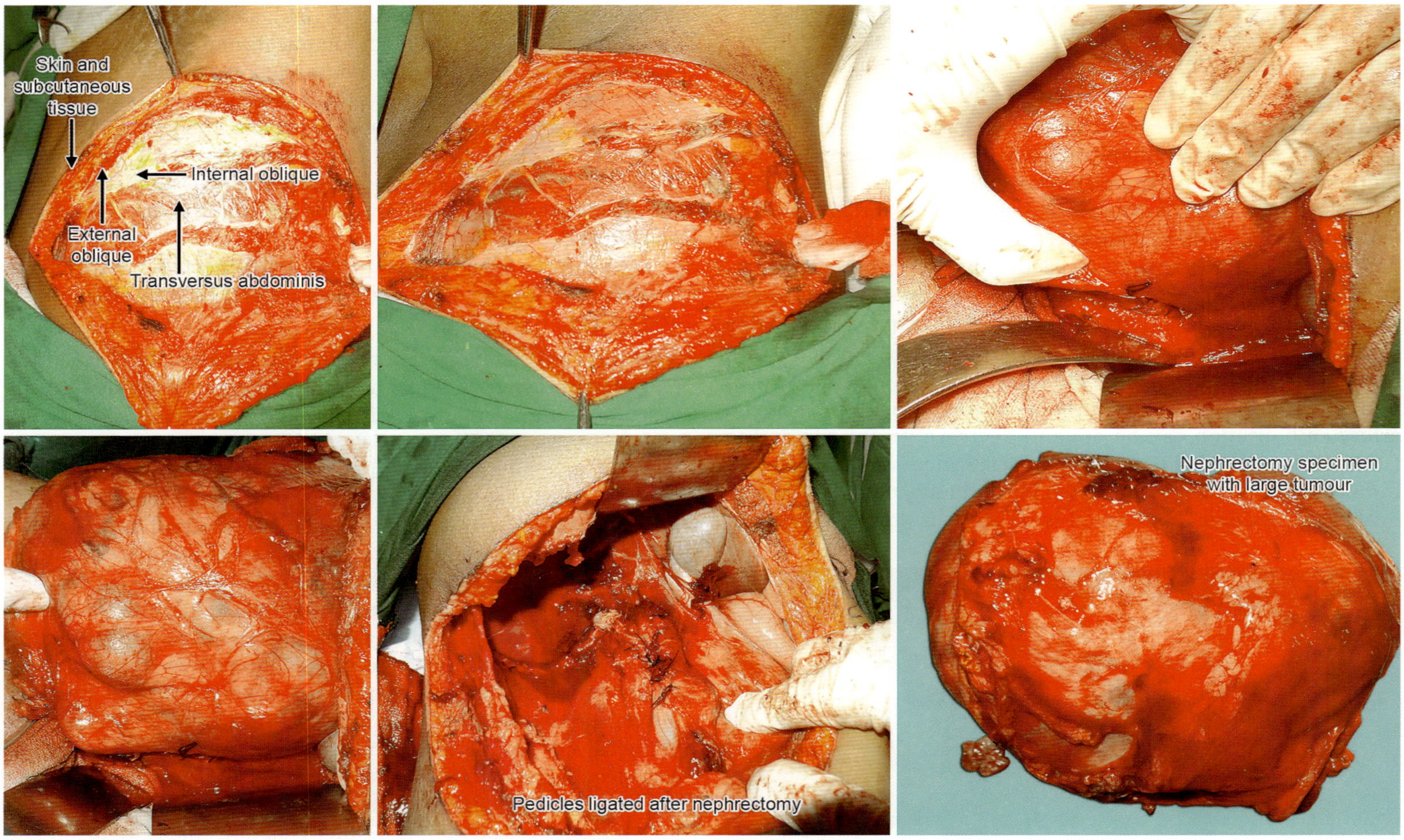

Skin and subcutaneous tissue
Internal oblique
External oblique
Transversus abdominis
Nephrectomy specimen with large tumour
Pedicles ligated after nephrectomy

Fig. 28-47: Large RCC—radical nephrectomy—approach and specimen.

Mayo's table
Position
Cleaning and draping
Marking the incision
Skin
External oblique
Internal oblique

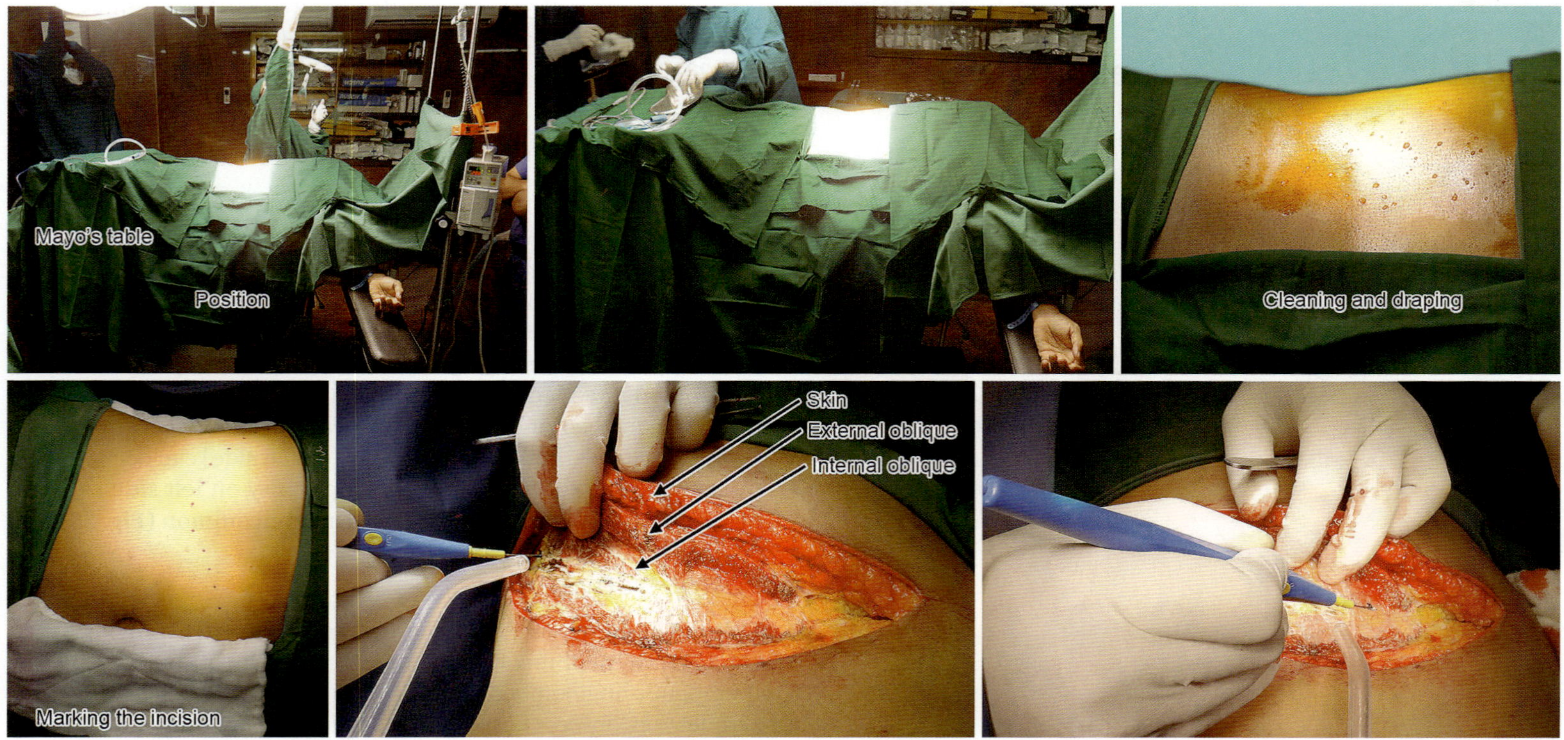

Figs. 28-48(1)

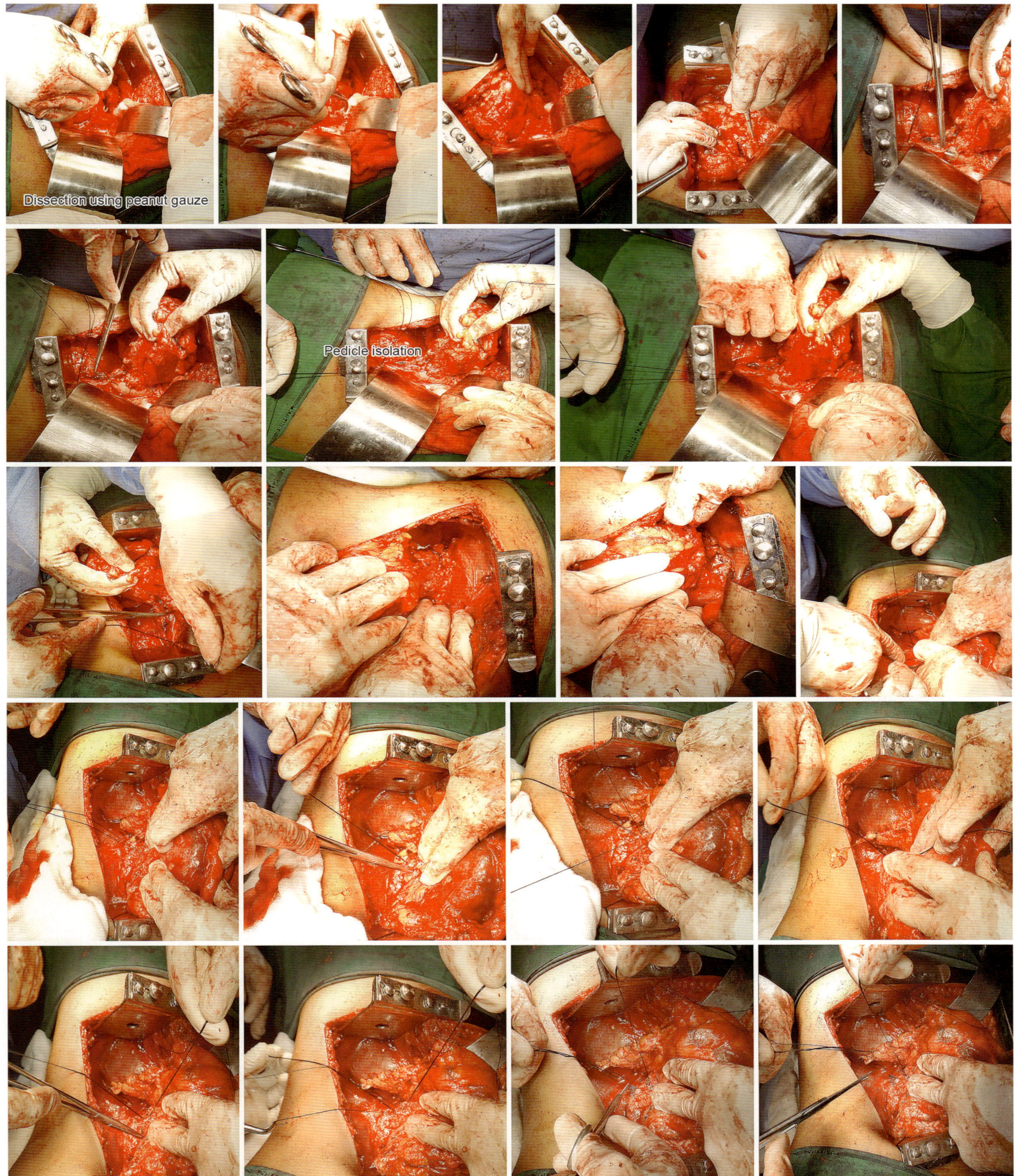

Figs. 28-48(2)

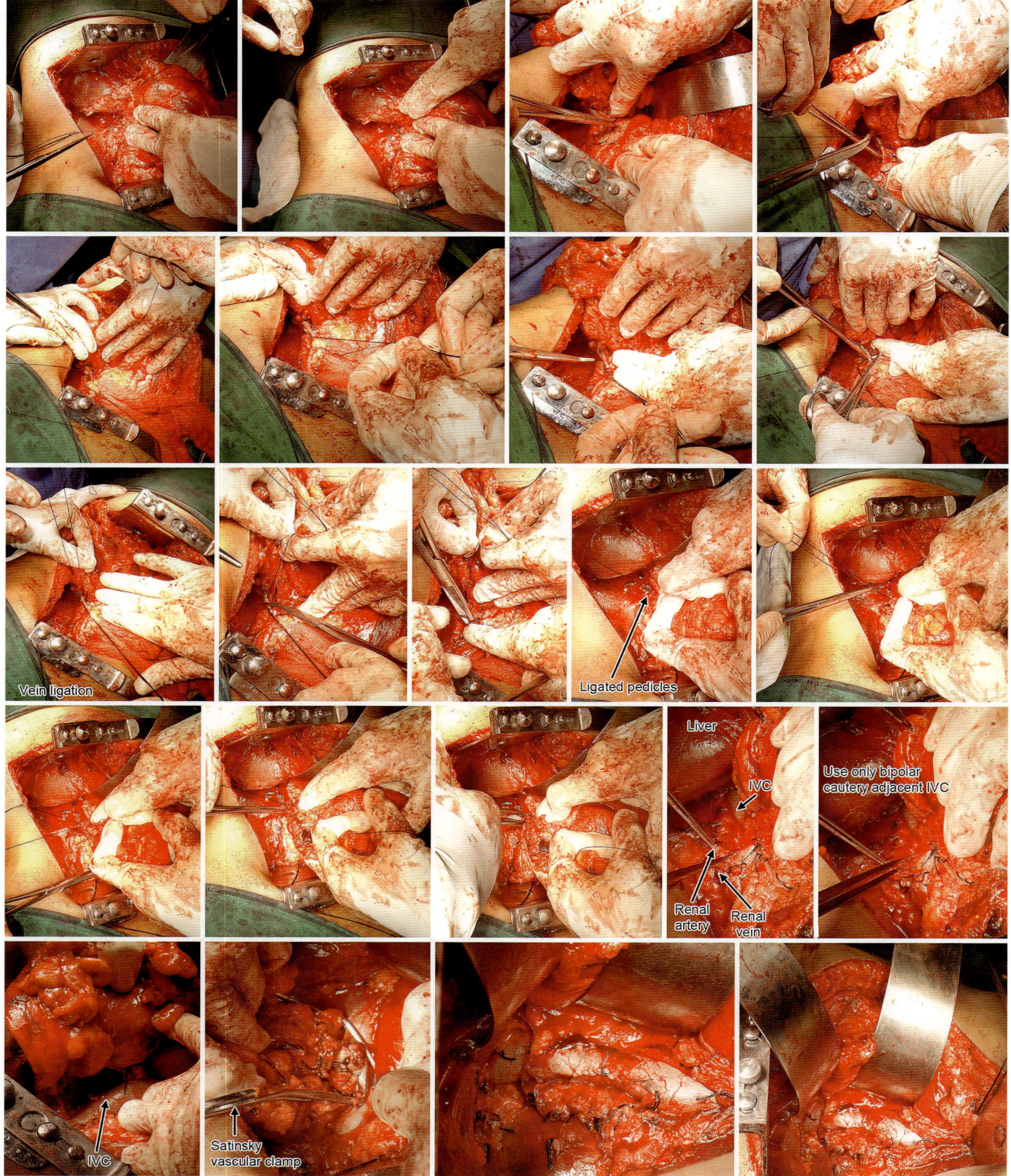

Figs. 28-48(3)

Figs. 28-48(1 to 3): Radical nephrectomy with IVC clamping to remove tumour thrombus in the vein.

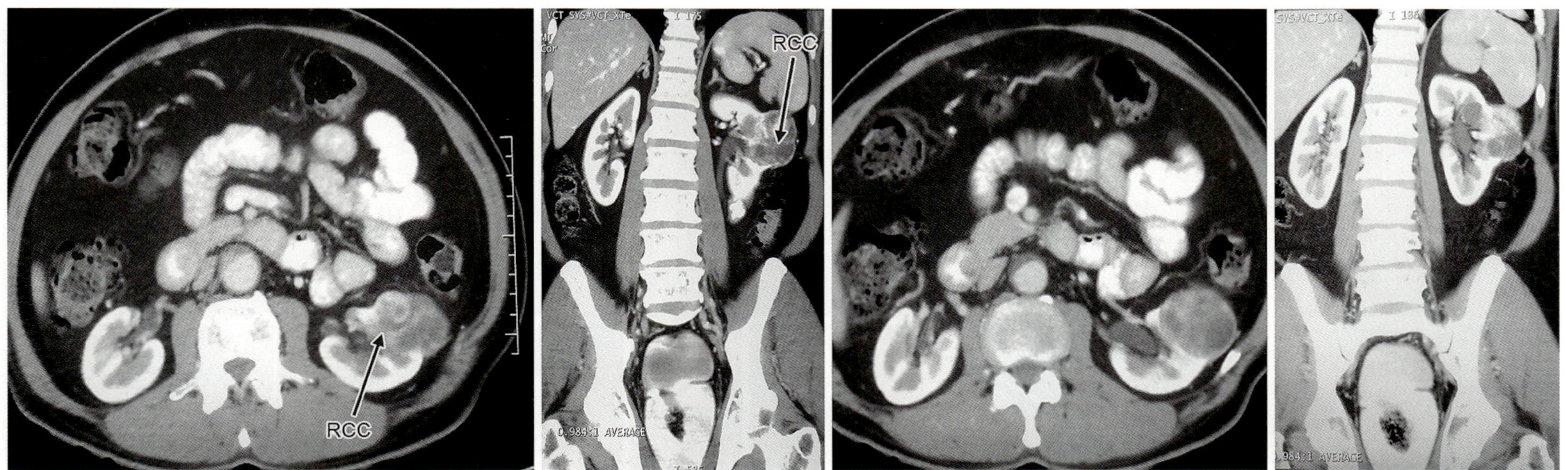

Fig. 28-49: CT pictures showing renal cell carcinoma.

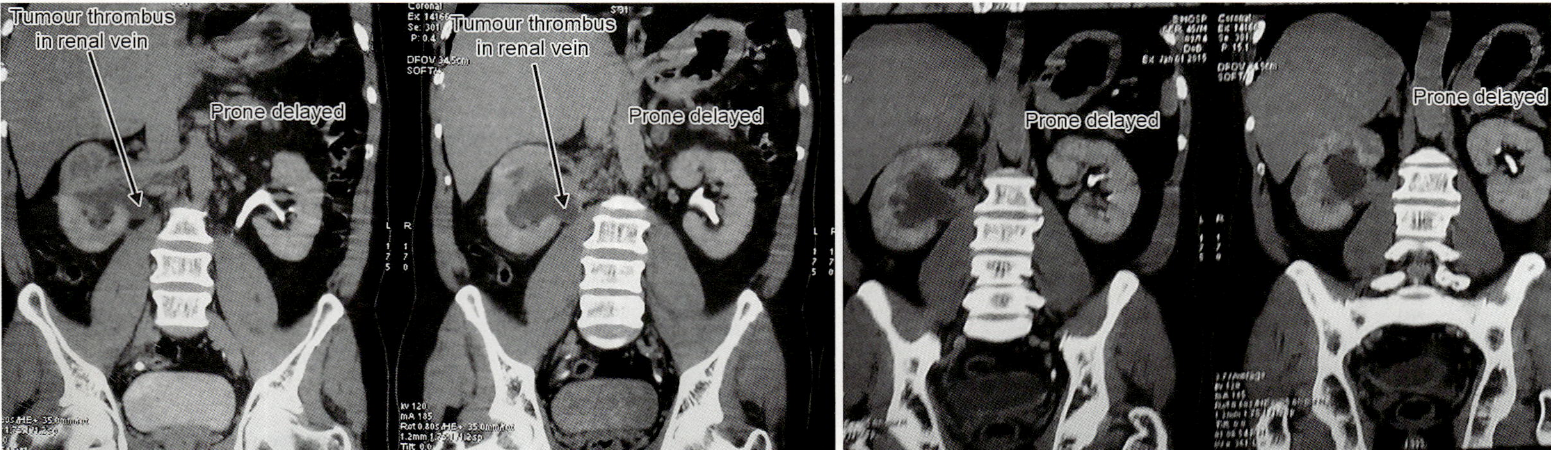

Fig. 28-50: CT scan showing RCC with thrombus in the renal vein extending into IVC.

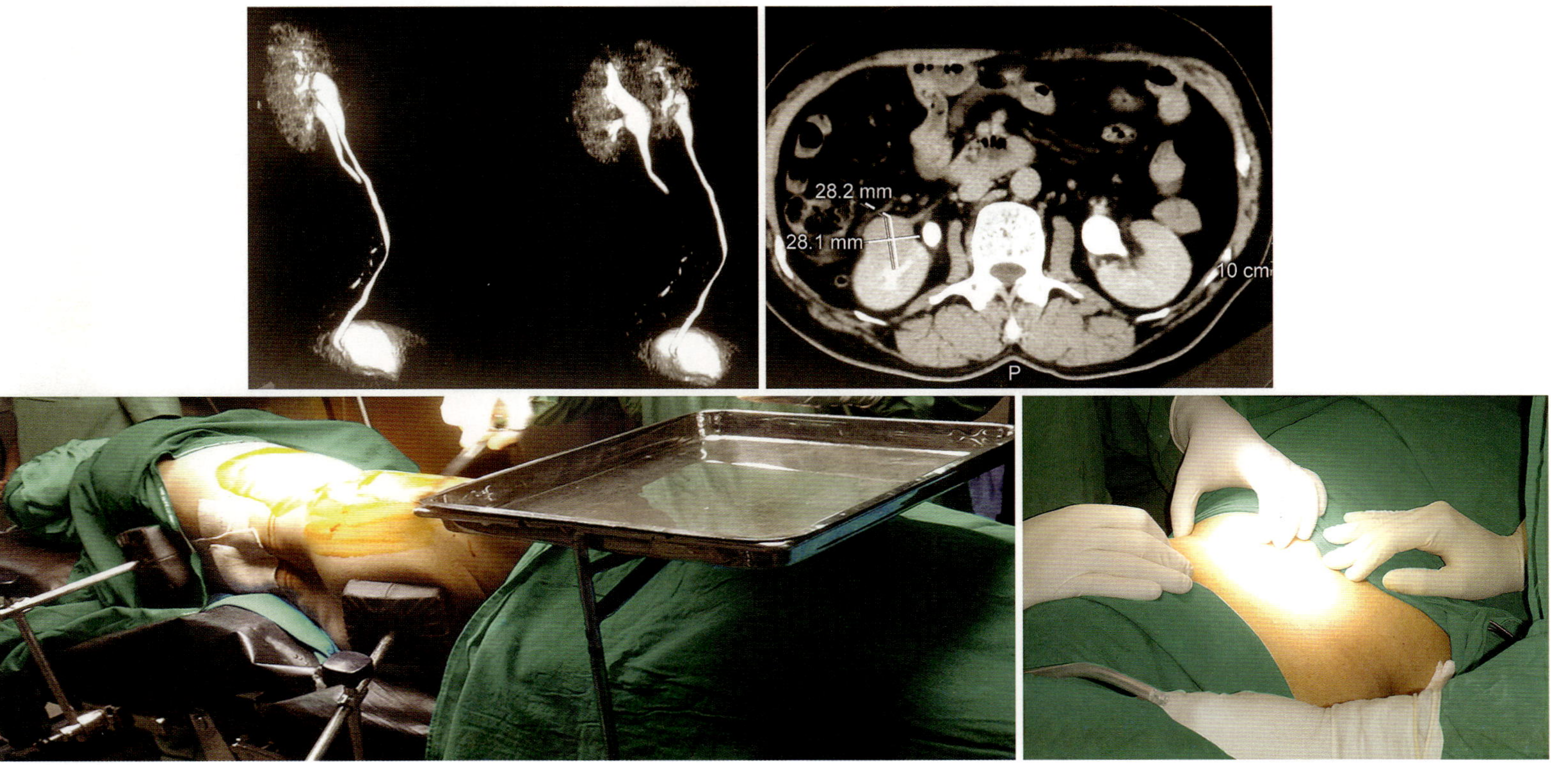

Figs. 28-51(1)

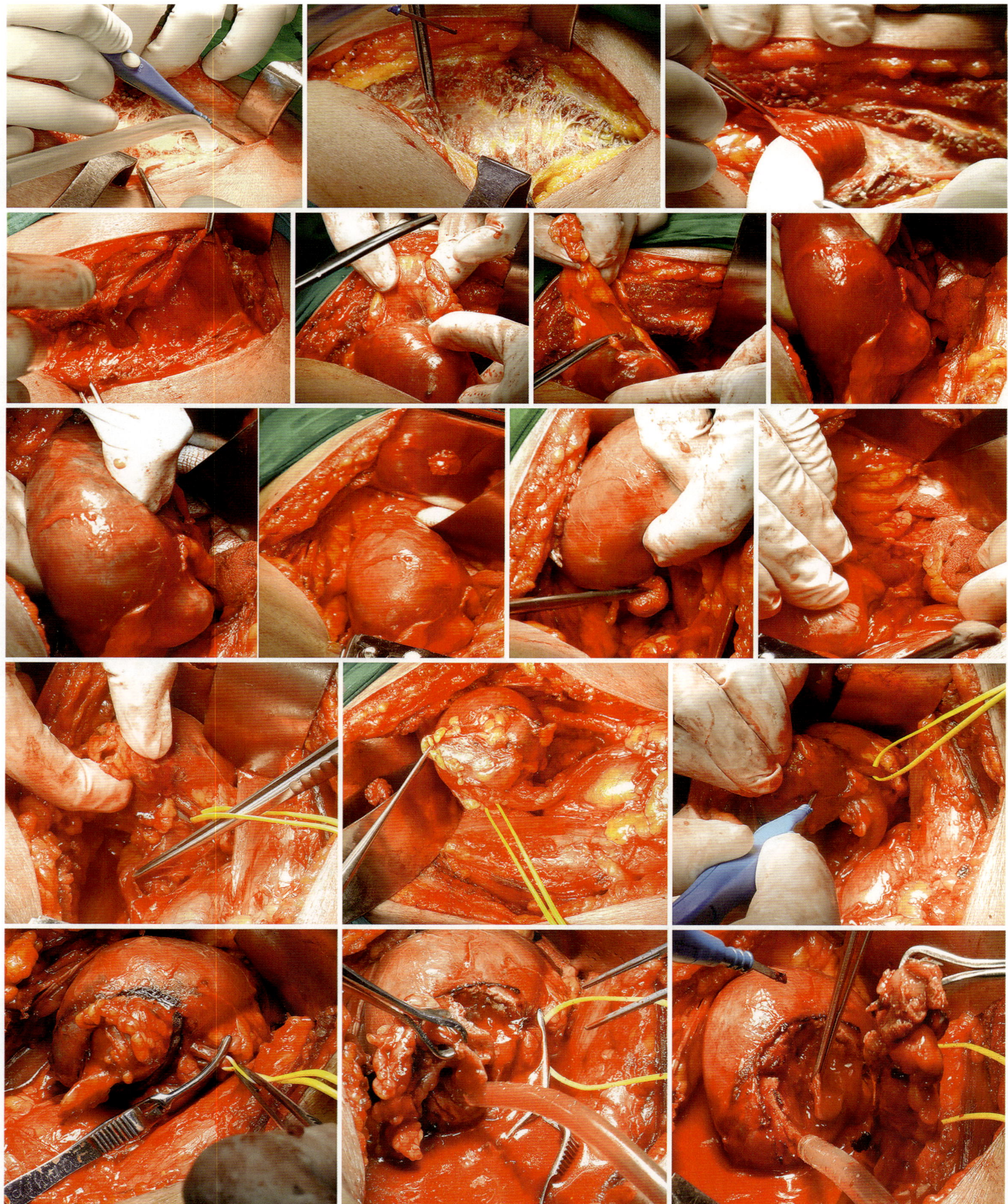

Figs. 28-51(2)

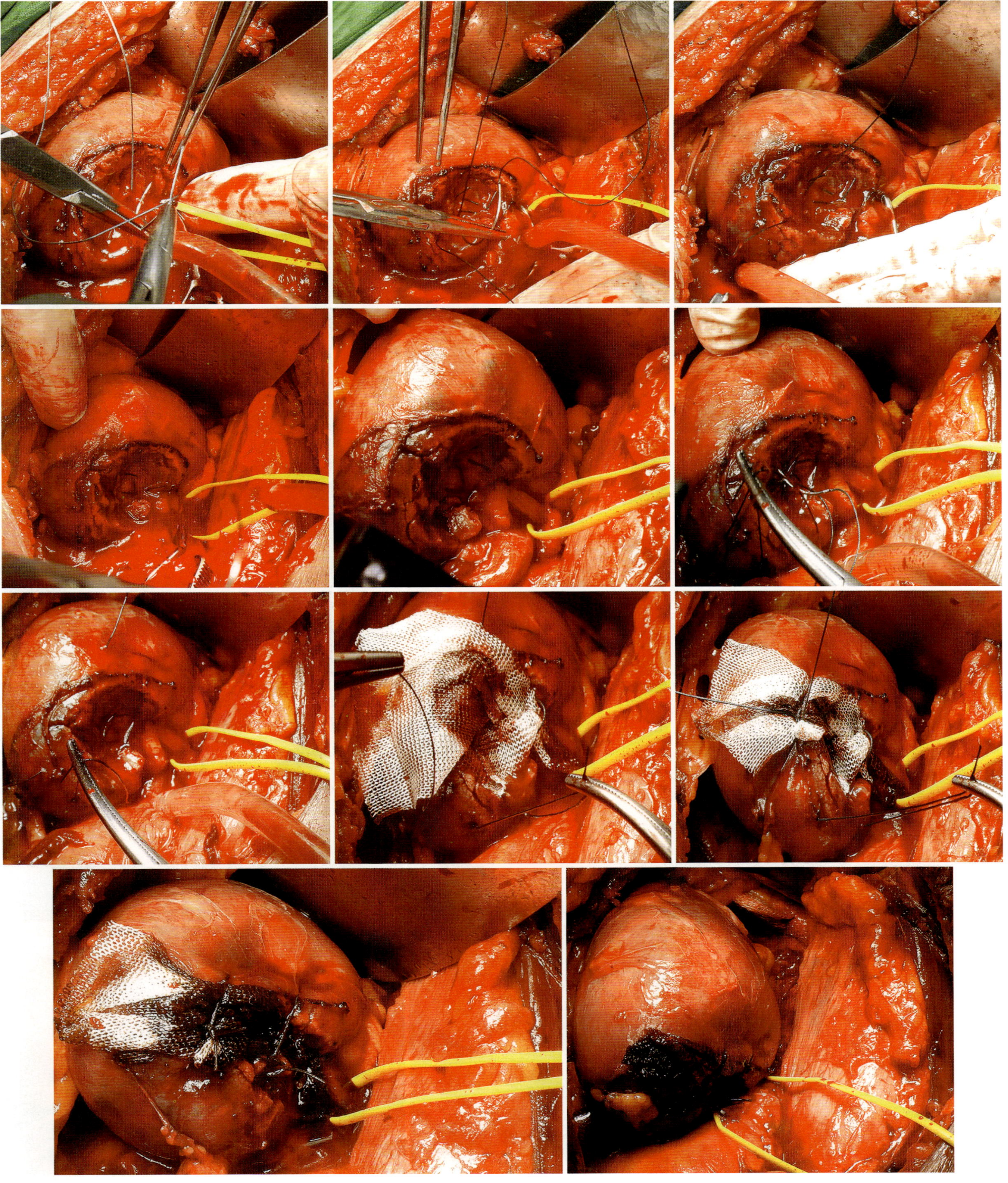

Figs. 28-51(3)

Figs. 28-51(1 to 3): Nephron sparing nephrectomy.

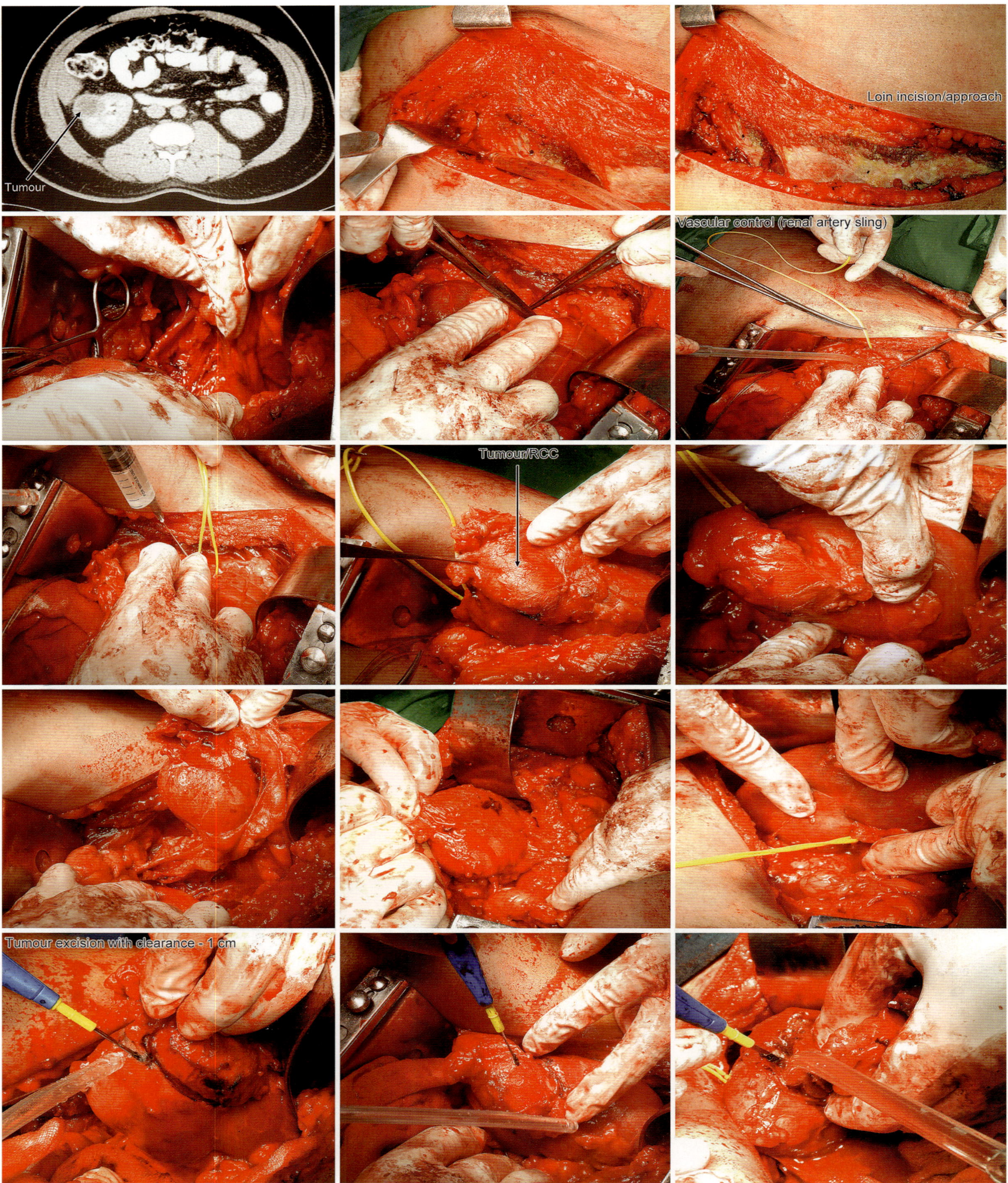
Tumour
Loin incision/approach
Vascular control (renal artery sling)
Tumour/RCC
Tumour excision with clearance - 1 cm

Figs. 28-52(1)

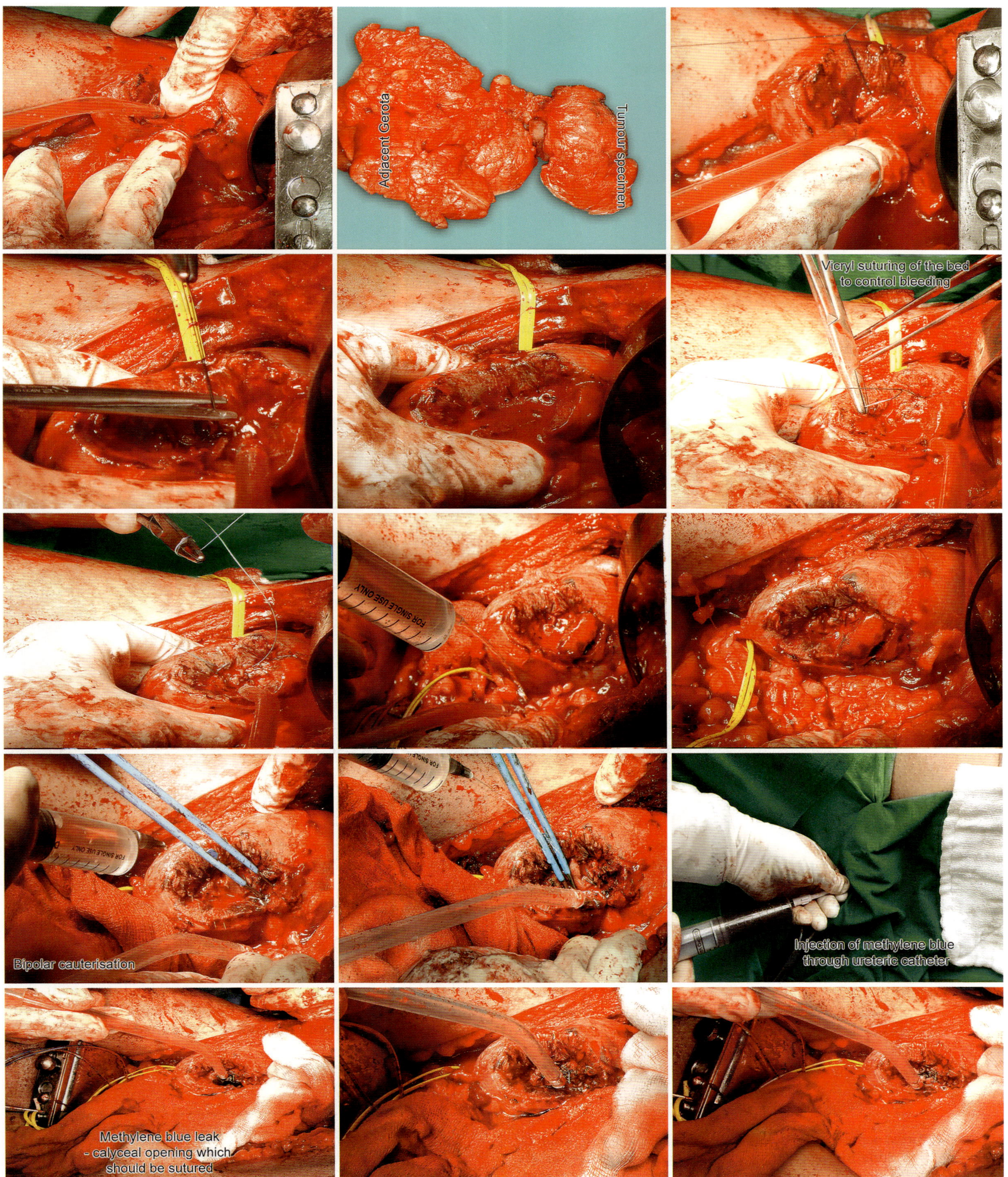
Adjacent Gerota
Tumour specimen
Vicryl suturing of the bed to control bleeding
Bipolar cauterisation
Injection of methylene blue through ureteric catheter
Methylene blue leak - calyceal opening which should be sutured

Figs. 28-52(2)

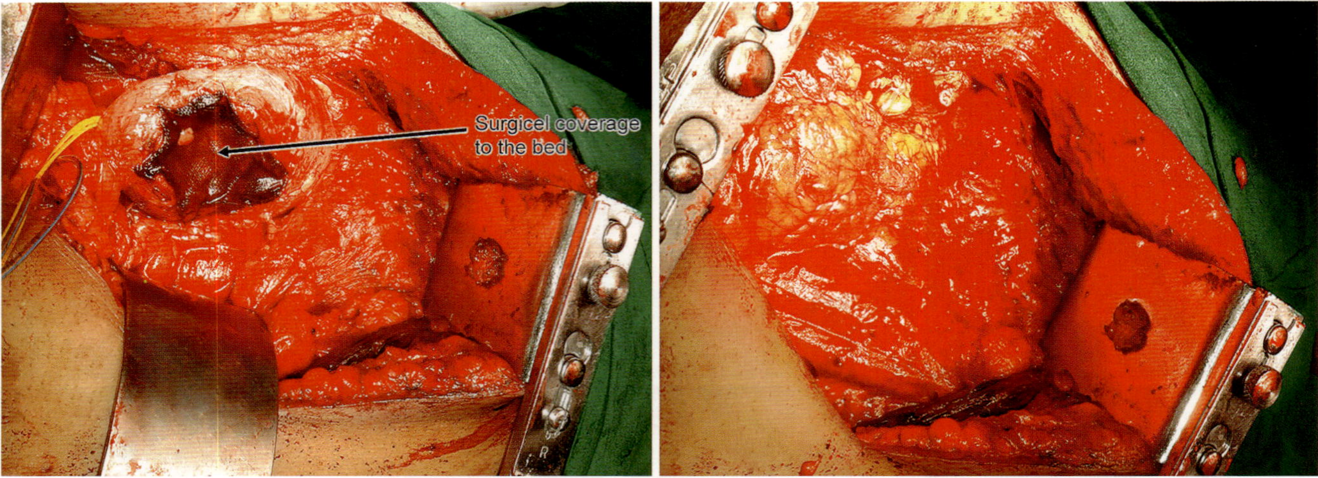

Figs. 28-52(3)

Figs. 28-52(1 to 3): Nephron sparing nephrectomy in a different patient with vascular control using a bull dog clamp.

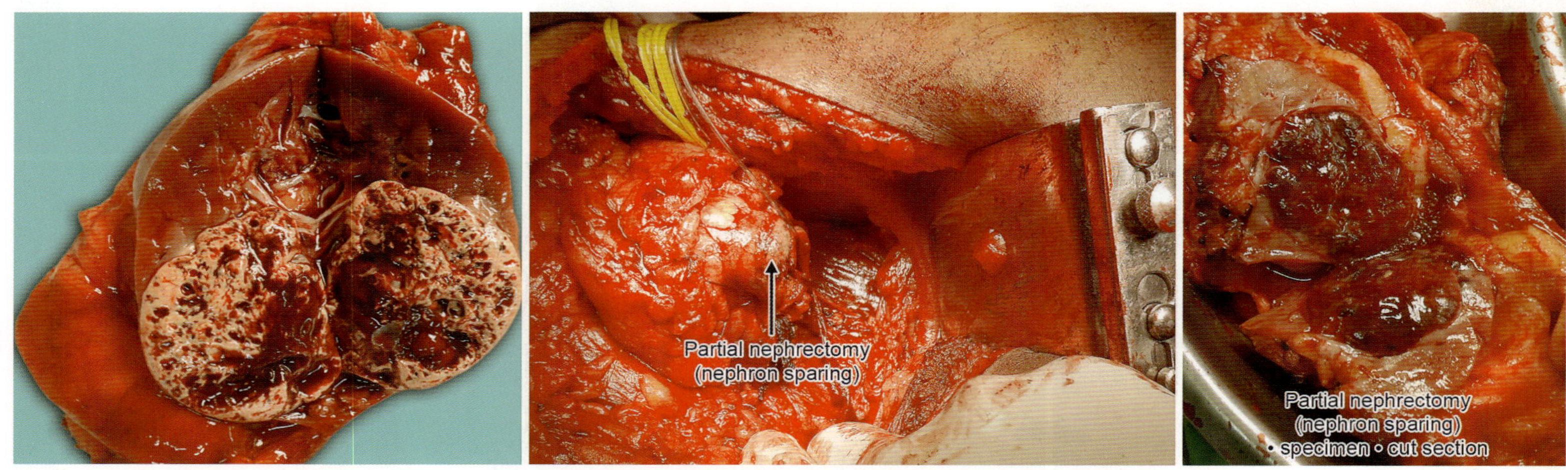

Figs. 28-53: Nephron sparing nephrectomy—resected specimen.

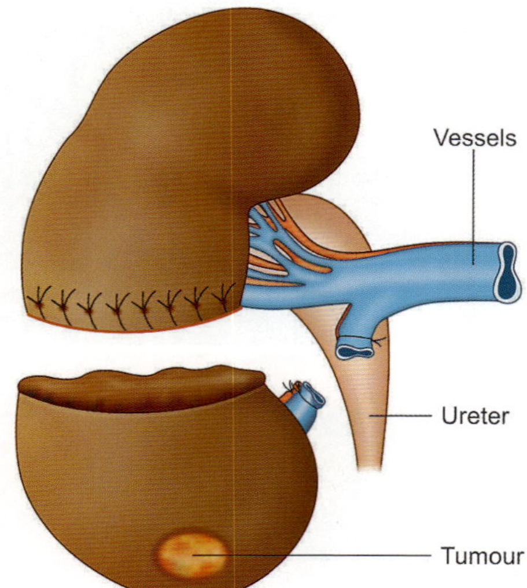

Fig. 28-54: Partial nephrectomy. Procedure is done through loin posterior approach. It is done for lower pole tumour. Segmental/polar vessels are ligated and kidney is divided; surface is sutured; surgicel is placed; J stent should be placed; wound is closed with a tube drain.

TREATMENT OF POLYCYSTIC DISEASE OF KIDNEY

Initially wait and watch policy. If one of the cysts overdistends causing pain, haemorrhage, infection, then surgical intervention is required. *Rovsing operation:* The kidney is exposed. The cyst is opened. The fluid is evacuated. The cut edge is marsupialised. Presently US-guided aspiration is done as a simpler approach. Laparoscopic/retroperitoneoscopic aspiration/de-roofing of the renal cyst is also commonly done. Once renal failure sets in, then initial haemodialysis followed by bilateral nephrectomy, is done and later renal transplantation should be planned for.

TREATMENT OF SOLITARY RENAL CYST

Kidney is exposed. The cyst is aspirated and a portion of the cyst wall is removed (*Kirwin's operation*) and cavity is filled with perinephric fat. Occasionally if the cyst is in one of the pole, partial nephrectomy is done. Laparoscopic approach is ideal.

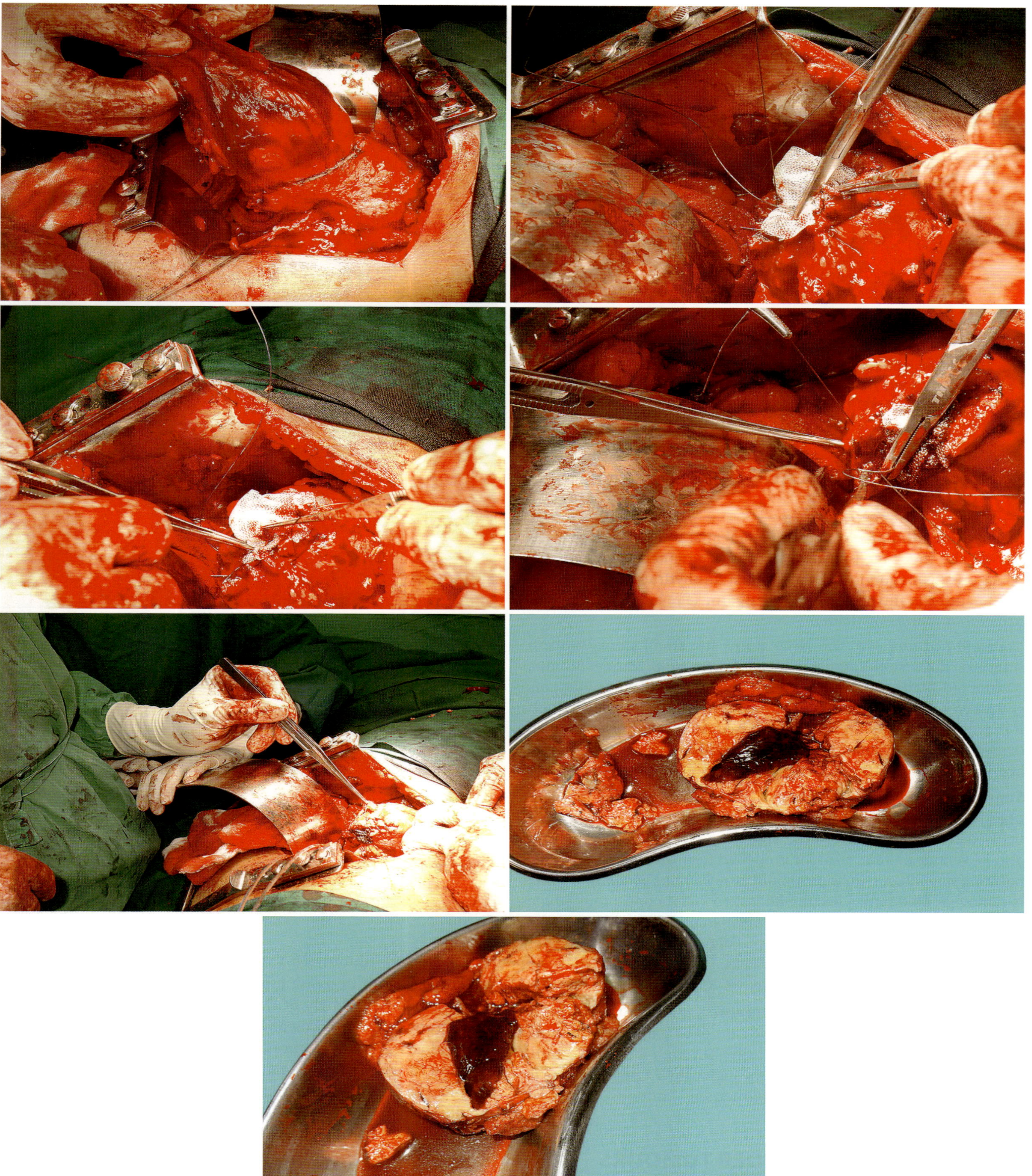

Fig. 28-55: Partial nephrectomy done for polar renal cell carcinoma (RCC).

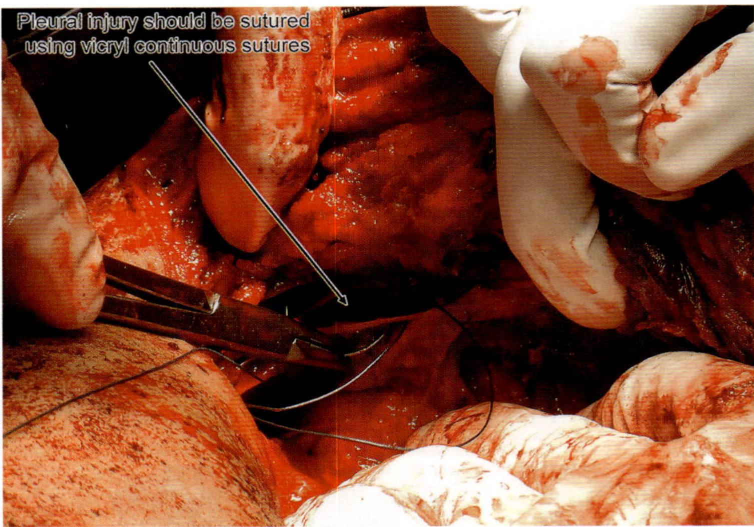

Fig. 28-56: Pleural injury can occur while approaching kidney. It should be sutured with vicryl continuous sutures. Anaesthetist should inflate the lung fully while taking the last bite from the pleura to inflate the lung properly.

TREATMENT OF BLADDER STONE (FIG. 28-57)

Cystoscopic litholapaxy: Under general anaesthesia, cystoscope is passed and the stone is visualised. It is fragmented by pneumatic, laser, electromagnetic waves or mechanohydraulic lithotripsy. The bladder is flushed using an irrigator (Freyer's evacuator or irrigator or Ellik's evacuator).

Contraindications are: Too large stone; too small stone, too soft stone, too many stones, stone in bladder diverticula, bladder tumour, contracted bladder, patient's age below 10 years. When patients general condition is poor, as the procedure takes a longer duration it is avoided and open removal is advised. However presently most of the stones can be removed through cystoscopy except very large and hard stone **(Fig. 28-58)**.

Suprapubic open cystolithotomy: Through Pfannenstiel incision, bladder is approached extraperitoneally. Bladder is identified by its detrusor muscle pattern, which has criss-cross pattern and also its venous pattern. Bladder is opened near the fundus vertically between stay sutures; incision should avoid venous plexus and stone is removed. Bladder is closed with 2-zero vicryl continuous single layer or two layers sutures. Often SPC is added using Malecot's/Foley's catheter but is not mandatory. Foley's catheter is passed per urethera which is removed after 3 weeks. Wound is closed in layers with a drain in retropubic space **(Figs. 28-59 to 28-62)**.

Suprapubic percutaneous litholapaxy: This procedure is becoming popular. When cystoscope cannot be passed per urethra, bladder is approached suprapubically. Through a needle, guide wire and dilators, a track is created through which a nephroscope is passed to remove the stone after fragmenting. The cause is treated **(Fig. 28-63)**.

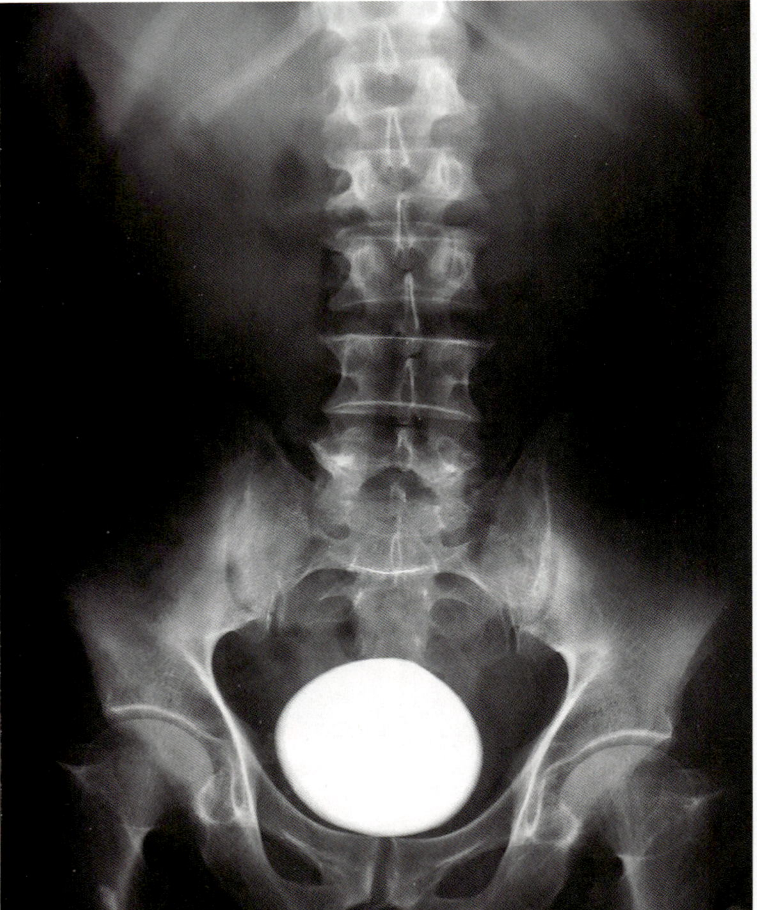

Fig. 28-57: X-ray showing bladder stone.

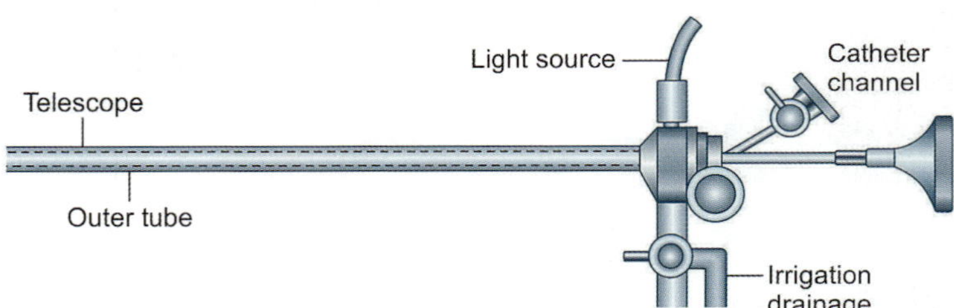

Fig. 28-58: Doing cystoscope as diagnosis and to remove bladder stone by fragmentation.

TREATMENT OF BLADDER TUMOURS

Non-invasive Tumour

Endoscopic resection of tumour is ideal. *Intravesical chemotherapy* using BCG (Dose: 120 mg in 150 mL of normal saline weekly for six weeks), mitomycin C, epirubicin, adriamycin, thiotepa, methotrexate can be given especially for carcinoma *in situ*. BCG is very useful. Very rarely *BCG provocation* can occur. Fever, joint pain, granulomatous prostatitis, sinus formation, disseminated tuberculosis are the features. Dysuria, frequency and urinary irritation can occur. BCG is *live attenuated vaccine*; its advertent IV entry can be *life threatening* and so if there is haematuria its infusion should be postponed. Mitomycin C causes skin desquamation and rash. *Systemic chemotherapy:* Using cisplatin, 5-FU, adriamycin, mitomycin.

Helmstein balloon degeneration for large papillary tumour. Balloon is passed into the bladder and inflated so as to cause pressure necrosis of the summit of the tumour. Later remaining part of the tumour can be resected easily through cystoscopy.

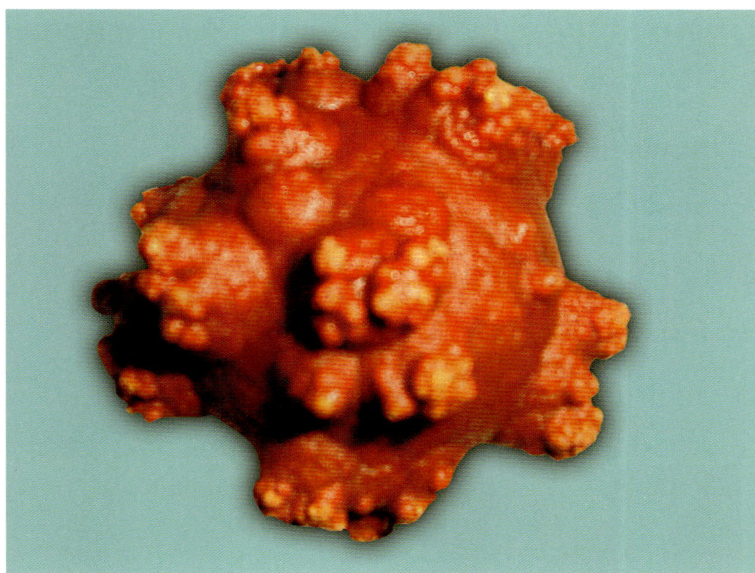

Fig. 28-59: Large oxalate stone removed from the urinary bladder.

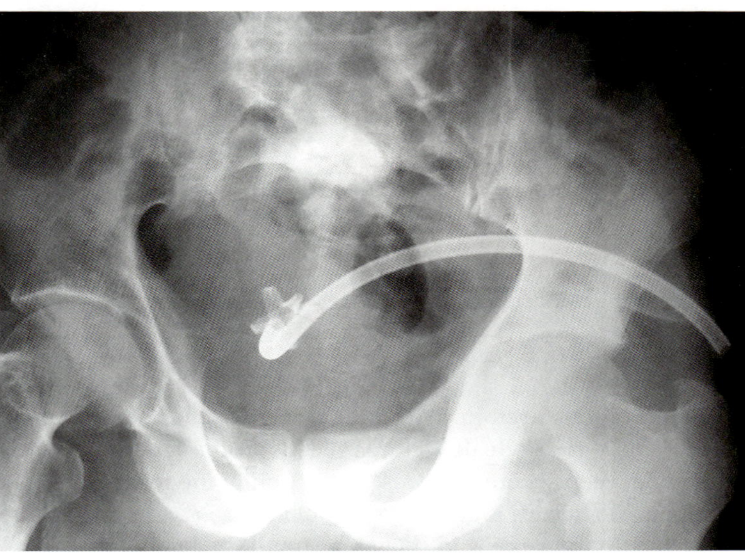

Fig. 28-60: X-ray showing SPC with Malecot catheter.

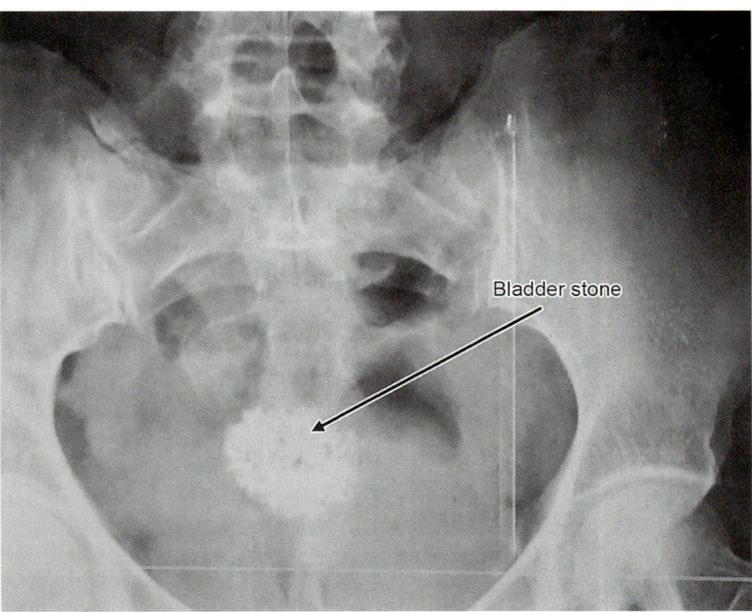

Fig. 28-61: X-ray showing bladder stone.

Invasive Bladder Tumour

Curative interstitial radiotherapy using implantation of radioactive gold grains (Au 198) (half life is two and half days), or radioactive tantalum wires (Ta 182) (half life is 4 months).

Radical deep external beam radiotherapy (45 Gy) using cobalt 60 is useful, as bladder is retained normal act of micturition and potency can be maintained. Complication is that it may eventually lead to formation of thimble bladder **(Fig. 28-64)**.

Surgery

Indications for surgery: Multiple bladder tumours, sessile tumours, recurrent tumours, poorly differentiated tumours, *in situ* carcinomas, squamous cell carcinoma, adenocarcinomas.

Partial cystectomy done when tumour is confined to fundus of the bladder and is single, with a margin of clearance of 2.5 cm. External beam RT and chemotherapy should be given. Partial cystectomy can be done through laparoscopy easily. Through cystoscopic guidance and laparoscopy tumour margin is marked on the bladder surface; resection is done through the laparoscopy; bladder wall is sutured by intracorporeal continuous vicryl sutures. Position and port sites are almost similar to laparoscopic hysterectomy. Partial cystectomy is also done often along with sigmoid resection, ileal resection or with hysterectomy whenever disease processes like diverticulitis, Crohn's disease or malignancy invades the bladder partially. Along with the resection of the primary tumour and organ, disc of urinary bladder attached to the colon or ileum is removed; primary suturing of the bladder wall is done using 2-zero vicryl sutures **(Fig. 28-65)**.

Radical cystectomy: CT scan is a must before doing radical cystectomy to see the pelvis and lymph node status. Here urinary bladder, urethra, paravesical tissues, lymph nodes (pelvic) are removed. In females hysterectomy with removal of part of the vagina is done. After surgery urinary diversion is done either by doing continent ileal conduit, or ureterosigmoidostomy or by creating rectal urinary pouch **(Fig. 28-66)**.

Intravesical chemotherapy by BCG, mitomycin C, adriamycin and interferons are used later.

Systemic chemotherapy by cisplatin, adriamycin, mitomycin, vinblastine—adjuvant therapy. Neoadjuvant cisplatin based chemotherapy is beneficial improving survival by 7%. MVAC regime is methotrexate; vinblastine; adriamycin and cisplatin.

Prognosis

Depends on type, differentiation, location, stage, invasion, number, lymph node status, pelvis involvement and response to treatment. TCC alone—85%; TCC with SCC or adenocarcinoma—6%; SCC/adenocarcinoma alone—3%; spindle cell carcinoma— 2%.

RADICAL CYSTECTOMY

It is done as a curative surgery for bladder carcinoma. Staging, cystoscopic biopsy, preliminary preparation for anaesthesia should be done.

Procedure is done under general anaesthesia in supine head down position. Head down (reverse Trendelenburg) position helps in keeping the bowel in the proximal abdomen away from the surgical field **(Fig. 28-67)**.

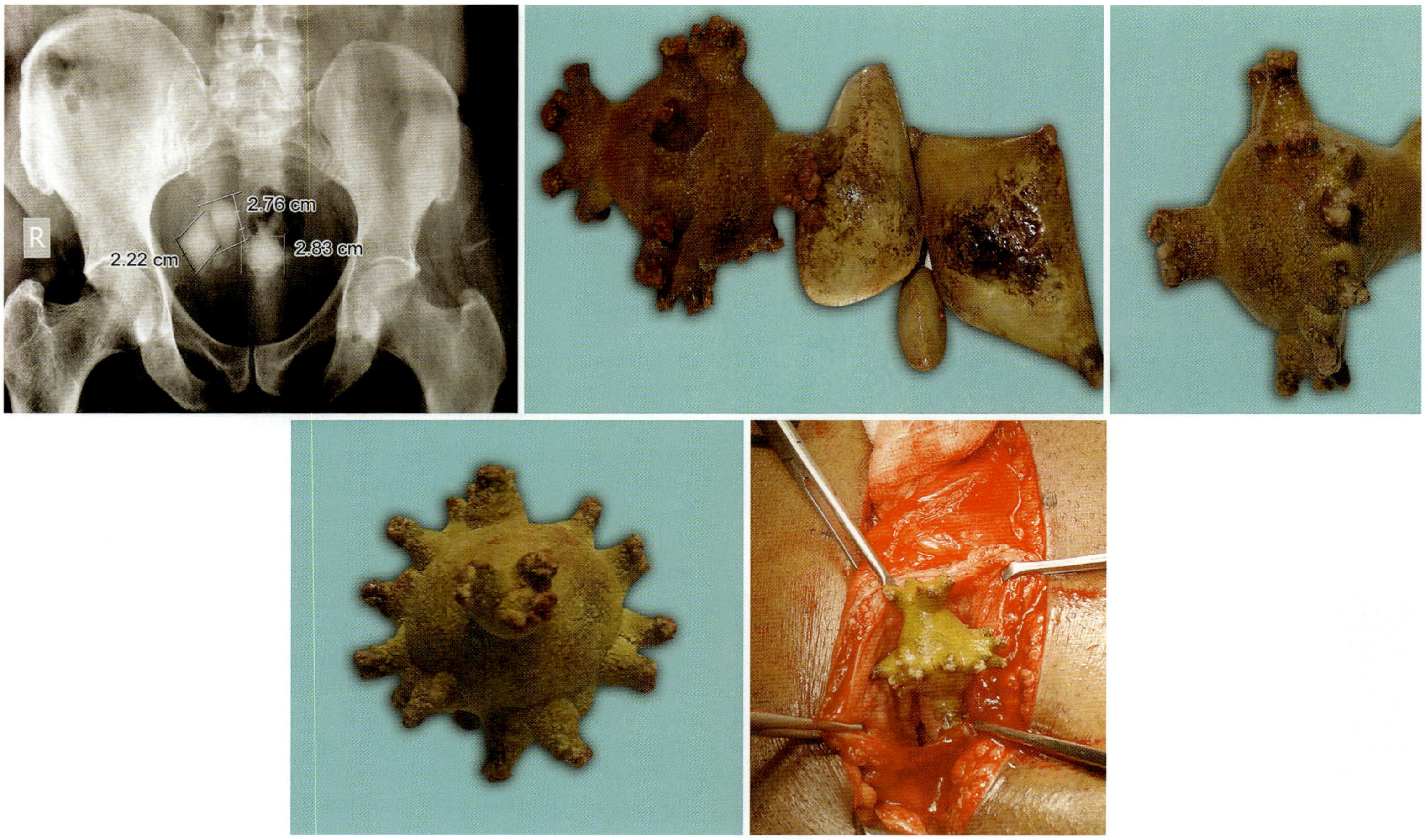

Fig. 28-62: Suprapubic cystolithotomy—oxalate stone in the bladder with X-ray look.

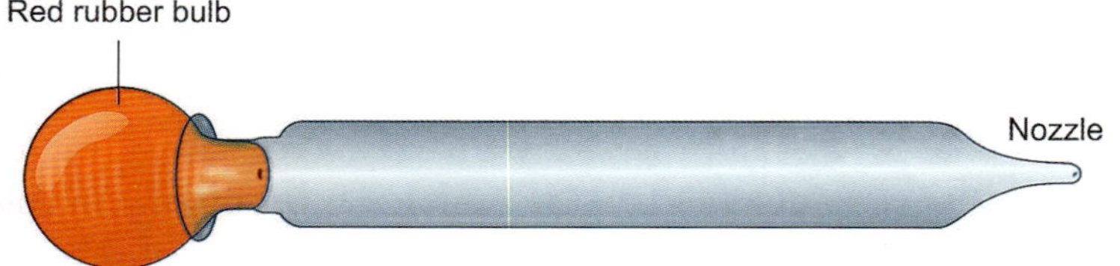

Fig. 28-63: Asepto syringe used for bladder wash in patients with urinary catheter which has been blocked; or when haematuria is noticed in the catheter. It is also used to fill the bladder with saline.

Technique

Lengthy midline incision is placed to open the abdomen. Incision extended above the umbilicus should be towards left side of the umbilicus. Abdomen is explored for liver, nodes and metastases in other areas. Median umbilical ligament is divided at umbilical level; it is dissected towards the dome of the urinary bladder. Lateral bladder dissection is done; vas deferens is identified, dissected, ligated and divided. Medial umbilical ligament is similarly dissected and divided between ligatures. Superior vesical artery (vessels) is ligated and divided. Posterior dissection is done in rectovesical plane after opening the peritoneum in rectovesical pouch. Fascia of Denonvillier's is dissected downwards. Dissection is done between rectum and urinary system. Neurological bundle of Walsh can be sacrified in radical surgeries. Seminal vesicles, prostate is identified; dissection is reached towards the apex of the prostate identifying the membranous urethra. With bipolar cautery harmonic scalpel ligation, vessels are dealt. Venous plexus in the lateral aspect is divided between secure ligatures. Dissection in the retropubic area in the space of Retzius is undertaken by blunt finger and sharp scissor dissection. Many vessels in this area should be ligated otherwise troublesome bleeding can occur. Dissection is done beyond the prostate. Both ureters are divided close to the trigone; cut end pieces of ureters are sent for frozen section biopsy. Lymph nodes are cleared from common iliac artery downwards along the iliac vessels up to Cloquet (Rosenmuller) lymph node which is cleared; posteriorly nodes are cleared up to obturator nerve. Lymph nodes on both sides are cleared according to template. Iliac and obturator lymph nodes are cleared completely.

Urethra distal to prostate is transected. 24 no. French sized Foley's catheter is passed per urethra from below and is inflated, pulled with traction; it gives compression to prostatic bed to prevent bleeding and also acts as drainage.

Reconstruction is planned. It is creation of neobladder and achieve drainage either by suturing the neobladder pouch to the cut end of urethra as orthotopic drainage; or neobladder is exteriorised after ureteral reimplantation into the created pouch.

Creation of Pouch

Two types of pouches are used. One pouch is ileal W pouch with creation of continent at its summit; summit is brought out with valve mechanism created in it through the right iliac fossa. Other pouch is

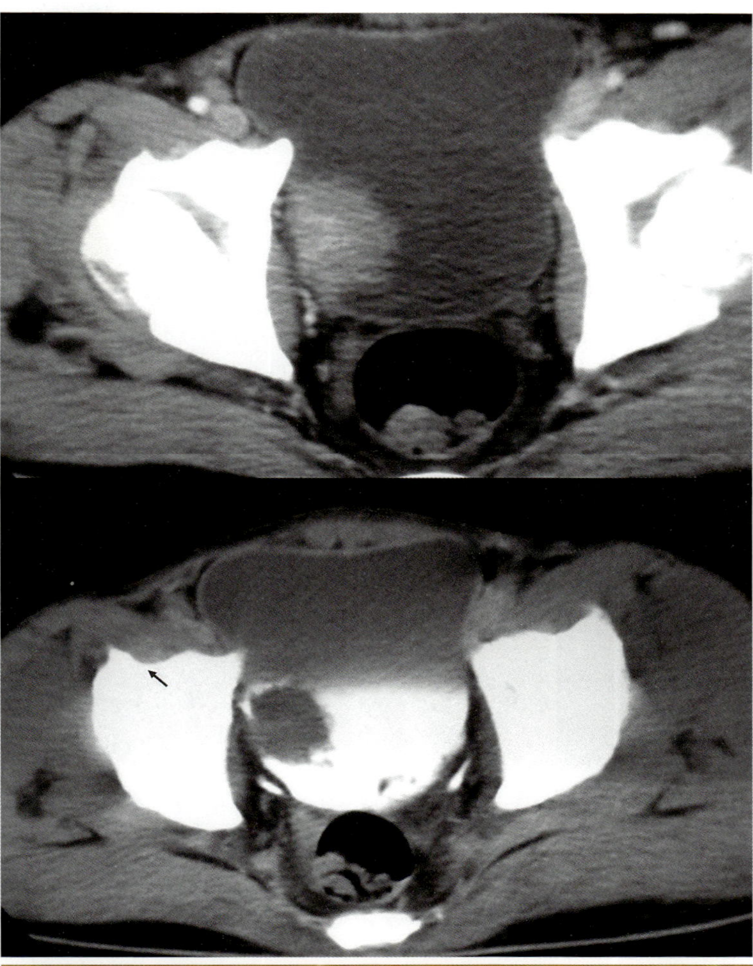

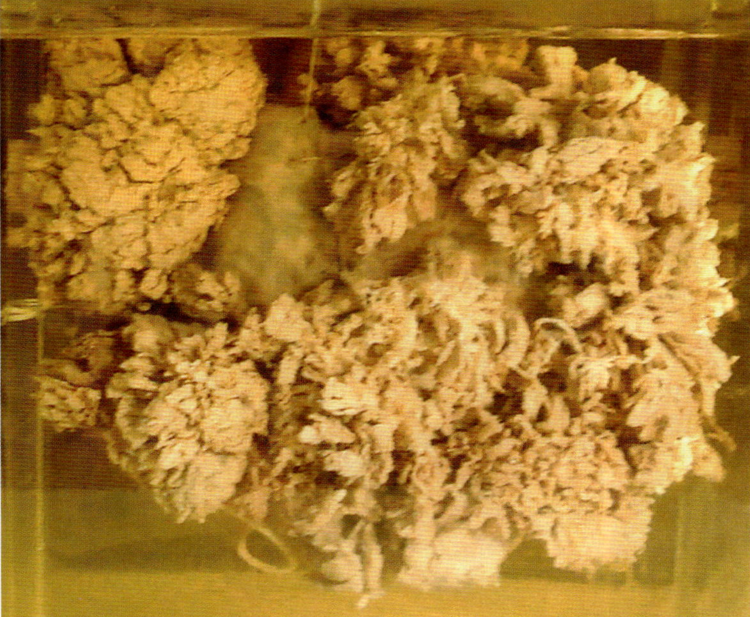

Fig. 28-64: CT picture showing bladder tumour. Specimen showing transitional cell carcinoma of bladder.

caecal and ascending colon pouch with terminal ileum as a passage with intussuscepted ileum towards the caecum as valve mechanism. Here 15 cm of terminal ileum is selected; additional further proximal 5 cm is also taken to create intussusception. Right colon is mobilised from right paracolic gutter, hepatic flexure, and right half of the transverse colon. Colonic mesentery is not ligated; right branch of the middle colic artery is ligated; left colic artery should be retained and also arcade of the terminal ileum. Ileum is transected either by stapler or with knife and cautery; right half of the transverse colon is transected; ileo transverse colon anastomosis is done. Mesenteric defect is closed. Harvested ileocolic segment is mobilised carefully towards right side without interrupting its blood supply; it is achieved by mobilising the mesentery up to the 3rd part of the duodenum. Ascending colon, part of the transverse colon in the harvested part is opened using scissor or cautery along the taenia. Ileocaecal valve is identified. Distal part of the harvested ileum is skeletonised for 5 cm which is intussuscepted towards ileocaecal valve; it is achieved by passing a long Babcock's clamp through the lumen and holding the ileal wall from inside at 5 cm from the ileocaecal junction and pulling it distally towards the caecum. Once it is intussuscepted its terminal mucosa is denuded for 2–3 cm and sutured again to prevent it retracting backwards; it functions like a valve. Foley's catheter 20 sized is passed from the cut end of the harvested ileum to confirm the patency and is placed in the caecum with inflation. Two ureteric catheters are passed through it towards caecum and kept. One of which is labeled or marked with tie to identify the side. Right side ureter is mobilised proximally for adequate length. Left side ureter is also mobilised adequately and is passed behind the mesentery from left towards right. Both ureters are reimplanted into posterior part of the caecum/ascending colon at around 1–2 cm gap. Small stab incision of 8–10 mm length is made in the right half of the caecum or proximal ascending colon; ureter is transected near its cut margin obliquely (fish mouth). Stent marked right is passed through right ureter into the pelvis. It is anastomosed to the caecal wall using interrupted 3-zero vicryl sutures with knots outside. Similarly left ureter is implanted into the caecum posteriorly on its left side. Opened ascending colon is closed horizontally to create a colonic pouch. An independent Foley's catheter is passed through the separate wound in front of the caecum to bring it as ostomy from the pouch to drain it. Length of the ileum is assessed to have adequate shortest distance from the pouch to reach right iliac fossa, the site of ostomy (stoma) which is permanent. Circular piece of the skin is excised in the spinoumbilical line in front of the rectus muscle. Either cruciate incision is made in the anterior rectus sheath or similar disc of the sheath is removed. Rectus muscle is split; peritoneum is opened; assistant will give counter pressure through a mop covered finger from inside while creating stomal opening. Care should be taken not to injure the inferior epigastric vessels. Cut ileal end of the harvested segment is brought out using a Babcock's clamp. 2 cm proximal from the cut end of the ileum seromuscular interrupted sutures are placed between the bowel and anterior rectus sheath using 3-zero vicryl. Even though it is not mandatory it is often practiced to fix the bowel to the peritoneum by interrupted vicryl sutured adjacent to stomal opening. Skin is sutured to the cut edge of the ileum; while initially taking seromuscular bites away from the cut edge then from the mucosa at the edge, then from the full thickness skin it is taken so as to create protrusion of the mucosa of stoma outwards—*Brooke's method of maturation of the urinary conduit.*

Gastrostomy may be done for feeding and aspiration purpose. Suction tube drains are placed one in the pelvis another in the right side abdomen. Abdomen is closed in layers.

Note: There are many methods of creating pouches—Mainz pouch (Ileo colic); Indiana pouch; orthotopic pouches like studer neobladder of ileum; Hautmann neobladder of ileum; Monti and spiral Monti types.)

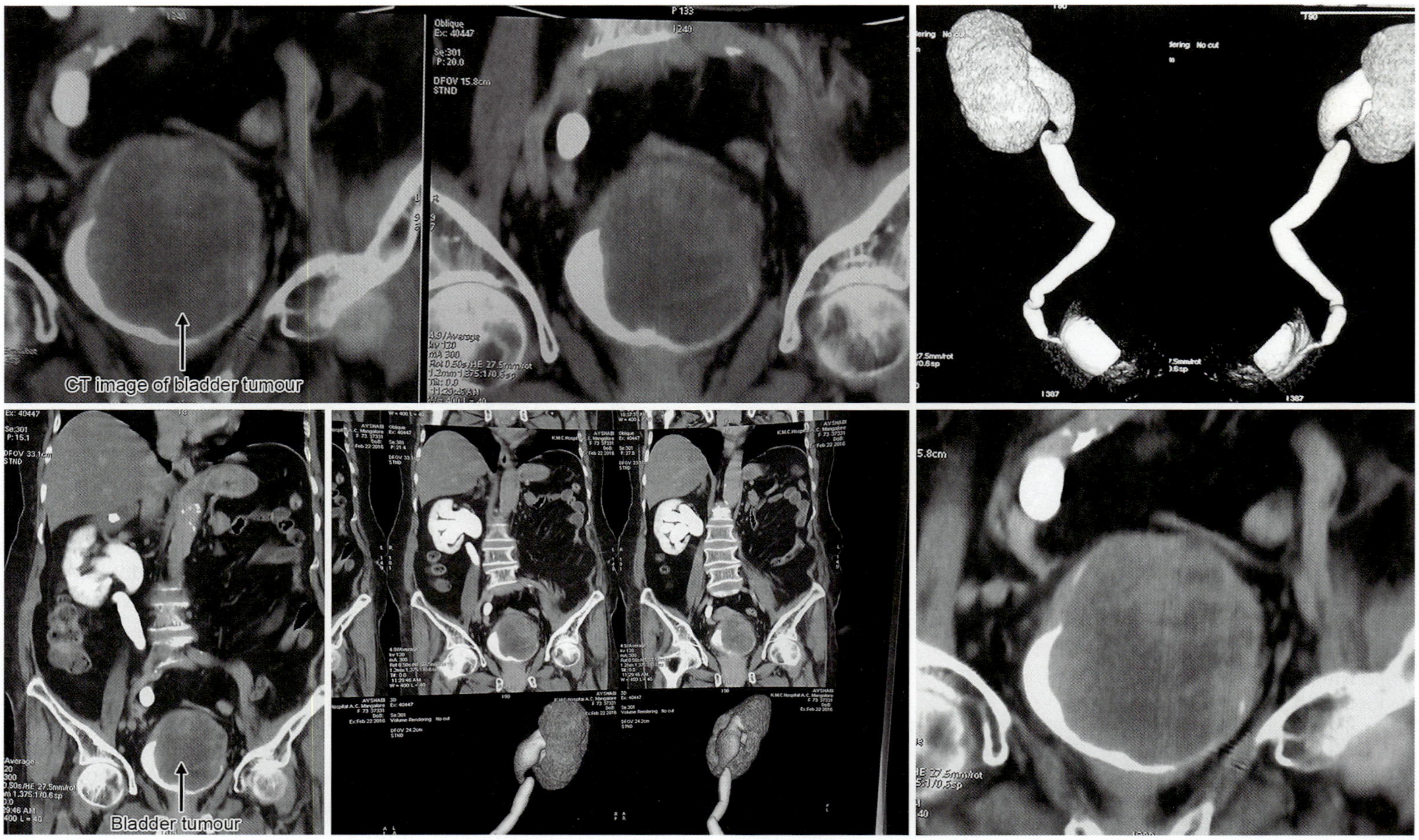

Fig. 28-65: CT images of urinary bladder tumour.

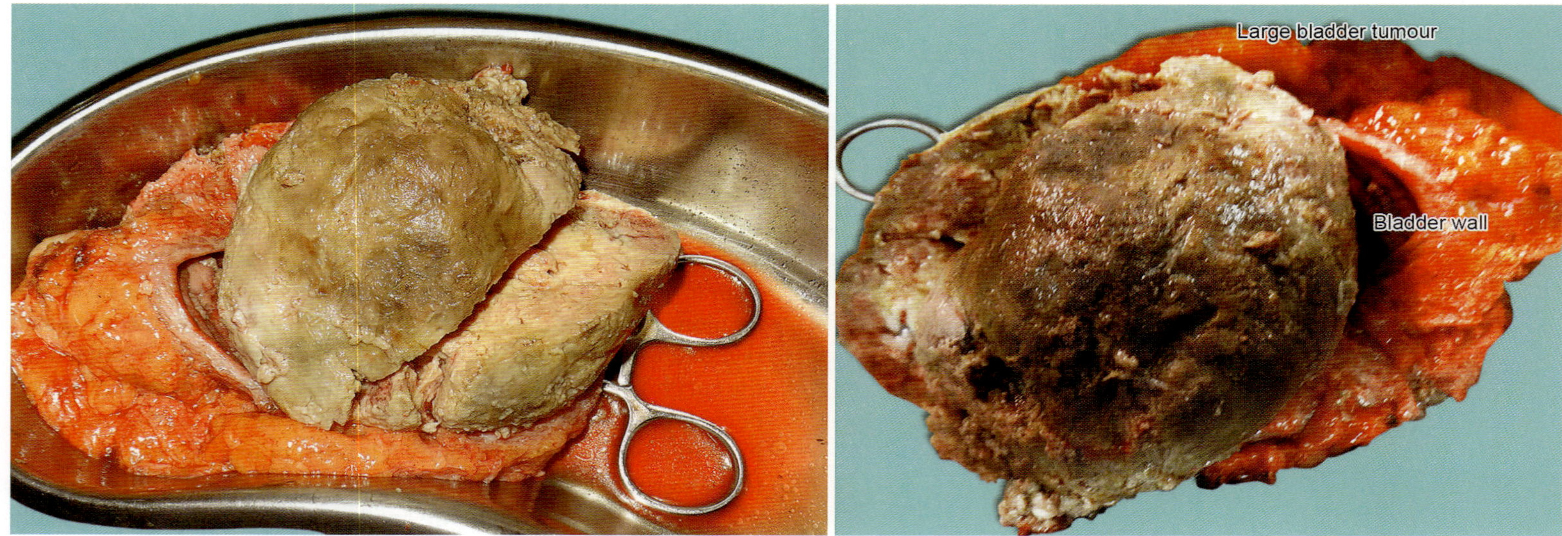

Fig. 28-66: Large bladder tumour—radical cystectomy is done.

URETEROSIGMOIDOSTOMY (HENRI CHAPUT, 1894, FRENCH SURGEON)

It is a procedure done for urinary diversion after radical cystectomy or as a permanent diversion for many other causes, e.g. bladder dystrophy. Left ureter is implanted to the sigmoid colon, right one to the upper rectum or rectosigmoid junction. Collecting system is not necessary here; but exposure of urinary tract to faecal infection is the real problem.

Different types of ureterocolic anastomosis are present. Fish like incision on the sigmoid by incising the seromuscular layer lengthier and mucosa is opened on the end of this incision to anastomose cut end of ureter on it. Coffey, Grey Turner, Nesbit, Cohen's, Cordonnier type; Leadbetter are different types. In Leadbetter (Boston, USA) type submucosal tunneling is done to prevent reflux.

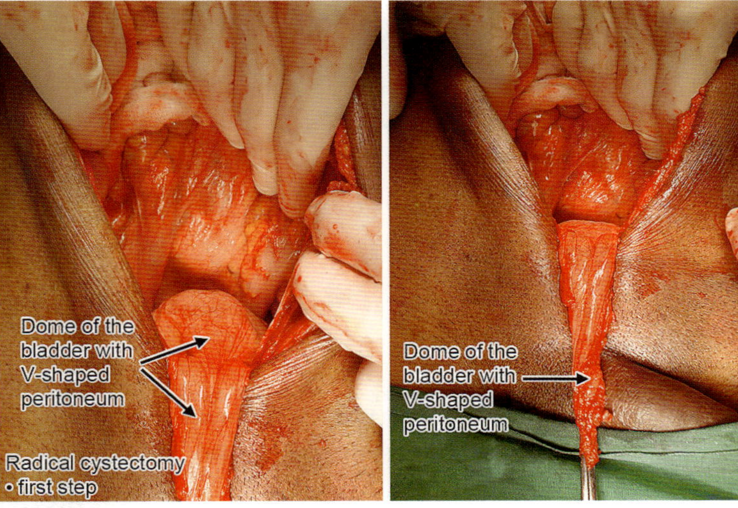

Fig. 28-67: Radical cystectomy—initial step. Lower midline incision is made; while opening the peritoneum, V-shaped peritoneum is included to clear the urachus from umbilical level towards the dome of the bladder. Foley's catheter should be in place in the urinary bladder. Ureter is identified and dissected from its insertion into the bladder proximally up to upper third for adequate tension free length. Vas deferens is identified ligated where it comes out of the internal ring towards the bladder; further dissection is done outer to the vas deferens so that it is included in the specimen along with seminal vesicles below. Medial umbilical ligament is ligated and divided; dissection is deepened into the pelvis; harmonic scalpel is used for in depth tissue dissection. Lateral ligament is dissected and cut using harmonic scalpel or after placing strong ligatures. Posterior dissection is done by separating the tissues from the rectum; rectum should not be injured; digital examination of the rectum may be done if doubt arises to confirm that rectum is safe. Anterior dissection is done distal to the prostate. Strong ligature using cutting needle is passed in front beyond the prostate to include the vessels in puboprostatic ligament which is secured by taking bite from the pubic bone in front; tissue is cut in between ligatures. Urethra distal to the prostate is opened to identify the Foley's catheter. Catheter is cut and further bipolar or harmonic dissection facilitates complete removal of the bladder. Iliac, obturator and Cloquet nodes are cleared on both sides. Haemostasis is achieved. Foley's catheter is passed per urethrally into the pelvis to keep it as a drain.

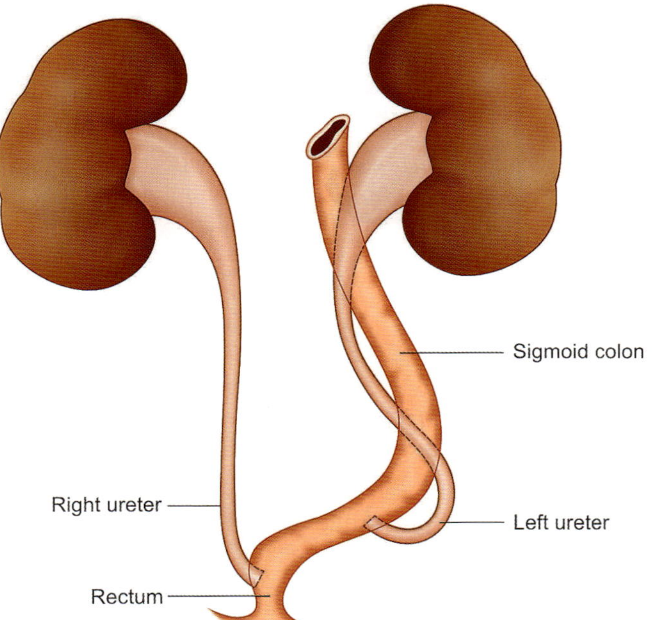

Fig. 28-68: Ureterosigmoidostomy.

Complications

Because the pressure in sigmoid colon is more, it causes *pyelonephritis* and recurrent upper urinary tract infection. due to diarrhoea *hypokalaemia occurs*. Because of reabsorption of chloride, *hyperchloraemic acidosis* occurs. *Treatment of complications*—IV sodium bicarbonate (8.4%) with slow IV potassium; IV antibiotics; Patient is advised to take potassium citrate and sodium bicarbonate and to avoid salt; in many cases conversion to *ileal conduit* may be required.

Stricture formation is common in ureterosigmoidostomy. Mucosa to mucosa anastomosis may prevent this **(Fig. 28-68)**

URINARY DIVERSION

It is diversion of urine temporarily or permanently, proximal to the site of obstruction. Temporary type is done in benign conditions and distal obstructions, to promote healing. Permanent type is done in advanced malignancies which block the urine flow distally, after radical cystectomy, and after radiotherapy with frozen pelvis, etc. **(Figs. 28-69 and 28-70)**.

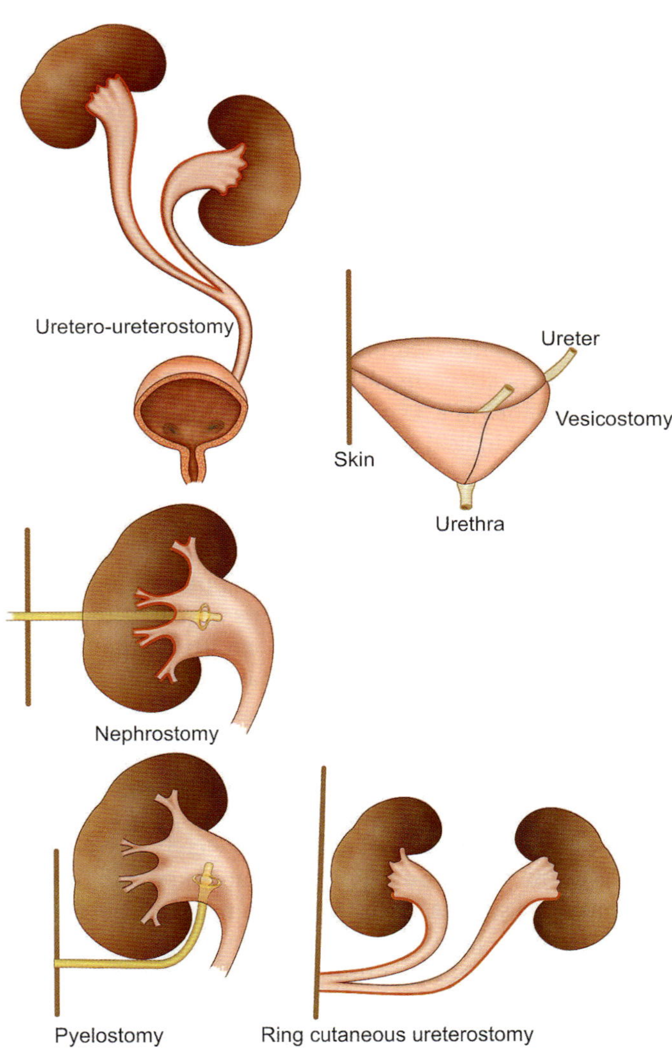

Fig. 28-69: Types of urinary diversions.

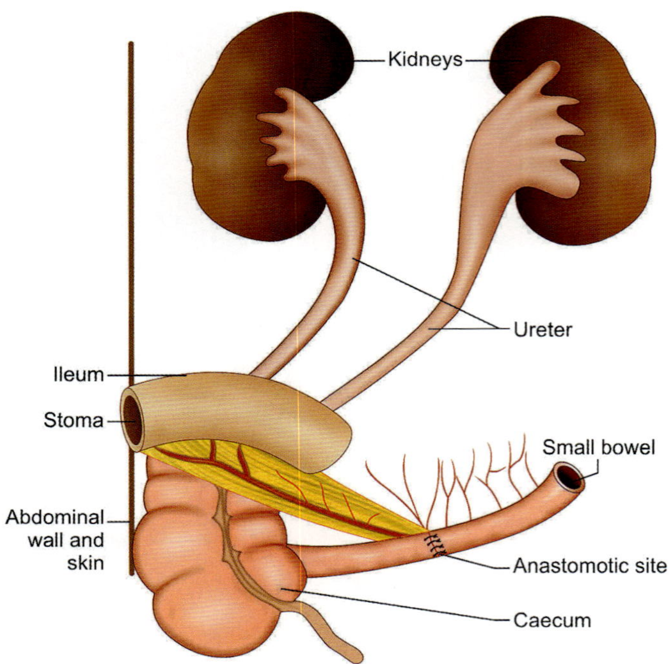

Fig. 28-70: Ileal conduit as urinary diversion.

Temporary Diversions

Suprapubic cystostomy (SPC); vesicostomy in children in ectopiae vesicae, epispadias, urethral anomalies; urethrostomies; nephrostomies in pyonephrosis and high obstructive uropathies; pyelostomies are other procedures; ureteral J stent is a method of internal temporary diversion which is kept maximum for 3 months.

Permanent Diversions

External Diversions

Non-continent ileal conduit

Here 20 cm of vascularised distal ileum (30 cm from IC valve) is prepared. Ureters are re-implanted over the ileum. Other end of ileum is brought out as a 3 cm stoma in right iliac fossa. Patient has to wear a bag over it. Ileal pouch can be created as a reservoir – J, S, W, etc.

Continent ileal conduit

It is similar conduit with creation of specialised valve (Koch's continent) within, using ileal mucosa or appendix. Patient has to empty the conduit by passing self catheters once in 6 hours. Instead of appendix, intussusception of distal 5 cm ileum into the caecum across the ileocaecal valve and denudation and suturing of the mucosa can create a continent conduit.

Mitrofanoff continent stoma of appendix

It is done in children with spina bifida with neurogenic bladder. Mesentery of appendix is retained (undisturbed). It is dissected at its base from caecum which closed with 2-zero vicryl. Base is mobilised without disturbing its blood supply and implanted into the bladder using 3-zero vicryl sutures. Tip is transected to get the needed lumen; warm saline wash is given into the lumen gently. Transected opened lumen is brought out through a stab incision into the skin in right iliac fossa and its mucosa (full thickness appendix wall) is sutured to skin to create a stoma; often local skin flaps are used to support the appendix and to achieve continence. Urine is drained

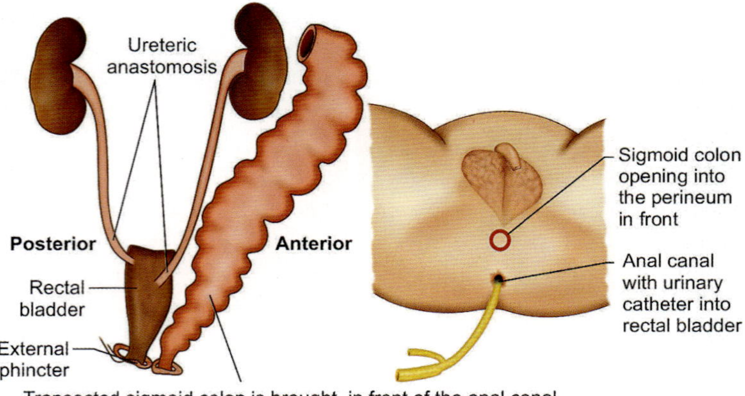

Fig. 28-71: Lowsley's rectal bladder.

from the urinary bladder by catheterisation across the appendix stoma. It is a continent cystostomy using pedicled appendix.

Lowsley's (urologist, New York) rectal bladder

Left side colon is mobilsed fully; rectosigmoid junction is transected; rectal stump is closed either hand sewn or with stapler. Distal cut end of the sigmoid is brought down through the perineum in front of the rectum and anal canal to anastomose to incised skin in front of the original anal canal. This new anal canal created acts as defecating organ. Rectal bladder behind acts as a urinary reservoir and normal anal canal acts as urination device. It is kept catheterised for few weeks **(Fig. 28-71)**.

Cutaneous ureterostomy/cutaneous ring ureterostomy are other options.

Internal Diversions

Ureterosigmoidostomy (Leadbetter-Palitano); rectal bladder creation; ileocystoplasty; caecocystoplasty/sigmoidocystoplasty; creation of neobladder (orthotopic) using ileum/caecum/sigmoid colon which is sutured to urethra.

Types of Urinary Diversions

Nephrostomy; pyelostomy; cutaneous ureterostomy; cutaneous ring ureterostomy; suprapubic cystostomy; vesicostomy in children; urethrostomy; ureterosigmoidostomy; rectal bladder; urinary ileal conduit (Koch's conduit).

Complications of Diversions

Urine leak, faecal leak, intestinal obstruction, sepsis; hyperchloraemic hypokalaemic metabolic acidosis; pyelonephritis; osteomalacia, growth retardation; calculi formation—4%; Continent failure, blockage of diversion stoma (stenosis); reflux of urine; vitamin B_{12} and folate deficiency due to absence of ileum; complications of stoma; renal failure; metaplasia and adenocarcinoma especially at uretero- sigmoidostomy junction.

URETERIC REIMPLANTATION

Ureter may often need to be reimplanted into the urinary bladder. Reimplantation is needed in stricture of distal ureter, ureteral tuberculosis, trauma to ureter which may be iatrogenic.

Usually oblique Gibson's loin incision extending to suprapubic area is ideal; Pfannenstiel incision also can be used.

Ureter is fully mobilised keeping its blood supply intact. Diseased part is excised. Urinary bladder is mobilised fully both in front, behind, and on opposite side to get adequate tension free length for anastomosis. Cut distal end is reimplanted into the urinary bladder. Ureter can be reimplanted directly or through tunneling depending on need and surgeons' choice. Mucosa to mucosal anastomosis is better.

Psoas hitch: Mobilised urinary bladder is fixed to psoas major muscle on its medial side adjacent to genitofemoral nerve without injuring it; 2-zero interrupted vicryl sutures are placed between muscular layer of bladder and psoas major muscle. Usually, three sutures are placed; this psoas hitch prevents urinary bladder getting retracted back into the pelvis and so keeps ureteric anastomosis tension free.

Boari flap: If psoas hitch seems inadequate to achieve tension free anastomosis, then superolateral part of the urinary bladder is elevated after incision as flap; it is tubularised to achieve extra needed length. Cut end of the ureter is sutured into that. This procedure is usually sufficient.

Isolated segmental ileal interposition is done whenever entire length of the ureter is lost. Isolated pedicled 30 cm ileum is harvested; bowel continuity is maintained by doing bowel anastomosis. Ileal harvested segment is washed thoroughly using warm normal saline. Proximal end is closed; just distal to this closed proximal end over the antimesenteric border 8–10 mm sized opening is made in the bowel; renal pelvis or proximal ureter is anastomosed to this ileal segment using 4–6 interrupted 3-zero vicryl sutures with knots placed on outside. Distal part of the isolated segment is sutured to the bladder using 2-zero vicryl as interrupted end to end anastomosis. Knots should be outside the lumen. Nephrostomy, J stent, cystostomy, nasogastric tube, peritoneal cavity tube drain and urinary catheterisation are also needed while finishing the surgery.

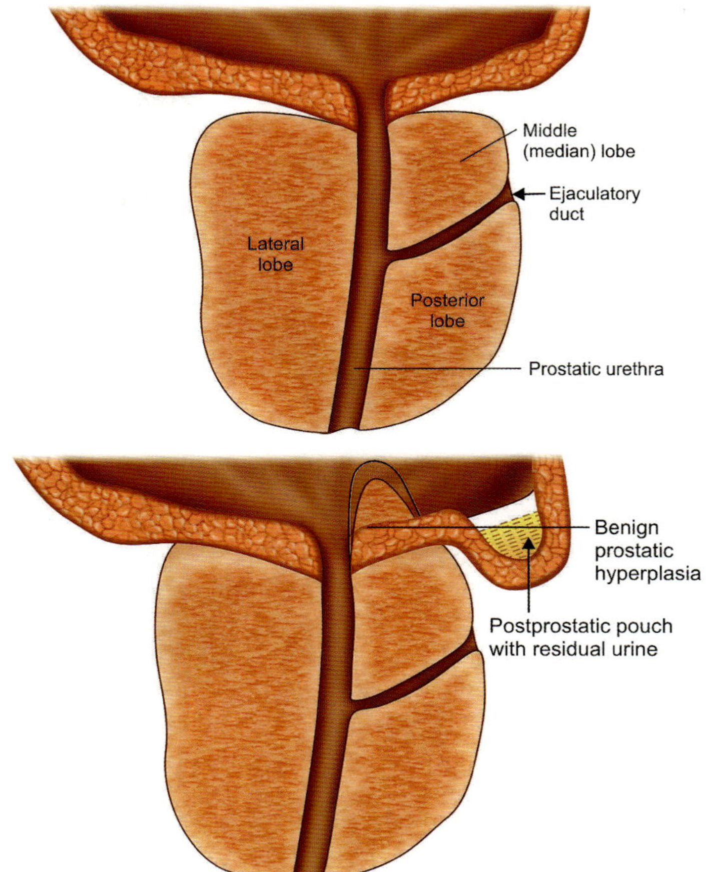

Fig. 28-72: Diagram showing normal prostate pattern and post-prostatic pouch with residual urine.

MANAGEMENT OF BENIGN PROSTATIC HYPERPLASIA (BPH)

Patient with *acute retention* of urine requires *urethral catheterisation*. If urethral catheterisation fails, then *suprapubic cystostomy (SPC)* is done. Trocar SPC is available which is technically easier to do and minimally invasive; but bladder should be full and is confirmed clinically by dullness in suprapubic region and by ultrasound. If bladder is not full chances of intraabdominal injury is high. If patient presents with *uraemia*, then urethral catheterisation is a must. That allows the kidney to function adequately and further obstructive damage is prevented. Serum electrolytes should be corrected properly in these patients **(Fig. 28-72)**.

Indications for Surgery

Prostatism (frequency, dysuria, urgency); acute retention of urine; chronic retention of urine with residual urine more than 200 mL; complications like hydroureter, hydronephrosis, stone formation, recurrent infection, bladder changes; haematuria.

Surgeries

Transurethral Resection of Prostate (TURP)

Using cystoscope with fluid like glycine irrigating continuously, enlarged prostate is identified and resected using a loop with a hand control. Resection is done using high frequency diathermy current, above the level of verumontanum. After surgery, continuous bladder irrigation using normal saline is done using three way Foley's catheter. Antibiotics should be given. Catheter is removed in 72 hours. ***Postoperative complications are:*** Water intoxication with congestive cardiac failure—TURP syndrome; hyponatraemia; haemorrhage; infection; incontinence; perforation of the bladder or prostatic capsule; stricture urethra; retrograde ejaculation and impotence; recurrence **(Figs. 28-73 and 28-74)**.

Transurethral resection of prostate

- No suprapubic incision
- Most common and popular method
- Done using resectoscope
- Recurrence may occur in large prostate
- TURP syndrome can develop
- Continuous postoperative irrigation using glycine solution is needed for 72 hours
- Faster recovery and early discharge is possible.

Freyer's Suprapubic Transvesical Prostatectomy

Before TURP, it was a popular and was the procedure of choice for enlarged prostate. Under spinal anaesthesia, through Pfannenstiel incision, rectus sheath is opened horizontally; recti are split; peritoneum is not opened; it is pushed upwards beyond the dome of the bladder. Urinary bladder is identified by its muscle pattern and lateral vesical venous plexus. Bladder is confirmed by aspirating urine. Stay sutures are placed one at the dome another at the lower part of the bladder. Urinary bladder is opened vertically; urine is sucked out. Deaver retractor is placed on the dome of the bladder. Prostate is felt by index finger. With finger dissection anterior plane

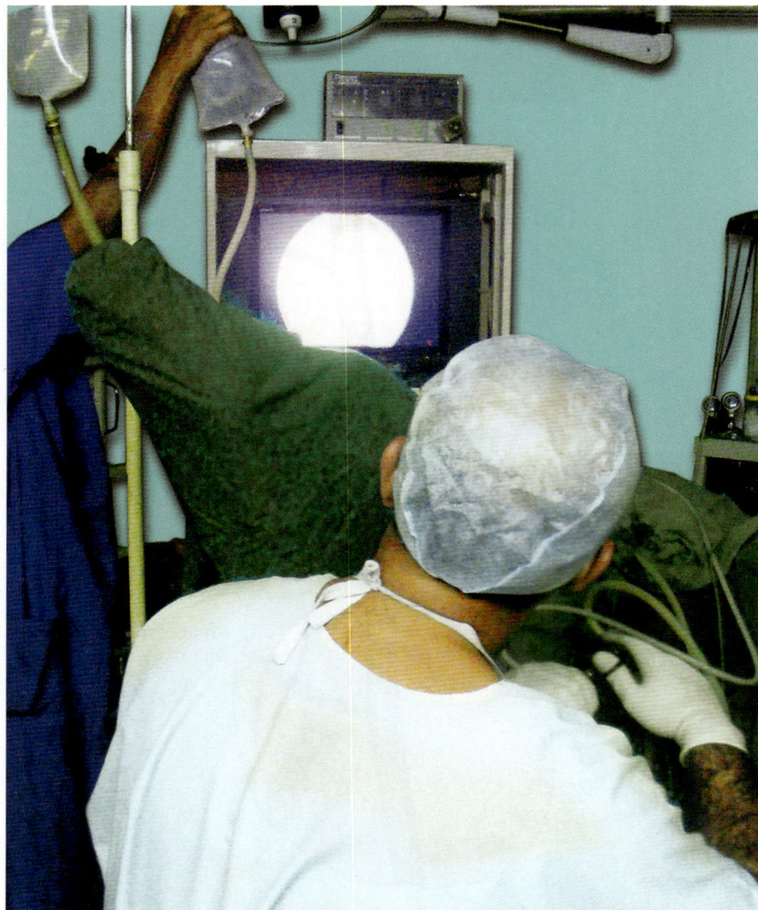

Fig. 28-73: TURP is done using cystoscope and resectoscope.

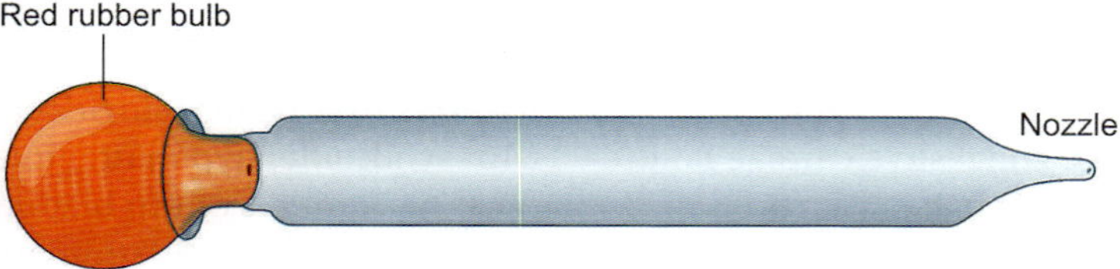

Fig. 28-74: Asepto syringe for bladder irrigation.

is created by opening the prostatic urethra anteriorly. Lateral lobes and median lobe are removed by finger dissection. Posterior lobe is not removed. Warm pack is kept on the prostate bed to control bleeding. Vicryl sutures are placed on either sides of the raw area to control bleeding. Often anterior and posterior wedge at the vesicourethral junction need to be excised to prevent later urinary obstruction. 24–30 F 3-way Foley's catheter is passed from urethra into the bladder; balloon is inflated adequately; traction is given to the catheter so that balloon creates tamponade and control of the haemorrhage. Malecot's catheter is placed through the bladder at a separate stab incision which is brought out through a separate stab wound at the abdominal wall. Bladder wall is closed using 2-zero vicryl sutures. Another tube drain is placed in the Retzius space. Recti are sutured; rectus sheath is closed; skin is closed. Complications are haemorrhage, infection, stricture urethra, incontinence, impotence, bladder neck contracture **(Figs. 28-75 and 28-76)**.

Millin's Retropubic Prostatectomy

Here urinary bladder is not opened; retropubic space is dissected to identify the prostate which is enucleated. Urethra is sutured; drain is placed and wound is closed. 3-way Foley's catheter should be placed in the bladder across the urethra. It is done without opening the bladder. Cystoscopy should be done before doing retropubic prostatectomy as bladder is not opened during surgery. Pfannenstiel extraperitoneal approach is used under spinal anaesthesia. Self-retaining retractor is placed. Supine head down position is used. Fat on the surface of prostate behind the pubis is gently cleared off. Bipolar or unipolar diathermy should be used as the area is vascular. Puboprostatic ligament is ligated and divided. Prostatic capsule is incised 1 cm below the bladder neck transversely. Stay sutures using 2-zero vicryl should be placed on both sides. Once prostate with adenoma is exposed, anterior commissure of the prostatic lobes are opened to enter the prostatic urethra. With finger dissection prostate is separated from the capsule entirely first on one side then on opposite side. Mop is placed over the area to control bleeding. Middle lobe is again excised using finger. Prostatic urethra may need to be divided above the level of verumontanum. 24 F Foley's 3-way catheter is passed per urethrally into the bladder; traction to that will control the bleeding. Capsule is sutured using 2-zero vicryl. Drain is placed in the retropubic space. Wound is closed in layers. Complications are—haemorrhage, infection, extravasation, urethral stricture, incontinence.

Young's perineal prostatectomy through perineal approach.

Other Methods

Treatment with microwave hyperthermia treatment with temperature of 45–50 degrees; laser treatment is becoming popular, using holmium laser; high energy electromagnetic treatment; placement of

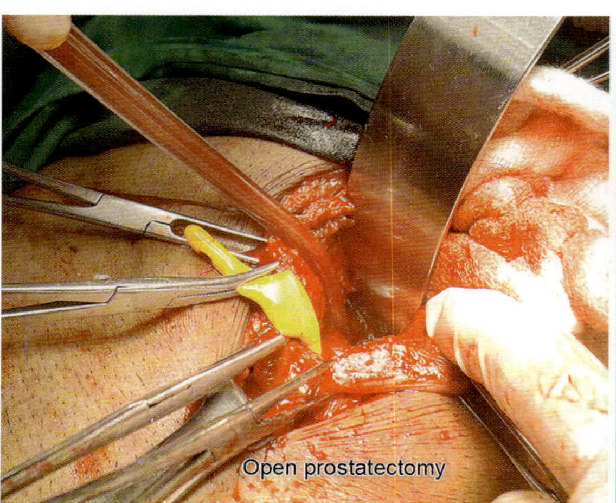

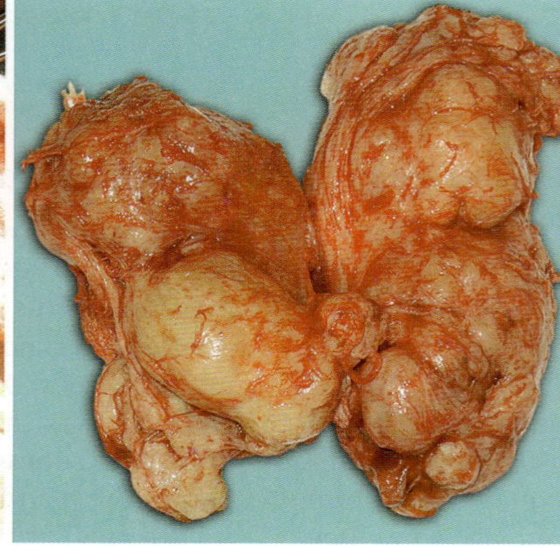

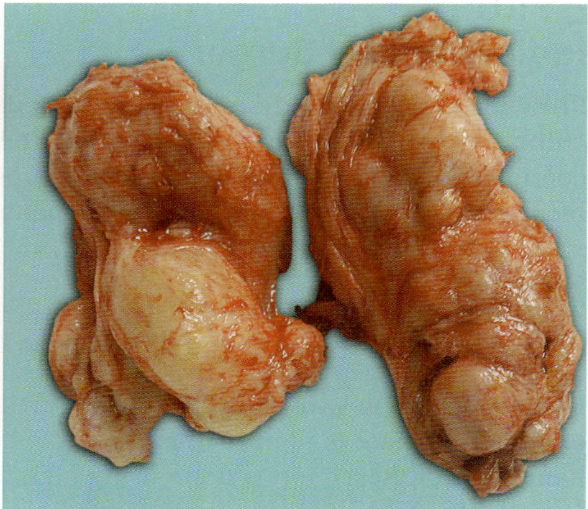

Fig. 28-75: Suprapubic open prostatectomy.

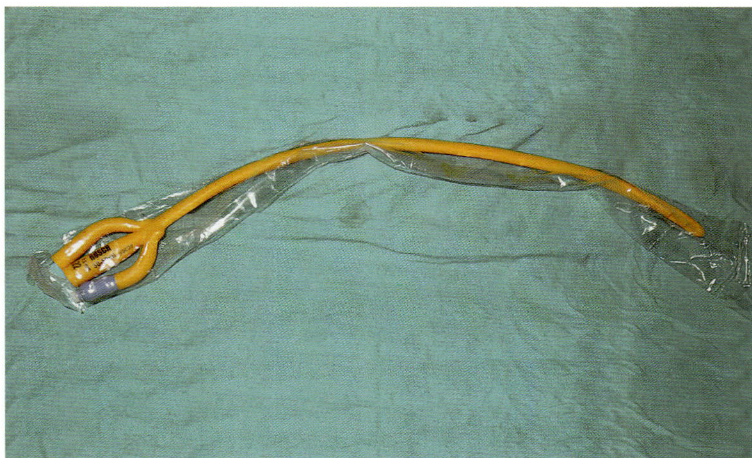

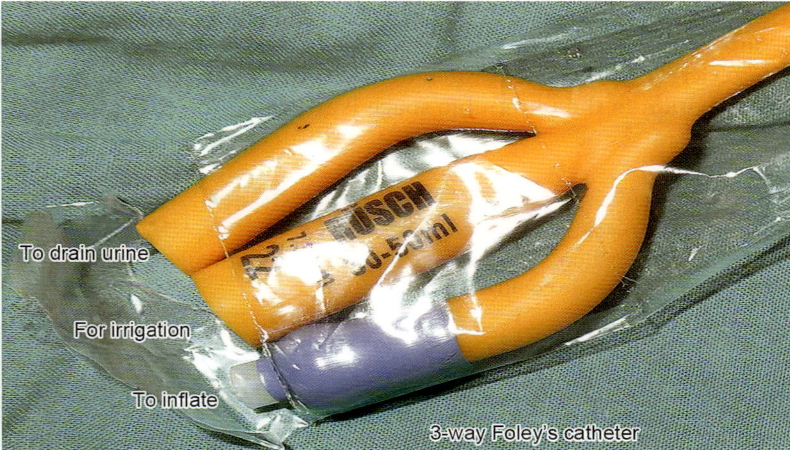

Fig. 28-76: 3-way Foley's catheter used after prostatectomy.

intraurethral stents at prostatic urethra; placement of extraurethral stents which are inert; transurethral balloon dilatation of the prostate; if patient presents with acute retention of urine, initial urethral catheterisation is done. If not possible then *suprapubic trocal cystostomy* ideally or formal open SPC is done. Once patient's obstructive uropathy is under control, TURP is done after 7–14 days after evaluation.

Specific Problems after Surgical Intervention of Prostate

Retrograde ejaculation—65%; erectile dysfunction—5%; failure, recurrence of symptoms and enlargement—10%; need for re TURP/ surgery in 10 years—15%; severe sepsis—6%; recurrent late urinary infection—20%; postoperative haematuria—3% needs transfusion; mortality in TURP is 0.5%.

Other methods used for BPH

- Transurethral incision of prostate—TUIP
- Laser ablation
- Transurethral microwave therapy—TUMT
- Transurethral needle ablation using high frequency radiowaves—TUNA
- High intensity US energy
- Water-induced thermotherapy—through a balloon placed in prostatic urethra
- Prosthetic stents
- Balloon dilatation

PROSTATIC ABSCESS

It is infection, suppuration and pus formation in the prostate gland. Presentation is fever, rigors, perineal pain, urinary disturbances, and tender soft fluctuant swelling in the prostate on rectal examination. Often presentation may be retention of urine. Total count will be increased. Urine microscopic examination will show pus cells. US is diagnostic. Ultrasound is often done over perineum also. Treatment is antibiotics; US-guided aspiration transperineally in lithotomy position or transperineal incision and drainage. Suprapubic cystostomy is better in case of retention of urine. After drainage antibiotics are needed for longer duration in weeks to prevent recurrent infection.

RADICAL PROSTATECTOMY

Radical retropubic prostatectomy is the treatment of choice in early carcinoma of prostate. Procedure can be done through laparoscopy or robotic assisted. Adenocarcinoma occurs in peripheral zone; not in central zone. Urethra passes through central zone.

Technique

Under spinal or general anaesthesia and patient is placed in supine with head down position. 30 F Foley's catheter is passed per urethrally and inflated with 30 cc distilled water. Lower midline incision is made. Anterior rectus sheath is incised; recti are retracted; space of Retizus is reached. Peritoneum is not opened. Blunt dissection is used to reflect the peritoneum above both sides to expose iliac vessels, obturator fossae and ductus deferens. Obturator and iliac lymph nodes are cleared from the bifurcation of the common iliac vessels above up to obturator nerve behind; below up to the pubic bone and along the obturator fossae on both sides. Bladder is retracted above with a retractor and by pulling up of the balloon of the Foley's catheter passed; endopelvic fascia is incised and puboprostatic ligament is divided. Superficial dorsal vein is divided. Bipolar cautery is used carefully. Deep dorsal vein is identified and securely ligated using no 1 vicryl by transfixation at two places to avoid injuring neurovascular bundle of Walsh (when nerve sparing dissection is planned). It is divided in between. Dorsal venous complex may extend posteriorly which is tackled better using harmonic scalpel. But care should be taken not to injure the nerve bundles and urethral sphincters by these energy sources. Judicious use of these instruments is needed. Ligation even though technically difficult and time consuming it often seems better. Once these veins are divided apex of the prostate and membranous urethra are exposed. Urethral wall is divided after placing four stay sutures at four angles (anchor sutures) on its wall which facilitates anastomosis later between bladder and urethra. Foley's catheter is divided after applying clamp on its balloon end side which prevents balloon getting deflated which is used for bladder traction later. Posterior wall is divided and rectourethralis. Denonvillier's fascia is identified which is divided in midline distal to apex of the prostate. In nerve sparing radical prostatectomy, dissection should be careful to preserve neurovascular bundle. Retrograde dissection once completed, ureteric orifices are identified by injecting the indigocarmine intravenously. Bladder neck posteriorly is dissected from the seminal vesicles to reach the isolated bladder neck which is transected. Bladder neck preservation by preserving the circular muscles will compromise the clearance of the tumour. Vas deferens, seminal vesicles are removed enbloc with the prostate.

Haemostasis is achieved by underruning the prostate bed using 3-zero vicryl sutures. Vesicourethral anastomosis is done using 3-zero vicryl or monocryl as water tight around 22 F Foley's catheter. Suction drain in the retropubic space is needed. Wound is closed in layers.

Complications

Bleeding, infection, septiacaemia, pelvic abscess formation, stricture or incontinence are complications.

TREATMENT OF STRICTURE URETHRA (FIG. 28-77)

Intermittent Dilatation

Gradual dilatation, initially with thin dilators, later with thicker dilators of increasing size. Dilatation should be done in operation theatre under aseptic precaution. One should avoid forcible dilatation or over dilatation. Dilatation is done *"Once a week for one month, once a month for one year, and later once a year.*

Dilators used: Lister's dilator [has got olive tip (blister)]; Clutton's dilator; Filiform bougies **(Fig. 28-78)**.

Complications of dilatation are—Infection and bleeding due to trauma; false passage; fistula formation.

Visual Internal Cystoscopic Urethrotomy or Stricturotomy

Here using cystoscope, stricture is visualised and is cut at 12 o'clock position, until it bleeds (fibrous tissue is cut completely). After that Foley's catheter is passed and kept in position for 48 hours **(Fig. 28-79)**.

External Urethrotomy

It is done by open method. Presently, it is not commonly done as cystoscopic urethrotomy is more popular. It is presently done as an initial stage surgery for urethroplasty (*Wheelhouse's operation*).

Urethroplasty

Stricture is excised and urethra is reconstructed using *prepuceal skin* or scrotal skin (*Johanson's urethroplasty*).

Problems in urethroplasty are: Staged procedure and so prolonged hospitalisation; infection; necrosis of skin flap; leak and fistula formation; restenosis.

Complications of stricture urethra

- Retention of urine
- Urethral fistula
- Infection—urethritis, cystitis, pyelonephritis
- Urethral diverticula
- Periurethral abscess
- Bilateral hydronephrosis
- Stone formation
- Renal failure
- Due to straining—hernia, haemorrhoids, rectal prolapse

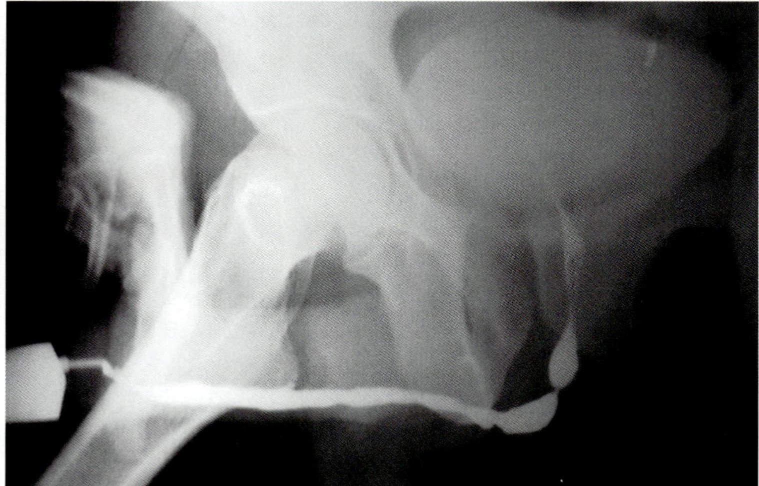

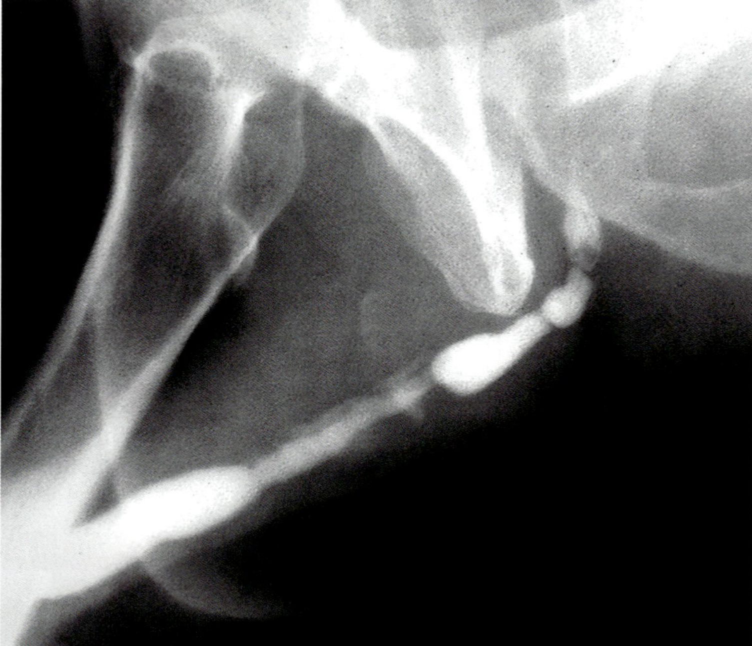

Fig. 28-77: Ascending urethrograms showing single and multiple strictures in two patients.

TREATMENT OF HYPOSPADIAS

Staged Procedure (Fig. 28-80)

I. At the age of one and half years, surgical correction of the chordee is done.
II. At the age of 5–7 years, reconstruction of urethra is done using *prepucial skin* (ideal) or scrotal skin if the patient has been circumcised. Best is prepucial skin. *Perineal urethrostomy is done for diversion.* Perineal urethrostomy should be there until reconstruction of urethra takes up well (*Denis-Browne procedure*).

Magpi repair: Meatal advancement glandular repair—for glandular hypospadias.

In hypospadias, circumcision is contraindicated as prepucial skin is required for future urethroplasty.

TREATMENT OF POSTERIOR URETHRAL VALVE

Micturating cystourethrography (MCU) is diagnostic. It shows dilated proximal urethra. U/S abdomen shows cricket ball bladder.

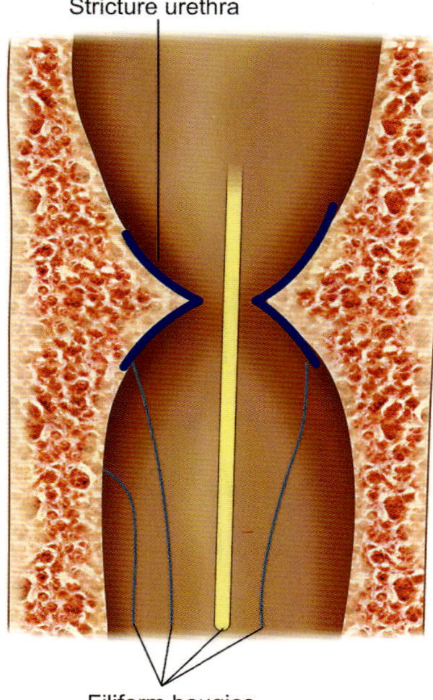

Fig. 28-78: Filiform bougies are used to dilate narrow stricture urethra. One of the bougies will be passed into the urethra (Faggot).

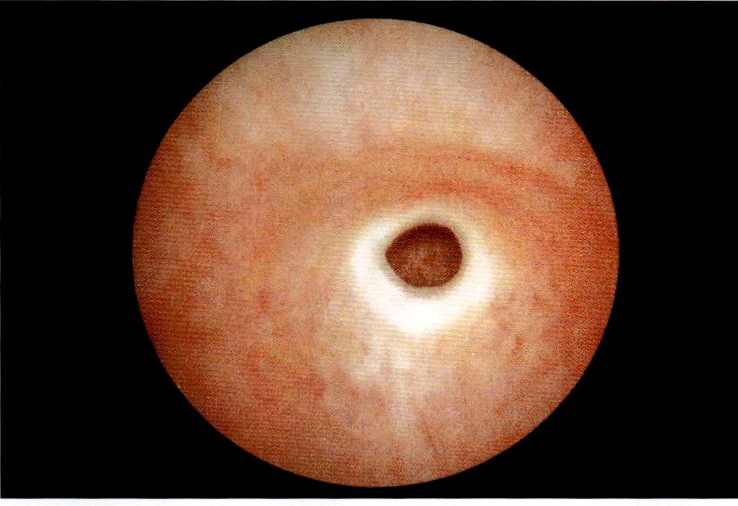

Fig. 28-79: Cystoscopic view of the stricture urethra which needs internal urethrotomy.

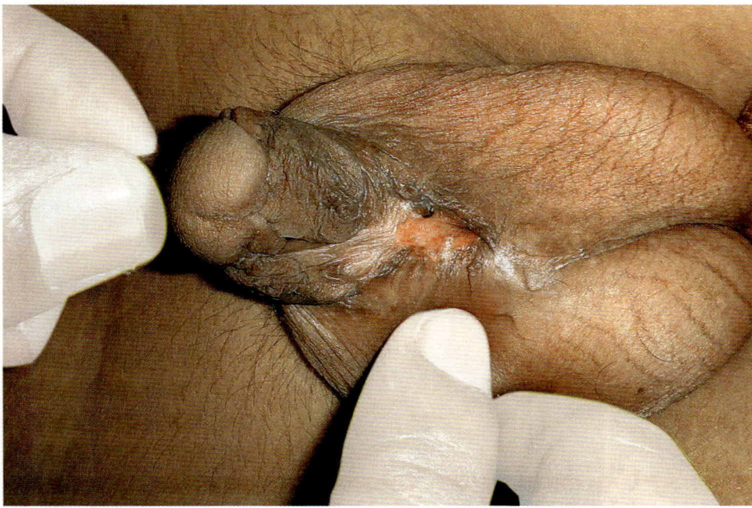

Fig. 28-80: Hypospadias which needs staged repair.

Blood urea and serum creatinine should be done. IVU may be needed. Antenatal US shows fetal urinary tract dilatation.

Differential diagnosis—*Marion's disease:* Bladder neck obstruction due to hypertrophied interureteric bar. MCU differentiates it from posterior urethral valve. Treatment is Y-V plasty *(Bonin's Y-V Plasty)*. Neurogenic bladder also mimics same.

Treatment

Initial SPC and later cystoscopic resection of the posterior urethral valve is done usually after several weeks.

TREATMENT OF URETHRAL STONES

If it is impacted in the external meatus or fossa navicularis, meatotomy and extraction of the stone is done (Meatotomy is cutting and widening of external meatus so as to have an easy stone extraction). If it is impacted in other parts of the urethra, urethroscopy and removal of stone from urethra is done or through a cystoscope the stone is pushed into the bladder and then extracted. In case of retention of urine, initial suprapubic cystostomy is required before removal of the stone. Diverticulum and stricture urethra should be treated accordingly.

Complications of urethral stones: Bleeding, stricture urethra and infection.

RENAL TRANSPLANTATION TECHNIQUE

Renal transplantation is commonly done transplantation worldwide. Advent of proper immunosuppression, donor laparoscopic nephrectomy (1994), good postoperative care has improved the results significantly in current years.

Kidney transplant which started in 1954 has become rapidly developing and currently it is safe and effective.

During pretransplant period, recipient is prepared with his general and specific assessment, nutrition, haemoglobin, cardiac and pulmonary functions.

Living donor is used. Transplant matching should be done; proper legal and judicial permission including consent should be taken. Both surgeries in donor and recipient are done together in two adjacent operation theatres by two urology teams. Nephrologist, immunotherapists, anaesthetists should be present as a team. Usually, left side kidney is taken as vessels are long and dissection is easier. Cold storage should be done after removal of the donor kidney.

Recipient dissection is done as heterotopic transplantation. Recipient diseased kidneys are usually not removed. Usually, right or left iliac fossa is used in the lower abdomen. Internal iliac artery when used end to end anastomosis is done between internal iliac artery and renal artery; if external iliac artery is selected then end of renal artery is sutured to side of the external iliac artery. Polypropylene 4-zero sutures are used or depends on the urologist or vascular surgeon's choice. Renal vein is sutured to the side of the external iliac vein. Ureter is sutured to the bladder like ureteric implantation.

Nephrologists manage the immunosuppression and post-operative care. Complications are—bleeding, infection, rejection, failure, anastomotic dehiscence, urine leak, complications of immunosuppression. Long-term complications are—changes in the kidney, failure, malignancies due to immunosuppression, recurrent sepsis **(Fig. 28-81)**.

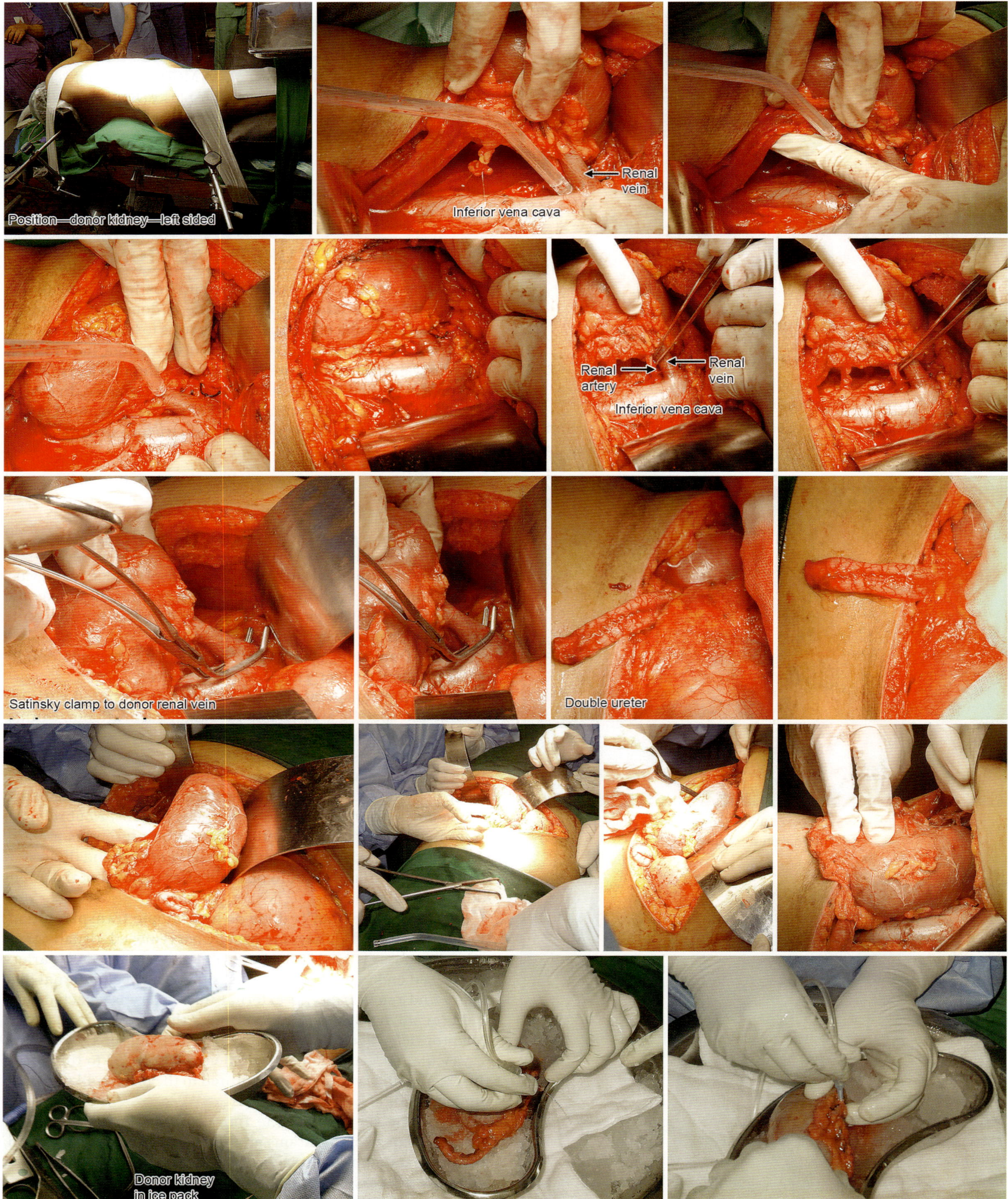
Position—donor kidney—left sided
Renal vein
Inferior vena cava
Renal artery
Renal vein
Inferior vena cava
Satinsky clamp to donor renal vein
Double ureter
Donor kidney in ice pack

Figs. 28-81(1)

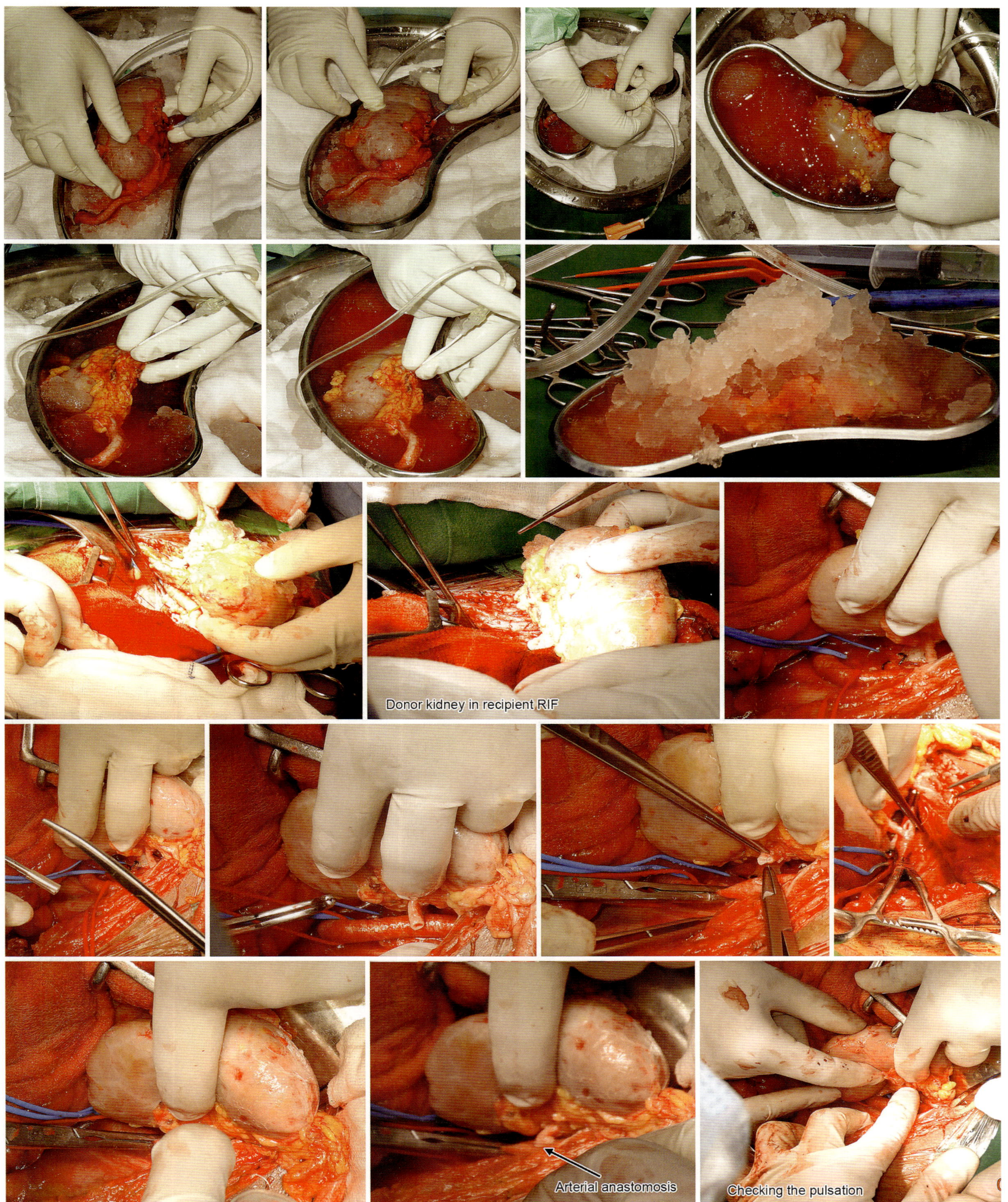
Donor kidney in recipient RIF
Arterial anastomosis
Checking the pulsation

Figs. 28-81(2)

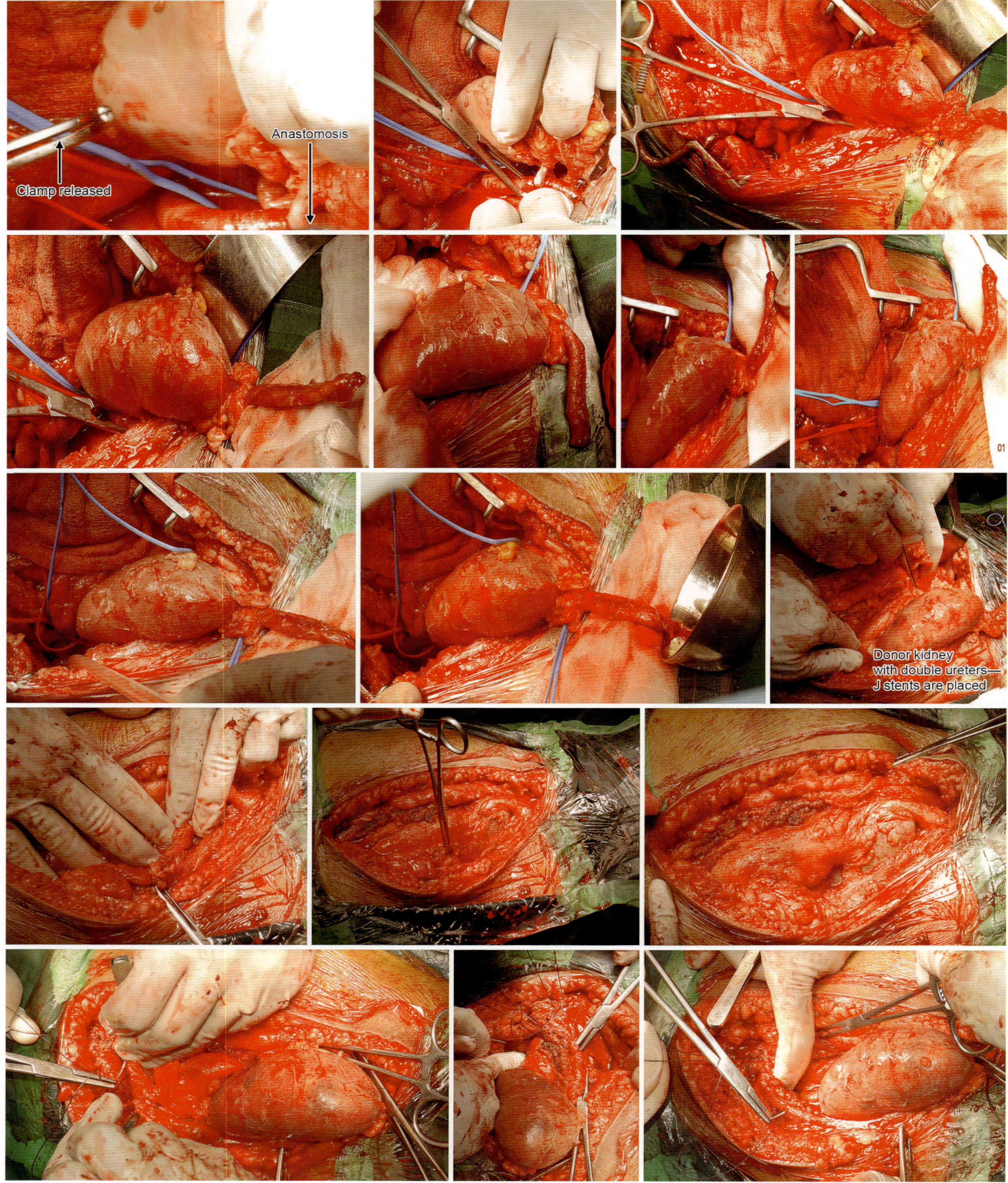

Figs. 28-81(3)

Figs. 28-81(1 to 3): Technique and steps of renal transplantation.

29

CHAPTER

Adrenal Gland Surgeries

ADRENAL GLAND SURGERIES

Adrenalectomy is the standard treatment for adrenal tumours, bilateral adrenal diseases like primary adrenal hyperplasia, incidentalomas more than 5 cm in size, and often metastases in adrenal gland.

Surgical Anatomy of Adrenal Glands

The adrenal glands are named in relation to the kidneys. The term "adrenal" comes from Latin—*ad* means "near"; and *renes* means "kidney". Suprarenal is derived from Latin—*supra* means "above" and *renes* means "kidney". Adrenal glands are essential endocrine glands.

Two suprarenal endocrine adrenal glands are located in the retroperitoneum along the upper pole and medial part of the kidneys in front of the crus of diaphragm opposite 12th rib and vertebral end of 11th intercostal space. Each adrenal gland is 5 × 3 × 1 cm in dimensions weighing 5 grams. Adrenal gland is within renal fascia but separated by a fascial septum from kidney. Right gland is *triangular* in shape (top hat); left one is *semilunar* (cocked hat). Gland is yellow or mahogany (reddish-brown) or *golden-orange* in colour. Right adrenal is relatively higher than left adrenal (right kidney is lower level than left kidney). Between two adrenal glands structures present are—crura, the aorta and coeliac arteries, coeliac plexus and inferior vena cava. Kidney may be ectopic or ptotic but adrenal will be in the original position. But fusion of kidney like horse shoe kidney may have fusion of adrenal glands also **(Figs. 29-1 and 29-2)**.

Right Adrenal Gland

It has got a base, an apex, anterior and posterior surfaces, anterior, medial and lateral borders. Anterior surface is related to inferior vena cava medially, bare area of the liver laterally, duodenum below. It is devoid of peritoneum. Posterior surface is related to right crus of diaphragm above and right kidney below. Hilum of right adrenal is near upper end. Apex is related to bare area; base is related to upper pole of right kidney. Three arteries supplying the right adrenal gland course behind the IVC. Right adrenal vein arises near upper part of the hilum. Right adrenal gland is not very close to right kidney (unlike left adrenal gland which is very closely attached to left kidney).

Left Adrenal Gland

It has got narrow upper end and round lower end. Upper end is related to posterior end of spleen; hilum of left adrenal gland is near lower end through which left adrenal vein exits. Anterior surface is related to cardiac end of stomach, splenic artery and pancreas. Gastric related part only is covered with peritoneum/omental bursa. Posterior surface is related to left kidney laterally, left crus of diaphragm medially. Medial convex border is related to left celiac ganglion, left inferior phrenic artery, left gastric artery. Lateral concave border is related to the stomach.

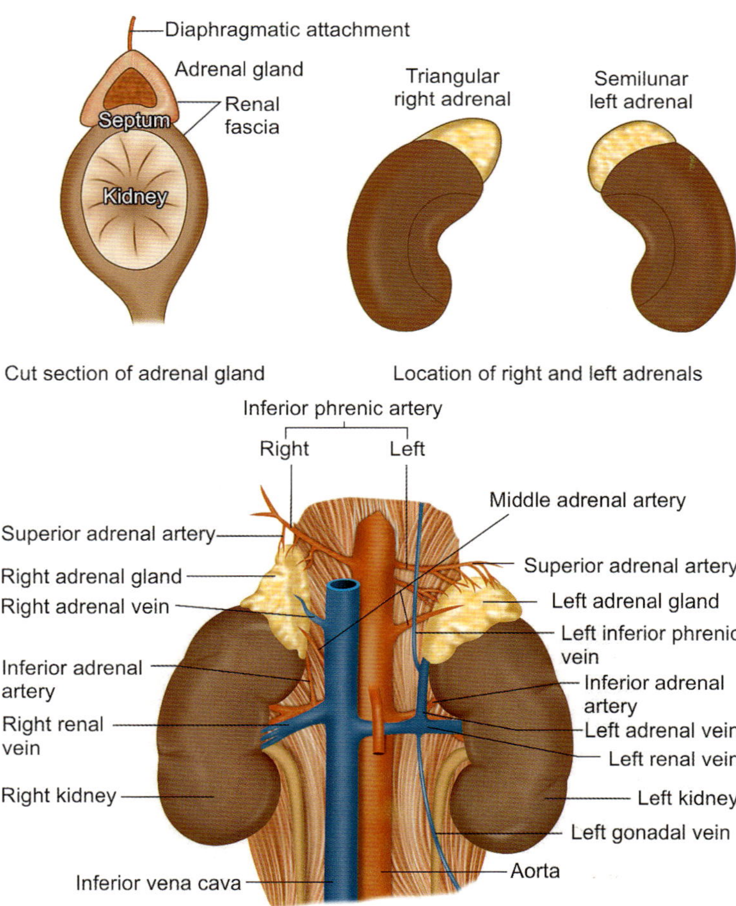

Figs. 29-1(1)

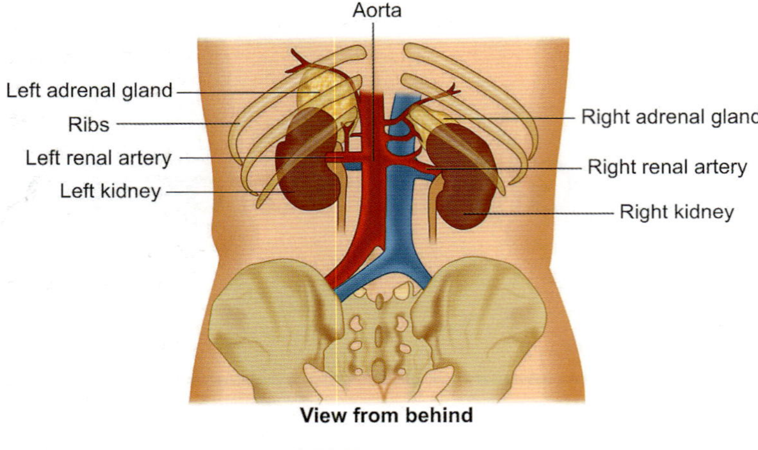

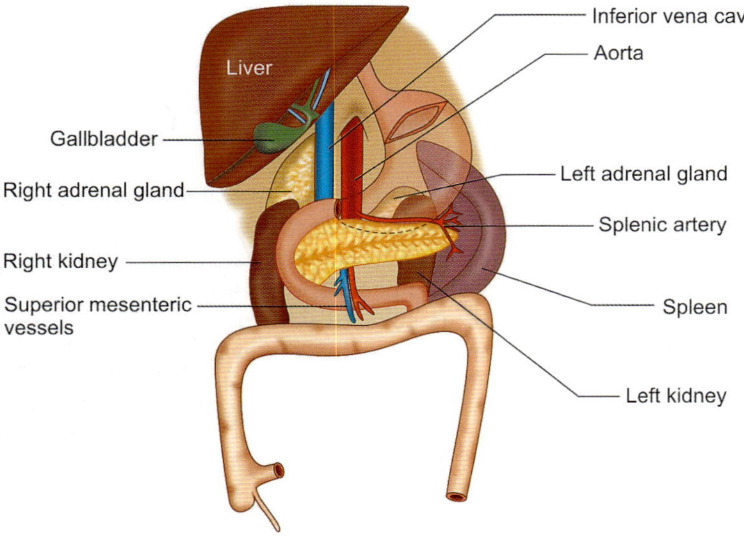

Figs. 29-1(2)

Figs. 29-1(1 and 2): Surgical anatomy of adrenal gland.

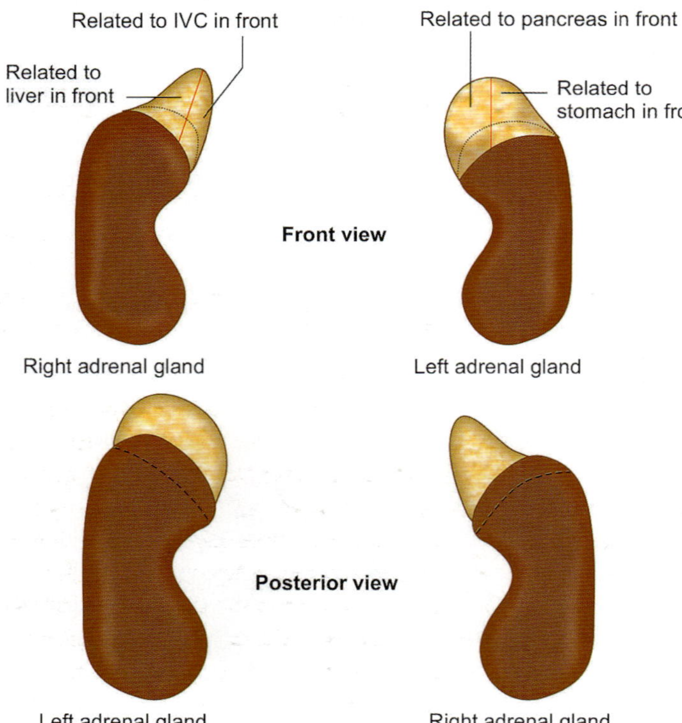

Fig. 29-2: Anterior and posterior views of adrenal glands.

Arterial Supply

Adrenal gland is one of the most vascular organ (gram of tissue) like thyroid (so metastases are common). It is supplied by—superior adrenal artery, a branch of inferior phrenic artery; middle adrenal artery, a branch of aorta; and inferior adrenal artery, a branch of renal artery. Main supply to right gland is superior adrenal artery; to left gland is middle adrenal artery. Inferior phrenic artery often gives group of 6–8 arteries separately instead of one superior adrenal artery. Middle adrenal artery arises from aorta at the level of origin of superior mesenteric artery; it may be single/multiple/often absent or supply perirenal fat. Left side, it is more commonly constant and predominant. Inferior adrenal artery is usually single but can be multiple arises from renal artery or from accessory renal artery or superior polar artery of kidney.

Venous Drainage

Venous drainage is not accompanied by adrenal arteries. Adrenal gland is drained by one single vein which begins at the adrenal hilum. *Right adrenal vein* is short <1 cm and stout drains from the anteromedial part of the gland from upper part of its hilum into inferior vena cava on its posterolateral aspect directed above downwards obliquely. Occasionally an *accessory right adrenal vein* may be present draining into IVC or hepatic veins above the level of right adrenal vein. Right adrenal vein may drain into right hepatic vein or right renal artery instead of IVC. *Left adrenal vein* is long and is directed downwards perpendicular to the renal vein and medially to drain into left renal vein after crossing the left renal artery in front. It is on the anterior surface of the gland. Left inferior phrenic vein joins left adrenal vein on its medial aspect at a point 1.5 cm above the junction of left renal vein and left adrenal vein. Variations like double adrenal veins may be present. Tearing or avulsion of adrenal vein from IVC or left renal vein can occur during dissection causing torrential haemorrhage.

Lymphatics

Adrenal gland is drained into lumbar and lateral aortic nodes. Lymphatic plexus are present under the capsule and in medulla. Subcapsular plexus drains with the arteries; medullary plexus drains with the veins. Right adrenal drains into para-aortic nodes, right renal nodes and nodes at right crus of diaphragm. Left drains into nodes adjacent to left renal artery and para-aortic nodes. Lymph may also drain into the posterior mediastinum through lymphatics along the inferior phrenic artery. Lymphatics from the upper pole of right adrenal gland may communicate with lymphatics of the liver.

Nerve Supply

Adrenal medulla has got myelinated preganglionic sympathetic fibres. Coeliac and renal plexus give branches to adrenals.

Structure

Adrenal gland has got outer thick cortex and inner thin medulla. Two are independent in development, structure and function. Cortex has got *outer* zona glomerulosa secreting mineralocorticoids; *middle* zona fasciculata secreting glucocorticoids; *inner* zona reticularis secreting sex hormones. Adrenal medulla contains chromaffin cells in groups, autonomic ganglion cells with capillaries.

Embryology

Adrenal cortex develops from *intermediate mesoderm* of coelomic epithelium; medulla is from *neural crest* cells. Foetal adrenal gland is 20 times larger in relation to body weight than adult adrenal gland. In foetus at 4 months of gestation, adrenal gland is 4 times larger than kidney size of that age. During birth adrenal gland becomes 1/3rd of the kidney size.

ADRENALECTOMY

Indications for Adrenalectomy

Unilateral

- Cushing's syndrome—cortisol secreting adenoma.
- Unilateral pheochromocytoma.
- Virilising tumours.
- Unilateral non-functioning tumour >4 cm in size.
- Adrenocortical carcinoma.
- Solitary adrenal metastasis (should be confirmed by PET scan to rule out other metastatic areas).

Bilateral Adrenalectomy

- Bilateral pheochromocytoma (10%).
- Bilateral nodular adrenal hyperplasia.
- Ectopic ACTH producing tumour.
- Cushing's disease (pituitary related).

Adrenal incidentalomas (4%) are identified on US/CT/MRI which are otherwise asymptomatic clinically. It can be functioning or non-functioning. Biochemical evaluation is a must to find out its functional nature if it is so. Incidentaloma more than 4 cm in size, progressive increase in size on repeated imaging, functioning tumour, suspicious of malignancy should be operated. Non-functioning cortical adenoma is the commonest type of adrenal incidentaloma.

Preoperative Preparation

CT imaging is the ideal one for diagnosis, to assess extent, involvement, nodal status. MRI is also used often. CT chest is done to check metastases.

In Functioning Tumours:
Relevant investigations like 24 hour urinary catecholamines and metanephrines and plasma metanephrine, VMA; for aldosteronoma ratio of plasma aldosterone concentration (PAC) to plasma renin activity (PRA) is assessed and it is greater than 20:25 with an absolute PAC more than 15 ng/dL, raised 24 hour urine aldosterone level >12 µg on a high sodium diet, raised urinary potassium excretion rate >30 mEq/24 hour; for Cushing's syndrome with cortical adenoma 24 hour urine free cortisol level estimation, dexamethasone test (1 mg dexamethasone is injected at 23.00 hours, morning 8 o'clock plasma cortisol level is assessed, in normal individual plasma cortisol level will be suppressed below 3 µg/dL whereas in Cushing's syndrome suppression will not be there) plasma ACTH level (if ACTH is raised MRI head for pituitary disease with inferior petrosal sinus blood sampling is done); for adrenocortical carcinoma 24 hour urine free cortisol and plasma DHEA (dehydroepiandrosterone) level estimation is done. Correction hypokalaemia and hypertension is important.

In Conn's syndrome correction of electrolytes and blood pressure is important. Oral potassium supplementation and spironolactone (200–400 mg daily for 3 weeks) are useful in aldosteronoma.

Hypertension in pheochromocytoma is corrected using α-blocker with phenoxybenzamine 10 mg twice daily up to a total dose of 60 mg/day inserted and increased if needed later. *Plenty of liquid (adequate hydration)* intake is essential while patient is in the hospital. Beta-blocker if at all is given only when the patient is fully undercover of alpha blocker for 4 weeks and usually given one week prior to surgery to control tachycardia and arrhythmias.

Preoperative intravenous steroid is needed in case of adrenalectomy for Cushing's syndrome. Contralateral gland may be *suppressed or atrophied* in Cushing's syndrome.

CVP line, arterial line, cardiac monitor, urinary catheterisation, nasogastric intubation are required.

Approaches for Adrenalectomy

Laparoscopic Approach

It is ideal for all unilateral adrenal tumours which are benign, less than 6 cm in size. It is the gold standard as access and dissection will be more precise in the depth. Gagner's transabdominal lateral approach is commonly (1962) is used. This gives a wider working space with better visualisation of abdominal contents. It is the preferred method. Anterior transabdominal laparoscopic approach is also used. Retroperitoneoscopic approach is direct approach to adrenal gland but working space is less. Retroperitoneoscopic approach allows lesser respiratory and haemodynamic complications.

Open Approach

It is advocated in tumours larger than 6 cm, previous upper abdominal surgery, malignant adrenal tumour, bilateral adrenal tumours.

Lateral Flank Open Approach:
It is used to reach the adrenal bed. It is like approaching the kidney and is more familiar to surgeons and urologists. Proper padding at different pressure points is important to reduce the chances of rhabdomyolysis and hyperextension neuropraxia **(Fig. 29-3)**.

Open Anterior Transabdominal Approach:
It is used in malignant tumours which are more than 8 cm size with extra-adrenal extension, with nodal spread and in case of previous upper abdominal surgery where bowel adhesions are common. Bilateral subcostal incision allows removal of both adrenal glands. This is commonly used approach for bilateral adrenalectomy **(Fig. 29-4)**.

Open Posterior Retroperitoneal (Lumbodorsal) Approach:
It is used in small tumours less than 6 cm which are not approachable through laparoscopy. This approach has become rare as most of these tumours when benign can be approached through laparoscopy. Tumour less than 6 cm which is malignant but not invaded is approached retroperitoneally. Patient is placed in prone position. Incision is placed along the 11th or 12th rib. 11th or 12th rib is resected. Two incisions on both sides allow bilateral adrenalectomy. Peritoneal opening is avoided in this approach. Postoperative ileus, infection wound dehiscence are less in this approach. Both sides can be approached in same prone position. But abdominal contents cannot be assessed for any pathology.

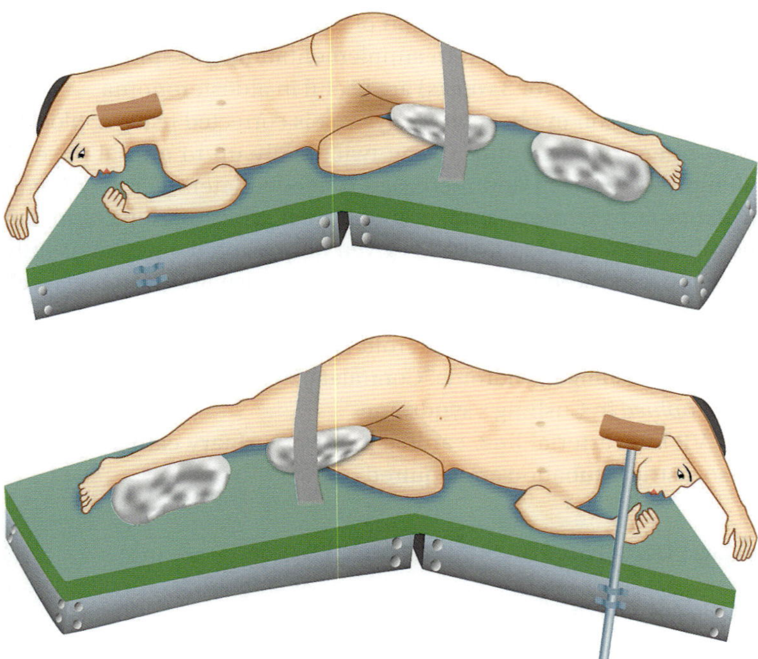

Fig. 29-3: Positions for lateral approach for left and right adrenalectomy.

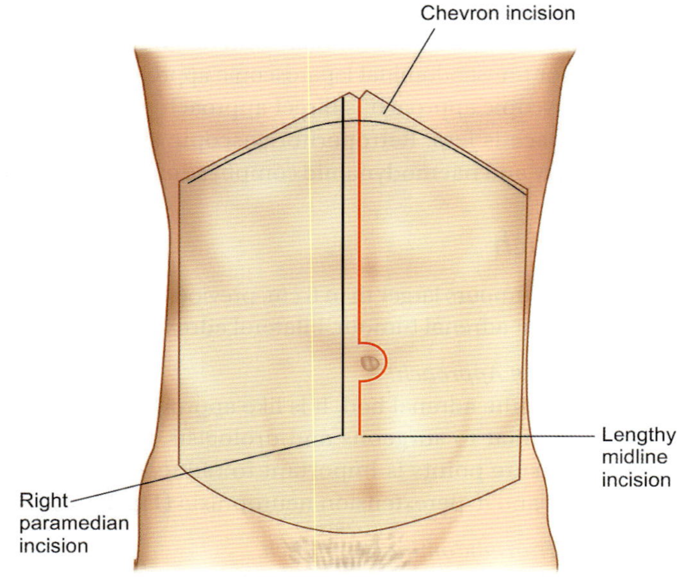

Fig. 29-4: Open abdominal approaches—Chevron incision for bilateral adrenalectomies; midline incision; right paramedian incision.

Hockey stick incision is another incision used for posterior approach which is placed from 10th rib extending downwards and then laterally towards iliac crest. Vertical incision also can be used. The latissimus dorsi muscle is divided with 12th rib resection subpleurally. Serratus posterior muscle is divided. Intercostal nerves (12th) are retained. Paraspinal muscles are retracted medially. Pleura is gently dissected from the diaphragm above; diaphragm is incised to reach Gerota's fascia. Gerota's fascia is incised; kidney is dissected downwards to expose the adrenal gland. Adrenal vein is identified, carefully dissected and doubly ligated. Adrenal arteries are also ligated to dissect the gland completely. Pleura if injured can be sutured with a small red rubber tube inside the pleural cavity which is removed after adequate inflation of lung during closure of the wound; otherwise intercostal tube drainage is done. Diaphragm is closed with sutures. Wound is closed in layers. Postoperative musculoskeletal pain, pleural injury and less access to adrenal vessels are the problems **(Fig. 29-5)**.

Thoracoabdominal Approach:

It is used when there is major vascular invasion like inferior vena cava or extensive upward dissection is needed. Patient is in semilateral position. Midline incision extending into the thorax through 9th or 10th rib to achieve thoracoabdominal exposure is used. Incision can also be used at the angle of the 9th to 10th ribs extending across the midline to the midpoint of the contralateral rectus muscle just above the umbilicus. Diaphragm is incised by taking care not to injure phrenic nerve. Liver, IVC and hepatic veins are exposed well. Dissection is carried out as usual **(Fig. 29-6)**.

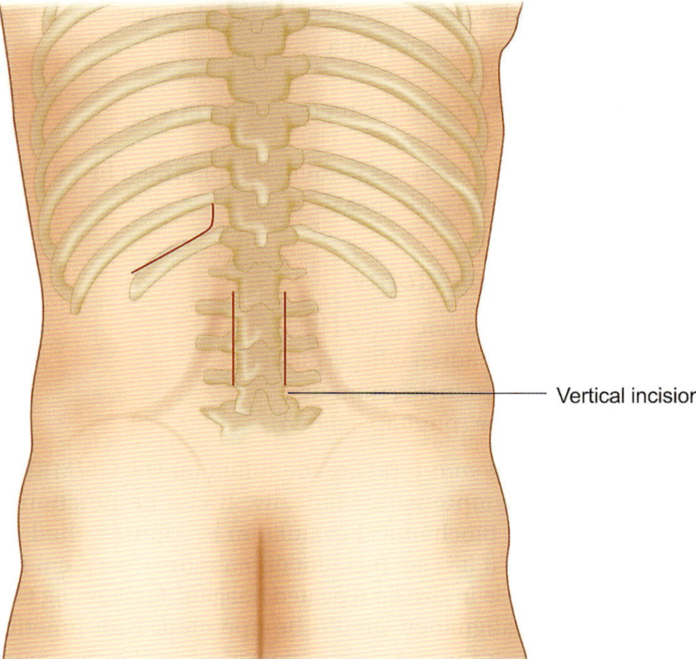

Fig. 29-5: Posterior approach for adrenal gland. It is rarely used now. It is useful in bilateral adrenalectomy.

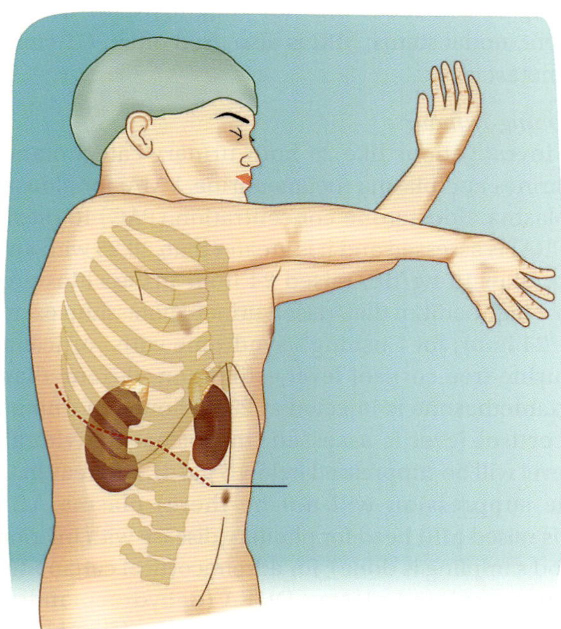

Fig. 29-6: Incision for thoracoabdominal approach.

TECHNIQUE OF OPEN ADRENALECTOMY

Open approach is done through lengthy subcostal incision. Bilateral subcostal incision is used to approach both adrenal glands. Anterior rectus sheath, rectus muscle medially and external and internal oblique and transversus abdominis muscles are divided to enter the peritoneal cavity.

Right Adrenalectomy

Hepatic flexure of the colon is mobilised medially and inferiorly. Triangular ligament of the liver is divided to retract liver medially to expose right adrenal area. Adequate Kocherisation of the duodenum medially is important to expose the IVC properly. Right adrenal gland will be deeper to inferior vena cava at its medial part and in front of the upper pole of right kidney below. Downward traction to right kidney improves the exposure. Resectability of the large tumour should be assessed. Encasement of IVC and liver metastases are contraindications for resection of the tumour. Lymph nodes should be assessed in malignancy and may require removal for radical clearance. Fascia between the right adrenal gland and IVC is incised carefully and dissected away from adrenal gland. While gentle lateral displacement of adrenal gland is done, right adrenal vein which is short and stout entering into the IVC identified. It is doubly ligated carefully or using clips. Right adrenal vein is divided. Often in large tumour right adrenal vein stretches over the tumour; in such situation right adrenal vein is ligated or stapled with appropriate device at its IVC junction. Rarely accessory right adrenal vein may be existing above the level of right adrenal vein which needs careful dissection and ligation or clipping. Arterial branches enter the gland on the medial side from deeper aspect of the IVC, which should be ligated or cauterised using bipolar cautery. Ultrasonic energy device can also be used. Laterally dissection is done between liver and adrenal gland and between kidney and adrenal gland. Right renal vein is safeguarded. Superior polar artery of right kidney will be often very close to the adrenal gland and should not be injured. If tumour involves adjacent structures then enblock removal of adrenal tumour with kidney, hepatic flexure of colon and part of the liver segment can be done. Partial infiltration of the IVC at one place may allow tumour resection by removing the small part of the wall of the IVC which will be repaired using 3- or 4-zero polypropylene suture material. One should not hold the adrenal gland/tumour as tumour spillage can occur. Only *periadrenal fat and thin fascia* should be held to facilitate the dissection. Dissection between adrenal gland and kidney should be done last, if done earlier, then adrenal gland will retract upwards and accessibility becomes difficult. Tumour spillage should be absolutely avoided. After tumour removal haemostasis is maintained. Irrigation with distilled water is done to adrenal bed. Drain is placed to the dissected area **(Fig. 29-7)**.

Left Adrenalectomy

Splenorenal ligament is divided; splenic flexure of the colon is mobilised adequately to retract it downwards. Peritoneum in left paracolic gutter (*Toldt's line*) is incised in its full length; incision is carried upwards through splenic flexure then towards left along the transverse colon in its upper part towards right up to ½ or 2/3rd of its length. Peritoneum in the lower border of the tail of the pancreas is incised. Spleen with tail of the pancreas is mobilised medially and upwards. Renal fascia is incised and superior pole of kidney is dissected. Adrenal gland is exposed. Often large left sided adrenal tumour may be adherent to the tail of pancreas and spleen and in such situation dissection of tail of pancreas and spleen is done through lesser sac by anterior approach. Left adrenal vein joins left renal vein vertically from above downwards after crossing the left renal artery in front. Left inferior phrenic vein joins left adrenal vein. Entire left renal vein should be dissected to have a proper visualisation in large tumour. Left adrenal vein is double ligated securely. It is better to ligate left inferior phrenic vein separately which joins left adrenal vein. Inferior mesenteric vein and splenic vein will be closer in large tumours which should not be injured. Newer energy sources like ultrasonic seal may be useful. Left renal artery runs horizontally just above and behind the left renal vein. Left inferior adrenal artery which arises from left renal artery is identified and ligated. Adrenal vein should be ligated first in functioning pheochromocytoma to prevent the release of catecholamines into the circulation. Periaortic lymph nodes with retroperitoneal fat and adjacent Gerota's fascia are removed along with the tumour in case of adrenal malignancies. Often enblock removal of left kidney, splenic flexure of colon and spleen with tail of the pancreas is done in large aggressive tumours. Occasionally inferior mesenteric vein may require to be ligated in large left adrenal tumour **(Fig. 29-8)**.

In primary hyperaldosteronism and pheochromocytoma, gland is hypervascular and friable. So gland should be held gently over periadrenal fascia using fine forceps. All small vessels should be clipped or haemostasis is achieved using bipolar forceps to prevent haematoma formation which will interfere with further dissection **(Fig. 29-9)**.

Postoperative Care

Respiratory physiotherapy, observation, pain control, prevention of sepsis, observation for bleeding are important. Acute adrenal insufficiency can occur in case of bilateral adrenalectomy which presents as sudden haemodynamic instability and circulatory failure. Prompt adequate steroid supplement is essential in these patients.

In adrenalectomy for pheochromocytoma, because patient is on phenoxybenzamine, more intravenous fluids are required after resection to maintain circulatory volume. During surgery sodium nitroprusside infusion (10 μg/kg/minute) is required. Circulating catecholamine/metanephrine/VMA level estimation and 24 hour urinary catecholamines estimation is needed postoperatively and later on yearly. *Hypertensive exacerbations* and tachycardia are likely to occur during induction of anaesthesia and during direct tumour handling. Intraoperative hypovolaemia, postoperative hypotension should be managed well. Central venous line with CVP monitoring and arterial line for monitor is a must.

In bilateral adrenalectomy postoperatively patient requires oral *steroid and mineralocorticoid* (fludrocortisone 100 μg/day) for lifelong. Even in Cushing's syndrome due to unilateral functioning cortical adenoma, oral steroid supplement is required for 2 years after unilateral adrenalectomy until hypothalamic pituitary adrenal axis which was suppressed earlier recovers to allow contralateral adrenal gland to function.

In adrenalectomy for aldosteronoma, postoperative hypotension, hyperkalaemia and acidosis can occur. It is corrected by intravenous infusion of normal saline infusion rapidly and intramuscular injection of deoxycorticosterone acetate (DOCA, 10 mg twice daily).

Regular blood sugar estimation is needed after adrenalectomy for functioning pheochromocytoma as sudden reduction in circulating catecholamine can cause hyperinsulinism and hypoglycaemia **(Fig. 29-10)**.

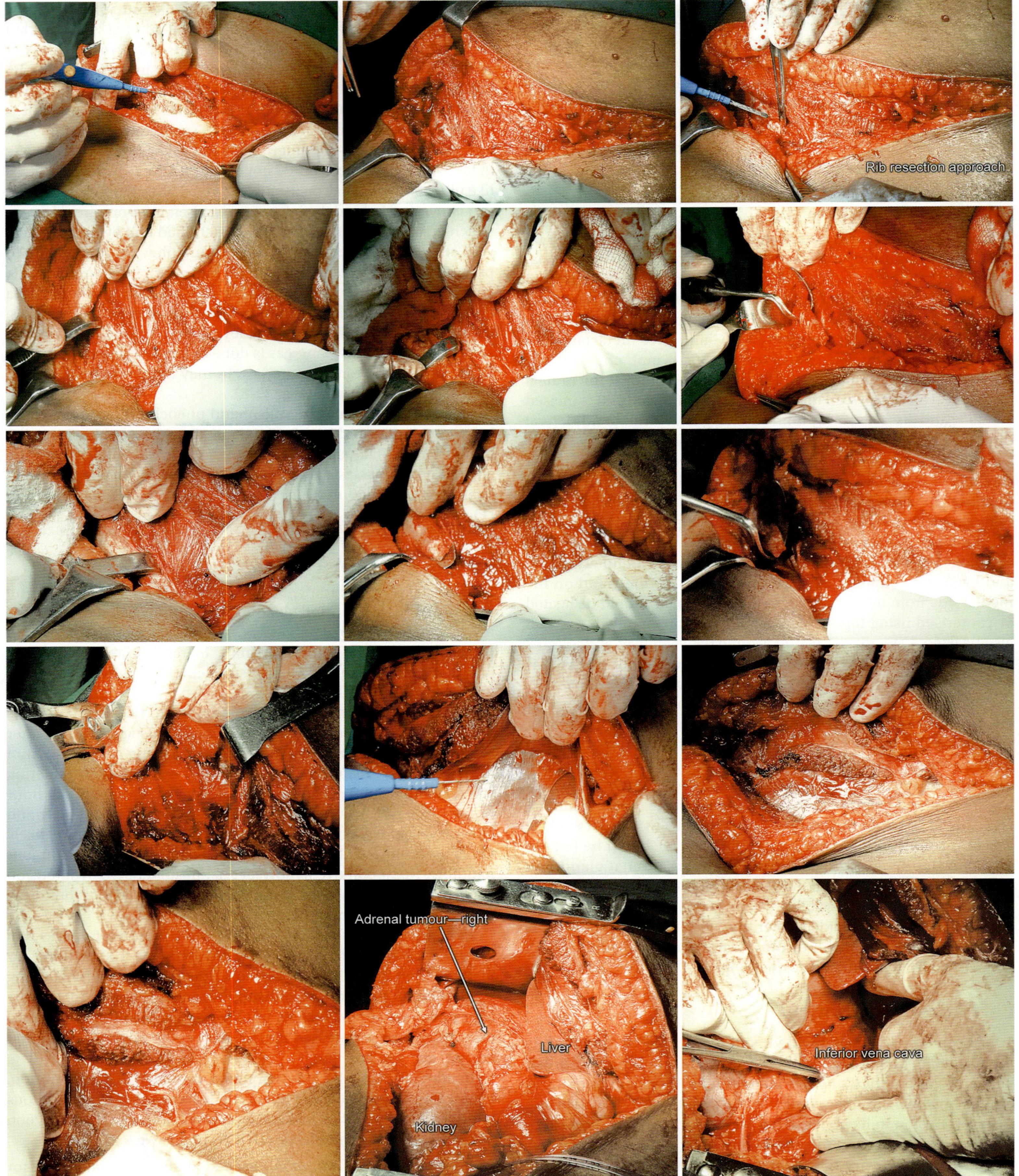
Rib resection approach
Adrenal tumour—right
Liver
Kidney
Inferior vena cava

Figs. 29-7(1)

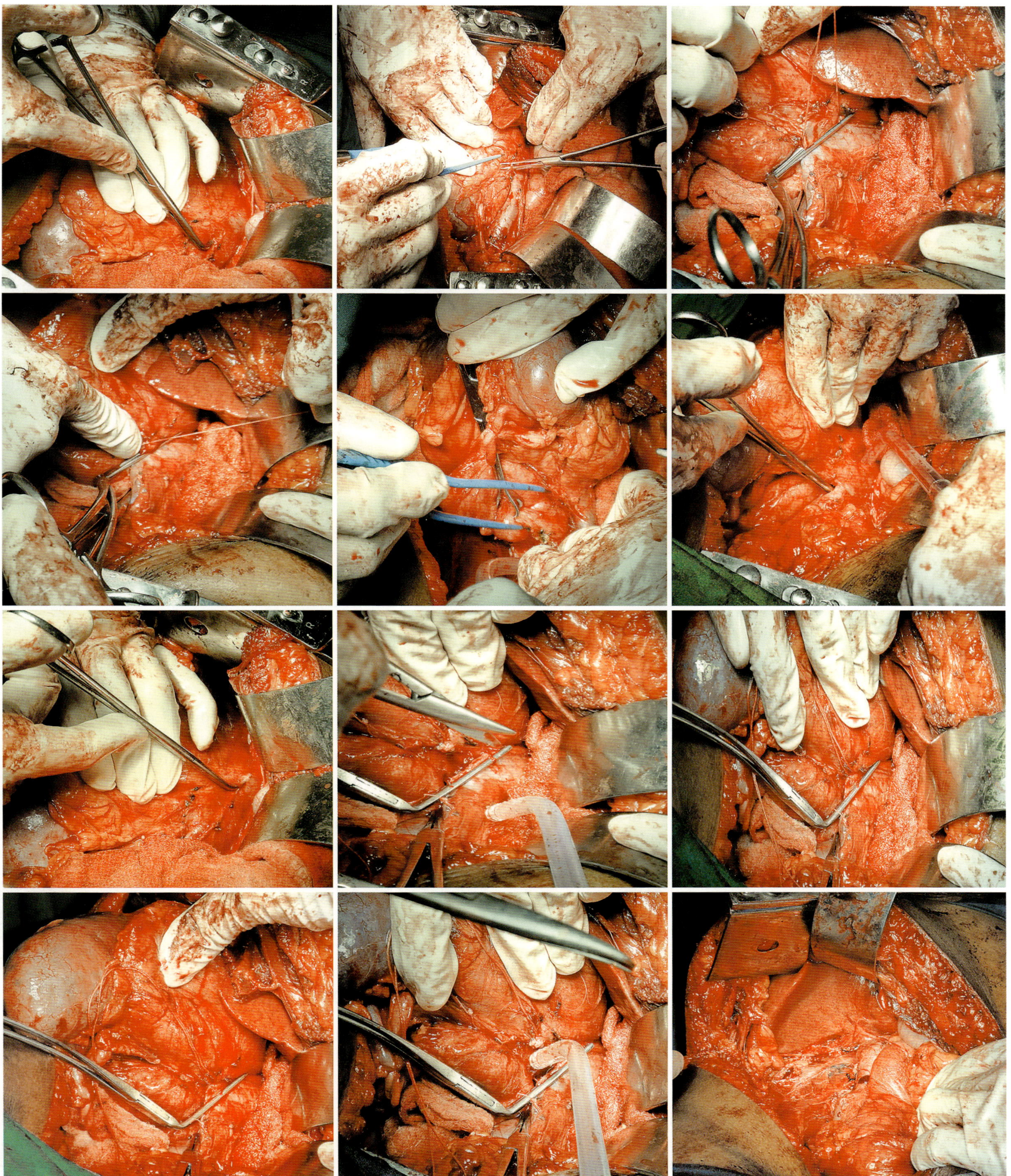

Figs. 29-7(2)

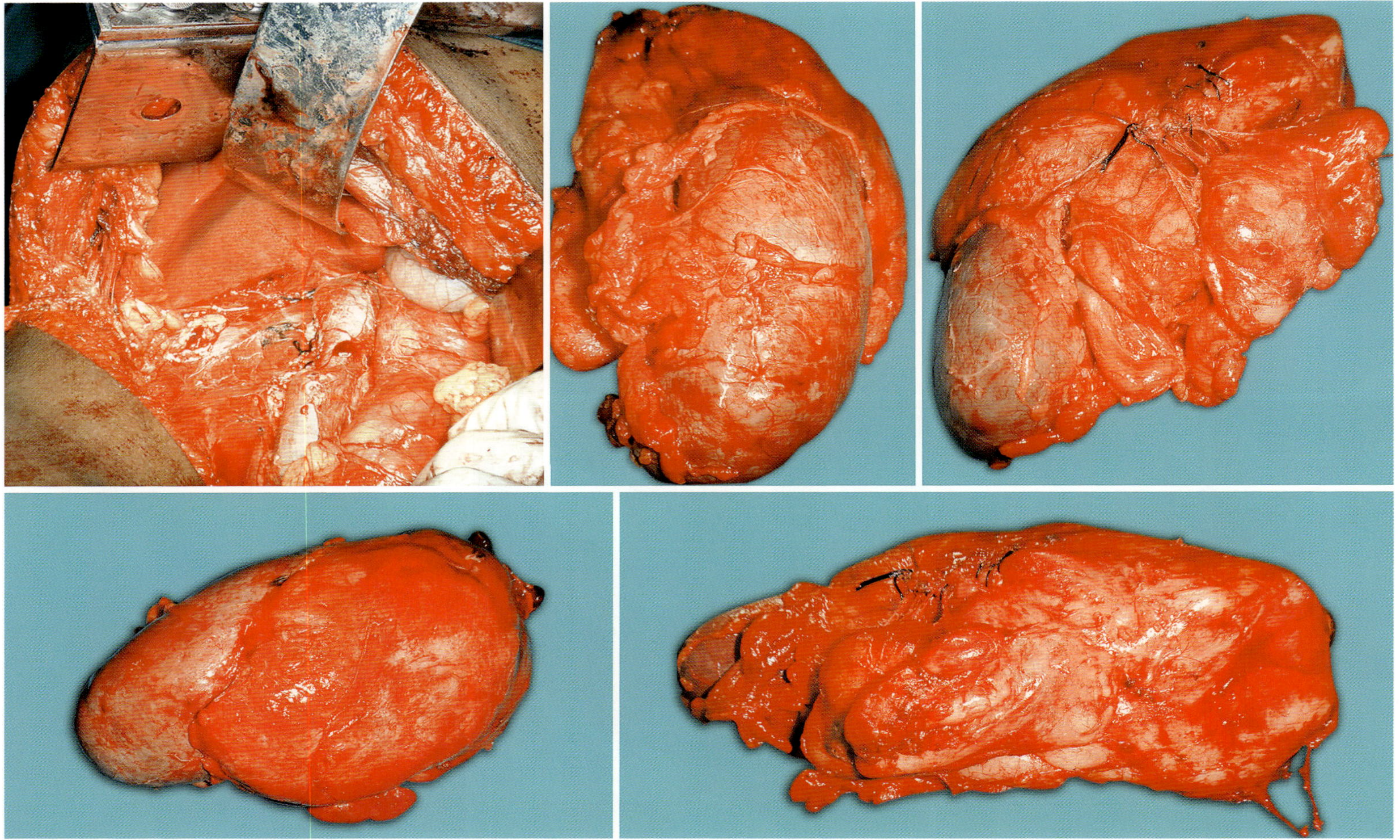

Figs. 29-7(3)

Figs. 29-7(1 to 3): Right-sided adrenal tumour; removed along with kidney while doing adrenalectomy.

Complications of Adrenalectomy

Bleeding which may life-threatening can occur from adrenal vein, inferior vena cava, renal vein, liver, spleen, pancreas and kidney tissue injury. Proper ligation of adrenal vein, reconstruction of the inferior vena cava or renal vein, suturing of the liver or kidney injuries is needed. Satinsky clamp is needed for proper suturing of the IVC. Central line, blood transfusion may be required. Haemorrhage is the most common complication after adrenalectomy.

Injury to pleura (pneumothorax) may warrant intercostal tube placement. On table chest X-ray may be needed after closure of the wound. Postoperative pulmonary collapse, pneumonia, ARDS can occur.

Injury to colon, pancreas and spleen can occur. Bowel injury may cause peritonitis, septicaemia. Injury may due to cautery or energy source or during scissor dissection.

Acute adrenal insufficiency may be fatal if steroid supplement is not started adequately.

Hypovolaemia on table and postoperative hypotension is common after resection of pheochromocytoma. Careful monitoring in critical unit is needed. *Postoperative hypotension* is common after adrenalectomy for functioning pheochromocytoma due to loss of α receptor mediated sympathetic tone which needs large quantity of intravenous fluids.

Rebound hyperinsulinism due to reduced inhibitory effect on insulin secretion by sudden reduction in circulating catecholamines (catecholamines inhibit insulin secretion thereby causing hyperglycaemia) leading into *hypoglycaemia.* Regular blood sugar estimation postoperatively is important in patients who underwent adrenalectomy for functioning pheochromocytoma. Weekly urinary catecholamine estimation initially and later yearly is important.

Other complications: Wound infection, sinus formation and postoperative wound pain are other problems.

Pheochromocytoma *in pregnancy* has got 50% maternal mortality; vaginal delivery is contraindicated in pheochromocytoma.

LAPAROSCOPIC ADRENALECTOMY

Gagner in 1992 started first laparoscopic transabdominal lateral flank approach which is commonly used. Transperitoneal anterior approach and retroperitoneal posterior approach (Mercan et al.) are other approaches used.

Laparoscopic adrenalectomy is the safe, effective '*gold standard'* operation for benign adrenal tumour of less than 6 cm in size. Approach, dissection, haemostasis, recovery, morbidity status, pain, hospitalisation are all factors in favour of laparoscopic adrenalectomy. Bilateral tumours are also better amenable through laparoscopy.

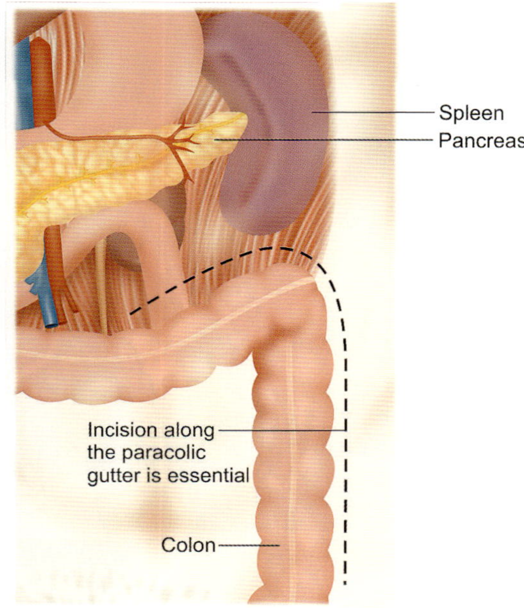

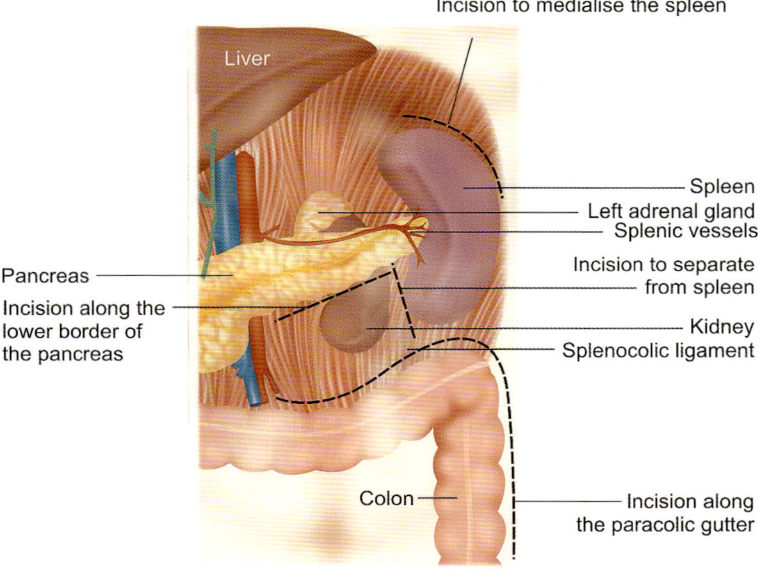

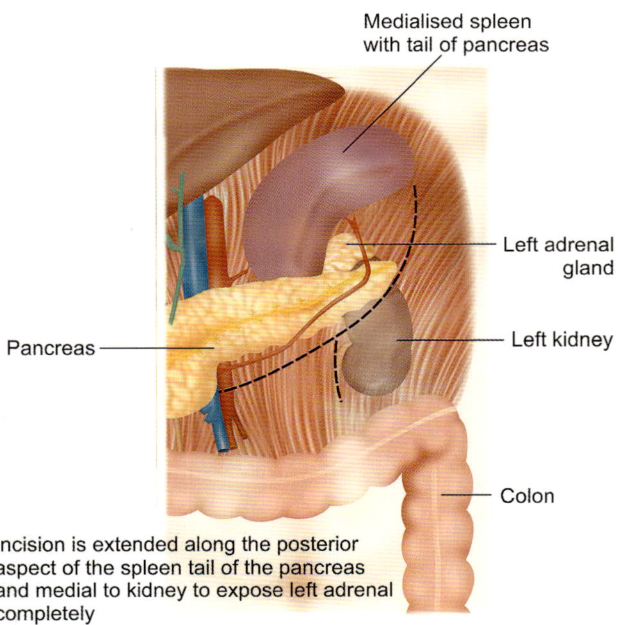

Fig. 29-8: Technique of left adrenalectomy.

Indications	*Contraindications*
♦ Cortisol producing adenoma, aldosteronoma ♦ Primary adrenal hyperplasia ♦ Pheochromocytoma ♦ Non-functioning cortical adenoma, incidentaloma ♦ Adrenal cyst, ganglioneuroma, myolipoma	♦ Adrenal cortical tumour more than 5–6 cm; >100 grams weight ♦ Malignant pheochromocytoma ♦ Adrenocortical carcinoma ♦ Any adrenal mass more than 8–10 cm ♦ Extensive previous upper abdominal surgery

Tumour more than 6 cm makes laparoscopic dissection difficult especially adrenal veins; causing higher chances of tear in IVC or left renal vein. Larger tumour is more likely to be adrenocortical carcinoma which is an indication for open surgery.

Approaches

Lateral flank transperitoneal approach: This position allows retraction of the adjacent organs by gravity to facilitate the exposure of the adrenal glands; adequate access to retroperitoneum as well as abdominal cavity; gives proper working space and triangulation; other organs in the abdominal cavity can be assessed properly. Additional procedures like gall bladder removal are possible. *Disadvantages:* postoperative ileus and mobilisation of colon is required. Opposite adrenal cannot be approached; if needed needs repositioning of the patient.

Transperitoneal anterior approach: It is done in supine position which allows access to both adrenal glands. But it is technically demanding with longer operative period. Mobilisation of viscera like colon, spleen, tail of pancreas, liver is needed. Usually left side adrenalectomy is done first; then right side. *Reason* is—left side is easier to approach by laparoscope and when once left side is over, right side can be addressed and in case if conversion is needed for right side (right side is difficult laparoscopically) it can be done by open conversion method.

Posterior retroperitoneal approach: It gives direct access to adrenal gland without opening the peritoneal cavity and without a need for mobilisation of other organs. It is also useful for bilateral adrenalectomy wherein change of position is not required in Cushing's syndrome, bilateral pheochromocytoma. But it gives less working space and minimum triangulation; orientation of anatomy from behind becomes difficult; on table inadvertent formation of pneumoperitoneum due to peritoneal tear limits the working space further; pleural injury may occur.

Patient is placed in prone/prone jackknife position. By open method through a small incision just below the tip of 12th rib followed by splitting the muscle layers retroperitoneum is reached. Through balloon or finger dissection space is widened. CO_2 insufflation can also be done using Veress needle under fluoroscopic guidance but it is difficult. Additional ports are placed as needed. Second port is in the loin at the level of inferior pole of the kidney just above the iliac crest 5 cm laterally below the 11th rib; 3rd port is at the level of midpoint of kidney just lateral to sacrospinalis; 4th port is 2 cm lateral to that. Further ports if needed may be placed. Retro-pneumoperitoneum pressure should be 20–25 mmHg which creates more working space and reduces the oozing. 30° telescope is used. Dissection is from lateral to medial first ligating the arteries and branches or sealing using harmonic. On right side, on deeper medial dissection IVC is identified; right adrenal vein is carefully dissected and clipped. On left side inferomedially, left renal vein with left adrenal vein entering the left renal vein is identified; left adrenal vein

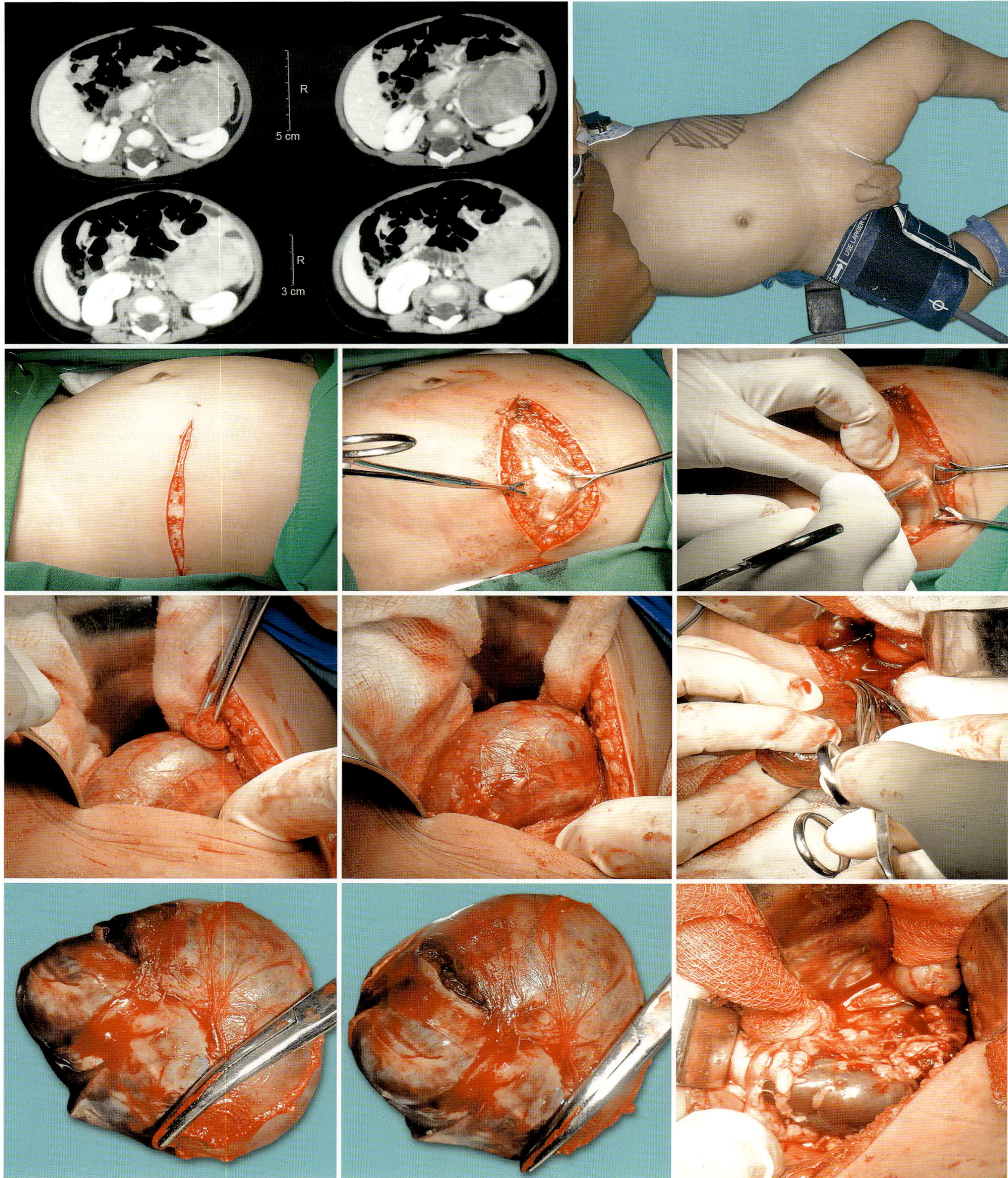

Figs. 29-9(1)

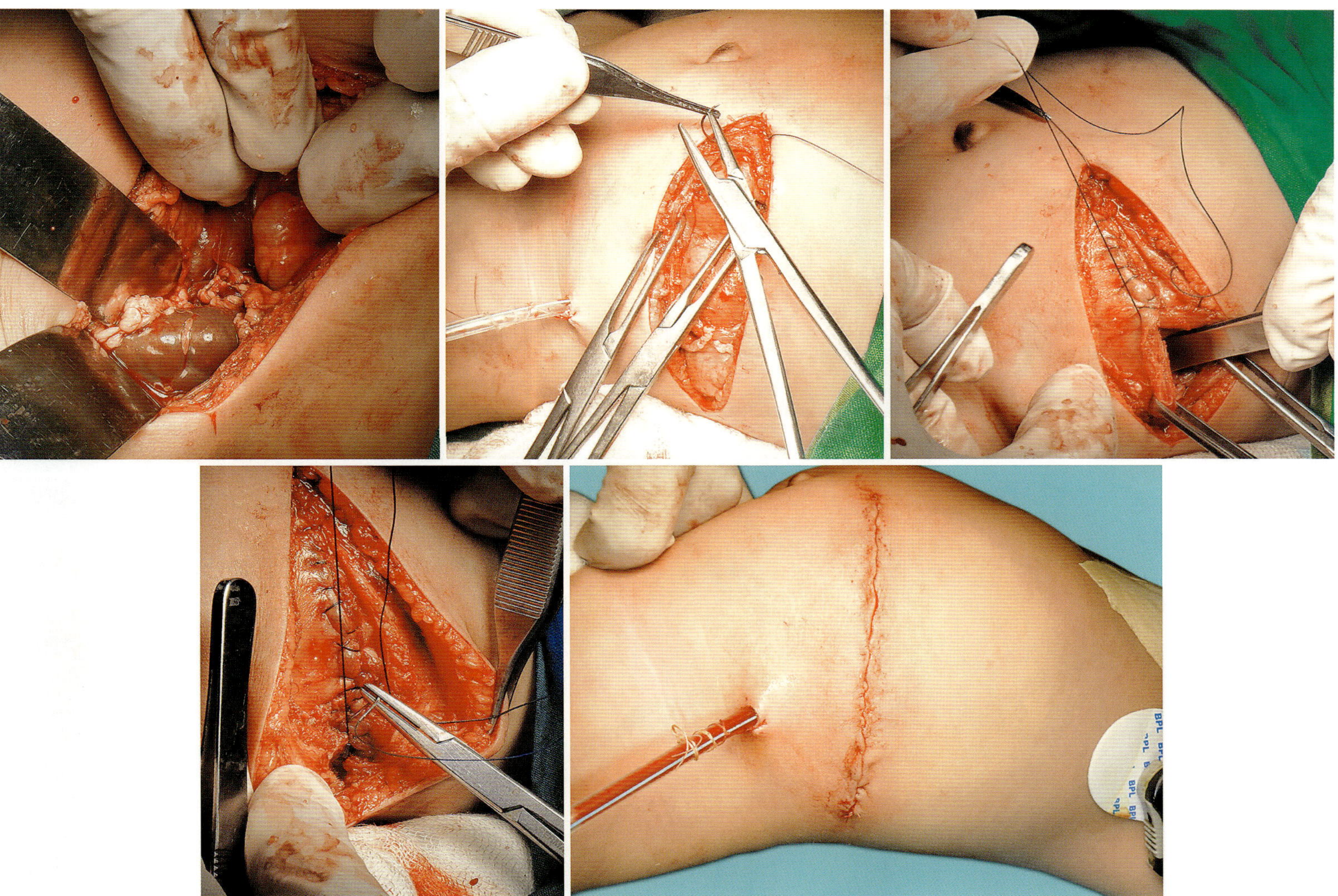

Figs. 29-9(2)

Figs. 29-9(1 and 2): Left-sided adrenalectomy in a child—neuroblastoma.

after careful dissection is clipped and divided. Remaining dissection is done using harmonic device. Haemodynamic and respiratory complications are less here.

Lateral retroperitoneal approach: Here retroperitoneum is approached in lateral position. Initial access port is placed in midaxillary line 3 cm above the iliac crest between latissimus dorsi and external oblique muscles. By open method retroperitoneum is reached; using finger or balloon space is created and widened. Additional ports are placed along the same line. Remaining dissection is same as posterior approach. Advantage here is conversion can be done when needed easily as transperitoneal approach.

Laparoscopic Right Adrenalectomy

Procedure is done under general anaesthesia with lateral decubitus position with right side upward (left lateral decubitus). Reverse Trendelenburg position (head up) is needed. Nasogastric tube and urinary catheterisation is used usually. Central venous line is needed. Right side up with knee adjacent to table is flexed. Safety straps with padding on all pressure pints and compression stockings to both legs are placed. Usually surgeon stands on the right side with camera operator on opposite side leg end or on the right side of the surgeon and assistant is opposite to surgeon. Position can be varied depending on the surgeon's choice and comfort **(Fig. 29-11)**.

Thirty degree telescope with high definition imaging system and medical monitor is needed. Energy source like harmonic sealer is also useful. Basic laparoscopic instruments, suction irrigation device, right angled instrument are all essential. A laparoscopic ultrasound may be useful often. Through Veress needle initial access is achieved at a point two fingerbreadth below the right costal margin medial to right anterior axillary line; through it one 10 mm port is passed for camera. Another 10 mm port is placed in the midaxillary line behind the first port. Two additional 5 mm ports are placed with a 5 cm gap between along the subcostal line in front. 15 mm pressure pneumoperitoneum is needed.

Right triangular ligament is divided using hook or harmonic energy device from IVC to diaphragm. Liver is rotated medially and superiorly. Liver is kept in retracted position using fixed retractor. Retroperitoneum is exposed. Subhepatic IVC, upper pole of the kidney and adrenal gland will be visualised by further careful dissection. Hepatic flexure if required may be reflected downwards by incising its peritoneal attachment. Duodenum is identified medially and in front to IVC. Duodenum is reflected in front and medially to expose IVC further. Peritoneum between adrenal gland and IVC is incised. Dissection between IVC and medial border of the adrenal gland is done for entire length carefully and meticulously. Adrenal gland is reflected away from IVC. *Right adrenal vein* is identified running into the IVC. It is less than 1 cm in length and stout. Adrenal gland is held

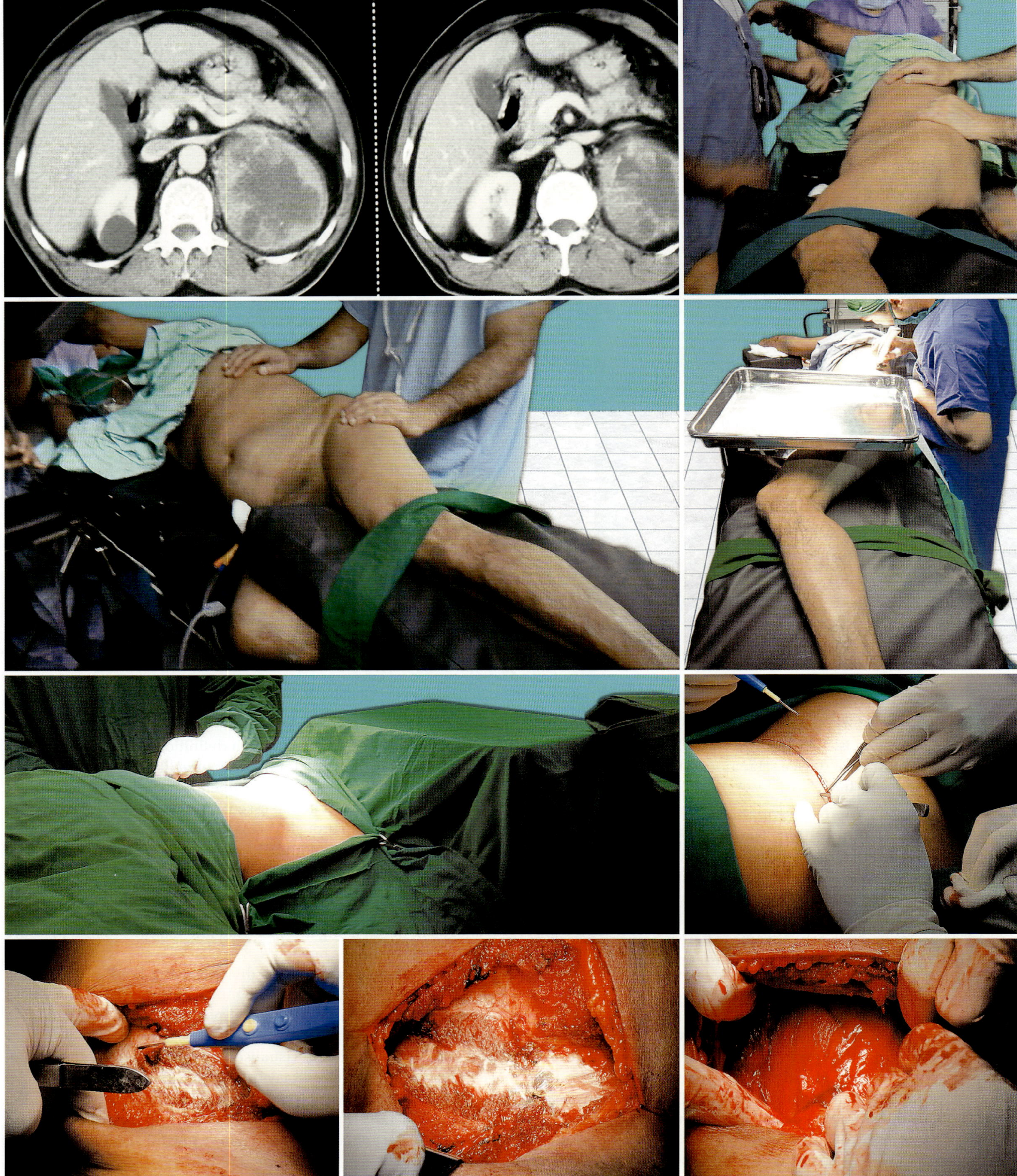

Figs. 29-10(1)

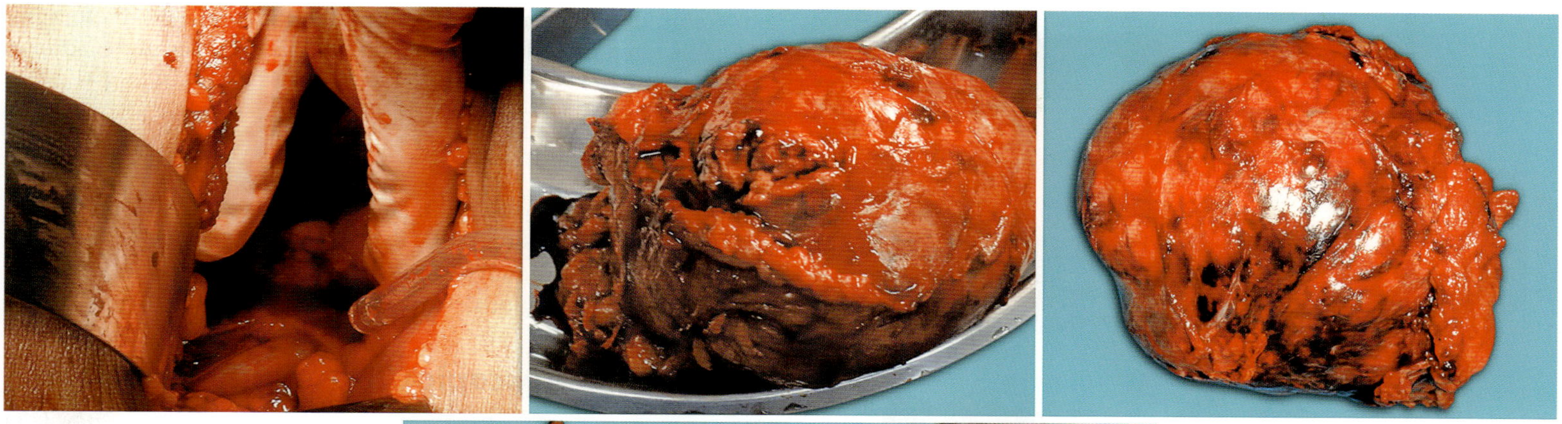

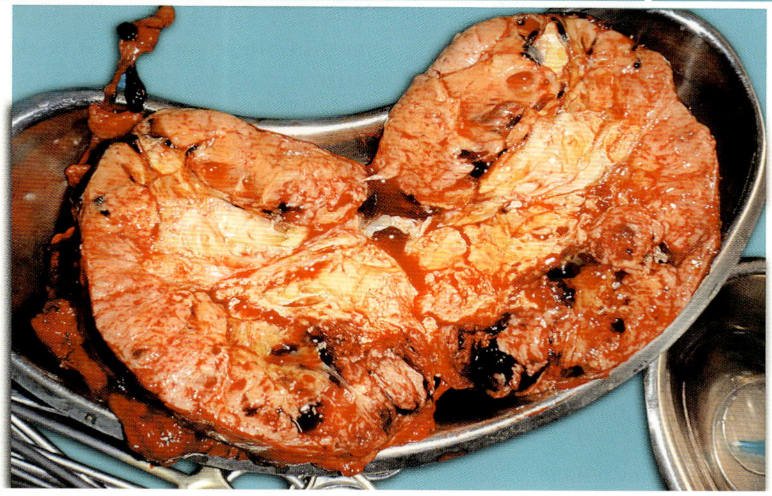

Figs. 29-10(2)

Figs. 29-10(1 and 2): Open left-sided adrenalectomy for left-sided adrenocortical carcinoma—non-functioning.

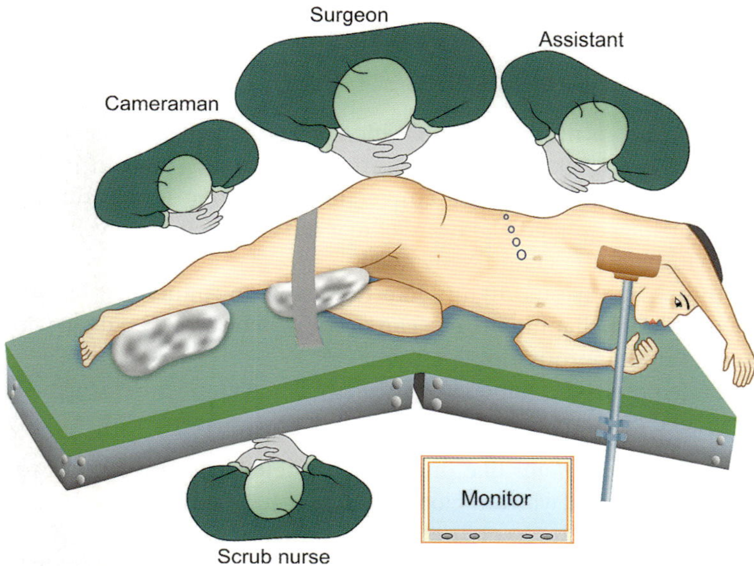

Fig. 29-11: Positions for laparoscopic right adrenalectomy.

carefully through its *periadrenal fat* and *thin fascia* and never on the gland substance as it may bleed and breach capsule causing tumour spillage. Right-angled dissector is used to isolate, separate and dissect the adrenal vein carefully. Endoclips are placed, 2 on the IVC side and one gland side. Right adrenal vein is cut to mobilise the gland from IVC. Endosutures or endovascular stapler can also be used.

Arterial branches are divided using clips or harmonic device. Anatomical *variation* of right adrenal vein which may drain at right hepatic or right renal vein instead of IVC should be remembered. Additional *right accessory adrenal vein* may exist above the level of right adrenal vein draining into right hepatic vein. *Arterial branches* are at lower level than adrenal vein and so often it is necessary to divide arterial branches first to facilitate the easier isolation of the right adrenal vein. But *in pheochromocytoma* adrenal vein should be ligated first to prevent early catecholamine release into the circulation. Adrenal gland is elevated off the IVC; posterior border is dissected off the diaphragm then lateral border. Adrenal gland is placed in impermeable pack to retrieve (retrievable bag). Adequate irrigation of adrenal bed using normal saline and also proper haemostasis is essential. Drain if needed is placed. Port sites are closed using vicryl in layers.

Laparoscopic Left Adrenalectomy

Lateral decubitus with left side upward position (right lateral decubitus) is used. Port position is similar counterpart of the right adrenalectomy. Often different port positions are advocated by many. Surgeon stands on the right side of the patient near hip region/abdomen side; camera operator left of the surgeon near left (lower) arm; assisting surgeon near head end above the left arm; staff nurse on extreme right near leg end. Camera operator can stand on the right side of the surgeon also if it seems convenient **(Fig. 29-12)**.

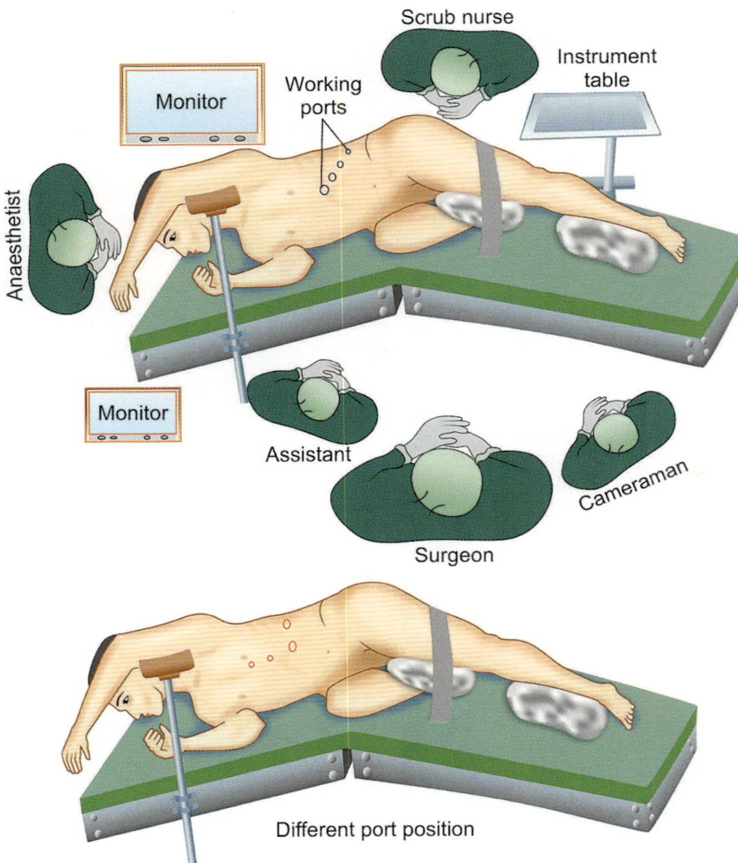

Fig. 29-12: Laparoscopic left adrenalectomy position, port placements.

Splenic flexure of colon is mobilised fully using hook or harmonic device with division of splenocolic attachment. Incision is needed along the entire length of the paracolic gutter along the *line of Toldt* and also along the upper left ½ to 2/3rd of transverse colon. Colon is reflected downwards and towards right. Splenorenal ligament is divided from lower pole of the spleen; splenic attachment to the diaphragm is divided to rotate the spleen and tail of the pancreas medially (rotated off the kidney and left adrenal gland—*open book method*). Short gastric vessels often require to be divided. Left side retroperitoneum is approached. Gerota's fascia is opened to reach the superior pole of the kidney which is dissected free of left adrenal gland.

Adrenal gland is identified between spleen and upper pole of kidney by its *golden orange colour* and fine granular texture. It is often difficult to differentiate adrenal gland (*golden orange*) from tail of the pancreas (*salmon coloured*). Laparoscopic ultrasound is useful to differentiate tail of the pancreas from adrenal gland. Adrenal gland is identified by gentle dissection. Inferomedial border of the gland is dissected first by principle. Inferior phrenic vein joins the left adrenal vein 1.5 cm above the level of the left renal vein. If dissection here found to be difficult then its upper, lateral and medial borders is mobilised first and later inferomedial border is addressed. *Left adrenal vein* is dissected using right angle instrument and doubly ligated or clips are applied. Renal vessels should be identified and safeguarded. Left renal artery is above and behind the left renal vein. Left adrenal vein joins left renal vein from above crossing the left renal artery vertically in front. Left inferior adrenal artery arises from left renal artery also to be clipped or ligated. Injury can occur to colon, diaphragm, spleen, tail of the pancreas and diaphragm. Drain is often placed after irrigation and haemostasis of the adrenal bed. Ports are closed in layers.

Conversion Rate

Cause for conversion is bleeding from adrenal vein during dissection. 5–10% is the conversion rate. Learning curve raises the conversion rate. When needed conversion should be postponed to minimise the further complications.

Role of Laparoscopic Ultrasound

It is very useful in identifying small tumours especially in left side and in obese patients. It is also useful in assessing the adjacent structures like renal vessels, IVC. Adrenal vein is difficult to identify through laparoscopic ultrasound. It is useful in identifying associated pathology in other organs and also while doing partial adrenalectomy.

Laparoscopic Partial Adrenalectomy/ Cortex Sparing Adrenalectomy

It is done *selectively* in a small peripherally located bilateral benign tumours or unilateral tumour (peripheral aldosteronoma) wherein opposite side adrenalectomy is already done. Tumour should not be lying close to or over the adrenal vein. Tumour is excised with a 0.5 cm margin of normal adrenal gland. Dissection is done using harmonic scalpel. Haemostasis is achieved using ligaseal or bipolar cautery. Adrenal vein can be preserved in this technique. *Problems* are—tumour spillage and recurrence of tumour even in benign lesion.

Complications and Problems of Laparoscopic Adrenalectomy

Haemorrhage is the main complication of laparoscopic adrenalectomy mainly during dissection of adrenal vein causing tear in IVC or left renal vein. Immediate conversion into open and control of haemorrhage is needed. Suring of tear in IVC or left renal vein after applying vascular clamp is the need.

Injury to various organs like liver, spleen, pancreas, kidney, colon, pleura, diaphragm, etc. can occur which should be dealt with accordingly appropriately.

Pancreatitis and pancreatic fistula may develop which is usually managed conservatively.

Respiratory problems like pneumonia, atelectasis, pneumothorax which is managed with antibiotic, intercostal tube drainage, antibiotics. Pneumothorax due to pleural injury and entry of CO_2 into thoracic cavity is specific problem related to laparoscopic adrenalectomy. In such situation patient if maintains the adequate saturation, laparoscopic procedure can be continued; otherwise conversion is needed.

Deep venous thrombosis, pulmonary embolism needs proper heparin prophylaxis.

Postoperative ileus, port site infection, port site hernia should be treated with antibiotics, conservative treatment and hernia repair.

Acute adrenal insufficiency may be fatal which should be treated with hydrocortisone of adequate dose.

Other complications are—nerve compression, compartment syndrome, renovascular hypertension, lymphocele, tumour recurrence, arrhythmias.

Variation in adrenal vein anatomy on the right side may confuse with right renal vein. Any vein which is not amenable to endoclip comfortably should be cautioned and differentiated from right renal vein.

On left side tail of the pancreas may be mistaken for adrenal gland. Often it may require laparoscopic ultrasound to differentiate. Adrenal gland is bright variegated dark yellow with fine granularity whereas pancreas is greyish white in colour. Upper pole segmental renal artery may be mistaken for adrenal artery. If adrenal artery is more than 0.5 mm in diameter then it is better to reconfirm its identity.

During retraction, liver or spleen may get lacerated during laparoscopy. Cautery injury to adjacent organs can also occur.

In *obese patients,* dissection of adrenal may be difficult due to large quantity of fat covering the adrenal gland. Laparoscopic ultrasound may be useful in such situation.

In *potentially curable adrenal malignancy,* laparoscopic approach is not advised until now.

Remember

- Careful selection of patient for laparoscopic adrenalectomy or open method is important.
- Laparoscopic adrenalectomy is the gold standard for benign adrenal tumours, tumours less than 6 cm sized.
- Malignant adrenal tumours, tumour more than 6–8 cm, previous upper abdominal surgery needs open adrenalectomy.
- Hormonal assessment is a must in all adrenal tumours to identify whether they are functioning or non-functioning tumours.
- In pheochromocytoma, on table hypertensive exacerbations are observed. After surgery, hypotension can occur which should be controlled. Postoperative hypoglycaemia is another complication after surgical extirpation.
- Adrenal vein should be ligated first ideally. Ligation of the adrenal vein is crucial step in adrenalectomy.
- Right adrenal vein is short and stout joins IVC posterolaterally. Right adrenal vein begins at the superior part of the hilum of the right adrenal gland. Right adrenal arteries runs from their origin behind the IVC to enter the right adrenal gland.
- Right adrenal gland is little more away and above than right renal vessels compared to left adrenal gland which is close to left renal vessels.
- During dissection adrenal capsule should not be breached to prevent tumour spill over. Gland should be held only over periadrenal fat and fascia using fine forceps.
- Ideally gland after removal should not be morcellated instead it should be retrieved using a retrieval impermeable bag.

30

CHAPTER

Surgeries of Penis, Scrotum and Testis

SURGICAL ANATOMY OF PENIS

Penis has got two parts—root and body.

Root of the Penis

Root of the penis is located in superficial perineal pouch containing two crura and one bulb. Each crus is attached to pubic arch and is covered by ischiocavernosus. Bulb is attached to perineal membrane in between crura and is covered by bulbospongiosus. Urethra pierces its deep surface traversing bulbospongiosus. Ischiocavernosus becomes corpus cavernosum (two in number one on each side); bulbospongiosus forms corpus spongiosum **(Fig. 30-1)**.

Body of Penis

It is covered by dark coloured thin skin, begins at pubic symphysis; contains two corpora cavernosa which are extensions of ischiocavernosa of both sides from the root and corpus spongiosum which is continuation of the bulbospongiosus located in the median plane.

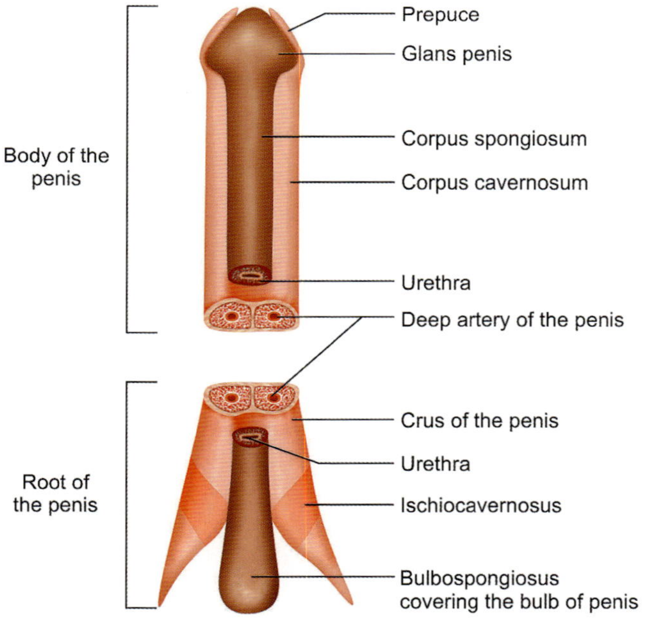

Body of the penis
Prepuce
Glans penis
Corpus spongiosum
Corpus cavernosum
Urethra
Deep artery of the penis
Root of the penis
Crus of the penis
Urethra
Ischiocavernosus
Bulbospongiosus covering the bulb of penis

Fig. 30-1: Parts of the penis—root and body.

Corpora cavernosa does not reach the end of the penis; each ends under cover of the glans. Tunica albuginea, a strong fibrous cover surrounds the corpora cavernosa of the penis; it has got superficial part which is longitudinal and covers both corpora; deep part which is circular surrounds each corpus separately with a median septum in between. Corpus spongiosum forms glans penis. Projecting margin at the base of glans is called as corona glandis with groove just proximal to it, which is neck of the penis. Dilated portion of the urethra within the root of the glans is called as navicular fossa **(Fig. 30-2)**.

Skin over the Penis

Skin over the glans continues as prepuce; it is foreskin which is freely mobile over the glans and has got two layers. On the ventral surface of the glans skin forms a fold called as frenulum. Preputial sac is a potential space between foreskin and glans. Numerous preputial sebaceous glands on the corona glandis and neck secrete smegma a sebaceous material which collects in the sac.

Fascia of the Penis

Inner Scarpa's membranous part of the superficial layer of the abdomen continues below over the penis as superficial fascia of penis which contains only areolar tissue and few muscle fibres without any fat (fat is totally absent). This superficial fascia contains superficial dorsal vein of the penis. Deep fascia of penis is actual fascia of penis called as Buck's fascia. Buck's fascia covers

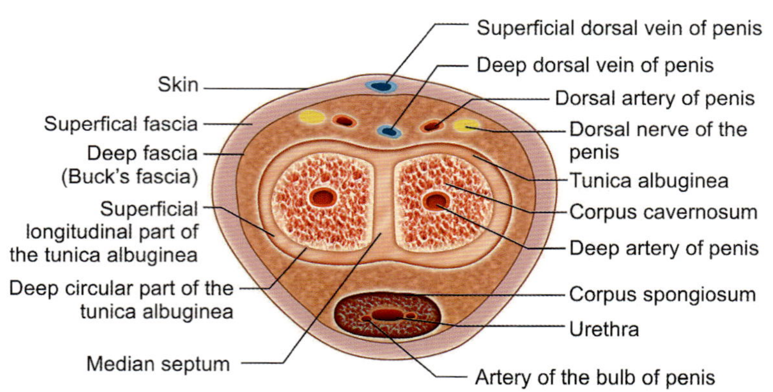

Fig. 30-2: Coverings and anatomy of penis (cross section).

both cavernosa and spongiosum; it does not extend into the glans. Deep dorsal vein, dorsal arteries, dorsal nerves are deep to Buck's fascia. Only proximally, it is covered with Dartos.

Ligaments of the Penis

Linea alba extends downwards as fundiform ligament of penis which splits to cover the penis. Deep to the fundiform ligament lies the suspensory ligament of penis, which extends from pubic symphysis and blends with deep fascia of the penis.

Arterial Supply of Penis

Internal pudendal artery supplies penis, which is a smaller terminal branch of anterior division of internal iliac artery. It runs downwards in front of the pyriformis, sacral plexus and inferior gluteal artery; pierces the pelvic fascia passing through the greater sciatic foramen below the pyriformis; from the gluteal region it enters the pudendal canal across the ischial spine. It gives three branches to penis. *Artery of the bulb* of penis supplies bulb and proximal half of the corpus spongiosum. *Deep artery of the penis* runs in the corpus cavernosum forming helicine arteries. *Dorsal artery of the penis* runs deep to deep fascia on the dorsum supplying distal part of the corpus spongiosum, glans penis, prepuce and frenulum. Skin and superficial fascia of the penis is supplied by the superficial external pudendal artery, a branch of femoral artery **(Fig. 30-3)**.

Venous Drainage of Penis

Single superficial dorsal vein lies in the superficial fascia; later divides into right and left branches draining into superficial external pudendal vein on each side. Deep dorsal vein is deep to deep fascia runs proximally between pubic symphysis and perineal membrane to drain into the prostatic plexus of veins. Dorsal vein, deep cavernosus vein, vein of the bulb drain to the internal pudendal vein.

Nerve Supply of the Penis

Sensory supply is from dorsal nerve of the penis and ilioinguinal nerve. Motor (to muscles) supply is by perineal branch of the pudendal nerve. Autonomic supply is from pelvic plexus through prostatic plexus (S2,3,4).

Pudendal Canal

It is the fascial tunnel just above the sacrotuberous ligament which travels forward on the lateral wall of the ischiorectal fossa 4 cm above the ischial tuberosity, leading from the lesser sciatic foramen posteriorly to the perineal membrane anteriorly. It contains internal pudendal vessels and pudendal nerve. It is formed by splitting of the fascia lunata with obturator fascia laterally and perineal fascia medially.

Pudendal nerve is derived from ventral divisions of S2, 3, 4 nerve roots leaving the pelvis (between pyriformis and coccygeus) to enter gluteal region medial to internal pudendal vessels and sciatic nerve through the greater sciatic foramen; crosses ischial spine to enter into the pelvis through lesser sciatic foramen and runs at the lateral wall of the ischiorectal fossa. It is the main nerve of the perineum and external genitalia. Branches—inferior rectal nerve supplies the external sphincter, levator ani, skin of the anal canal and anus. Anus also gets its nerve supply from perineal branch of 4th sacral nerve, perforating cutaneous branches of the 2nd and 3rd sacral nerves and gluteal branches of posterior cutaneous nerve of the thigh. Perineal branch (larger terminal branch) gives medial and lateral posterior scrotal/labial branches and supplies urogenital diaphragm. Dorsal nerve of the penis or clitoris is purely sensory. It supplies skin of the body of penis and glans or clitoris **(Fig. 30-4)**.

Pudendal nerve block is done by blocking the nerve with local anaesthetic agent where it crosses the ischial spine. Ischial spine is palpated per vaginally. Sensory branches of the perineal skin are also derived from ilioinguinal nerve, perineal branch of posterior cutaneous nerve of the thigh and genital branch of genitofemoral nerve.

Pudendal artery is branch of internal iliac artery. From its origin it follows same path as the pudendal nerve on its medial side to supply perineum. It gives inferior rectal artery, perineal artery and artery of penis or clitoris. In females it is much smaller.

TREATMENT OF CHORDEE

Chordee due to hypospadias is corrected by staged procedure. In chordee following circumcision, initially stilbestrol 6 mg is given daily. Later chordee is corrected surgically by excising fibrous

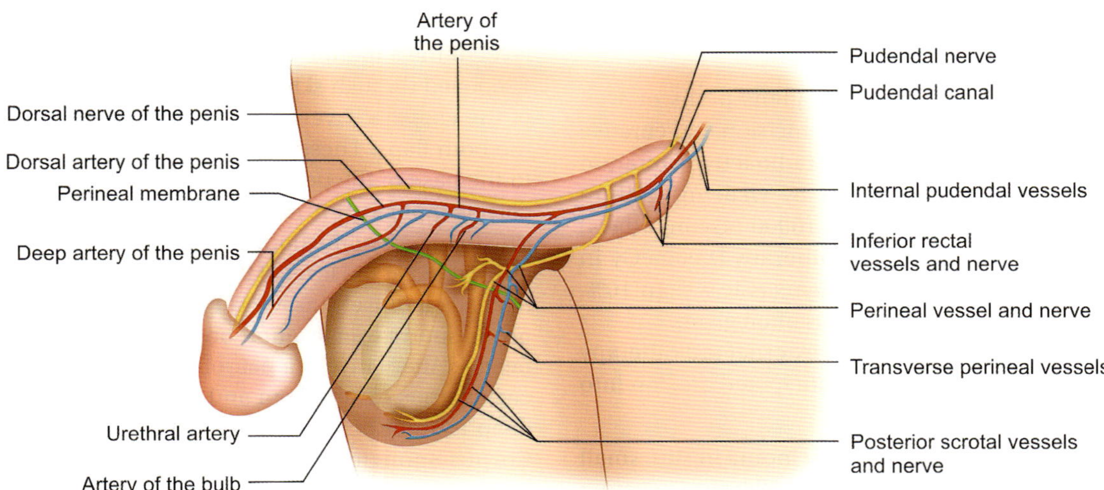

Fig. 30-3: Blood and nerve supply of penis.

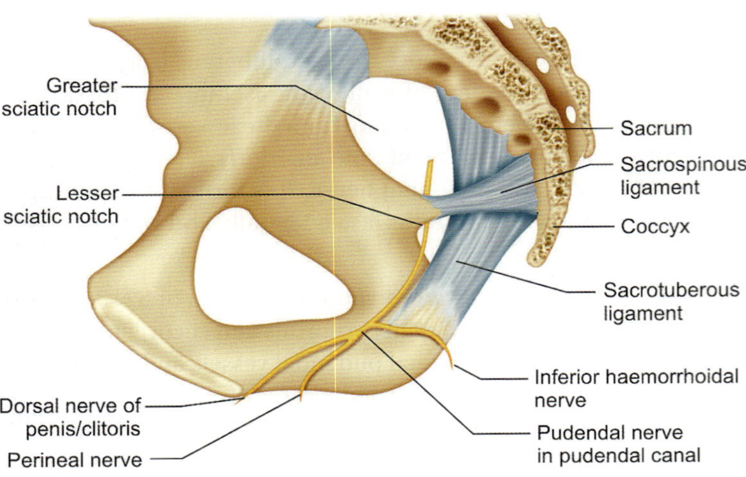

Fig. 30-4: Anatomy of pudendal nerve.

tissue followed by skin grafting. More often they require surgical intervention.

TREATMENT PEYRONIE'S DISEASE (INDURATIO-PENIS PLASTICA)

Some cases resolve spontaneously. Drugs—steroids; vitamin E; potassium aminobenzoate 12 mg/day; tamoxifen 20 mg daily; terfenadine and fexafenadine; colchicine therapy; intralesional injection of verapamil 10 mg once in 2 weeks—12 injections.

Surgery is needed in many cases. Excision and plication to opposite side is done—*Fitzpatrick operation*. Multiple incisions over the fibrous plaque and temporal fascia bridging gives often good success—*Gelhard's operation*. Excision of fibrous plaque and corporotomy is covered with overlay flap like tunica vaginalis flap (*Lockhart's*)/ dermal flap (*Devine and Horton's*). Intracorporeal penile prosthesis placement is often needed.

TREATMENT OF CARCINOMA OF PENIS

Sentinel lymph node biopsy: ***Cabana sentinel node*** is located above and medial to the junction of saphenous and femoral vein. It is the first node to get involved in carcinoma penis. So this sentinel lymph node biopsy (SLNB) after isosulphan blue dye injection into the primary is done to decide for the necessity for ilioinguinal block dissection. In operable cases surgery is the prime and initial method of treatment.

In case of carcinoma in situ, T1 lesion of glans penis or well differentiated tumour in young individual, circumcision and curative radiotherapy to the penis can be given using radioactive tantalum wire implantation (6000 cGy in 7 days) or by wearing radium penile mould continuously or intermittently (6000 cGy in 7 days) or by linear accelerator external beam radiotherapy (6000 cGy in 5 weeks). Involvement of nodes in these patients is less than 10%. Postoperative radiotherapy to inguinal region is often given.

In advanced fixed inguinal nodes palliative external radiotherapy is given. It is to palliate pain, fungation and anticipated erosion into femoral vessels.

Role of radiotherapy in carcinoma penis: Carcinoma in situ; small lesion less than 2 cm; lesion confined to glans; small lesion in young individual; advanced inoperable disease; palliation to inoperable inguinal nodes in groin; postoperative RT.

Staging of carcinoma of penis

Jackson's staging of carcinoma penis:

Stage I – Tumour involving only 90% five-year glans/prepuce/both survival
Stage II – Tumour extending into 70% body of penis
Stage III – Tumour having mobile 50% inguinal nodes
Stage IV – Tumour spreading to 5% adjacent structures/fixed nodes

TNM staging:

T_0 – No primary tumour
Tis – Carcinoma in situ
T_1 – Tumour <2 cm without deep invasion
T_2 – Tumour between 2 cm and 5 cm with minimal deep invasion
T_3 – Tumour >5 cm with deep invasion/urethral spread
T_4 – Tumour spread to adjacent tissues
N_0 – No nodal spread
N_1 – Mobile regional nodes—unilateral
N_2 – Mobile regional nodes—bilateral
N_3 – Fixed regional nodes
M_0 – No distant spread
M_1 – Distant spread present

Topical 5 FU cream or Nd:YAG laser photoirradiation is useful in carcinoma in situ.

Chemotherapy: 5 FU; methotrexate, bleomycin, cisplatin and vincristine are useful. MBP/VBM combinations are used. Bleomycin is a radiosensitiser and so beneficial if RT is planned later.

Partial Amputation of the Penis

If growth involves the glans or prepuce without extending into the proximal part of shaft of the penis, then *partial amputation of the penis* is done. In olden days if growth is extending to the body then partial amputation was not done; instead total amputation was done. A length of 2.5 cm stump is retained. Clearance of 2 cm from the proximal extended part of the tumor is needed. Advantage is proper streaming of the urine is possible.

Under spinal anaesthesia, in supine position cleaning and draping is done including both groins. Red rubber catheter is passed per urethrally which facilitates the easier identification and dissection of the urethra in the corpus spongiosum. A rubber tourniquet to the base of the penis may be used. Incision is by flap method. Two flaps are used. Dorsal/superior flap is 2.5 cm from the root of the penis; ventral or inferior flap is longer by 1 cm so that urethra is brought out through this flap in its centre and closed wound will come on the end of the dorsal part. Inferior flap is incised through skin, subcutaneous tissue up to the fascial sheath and is initially elevated up to the level of the superior dorsal flap which is more proximal. Incision is deepened through skin and subcutaneous tissue to the fascial sheath of the corpora cavernosa and corpus spongiosum all round along the both flaps. These flaps are elevated using scissor proximally up to the base of the penis to expose the entire corpora cavernosa and corpus spongiosum. Monopolar cautery is better avoided as retained proximal part of the body may undergo necrosis. Corpora cavernosa are divided at the level of the beginning of the superior dorsal flap; as it bleeds profusely (as it is very vascular) proximal corpora cavernosa needs suture transfixation on each side using no. 1 vicryl in cutting needle. Alternatively, a pair of Kocher's clamps can be placed on the each corpus cavernosum and divided distally; transfixation are done deep to the Kocher's clamps which is released after transfixation. Corpus spongiosum with urethra is dissected, isolated carefully (prior passed red rubber catheter facilitates the easier dissection). Red rubber catheter is removed. Urethra with corpus spongiosum is divided 1.5 cm distally. Tourniquet if placed at the root of the penis should be removed now. Site of urethral passage through the ventral inferior flap is marked; stab incision is made; cut end of the urethra is passed through it. Emerged cut end of the urethra is split vertically for 1 cm; each side of the split urethra is sutured not to the edge of the stab wound of the skin but skin just beyond it to facilitate protrusion of the urethral mucosa so as to reduce the chances of stricture formation. Foley's catheter 18 F sized is passed and is kept in situ for 7 days. If stricture develops then regular dilatation of the urethra is needed.

Partial amputation of penis with bilateral ilioinguinal lymph node block dissection is called as *Young's operation* **(Figs. 30-5A to C)**.

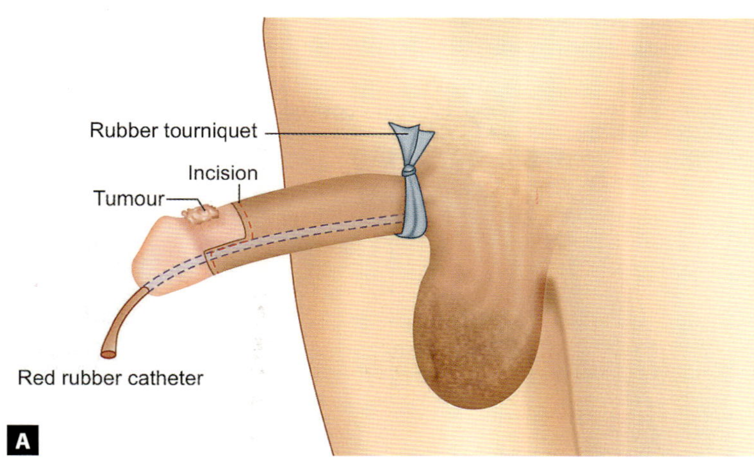

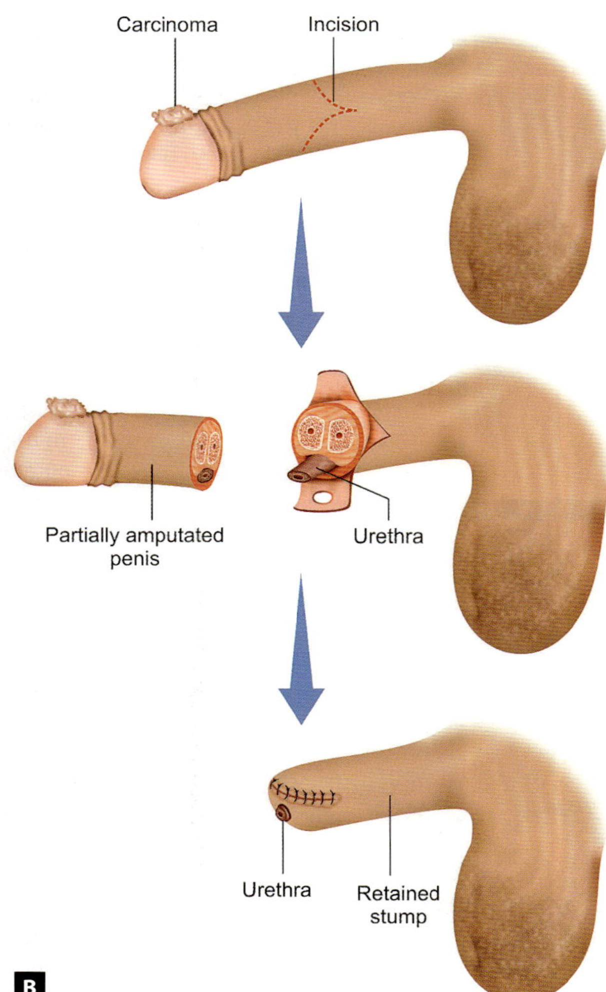

Figs. 30-5A and B

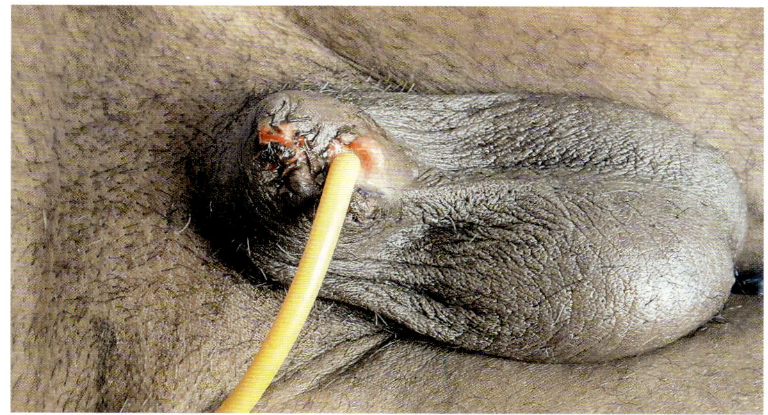

Fig. 30-5C

Figs. 30-5A to C: Partial amputation of penis with catheter in situ.

Total Amputation of Penis

If tumour involves the proximal part of the body of penis or if it is anaplastic/poorly differentiated tumour *total amputation of penis* is done with *perineal urethrostomy*. It is done when body of the penis involved and when there is impossible to do partial amputation of the penis. It is done under spinal anaesthesia **(Figs. 30-6A and B)**.

Lithotomy—Trendelenburg position is used. Red rubber catheter is passed per urethra or a metal bougie or male metal catheter can also be used for this purpose. Penile growth is covered with a sterile glove and sterile band or tie is used to fix it the body of the penis. A racquet shaped incision is made covering the penis; it begins as a vertical midline from the pubis downwards encircling the root of the penis again joining on the ventral aspect and extending downwards in the midline scrotal raphe and towards the perineum 3 cm in front of the anus. Scrotum is split into two halves; retracted laterally. Anteriorly fundiform and suspensory ligaments of the penis are split. Dorsal vessels are dissected and ligated. With blunt and sharp dissection and also using cautery perineal incision is deepened. Both crura and bulb are exposed; dissected. Bulb is separated from the perineal membrane; crura are detached from the pubic arch. Urethra is dissected from the muscular component of the bulb; red rubber catheter is removed. Urethra is transected 5 cm distal to the perineal membrane through which it passes out. No. 18 Foley's catheter is passed and inflated. Haemostasis is achieved using cautery **(Fig. 30-7)**.

Often if detachment of the crura from the pubic arch is difficult then a Kocher's clamp is applied one on each side of the corpora and is transfixed each side using thick no. 1 vicryl with cutting needle. It is impossible to transfix the corpora using round body needle.

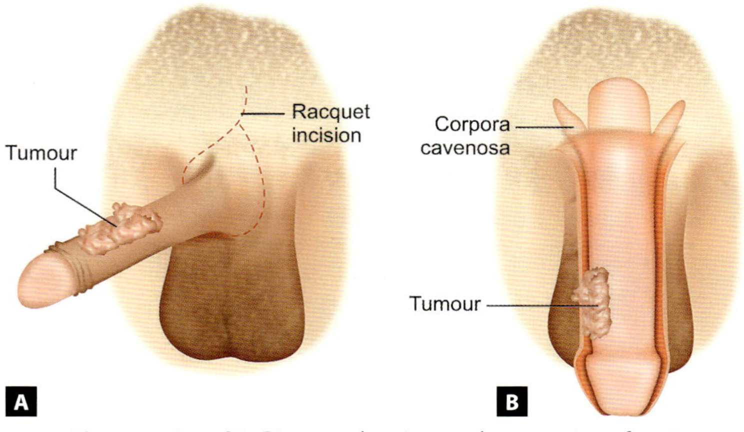

Figs. 30-6A and B: Diagram showing total amputation of penis.

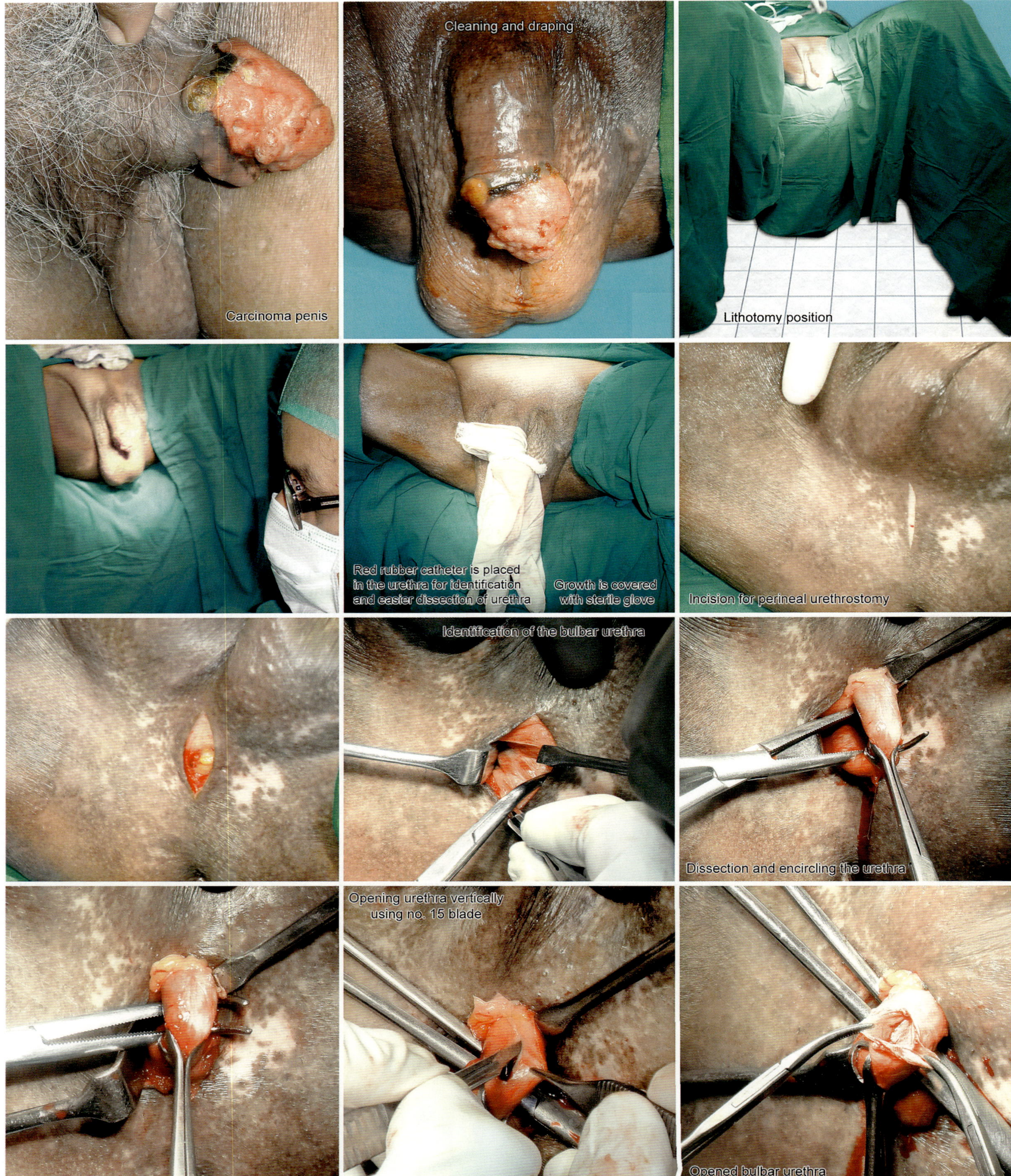
Carcinoma penis
Cleaning and draping
Lithotomy position
Red rubber catheter is placed in the urethra for identification and easier dissection of urethra
Growth is covered with sterile glove
Incision for perineal urethrostomy
Identification of the bulbar urethra
Dissection and encircling the urethra
Opening urethra vertically using no. 15 blade
Opened bulbar urethra

Figs. 30-7(1)

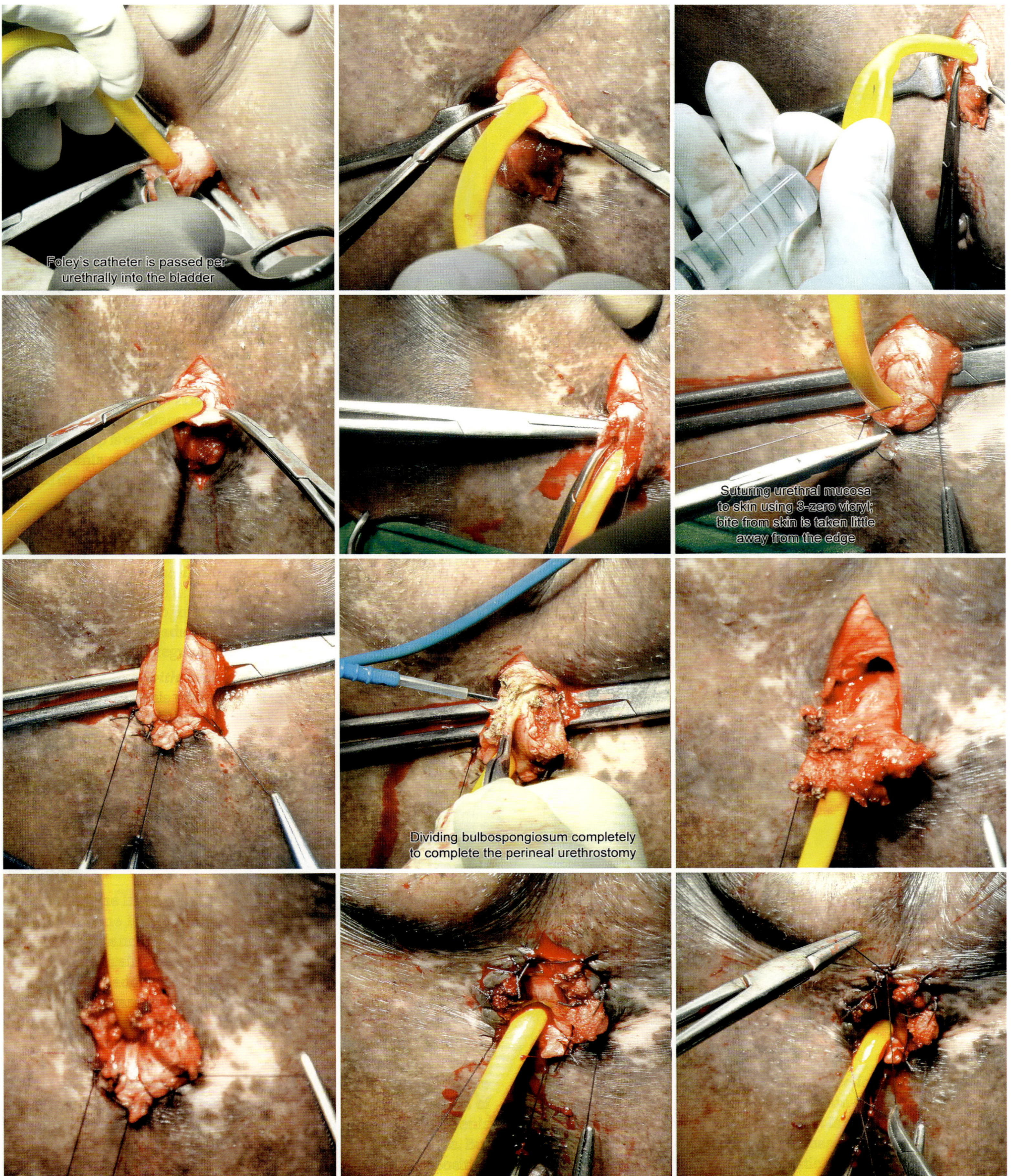
Foley's catheter is passed per urethrally into the bladder
Suturing urethral mucosa to skin using 3-zero vicryl; bite from skin is taken little away from the edge
Dividing bulbospongiosum completely to complete the perineal urethrostomy

Figs. 30-7(2)

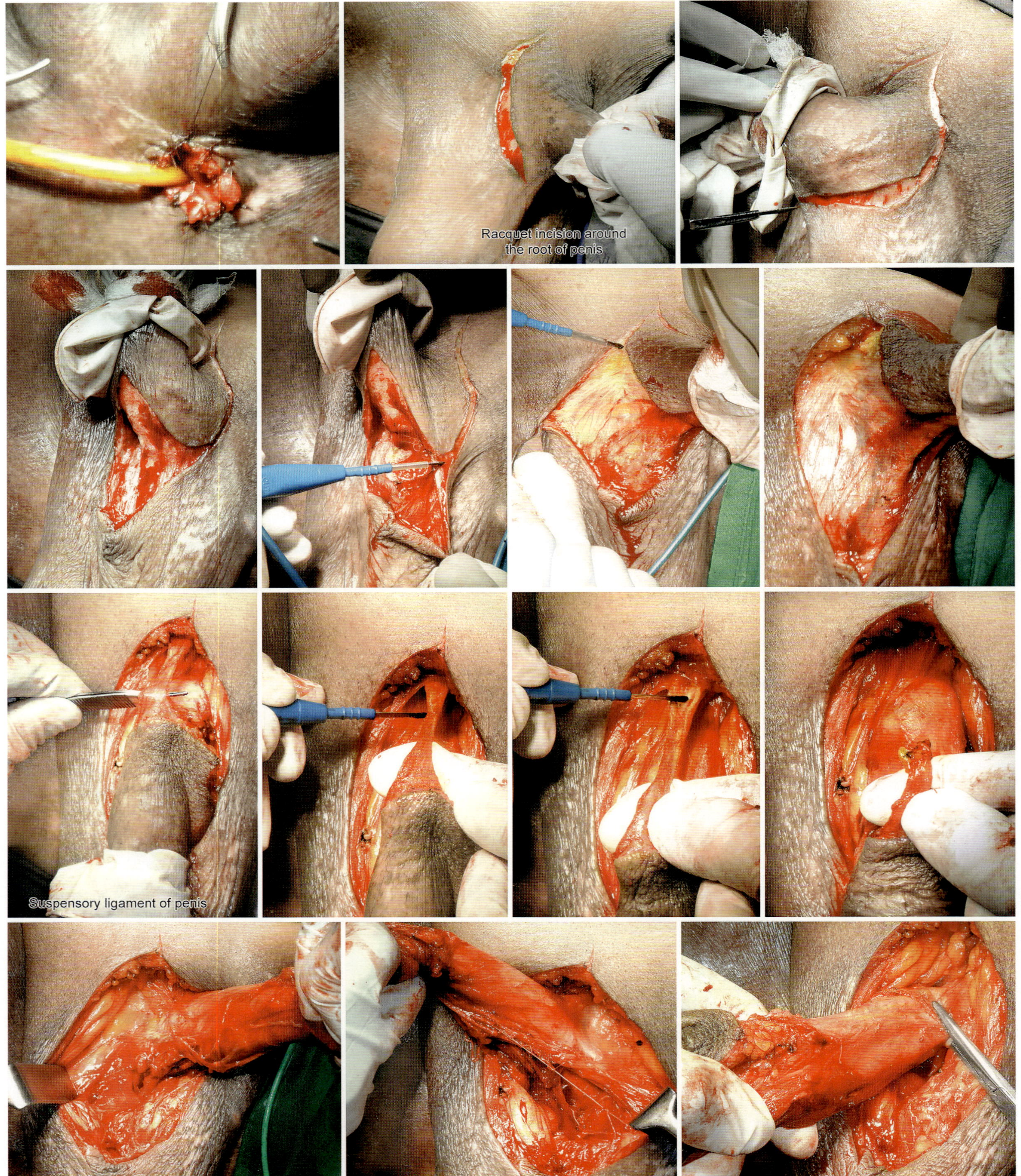
Racquet incision around
the root of penis
Suspensory ligament of penis

Figs. 30-7(3)

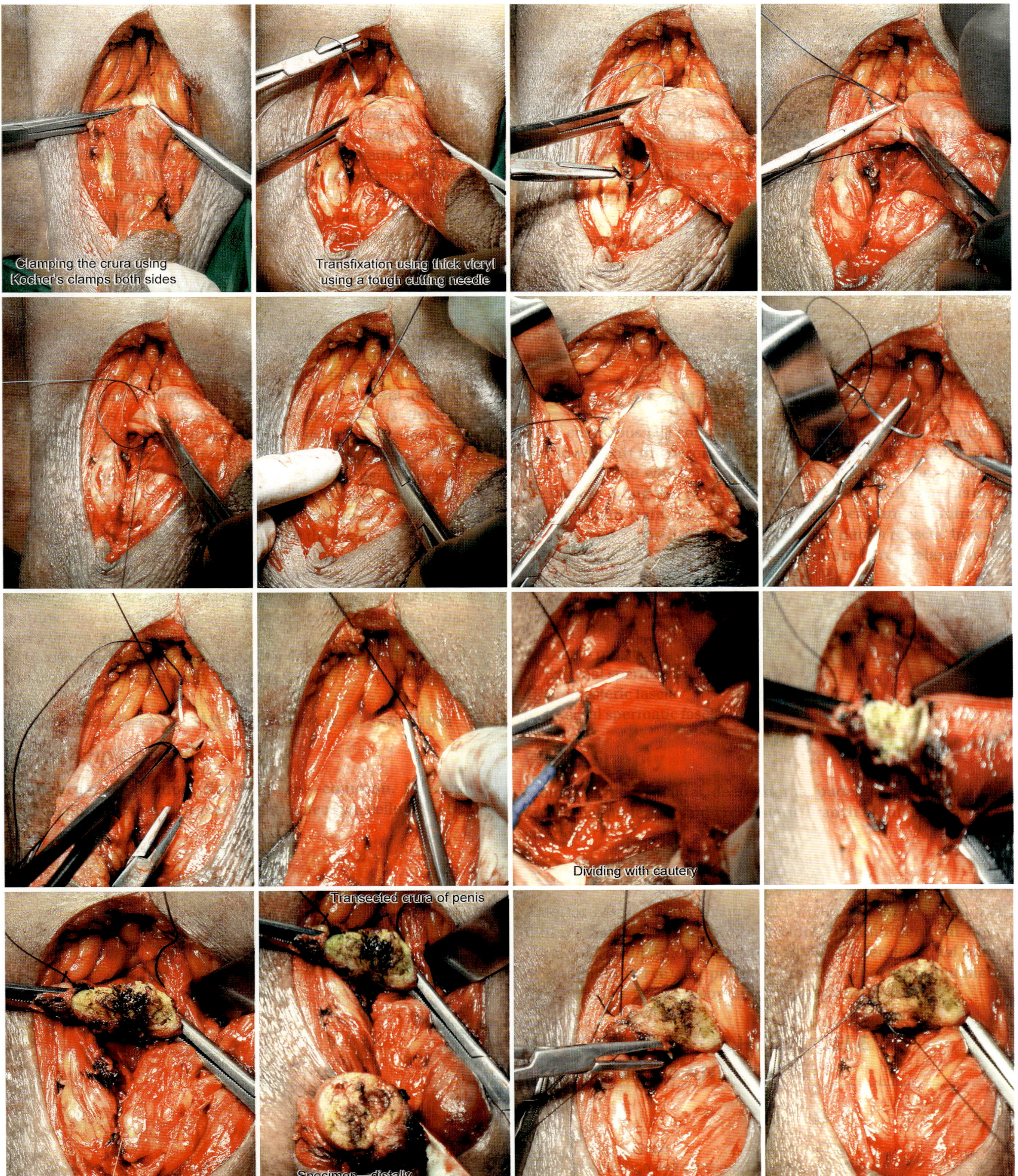
Clamping the crura using
Kocher's clamps both sides
Transfixation using thick vicryl
using a tough cutting needle
Dividing with cautery
Transected crura of penis
Specimen—distally

Figs. 30-7(4)

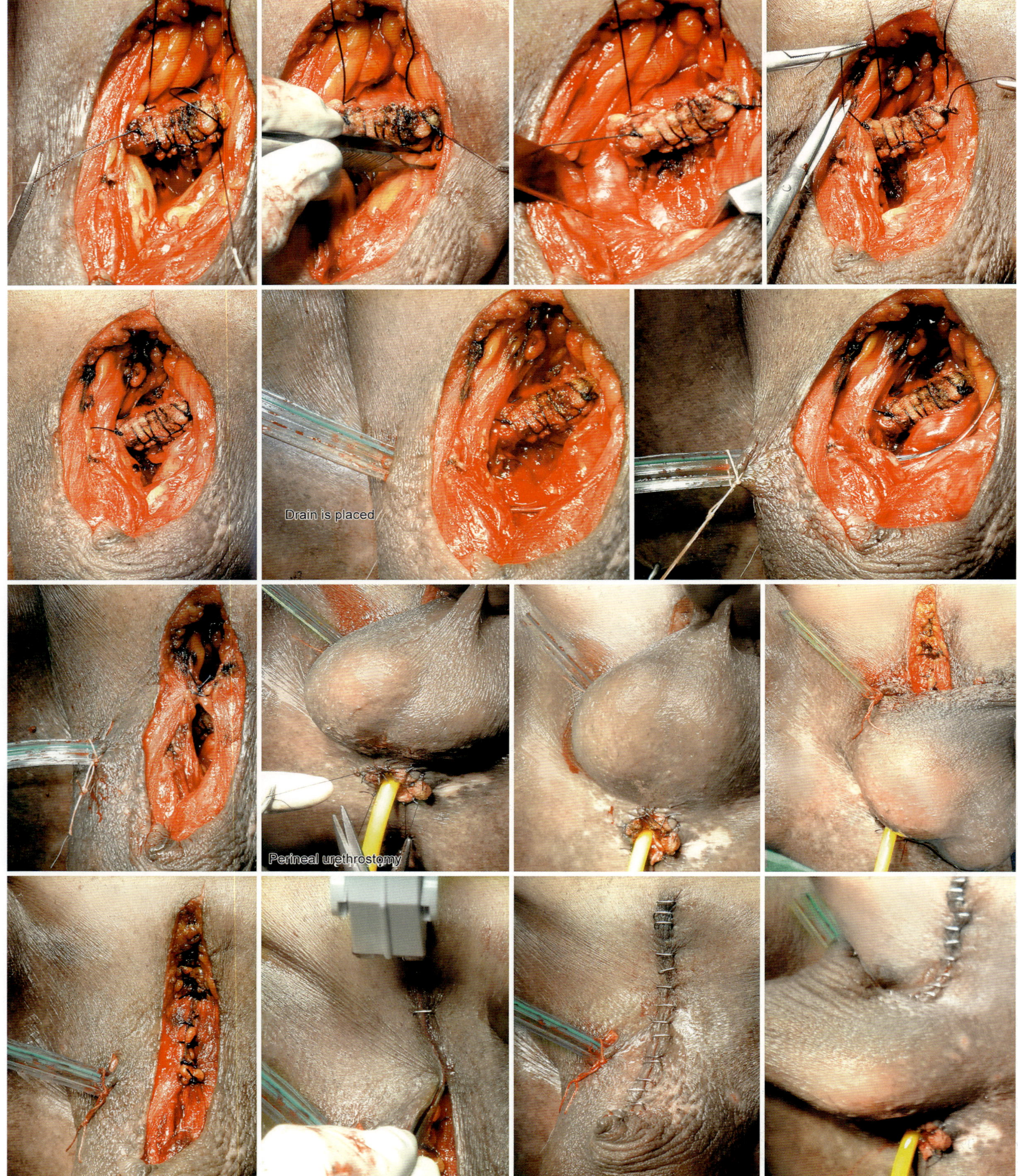

Figs. 30-7(5)

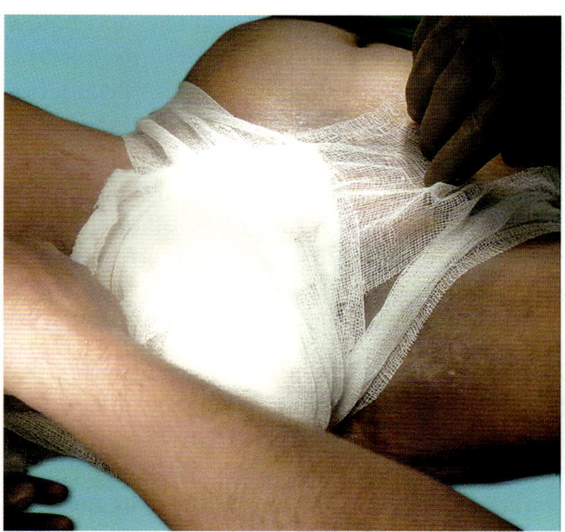
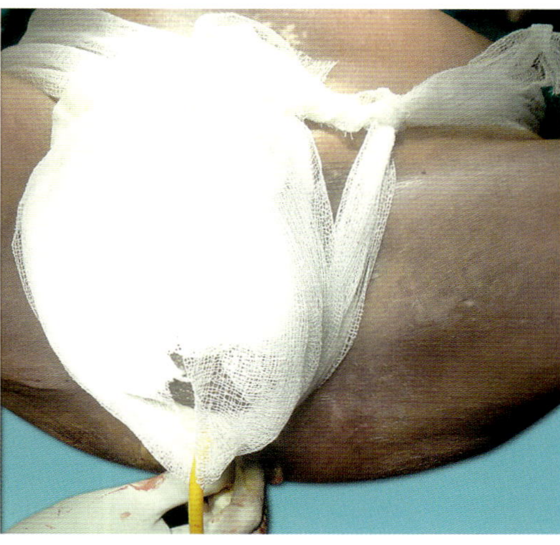
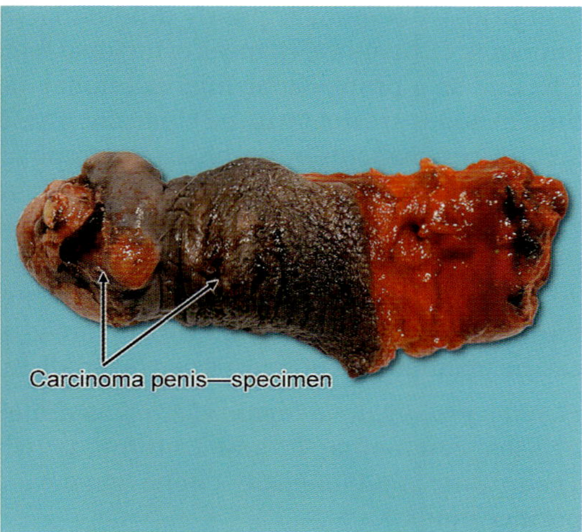

Figs. 30-7(6)

Figs. 30-7(1 to 6): Technique of total amputation of penis.

Drain is placed on the anterior part of the wound. Skin is closed vertically leaving space posteriorly for perineal urethrostomy. Urethral stump is split longitudinally for 5 mm both in front and behind (this prevents stricture formation) and is sutured to the skin little beyond the cut margin of the skin using 3 zero interrupted vicryl sutures.

Alternatively perineal urethrostomy is done first in lithotomy position. Urethra distally is transected. Racquet incision is placed around the root of the penis. And total amputation of the penis is done in same way.

Problems with perineal urethrostomy are scrotal skin ammoniacal dermatitis and stricture at urethrostomy site. Dermatitis is prevented by asking the patient to urinate in sitting position lifting the scrotum upwards. Stricture needs dilatation. Stricture of the urethra is not uncommon. It needs regular urethral dilatation **(Fig. 30-8)**.

Total scrotectomy with orchidectomy is done along with total amputation of the penis with perineal urethrostomy—*Sir Piersey Gold operation*. This avoids ammoniacal dermatitis and lymphoedema of the scrotum, a sequelae which may occur after inguinal node dissection. It also reduces the sexual desire.

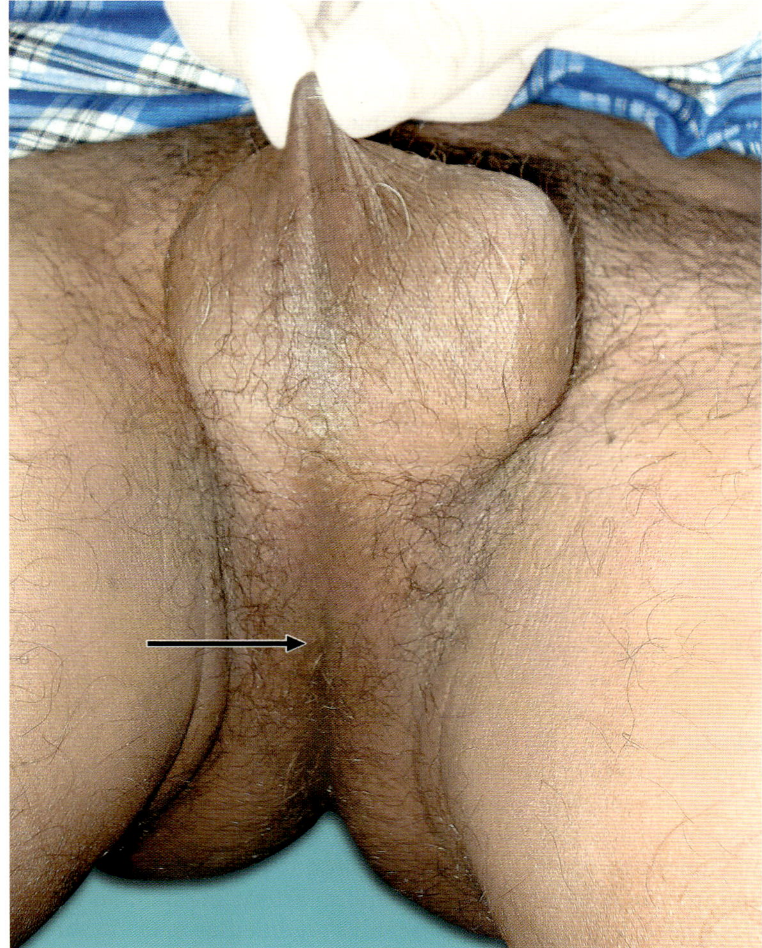

Fig. 30-8: Perineal urethrostomy with stricture in the created urethra.

INGUINAL BLOCK DISSECTION—RADICAL GROIN DISSECTION

Principles

It is clearing the inguinal nodes with fat and fascia en bloc from the groin. It is done in carcinoma penis, skin carcinomas of the limb including melanoma and squamous cell carcinoma, carcinoma anal canal or drainage areas like scrotum/vagina, etc. Dissection is done between adductor longus, sartorius, base of femoral triangle and inguinal ligament; with clearing fat and fascia 5 cm above the inguinal ligament in front of the external oblique aponeurosis. Long saphenous vein is ligated and divided 10 cm below the saphenofemoral junction. It covers the *Dresslers quadrangle*.

Presence of metastatic inguinal node even though is a more important prognostic factor than tumour grade. Even the 50–55% of patients present with palpable inguinal nodes in carcinoma penis only 50% of these patients will have histologically positive nodes. But 25% of patients without clinically palpable nodes will have positive metastatic nodes. When lymph nodes are involved on one side, contralateral nodes are involved in 50% of cases and iliac nodes are involved in 30% of cases. When lymph nodes are involved and are mobile, *bilateral ilioinguinal nodal dissection* is done. *Primary inguinal block* is doing block dissection within 4 weeks of surgery for primary tumour. *Secondary inguinal block* is doing block dissection after 4 weeks of surgery for primary disease. Only 50% of palpable inguinal nodes are involved by metastatic spread. So often a course of antibiotic is given and waited for 6 weeks. Complications of ilioinguinal block dissection are *flap necrosis*, lymphoedema of lower limb, femoral blow out, infection, lymphorrhoea and haemorrhage.

If primary tumour is poorly differentiated (high grade), and if tumour is T2 or above, chances of inguinal nodal spread is more than 50% and so a prophylactic inguinal nodal dissection is done even though nodes are not involved clinically. 5-year survival improves by 50% in these patients by prophylactic lymphadenectomy.

Often, involvement of inguinal nodes may be due to infection. So a trial of antibiotic therapy is given for 6 weeks to reduce the size of the inguinal node.

Removal of iliac nodes (pelvic lymphadenectomy) does not alter the outcome. It is done to confirm the spread, so that further therapy can be planned and prognosis can be predicted.

Elective prophylactic inguinal block is done in high-risk group—invasive carcinoma; T2 and T3 tumours; with vascular invasion. *Therapeutic inguinal block* is done whenever FNAC of node shows positive tumour.

Superficial lymph node block is dissected superficially to fascia lata in N0 disease. It should undergo frozen section biopsy. If nodes are positive, then formal block dissection should be done.
Standard inguinal lymphadenectomy—is classical block dissection.

Modified inguinal block dissection (Catalona): Small incision, limited dissection, preservation of saphenous vein—this reduces the morbidity and lymphoedema of the limb. However, there is not much evidence to confirm its advantages.

Surgical Anatomy of Femoral Region

It is a triangle shaped space in front of the upper 1/3rd of thigh immediately below the inguinal ligament; it is bounded laterally by the medial border of the sartorius medially by the medial border of the adductor longus, base is by inguinal ligament apex is below at a point of joining of sartorius and adductor longus. Roof is formed by skin, superficial fascia, superficial inguinal nodes, femoral branch of the genitofemoral nerve, branches of the ilioinguinal nerve, superficial branches of the femoral artery and associated veins, upper part of long saphenous vein, deep fascia, saphenous opening and cribriform fascia. Floor is formed by adductor longus, pectineus, iliacus and psoas major from medial to lateral. *Contents are*—femoral artery and branches (superficial external pudendal, superficial epigastric, superficial circumflex iliac; deep branches are profunda femoris, deep external pudendal and muscular); medial and lateral circumflex branches of the profunda femoris artery; femoral vein and its tributaries (vein is medial and posteromedial to artery); femoral sheath extends 4 cm along the femoral vessels; femoral nerve is lateral to artery in the iliopsoas groove; nerve to pectineus, femoral branch of genitofemoral nerve, lateral cutaneous nerve of thigh and deep inguinal lymph nodes. *Tributaries of the femoral vein are*—great saphenous vein; veins along the profunda femoris, deep external and muscular branches of the femoral artery; medial and lateral circumflex femoral veins; descending genicular vein. Branches at saphenofemoral junction are—lateral and medial circumflex femoral, external pudendal, superficial and deep circumflex iliac, superficial epigastric veins **(Fig. 30-9)**.

Femoral nerve is about 2 cm in length. It divides into anterior and posterior divisions. Anterior division supplies sartorius and gives medial and intermediate cutaneous nerves of the thigh; posterior division supplies rectus femoris, three vasti and gives saphenous nerve branch the only cutaneous one. Nerve also gives articular and vascular branches **(Fig. 30-10)**.

Superficial external pudendal artery pierces the cribriform fascia travelling medially in front of the spermatic cord supplying the external genitalia; superficial external pudendal vein lies below and medial to artery. Superficial epigastric artery pierces the cribriform fascia travels upwards towards umbilicus to supply anterior abdominal wall. Superficial epigastric vein is medial to artery. Superficial circumflex iliac artery pierces the fascia lata lateral to the saphenous opening travel upwards below the inguinal ligament anastomose with branches of the deep circumflex iliac, superior gluteal, lateral circumflex femoral arteries at the level of anterior superior iliac spine. Superficial circumflex iliac vein is below and lateral to the artery.

Dresslers quadrangle—upper border is formed by line joining anterior superior iliac spine and pubic tubercle; laterally line joining anterosuperior iliac spine and a point 20 cm below it; medially pubic tubercle and a point 15 cm below it. Nodal block dissection for carcinoma penis should cover this area adequately **(Fig. 30-11)**.

Deep fascia of thigh also called as fascia lata; is attached anteriorly to inguinal ligament, laterally to iliac crest, behind through gluteal fascia to sacrum, coccyx and sacrotuberous ligament, medially to the pubis, pubic arch and ischial tuberosity. Below it is attached to bone and knee joint and continues as popliteal fascia posteriorly. Lateral thickened 5 cm wide band called iliotibial tract splits above into superficial lamina which is attached to tubercle of iliac crest and deep lamina attached to capsule of the hip joint. Below it is attached to the anterior part of the lateral condyle of tibia. Tract stabilises the knee joint and has got insertions of gluteus maximus and tensor fascia latae in its upper part.

Saphenous oval opening in the fascia lata is 4 cm below and lateral to pubic tubercle; it is vertically 2.5 cm and transversely 2.0 cm (vertically oval); it is directed down and lateral. Its lateral crescentic sharp margin lies in front of the femoral sheath; its medial margin is deeper and is formed by pectineal fascia.

Funnel-shaped femoral sheath encloses upper 4 cm of femoral vessels; its anterior wall is formed by downward extension of transversalis fascia; its posterior wall is formed by the fascia iliaca. Sheath is asymmetrical with vertical lateral wall and oblique medial wall directed below and laterally. Sheath is divided into lateral arterial, intermediate venous and medial lymphatic compartments by two septa. Medial one is called as femoral canal 1.5 × 1.5 cm at base above (femoral ring) and narrow below. Femoral ring is bounded by fascia over pectineus behind, lacunar ligament medially, septum laterally and inguinal ligament in front **(Fig. 30-12)**.

Femoral canal contains lymph node of Cloquet (one of the deep inguinal nodes); femoral hernia can occur through it; abnormal obturator artery arising from the inferior epigastric artery or pubic branch of obturator artery may communicate with the pubic branch of inferior epigastric artery. Any of these may run on the lacunar ligament on the medial wall of the femoral canal injury of which during surgery may cause torrential haemorrhage.

Inguinal Lymph Nodes

Superficial lymph nodes drain from skin and fascia of the lower limb, perineum and trunk below the watershed umbilical line. It is classified as lower vertical; upper lateral and upper medial. Upper medial and lateral group is often called as horizontal group. *Lower vertical group (4–5)* is located along both sides of the saphenofemoral junction which drain from the lower limb except buttock. 2–3 upper lateral nodes are located below the lateral part of the inguinal ligament draining skin and fascia of lateral thigh, buttock, flank and back below the umbilical line. *2–4 upper medial nodes* are located below and medial part of the inguinal ligament; few nodes lie above the

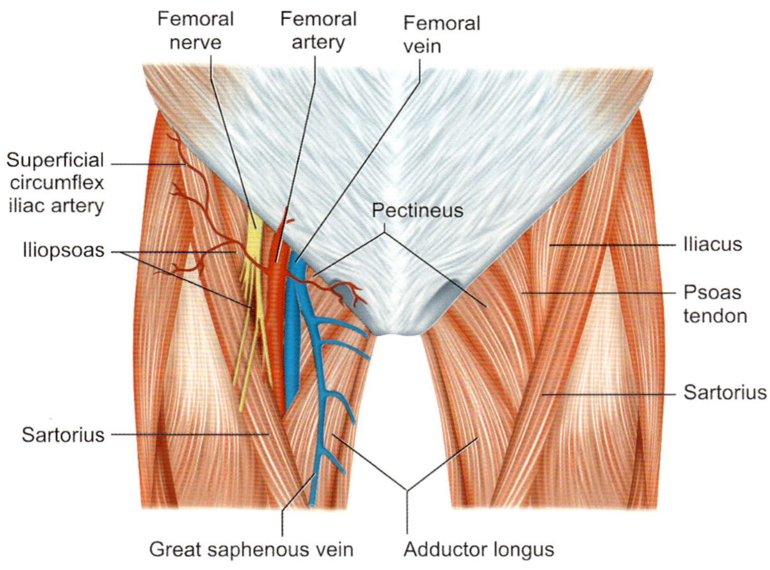

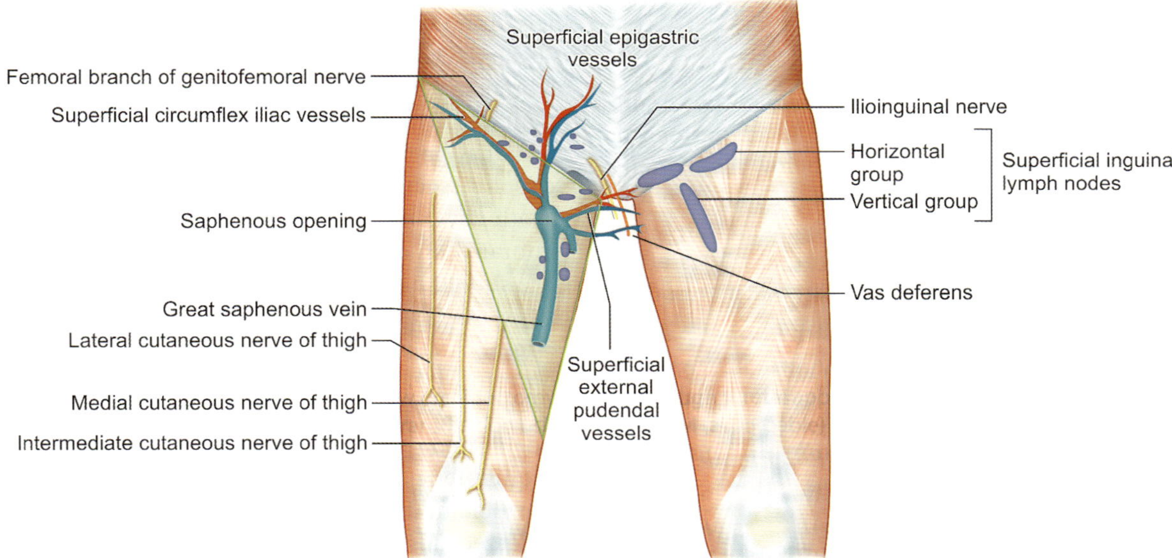

Fig. 30-9: Surgical anatomy of femoral triangle—boundaries; floor, relations; contents; inguinal lymph nodes.

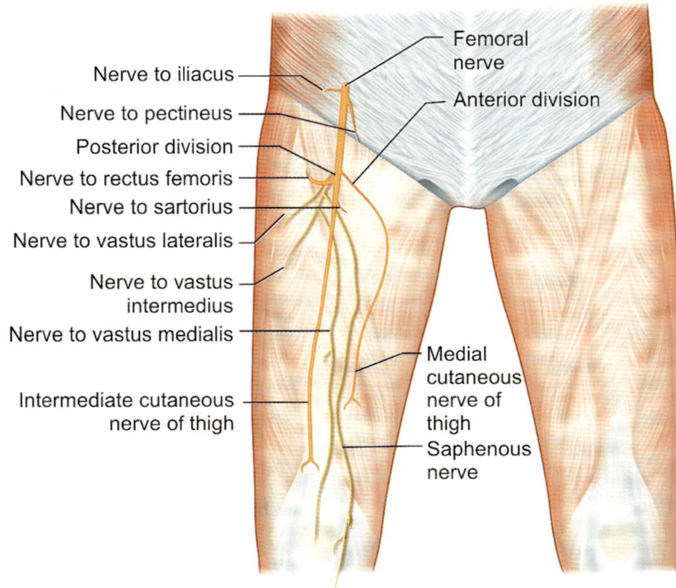

Fig. 30-10: Anatomy of femoral nerve in the thigh.

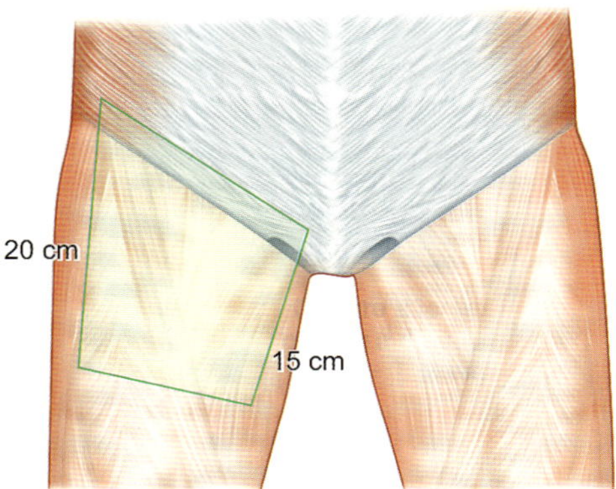

Fig. 30-11: Dressler's quadrangle.

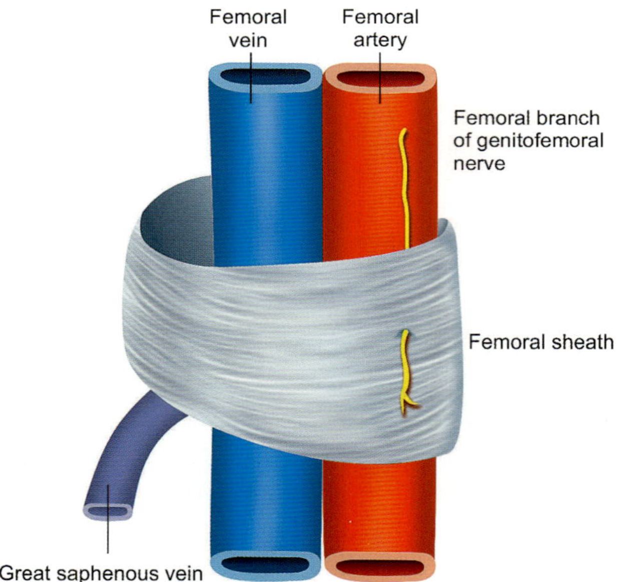

Fig. 30-12: Femoral sheath—anatomy.

inguinal ligament along the superficial epigastric vessels. They drain the anterior abdominal wall below the umbilical level; perineum with anal canal below the pectinate line, vagina below the hymen, with external genitalia except glans, penile part of the male urethra superolateral angle of the uterus through round ligament. Efferents from superficial nodes drain into the deep inguinal nodes after piercing cribriform fascia; few drain directly into external iliac nodes.

Deep inguinal nodes (4–5) are located medial to the upper part of the femoral vein. They receive afferent from superficial inguinal nodes, popliteal nodes, glans penis/clitoris and deep lymphatics of the lower limb. Efferent from deep nodes reach external iliac nodes. Proximal most deep node is called as *Cloquet/Rosenmuller* node which is located in the femoral canal.

Technique of Inguinal Block Dissection

It is properly called as *inguinofemoral lymphadenectomy*. If pelvic lymphadenectomy is added then it is called as *ilioinguinal lymphadenectomy* (Ilioinguinal block dissection).

Preoperative antibiotics are given (1 hour before surgery); heparin prophylaxis is also recommended.

It is done under spinal anaesthesia. Supine, with hip slightly abducted and knee flexed, position is used. Lower abdomen, groin, entire thigh is prepared and draped.

Different incisions are used—S; two incisions one vertical and one horizontal; two parallel incisions suprainguinal and infrainguinal; vertical L; oblique with elliptical excision (3 cm wide) of skin over the femorals **(Fig. 30-13)**.

Flap is elevated with retaining some amount of fat in the skin otherwise necrosis of skin flap will occur. 5 cm above the inguinal ligament fat and fascia is dissected towards the inguinal ligament. Flap is elevated laterally over the sartorius; medially above over the pubic tubercle to expose the cord structures and external ring; medially and below over the adductor magnus up to the apex of the femoral triangle. Great saphenous vein is identified at the apex and ligated. Fascia over the sartorius adductor magnus and pectineus can be removed along the specimen. Fascia over the sartorius is incised and swept medially; near the apex long/great saphenous vein is ligated. Dissection begins from lateral aspect extended medially; all branches of the femoral vessels are ligated, divided or clipped or fulgurated. Bipolar cautery is better otherwise branches of femoral nerve may be injured especially motor nerves (if monopolar is used). Scissor dissection offers good mobilisation of the tissues. Femoral sheath covering the femoral vessels is incised to expose the both femoral vein and artery; femoral vein is posteromedial to artery. Care should be taken not to injure the vein. Small direct branches of the vessels are ligated securely after meticulous dissection. Above femoral canal is identified and Cloquet's lymph node is dissected and removed. When saphenofemoral junction is reached, great saphenous vein is again ligated with transfixation. Cloquet node is bridging node between inguinal and pelvic nodes; if on frozen section Cloquet node is positive then pelvic lymphadenectomy is done to clear iliac nodes. All nodes in front of the femoral vessels should be cleared. It is better to place a retractor under the inguinal ligament and remove uppermost lymph nodes of the groin. Distilled water wash is given to the wound. Femoral canal is closed with interrupted non-absorbable sutures between lacunar ligament and inguinal ligament **(Fig. 30-14)**.

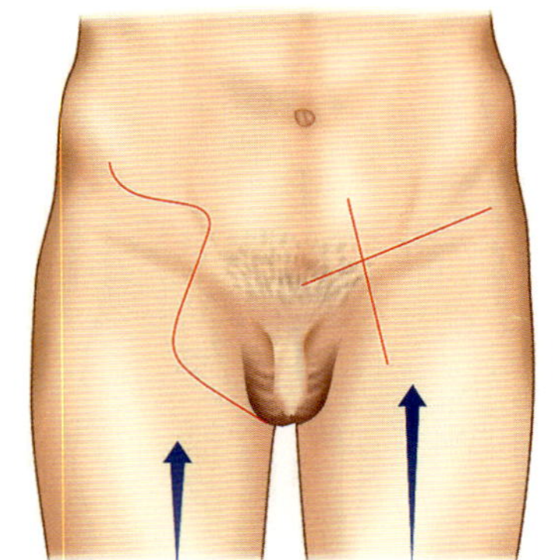

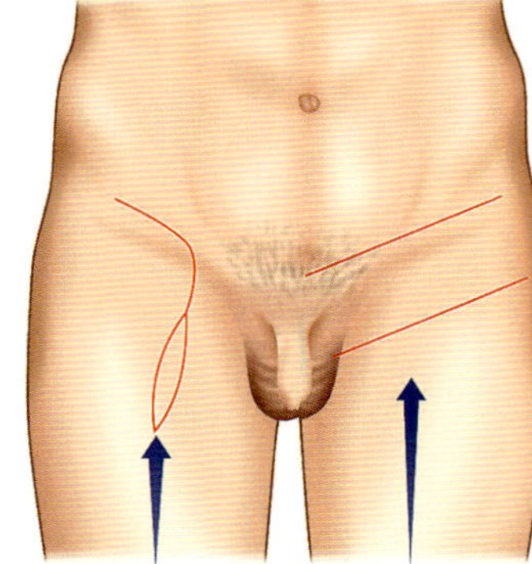

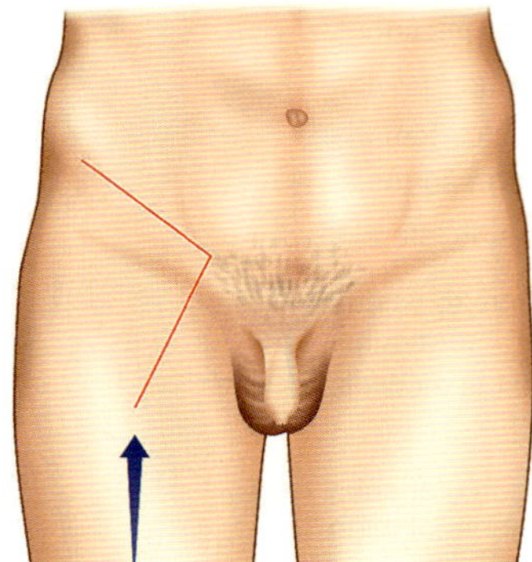

Fig. 30-13: Different incisions which can be used for inguinal block dissection.

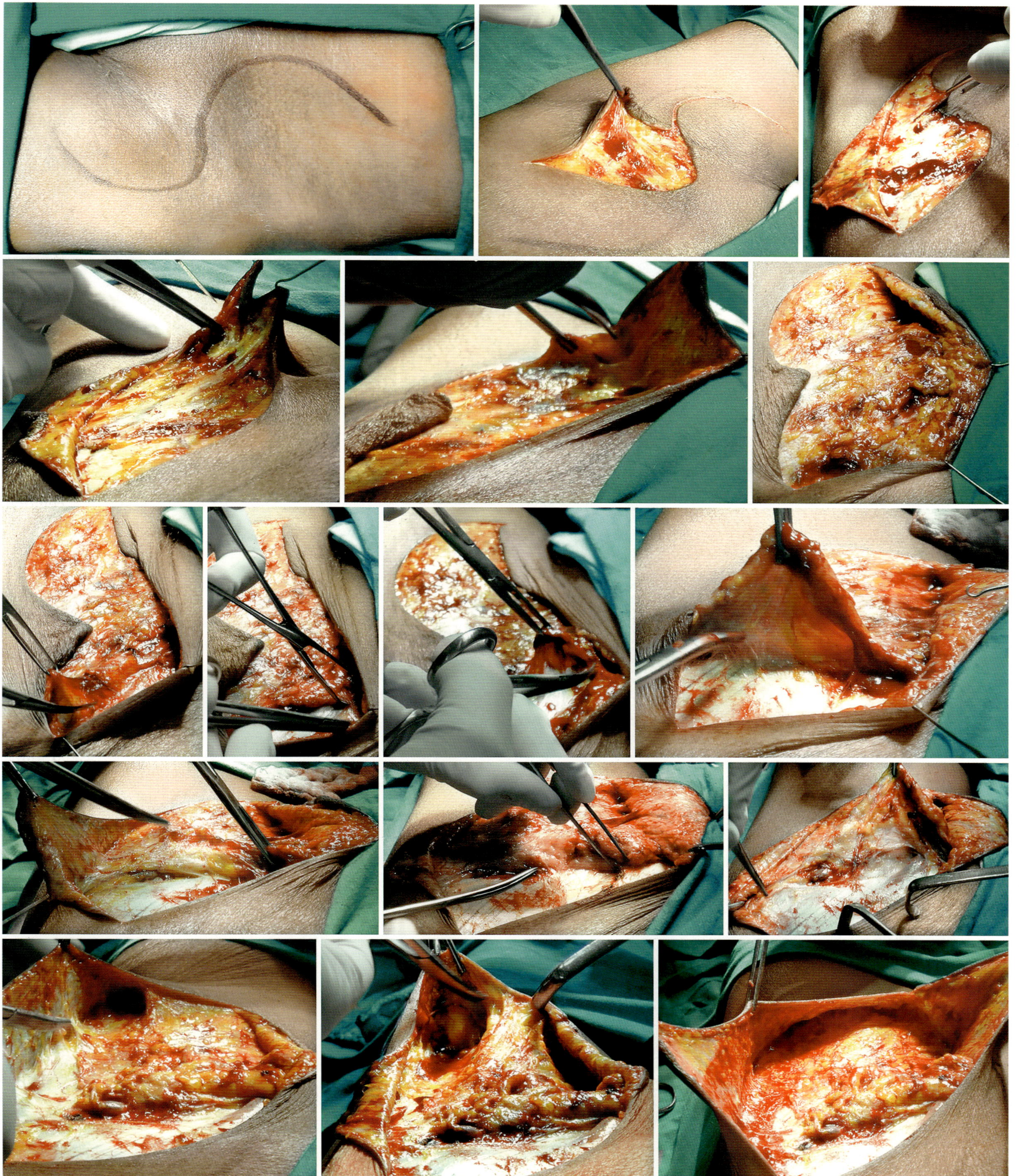

Figs. 30-14(1)

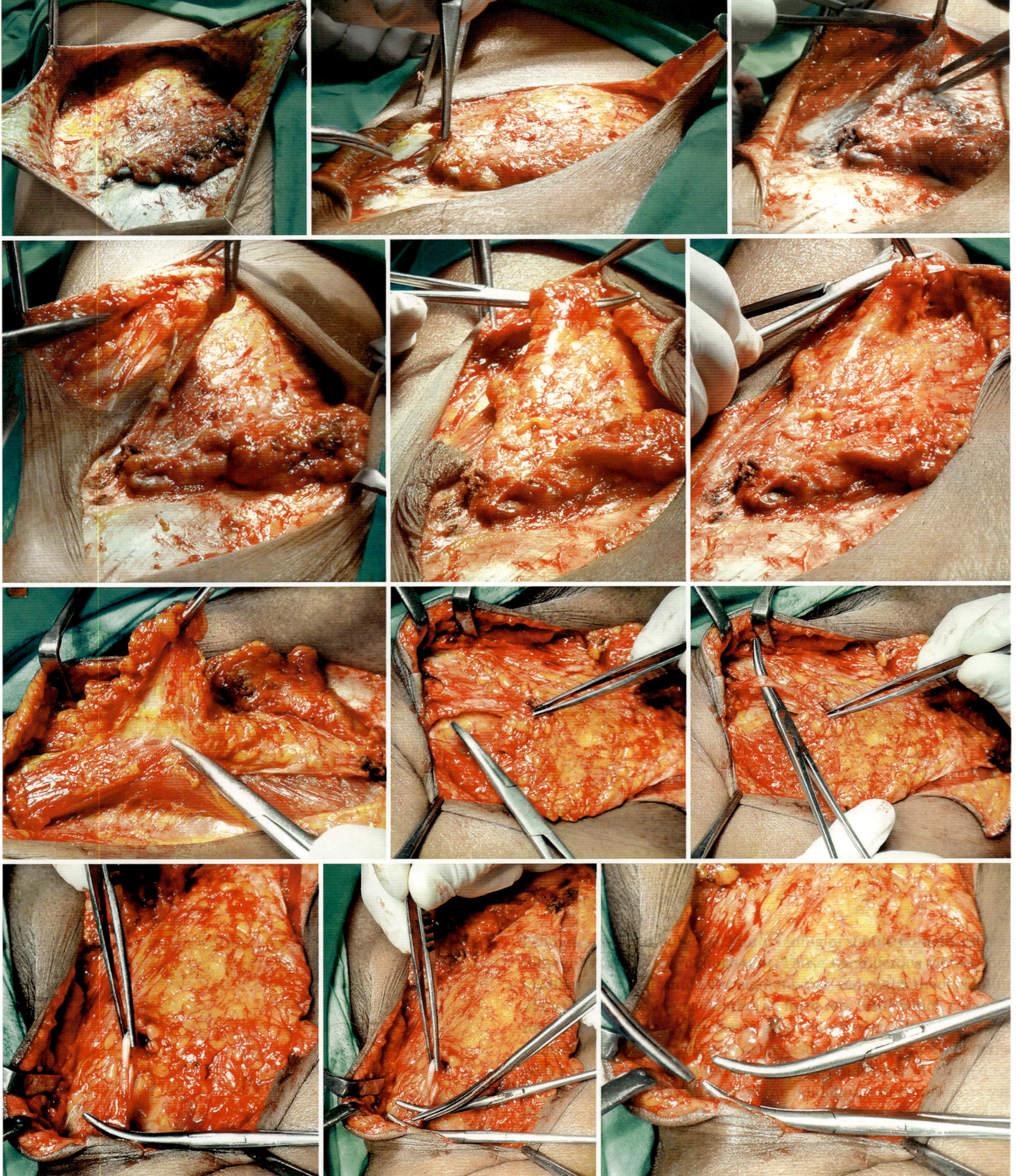

Figs. 30-14(2)

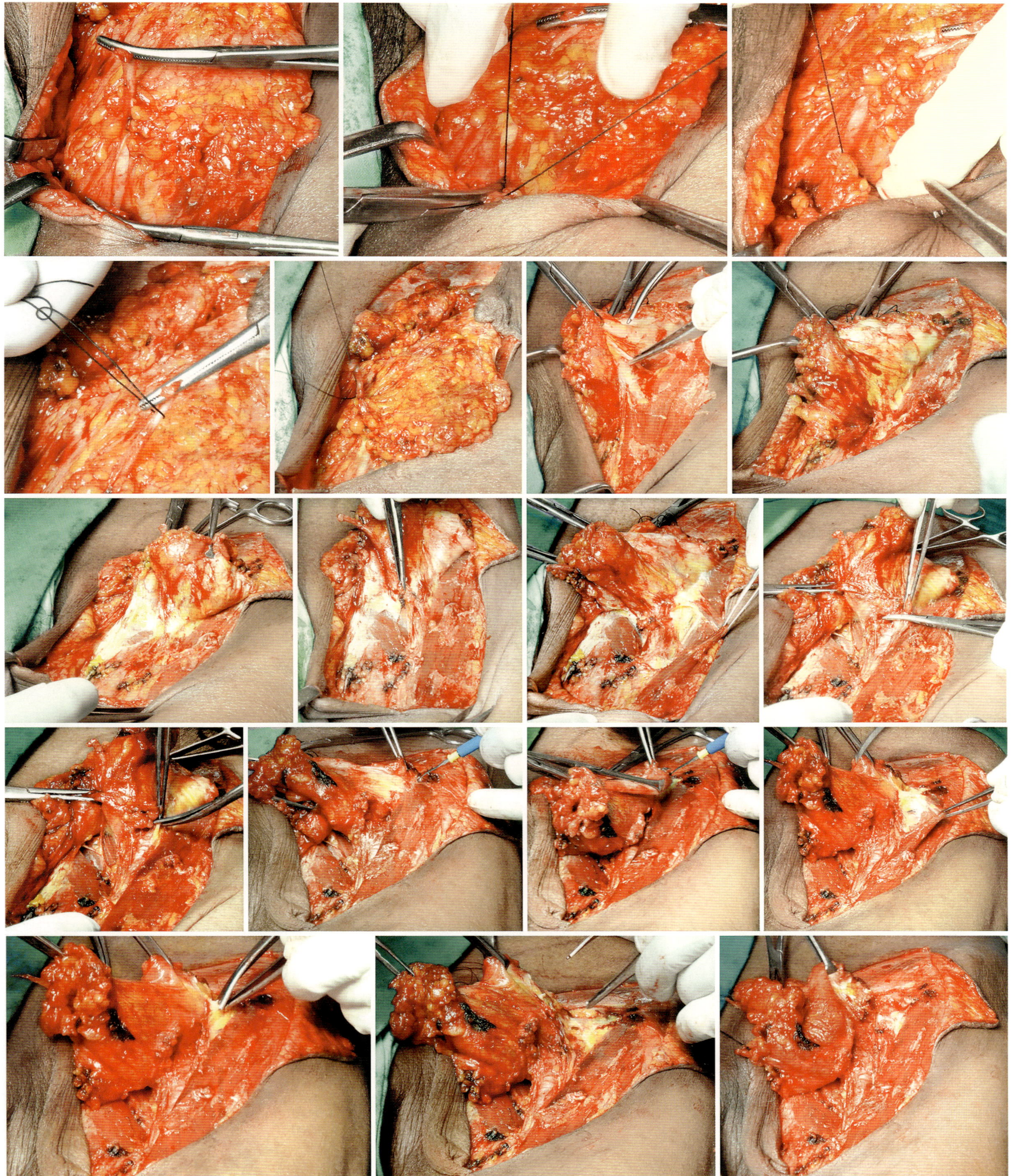

Figs. 30-14(3)

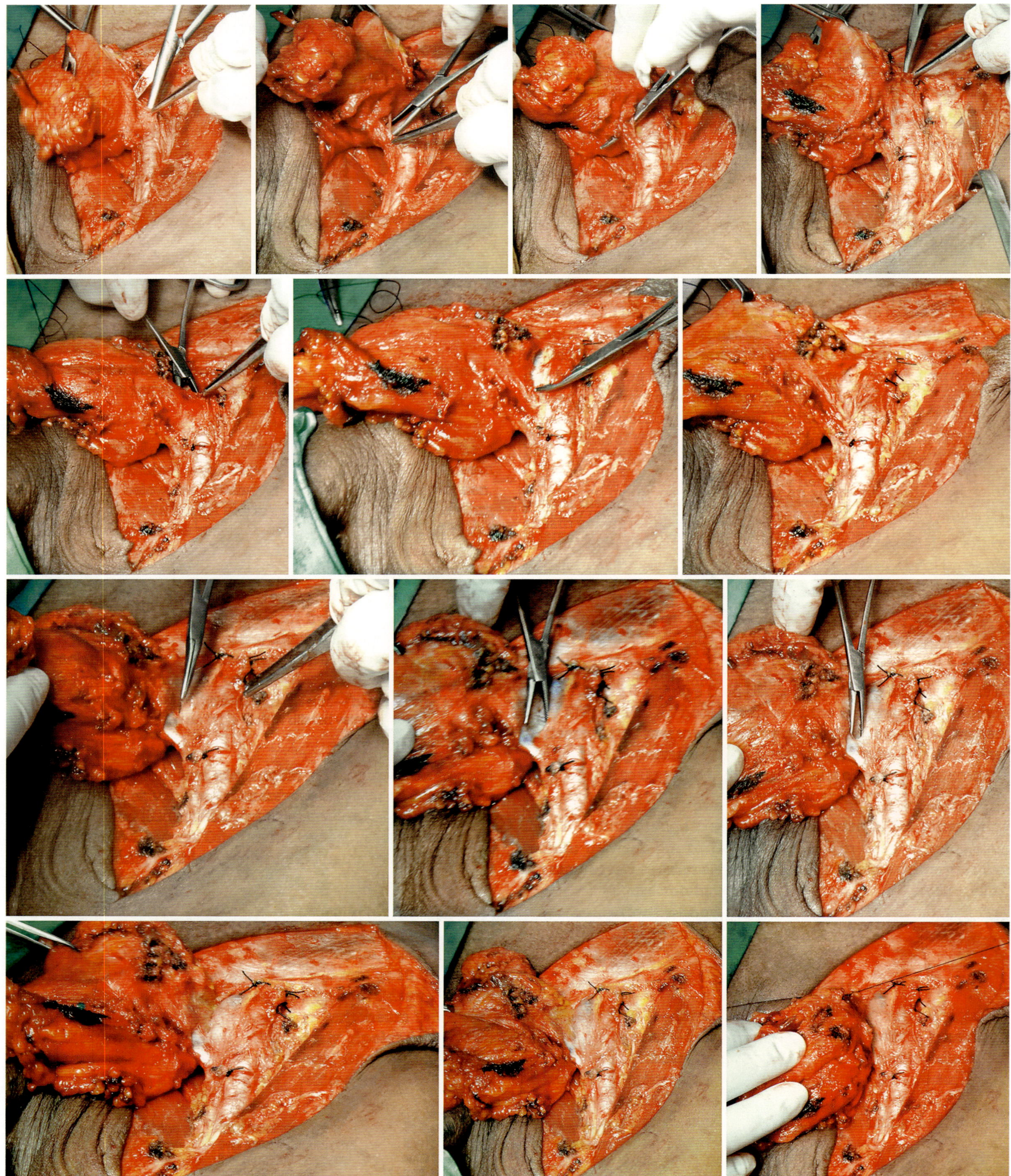

Figs. 30-14(4)

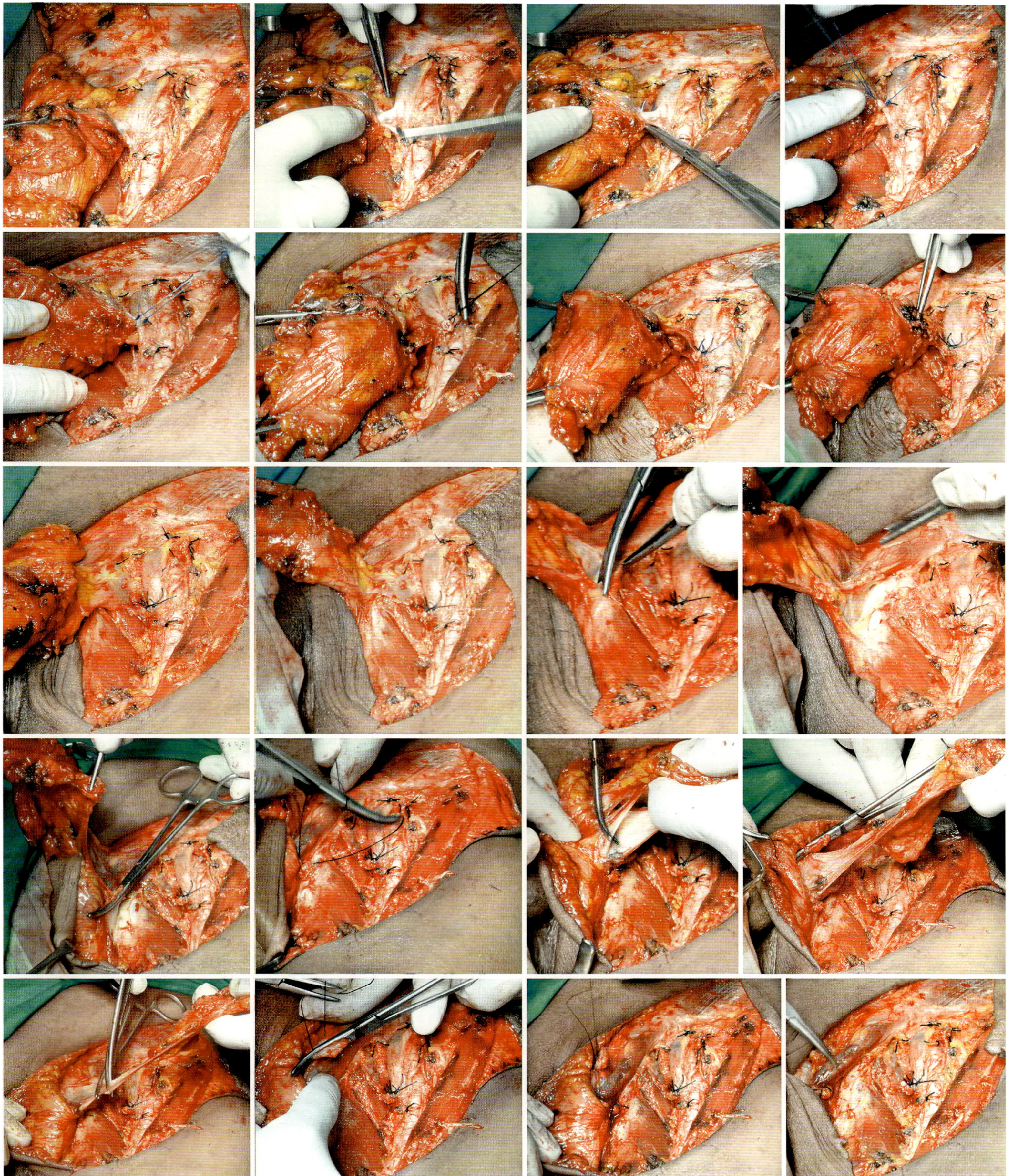

Figs. 30-14(5)

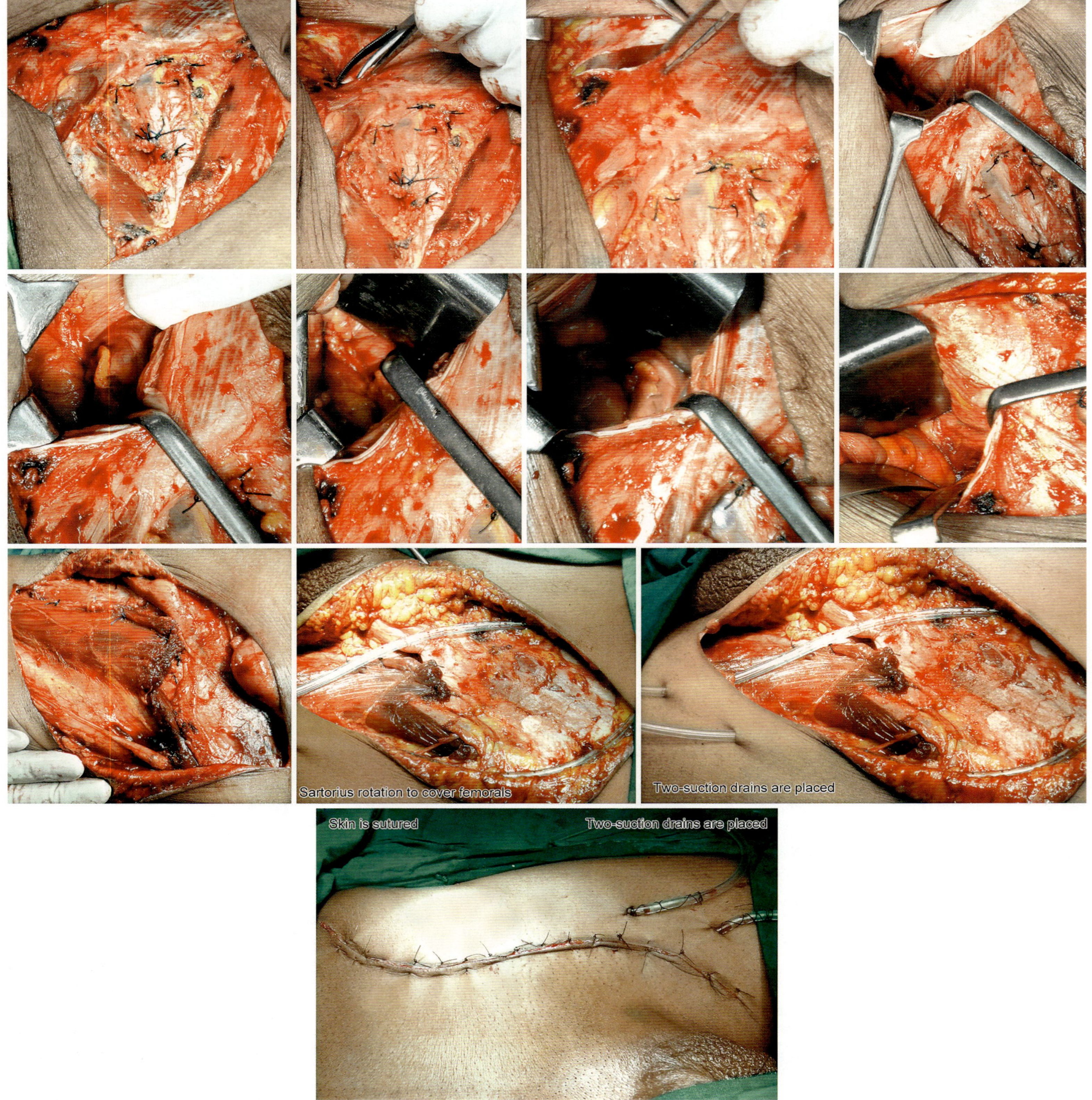

Figs. 30-14(6)

Figs. 30-14(1 to 6): Technique of ilioinguinal block dissection done for carcinoma penis. 'S' incision is used here. 5 cm above the inguinal ligament is cleared. Pelvic lymphadenectomy (ileo-obturator/iliac) is also done; sartorius rotation is done; two drains are placed.

Deep Ilio-obturator (Pelvic) Lymphadenectomy

It is done by extending the groin incision upwards and laterally. Inguinal ligament is divided after placing a flat instrument or finger over the femoral vessels. Skin, superficial fascia and external and internal oblique muscles are incised; transversus abdominis is split. Peritoneum is swept medially towards midline with blunt finger dissection to expose the common iliac vessels and pelvis. Peritoneum should not be opened. Peritoneum with its contents is retracted using broad Deaver retractor. Alternatively self-retaining retractor may be used. Pelvic lymph node dissection begins from common iliac vessels downwards; laterally from genitofemoral nerve towards medially. All nodes along the common iliac vessels are cleared; nodes in front and in between the external iliac vessels (between external iliac artery and vein) should be properly dissected and removed. Dissection proceeds downwards and medially along the internal iliac vessels (hypogastric vessels) by clearing all nodes. Obturator nerve (thick nerve) is identified in the triangle formed by external and internal iliac vessels. Branches of the internal iliac arteries may be identified. All fat, tissues and lymph nodes are cleared from the endopelvic fascia preserving obturator nerve and important branch vessels from bladder medially, obturator foramen below, above towards the external iliac vessels and inguinal ligament. Haemostasis is achieved by bipolar cautery. Drain may be placed in the pelvis.

Closure

Internal oblique and external oblique muscles are closed using 2-zero vicryl. Femoral canal is closed with interrupted non-absorbable sutures. Often it is necessary to place a mesh between the groin and retroperitoneum to prevent hernia formation. Lateral attachment of the sartorius in the anterior superior iliac spine is divided and is rotated over the femoral vessels keeping its blood supply intact. Mobilised/transposed sartorius is sutured to inguinal ligament above and adductor magnus muscle medially using interrupted 2-zero vicryl sutures (*Sartorius muscle transposition, its blood supply is segmental*). It covers the femoral vessels and so gives protection to them; also it seals the large defect under the groin thus preventing herniation of the abdominal content. Alternatively, if sartorius is not adequate or is removed for clearance purpose then *rectus abdominis flap or tensor fascia lata flap* will be very useful. Skin grafting may be needed over the possible necrosed area which is excised **(Fig. 30-15)**.

Closed suction drain should be placed until drain fluid becomes less than 50 mL/day; usually in 3 weeks.

Complications of Inguinal Block Dissection

Early Complications

Haemorrhage, infection, flap necrosis—common. Infection is common in the wound. It may be skin infection, cellulitis, abscess formation. Sutures are removed if there is collection inside. Thorough irrigation with normal saline is done. Discharge is sent for culture and sensitivity. Antibiotics and drainage under anaesthesia is often required in such situation. Usually wound will granulate and heal in 6 weeks. Once it granulates well occasionally skin grafting may be required. Postoperative DVT is not uncommon. Venous Doppler will confirm the diagnosis. LMWH should be started immediately. Lymphorrhoea is lymph ooze from the wound; usually occurs in 6 weeks, often persists for long time. It is due to disruption of lymphatic drainage.

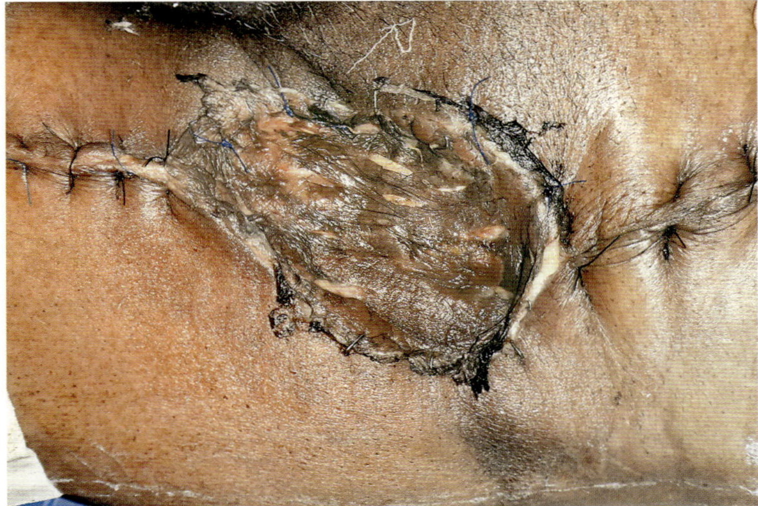

Fig. 30-15: Split skin graft is often placed on the centre of the wound with excision of the skin over the femoral area around 3 cm with which avoids flap necrosis.

Late Complications

Lymphoedema is a distressing complication. It is more common in obesity, old age, after additional adjuvant RT, deeper node clearance and saphenous vein ligation (not proved). Limb elevation, manual massaging, stockings, avoiding injury, prevention of recurrent infection are the therapeutic methods used.

SURGICAL ANATOMY OF SCROTUM

It is a cutaneous bag containing the right and left testis, epididymis and lower part of spermatic cord. It is divided into right and left half by a raphe which is continued in front along the penis and backwards along the perineum towards anus. Left hemiscrotum is lower than right. In cold environment scrotum is contracted, short and corrugated due to contraction of dartos muscle. In warm environment, it is flaccid and elongated due to dartos relaxation.

Layers of the Scrotum (From without Inwards)

1. Skin
2. Dartos muscle
3. External spermatic fascia
4. Cremasteric fascia
5. Internal spermatic fascia

Blood Supply

From external pudendal, deep external pudendal scrotal branches of internal pudendal and cremasteric branch of inferior epigastric arteries.

Nerve Supply

Anterior 1/3rd portion is supplied by (segment L1 of spinal cord) ilioinguinal nerve and genital branch of genitofemoral nerve. Posterior 2/3rd portion is supplied by (S3) posterior scrotal branch of pudendal nerve and perineal branch of posterior cutaneous nerve of thigh. Dartos is supplie d by sympathetic nerve.

TREATMENT FOR HYDROCELE (FIGS. 30-16 AND 30-17)

Surgeries

- Sub-total excision
- Partial excision and eversion (Jabouley's operation)
- Evacuation and eversion
- Lord's plication
- Sharma and Jhawer's technique

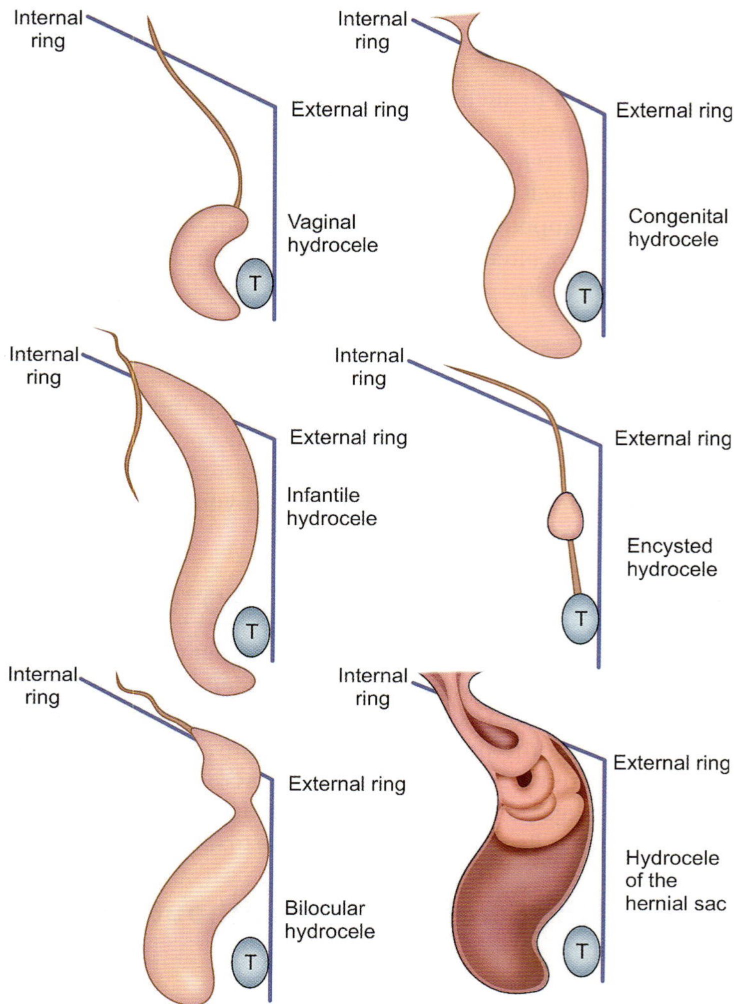

Fig. 30-16: Different types of hydrocele.

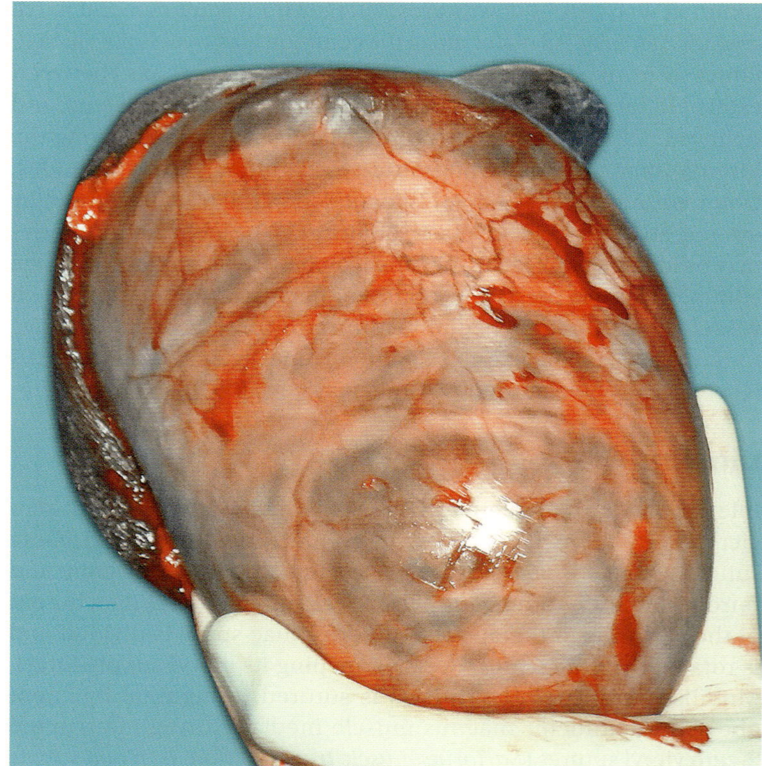

Fig. 30-17: Bluish coloured sac of the large hydrocele.

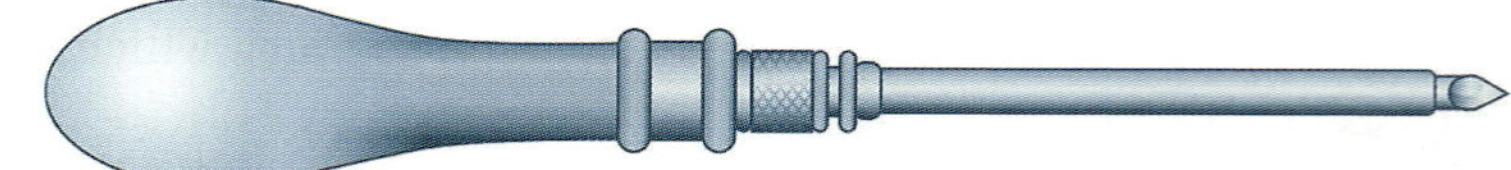

Fig. 30-18: Trocar and cannula used to evacuate the hydrocele fluid.

Procedure

Under general anaesthesia or spinal or local anaesthesia (cord block), after cleaning and draping, vertical incision of about 6–8 cm in length is made over the scrotum, anteriorly 1 cm lateral to the median raphe. Skin, dartos, external spermatic fascia, internal spermatic fascia are incised. *Bluish* hydrocele sac is identified, i.e. parietal layer of tunica vaginalis of testis (it is bluish due to congested venous network over the stretched sac). Fluid is evacuated using trocar and cannula. Sac is opened. Monopolar cautery should be used with care otherwise testicular artery goes for spasm causing testicular atrophy. It is better to use bipolar cautery or fine ligatures for these bleeders **(Fig. 30-18)**.

If the sac is small, thin and contains clear fluid, Lord's plication can be done, i.e. tunica is bunched into a "ruff" by placing series of multiple interrupted chromic catgut/vicryl sutures so as to make the sac to form fibrous tissue (It is relatively avascular and so haematoma will not occur).

Evacuation and eversion of the sac behind the testis also can be done if sac is thin and fluid is not infected. After eversion, everted sac is sutured with chromic catgut/3-0 vicryl by continuous sutures **(Fig. 30-19)**.

If the sac is thick, in large hydrocele and chylocoele, subtotal excision of the sac is done (as tunica vaginalis is reflected on to the cord structures and epididymis posteriorly, total excision leads to orchidectomy with division of cord). It is also called as *radical cure or hydrocelectomy*. It is ideal procedure for hydrocele with least complications and recurrence **(Figs. 30-20 and 30-21)**.

Alternatively, the sac is excised partially and then eversion is done and everted edges are sutured together, which is called as *Jabouley's* operation.

After evacuation, the sac with the testis can be placed in a newly created pocket between the fascial layers of the scrotum—*Sharma and Jhawer's technique*.

A drain is placed near the root of the scrotum on the lateral aspect because it becomes the most dependent portion, when scrotal support is given. Scrotal support is given to reduce the scrotal oedema. Routinely, it may not be necessary but in large hydrocele, and in infected hydrocele it is better to keep a drain. Corrugated drain is commonly kept.

Wound is closed in layers, inner dartos with absorbable; outer skin with interrupted non-absorbable sutures. *Presently* skin with dartos is closed as single layer with interrupted non-absorbable monofilament sutures. Scrotal support is given to elevate the scrotum so that oedema of the scrotum will reduce and so also pain. Drain is removed in 48 hours **(Fig. 30-22)**.

In bilateral hydrocele, each side is dealt separately by two separate incisions on each hemiscrotum and two drains are kept. In small bilateral hydrocele both sacs can be approached through median raphe and treated with evacuation, excision and eversion the sac

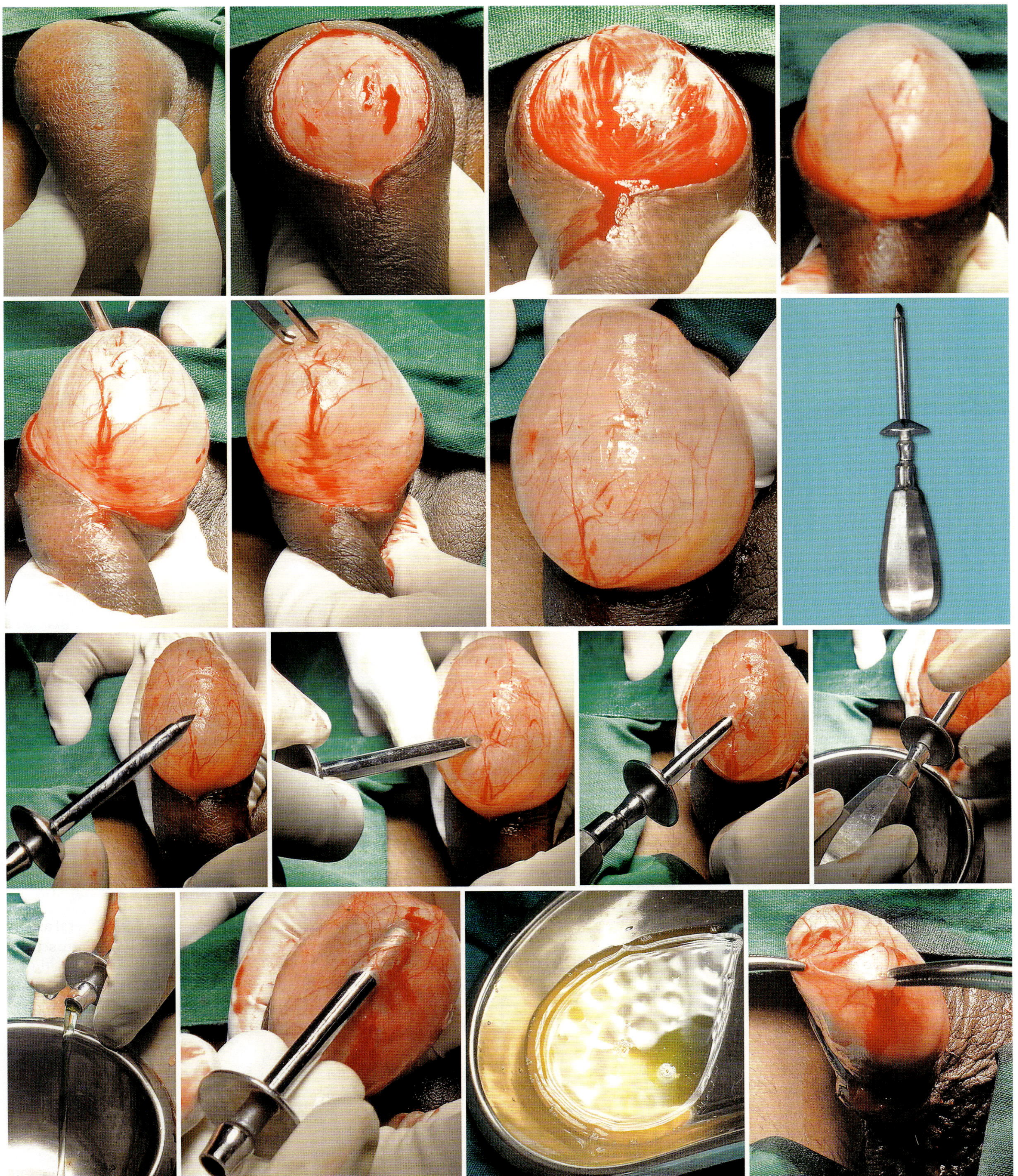

Figs. 30-19(1)

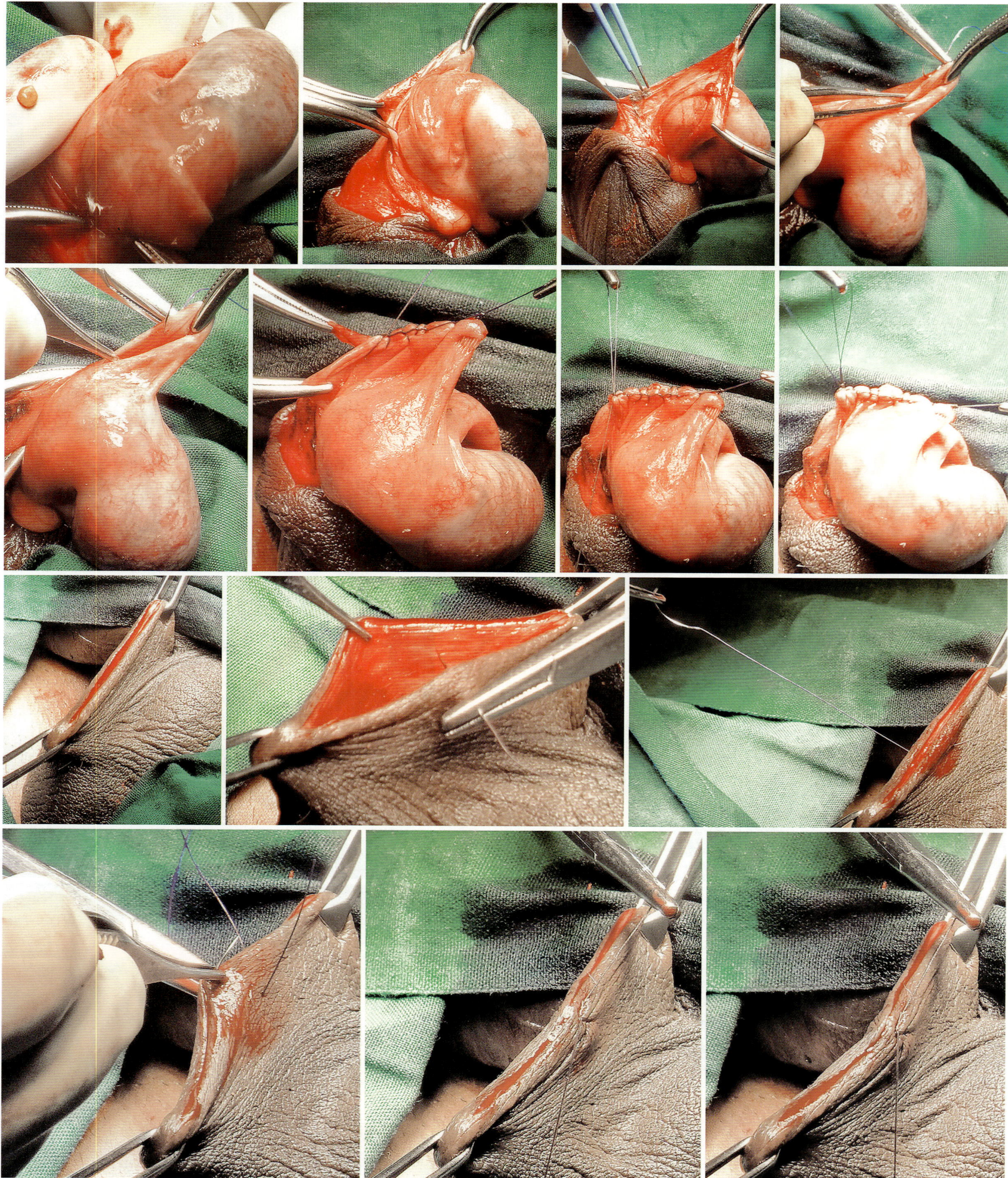

Figs. 30-19(2)

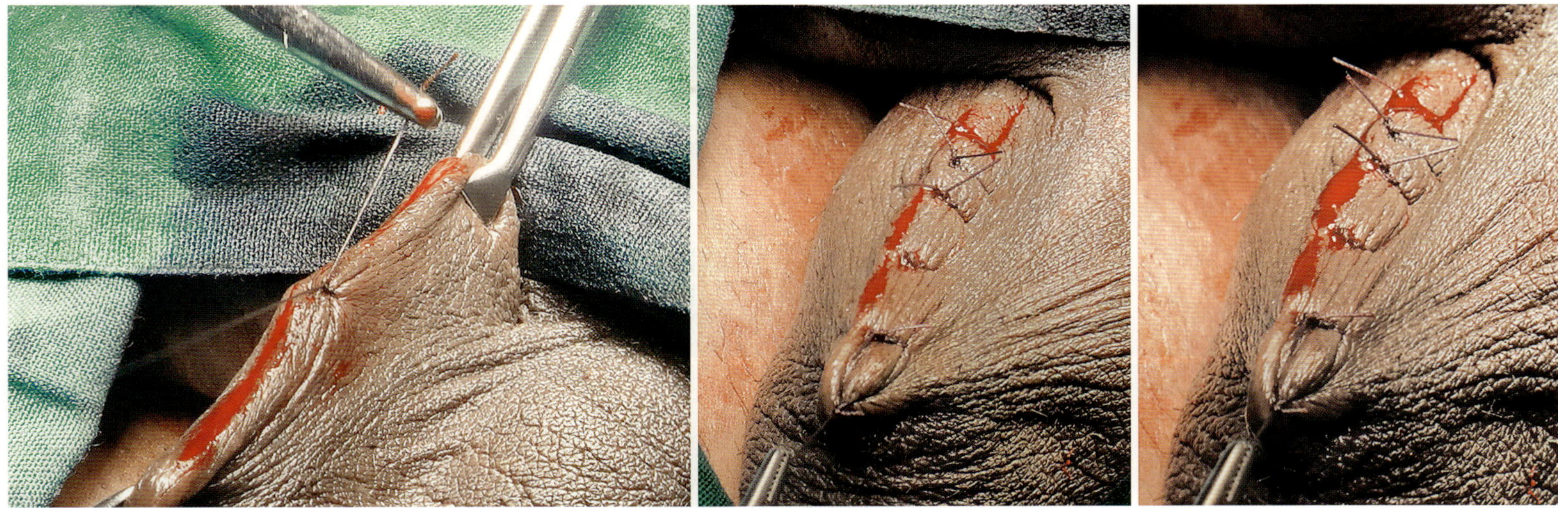

Figs. 30-19(3)

Figs. 30-19(1 to 3): Technique of evacuation and eversion for hydrocele surgery.

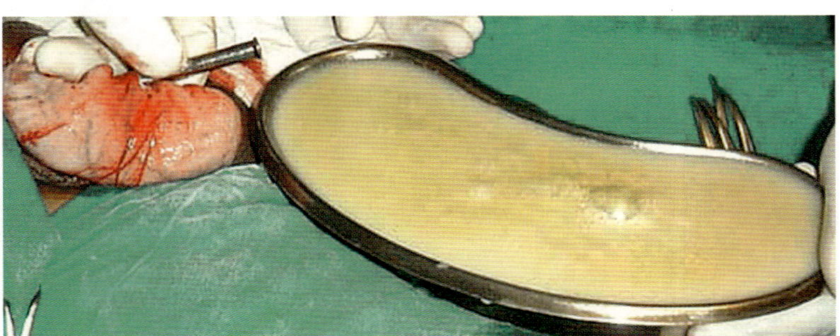

Fig. 30-20: Chylocele.

(*single layer procedure*). However, in bilateral large hydroceles median raphe approach is not advisable **(Fig. 30-23)**.

Note

Aspiration must be avoided as much as possible as it is only a temporary measure (recurrence occurs very early) and chances of haematocele, infection are higher.

Encysted hydrocele of the cord: It is located in the root of the scrotum. It is brilliantly transilluminant; traction test is positive; mimics epididymal cyst. It is treated by excision of the encysted hydrocele through scrotal approach. Normal tunica vaginalis is also usually opened and everted **(Fig. 30-24)**.

Multiloculated hydrocele is known to occur. If found each loculi should be opened and their sacs are removed **(Fig. 30-25)**.

Complications of Surgery

Reactionary haemorrhage is common. It causes haematoma formation with swelling, pain, distress. Small haematoma can be left alone, as it will resolve spontaneously. If haematoma is large it is evacuated after re-exploration, bleeders are ligated using vicryl. Wound is closed with a drain.

Infection is not uncommon. It may lead into wound disruption, sinus formation, and orchitis. Suitable antibiotics control this problem.

Pyocele can occur due to severe infection especially in diabetics. It is treated by proper drainage under general anaesthesia with warm saline irrigation and suitable antibiotics. On table Doppler can be used to check the viability of the testis. Orchidectomy can be postponed at a later period if needed during reinspection of the wound and testis under general anaesthesia.

Sinus formation—persistent sinus may be due to suture material reaction, or focus of infection or retaining of the thick diseased sac. So, it is always better to excise the sac if it is thick, infected and diseased. Rarely need may arise to re-explore the sinus for complete excision. Specific disease like tuberculosis of the epididymis has to be thought of. Sinus track excised should be sent for histology.

Recurrent hydrocele is due to retained sac, formation of another sac or loculated sacs if present. It should be treated by resurgery again.

Conditions Where Orchidectomy is Done in Hydrocele

Pyocele with testicular destruction; Clotted haematocele with testicular destruction. Doppler study is a must before doing orchidectomy. Consent has to be taken. Doppler study of the opposite side also should be done. Low orchidectomy is done **(Fig. 30-26)**.

TREATMENT OF HAEMATOCELE

Acute haematocele is treated by incision and drainage under general anaesthesia. Chronic clotted organised haematocele is treated with low orchidectomy **(Fig. 30-27)**.

TREATMENT OF PYOCELE

Antibiotics are started. Under general anaesthesia, scrotum is explored immediately and pus is evacuated. Viability of the testis is checked. On table Doppler study is ideal. If viable, pus is evacuated and sent for culture, wound is loosely closed with a drain or *ideally* left open and at a later date examination is done under anaesthesia to check for viability and secondary suturing is done with placing a drain if testis is viable. If the testis is not viable, then *orchidectomy* is done (after taking consent). When in doubt, always testis is left in place and observed. Often, testis will show signs of viability. If not, then low orchidectomy is done at a later stage **(Fig. 23-28)**.

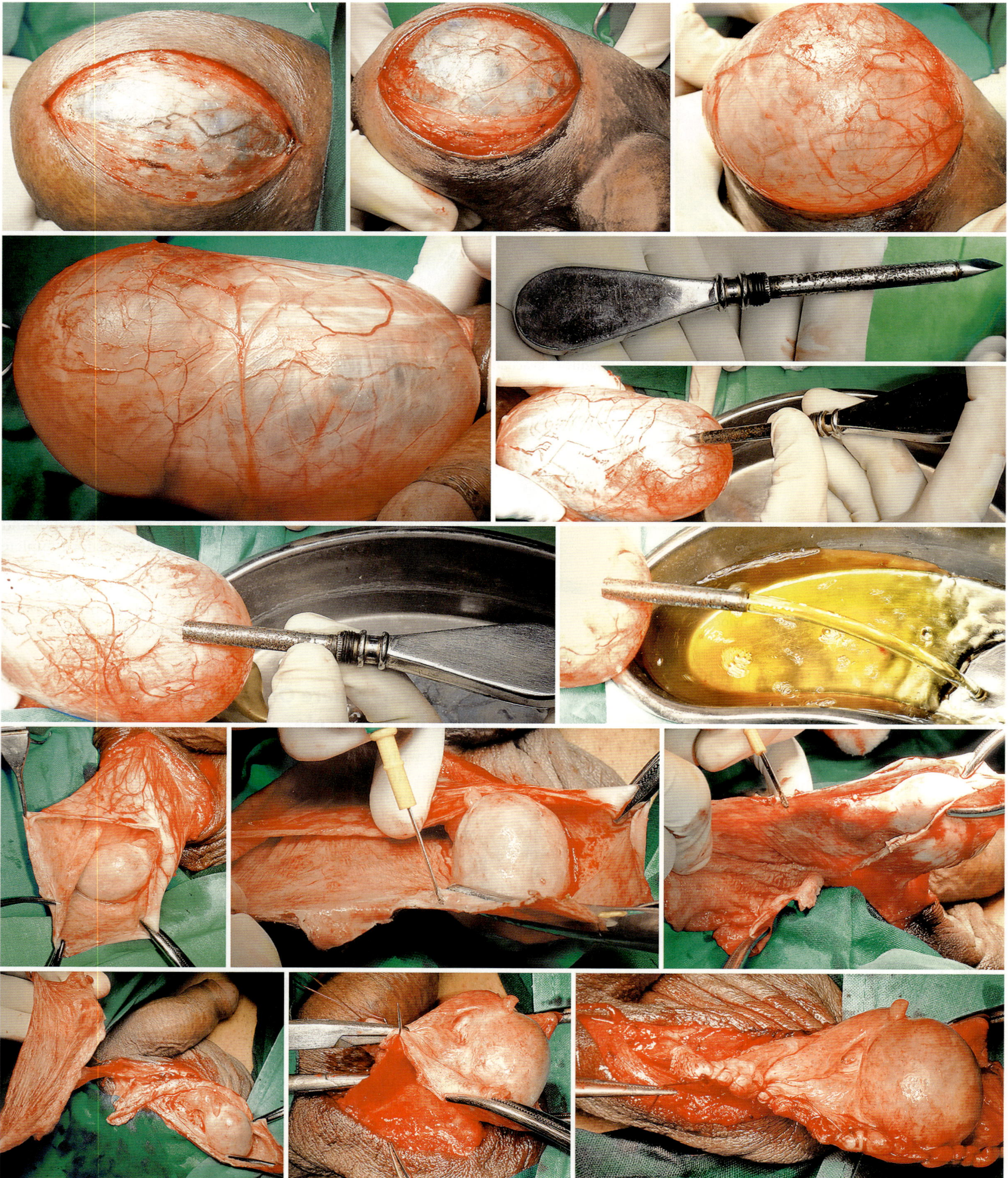

Figs. 30-21(1)

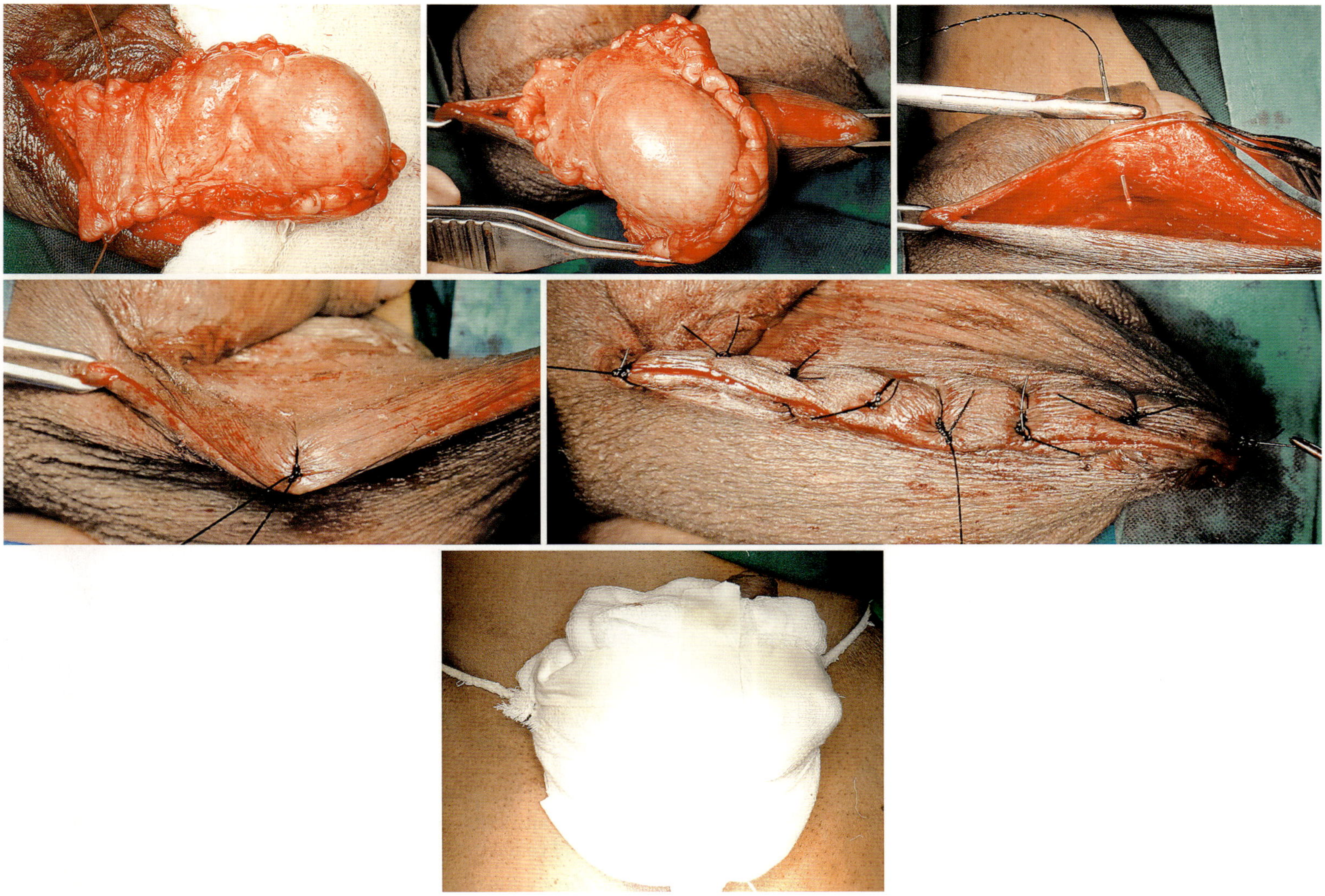

Figs. 30-21(2)

Figs. 30-21(1 and 2): Radical cure/hydrocelectomy/subtotal excision of the sac for large hydrocele.

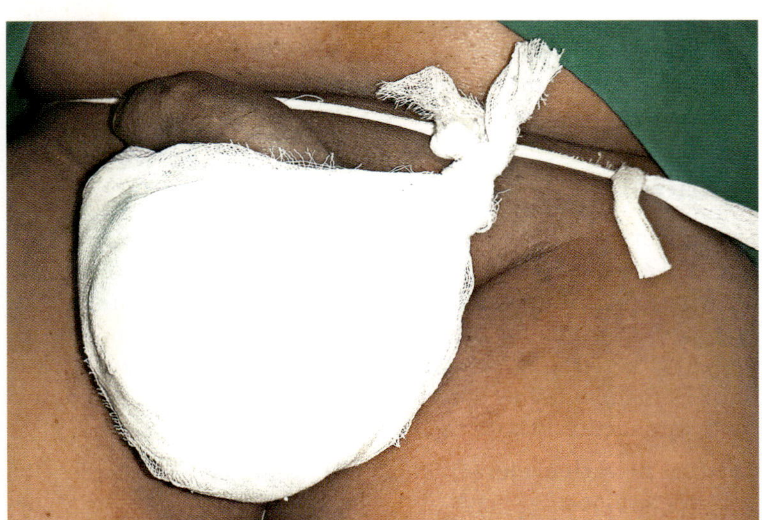

Fig. 30-22: Scrotal support is used in all scrotal surgeries to reduce oedema and pain.

VARICOCELE

It is dilatation and tortuosity of the pampiniform plexus of veins and so also the testicular veins. Normally, there will be numerous plexus of veins (pampiniform) in the scrotum, which all join together to form about 4–8 veins in the inguinal canal. Above, in the abdominal cavity, in the posterior abdominal wall all join to form a single testicular vein. On left side, it drains into left renal vein; on the right side, it drains into inferior vena cava.

Varicocele is common in *tall, thin young men*. More common on the *left side*, but often can be bilateral **(Fig. 30-29)**.

Commonly, it is idiopathic in origin, may be due to absence or incompetent valve at the junction of left testicular vein and left renal vein causing inefficient drainage of blood. Other reason is, due to perpendicular (right angle) entry of the left testicular vein into the left renal vein. In left-sided renal cell carcinoma, tumour proliferates into the left renal vein and blocks the entry of left testicular vein causing varicocoele on left side which is *irreducible*. Varicocele causes increased temperature in the scrotum which depresses

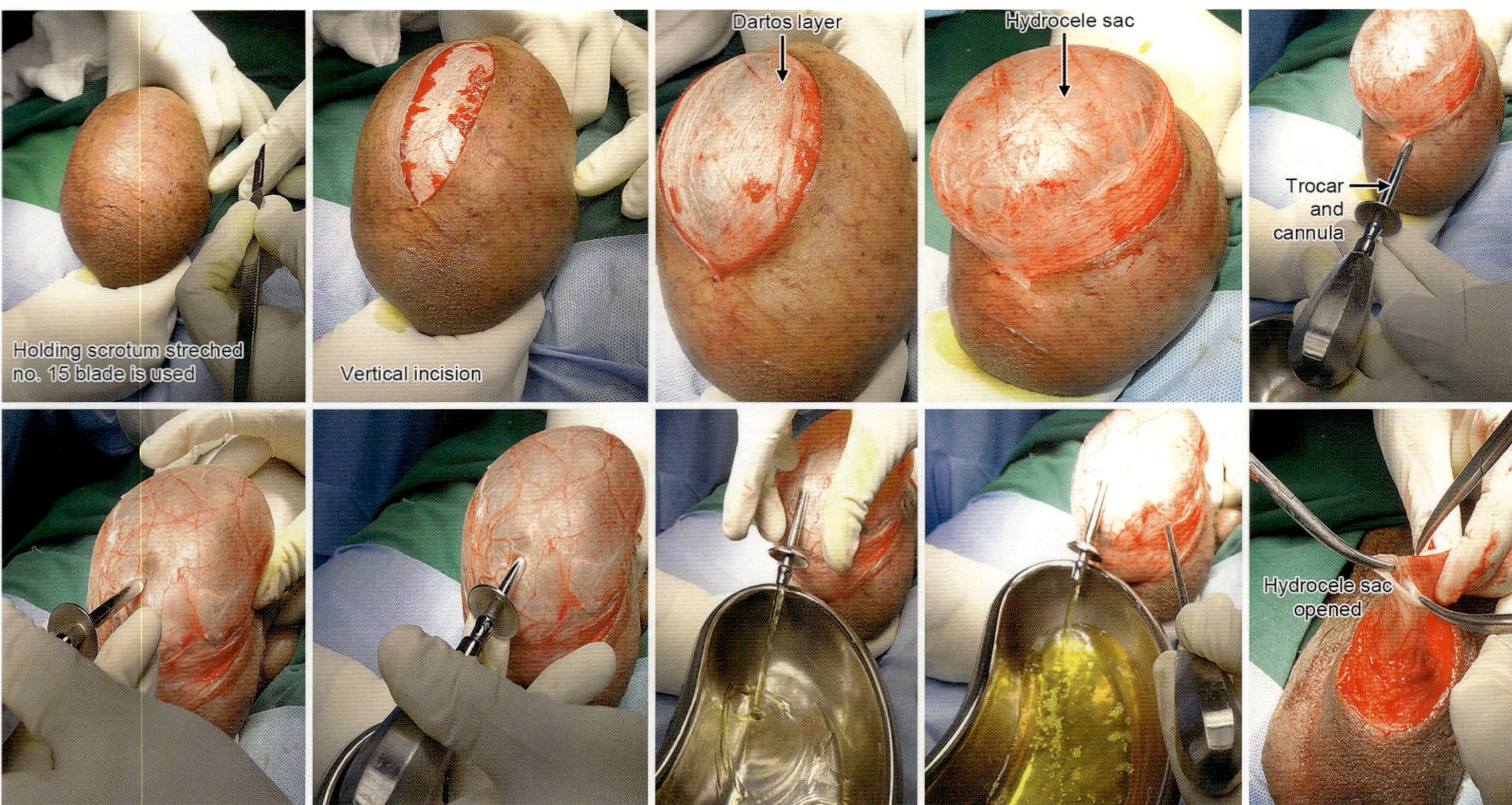

Fig. 30-23: Approach to hydrocele sac—incision, layers, trocar and cannula.

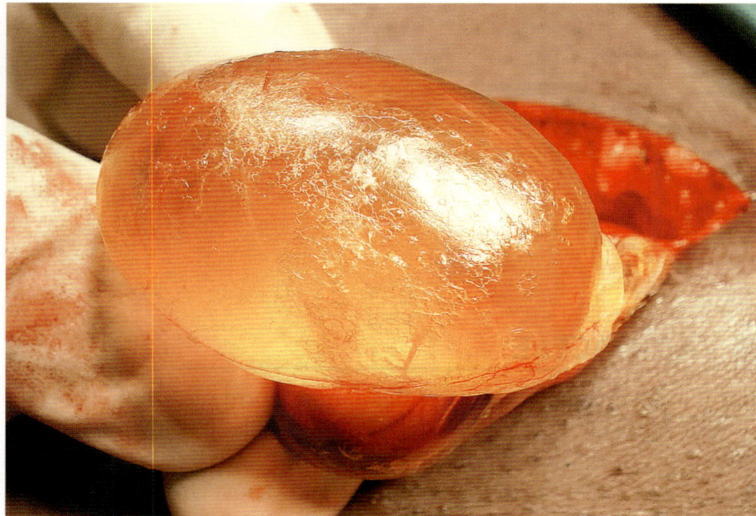

Fig. 30-24: Encysted hydrocele of the cord.

the spermatogenesis and so causes *infertility* (correctable infertility) **(Fig. 30-30)**.

Types of Varicocele

Primary/idiopathic—95%: No cause is found. There is incompetence of valves of the testicular vein. It is common on left side because left testicular vein joins left renal vein perpendicularly and left side vein is longer and liable to get compressed by loaded sigmoid colon. Left renal vein is often compressed between aorta and SMA.

Secondary—due to specific cause like left-sided renal cell carcinoma with a tumour thrombus in left renal vein causing obstruction to venous flow of left testicular vein. *Subfertility/infertility* are observed even in unilateral varicocele. It is a debate whether it really causes subfertility. Possible causes are: Altered heat exchange mechanism of the scrotum due to varicocele; hyperthermia; inhibition of spermatogenesis; increased blood flow; increased temperature in the testes; increases the metabolic activity using glycogen storage; depletion of glycogen → injury of parenchyma of testes; oligospermia; hypoxia of testes; same cause leads into Leydig cell dysfunction, decreasing testosterone levels. Final effect is maturation arrest and poor spermatogenesis.

Features

Swelling in the root of the scrotum; dragging pain in the groin and scrotum; a feel of "*Bag of worms*" on palpation impulse on coughing; on lying down it gets reduced (except in renal cell carcinoma); *Bow sign:* After holding the varicocele between thumb and fingers, patient is asked to bow. Varicocele gets reduced in size. Bowing reduces the blood flow of testicular vein and pampiniform plexus causing reduction in size.

Grading of varicocele: (I) Small; (II) Moderate; (III) Large; (IV) Severely tortuous.

Investigations: Venous Doppler of the scrotum and groin; ultrasound abdomen to look for kidney tumour; semen analysis.

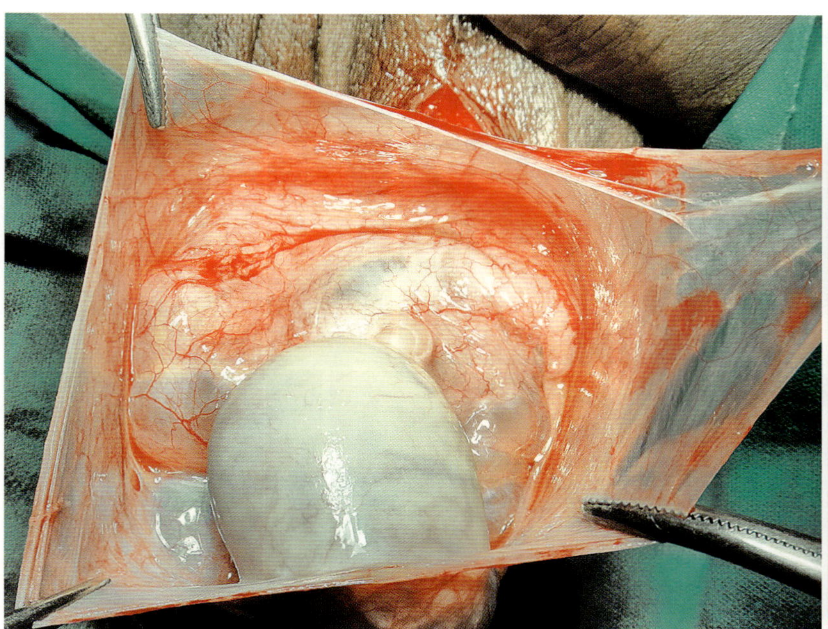
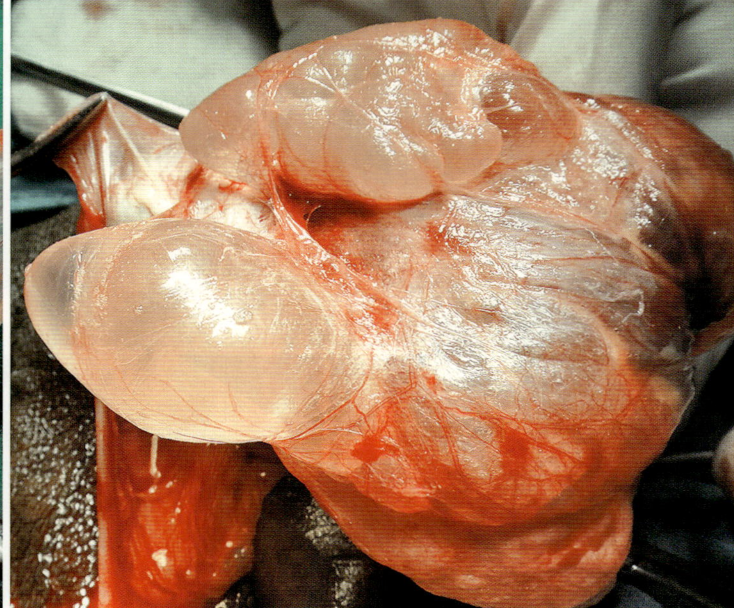

Fig. 30-25: Multiloculated hydrocele.

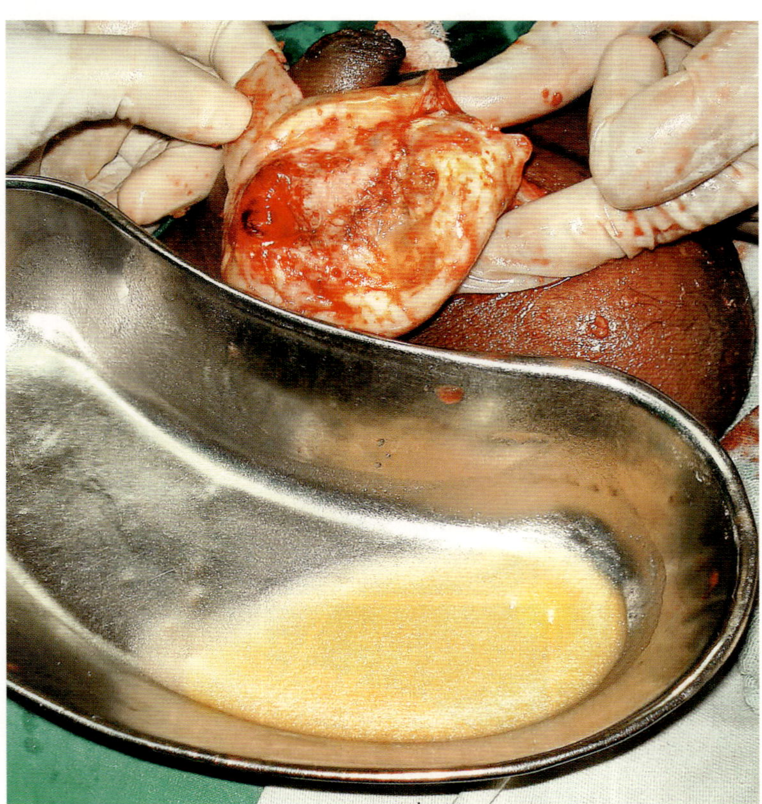

Fig. 30-26: Pyocele with non-viable testis is an indication for low orchidectomy.

Treatment

Indications for Surgery

Pain; Oligospermia—usually in 6–12 weeks oligospermia improves very well and also the conception rate.

Surgeries

Palomo's operation: Suprainguinal extraperitoneal ligation of testicular vein. Under spinal anaesthesia, above the inguinal canal in the line of anterior superior iliac spine lateral to the rectus muscle, horizontal incision is made; skin superficial fascia, external oblique are incised; internal oblique and transversus abdominis is split to reach extraperitoneal space. By careful blunt dissection the testicular vein is identified which runs upwards towards IVC on right side and towards left renal vein on left side. Testicular vein is dissected using right angle instrument, ligated and divided.

Inguinal approach (Ivanissevich approach): Easier and safer. It is same as approaching for inguinal hernia by open method. After opening the external oblique, cord is mobilised and cremaster is opened; pampiniform veins are observed; dilated veins are individually dissected and ligated securely using silk or vicryl. There is no indication to do any repair of the posterior inguinal canal in this procedure.

Subinguinal approach (Marc-Goldstein): It is subinguinal approach at superficial inguinal ring outside the external oblique aponeurosis without opening the external oblique aponeurosis. Here cord is easily identified through a small incision. Under local anaesthesia, pubic tubercle is marked. Cord after exiting though the external ring passes in front of the pubic tubercle before entering into the root of the scrotum. A small horizontally oblique incision is made directly on the pubic tubercle. Gentle careful dissection directly visualises the cord. Cord is dissected all around for a short distance. Ilioinguinal nerve lies outside the cord very closely which should not be injured. Fine haemostat is passed underneath the cord structure to stabilise the cord. Cord is dissected by opening the overlying cremaster; dilated veins are individually dissected and ligated securely. One should not allow tear of the vein, if it happens upper part will retract and bleed which is difficult to identify and ligate. Skin is closed using absorbable sutures (subcuticular/interrupted). It is technically easier; inguinal canal is not opened **(Figs. 30-31 and 30-32)**.

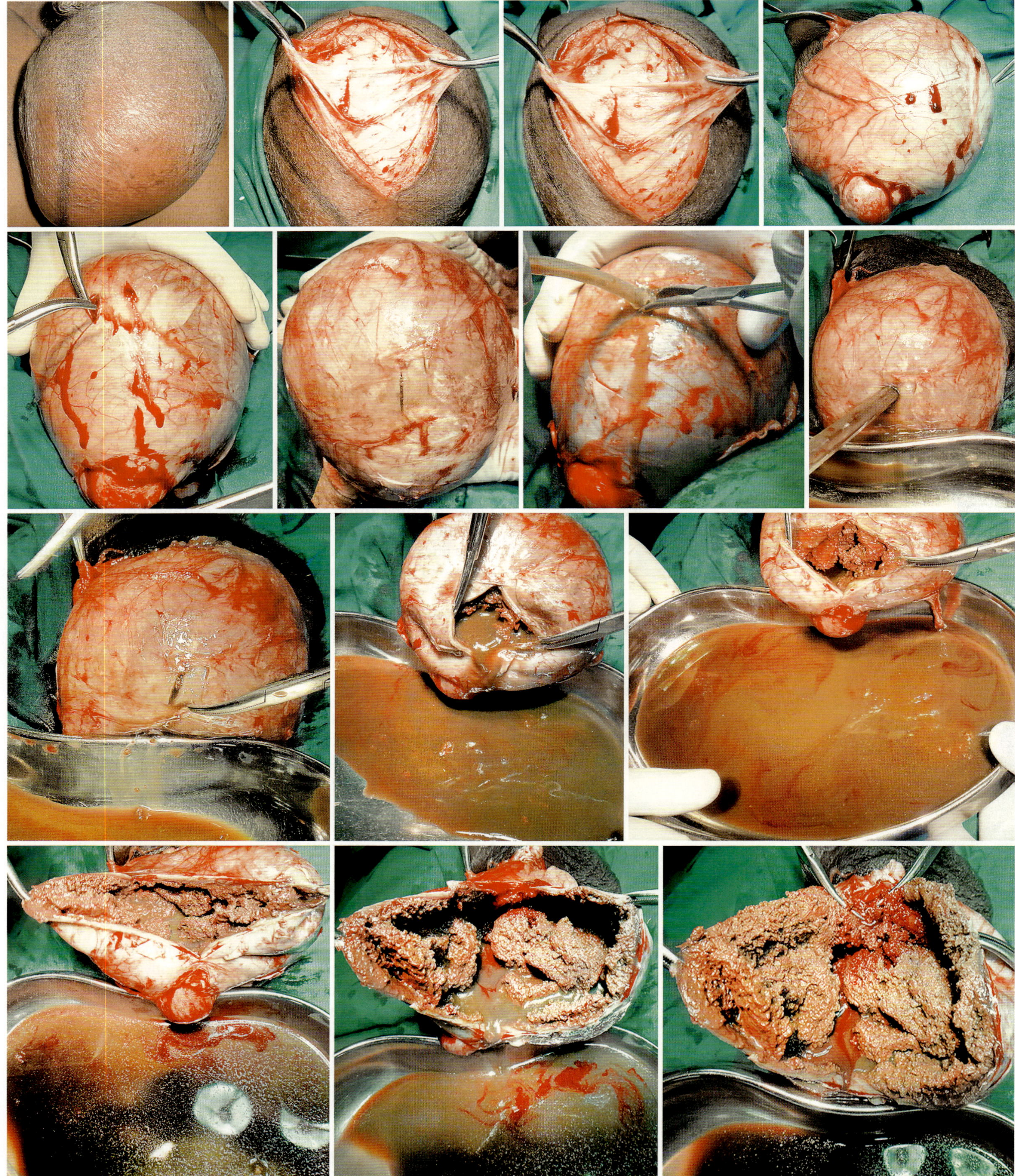

Figs. 30-27(1)

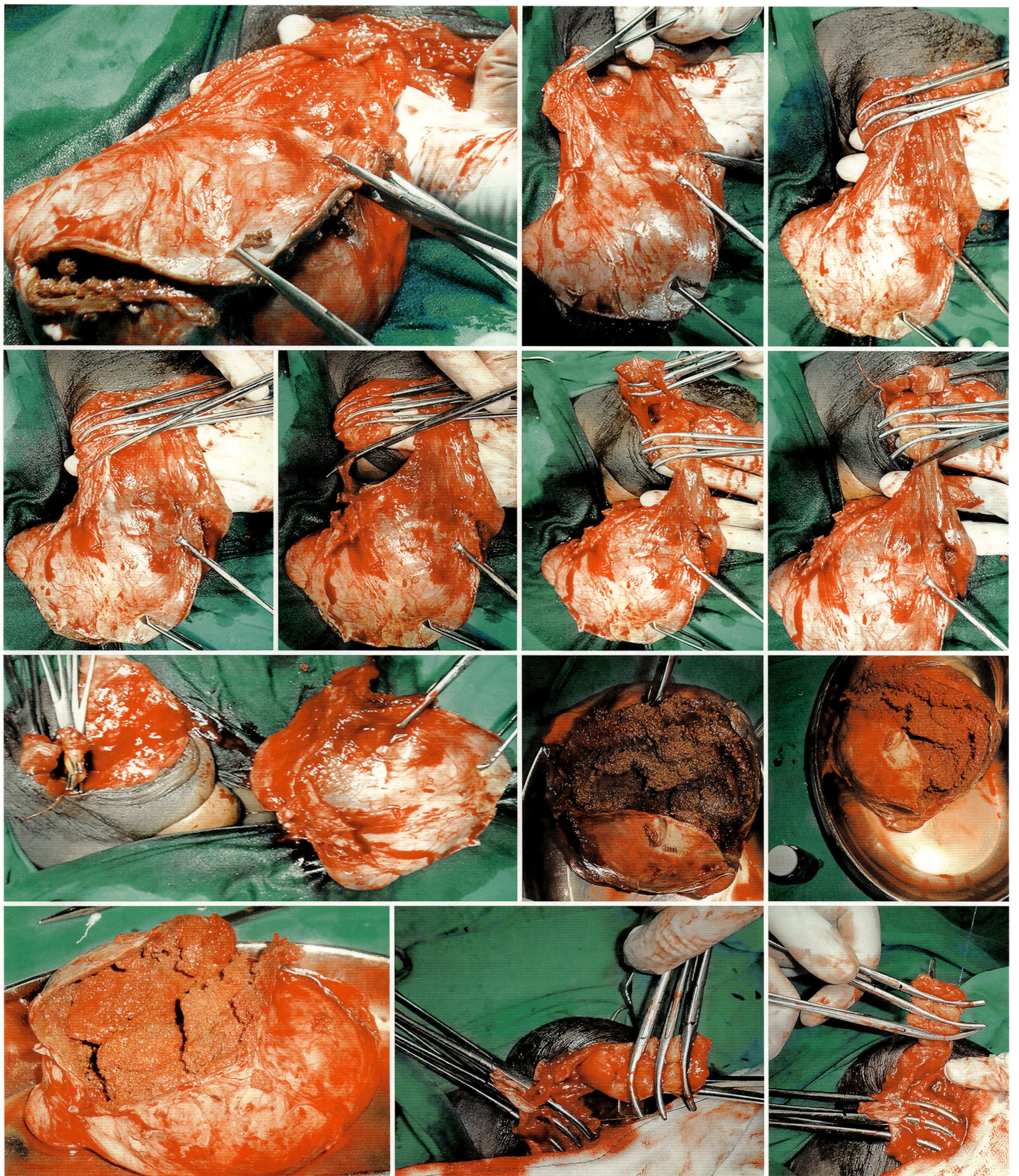

Figs. 30-27(2)

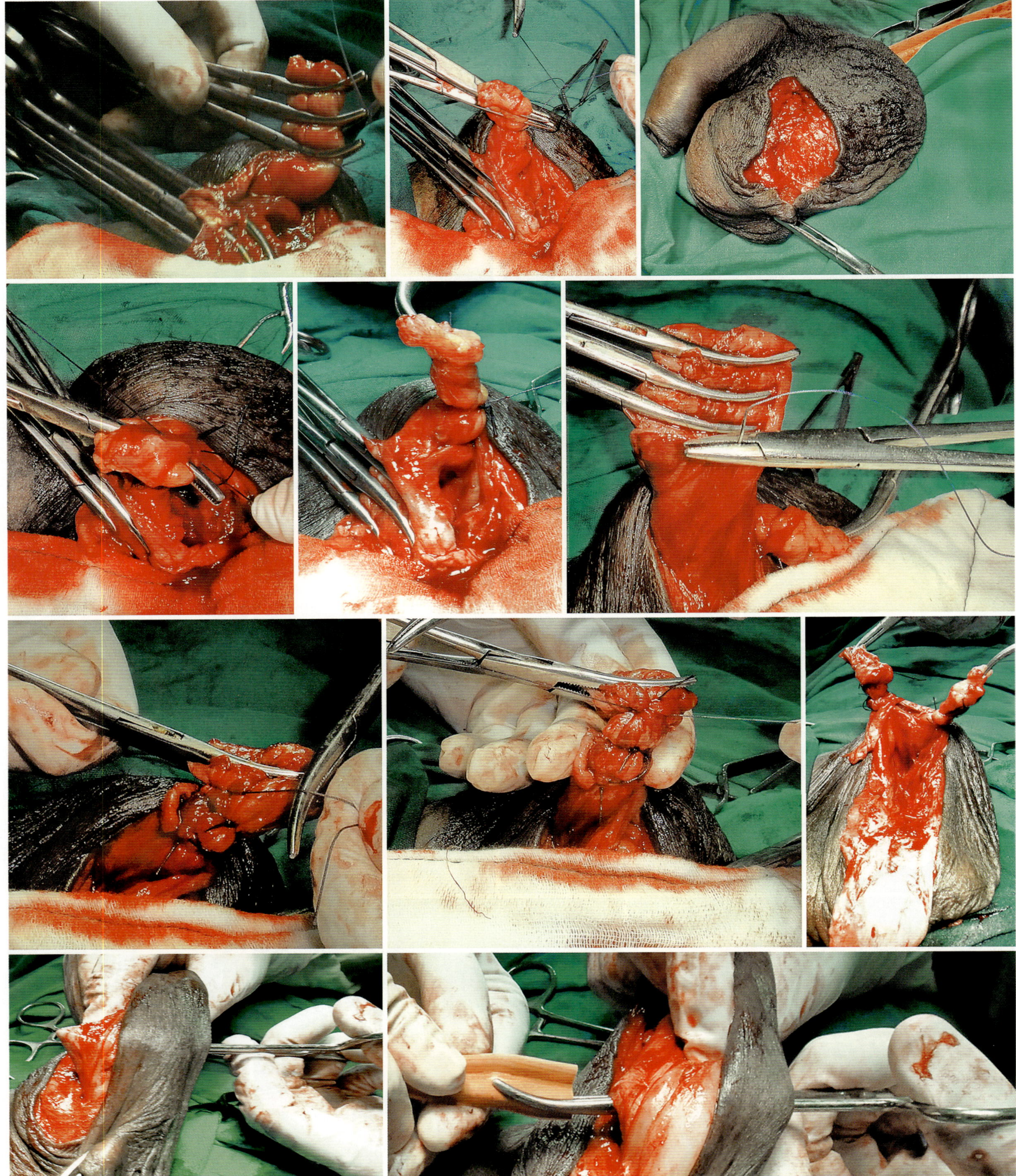

Figs. 30-27(3)

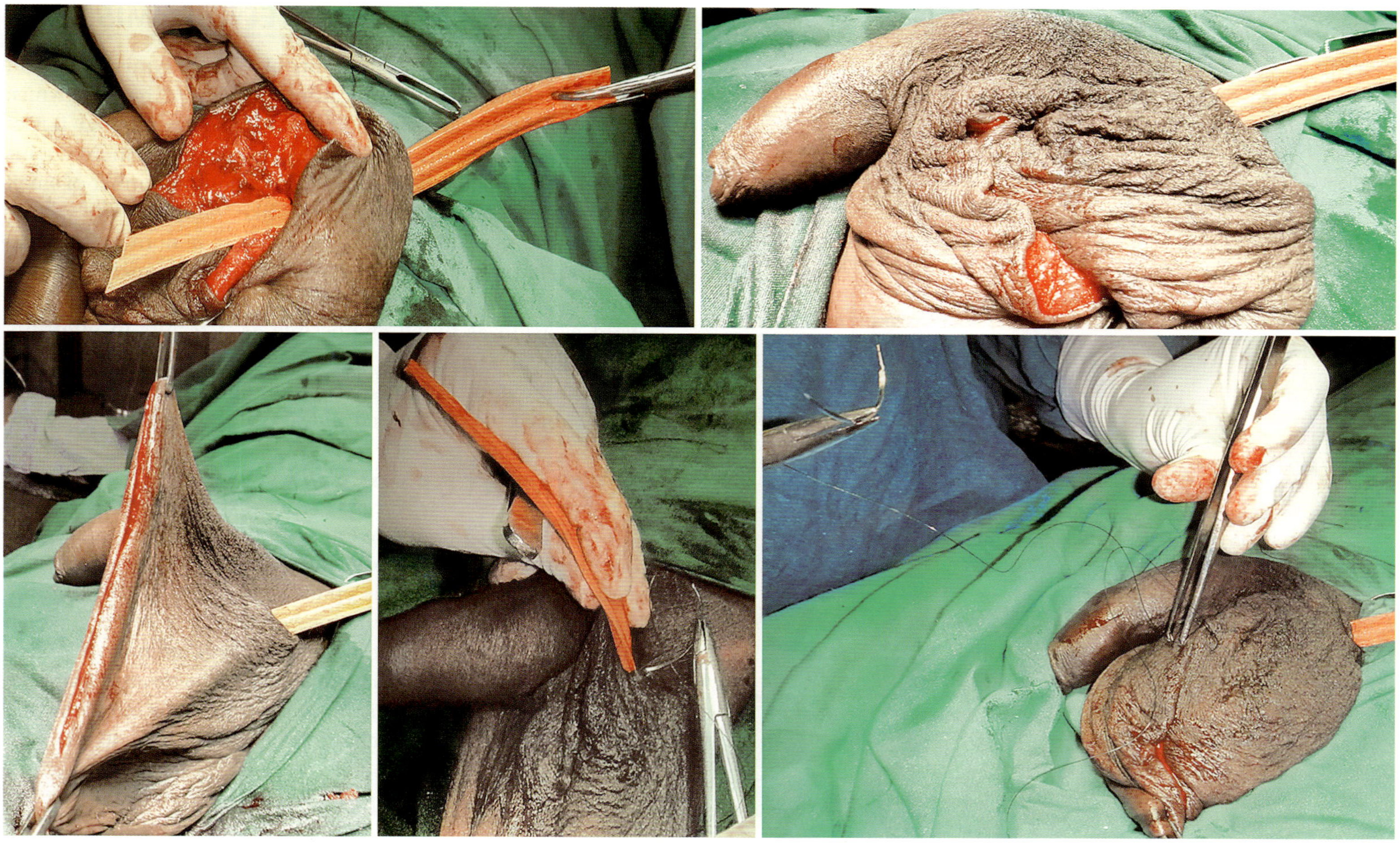

Figs. 30-27(4)

Figs. 30-27(1 to 4): For chronic haematocele low orchidectomy is done through scrotal approach. Cord is divided between clamps and ligated by transfixation using 1-zero vicryl (absorbable) suture.

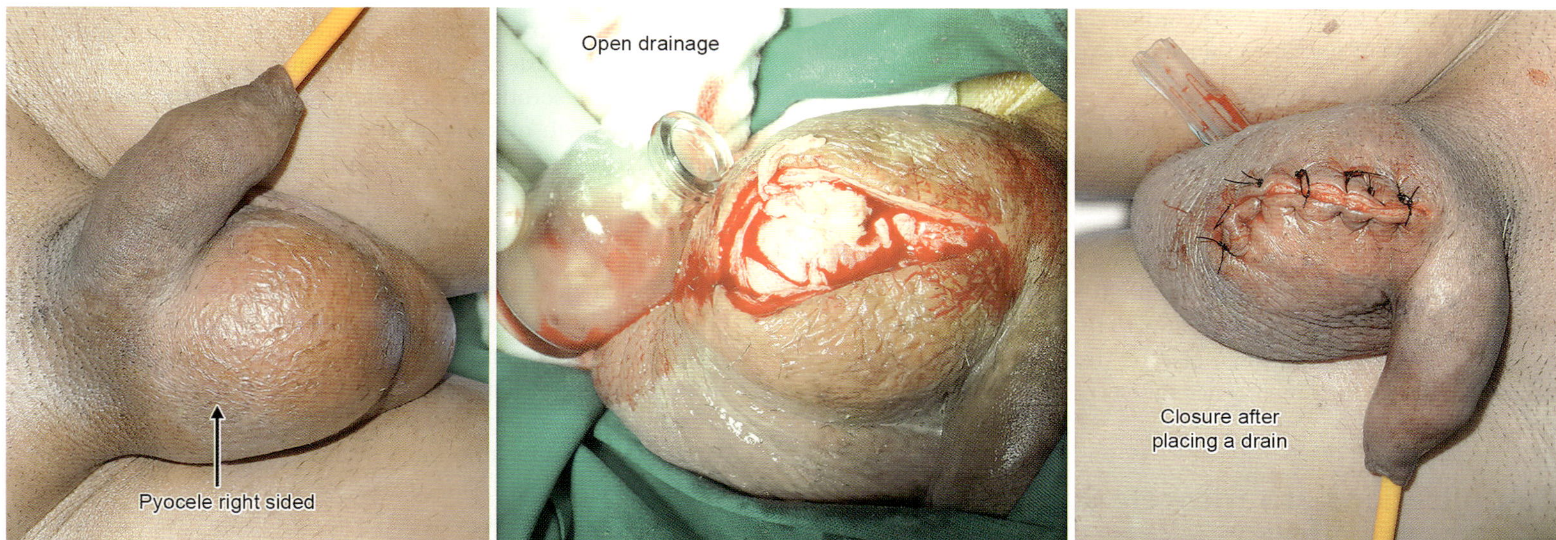

Fig. 30-28: Drainage of pyocele; if testis is not viable low orchidectomy is done after taking consent.

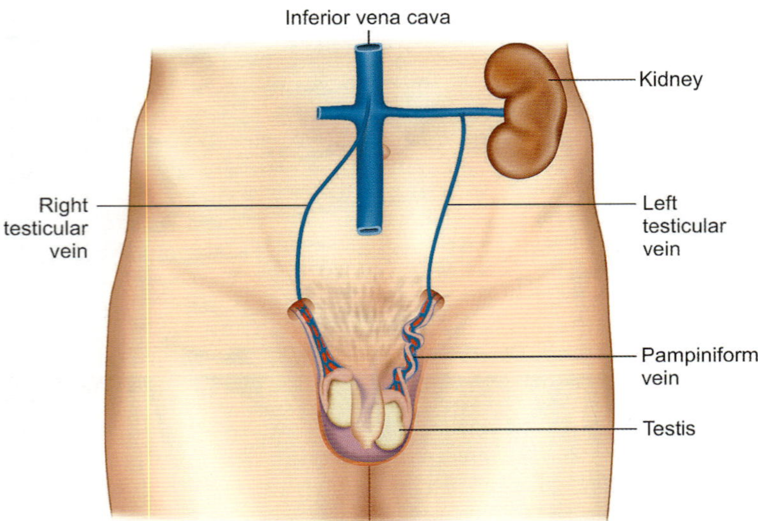

Fig. 30-29: Anatomy of testicular veins. Left testicular vein joins into left renal vein in perpendicular fashion. Right vein joins IVC directly.

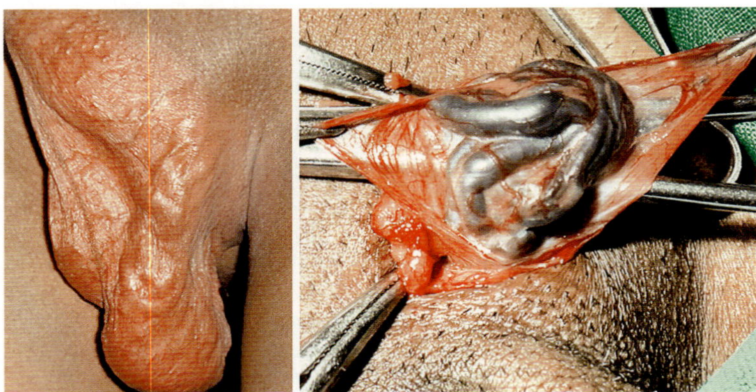

Fig. 30-30: Varicocele—it is common on left side—'bag of worms' look. Note the on table look of dilated veins.

Scrotal approach: In case of grade IV, veins have to be excised through this approach. Vertical paramedian incision is made in the scrotum, cord is identified and dilated veins are dissected and securely ligated with vicryl. Often tunica vaginalis sac is opened and everted to prevent possible chance of developing hydrocele due to lymphatic disruption.

Laparoscopic approach: Earlier it became very popular as technically, it was very easy. Under general anaesthesia, with head down position, after creation pneumoperitoneum, laparoscope is passed through umbilical port. Additional 5 mm or 10 mm ports are placed. Testicular veins are identified on both sides which run retroperitoneally upwards and medially. Peritoneum is incised; vein is dissected and clipped; alternatively bipolar fulguration or intracorporeal ligation can also be done. Once a enthusiastic procedure due to high recurrence rate its efficacy and acceptance is slowly going way.

Complications of Varicocele Surgery

Haemorrhage and scrotal haematoma; infection, pyocele; injury to testicular artery; injury to ilioinguinal nerve and pain; recurrence—5–10%.

TREATMENT OF CYST OF EPIDIDYMIS

It is due to the cystic degeneration of: Paradidymis (organ of Geraldes)—is the most common cause; appendix of the epididymis; appendix of the testis; the vas aberrans of Haller. Eventhough it is of congenital origin, it occurs in middle age. It is tensely cystic, contains clear fluid; often bilateral. They are aggregation of number of small cysts and so *multiloculated*. They feel like *'bunch of tiny grapes'* situated behind the body of the testis. Because of numerous septae they are finely tessellated and so are brilliantly transilluminant, appear like *'Chinese lantern pattern'* **(Figs. 30-33A and B)**.

Avoid excision as much as possible as it results in infertility in young individual as it may block the sperm transfer. In old age, excision can be done. Approach (scrotal) and technique is similar like for hydrocele. Cyst is excised and scrotal wound is closed.

TREATMENT OF SPERMATOCELE

It is a *unilocular, acquired retention cyst* derived from blockage of some portion of the sperm conducting mechanism of the epididymis. It is situated in the head of the epididymis, above and behind the body of the testis. Swelling contains *barley water like fluid,* which contains spermatozoa. It is soft, cystic and transilluminant. It is often considered by the patient as having an additional testis. Aspiration cytology confirms the diagnosis. *Treatment:* It can be left alone. If it is large, excision is done through scrotal approach **(Fig. 30-34)**.

SURGICAL ANATOMY OF TESTIS

It is the male gonad. It is suspended in the scrotum by the spermatic cord. It lies obliquely such that its upper pole is tilted forwards and laterally. It is 4 cm long, 2.5 cm broad, 1.8 cm thick with a weight 15 grams (adult). Epididymis lies along the lateral part of the posterior border **(Fig. 30-35)**.

Descent of Testis

Testis develops from mesonephros at T10,11,12 segments. Both side they descend downwards towards scrotum. It appears in 2nd month of intrauterine life; reaches iliac fossa in 3rd intrauterine month; between 4th to 7th month rests in deep inguinal ring; 8th month reaches external ring; at 9th month before delivery reaches to bottom of the scrotum. Factors are hormones, gonadotrophins, differential growth of body wall; action of gubernaculum; intra-abdominal pressure and temperature **(Fig. 30-36)**.

Coverings of the Testis

1. Tunica vaginalis—lower persistent portion of processus vaginalis.
2. Tunica albuginea—dense, white fibrous coat covering the testis; the posterior border of which is thickened to form the mediastinum testis. Numerous septa extend from it into the inner surface to create around 300 lobules.
3. Tunica vascularis is innermost vascular layer lining the lobules.

Structure of Testis

Testis contains 200–300 lobules, each containing 2–3 seminiferous tubules. Each tubule is 60 cm in length but heavily coiled.

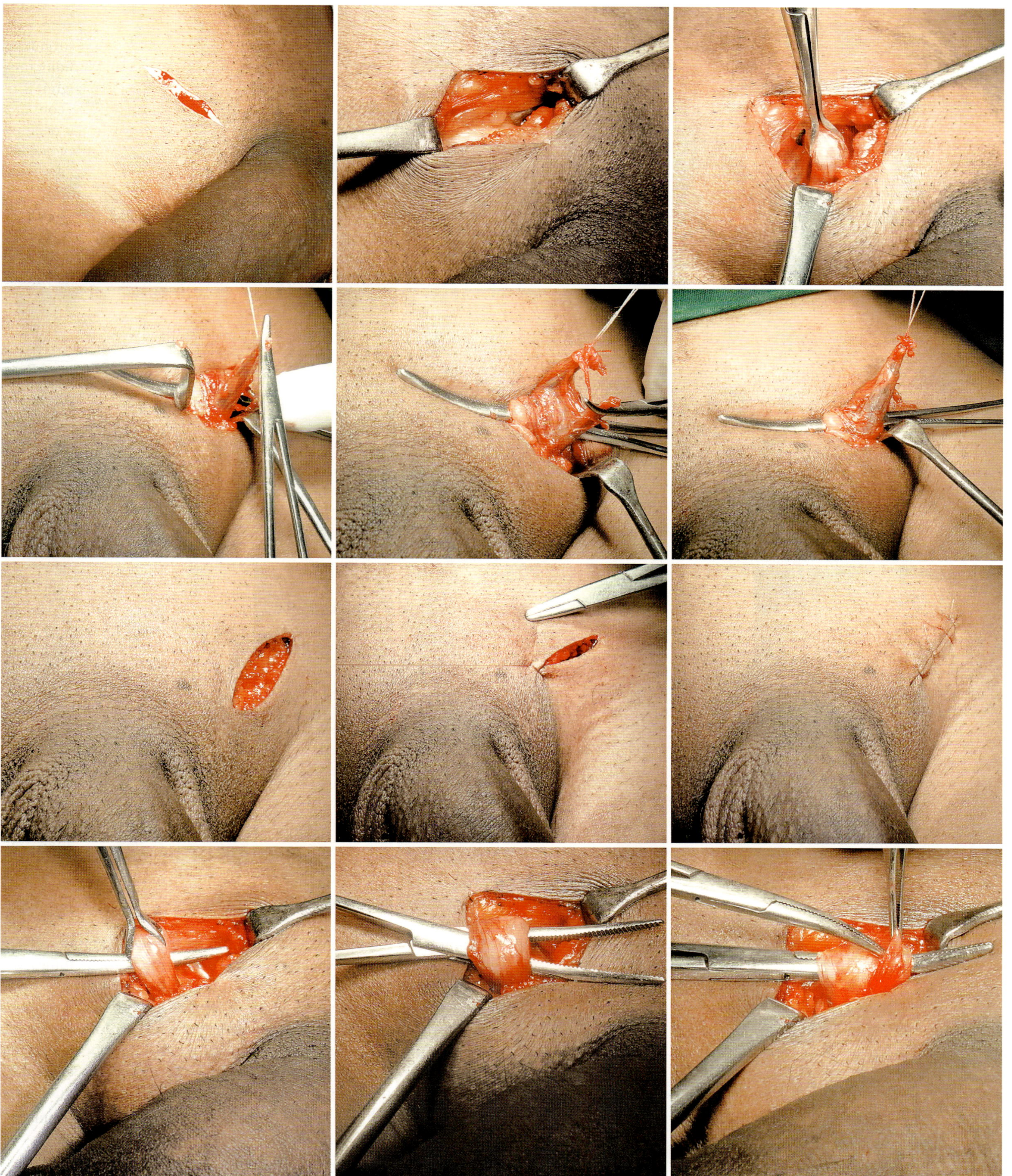

Figs. 30-31(1)

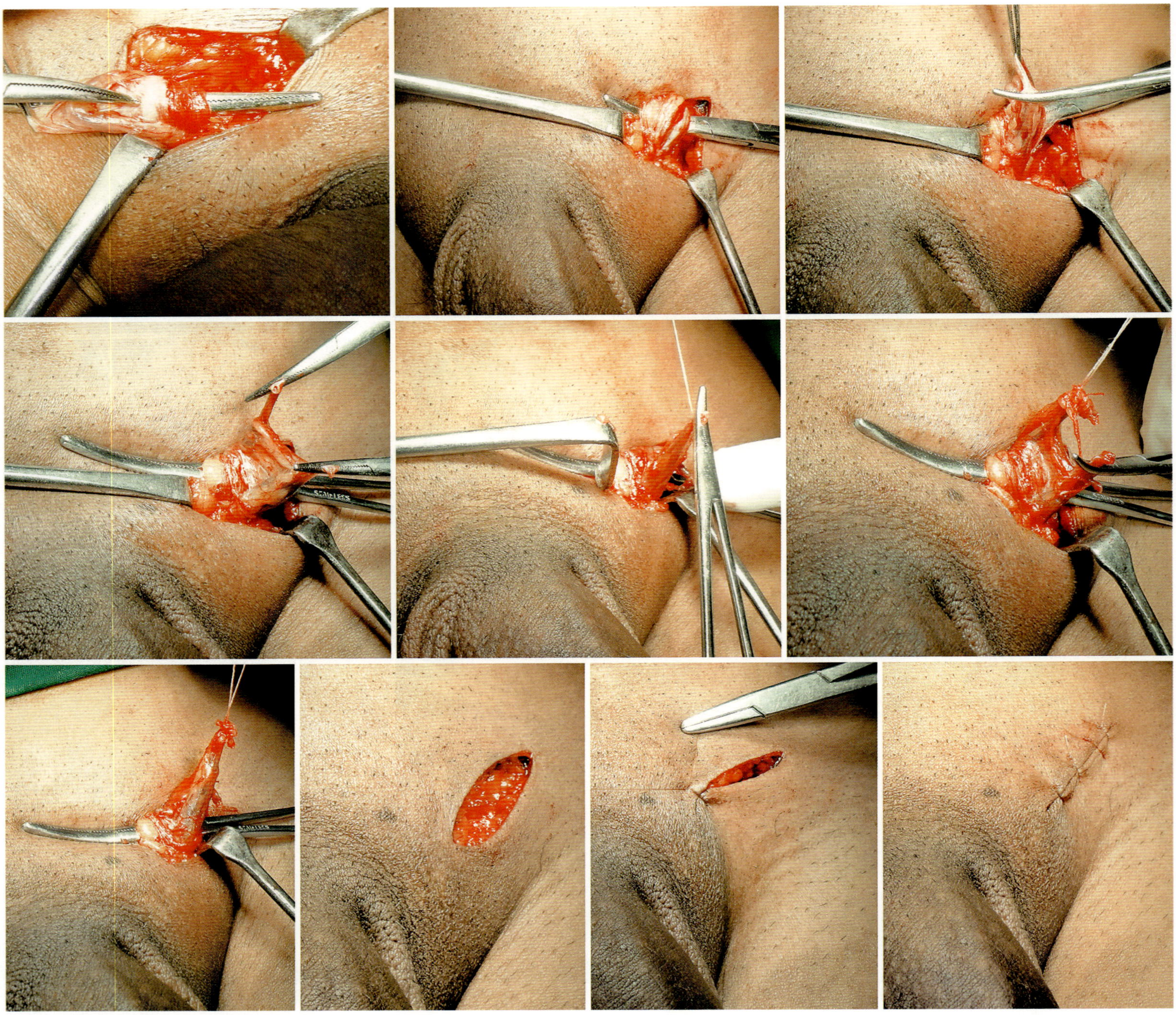

Figs. 30-31(2)

Figs. 30-31(1 and 2): Technique of subinguinal varicocele repair.

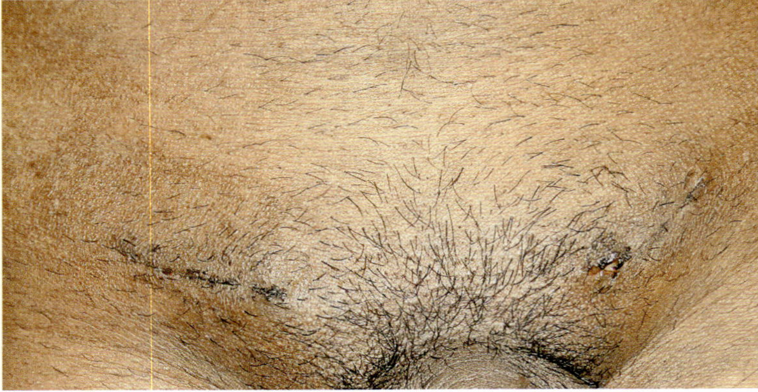

Fig. 30-32: Subinguinal incision both sides for bilateral varicocele ligation of veins.

Diametre of the tubule is 0.2 mm. Lining of tubule contain cells of different stages of spermatogenesis. These seminiferous tubules join together to form around 30 straight tubules; they enter mediastinum of testis; after joining each other to form rete testis which contains network of tubules. Rete testis gives 30 efferent ductules which comes out at the superior pole of the testis and enters the epididymis with a coiled ductules to form head of the epididymis. A single duct is formed in the body and tail of the epididymis to continue as vas deferens at the lower pole of the testis.

Arterial Supply

Testicular artery, a branch of abdominal aorta arises at the level of 12th vertebra a little below the origin of renal arteries;

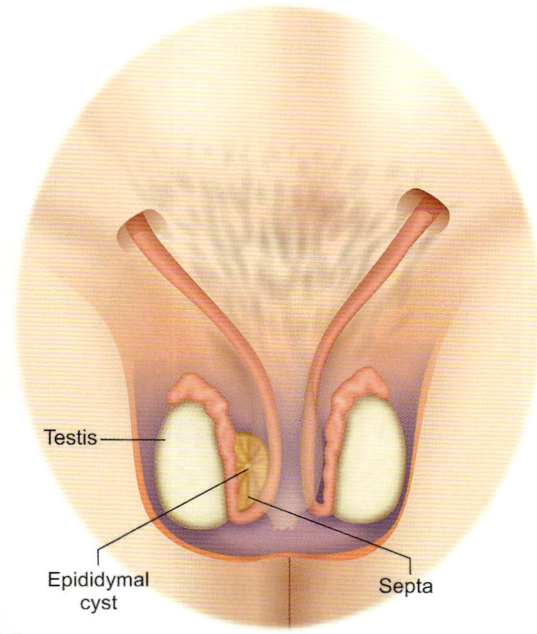

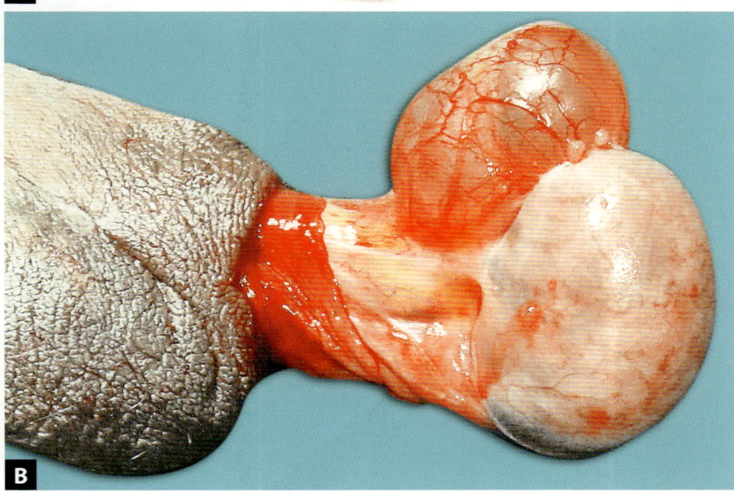

Figs. 30-33A and B: Epididymal cyst.

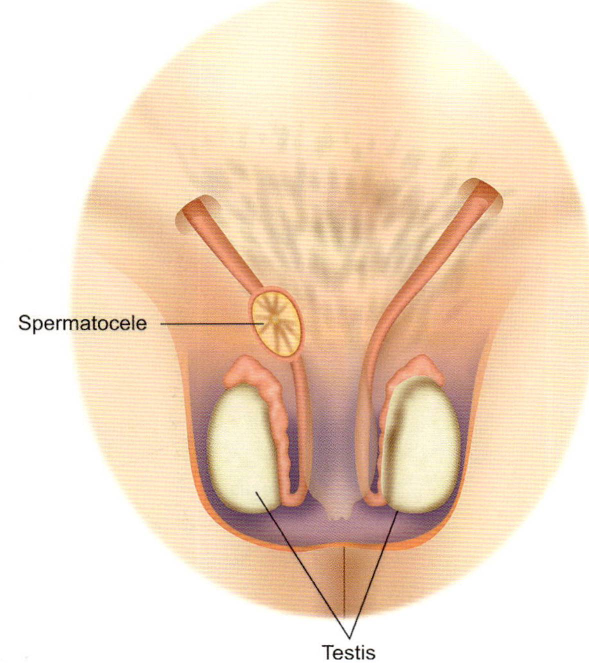

Fig. 30-34: Diagram showing position of spermatocele.

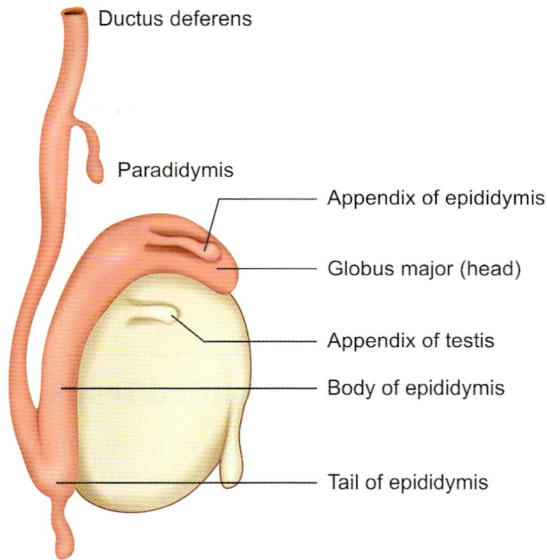

Fig. 30-35: Anatomy of the testis.

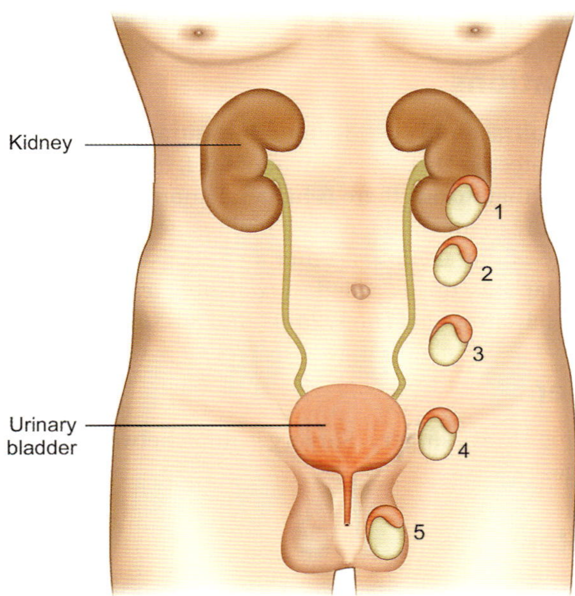

Fig. 30-36: Stages of testicular descent.

runs downwards and laterally on the psoas major in the posterior abdominal wall crosses the IVC, ureter and genitofemoral nerve on the right side. On right side, it is deep to the ileum (small bowel, terminal ileum). On the left side, artery crosses the left ureter, left genitofemoral nerve running on the left psoas major lying deep to colon. It travels downwards to enter the internal inguinal ring and inguinal canal. It runs in the spermatic cord (within the cord anterior to the vas deferens) to reach the posterior border of the upper pole of the testis. It divides into smaller and larger branches. Medial and lateral branches pierce the tunica albuginea to reach tunica vasculosa.

Venous Drainage

It is by forming pampiniform (*like a vine*) plexus of veins which ultimately fuse to form single vein, which drains into IVC on right side, left renal vein on left side. In the scrotum, its anterior part is around the testicular artery; middle part is around vas deferens and testicular artery; posterior part is isolated. It forms four veins at external ring; two veins at internal ring; single vein at retroperitoneum.

Lymphatic Drainage

It is into para-aortic and pre-aortic group of lymph nodes at the level of L2 vertebra.

UNDESCENDED TESTIS

Complications of Undescended Testis

Sterility; trauma and pain; an associated indirect inguinal hernia (70%); torsion testis; epididymo-orchitis (as the pain will be high up it mimics acute appendicitis); testicular atrophy; *malignant transformation in undescended testis is 20 times more common* than normally descended testis. It is higher in abdominal than in inguinally located testis. *Seminoma* is the most common malignancy in undescended testis. The testis which has normally descended on other side (in case of unilateral undescended testis), is also more prone for malignant transformation than normal individual.

Investigations

Abdominal ultrasound (US) is done but intra-abdominal testis is difficult to detect in U/S. Assessment of FSH, hCG. If FSH is high in a young boy, that means there is bilateral anorchia. CT scan can be done probably to locate the abdominal testis; gonadal venogram; laparoscopy—quiet useful and therapeutic also; blind ending *vas deferens* in laparoscopy is called as *vanishing testis*. It means testis has completely atrophied **(Figs. 30-37 and 30-38)**.

Treatment

Treatment is always surgery. Surgery is done between two and four years of age.

Principles

Mobilisation of cord to achieve adequate length is important. Repair of associated inguinal hernia is essential as it is a very common association. Finally needs adequate scrotal fixation without tension which will keep the testis in place and prevents its retraction into the groin during healing.

Mobilisation of Spermatic Cord

Under general anaesthesia in children, spinal in adult after cleaning and draping, inguinal canal is opened with lengthy incision like for inguinal hernia. Hernial sac is identified; often cord will be less developed and testis will be smaller than normal. Unless sac or tunica vaginalis is opened it is often difficult to identify the undescended testis. Herniotomy is done. Inferior epigastric vessels are ligated to lengthen the cord. If length is still required, vas and testicular vessels are mobilised retroperitoneally. If further length is required then a soft clamp is applied to the testicular artery and the viability of testis is checked. If it is viable that means it is also receiving blood supply from the artery of vas or cremaster vessels. Then testicular artery can be ligated safely so that adequate length can be achieved to bring down the testis to the scrotum—*Stephen-Fowler's technique.*

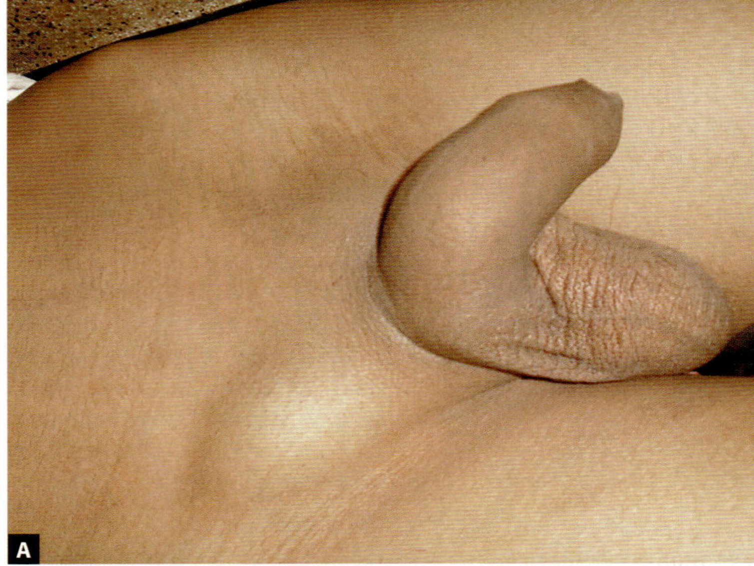

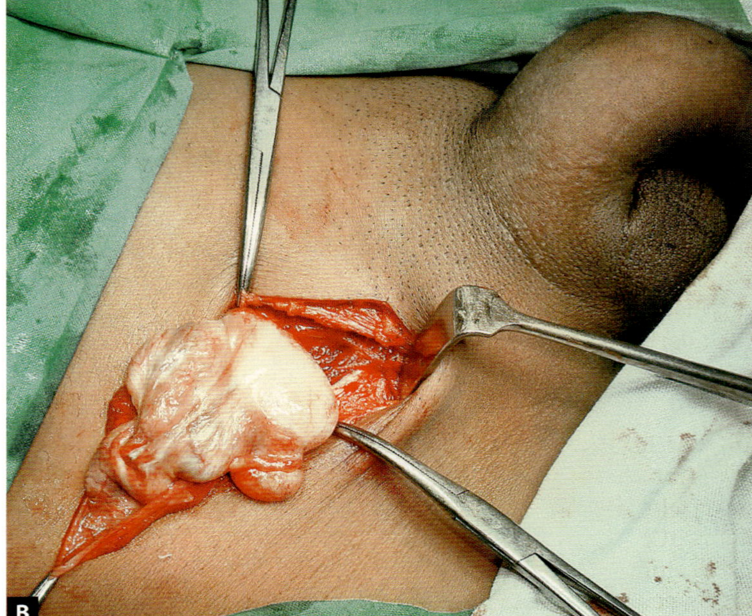

Figs. 30-37A and B: Undescended testis; on table finding.

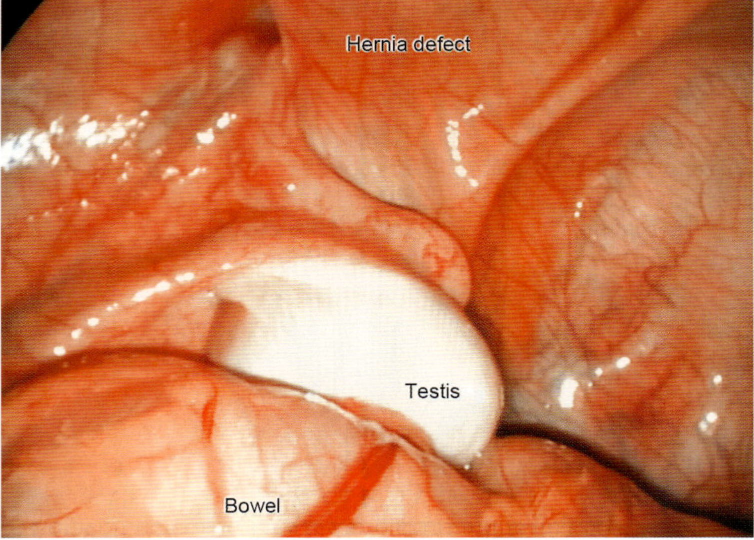

Fig. 30-38: Laparoscopic view of undescended testis adjacent and deep to internal ring.

Fixation of the Testis

Proper scrotal pouch is created by finger dissection. Fixation of the testis into the scrotum is done using non-absorbable interrupted sutures (polypropylene). A small scrotal incision is made at the bottom of the scrotum. Long haemostat is passed through the scrotal wound across the scrotum to inguinal wound; stay suture placed at the gubernaculum is held with haemostat and pulled gently out towards the scrotal wound. Interrupted bites are taken between tunica albuginea and scrotal wall; usually three bites are taken from below upwards using 3-zero polypropylene suture. Knots are tied at the end. Scrotal wound is sutured. Inguinal wound is closed in layers.

In bilateral cases, testis is passed into the opposite scrotum through an opening in the scrotal septum—*Ombredanne's operation* **(Fig. 30-39)**.

If the testis is totally atrophied, *orchidectomy* should be done after taking consent, because even though this is a non-functioning testis, it is highly prone for malignant transformation. Removed testis should be sent for histology.

Laparoscopic orchidopexy: Laparoscopic mobilisation of the testis is very useful. Under general anaesthesia, head down position, ports are placed on both sides at the level of the umbilicus. Gonadal vein is identified and traced downwards to reach the testis. Usually it will be very close to the internal ring. Peritoneum is incised close to the cord and the testis and mobilised. Hernial sac is dissected like in laparoscopic hernia repair. Once adequate mobilisation is done like in open method small scrotal incision is made and through a long haemostat mobilised testis is pulled down to scrotum to fix it similarly. Inferior epigastric vessels can be clipped and divided through laparoscopy safely which will add on to the extra length of the cord.

Role of hormone therapy: Not much. Only indications are cryptorchidism associated with hypogenitalism and obesity and doubtful retractile testis. It should be given at or after the age of eight. hCG (Chorionic gonadotrophin) 1000 I/U—twice weekly for maximum of ten weeks (not more than 10 weeks). It stimulates Leydig cells to produce testosterone. GnRH—1.2 mg/day as nasal spray for one month.

Note: In bilateral case surgery is done with an interval of 6 months.

Ladd and Gross procedure: After placing the testis in the scrotal pouch, it is fixed by a polypropylene suture into tunica albuginea, across scrotal skin and into the thigh skin outside. This suture is removed in 14 days.

Keetley–Torek procedure: Testis is mobilised and is brought into the scrotal pouch first. Then it is brought out through scrotal skin. A pouch is created on the medial aspect of the thigh outer to fascia lata, deep to thigh skin after making skin incision. Testis delivered from scrotal pouch is placed into the thigh pouch. Scrotal and thigh incisions are sutured around the cord inside. After 6 months scrotal sac with cord and testis is separated and placed in the scrotal pouch.

Laparoscopic approach: Orchidopexy has become popular and accepted method.

Orchidopexy may not alter the chances/risk of developing carcinoma of testis. But it makes early observation and evaluation by ultrasound easy to detect the possible changes.

Orchidectomy is considered if there is atrophy; torsion; inability to bring down abdominal testis.

Testicular biopsy in infertility to study spermatogenesis is sent in *Bouin's fluid*—picric acid (75%); acetic acid (25%). It should not be sent in usual formalin.

Surgeries in undescended testis

- External anchorage—Ladd and Gross
- Ombredanne's procedure
- Denis–Browne's operation—narrowing of the neck and external anchorage
- Keetley–Torrek procedure into the thigh
- Dartos pouch creation and placing the testes
- Stephen–Fowler's technique
- Silbar procedure—autotransplantation with microvascular anastomoses into inferior epigastric vessels

ECTOPIC TESTIS

Lockwood theory: Even though there are multiple gubernaculum, scrotal tail normally gets activated better and so testis is brought down to the scrotum. In ectopic testis, scrotal tail weakens or ruptures and so one of the other accessory tails will act and pulls the testis in direction according to its site.

Different Sites

Superficial inguinal pouch; perineum; root of the penis; femoral triangle (thigh) **(Fig. 30-40)**.

Testis, here functions normally and is of normal in size. It is more prone for trauma and can cause psychological problem.

Superficial inguinal pouch is a space between external oblique and Scarpa'a fascia. On raising the legs, ectopic testis in superficial inguinal pouch becomes more prominent but not in case of undescended testis located in inguinal canal.

Treatment

Mobilisation and creation of a new scrotal pouch to place and fix the testis to scrotal pouch using polypropylene interrupted sutures.

TREATMENT OF TORSION TESTIS

Emergency exploration of the scrotum and untwisting of the torsion testis is done. Then viability of testis is checked. Arterial Doppler of both sides is essential. Twisted testis will be viable only for 6 hours—critical period/golden period, so urgent correction of twist and fixation is essential **(Figs. 30-41 to 30-43)**.

Once viability is confirmed, the testis is fixed to the scrotal sac using three interrupted non-absorbable sutures (3-0 polypropylene). Fixation should be done using only non-absorbable sutures, never absorbable sutures. If surgery is done within 6–12 hours, viability of the testis may be retained. If delayed, testis becomes gangrenous and *orchidectomy* is done after taking informed consent. *When in doubt, testis is retained and orchidectomy can be postponed to later period* so as to give a chance to have a viable testis. Here *early exploration is an important aspect.* When diagnosis is in doubt, exploration is advised.

Postoperatively, a repeat Doppler study helps to confirm the viability. As often the condition is *bilateral, other side testis should*

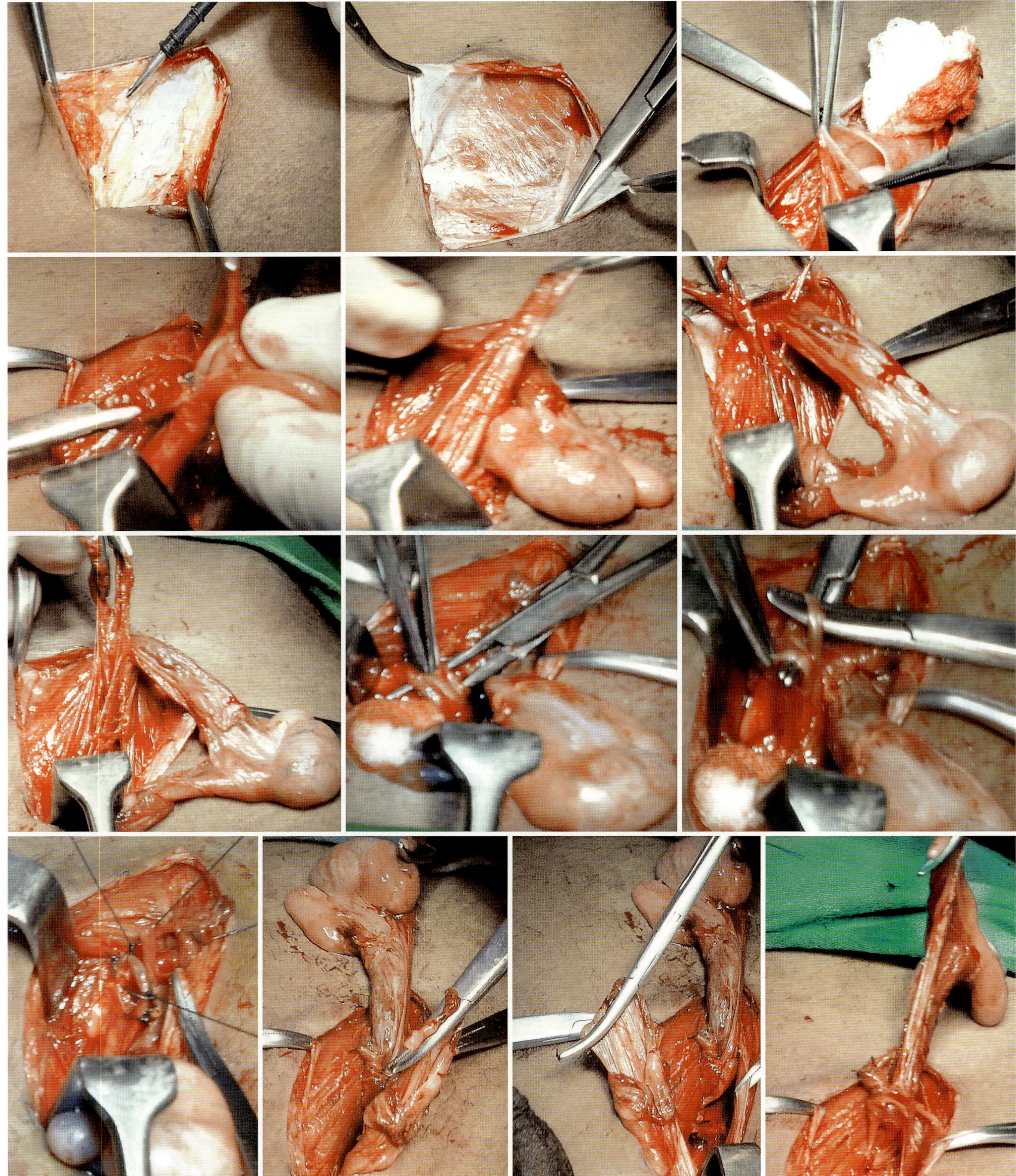

Figs. 30-39(1)

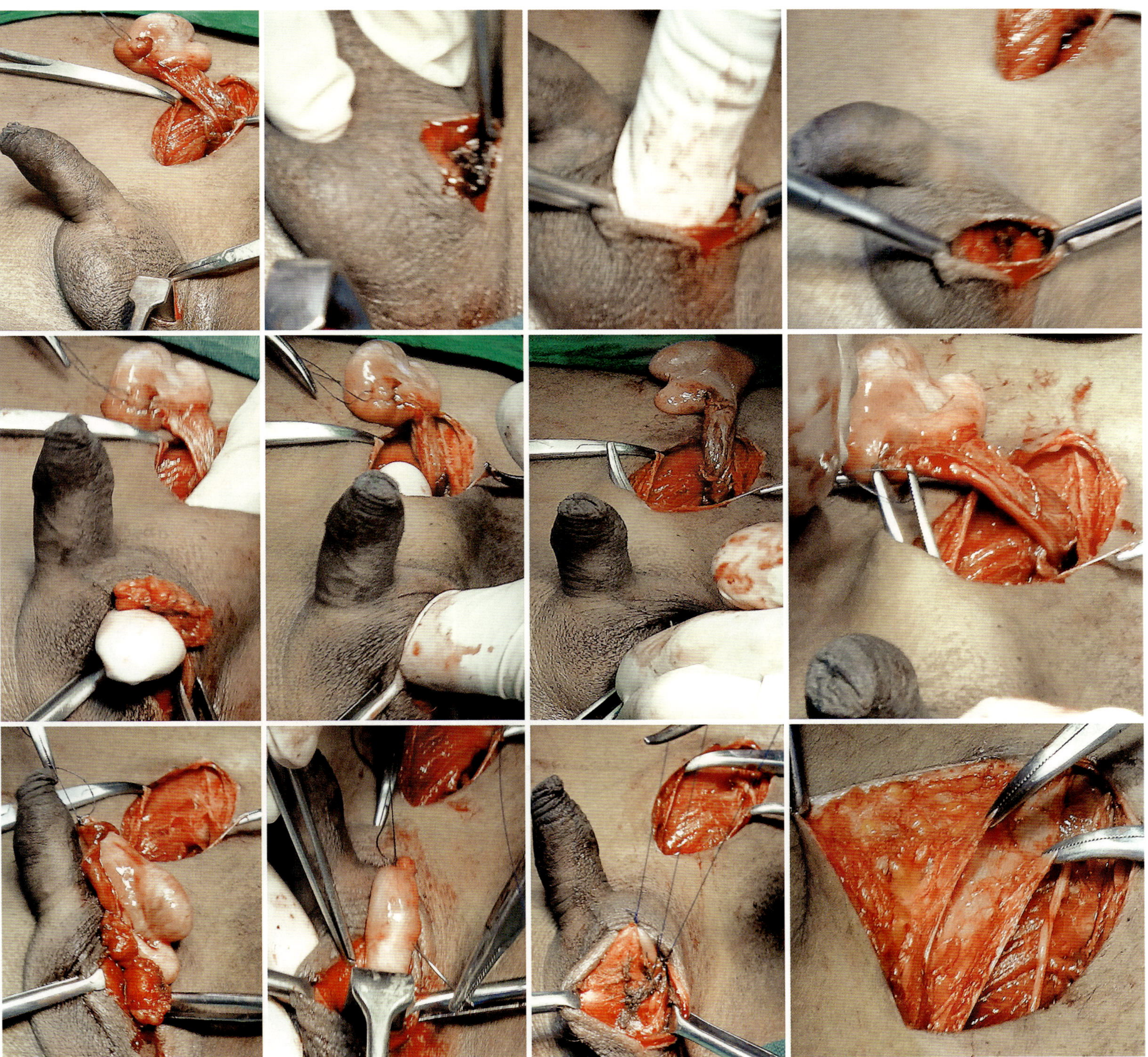

Figs. 30-39(2)

Figs. 30-39(1 and 2): Orchidopexy—technique in undescended testis.

also be fixed to prevent the torsion. Approach to other side should be separate through other side hemiscrotum. It is better to avoid approaching other side through same ipsilateral incision.

TESTICULAR BIOPSY

It is done in infertility with low sperm count. It is usually done under local anaesthesia. Only one side is done. After injecting local anaesthesia xylocaine without adrenaline (plain), skin, dartos, spermatic fasciae are incised. Tunica vaginalis is incised. Testis is exposed. With no. 15 blade small incision is made on the tunica albuginea. Protruding seminiferous tubules less than 5 mm size is excised. Tunica albuginea is sutured using 3 zero vicryl or monocryl continuous sutures. Tissue is placed in *Bouin's fluid*—picric acid (75%); acetic acid (25%). It is sent for spermatogenesis assessment. Skin is closed **(Fig. 30-44)**.

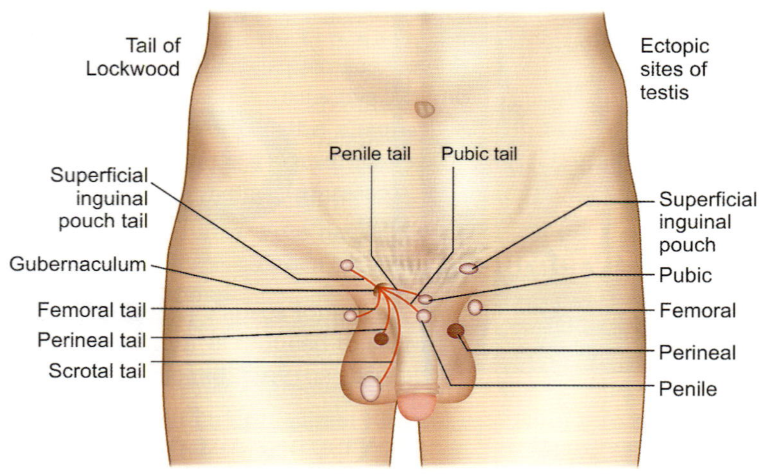

Fig. 30-40: Tails of Lockwood and ectopic testes.

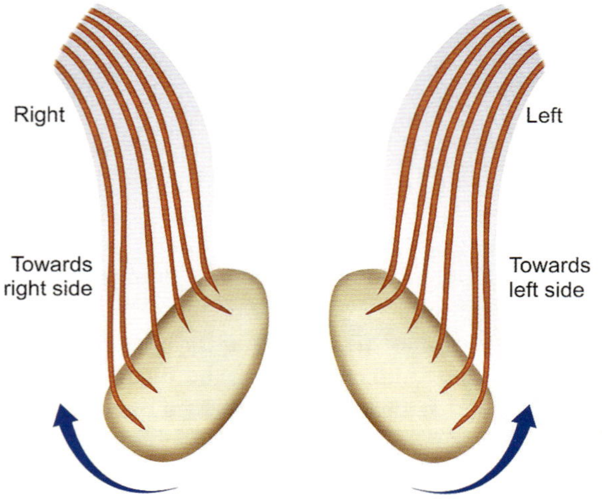

Fig. 30-41: Direction of torsion of testis is always outwards.

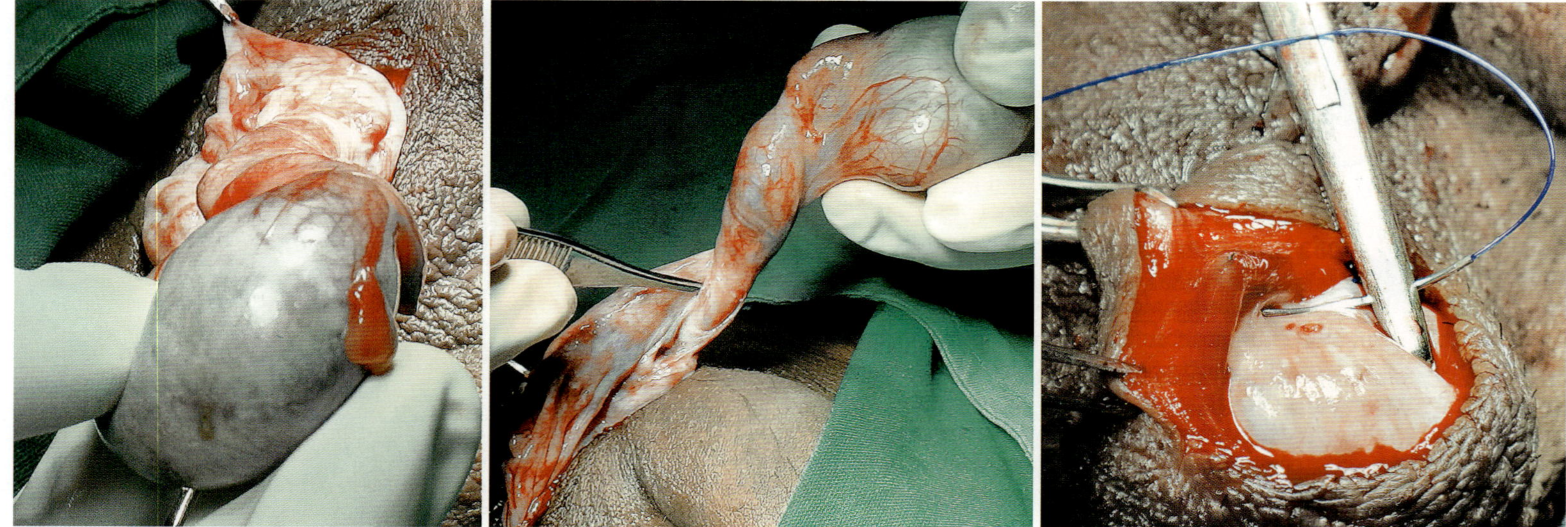

Fig. 30-42: Torsion testis—early intervention shows viable testis. It should be fixed to scrotal wall; opposite testis is also fixed using non-absorbable interrupted sutures.

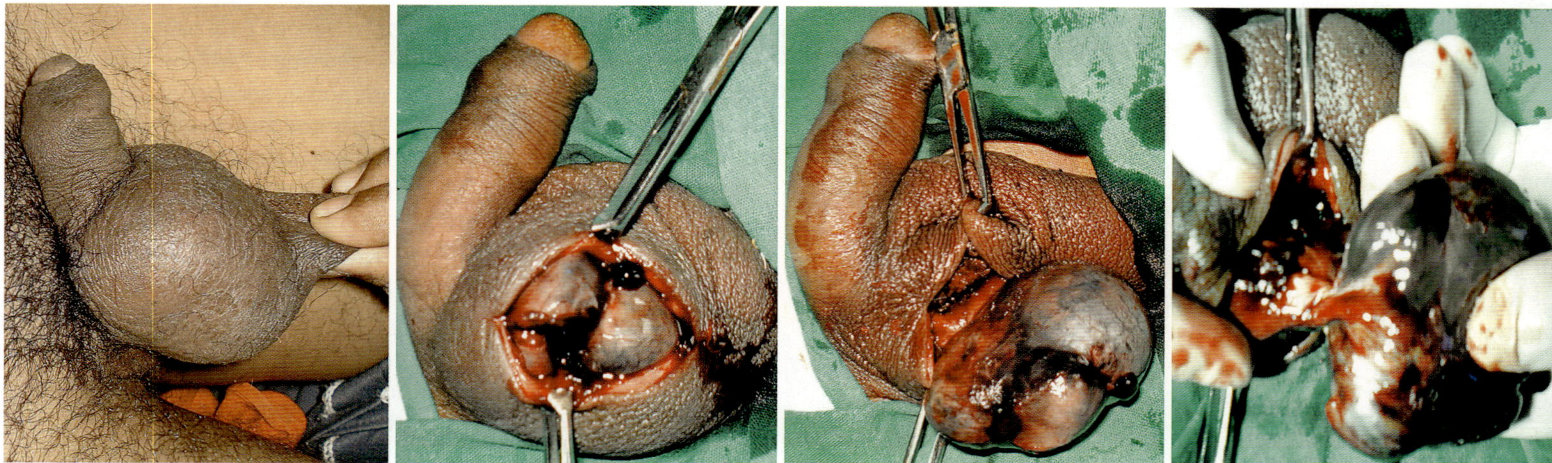

Fig. 30-43: Testicular torsion with gangrene testis. This testis is not viable; so needs orchidectomy.

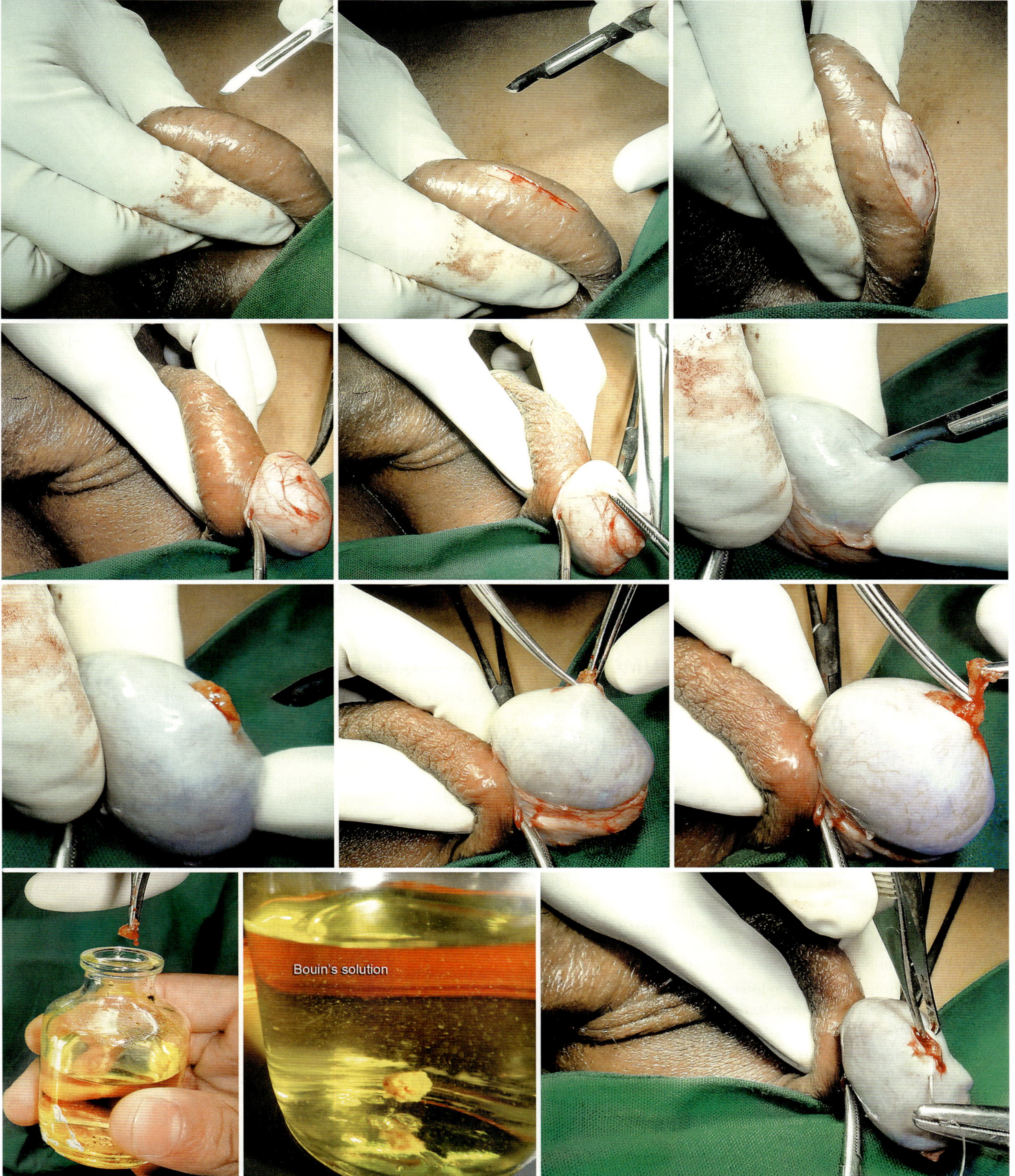

Figs. 30-44(1)

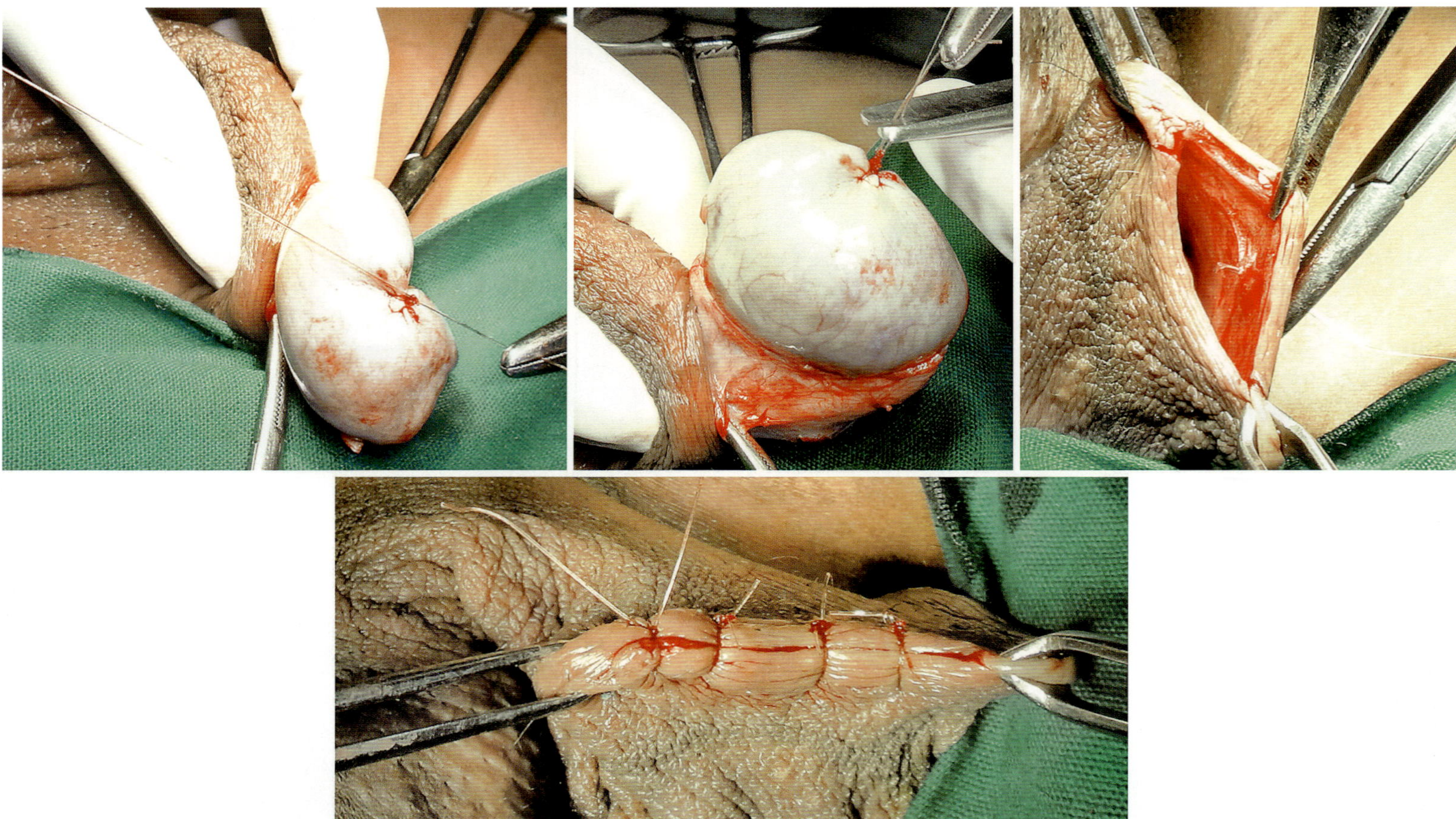

Figs. 30-44(2)

Figs. 30-44(1 and 2): Testicular biopsy is done to study stages of spermatogenesis in infertility with low sperm count. Bouin's fluid is used. Only one side is done.

TREATMENT OF TESTICULAR TUMOUR

Spread of Testicular Tumour

Local

To epididymis, cord, tunica albuginea, scrotum and so inguinal nodes.

Lymphatic Spread

Lymphatics drainage of testis is through its mediastinum along the gonadal vessels to para-aortic and retroperitoneal nodes. Through the lymphatics along the medial side of testis may run with the artery of vas draining into the common iliac nodes at the bifurcation of common iliac artery. Spread mainly occurs to ***para-aortic***; often to retroperitoneal and common iliac nodes. Malignancy spreads to inguinal nodes, only if scrotal skin is involved.

Right testicular tumour spreads to interaortocaval nodes immediately below the renal vessels as *primary landing zone* (L2 level), then to para-aortic nodes. Paracaval, preaortic, common iliac nodes can be involved.

Left testicular tumour spreads to true para-aortic nodes to begin with just below the renal vessels; then to preaortic and common iliac nodes.

From retroperitoneal and para-aortic nodes spread occurs to left supraclavicular nodes and posterior mediastinal nodes. Seminoma mainly spreads through lymphatics than teratoma.

Extranodal Spread

It occurs to lungs, liver, brain, bone, kidney, adrenals in order of frequency.

Investigations

No FNAC; No scrotal approach; No incision biopsy.

Through inguinal approach, cord and testis are exposed. A soft clamp is applied to the cord at or above the level of the deep ring so has to prevent dissemination through blood. Frozen section biopsy is done from the suspected area. If tumour is positive, *high orchidectomy is done (Chevassou manoeuvre).*

Measurement of tumour markers (hCG, AFP, LDH) are important. AFP and hCG are elevated in non-seminomatous germ cell tumours (teratomas)—65%. Raised AFP always indicates teratomatous tumour. *AFP level increase is not seen in pure seminomas.* hCG may be elevated in *advanced* cases of seminomas (10%). LDH level depends on growth rate/cellular proliferation/tumour burden. LDH is increased in 80% of advanced seminomas and 60% of non-seminomatous germ cell tumour. hCG is never found in normal individual. It is secreted by syncytiotrophoblasts. Half life is 18–36 hours. It is increased in choriocarcinoma (100%); embryonal carcinoma (65%); teratoma testis; recurrent or residual disease in testicular tumour after therapy. Placental alkaline phosphatase (PLAP) is increased in seminoma.

Chest X-ray is done to look for lung secondaries. HRCT scan is ideal. *Ultrasound abdomen* is done to see nodal status like para-aortic nodes and liver secondaries. *Ultrasound scrotum to see* echogenicity of testis and tumour within is essential.

CT scan abdomen and pelvis is to look for secondaries, iliac and para-aortic nodes. CT chest is needed to confirm lung secondaries.

Based on presence of AFP; hCG; LDH; non-pulmonary visceral secondaries (bone/liver/brain), germ cell tumour risk group

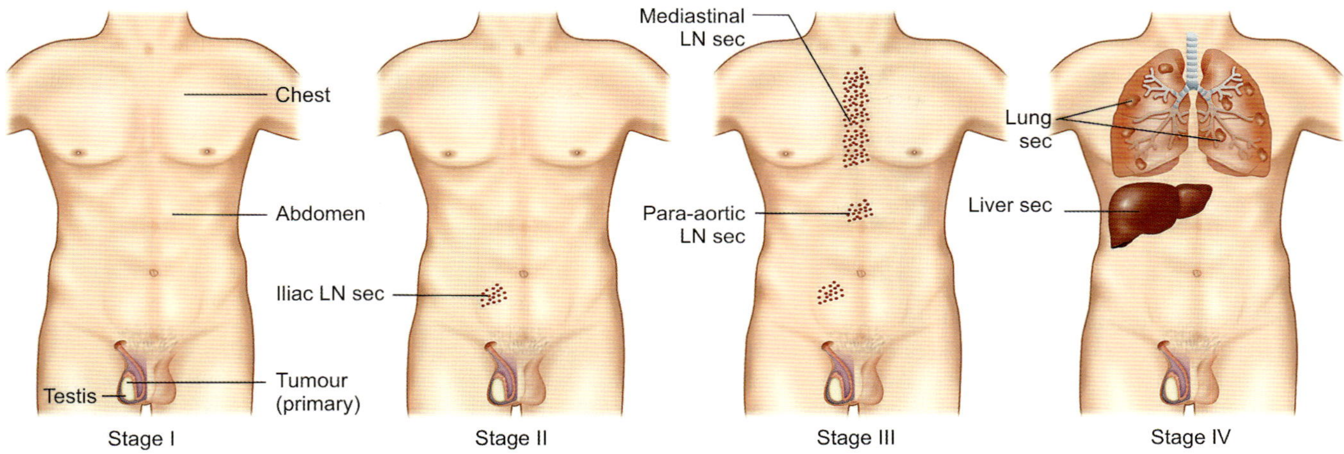

Fig. 30-45: Staging of testicular tumours

classification is done to both seminomatous germ cell tumour (SGCT) and also to non-seminomatous germ cell tumour (NSGCT).

Good risk and intermediate risk group for SGCT.

Good risk; intermediate risk and poor risk for NSGCT **(Fig. 30-45)**.

Staging of testicular tumours

I. Lesion confined to testis
II. Nodes involved below the diaphragm
III. Nodes involved above the diaphragm
IV. Distant (blood) spread

TNM staging

T_0 – No evidence of tumour
Tis – Carcinoma in situ
T_1 – Tumour limited to testis and epididymis. Vascular/lymphatic invasion not present. Tumour may invade tunica albuginea but not tunica vaginalis
T_2 – Tumour limited to testis and epididymis with vascular/lymphatic invasion. Or tumour extends through the tunica albuginea with involvement of tunica vaginalis
T_3 – Tumour invades to spermatic cord with or without vascular/lymphatic invasion
T_4 – Tumour invades to scrotum with or without vascular/lymphatic invasion
N_0 – Regional lodes not involved
N_1 – Single/multiple nodes—not more than 2 cm in size
N_2 – Regional nodes—between 2 cm and 5 cm
N_3 – Regional nodes >5 cm
M_0 – Distant spread not present
M_1 – Distant spread present
M_{1a} – Distant spread to non-regional nodes or to lungs
M_{1b} – Distant spread to other than non-regional nodes or lungs

Serum tumour markers (S)

S_x – Marker study not done
S_0 – Normal marker study
S_1 – LDH <1.5 × N (upper limit of normal) and hCG <5000 mIU/mL and AFP <1000 ng/mL
S_2 – LDH 1.5–10 × N or hCG 5000–50000 mIU/mL or AFP 1000–10000 ng/mL
S_3 – LDH >10 × N or hCG >50000 mIU/mL or AFP >10000 ng/mL

Treatment

Initially high orchidectomy is done in all patients through inguinal approach by ligating and dividing the cord at internal ring level **(Fig. 30-46)**.

Seminomas are radiosensitive. So after high orchidectomy, *radiotherapy* is given to increase the cure rate and also to reduce relapse. It is *the treatment of choice* in stage I seminomas. Opposite testis should be shielded during radiotherapy. Seminomas with high levels of tumour marker are treated as non-seminomatous tumours.

Chemotherapy is also effective. *Cisplatin* is very useful drug in seminoma. *In teratoma, retroperitoneal radical lymph node Dissection (RPLND)* is beneficial after high orchidectomy. Even in stage I disease, chances of existing retroperitoneal spread is 30%. So RPLND (infrahilar) has a major role especially in teratomas which are relatively radioresistant. It involves removal of precaval, retrocaval, paracaval, interaortocaval, retroaortic, para-aortic, common iliac nodes along with removal of gonadal vein and adjacent fibrofatty tissues from internal ring level to its insertion into renal vein on left side and inferior vena cava on right side. Commonly bilateral RPLND is done as contralateral nodes also can be involved. Mortality in RPLND is only 1%. RPLND may cause ejaculatory problems. Nerve sparing RPLND is ideal if technically possible. Nerve sparing dissection is done on opposite side of the tumour. Laparoscopic RPLND is also advocated safely.

Note:

Please refer Chapter 27 Retroperitoneal Surgeries for description of RPLND.

Modified RPLND is same side lymph node dissection both above and below the inferior mesenteric artery (IMA); opposite side dissection is limited to above the level of IMA so that sympathetic chain on opposite side is preserved to retain ejaculation.

Complications of RPLND: Haemorrhage; injury to main structures like major vessels/ureter/bowel; chylous ascites; lymphocele; retrograde ejaculation.

Chemotherapeutic drugs for teratoma are *cisplatin, bleomycin,* vinblastine, *etoposide,* ifosfamide, mesna, paclitaxel. BEP regime is commonly used (Bleomycin, etoposide, cisplatin).

ORCHIDECTOMY

Testis is removed for variety of reasons. However, formal written consent should be taken before doing orchidectomy. It is done in pyocele, chronic haematocele, testicular tumour, undescended testis where testis is atrophied. Bilateral orchidectomy is done in carcinoma prostate to achieve hormone control.

Types

- Low orchidectomy.
- High orchidectomy.
- Subcapsular orchidectomy.

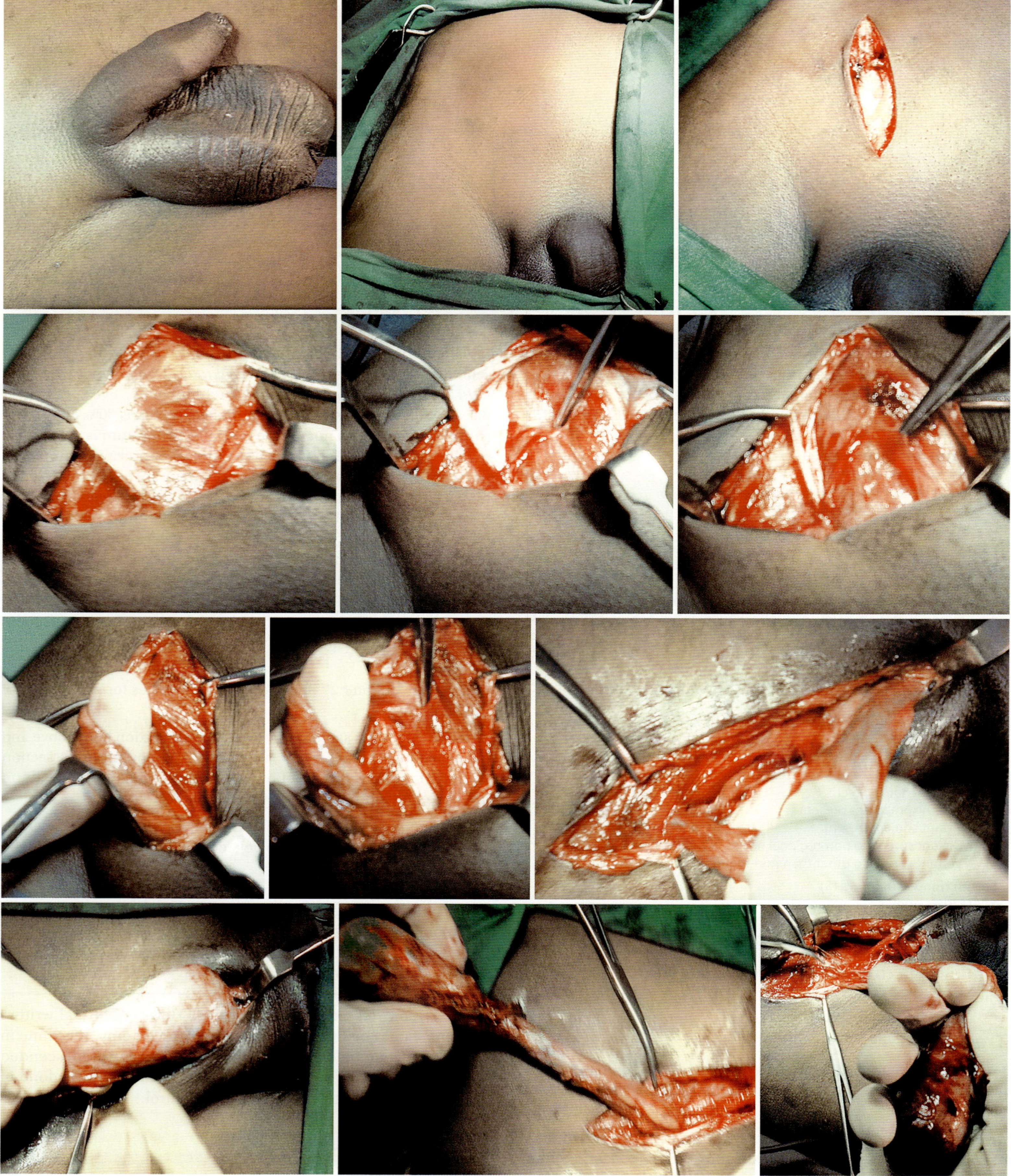

Figs. 30-46(1)

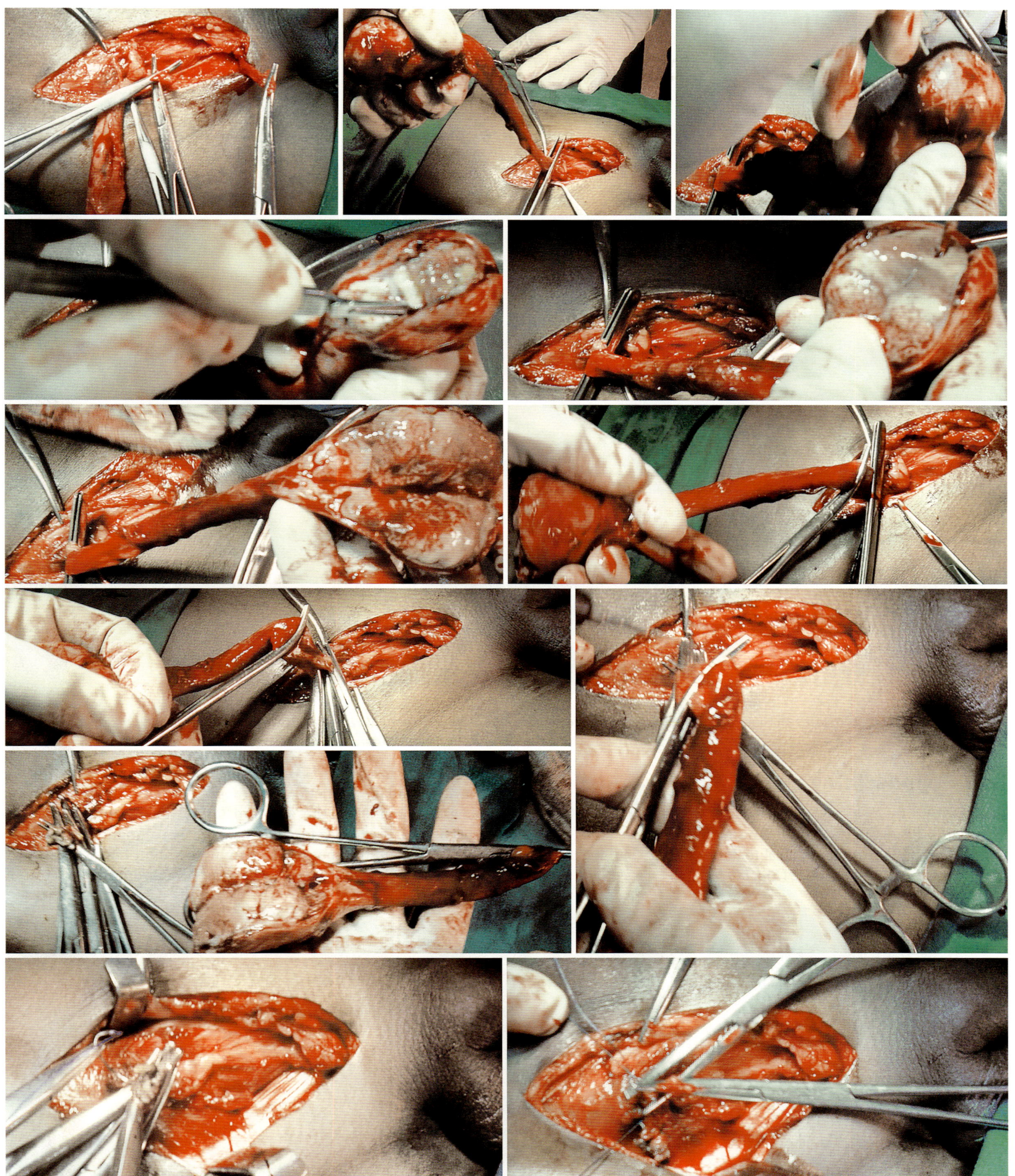

Figs. 30-46(2)

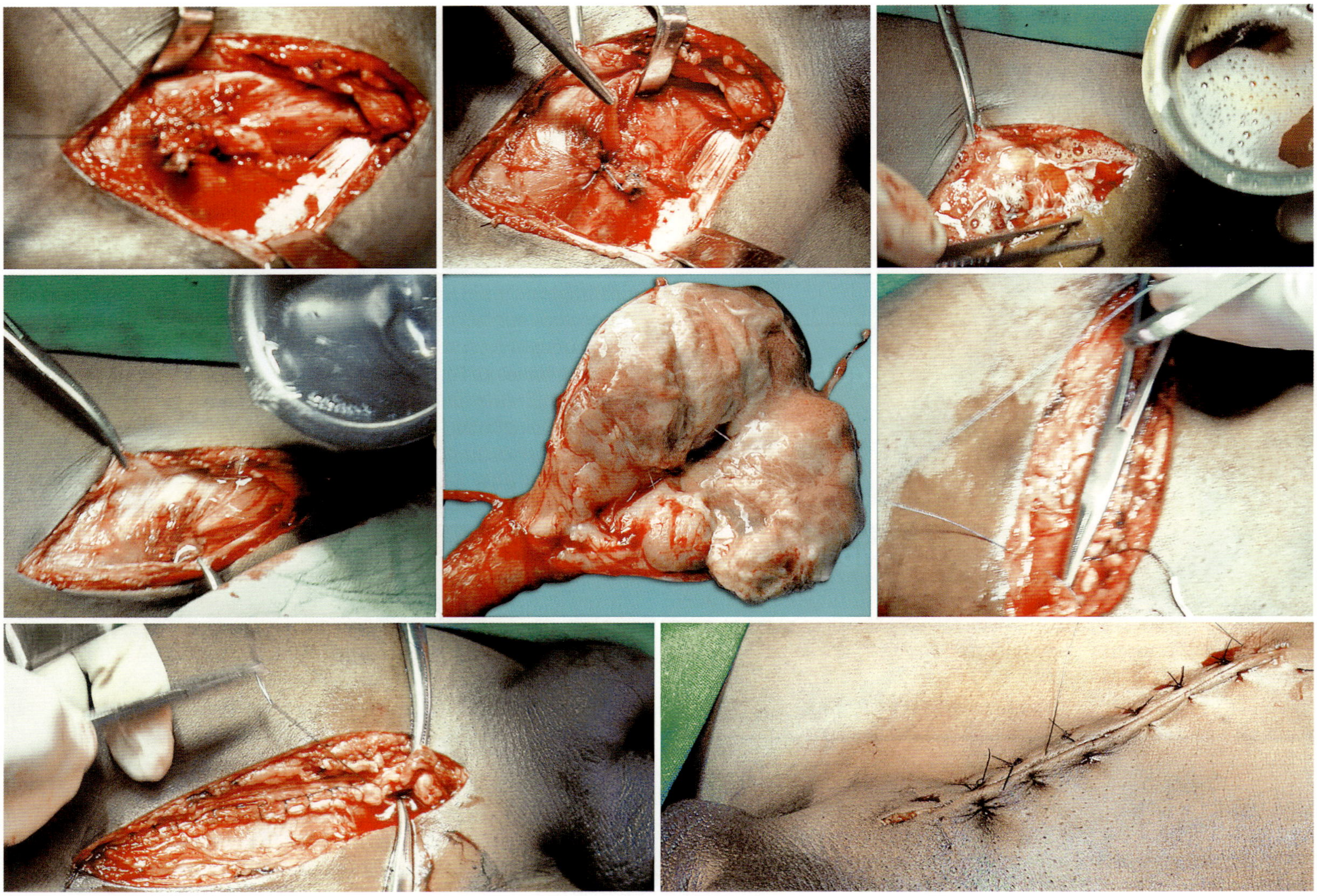

Figs. 30-46(3)

Figs. 30-46(1 to 3): High orchidectomy is done for testicular tumour through inguinal approach. Not through scrotal incision. Cord is ligated at the level of the internal ring.

Low Orchidectomy

It is done in pyocele, old clotted chronic haematocele. Arterial Doppler is a must to confirm the non-viability of testis. In case of pyocele, on table Doppler is ideal to confirm non-viability and also to document for legal purpose **(Fig. 30-47)**.

Under spinal or general anaesthesia after cleaning and draping incision is made on the scrotum lateral to the median raphe. Skin, dartos, spermatic fascia is incised. Non-functioning testis is mobilised up to the root of the scrotum by blunt finger dissection. Cord is mobilised for adequate length. At the root of the scrotum

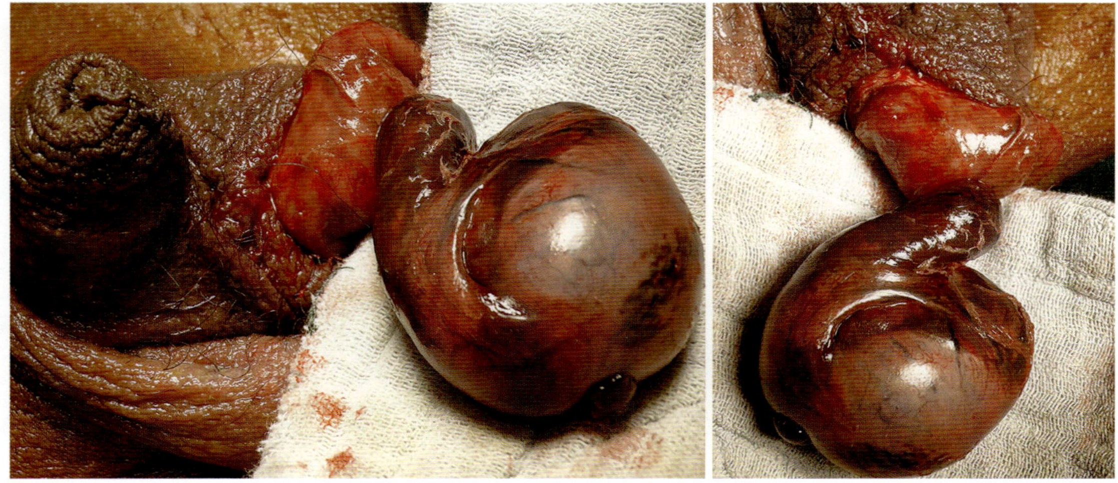

Fig. 30-47: Typical torsion testis. Low orchidectomy is needed.

cord is clamped using three strong clamps or Kocher's forceps. Distally one more haemostat is applied **(Fig. 30-48)**.

Cord is divided and testis is removed and sent for histology. Transfixation suture is placed using 1-zero vicryl or chromic catgut **(Fig. 30-49)**. Non-absorbable suture material like polypropylene is not used as it may cut through the tissues. It is also not possible to dissect the cord structures to isolate the vessels and ligate independently.

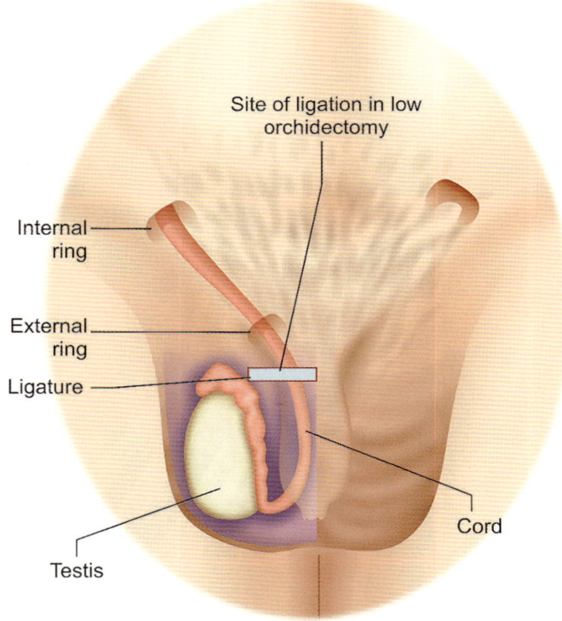

Fig. 30-48: Site of clamping for low orchidectomy.

Clamps should not slip as if it happens vessels retract proximally into the groin causing torrential bleeding and it is difficult to identify the bleeder from the retracted vessel. Alternatively after mobilisation of the cord, first transfixation is done proximally using vicryl and clamps are applied to divide the cord which prevents retraction and possible bleeding of the vessel.

Corrugated or suction drain is placed which is removed in 48 hours. Skin with layers is sutured with interrupted sutures. Sutures are removed 7–10 days **(Fig. 30-50)**.

High Orchidectomy

It is done classically for testicular tumour. It is also done in undescended testis. Lengthy inguinal incision is placed. Inguinal canal is opened. Testis with cord is dissected, mobilised fully up to or proximal to the internal ring. A soft occlusion clamp is placed over the cord at internal ring level. Testis is palpated for confirmation of the tumour. Often it is transected partially and seen; biopsy is done from the suspected area and confirmation is done by frozen section. If biopsy is negative then testis capsule is sutured back and testis is placed in the scrotum **(Fig. 30-51)**.

Once frozen section confirms the malignancy, clamp is not released; transfixation of the cord is done just proximal to the clamp using silk or vicryl and distally cord is divided to complete the orchidectomy. Double ligation of proximal cord stump is needed. Wound is closed with a suction drain. Testis specimen should be sent for histology. Often it is a practice to place prosthesis in the scrotum in young individual. It is also often practiced to do biopsy of opposite side as malignancy can be bilateral. But nowadays due to good imaging (ultrasound) this technique it is not practiced.

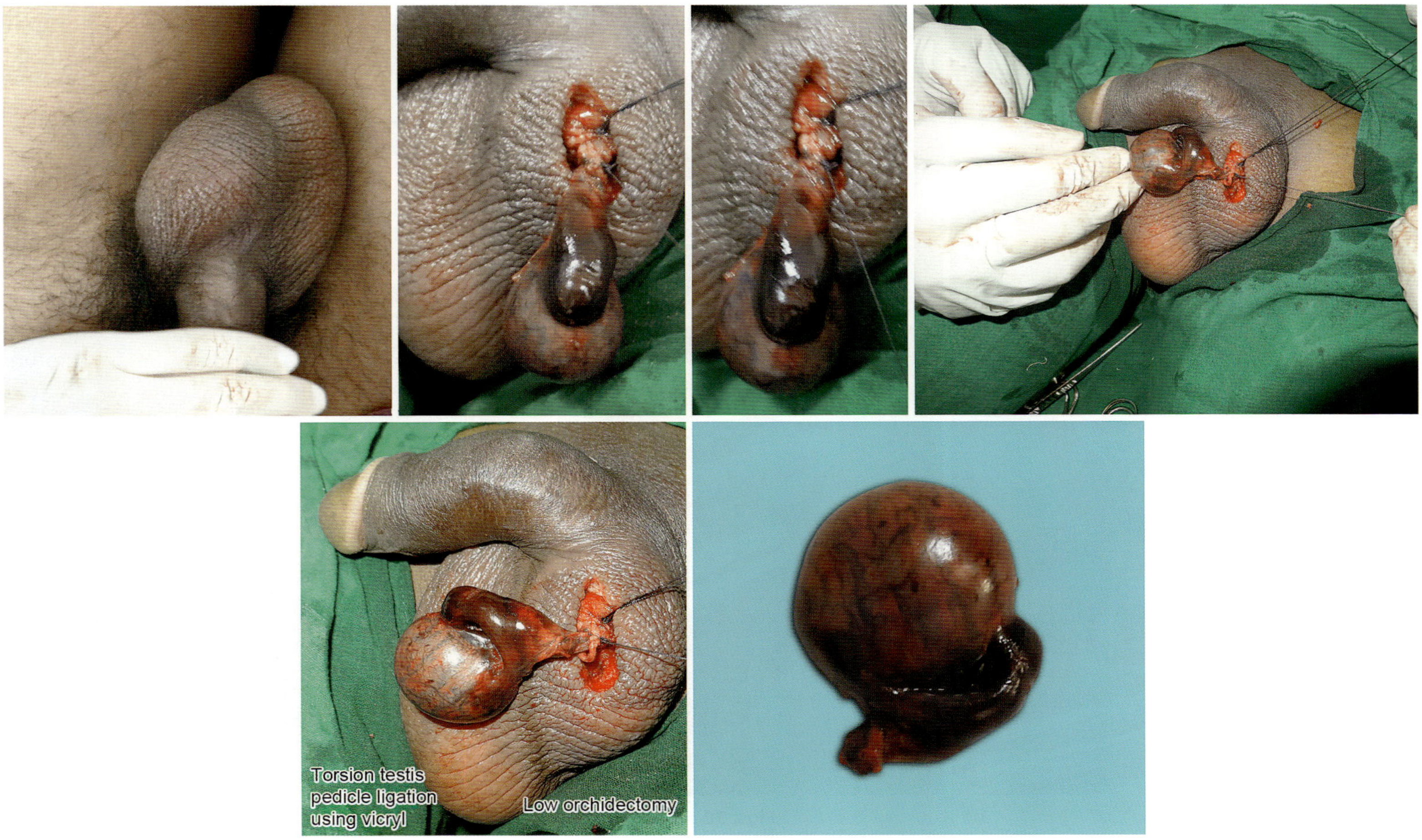

Torsion testis pedicle ligation using vicryl

Low orchidectomy

Fig. 30-49: Torsion testis—low orchidectomy is done. Testis is gangrenous.

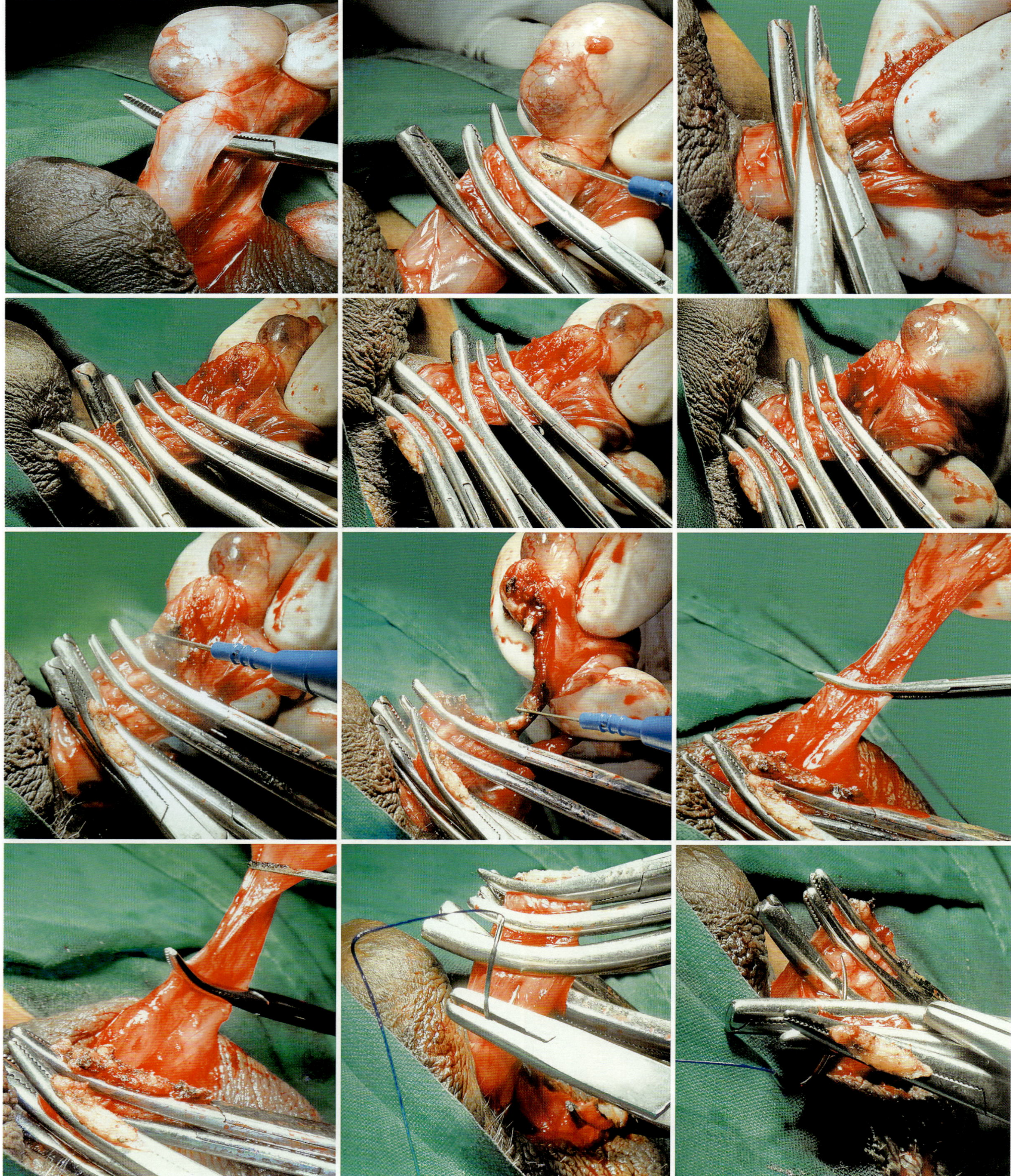

Figs. 30-50(1)

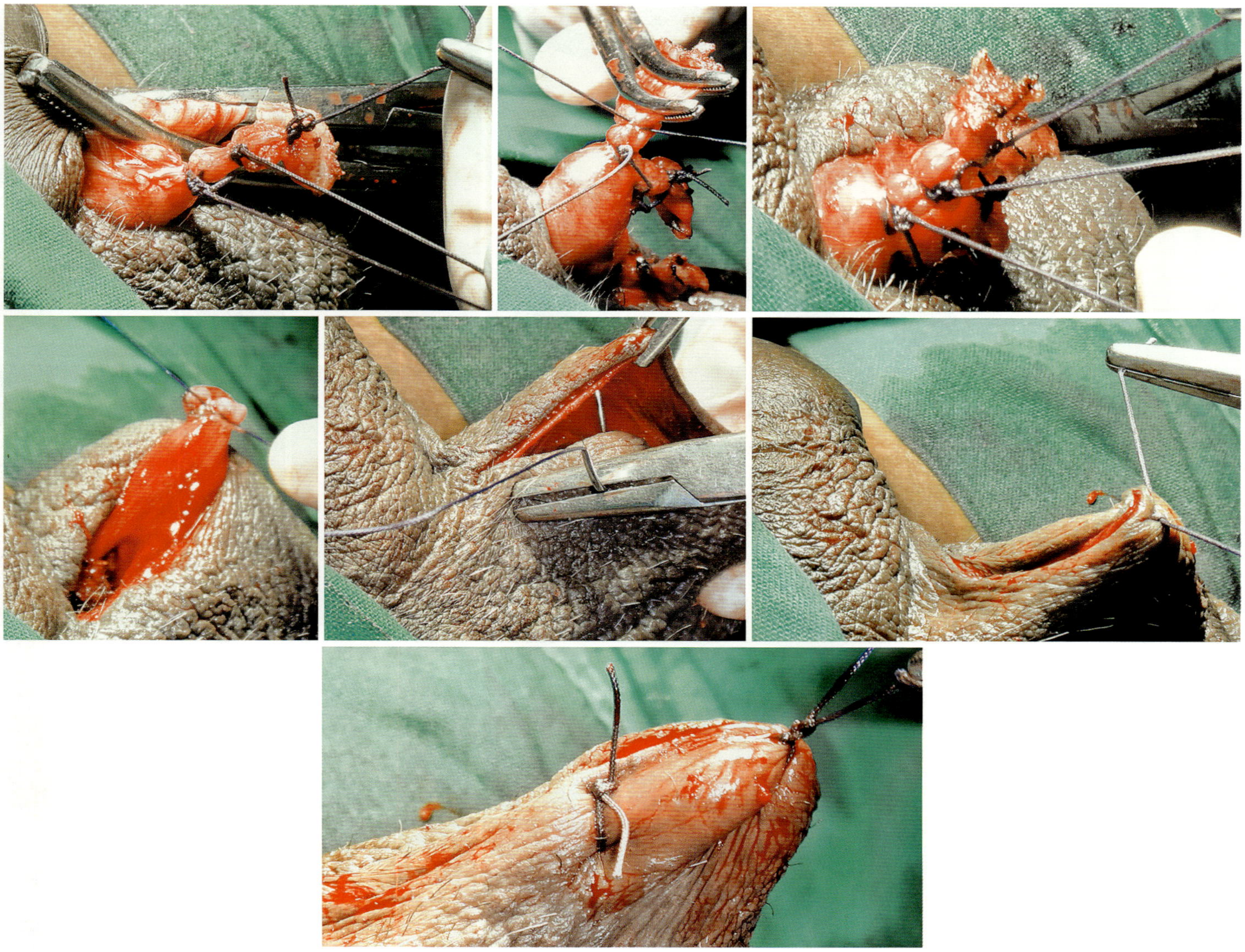

Figs. 30-50(2)

Figs. 30-50(1 and 2): Low orchidectomy is done for pyocele; haematocele. In this old aged patient while doing hydrocele surgery, firm lesion was found in the testis and so through scrotal approach only low orchidectomy was done. Biopsy report was inflammatory mass. Ideally scrotal wound should have been closed; new separate inguinal incision should have been made through which testis with cord is delivered into the groin high up to deep ring and cord is ligated at deep ring to achieve high orchidectomy. On table ultrasound will be very useful.

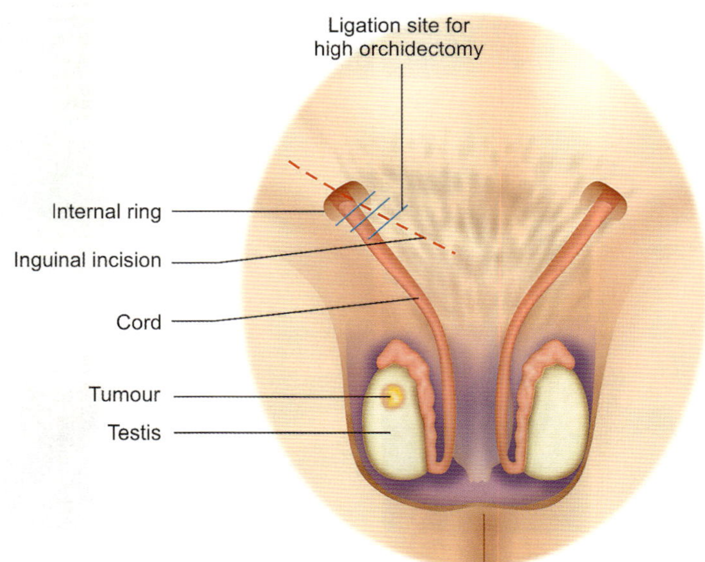

Fig. 30-51: Site of ligation in high orchidectomy (Chevassou manoeuvre).

Subcapsular Orchidectomy

It is done in carcinoma prostate to achieve hormonal control. So it is done always bilateral. It is done under spinal anaesthesia or local anaesthesia. Single midline median raphe incision is sufficient. If surgeon is not comfortable then two separate vertical incisions one in each hemiscrotum may be placed **(Fig. 30-52)**.

Testis is reached; tunica albuginea is incised longitudinally using no. 15 blade or cautery. All seminiferous tubules are removed using finger and scoop. Small bleeders in the inner wall of the testis are fulgurated using bipolar cautery. Tunica albuginea is sutured using 3-zero vicryl. Procedure is repeated on the other side. Skin wound is closed using non-absorbable interrupted sutures. Presently urologists prefer to do low orchidectomy rather than subcapsular one.

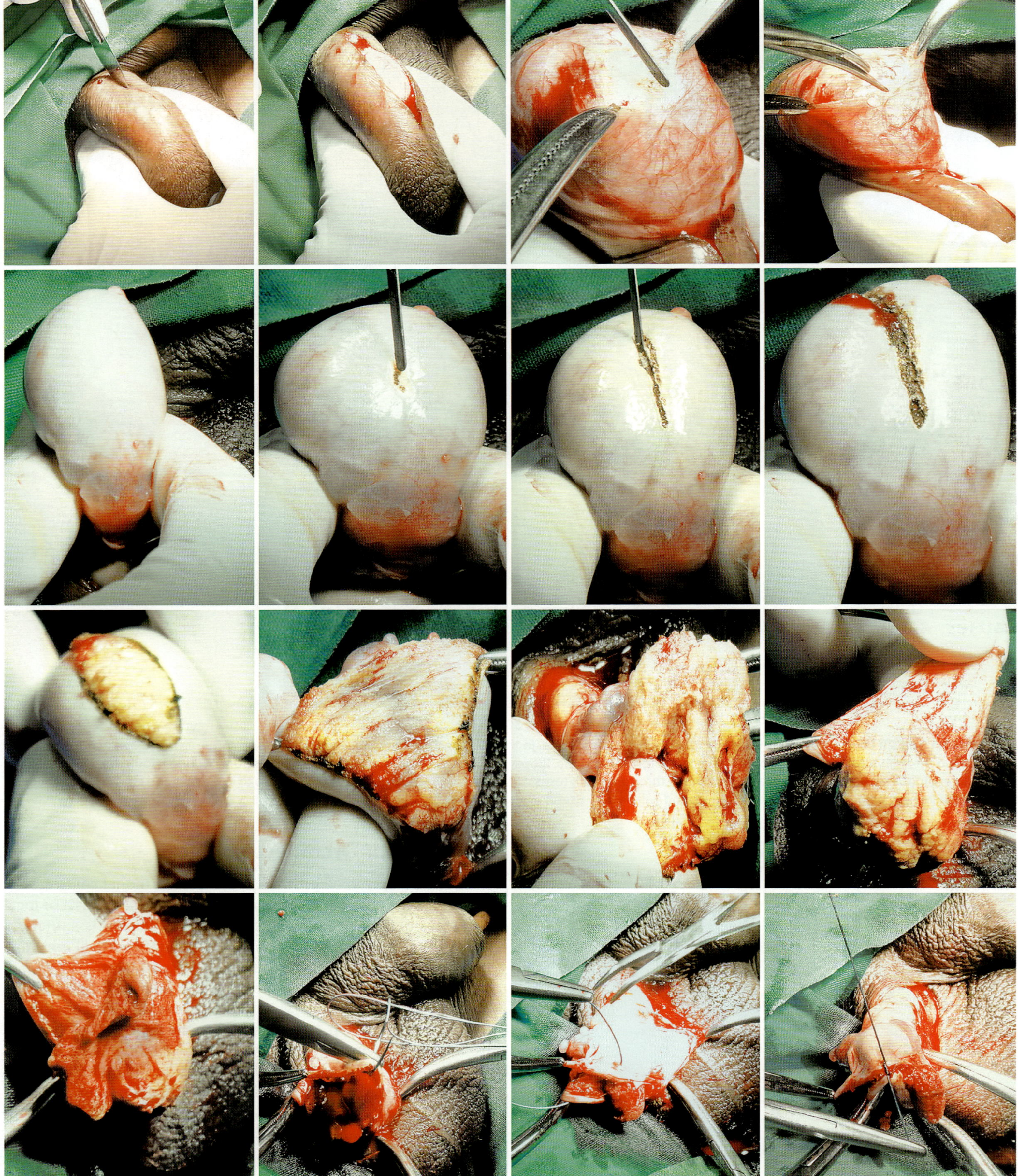

Fig. 30-52: Technique of subcapsular orchidectomy.

31

CHAPTER

Obesity and Morbid Obesity

OBESITY AND MORBID OBESITY

Obesity is weight more than 20% above the normal. Body mass index (BMI) is weight in kilogram divided by height in meters squared [wt in kg/(Ht in meters)^2].

Morbid obesity is a condition wherein BMI is more than 40 kg/m^2. It is often also defined as weight 100 lbs or more; or 100% over ideal body weight.

Weight more than double the expected weight to that age and height of the individual is also often called as *morbid obesity*. If body weight exceeding BMI 50 kg/m^2 is called as *superobesity*.

Causes of Obesity

- Familial, hyperinsulinism, hyperadrenocorticism, hypogonadism.
- Abnormal eating behaviour—Hormones which control eating are—ghrelin from stomach; insulin from pancreas; leptin from fat; PYY 3-36 from colon. Hypothalamus is the center in CNS which controls eating.

Nutritional status	*BMI (kg/m^2)*
♦ Underweight	♦ <18.5
♦ Normal	♦ 18.5–24.9
♦ Overweight (Preobesity)	♦ 25.0–29.9
♦ Obesity	♦ >30
– Class I	– 30.0–34.9
– Class II (Moderate)	– 35.0–39.9
– Class III (Severe/Morbid)	– 40.0
♦ Superobesity	♦ >50
♦ Super superobesity	♦ >60

Complications of obesity	*Obesity and surgery*	*Treatment for obesity*
General: Difficulty in work, fatigue, depression, back pain, arthritis and gout *Cardiovascular:* Hypertension, stroke, thrombophlebitis, pulmonary embolism *Pulmonary:* Hypoventilation, poor respiratory effort *GIT:* Hiatus hernia with reflux, changes in liver, pancreatitis, gallstones *Endocrine:* Diabetes mellitus	♦ Hernia and gallstones are more common in obese individual. ♦ Burst abdomen, incisional hernia are more common in obesity ♦ Delay in recovering from anaesthesia ♦ Infertility is more common	*General:* Dieting, exercise *Drugs:* Orlistat, Sibutramine *Surgeries:* ♦ *Restrictive* – Vertical banded gastroplasty – Laparoscopic adjustable gastric banding (LAGB) – Jaw wiring ♦ *Malabsorptive* – Biliopancreatic diversion (BPD) – Biliopancreatic diversion with duodenal switch (BPD – DS) – Jejunoileal bypass ♦ *Combined* ♦ Roux-en-Y gastric bypass (RYGB) open or laparoscopic

Obesity is more common in young women. Child of a normal weight parents has 10% chance of become obese. If both parents are obese then child has got 80% chances to develop obesity.

Problems with Morbid Obesity

Obstructive sleep apnoea, degenerative joint disease, back pain, hypertension, GERD, gallstones, type II diabetes, hyperlipidaemia, arrhythmias, venous diseases, DVT, skin diseases, urine incontinence, infertility, ventral hernias, obesity hypoventilation syndrome, polycystic ovarian disease, hirsutism, gynaecomastia, steatohepatosis, malignancies—are common problems. All these conditions are called as *comorbidities.*

Infertility is common in married morbid obese women due to improper ovulation, polycystic ovary disease. Urinary incontinence is common in morbid obese women (stress incontinence and detrusor instability). Pregnancy in morbid obese patient is considered as high risk pregnancy. Gestational diabetes, hypertension, are common. It is better these women to undergo bariatric surgery prior to pregnancy which definitely reduces the complications during pregnancy. Such individual after bariatric surgery needs more iron and vitamin supplements.

Evaluation of the patient—cardiac, respiratory assessment, lipid profile, blood glucose, renal and liver status assessment, anaesthesia risk assessment.

Medical Management

- *General:* Diet, lifestyle changes, exercise.
- *Drugs:* (1) Orlistat is a selective inhibitor of gastric and pancreatic lipases that reduces the absorption of lipids from intestine. (2) Sibutramine is a noradrenaline and 5 HT reuptake inhibitor which act as appetite suppressor.

Surgical Treatment (Bariatric Surgery)

Bariatric surgery causes long term durable weight loss. Patient's eating behaviour is reduced to slow ingestion of small boluses of food and or also reducing the absorptive surfaces.

Types of Bariatric Surgery

1. *Restrictive* wherein caloric intake is reduced. Purely gastric restrictive procedures are vertical banded gastroplasty (VBG) and laparoscopic adjustable gastric banding (LAGB).
2. *Malabsorptive* wherein absorption of calories and nutrients from food is reduced. Biliopancreatic diversion (BPD) and biliopancreatic diversion with duodenal switch (BPD–DS) are malabsorptive procedures.
3. *Combined* wherein both methods are used. Roux-en-Y gastric bypass (RYGB) is both restrictive and malabsorptive types. Gastric bypass reduces GI polypeptide ghrelin level secreted from fundus of stomach and duodenum. Ghrelin acts on specific receptor in CNS—hypothalamus to initiate appetite. This stimulation is reduced to decrease appetite. In restrictive only procedure ghrelin level raises and so appetite stimulation is not controlled.

Indications for Bariatric Surgery

BMI more than 40 kg/m^2 or BMI more than 35 kg/m^2 with comorbidity is indication for bariatric surgery. American Association of Bariatric Surgery (ASBS) published indications and approved surgeries.

Contraindications

Patients who are unfit for general anaesthesia (cardiac/renal/respiratory/hepatic) or who are unable to adjust postoperative life styles or psychiatric patients are contraindications for bariatric surgery.

Preoperative preparations and evaluations are:

- Complete cardiac, respiratory/renal/hepatic evaluation.
- Lipid profile and blood glucose assessment.
- Obstructive sleep apnoea in obese patient should be assessed using polysomnography and be treated.
- Risk assessment for DVT should be done.
- If GERD symptoms are present gastroscopy should be done.
- USG abdomen to identify gallstones should be done; if gallstones are present it is of usual practice to do cholecystectomy along with bariatric procedure.
- Nutritional evaluation and dietician advice for preoperative and postoperative diet management.
- Psychological screening is needed to all patients to counsel their postoperative care and diet.
- Separate theatre table is needed for morbid obese patient. Equipment should be long and flexible. In laparoscopic surgery, special ports and instruments are needed.

DIFFERENT SURGERIES

Vertical Banded Gastroplasty (VBG); Mason (1982)

It is a purely restrictive type with creation of a calibrated stoma in the lesser curvature which is reinforced by an encircled mesh with a proximal gastric pouch. After laparotomy Ewald's stomach tube is passed per orally to place against lesser curve. A 2.5 cm circular window is created in the body of stomach near lesser curvature 8 cm below the *angle of His*. After this, four lines of linear vertical stapling are done from circular opening towards angle of His. This staple line ideally should be divided using another cutting linear stapler to reduce chances of dehiscence. This creates a 50 mL proximal gastric pouch. A 1.5 × 7 cm polypropylene mesh is placed around the lesser curve through circular opening and sutured to create a 5 cm collar stoma **(Fig. 31-1)**.

VBG causes only medium term weight loss; its efficacy is less compared to other procedures. *Complications of VBG are*—stricture at stoma (20%), vomiting (30%), reflux (20%), staple line dehiscence (40%), conversion into other procedures. Mortality is 0.3%.

VBG is technically easier to do; it has got very less chances of long term metabolic and nutritional deficiencies.

Laparoscopic Adjustable Gastric Banding (LAGB)

It is also a restrictive type (1992, Guy Bernard) to create a narrow stoma just below the OG junction. It is used in adolescents and elderly. It is contraindicated in hiatal and paraoesophageal hernias. It is done using *laparoscopy*.

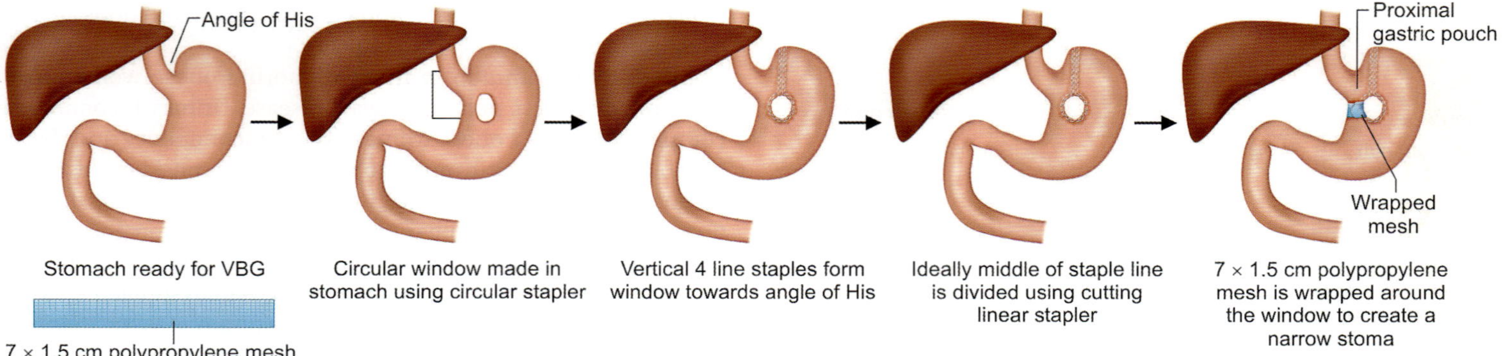

Fig. 31-1: Vertical banded gastroplasty (VBG).

Under general anaesthesia, with patient in reverse Trendelenburg position six laparoscopic ports are placed. Using pars flaccida method, retrogastric tunnel is created; a silicone band is passed through the tunnel to encircle the cardia just below the OG junction; tail of the band is buckled and locked. Stoma diameter is determined by inserting a calibration tube. Stomach over the band is imbricated using interrupted sutures except the buckle area. Silicone tube end is brought out through the abdominal wall to connect access port. It is used for band volume adjustment by injecting or withdrawing the saline.

Gastrograffin study is done on 1st postoperative day to assess band position and lumen patency. Patient is advised to have liquid diet for one month. Band adjustment is done under fluoroscopic guidance in 2 months. Adjustment is done to achieve weight loss at a rate of 2 kg/week. Efficacy of LABG is 55% **(Fig. 31-2)**.

Complications of LABG are—spleen/stomach injury; bleeding; band slippage (10%); band erosion (7.5%); tube-related complications; vomiting; pouch dilatation; reflux. Conversion rate is 3%; mortality is less than 0.5%.

Jejunoileal Bypass

It was the first malabsorptive procedure done for obesity. Now this technique is not done due to high incidences of complications.

Proximal jejunum is divided and proximal cut end is anastomosed to distal ileum just proximal to ileocaecal valve to reduce the absorptive surface area of small bowel **(Fig. 31-3)**.

Complication rates were higher and so procedure is not practiced. Colon in these patients absorbs high level of oxalate causing nephrocalcinosis. Bypassed bowel promotes bacterial growth causing endotoxin induced liver injury, cirrhosis, liver failure. Complications like protein, vitamin K, vitamin B_{12} deficiencies; gallstone formation; enteritis and diarrhoea; arthritis, osteoporosis are common.

Roux-en-Y Gastric Bypass

It is commonly done combined procedure. It can be done by open or laparoscopic method. Proximal stomach is dissected between 1st and 2nd branches of left gastric artery. Vagii nerves and *nerves of Latarjet* are retained carefully. Stomach is transected at this proximal site to create a proximal gastric pouch (15 mL if BMI is >50; 30 mL if BMI is 40–50). It is usually carried out through linear stapler. Jejunum is transected 45 cm from *ligament of Treitz*. A side to side jejunojejunal anastomosis is done using stapler 75 cm distal to the distal cut end. Proximal Roux part of the distal jejunal cut part (75–150 cm, based on patient's preoperative weight) is brought out through the transverse mesocolon towards the created proximal gastric pouch and gastrojejunostomy is done to this proximal gastric pouch. Mesenteric defect is closed. Stomal integrity is checked on table by air distension and methylene blue infusion. Gastrograffin study is done in 24 hours to assess pouch size, stomal patency and distal obstruction. Oral food is started in 24 hours and patient is discharged in 4 days **(Fig. 31-4)**.

RYBG is more useful in weight loss compared to purely restrictive types. 5-year weight loss is 60–75%. It also prevents progression of non-insulin dependent diabetes mellitus, controls hypertension, sleep apnoea, hyperlipidaemia, asthma, arthritis, GERD.

Complications are—Roux obstruction, anastomotic leak, acute distal gastric dilatation, stomal stenosis, marginal ulcer, dumping syndrome, internal hernias, vitamin B_{12} deficiency, iron deficiency anaemia. Distal gastric dilatation needs emergency intervention which is usually due to jejunojejunal obstruction.

Laparoscopic RYGB (1994, Wittgrove, Clark, Trembly)

Technique is similar to open RYGB. Anastomoses are done using endoscopic stapler. GJ between gastric pouch and Roux jejunum is done either using linear stapler through laparoscopic port after making a gastrotomy in the pouch which is later sutured after staple firing; or by using circular stapler anastomosis is done wherein anvil is initially passed transorally often under endoscopic guidance across the pouch into the Roux jejunum; or by using hand sewing with absorbable sutures. Omentum is released from the colon and is covered over the GJ. Mesenteric defect and *Patterson Brown defect* are closed. A *Brolin antiobstructive stitch* is placed between Roux and biliopancreatic limbs. Integrity of anastomosis is checked using insufflation of air, methylene blue. *Complications* are similar to open RYBG. Conversion rate is 9%. *Advantages* of LRYBG to open RYBG are—faster recovery, less postoperative pain, less wound related complications, less morbid one. *Disadvantage* of LRYBG is availability of facility, technical expertise, and steep learning curve.

Now technique is modified to antegastric, antecolic one which has become popular (Gagner).

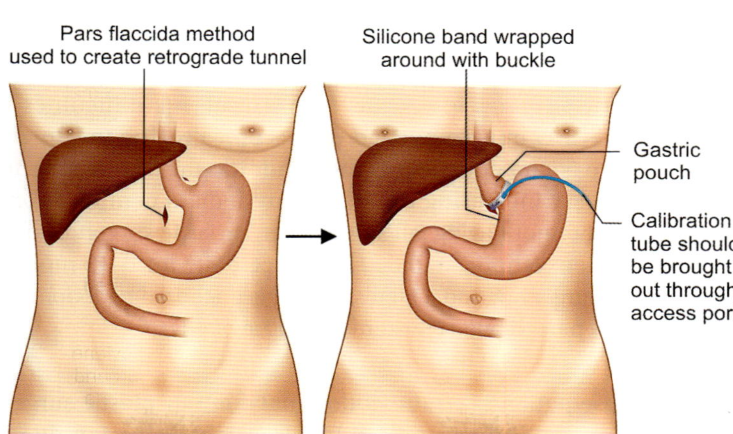

Fig. 31-2: Laparoscopic adjustable gastric banding (LAGB).

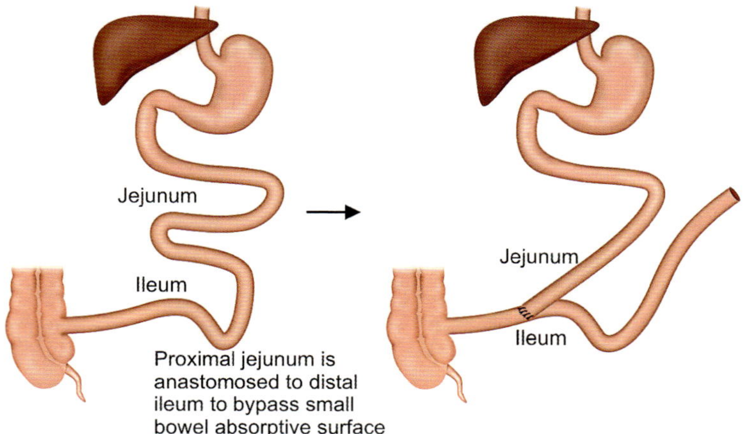

Fig. 31-3: Jejunoileal bypass procedure (JIB).

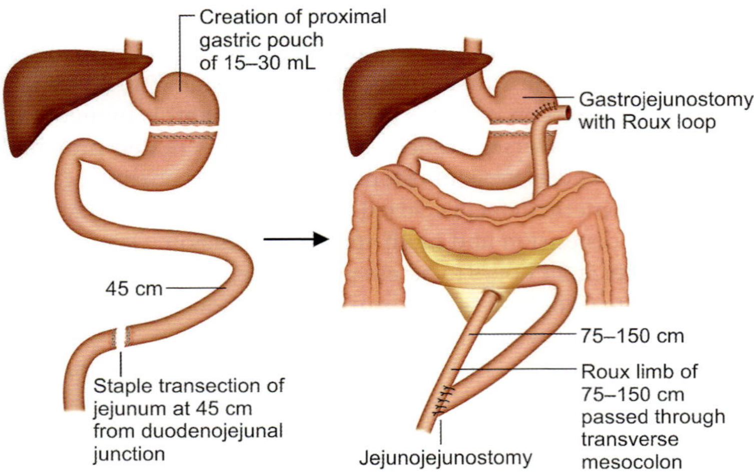

Fig. 31-4: Roux-en-Y gastric bypass procedure (RYBG).

Biliopancreatic Diversion (BPD) (Nicola Scopinaro, Italy)

It is done in patients who had failed restrictive procedure or who are superobese.

Distal subtotal gastrectomy is done with formation of proximal gastric pouch (of 400 mL in BMI 40–50; 200 mL in BMI >50). Ileum is transected 250 cm proximal to ileocaecal valve; distal ileal segment is brought up to anastomose into the proximal gastric pouch. Proximal biliopancreatic jejunoileal limb is anastomosed into distal ileal segment 50 cm proximal to ileocaecal valve as end to side stoma. Additionally cholecystectomy should be done **(Fig. 31-5)**.

Modification of BPD with duodenal switch (BPD-DS) has become more popular. Here sleeve gastrectomy along the greater curvature is done to create gastric reservoir (200 mL) along lesser curve. Duodenum just distal to first part is divided using stapler; proximal cut end is sutured to proximal upward pulled end of the distal ileal segment of earlier transected ileum, 250 cm from ileocaecal valve.

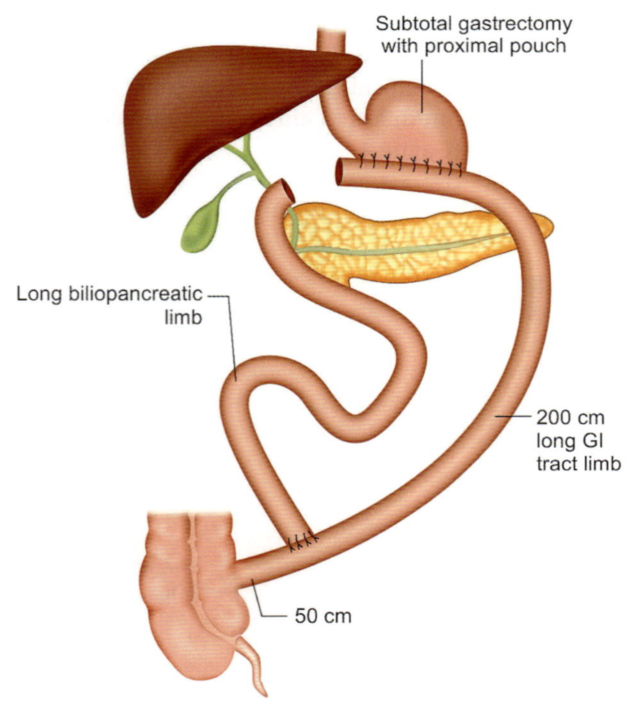

Fig. 31-5: Biliopancreatic diversion procedure (BPD).

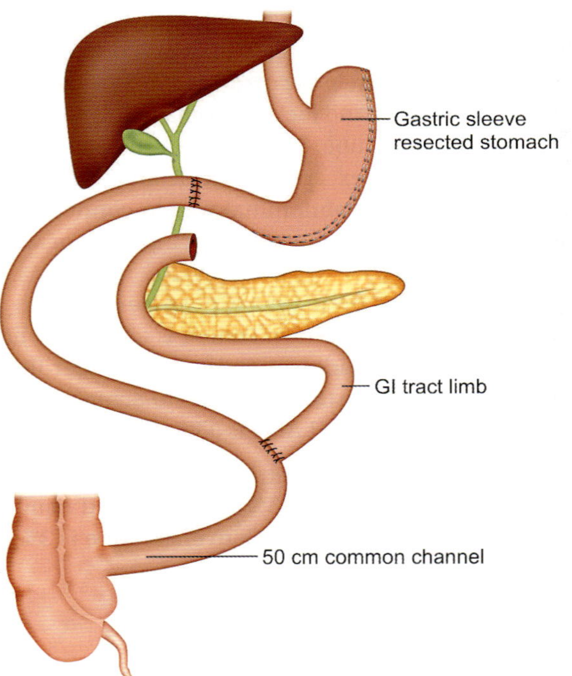

Fig. 31-6: Biliopancreatic diversion with duodenal switch procedure (BPD–DS).

Biliopancreaticoduodenal with proximal jejunoileal segment is later stapled to distal ileum 50 cm proximal to ileocaecal valve. Duodenal switch reduces the marginal ulcer rate and dumping syndrome.

Results of BPD/BPD-DS are excellent for weight reduction compared to restrictive procedures. But they need lifelong supplement of vitamins, fat soluble vitamins, calcium, and iron. Technically BPD is easier to do when compared to BPD–DS **(Fig. 31-6)**.

Complications of BPD/BPD-DS are—anaemia (30%); protein deficiency (20%); dumping syndrome; marginal ulcer (in BPD 10%; in BPD-DS it is 1%); osteoporosis; night blindness; biliopancreatic limb obstruction; staple line leak; staple line bleed; DVT; subphrenic abscess. Vitamin B_{12} deficiency is specific.

Cholecystolithiasis after Bariatric Surgery

Gallstone formation is common after bariatric surgery (50%). It is due to rapid weight loss. If gallstones are present at the time of bariatric surgery it is essential to do laparoscopic cholecystectomy during bariatric procedure. It is controversial about doing prophylactic cholecystectomy during bariatric surgery even though it is practiced in many places. Advantages are—it prevents future gallstone formation after bariatric surgery (loss of access); it prevents difficulties in approaching CBD in case needed endoscopically due to surgery. Disadvantage is cholecystectomy adds additional 1 hour time for bariatric surgery increasing the risk of immediate complications. Patients who are not having gallstones after bariatric surgery should receive ursodeoxycholic acid 300 mg twice daily for 6–12 months postbariatric surgery period. Often stomach is anchored to abdominal wall as access part to biliary system for future need.

Note:
Many of these patients require abdominal contour plastic surgery (panniculectomy, abdominoplasty) after weight reduction due to bariatric surgery.

Bariatric Surgery

Only effective therapy for severe obesity is bariatric surgery.
80% of bariatric surgeries are gastric bypasses specifically laparoscopic approach.
Original gastric pouch was of 150 mL volume with loop gastrojejunostomy which is later changed to a pouch of <20 mL volume with Roux-en-Y gastrojejunostomy.
Indications are—BMI more than 40 kg/m^2 or BMI more than 35 kg/m^2 with comorbidity (diabetes, hypertension), sleep apnoea, obesity hypoventilation syndrome.
Management needs—bariatric surgeon, nutritionist, physician, pulmonologist, cardiologist, endocrinologist, psychiatrist, psychologist and anaesthesiologist.
Principle—bypassing the gastroduodenum blocking the neurohumoral effect; rapid delivery of food to hindgut; early satiety; malabsorption. Usually 75 cm Roux limb is used; longer limb of 150 cm Roux limb is used for BMI more than 50 kg/m^2.

Technique:
Access: Supine position; operating surgeon stands on the right side; 5 mm optical viewing trocar; left upper quadrant Veress needle and trocar; 5 mm liver retractor, is placed and anchored to the bed with a self-retaining device; wider trocar for endostapler (12 mm).

The Roux limb creation: The transverse colon and omentum are placed towards the upper abdomen; ligament of Treitz is identified; proximal jejunum is oriented as proximal and distal parts by C configuration; jejunum is divided 50 cm distal to the ligament of Treitz using linear cutting stapler; the mesentery of the jejunum divided using two stapler firings; sufficient length of mesentery is created to achieve adequate tension-free passage Roux limb; the Roux limb is marked. Roux limb is measured distally for 75 cm from the marker; bowel should be straightened (not stretched) while marking; side to side jejunojejunostomy anastomosis is done after doing jejunotomies using harmonic scalpel between the biliopancreatic and the Roux limb using linear stapler; jejunotomy ends are closed using another lineal stapler firing. Reinforcing sutures may be placed using 3-0 silk. One reinforcing stitch is placed between the stapled end of the biliopancreatic and the Roux limb—*Brolin stitch*. One more is placed proximally at the crotch between the biliopancreatic and Roux limb. The mesenteric defect (*Patterson Brown defect*) between the biliopancreatic and Roux limb is then closed with a continuous vicryl or silk 3 zero suture.

Greater omentum is divided at the level of the midtransverse colon using the harmonic scalpel. The Roux limb is passed upward between the leaves of the divided omentum to the gastric pouch in the *antecolic* and *antegastric* approach.
Creation of gastric pouch: The patient is placed in the steep reverse Trendelenburg position; window is created in the gastrohepatic ligament with the harmonic scalpel. Linear stapler is fired toward the gastric lesser curvature to divide the lesser omentum and descending branch of the left gastric artery but the main left gastric arterial trunk should be preserved which is the main blood supply of the gastric pouch. Gastric pouch of 15–20 mL is created by sequential firing using lineal staplers from lesser curve towards the angle of His. Gastric pouch is dissected off from left crus to achieve pouch mobility and to reduce tension while creating GJ; pouch is also properly separated from gastric remnant below to avoid gastrogastric fistula.

Creation of GJ—linear: Posterior suture line between gastric pouch and Roux limb → gastrotomy and jejunotomy creation using harmonic scalpel → GJ is done using lineal stapler → stapler entry common opening is sutured using 3-zero silk with endoscope in place → GJ is checked for leak and bleeding (*bleed and leak test* by insufflation using endoscope). *Transoral circular stapler method*—gastroscope is passed into the pouch → snare is pushed through a small gastrotomy → guidewire is passed through a laparoscopic port which is grasped by the snare to pull out through the mouth → anvil of the stapler is attached to the guidewire and pulled antegrade into the gastric pouch → the circular stapler is passed in the open end of the Roux limb → the stapler and anvil are connected → the stapler is fired to create a circular stapled GJ anastomosis → the open Roux limb is closed with a linear stapler. *Circular transabdominal and hand sewn* are other methods.

Jackson Pratt *drain* is placed behind the pouch; omentum is placed and sutured on the GJ as Schauer cap. Roux limb may be stitched (one stitch) to the gastric remnant to avoid its twist.

Leak test: It is done by initially occluding the Roux distal limb with a clamp and by submerging the GJ with warm normal saline and pouch is insufflated with air through endoscope.
At the end *cholecystectomy* is done; if not patient is put on ursodeoxycholic acid for 6–12 months. Additional core needle biopsy performance is a controversial.
Postoperative management: Pain control; antiemetics; essential preoperative medications are continued as IV until the patient is started on liquids; incentive spirometry use; nil orally on the night of surgery; gastrografin swallow study on 1st postoperative day (must); if the swallow study does not show any leak or obstruction, then oral clear fluid is started; monitoring; cardiac evaluation; psychiatrist counseling; drain removal on 7th day.

Complications: Gastric leak (1–5%), sepsis, pulmonary embolism (1%) are major complications. Fever, tachycardia, tachypnoea are probable features of leak. Acute dilation of the gastric remnant is less than 1% in incidence but life threatening; it is due to obstruction of the biliopancreatic limb; presents as severe epigastric pain with gastric distension; plain X-ray is useful; CT scan is diagnostic; it is treated with emergency decompression by percutaneous gastrostomy; the biliopancreatic limb obstruction is managed surgically only once the patient has stabilised. Wound infection rate is 10%. Infections of laparoscopic trocar sites can occur.

Late complications are: Marginal ulceration at GJ site (10%) is due to ischemia, smoking, gastrogastric fistula, large pouch size, retained anastomotic suture, NSAID; *Helicobacter pylori* infection. Late bowel obstruction can occur which is due to an internal hernia 1–10%; if episodic abdominal pain or recurrent partial small bowel obstruction, laparoscopic exploration is performed; often obstruction is due to intermittent bowel herniation through a mesenteric defect. Anastomotic stricture at GJ can occur due to tension on the Roux limb or pouch ischaemia or chronic marginal ulcer, usage of circular stapler; strictures occur 1–3 months after surgery; present with dysphagia, vomiting; treated with endoscopic balloon dilations in 2–3 times. Nutritional deficiencies like deficiency of iron (30%); folate (35%); vitamin B_{12} (25%); anaemia (up to 54%) can occur. Very late long term complications like severe protein calorie malnutrition requires revision surgery to lengthen the common channel.

32 CHAPTER

Basic Surgeries in Obstetrics and Gynaecology

General surgeons frequently encounter with gynaecological problems in females. Previously before the advent of ultrasound and CT scan there would be lots of confusion with diagnosis and the surgeon would be surprised with a gynaecological condition on table as the clinical features of some surgical conditions overlap with those of gynaecological conditions. Current investigative methods have reduced the surprises for the surgeons. But still it is wise for a surgeon to know common gynaecological conditions and their operative treatments.

SURGICAL ANATOMY OF FEMALE GENITALIA

Female genitalia are broadly classified into *external* and *internal genitalia*.

External Genitalia

It is also termed as *vulva* or *pudendum*. It is an ill-defined area bounded by *mons veneris* anteriorly, *labia majora* laterally and *perineum* posteriorly.

Mons veneris is a pad of subcutaneous adipose tissue over the pubis, covered by hair in adult females.

Labia majora consists of folds of skin with underlying subcutaneous fat extending on either side from mons in front to end in skin of perineum posteriorly. It is prominent in reproductive age group, covered with hair on outer aspect, whereas the inner aspect is hairless, moist and pinker than outer surface. Labia majora is covered with stratified squamous epithelium, contains hair follicles, sweat glands, sebaceous glands and a specialised sweat glands called apocrine glands whose secretions give the characteristic aroma. So presence of all these structures makes labia majora prone for folliculitis, boils, and sebaceous cysts. Labia majora are homologous ith scrotum in males.

Labia minora are two thin folds of skin devoid of fat lying on either within the labia majora, which divide anteriorly to enclose the ris forming *prepuce* on upper surface and *frenulum* on under e; posteriorly unite together to form a fold of skin in midline *ourchette*. It is devoid of hair follicle but contains erectile muscle umerous sebaceous glands, vessels and nerve endings.

's is cylindrical erectile body consists of a glans, covered by nalogue to the penis in male but here it is entirely separate ra, attached to the undersurface of symphysis pubis ry ligament. It is extremely sensitive with numerous nerve endings, plays considerable part during sexual intercourse in inducing orgasm in females.

Bartholin glands are a pair of pea-sized glands situated on either side at the junction of middle and posterior thirds of labia majora deep to bulbospongiosus muscle. They are compound racemose type of glands, secrete abundant lubricating mucus during sexual excitement. Duct is 2 cm long, opens below the level of hymen at the junction of anterior 2/3 and posterior 1/3. It is lined by columnar epithelium but by stratified squamous epithelium near the opening. Gland which is otherwise not palpable becomes enlarged by inflammation. Pus can be expressed through the duct opening on applying pressure on the gland when infected in acute gonorrhoea.

The space between the anterior and inner aspect of the labia minora is the *vestibule* which is bounded posteriorly by the vaginal introitus. *Urethral meatus* lies in the midline just below the clitoris. *Vaginal orifice* lies posterior to the urethral meatus, bounded by a thin membrane called *hymen* in virgins, which contains an eccentrically placed opening. Hymen gets ruptured by coitus which may sometimes cause brisk haemorrhage. It is lined on either side by stratified squamous epithelium.

Vestibular bulb are bilateral elongated masses of erectile tissue that lies beneath the mucous membrane of the vestibule, on either sides of the vaginal orifice in front of the Bartholian gland, which may get injured during childbirth resulting in brisk haemorrhage.

Arterial supply of external genitalia is by branches of internal pudendal arteries and femoral arteries. *Venous plexus* formed drain into internal pudendal vein, vesical venous plexus and long saphenous vein. Varicosities that occur in these venous plexus during pregnancy may spontaneously rupture or cause haematoma formation. *Nerve supply* is by cutaneous branches of ilioinguinal and genital branches of genitofemoral nerve and pudendal branches of posterior cutaneous nerve of the thigh. *Lymphatics* drain bilaterally into superficial inguinal lymph nodes, lymph node of Cloquet and external and internal iliac nodes.

Internal Genitalia

It includes vagina, uterus, fallopian tubes and ovaries.

Vagina is the channel that communicates uterus with the exterior at vulva. The canal is directed upwards and backwards making an angle of 45° with the horizontal in erect posture. Though, it is distensible its diameter is wider at its upper part, narrow at its lower part. It is attached to the cervix slightly at a higher level on the posterior aspect making the posterior fornix deepest of the all. This part of the vagina is indirect contact with the peritoneum of the pelvic floor and is the thinnest area in whole of the peritoneal cavity. Pointing pelvic abscess can be drained through the posterior fornix. Herniation of coils of intestine or *enterocele* can occur through this fornix. Ureter lies 12 mm anterolateral to the lateral fornix. Vagina is related to base of the bladder and urethra in front, ampulla of rectum and *pouch of Douglas* behind. Vaginal secretion is derived from cervix and from transudation across the epithelium. Its acidic nature (pH is 4.5) is due to the presence of lactic acid formed by the bacterial (*Doderlein*) activity on the glycogen of the epithelial cells which is also estrogen dependent. This acidic nature is protective and inhibits the growth of pathogenic organisms and also explains the growth of mixed organisms before puberty and in menopausal age group where the influence of estrogen is low. It is supplied by the cervicovaginal branch of uterine artery, branches of internal iliac artery, and middle rectal with internal pudendal artery. Vaginal veins form plexus that drain into internal iliac vein. Lymphatics from lower 1/3rd vagina drain along with external genitalia into superficial and deep inguinal lymph nodes; middle 1/3rd into internal iliac nodes upper 1/3rd into external iliac nodes.

Uterus is a pyriform-shaped muscular organ that lies in the pelvis between bladder in front and rectum behind. It measures 8.5–9 cm in length 6.5 cm in breadth and 3.5 cm in thickness, flattened antero-posteriorly, lies in anteverted, anteflexed position, slightly deviated to right. It is divided functionally and anatomically into body and cervix with isthmus being the line of demarcation. It is at this level, the peritoneum gets reflected from the bladder onto the body of the uterus and this loose peritoneal fold is called the *utero-vesical* fold of peritoneum. Uterine artery, at this level changes its horizontal course into vertical, along the lateral surface of the body. Uterus consists of corpus or the body and cervix. *Fundus* is that part of the body above the attachment of fallopian tubes. *Cornu* is the junction of attachment of tubes to the uterus. *Isthmus* is the constricted portion that lies between the body and the cervix that forms the lower uterine segment during pregnancy. *Cervix* is the cylindrical lower part of the uterus that opens into the vagina. The endocervical canal is 2–3 cm in length that continues with the endometrial cavity at the isthmus. The exocervix is lined by stratified squamous epithelium whereas the endocervix by mucus secreting columnar epithelium, their junction of transformation is the squamocolumnar junction which is the site of initiation of dysplasia.

Peritoneum covers most part of the uterus except over the anterior aspect of the cervix, and laterally at the sites of attachment of tubes, round ligament and ovarian ligament. Posteriorly, the peritoneum covers whole of the uterus, supravaginal cervix, upper part of the vagina and then reflects onto the anterior surface of the rectum thus forming the *pouch of Douglas* that consists of coils of intestine. The two sheets of peritoneum form the *broad ligament* on either side of the uterus which extends to lateral pelvic wall. Fallopian tubes lies in the medial 3/4th of the superior free border, where the lateral 1/4th forms the *infundibulopelvic* ligament which contains the ovarian vessels. *Mesovarium* is a fold of peritoneum that attaches ovary to the posterior layer of broad ligament. *Round ligament* is attached to the uterine cornu reaches the internal abdominal ring. The *ovarian ligament* attaches inner poles of the ovaries to the uterine cornu below the fallopian tubes.

Fallopian tubes are a pair of hollow muscular tubes, 10 cm long, attached to uterine cornu at one end and opens into the abdominal cavity on the other end, the opening of which is surrounded by radiating fimbria, *ovarian fimbria* being the longest is attached to ovaries. Interstitial portion is the narrowest portion of the tube, ampullary is the widest.

Ovaries are paired gonadal structures measuring 5 × 3 × 3 cm, that is suspended in the pelvis by the infundibulopelvic ligament laterally and ovarian ligament medially; mesovarium attaches the hilar surface of the ovary to the posterior surface of the broad ligament. It receives blood supply mainly from branches of ovarian artery and also branches of uterine artery.

Uterine artery, the branch of anterior division of internal iliac artery, supplies chiefly the uterus, tubes, and vagina. Once it reaches the parametrium, it runs medially to reach the internal os, where after giving a vaginal branch it turns upwards along the lateral border of the uterus, running a tortuous course ends near the cornu after anastomosing with ovarian artery. Uterine artery during its course towards internal os crosses over the ureter where it pierces the Mackenrodt's ligament. The vaginal branch of the uterine artery reaches the lateral fornix traversing the parametrium, has to be separately ligated during hysterectomy, which otherwise may lead into severe postoperative haemorrhage.

Ovarian artery arises from the abdominal aorta below the renal vessels; enter the infundibulopelvic ligament, ends by anastomosing with the uterine artery after giving branches to tubes, ovary, broad ligament and uterus. Veins form plexus which lie between layers of broad ligament that drain into renal vein on the left side, into inferior vena cava on the right side.

Lymphatics from the fundus and adjoining uterine corpus drain into para-aortic nodes along the ovarian vessels, from the cornu along the round ligament into superficial inguinal lymph nodes, from the lower part of the corpus into external iliac nodes; lymphatics from the cervix drain into external and internal iliac group, obturator group, paracervical and sacral group of nodes. Lymphatics from these entire groups ultimately drain into para-aortic group of lymph nodes. The lymphatic vessels of the ovary drain in three directions. The main group accompanies the ovarian vessels in the infundibulopelvic ligament, eventually reaches the periaortic nodes near the kidney. Other lymphatic channels communicate with channels of the opposite ovary by crossing the fundus of the uterus through the ovarian ligament. Some channels drain through the ovarian and round ligaments into the superficial inguinal lymph nodes in the groin.

Anatomy of Pelvic Floor

Pelvic floor consists of all structures from the skin of perineum below to the facial covering of the levator ani muscle above. It is pierced from before backwards by the urethra, vagina, and anal canal. Pelvic floor not only supports these canals but also the pelvic organs. Normal physiological function of the pelvic organs depends on the anatomic integrity of this pelvic support. Pelvic organ prolapse, urinary and anal incontinence sexual voiding and defecatory dysfunction can result defect in pelvic support. A proper knowledge of the pelvic support helps to treat pelvic floor dysfunction.

Pelvic Floor Supports

1. Levator ani muscle support
2. Perineal membrane
3. Perineal body
4. Pelvic connective tissue

Levator ani is a paired muscle that forms the main muscular component of the pelvic floor. It is also called as *pelvic diaphragm* and is composed of 3 components—iliococcygeus, ischiococcygeus, pubococcygeus. Normally levators maintain a constant state of contraction, thus an active floor is provided that supports the weight of the abdominopelvic organs against the forces of intraabdominal pressure. This helps to prevent excessive strain over the ligaments. Type 1 muscle (slow twitch) fibres are predominant in these levators which bring about this normal resting contraction of these levators. This helps to keep the urogenital hiatus closed and draw the distal urethra, vagina and rectum towards pubis. The reflux contraction of these muscle elicited by the sudden increase in the intra-abdominal pressure is brought about by the type 2 muscle fibres. Relaxation of the levators occurs for a brief intermittent period at the time of voiding, defecation and parturition. Other muscles which form the important component of pelvic floor are bulbospongiosus and ischiocavernosus, superficial transverse perineal muscle of superficial perineal pouch, sphincter urethrae and deep transverse perineal muscle of deep perineal pouch, and external anal sphincter. Levators receive efferents from S_2–S_5 nerve roots; the urethral and external anal sphincters by pudendal nerve.

Mass of dense connective tissue between the distal third of the posterior vaginal wall and the anus below the pelvic floor formed primarily by the connection between the halves of the perineal membrane in the midline forms the *perineal body*. It supports the distal vagina and rectum.

Uterus is supported in its position of anteversion and anteflexion in the pelvis by uterine ligaments, pelvic floor and pelvic cellular tissues. *Endopelvic fascia* is the connective tissue covering of the vagina, supravaginal cervix, uterus, bladder, urethra and rectum. *Pelvic cellular tissue* is the loose areolar tissue that acts as a packing material filling the space between the pelvic peritoneum and the fascia covering the pelvic floor. It condenses into bands that radiate from these organs to lateral pelvic wall laterally, sacrum posteriorly and pubic bones anteriorly. The anterior band which is attached to the anterolateral aspect of cervix, anterior vaginal vault and back of pubic bone is the *pubovesicocervical ligament*. The lateral band called the *Mackenrodt's ligament* or *cardinal ligament* extends from the supravaginal cervix and upper part of the vagina to the lateral pelvic wall, consists of ureteric canal 1 cm lateral to cervix through which passes the ureter, supports the uterus preventing it to be dragged through the vagina when there is increased intra-abdominal pressure. The posterior band is the *uterosacral ligament* that extends from the uterine isthmus to the level of junction of 2nd and 3rd sacral vertebra, lateral to rectosigmoid, below the fold of peritoneum, acts as support of the uterus, maintaining it in its anteverted position. Mackenrodt's and uterosacrals constitute an important support (*level 1*) to the cervix and upper vagina, whose defects leads to post-hysterectomy vault prolapse. The lateral walls of the midvagina are attached on each side to the pelvic walls. The anterior wall of the vagina is attached on its lateral aspect to arcus tendinosus and to the medial aspects of levator ani muscle (*level 2 support*). Clinical manifestation of defects in these support results in prolapse of anterior and posterior vaginal wall and stress urinary incontinence. The distal third of the vagina is attached to the urethra anteriorly, pubovaginalis muscle and perineal membrane laterally, to the perineal body posteriorly (*level 3 support*). Defect in these support results in distal rectocele or perineal descent. While treating genital prolapse it is very important to know and understand the integrity of these supports.

As pelvic cellular tissue extends into the gluteal region through sacrosciatic foramen, obturator region through obturator foramen, femoral triangle through femoral canal, perirenal region along the ureter, labia majus along round ligament, any inflammatory processes in pelvis can spread to any of these regions.

Anatomy of Pelvic Part of Urinary Apparatus in Females

It is important to know the *course of ureter* in pelvis as its course is altered in large broad ligament tumours or myomas. It needs to be dissected during Wertheim's operation. It crosses the bifurcation of common iliac artery beneath the peritoneum, to enter the pelvic brim where it is crossed by the ovarian vessels; and on left side also by mesosigmoid. It forms the posterior boundary of ovarian fossa, lies medial to the structures on the lateral pelvic wall along the anterior margin of greater sciatic foramen. It further progresses downwards, and at the level of ischial spine turns medially and forwards to enter into the ureteric canal in Mackenrodt's ligament, where it is crossed from above by the uterine vessels. After its exit from the canal it progresses forwards and medially to reach the bladder, where it lies from the cervix at a distance of 1–2 cm. Pelvic ureter is supplied from its lateral aspect by branches of internal iliac artery, vaginal artery, vesical and middle rectal arteries which form plexus on its outer fibrous sheath.

Urinary bladder is a hollow muscular organ, which when empty lies in the pelvis in front of vagina and uterus. When filled and gets distended rises above the pelvic brim to become palpable per abdomen. Uterovesical fold peritoneum lies above the bladder base at the level of internal os. Bladder is firmly attached to supravaginal portion of cervix at its base above and to the middle of the anterior vaginal wall at its neck below, but bladder base is separated from the upper part of anterior vaginal wall by a loose areolar tissue that forms the plane of cleavage between the two. It is through this plane where the bladder is separated off the cervix and anterior vaginal wall during hysterectomy and caesarean section. Bladder is supplied by superior and inferior vesical branches of internal iliac arteries. Veins form plexus around bladder neck that drain into internal iliac veins.

Urethra from the base of the bladder passes downwards and forwards behind the symphysis pubis, measures 3.5 cm in length, opens out at the *external urinary meatus* below the clitoris. There is pair of *paraurethral gland of Skene* along the floor of the urethra, the duct of which opens near the external meatus, can get infected to form an abscess or cyst.

SURGERIES IN FEMALE GENITAL TRACT

Preoperative Preparation

Minor surgical procedures of vulva and vagina, dilatation and curettage, cervical biopsy which are done under local anaesthesia can be done as outpatient procedures. Major surgeries of vagina, abdominal operations, needs admission one or two days prior to the procedures.

Patient is assessed by taking detailed history pertaining to her menstruation, pregnancy and postpartum period, other medical illness like hypertension, diabetes, bronchial asthma and epilepsy, tuberculosis, and any surgeries done in the past.

In detail, medical examination is done before major surgeries to rule out hypertension, diabetes and ischaemic heart disease. Chest X-ray is taken in case of chronic cough to rule out emphysema, tuberculosis. ECG and ECHO are done to assess the cardiac status.

Antihypertensives are started for hypertension, insulin for diabetics, antibiotics sometimes with bronchodilators for chest infections. Bleeding tendencies are ruled out by doing bleeding time, clotting and prothrombin time. Blood grouping is done and required amount of blood is kept ready for transfusion. Anaemia with HB% <10 g needs preoperative transfusion of blood or packed cells in emergency. Urine routine examination is done to rule out urinary tract infection which has to be actively treated prior to surgery. Renal functions are assessed by doing blood urea and serum creatinine levels. Caries tooth and gum sepsis must be managed.

Preparation of the part: The operating site over the abdomen, vulva and perineum must be shaved for all major surgical procedures. Shaving is done with a sharp disinfected razor blade using soap or cream to prevent any injuries to the skin. Vaginal douche must be given for few days prior to abdominal surgeries and vaginal surgeries. For minor surgeries, no vaginal preparation or shaving is required.

Preparation of the bowel is essential for all major abdominal and vaginal surgeries. Bowel wash or enema may be given on the previous day evening. Minor vaginal procedures require no enema. Patient kept fasting for 8 hours for all major surgeries done, with light food intake on the previous day.

Premedications like injection Pethidine 50 mg injection. Phenergan 25 mg with injection atropine or any other drug is given 1 hour prior to the surgery as per anaesthetists instructions. Preoperative antibiotics are given 1 hour prior to surgery.

Patient is made to empty the bladder prior to minor surgeries. But for major abdominal surgeries catheter is inserted and left *in situ*. For vaginal procedures bladder is initially catheterised and later left *in situ* after the surgery.

Informed consent of the patient is taken for all major and minor procedures explaining the nature of the procedures, its after effects and care.

Patient is placed in Trendelenburg position for abdominal surgeries and in lithotomy position for vaginal surgeries.

For abdominal surgeries, vagina is initially cleaned with iodine preparation and later abdomen is painted with iodine preparation and spirit from mid chest to mid thighs. For vaginal surgeries whole of perineum, thighs and lower abdomen is painted with antiseptic solution. Later, vulva is initially swabbed followed by vagina. Later, the painted area is draped with sterile linen, except the area to be operated is exposed.

Routine bimanual examination under anaesthesia is very beneficial in all vaginal and abdominal surgeries.

DILATATION AND CURETTAGE (D & C)

It is done for diagnostic purpose:

- As a part of investigation and treatment of menstrual disorders
- As a part of initial workup in infertility
- In postmenopausal bleeding.

As a part of treatment in:

- Dysfunctional uterine bleeding
- To remove retained products of conception
- To remove retained intrauterine contraceptive device (IUCD)
- To remove endometrial polyps.

Only cervical dilatation done in:

- Cervical amputation
- For intrauterine radium insertion
- For insertion of LNG-IUCD
- For drainage of pyometra
- For cervical cautery.

This procedure is deferred in the presence of active infections of vagina, cervix, fallopian tubes and endometrium.

D&C is done as an outpatient procedure with the patient instructed to fast for 4–6 hours. It can done under general anaesthesia, but doing under local paracervical block and IV sedation (petidine/diazepam and fortwin along with atropine) would be ideal. Prior to the procedure preparing the local area by shaving is not an absolute necessity. Patient is asked to void urine just before the procedure. Patient is placed in the lithotomy position with buttocks protruding slightly beyond the edge of the table. Vulva, vagina and perineum is cleaned with suitable antiseptic lotion (savlon). Bimanual examination is done to assess the position of the uterus, size of the uterus, its mobility, and to assess any other pelvic pathology. Labia is gently drawn apart and *vaginal speculum* (Sim's or Auvard's) of appropriate size is inserted into the vagina. Anterior lip of cervix is held with *volsellum*. If there is difficulty in visualising the cervix, one can use *anterior vaginal wall retractor* to lift up the bladder. The cervix that is held is drawn towards introitus by gentle traction. By doing this the endocervical canal is straightened thereby allowing easy passage of instrument into the uterine cavity. *Uterine sound* held lightly between thumb and fingers is passed gently through the cervix to note the uterocervical length and also to confirm the position of the uterus whether retroflexed or anteflexed. This has to be done very carefully as any forceful introduction of sound will cause false passages in the endocervical canal.

Dilatation of Cervix

Cervix is now gradually dilated using *graduated metal dilators* (Hegar's or Hawkin's-Amblar's) starting from lowest size close to that of the sound. It is gently pushed into the cervical canal with steady pressure, the tip of which should go well beyond the internal os. The distance to which the dilator is pushed should not be beyond that of the uterocervical length determined by the uterine sound. And the pressure to be used on the dilator comes by repeated practise. Uterine perforations are more common with smaller dilators than larger ones. The degree dilatation depends on the type of procedure to be done. For simple curettage, it is sufficient to dilate up till 7 mm so to allow the passage of a *curratte*, whereas for suction in termination of pregnancy it can be dilated maximum up to 10 mm. Overdoing in nulliparous will cause damage to cervix leading to incompetence.

Curettage of Endometrium

A small sharp curette of 7 mm width is inserted into the uterine cavity. Holding its sharp concave edge firmly against anterior uterine wall curetting is started from 12 o'clock position in anteclockwise direction with stroke done from fundus to the cervix. Pressure used should be optimum enough to scrape off the endometrium but not too excess to cause uterine perforation. This gauging of pressure comes only by practice. All the anterior wall, posterior wall, cornual ends and fundus must be optimally scraped and are collected on sterile gauze. Endometrial curettings that is scraped off is collected in a bottle containing 10% formalin saline and is sent for histopathological study. In *fractional* curettage, the samples collected from anterior wall, posterior wall, cornual ends and endocervix are separately collected and sent in separate bottles with proper labelling. The sample has to be sent in normal saline to rule out endometrial tuberculosis.

The speculum is removed off the vagina after ensuring the haemostasis. After the patient recovers from anaesthesia she is discharged with a course of antibiotics and analgesics.

Complications

Cervical tear—common at the time of dilatation during earlier days. But now with the use of prostaglandins (vaginal misoprostol 400 mcg 3-4 hours prior to procedure) which aids in softening the cervix and help in favourable dilatation. If cervical tear has occurred it has to be sutured without fail. Sometimes, the tear may extend upwards involving the descending cervical arteries causing profuse haemorrhage. This can be controlled by a deep lateral stitch on the cervix. It may sometimes necessitate opening the abdomen if there is a tear of the cervix involving the uterine artery above which needs to be ligated.

Uterine perforation—this can be produced by uterine sound, dilators or curette. Sudden loss of resistance while sounding the uterus, dilating the cervix or curetting the uterus should one suspect perforation. The procedure is abandoned at this point and laparoscopy is done to confirm the perforation. The perforation may be simple involving only the uterus or may injure the bladder, omentum, vessels and intestines. If it is simple uterine perforation without involving adjacent viscera, patient is admitted and observed for 24 hours with antibiotics, monitoring pulse, temperature and respiration. If she is stable she may be discharged. Laparotomy is required when there is visceral injury, big uterine perforation, vessel injury and peritonitis. Uterine rent is sutured, bleeding vessel is ligated. Hysterectomy is done when there is extensive uterine injury with haemorrhage or broad ligament haematoma. Bowel is inspected from jejunum to rectum including omentum. Simple bowel perforation can be sutured in 2 layers using vicryl sutures. Bowel resection with end to end anastomosis is required in case of multiple perforations along with avulsion of mesentery. Bladder injury if present should be identified and sutured with 2 layers of 2-zero vicryl sutures and catheter should be left *in situ* for 7–10 days.

Infection—may be immediate or late; may be localised to pelvis and uterus or may extend to the general peritoneal cavity causing peritonitis. Local pelvic infection is treated conservatively with higher antibiotics. Generalised peritonitis require proper management of fluid and electrolytes, higher antibiotics, laparotomy, pus drainage, hysterectomy if necessary.

Remote complications are secondary amenorrhoea, infertility due to secondary sepsis.

MEDICAL TERMINATION OF PREGNANCY

Induced abortions in India are been liberalised and was brought under *Medical Termination of Pregnancy Act* passed by the parliament which came into force on April 1, 1971. The law specifies:

1. The condition under which pregnancy can be terminated.
   a. *Medical grounds* where the continuation of pregnancy (i) may endanger the life of pregnant woman (ii) cause grave injury to the physical and mental health of the woman as in cardiac diseases (severe grade III and grade IV types, pulmonary hypertension, cardiac enlargement, left ventricular hypertrophy, ECG changes showing myocardial ischemia) renal diseases (CRF),uncontrolled hypertension and diabetes, ongoing psychiatric diseases (like schizophrenia, severe depression), malignancies of cervix or breast, severe degree of hyperemesis not responding to any conservative management.
   b. *Eugenic grounds* where there would be a risk of physical and mental disability in foetus when the mother has been exposed to teratogenic drugs, radiation, viral infections (rubella), at the time of organogenesis (First 8 weeks of gestation); risk of chromosomal abnormalities (trisomy 21, 18) and inborn errors of metabolism in foetus picked up by amniocentesis done after 14 weeks, sonar study done at 18–20th week revealing neural tubal defects (spina bifida, anencephaly) in foetus.
   c. *Social grounds* to prevent grave injury to the physical and mental health of the pregnant woman, where the woman has to undergo an unplanned pregnancy resulted from contraceptive failure or rape.
2. The abortion procedure can be performed by:
   a. Registered Medical Practitioner who has assisted at least 25 MTP's in an authorised centre and having a certificate.
   b. One who had 6 months house surgeon training in obstetrics and gynaecology.
   c. MD/diploma holder in obstetrics and gynaecology.
3. This procedures can be done at government hospitals or places maintained by the government or at places approved by the government.

Written consent of only the patient is sufficient; in case of minor or lunatic consent of the parent or the legal guardian can be taken.

Termination is legally permitted up to 20 weeks, beyond 12 weeks opinion of two medical practitioners is necessary.

Methods of Termination

Prior to termination, it is essential to assess Hb%, blood grouping and Rh typing, urine analysis and blood sugar estimation. If patient is Rh negative blood group, it is essential to give injection. Anti-D 50 µg within 72 hours of the procedure. USG to confirm period of gestation.

First Trimester (up to 12 weeks)

Medical Method

Mifepristone (RU486) and misoprostol—Mifepristone an analog of natural progesterone blocks its effect and misoprostol (PGE_1) helps in expulsion of conceptus by bringing about powerful uterine contraction. Recommended dose of 600 mg of mifepristone orally on day 1 followed by 400 µg of misoprostol orally on day 3 is effective when used within 50 days of gestation. 200 mg of mifepristone orally with 800 µg of misoprostol vaginally is also equally effective.

Problems:

- Incomplete expulsion (2–3%), confirmed by USG done after 2 weeks, needs surgical evacuation.
- Non-responders (1%), where the above protocol has failed to bring about abortion, requires surgical evacuation.

Other regimens:

- Methotrexate 50 mg/m^2 IM followed by misoprostol 800 µg vaginally after 7 days.
- Tamoxifen 20 mg orally for 4 days followed by 800 µg of misoprostol vaginally.

Surgical Method

- Menstrual regulation
- Dilatation and suction evacuation

- Dilatation and curettage.
  - *Menstrual regulation:* This involves aspiration of uterine cavity within 2 weeks of last missed period without confirming the pregnancy. The contents of uterine cavity is aspirated using a special plastic syringe of 60 mL capacity with a non-return valve attached to a flexible plastic cannula (Karman) of 6–12 mm diameter. The syringe can be used 65–75 times and the cannula for 10–12 times. The vacuum created in the syringe is similar to that in an electrical apparatus, up to 660 mm of mercury. The procedure can be done as an outpatient procedure without anaesthesia but may sometimes require paracervical block.

    Under aseptic precaution, speculum is inserted into the vagina, cervix is visualised and held with Allis forceps or small-sized vulsellum. The cervix is dilated up to the required size. The cannula is inserted into the cavity. It is attached to the syringe. The valve of the syringe is closed and the piston is pulled back to create a vacuum before attaching it to the cannula. Once the cannula is inserted into the uterine cavity the valve is released. The cannula is moved to and fro gently until whole of the endometrial contents are aspirated or the syringe gets completely filled with contents. The cannula is detached from the syringe and the aspirated contents are inspected by pouring it over basin filled with water. The procedure may be repeated until no contents fill the syringe, or you see air bubbles in the syringe or when you feel the gripping sensation of the uterus and uterine cavity feels empty. The vacuum must be repeatedly created as mentioned above before attaching it to the cannula.

    Problems: The procedure may be inadequate in pregnancies beyond 7 weeks. There is risk of continuation of pregnancy (5%) and also a possibility of missing ectopic pregnancy. Other risks are uterine perforation (05%) though rare do can occur. Incomplete abortion, haemorrhage due to retained products of conception, cervical tear and perforations are the other problems that can be encountered.
  - *Dilatation and suction evacuation:* This procedure involves sucking of products of conception with the help of a cannula attached to a suction apparatus.

    This method is useful in termination of pregnancy less than 12 weeks, in incomplete abortion, inevitable abortion, and molar pregnancy. It can be done as an outpatient procedure under paracervical block and IV sedation (injection diazepam 10 mg and atropine 0.6 mg). General anaesthesia may be required in apprehensive patients.

    Prior to the procedure a gentle vaginal examination is done to note the size, position of the uterus with patient in lithotomy position, perineum is cleaned with any antiseptic solution. Draping is done. Posterior vaginal speculum of appropriate size is inserted. Cervix is visualised and held with vulsellum or Allis's forceps. Paracervical block given uterine sound is inserted into the uterine cavity to know the uterocervical length and the direction of the uterine cavity. The cervix is dilated with the help of dilators as mentioned in the previous topic to a size less than the size of the cannula which has to be used. The dilatation can be made easy by the use of vaginal misoprostol 400 μg 3 hours prior to the procedure or parenteral carboprost (15 methyl $PGF_{2\alpha}$). Once the dilatation is done cannula is inserted into the uterine cavity. Noting the uterocervical length, it should not move beyond that length. With a help of rubber tubing or plastic tubing, it is connected to a suction apparatus. The pressure of the suction apparatus is maintained at 400–600 Hg. Injection methergine 0.2 mg is given intravenous. By to and fro movements of the cannula the contents of the uterine cavity are aspirated which gets collected in the bottle of the suction apparatus. The suction can be regulated by placing a finger over the hole at the base of the cannula. The suction is said to be complete when no contents are aspirated from the uterine cavity, air bubbles are seen in the cannula, when one feels the gripping sensation over the cannula by the contracting uterus, and the typical grating sensation. The vacuum has to be broken by detaching the tubing before the cannula is removed. The cavity is gently curetted with a curette. The cannula may be re-inserted to aspirate any leftover contents. At the end of the procedure cervical os is examined for any bleeding. A sterile vulval pad is placed.
  - Problems:
    - Cervical injury and laceration (already discussed in dilatation and curettage).
    - Perforation (already discussed in dilatation and curettage). Can be minimised with the use of plastic cannula.
    - Infection can be reduced and/controlled with the use of proper antibiotics before and after the procedure.
  - Drawbacks: Not beneficial in gestation beyond 10 weeks as the products are big to be sucked into the cannula.
  - *Dilatation and curettage:* The steps are similar as described before. But as the products of conception has to be removed the cervix needs to be dilated to 10–12 mm even for 8 weeks gestation,14–15 mm for 11–12 weeks gestation. The cervix needs to be softened prior to the procedure by vaginal misoprostol (inserted 3 hours before) or intramuscular carboprost (given 2 hours before). Dilatation must be carried out gently and smoothly to avoid cervical tear.

    As the pregnant uterus will be soft intravenous methergine 0.2 mg has to be given once the dilatation is complete and curettage is begun in order to contract the uterus and make it hard. Alternatively oxytocin 5U can be given intravenously as methergine causes undesirable vomiting.

    Uterine sound is passed to know the uterocervical length. Sponge holding forceps or ovum forceps of appropriate size is inserted through the dilated cervix and advanced towards fundus. The sac is ruptured allowing the fluid to flow out. The blades of the forceps is opened and the products are held with the blades and gently pulled out through the cervix. The procedure is repeated until all products are pulled out. Undue traction should be avoided while pulling out the products. If resistance is felt then the products are pulled in small bits until the cavity is felt empty. A blunt curette can now be inserted into the cavity and curettage is done to loosen the tissues. The ovum forceps is re-inserted to remove any more bits left especially from the cornual ends. Cavity can be curetted gently until you feel the grating sensation of endometrium and no blood trickles through the cervical os ensuring the completeness of the procedure. Antibiotics are always given for 5 days to prevent any infection.

Second Trimester Termination

- *Surgical evacuation:* Dilatation and evacuation, aspirotomy
  It is suitable up to 13–15 weeks of pregnancy.
- Intra-amniotic instillation of drugs: Hypertonic saline, urea, prostaglandins.
- Extra-amniotic instillation of drugs: Ethacridine lactate, prostaglandins and hypertonic saline.
- Hysterotomy.

Combining the use of oxyrocic drugs augments the myometrial activity and thereby help to shorten the induction-abortion interval. Vaginal misoprostol 400 mg can be used prior to the above procedure which will help in cervical softening and dilatation thereby preventing cervical tears.

Dilatation and evacuation: Patient is in lithotomy position. Vulva is cleaned with antiseptic solution and draped with sterile clothes. Posterior vagina is depressed with Sim's speculum. Cervix is visualised and held with sponge holding forceps or vulsellum. Paracervical block given. Cervix is dilated as described before up to no. 12. Sac is ruptured and the liquor amnii is aspirated with a large-bore suction cannula. A special forceps called the aspirotomy forceps which has long blades, strong jaws measuring 7–12 mm across and no ratchet is inserted into the cavity. The foetal parts are crushed with it and extracted out through the cervix. Injection methergine 0.2 mg IV is given at the time of evacuation to contract the uterus so as to make it hard to avoid perforation and also to minimise the bleeding. Placental parts are also removed with the forceps. Cavity is curetted with blunt curette.

With expert hands this method helps to evacuate the uterus with minimal bleeding and no hospitalisation.

Intra-amniotic instillation of drugs: This method is employed beyond 16 weeks up to 20 weeks. It requires hospitalisation. Drugs instilled into the amniotic cavity may be $PGF_{2\alpha}$ alone or combination of PGE_2 and hypertonic urea solution or hypertonic saline solution. USG is necessary to confirm the placental site. Coagulation profile, cardiac and renal status, are checked.

The prostaglandin solution to be injected is freshly prepared before use by diluting 40 mg of $PGF_{2\alpha}$ in 20 mL syringe containing physiological saline. Combination of hypertonic urea solution and PGE_2 is prepared by dissolving 80 g of 40% urea in 150 mL of physiological saline and mixing it with 10 mg of PGE_2 in 50 mL syringe. 2 mg of 15 methyl $PGF_{2\alpha}$ (carboprost) can also be used with urea solution. Amount of hypertonic saline required is 10 mL per weeks of gestation.

Patient is placed in dorsal position after emptying the bladder. 5 mL 1% lignocaine is used to infiltrate the skin over the chosen site far away from placenta. 19-gauge needle is used to inject the local anaesthetic agent into the rectus muscle and peritoneum. An 18-gauge spinal needle or Tuhey needle is inserted into the uterus with the tip in a clear pocket of amniotic fluid. About 20 mL of fluid is withdrawn to ensure the correct placement. If blood comes out of the needle, then probably the needle placement may be incorrect or it may have pierced some blood vessel. The needle is withdrawn and reinserted in another site till clear amniotic fluid is aspirated.

The drugs to be instilled are injected slowly through this needle. As the volume injected may lead to over distension of uterus causing discomfort to the patient, sufficient amount of amniotic fluid (at least 50 mL) must be aspirated prior to instillation. When hypertonic saline is used, it is safer to infuse by means of drip set taking at least 5–10 minutes to infuse it. Vital signs should be recorded immediately after the procedure. Patient should be under close observation at least for 2 hours. Antibiotic coverage is given.

The patient may feel severe pain if the drug is injected into the myometrium or into the peritoneal cavity at when the procedure may be abandoned. When hypertonic saline is used as the instillating agent the patient may experience severe thirst, headache, flushing hypertension, chest pain, bradycardia, apnoea, tingling of fingers and severe pain, if the solution is accidently injected into the blood vessel. The procedure should be immediately abandoned and 1000 mL of dextrose solution should be rapidly infused with intravenous diuretics. This may sometimes also cause anuria, cerebral oedema.

Uterine contraction usually commences within 2–6 hours. If at all no satisfactory contraction is seen then the dose of prostaglandins can be repeated without urea solution. One should withhold the use of syntocin infusion to avoid uterine hyperstimulation, cervical laceration and rupture uterus and fluid overload.

Induction-abortion interval is 36–48 hours in 95% of cases when hypertonic saline is used; whereas it is 13–16 hours in 90% of cases when the combination of urea and prostaglandins are used.

Complications

- Nausea, vomiting, diarrhoea (more when PG's are used).
- Intense abdominal pain due to hyperstimulation of uterus.
- Cervical tear and laceration leading to profuse haemorrhage.
- Incomplete expulsion with retained products of conception which might require exploration and evacuation under anaesthesia.
- Intrauterine infection leading to severe sepsis which can be checked with proper usage of higher antibiotics.
- Hypernatraemia due to accidental infusion of hypertonic saline into a blood vessel.
- Uterine necrosis, rupture, pulmonary and cerebral oedema, consumption coagulopathy, and renal failure are hazards more common with hypertonic saline infusion.
- Accidental infusion of saline into bladder wall or myometrium or peritoneal cavity or ovaries can cause severe irritation and tissue necrosis.

Contraindications:

- Hypertonic saline is better avoided in pre-existing cardiovascular disease, hypertension, sickle cell anaemia, renal disease and severe anaemia (as hypernatraemia can cause haemolysis).
- PG's are better avoided in patients with known history of bronchial asthma.

Late sequelae: Menstrual disturbances due to chronic endometritis, secondary infertility due to cervical incompetence and tubal block, chronic pelvic inflammatory disease, ectopic pregnancy.

Extra-amniotic instillation of drugs: Drugs used—0.1% ethacridine lactate (10 mL per week but maximum is 150 mL) $PGF_{2\alpha}$ 200-500 μg or PGE_2 200 μg.

Patient is placed in lithotomy position after emptying the bladder. After cleaning with antiseptic lotion, perineum is draped. Vagina is cleaned with antiseptic solution, cervix is visualised with the help of Sim's speculum and held with tenaculum. A no. 16 Foley's catheter is pushed through the cervix well beyond the internal os up to 10 cm between uterine wall and membranes. The balloon of Foley's is inflated with 10 mL saline or distilled water. This will fit at the internal os there by preventing the fall of the catheter.

Now the drug either ethacridine lactate or prostaglandins is injected to the extra-amniotic space through this catheter. The required dose of prostaglandin is taken and dissolved in physiological saline to make 100 mL solution. This solution is injected through the catheter to the extra-amniotic space. The dose of prostaglandins can be repeated every 2 hours or can be be given as a continuous infusion through the catheter. Usually, contraction starts within 1–2 hours and induction - abortion interval is around 16–18 hours in 90% cases. Patient should be monitored continuously for vital signs, uterine contraction and cervical dilatation. The catheter gets expelled with dilatation of cervix followed by expulsion of the foetus.

Placenta is frequently retained which needs to be evacuated under anaesthesia.

Complications

- Infection due to indwelling catheter. So some prefer to remove the catheter within 4 hours. antibiotics coverage should be started at the earliest.
- Intolerance to prostaglandins—fever, severe nausea, vomiting, diarrhoea, uterine hyperstimulation.
- Cervical tear and laceration leading to profuse bleeding.
- Expulsion of live foetus giving an uncomfortable feeling.
- Retention of placenta needing evacuation under anaesthesia.
- Menstrual disturbances due to chronic endometritis, secondary infertility due to cervical incompetence and tubal block, chronic pelvic inflammatory disease are the late sequelae.

Hysterotomy

This is not routinely done for medical termination of pregnancy. It is done if all the other methods for midtrimester abortion fails and is usually combined with tubal sterilisation whenever necessary. The procedure is usually done through abdominal route but can also be done vaginally.

The patient is prepared as for any abdominal surgery. The procedure can be done under general or spinal or epidural anaesthesia. The abdomen is painted with antiseptic lotion, draped with sterile drapes. Abdomen is opened by Pfannenstiel incision. After opening the peritoneum uterus is drawn out of the incision and the abdomen is packed with sterile mops to prevent the spillage of uterine contents into the peritoneal cavity (to prevent scar endometriosis). The loose uterovesical fold of peritoneum is opened and bladder is pushed down. A vertical incision of 5 cm is made on the myometrium as low as possible, deepened until the membranes are visible. As the isthmus is narrow in early pregnancy, transverse incision may cause injury to uterine vessels. Injection Methergine 0.2 mg is given intravenously. The products of conception are gently removed from the uterine cavity. Cavity is cleaned with a gauze gently. The uterine incision is closed by apposing the muscle in 2 layers by continuous sutures, with 1-zero chromic catgut in round bodied needle.

Alternatively, uterus can be opened in the upper segment without opening the UV fold of peritoneum, but the incision is made as low as possible. This approach is usually followed by tubal ligation to prevent rupture uterus in future pregnancy.

Abdominal packs are removed. Abdomen is closed in layers after a peritoneal wash with saline.

Patient is kept nil oral till the bowel movements are heard. Hydration is maintained with IV fluids. Sepsis is prevented with proper antibiotics. Patients is watched for vaginal bleeding, and sepsis. Patient is discharged on 5th day from the hospital.

Complications

Sepsis peritonitis, uterine bleeding, anaesthetic hazards are the immediate complications. Menstrual irregularities, scar endometriosis, rupture of hysterotomy scar in future pregnancy are the delayed complications.

Vaginal Hysterotomy

Patient is placed in lithotomy position. Cervix is exposed with Sim's speculum and anterior wall retractor. It is held with vulsellum. Anterior vaginal skin above the cervix is infiltrated with 10 mL 1:200,000 adrenaline to reduce the bleeding. A horizontal incision is made on the vaginal epithelium at its junction with the cervix. Bladder is identified and pushed up with finger and guaze to expose the cervix and the lower segment. Uterine wall is incised 3 cm on the lower segment; products of conception are removed with ovum forceps. Later the uterine wall is closed followed by the closure of the vaginal epithelium.

This procedure avoids all the hazards of abdominal procedure.

BARTHOLIN CYST AND ABSCESS

Bartholin's cyst is a rounded swelling on the inner aspect of labium majus at the junction of anterior 2/3rd and posterior 1/3rd due to blockage of duct orifice following chronic inflammation. Cyst is asymptomatic but may cause slight vulvar discomfort, dyspareunia.

Cyst may sometimes rupture spontaneously which then may require sitz bath and a course of antibiotics. Persistent cyst needs excision which can be done under general anaesthesia with the patient placed in lithotomy position. Vulva and perineum is painted with antiseptic lotion and draped. A vertical incision is made over the outer aspect of the cyst not extending upwards too much as it may cause damage to vestibular bulb containing venous plexus. A plane of cleavage is dissected between the cyst wall and the vaginal mucosa and skin. As the cyst is thin walled and the tissues around the cyst wall are thickened and vascular, the cyst is likely to rupture during the dissection. Sharp dissection helps to enucleate the cyst completely. Duct also should be removed along with the cyst. Bleeding vessels has to be cauterised or ligated. Cavity is obliterated with interrupted sutures. A silastic drain can be kept in the cavity if there is excess oozing. The skin is trimmed and closed with interrupted sutures. Drain may be removed on the 2nd day. Patient is discharged with a course of antibiotics **(Fig. 32-1)**.

Acute inflammation of the Bartholin gland leads to bartholinitis and abscess formation. Abscess is very painful causing the patient difficult to sit, and walk. Incision and drainage of the abscess is done under general anaesthesia. A vertical incision is done on the outer aspect of the abscess. Pus drained is sent for culture and sensitivity. Finger is inserted into the cavity and explored. Gauze plug soaked with betadine solution is kept in the cavity. Daily dressing is done till cavity heels. Antibiotics are given. Alternatively *marsupialisation* can also be done for Bartholin abscess. Under general anaesthesia a vertical incision 2.5 cm is made over the vaginal aspect of the labium. The skin is separated from the underlying abscess. The abscess cavity is opened with scalpel. Pus drained is collected and sent for culture and sensitivity. The edges of abscess cavity and skin is trimmed and apposed with 3-zero interrupted catgut sutures. No drain is required. Even though, it is practiced to suture the skin if infection is severe, pack can be kept and dressing can be done. As if it is severely infected area, it will not granulate if sutured. Non-suturing may lead into wide scar. When healing occurs a small permanent opening will remain **(Fig. 32-2)**.

ECTOPIC PREGNANCY

It is an abnormal pregnancy where the fertilised ovum implants and develops outside the normal uterine cavity.

Sites of Ectopic Pregnancy

Fallopian tubes—98% (ampullary portion commonest)
Ovaries—0.15%
Abdominal cavity—1%
Cervix

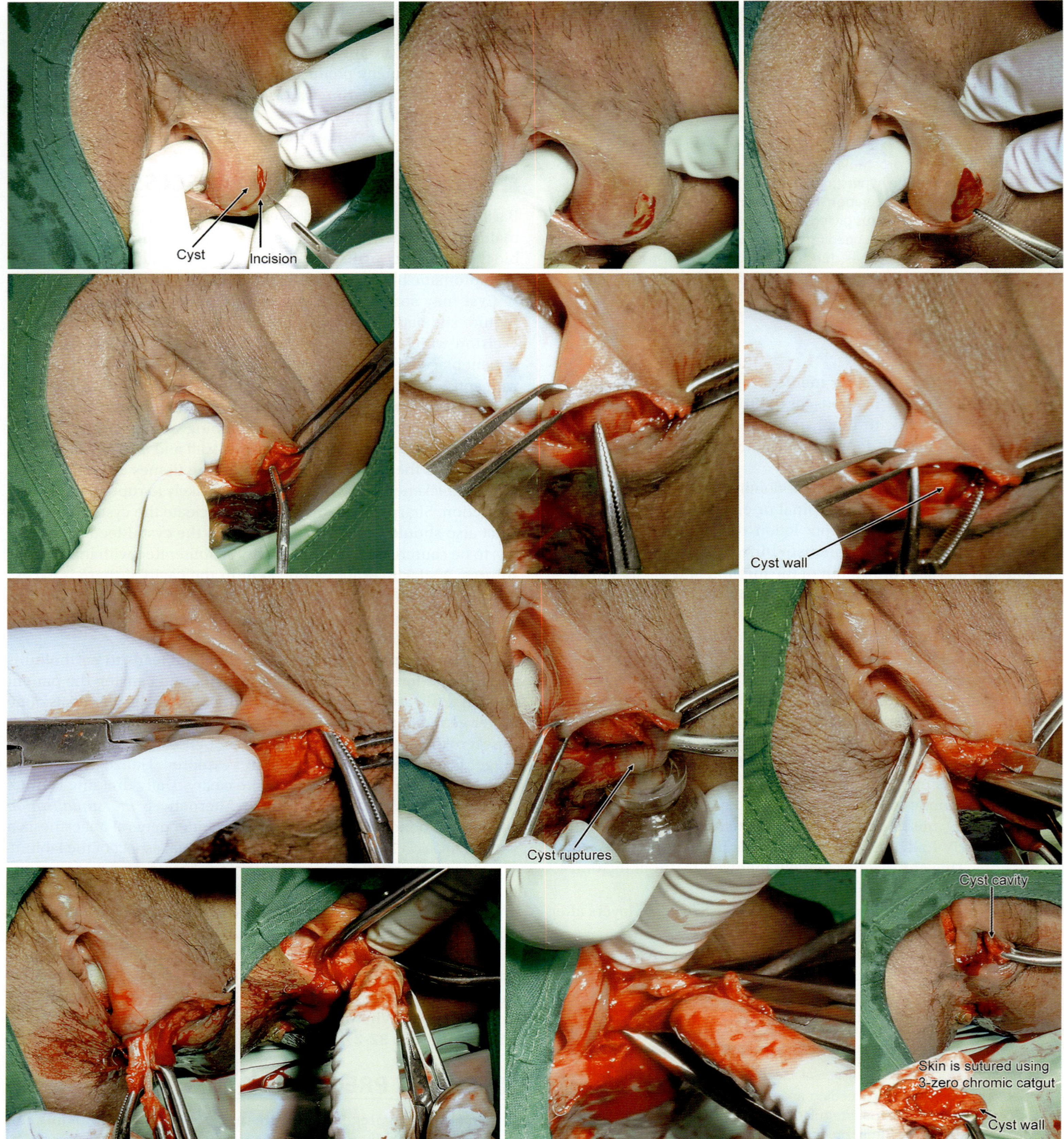

Fig. 32-1: Bartholin cyst excision—technique.

Clinical Features

Patient with ectopic pregnancy presents with variable degrees of abdominal pain (may be severe, acute or dull aching type); short period of amenorrhoea (may or may not be present, may have on and off spotting); fainting episodes (typical of ectopic), feeling of nausea and vomiting with pain. Some patients may present with profound shock with a characteristic pallor out of proportion to visible vaginal bleeding. Tenderness in lower abdomen and the

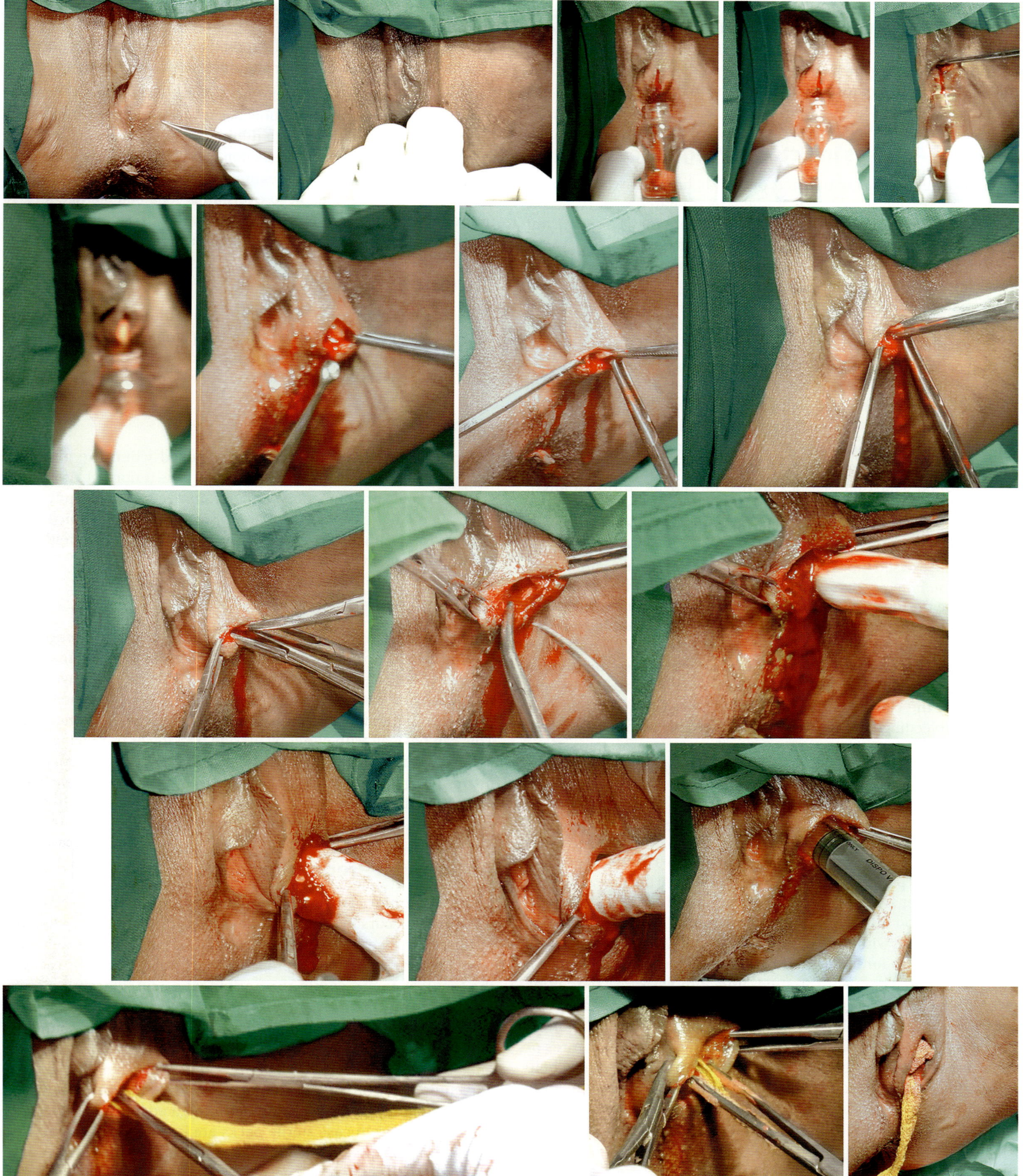

Fig. 32-2: Bartholin abscess drainage.

typical tender uterine movement, raised serum β-hCG, ultrasound abdomen and pelvis may show free fluid in pelvic cavity along with absence of intrauterine gestation with presence of gestational sac outside the uterine cavity—all help in coming to a diagnosis. In doubtful cases, laparoscopy can be done to diagnose and proceed with ectopic gestation.

Surgical Aspects in Ectopic Pregnancy

Once the diagnosis is confirmed patient is immediately taken up for surgery. Patient in shock is initially resuscitated with IV fluids. Minimum 2 points of blood is arranged as there may be significant intra-peritoneal haemorrhage. IV antibiotics are given.

Abdomen is opened by a large incision either by Pfannenstiel or lower midline so as to have adequate access to ectopic site and also there may be adhesions which may have to deal with. Blood in the peritoneal cavity is cleared off with suction. Ectopic site is identified.

In tubal ectopic gestation, *salpingectomy* is done when future fertility is of no concern, when there is rupture with major intra-peritoneal haemorrhage, or when the tube is extensively damaged. One pair of long haemostatic clamps (Kocher's long and straight clamp) are placed on the medial end of the fallopian tube including the mesosalpinx close to the tube so as to conserve the ovarian vasculature. Second pair is placed on the lateral aspect on the mesosalpinx. The tips of the clamps should be approximated. If the adjacent ovary need to be removed the second pair of clamp is placed over the infundibulopelvic ligament. The divided pedicles are transfixed and ligated with 1-zero vicryl sutures before releasing the clamps. The excised tubes are sent for histopathological examination.

Partial salpingectomy/segmental resection is done when one wants to conserve the tube for fertility. Only that part of the tube damaged by ectopic pregnancy is removed, leaving behind considerable amount of tube for reanastomosis in later period. Clamps are applied on either side of the ectopic. Before applying clamps, it is essential to note vessel free area in the mesosalpinx which appears transilluminant. The tips of the clamps should be placed close to each other. This will avoid bleeding from any blood vessels when sutures are applied. The pedicles include the cut end of the tubes and mesosalpinx. If the patient does not wish for future fertility tubal ligation (by *Pomeroy's method*) is done on the other tube.

Conservative Surgery in Ectopic Pregnancy

Salpingostomy/Salpingotomy: In case of un-ruptured ectopic pregnancy, this procedure can be done to conserve the tube. The tube is held on either side of the ectopic gestation with Babcock's forceps. A linear incision on the antimesenteric border, running parallel to the tube is done with knife/needle tip cautery/laser, at the site of ectopic gestation for about 2/3rd of the length of the swollen part. Prior to the incision over the tube, injection vasopressin may be given to the tube so as to reduce bleeding. Products of conception are flushed out with suction irrigator or removed with non-toothed dissecting forceps. Bleeding points are ligated with fine sutures or cauterised. Lavage of the tube with Hartmann's solution may help in identifying the bleeding points. If the tube is not very healthy with fimbria partly occluded, it is left open (*salpingostomy*) without suturing to heel by itself, which usually occurs in 3–6 weeks. The incision may be closed in one layer with fine 6-zero prolene if the tubes look healthy (*salpingotomy*).

The success of conservative surgery depends on:

- One should not use catgut as it may cause inflammatory reaction in the tube leading to decreased fertility.
- Tubes are to be handled gently using atraumatic instruments and sutures.
- Peritoneal cavity must be cleared off blood clots so to reduce the adhesion formation. Proper haemostasis should be ensured.

Laparoscopic surgeries for ectopic pregnancy is done in haemodynamically stable patient, is now becoming immensely popular as the healing time is quicker with minimal adhesions. Salpingectomy, salpingostomy or segmental resection can be done laparoscopically. In salpingectomy, the tubal segment to be removed is coagulated with bipolar forceps. The meso-ovarium is coagulated and cut close to the tube. The specimen can be retrieved by a small suprapubic stab incision. Haemostasis can be obtained with diathermy.

Chronic Ectopic

Here the patient has passed the acute phase of the ectopic presentation. Due to continuous slow bleed from the ectopic site haematoma is formed which organises to form a mass in the lower abdomen with significant adhesions with the adjacent bowel, omentum and bladder.

Ovarian Pregnancy

Ectopic pregnancy in ovaries is diagnosed when the gestation occupies the region of ovary and that side tube is normal. As rupture is an inevitable phenomenon *oophorectomy* is done. Presently many have advocated cystectomy as the procedure of the choice. Only the portion of the ovary involved by ectopic is removed either by laparotomy/laparoscopy.

Cervical Pregnancy

When the implantation occurs in cervix it leads to cervical pregnancy. It mimics inevitable abortion. But here the uterine size is smaller for the gestational age with internal os closed. Uterine curettage shows no placental tissue. When suction curettage is done to evacuate the pregnancy, one may encounter with mild to severe haemorrhage. This can be dealt with either by uterine packing or by placing lateral cervical suture to ligate the lateral cervical vessel. Cervical encirclage or applying tamponade with Foley's catheter or angiographic embolisation are other methods tried to control bleeding. In severe cases one may need hysterectomy.

Abdominal Pregnancy

It can be *primary* (when the implantation of the fertilised ovum exclusively occurs in the peritoneal cavity) or *secondary* (when the fertilised ovum escapes into the peritoneal cavity either following tubal abortion or through uteroperitoneal fistula). Amniotic sac with the foetus is found within the peritoneal cavity. Placenta may be attached to any of the organs receiving blood supply from it. Empty uterine cavity with abnormal position of the foetus on ultrasound will help one to come to a diagnosis. Laparotomy is done immediately once the diagnosis is made. Foetus is removed out after clamping and cutting the cord close to the placenta. Placenta can be removed if its vascular supply can be identified and ligated. But severe bleeding can occur wherein case sterile packs are kept for 24–48 hours and closed. Angiographic embolisation can be tried to stop the bleeding. Alternatively or in case the vascular supply cannot be identified or the placenta is stuck to a vital organ, it is left *in situ* and abdomen is closed. Higher antibiotics are given to prevent infection. Follow-up with serial ultrasound and serum β-hCG is done to look for the shrinkage of the placenta which can occur by aseptic autolysis. Bowel obstruction, sepsis and fistula formation are the likely complications.

CAESAREAN SECTION

It is an important operative procedure where in foetus after 28 completed gestational week is removed from the uterine cavity by an incision over the abdominal and uterine walls.

When it is done for the first time, it is called as *primary caesarean section*, when done on subsequent pregnancies, it is called *repeat caesarean section*.

Types

Classical caesarean section: Where the incision made over the uterus is in the upper segment.

Lower segment caesarean section: Where the incision made over the uterus is in the lower segment.

Although caesarean section started as the 'classical type' it is now been totally replaced by 'lower segment caesarean section', as postoperative complications like adhesions, peritonitis and sepsis are more with classical type and also because of the poor integrity of the scar in classical type giving high chances of rupture uterus. Now classical type is totally out of practice.

Emergency caesarean section: When an unforeseen complication arises either during pregnancy or during labour that may endanger mother's or baby's condition, an emergency section is resorted to.

Elective caesarean section (Planned C-section): The caesarean is planned and done on a specific date during pregnancy (patient not in labour) chosen by the patient and the doctor after assessing the maturity of the baby.

Indications

Elective indication:

- Previous caesarean section done for a recurring cause like contracted pelvis, CPD
- Previous 2 caesarean section
- Malpresentations
- Severe degrees of placenta previa
- Severe diabetes mellitus, severe hypertension, severe degrees PIH, cardiac disease not fit for induction of labour
- Bad obstetric history
- Elderly primigravida
- Foetal macrosomia with birth weight >4 kg
- Advanced carcinoma cervix
- Pelvic tumours, impacted ovarian cysts not allowing a vaginal delivery
- Previously repaired VVF
- HPV infection in mother
- Maternal request.

Emergency indication:

- Complications of labour—prolonged labour or a failure to progress (dystocia)
- Foetal distress
- Cord prolapse
- Uterine rupture
- Increased maternal blood pressure after amniotic membrane rupture
- Maternal or foetal tachycardia after amniotic membrane rupture
- Placental problems (placenta praevia, placental abruption or placenta accreta)
- Failed labour induction
- Failed instrumental delivery (by forceps or ventouse)
- Umbilical cord abnormalities (vasa praevia, multilobate including bilobate and succenturiate-lobed placentas, velamentous insertion).

Preoperative Preparation

For elective caesarean section, it is advisable to keep the patient fasting for 6 hours. But if the patient is in labour as for emergency C section, it is not possible to keep the patient fasting. To prevent acid aspiration injection ranitidine 150 mg, antiemetic metoclopramide is injected an hour before the surgery. Abdomen and perineum up to mid-thigh is shaved. Injection atropine 0.6 mg is administered IV. Bladder is catheterised. Before giving anaesthesia, it is always advisable to hear the foetal heart sound and do a pelvic examination (especially in patients who were in labour). Some indications like placenta previa, placenta accreta, previous caesarean section, twin pregnancy, rupture uterus require cross-matched blood to be kept ready. Paediatrician should be called for to attend the baby soon after extraction.

Anaesthesia

It may be general/spinal/epidural. It depends on the indication and the experience of the anaesthetist. Most of the elective C section is preferably done under epidural/spinal. General anaesthesia is given when spinal anaesthesia is contraindicated or not possible.

Positioning of the Patient

Patient is positioned in dorsal position with left lateral tilt of 15° to avoid *supine hypotension syndrome*. Under anaesthesia due to direct pressure of the gravid uterus over the inferior vena cava, there would be fall in cardiac output and uterine perfusion which can be prevented by giving a 15° tilt on the lateral aspect with a sandbag or firm pillow.

Antiseptic cleansing with iodine or savlon solution is done followed by draping of the abdomen.

Incision

Before putting an incision over the abdominal wall the lie, presentation of the foetus is confirmed.

The incision may be midline or paramedian or *Pfannenstiel*. *Midline incision* extends from upper border of the pubes to 2 cm below the umbilicus. But its extent depends on the foetal size or configuration of the abdomen. The incision is deepened through the rectus sheath. Peritoneum is opened in the upper third so as to avoid injury to the bladder. Alternatively *Pfannenstiel* incision is used which is now very popular and in wide use, as the wound healing is better and postoperative discomfort, wound disruption is less with this incision. This transverse skin incision is approximately 12 cm long, placed 2–3 cm (2 fingers breadth) above the symphysis pubes. *Joel-Cohen* incision is another transverse incision that could be alternatively used, placed slightly higher, 3 cm below the line joining the anterior superior iliac spine. The incision is deepened through the subcutaneous tissues, haemostasis is obtained with diathermy. Rectus sheath is incised in midline and the incision is extended laterally with scissors. Rectus sheath held with Allis forceps or Lane's tissue holding forceps and dissected upwards. Bleeders are secured with diathermy. The parietal peritoneum is identified, held with two artery forceps and opened with knife or scissors after confirming that there is no structure in the underlying the peritoneum. The peritoneal incision is extended upwards; downward extension must be done carefully due to the presence of bladder which may have displaced unexpectedly high.

The lateral recesses of the wound may be packed with taped abdominal packs to prevent the soiling of the peritoneal cavity with liquor or meconium. Free packs should be avoided as they may get lost in the abdominal cavity leading to medicolegal issues and other complications.

Any rotation (*dextrorotation* commonly) in the long axis of the uterus is noted by the position of the round ligament. This is very important, as if not corrected now; when the uterine incision is done, there will be unnecessary lateral extension into the uterine vessels causing bleeding.

Exposing the Lower Uterine Segment

A Doyen's retractor is inserted on the pubic side of the incision. Lower segment is identified. This may not be well formed if is preterm gestation. The loose uterovesical fold of peritoneum is identified. It is held with non-toothed forceps and opened with scissors. It is extended transversely all along the fold. And the bladder is pushed down away gently by fingers from the site of uterine incision. Fingers are kept towards uterine side rather than bladder. In case of previous caesarean section where there is adhesion of bladder to the lower segment one may have to do sharp dissection with scissors or else it may result in bladder injury. The retractor is advanced further to retract the bladder away from the lower segment.

Uterine Incision

A small transverse incision is made over the lower segment, deepened carefully till one sees the amniotic membrane. The level of the incision depends on the level of the head, such that its widest diameter can be easily brought out. It is usually put 2–3 cm above the bladder base. In unengaged floating head, when the lower segment has not formed and thick as in preterm pregnancy it is better to put the incision slightly higher or else it may extend laterally into the base of the broad ligament involving the vessels. Alternatively low midline, ⊥-shaped or J-shaped incision is used. When caesarean section done in advanced stages of labour where the lower segment is stretched incision is placed slightly higher or else the incision may extend into the bladder or into the vagina. It is also better to put a stay stitch in the midline so that the lower uterine flap will not get lost behind the bladder and will help to identify during subsequent suturing.

If the amniotic membrane is not ruptured during uterine incision, it is done and the gushed out fluid is sucked out with the suction. The incision is widened on either side by stretching it with forefingers. This may give ragged edges thereby suturing the uterine edges may give poor quality scar. So, some prefer to widen the uterine incision using scissors, keeping the index and middle fingers underneath the incision for guiding and protection.

Extraction of the Foetus

Four fingers of the hand are inserted below the presenting part. In cephalic presentation, the head is gripped with the fingers. The Doyen's retractor is removed. The head is delivered out through the incision which is assisted by the pressure applied over the fundus by the assistant. If the head is deeply jammed in the pelvis, it has to be pushed up by an assistant with sterile gloved hand inserted into the vagina. Once the head is out the secretions in the mouth and nostrils are cleared with hand suction. Shoulders are delivered by insinuating fingers in the axilla; meanwhile the assistant has to retract the upper uterine flap. Once the shoulders are freed the baby will come out freely. The cord is clamped with two artery forceps and cut between the two. Baby is handed over to the paediatrician. Meanwhile injection Methergine 0.2 mg is given to the mother either IV or IM at the time of delivery of the shoulders to prevent postpartum haemorrhage. Alternatively 5 units of oxytocin may be used in the infusion fluid to prevent bleeding.

In case of high floating head where the delivery of the head through the incision is difficult, one can use outlet forceps or ventouse to extract the head.

In case of breech presentation, the breech is first extracted first through the incision later followed by shoulders and head.

Removal of Placenta

Once the baby is delivered out, the lateral angles of the uterine incision is secured with Green-Armytage clamps. The uterine incision is observed for any bleeding sinuses which are secured with the clamps. Identifying the lower margin of the incision is important as most of the time it gets retracted below and behind the bladder, getting hidden by the pool of blood. It is traced from its lateral angle and held up with Green-Armytage clamps. The stay sutures applied before uterine incision will now come into role to identify the lower margin.

It is always better to wait for placental separation rather than forceful extraction. Once the placenta is found to have separated, it is extracted by controlled cord traction, meanwhile applying pressure over the fundus in upward direction. Along with the placenta, the membranes are to be carefully stripped off, even from the lower uterine segment. This may require the clamps applied to the margins and the angle to be removed and reapplied.

Complete removal of placenta is ensured by observing for the cotyledons. The uterine cavity may be cleaned gently with sterile gauze. If the patient was not in labour the cervical canal may need to be widened with finger for the outflow of uterine discharge **(Fig. 32-3)**.

Closure of the Uterine Incision

Uterus is closed with atraumatic round bodied needle using 1-zero chromic or 1-zero vicryl needle.

Uterine wound is well visualised. Doyen's retractor is re-inserted to retract the bladder. The suturing is started from the angle far from the operator. The first stitch is taken slightly beyond the angle so as to secure the vessels near the angle. This stitch is very important as sometime the incision may extend laterally tearing the uterine vessels. The suturing is continued taking full thickness of uterine muscle excluding the decidua. Continuous locking suture are used to secure haemostasis. Need of second layer suturing has become a controversy. Some prefer to put a second layer of continuous suture to invert and strengthen the first layer. If haemostasis is well maintained with one layer suturing, then some prefer to avoid second layer suturing. The uterus is palpated to see whether it has contracted or not. Sometimes, it may require continuous massage to make it contract and become hard as a cricket ball. UV fold of peritoneum is usually left as such as spontaneous healing is known to occur.

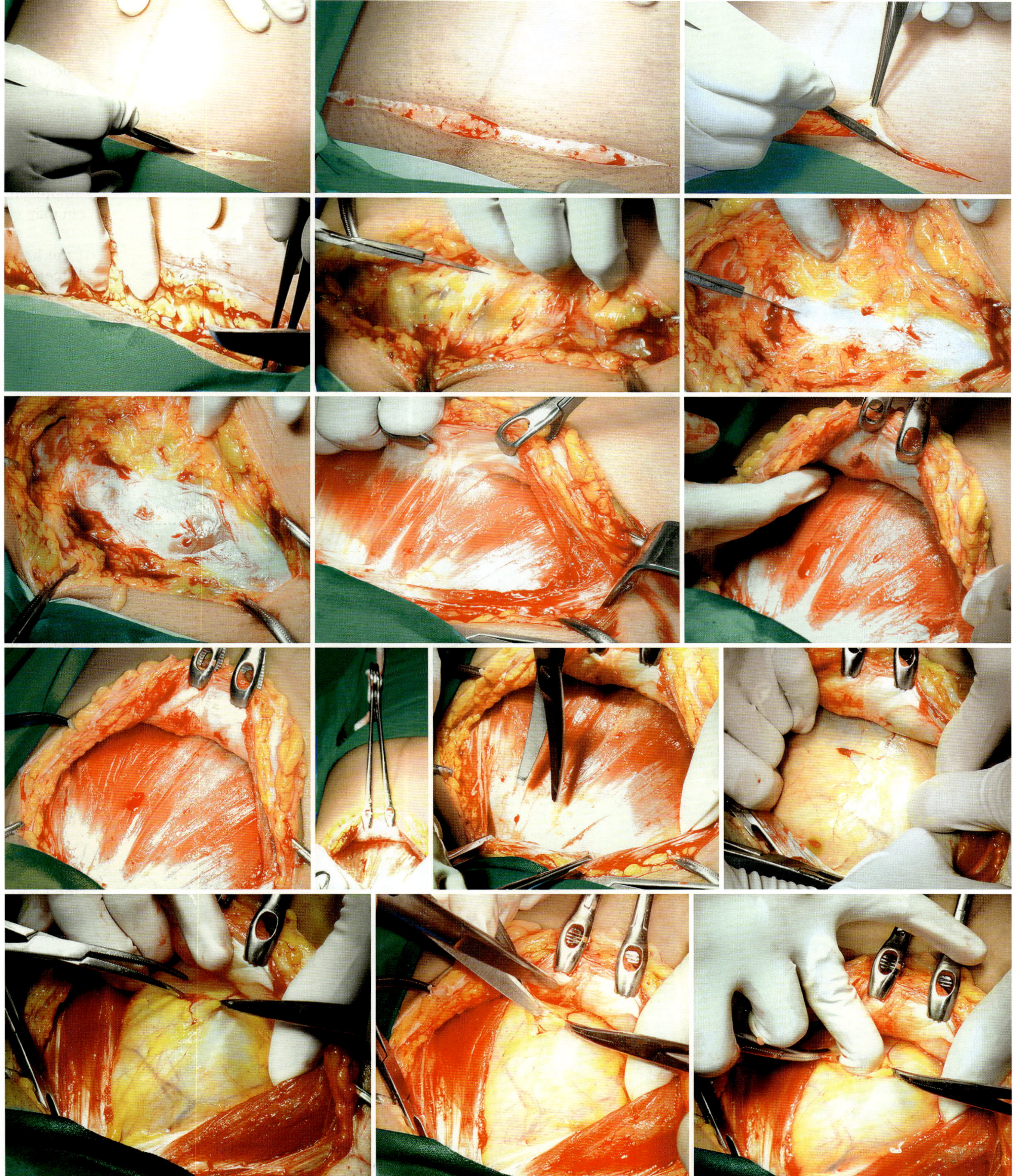

Figs. 32-3(1)

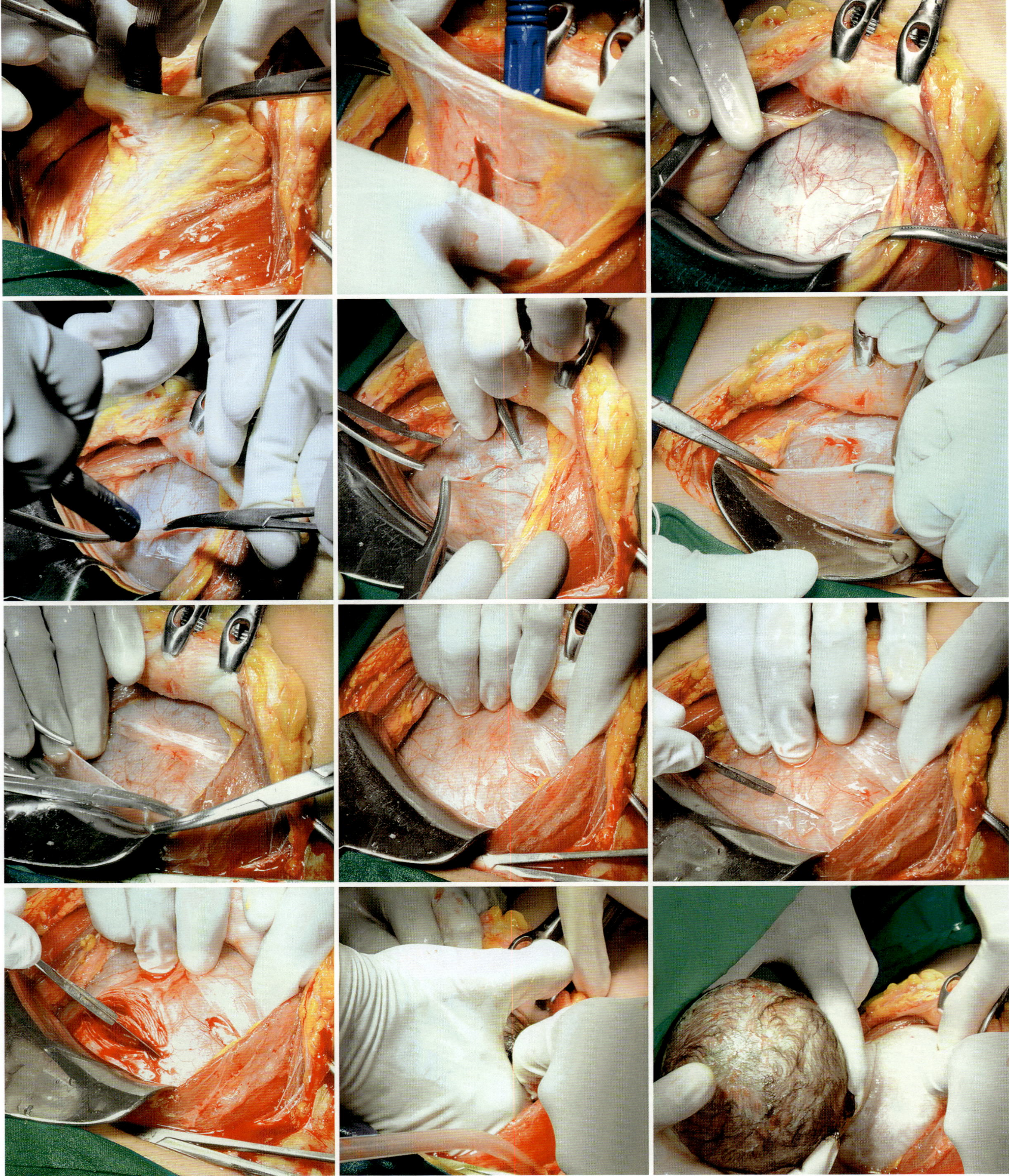

Figs. 32-3(2)

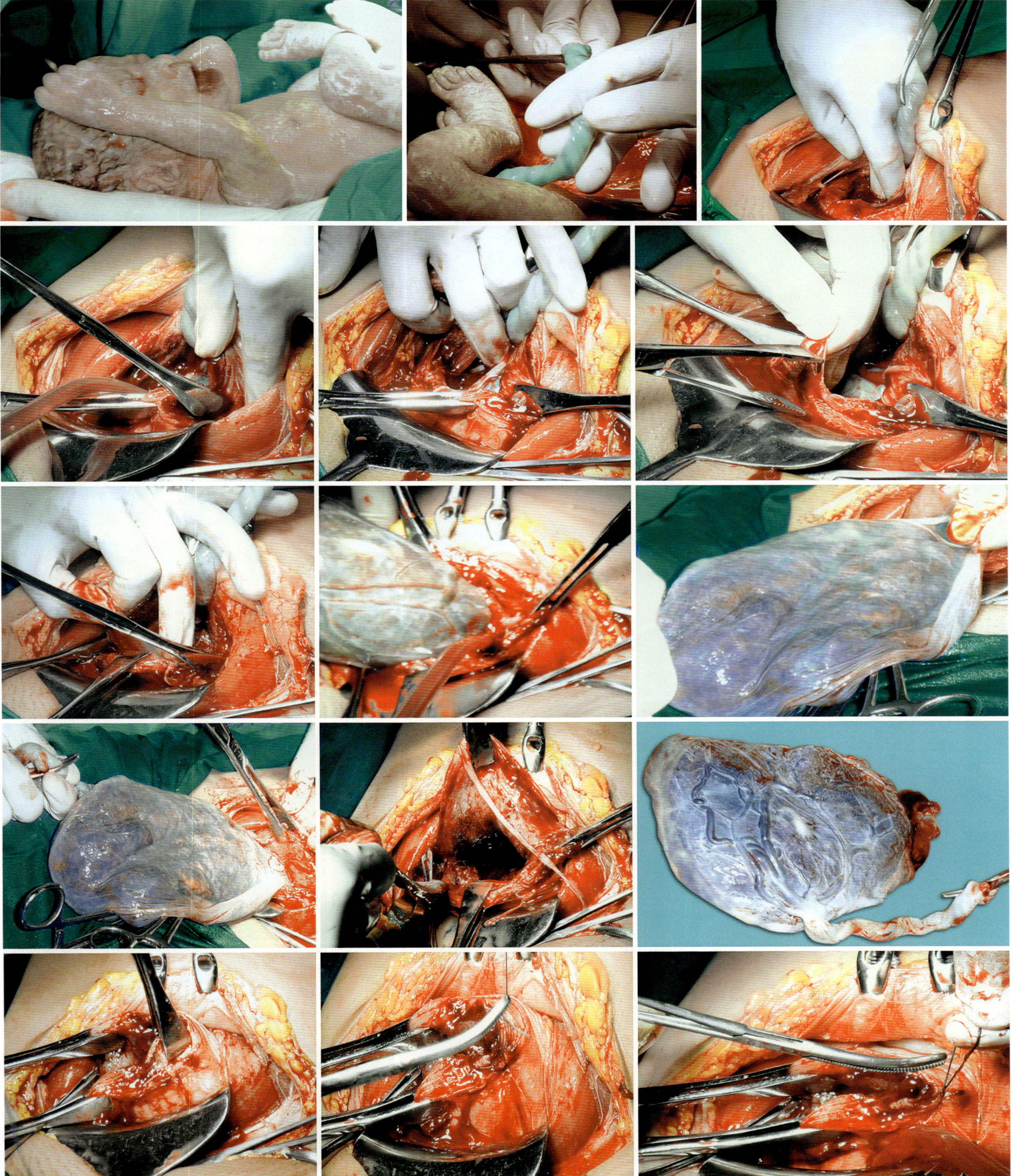

Figs. 32-3(3)

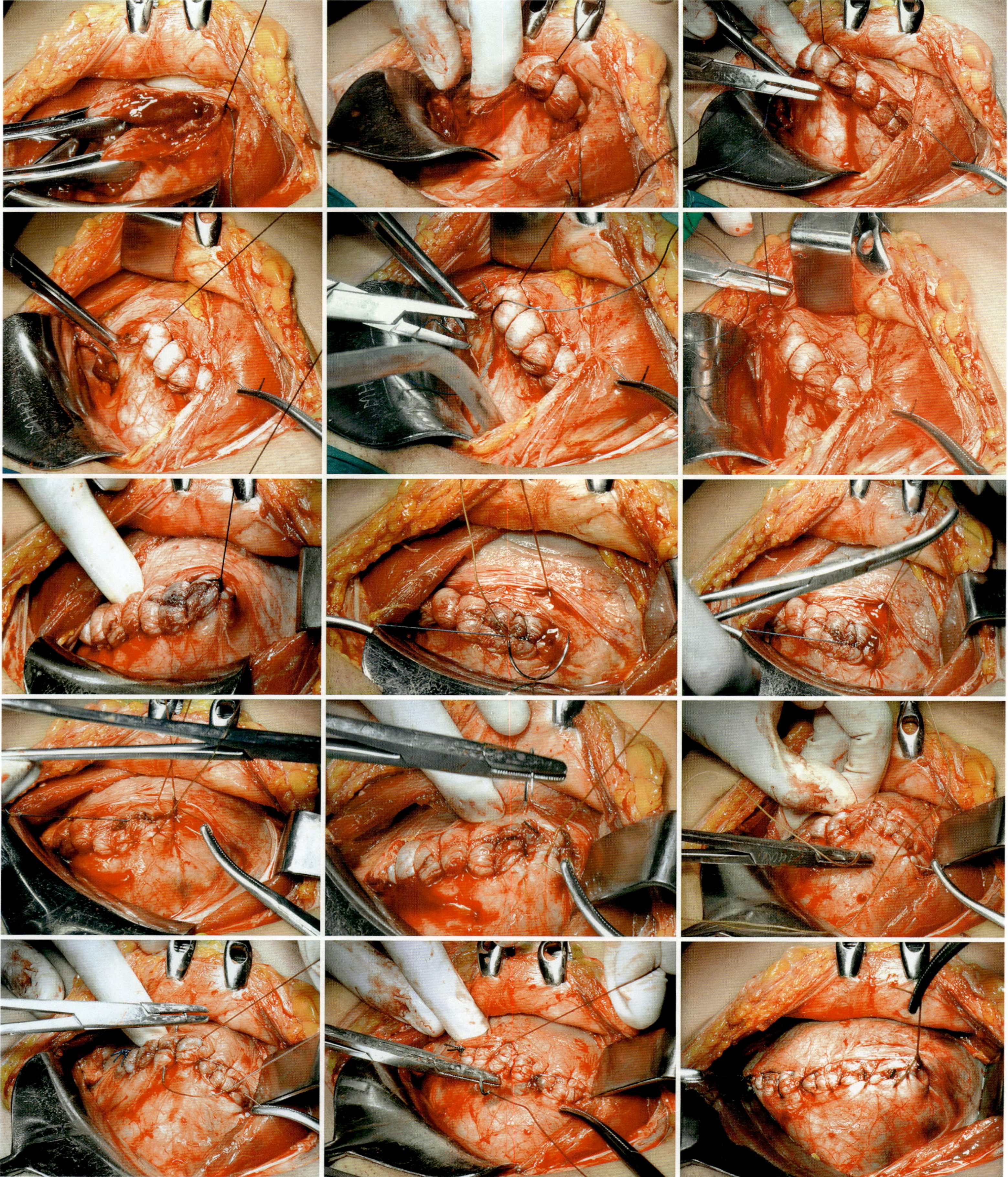

Figs. 32-3(4)

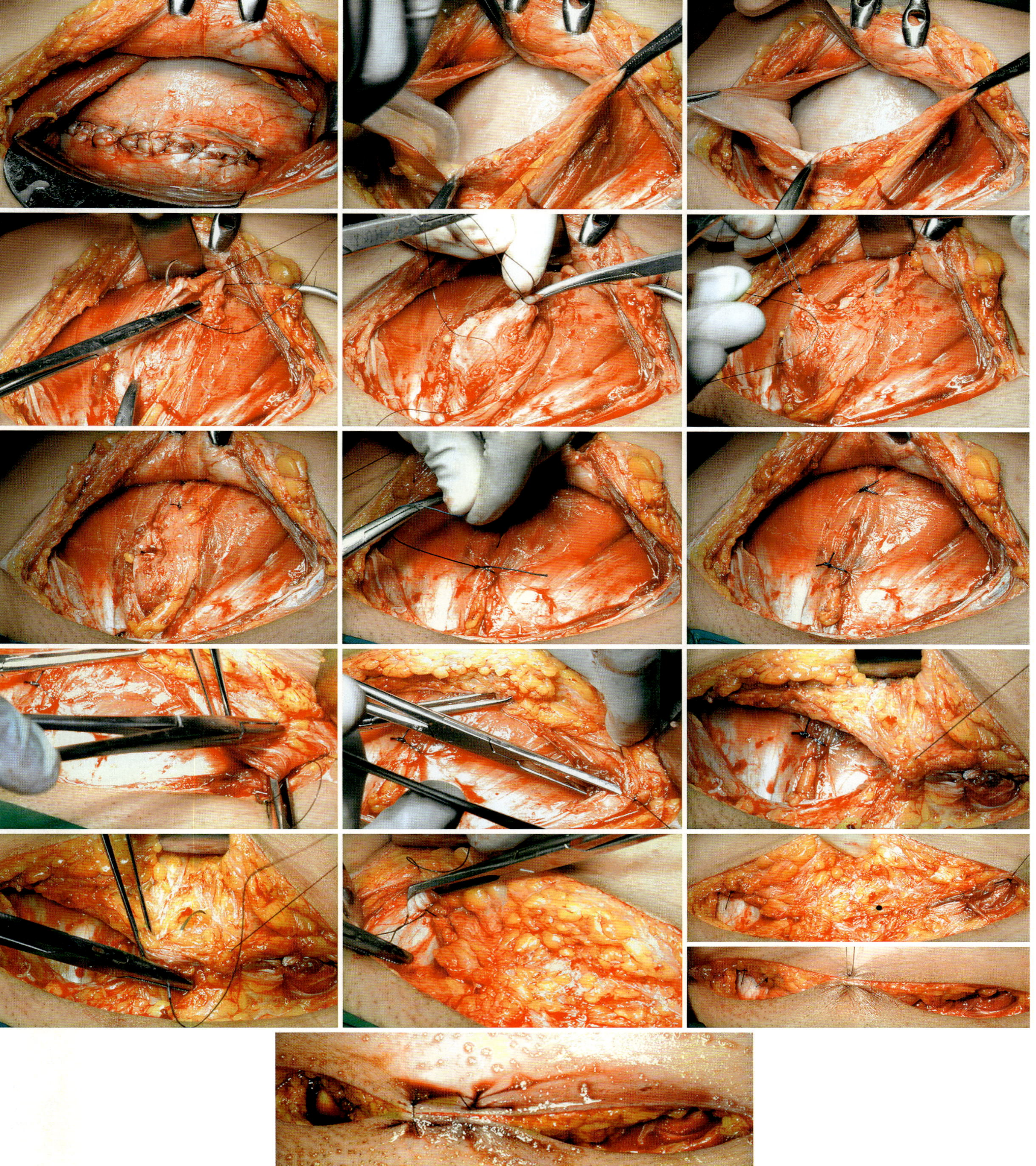

Figs. 32-3(5)

Figs. 32-3(1 to 5): Lower segment caesarean section—technique.

Any major bleeding from the bladder base is identified, may need securing with sutures. Ovaries and tubes on both sides are visualised for any abnormalities. The abdominal packs if kept prior to the procedure are removed. The paracolic gutters are cleared off clots, and meconium. Irrigation with saline may be used if needed.

Closure of the Abdomen

Once haemostasis is ensured, instruments and mop count are cleared from the theatre nurse; the abdomen is closed in layers. Initially peritoneum with continuous 1-zero vicryl sutures, followed by the rectus sheath with continuous 1-zero vicryl sutures. The subcutaneous fat if thick may need to be sutured with 2-zero plain catgut or 3-zero vicryl. The skin is closed with subcuticular sutures with 3-zero monocryl or 2-zero ethylon or with clips.

- Vagina is cleaned off clots.
- Catheter is placed *in situ* for 24 hours.
- Patient is kept nil oral for 18–24 hours.
- Breastfeeding of the baby is started as soon as possible when the mother is able to hold it against the breast.
- Parenteral antibiotics given for 24–48 hours followed by oral preparation.

Complications of Caesarean Section

Maternal Complications

a. *Haemorrhage:* It is common in emergency caesarean section done in patient who was in labour for long hours, multiple pregnancy, and placenta praevia, placental abnormalities (increta, percreta, and accreta).

It may be primary or secondary. Primary haemorrhage is due to bleeding from placental bed, uterine sinuses, uterine vessels, or atonic PPH. Bleeding from lacerated uterine vessels and sinuses can be controlled by taking appropriate stitches. Bleeding from placental bed is controlled by giving bimanual uterine compression with warm mops. Occasionally may require figure of eight sutures. When caesarean section is done for placenta previa, where the placental attachment is over the lower segment whose retraction is not sufficient to control the bleeding, careful application of simple or box stitches or figure of eight sutures over the bleeding sinuses will control the bleeding. Compression sutures of lower anterior and posterior segment can be tried. Alternatively lower segment can be packed with a sterile pack; the end of it should be passed through the cervix into the vagina so that it can be pulled out after 18–24 hours. In *atonic PPH* intramyometrial injection of prostaglandin can be tried after parenteral uterotonics. Continuous bimanual compression is tried. If by bimanual compression the bleeding gets controlled then this patient will benefit with B-Lynch sutures.

Technique of B-Lynch suture: With vicryl no.1 or monocryl mounted on 70 mm round bodied needle the uterus is punctured 3 cm below the right lower edge of uterine incision 3 cm from right lateral border. The suture is brought out from within the uterus puncturing at a point 3 cm above the right upper edge of the incision, 4 cm from the right lateral margin. The suture is now passed above the fundus 3–4 cm from right corneal border. Sutures can be fixed here so as to prevent the slippage of the sutures. The suture is pulled back posterior under moderate tension. It is now brought into the uterine cavity piercing the posterior uterine wall at the same surface points as that of anterior. The suture is then brought back to the posterior aspect of the uterus piercing the posterior wall 4 cm from its left lateral margin. It is passed round the fundus 4 cm from the corneal end. The suture is brought near the left side of the uterine incision in similar fashion as on the right side. With the assistant giving bimanual compression of the uterus the sutures are tightened. One has to confirm that the vaginal bleeding has stopped. Once it is confirmed that bleeding has stopped the uterine incision is closed as explained before.

This procedure will save the uterus from unnecessary hysterectomy. But this procedure will help only if bleeding reduces by bimanual compression. This procedure can also be done in atonic PPH following vaginal delivery, but the uterus need to be opened as in lower segment caesarean section.

Uterine artery ligation: Ligation of uterine artery on both side will reduce the bleeding by 90%. Uterus is grasped and held to expose the vessels in the broad ligament. With vicryl 1-zero on a round bodied needle uterus is pierced 2 cm below the lateral end of the incision. The needle should pass though the full thickness of myometrium so that both uterine artery and vein should be included in the ligation. Then the needle is passed from behind through an avascular portion of broad ligament and tied anteriorly. Effective ligation will result in blanching of the uterus.

Uterine artery embolisation may be tried to occlude the uterine vessels. Meanwhile blood test for coagulation profile is done. Replacement of blood volume with packed cells and FFP is done.

b. *Injury to bladder, ureter, intestines:* Bladder wall may get opened while opening the peritoneum due to upward pull of the bladder as seen in prolonged labour or obstructed labour or previous history of caesarean section. It may also get injured while pushing the bladder away from the lower segment. When caesarean section is done in 2nd stage of labour, bladder is likely to be injured during extraction of the foetus. The damaged area is identified and sutured with vicryl 2/0 in two layers. Catheter is kept for 7–10 days.

Ureters are likely to get injured or ligated while suturing the uterine incision. This occurs quite commonly when the pelvic architecture is distorted as in previous surgeries. Complete ligation is rare. Ureter may get kinked due to placement of suture into the paraureteral tissue or partially ligated if the suture passes though its wall partially. When the ureters are kinked due to placement of suture in paraureteral tissue, ureterolysis is done; but one has to be assured that one stays out of the adventitia. If the ureters are partially or totally ligated, the ligatures are removed. Viability of the ureters is checked by looking for peristalsis, absence of blanching and discolouration. In case of doubt on viability, that particular segment is resected and re-anastomosed with 3-zero vicryl sutures. J-stent has to be kept *in situ* which is removed after 6-12 weeks through cystoscopy.

Intestine injuries are rare during caesarean section but do can occur. The caecum on right side and sigmoid colon on left may get injured. If injury is small, it is sutured with 3-zero silk or vicryl with a drain in the peritoneal cavity. If the injury is large, it requires diversion colostomy for sigmoidal injuries, ileostomy for caecal injuries. Though, these injuries are rare, prompt recognition and early treatment is very essential to prevent sepsis, fistula formation, renal failure and so on.

c. *Sepsis:* Infection in the urinary tract, lungs, abdominal wound, uterus, and peritoneum is known to occur. Usage of appropriate prophylactic antibiotics have reduced their incidence.

Postoperative atelectasis (partial lung collapse) can sometime occur in CS. Postoperative peritonitis, wound dehiscence, burst abdomen is quite common, often associated with premature rupture of membrane, severe anaemia, poor nutritional status. The incidence of wound infection in caesarean section is high (2.5%—16%) which needs active management.

d. *Amniotic fluid embolism:* Though extremely rare, is known to occur which has 60-80% mortality. The amniotic fluid, foetal cells, hair enter maternal circulation through placental bed trigger an allergic reaction in the mother resulting in cardiorespiratory collapse and DIC.
e. *Anaesthetic hazards:* As most of the time when patient is taken up for emergency caesarean section, she is unlikely fasting for 6 hours. This can lead to aspiration of stomach contents especially when under general anaesthesia leading to atelectasis, aspiration pneumonitis.
f. *Thromboembolism:* Thrombus is more likely to occur in lower limb and pelvic veins. Common in obese patients. If gets dislodged and can precipitate pulmonary embolism. Therefore, proper hydration in postoperative period, and early ambulation is necessary.
g. *Shock:* Due to haemorrhage, amniotic fluid embolism or sepsis.
h. *Paralytic ileus:* Control of sepsis, maintenance of electrolyte balance is necessary.
i. *Intestinal obstruction—due to adhesions.*
j. *Poor healing of the uterine scar leading to scar dehiscence and rupture in future pregnancy or delivery.*
k. *Increased risk of placenta praevia, placenta accreta, placenta increta, placenta percreta in future pregnancy necessitating hysterectomy.*

Foetal Complications

Respiratory distress, prematurity, birth injury while extraction are some of the common problems seen in the babies born by caesarean section.

CAESAREAN HYSTERECTOMY

It is the removal of uterus at the time of caesarean section.

Indications

- Abnormal placentation—placenta increta, placenta percreta, placenta accreta.
- Atonic PPH—when all other methods (both medical and surgical) of arresting the bleeding have failed.
- Rupture uterus—where the damage to the uterus is beyond repair.
- Carcinoma cervix diagnosed during pregnancy.

It can be called as *postpartum hysterectomy* if done immediately after vaginal delivery.

After caesarean section, once hysterectomy is decided, the surgeon has to inform the anaesthetist and the patient's relatives. Patient's consent should be taken in planned hysterectomy. In emergency situation when the patient is not in a position to give consent, the consent of the patient's husband or the close relative is taken.

Precaution

Pelvic architecture is altered in pregnancy. So it may not be as easy as in non-pregnant uterus. Blood vessels are engorged and tortuous and tissues are edematous. So, careful clamping and ligating the pedicles is necessary. The vessels may otherwise retract leading to severe bleeding which may be difficult to control. The pelvic anatomy may get distorted in conditions like rupture uterus. Proper identification of the structures followed by their repair, and control of bleeding is very essential.

Incision

If it is a planned hysterectomy, midline vertical is ideal as it gives good exposure and also helps to access the upper abdomen. But most of the caesarean section is started with *Pfannenstiel incision* where most of the time the exposure is not adequate enough for hysterectomy. One may need to put a vertical incision converting it into an inverted T-shaped incision which gives a cosmetically bad scar and more postoperative pain. A transverse incision can be converted into a *Cherney incision* by transecting the rectus muscle at its insertion which can provide adequate exposure. An alternative approach is division of the rectus muscle converting a standard Pfannenstiel to a modified *Maylard incision.*

Procedure

The fundus of the uterus is grasped, removed from the pelvis and placed on the abdominal wall. The uterus should be kept under upward traction so as to diminish blood loss by constricting the uterine vasculature.

The uterine incision may be closed with single continuous sutures before proceeding to hysterectomy as this will reduce the bleeding. In atonic PPH uterus may be packed with sterile gauze so as to prevent continuous bleeding from placental site till the hysterectomy is complete. In abnormal placental attachment like placenta accreta, percreta, severe bleeding will occur by forceful removal of placenta. So cord is cut short and tied and proceeded with hysterectomy without removing the placenta. When the uterus need to be saved placenta may be left back with cord cut short covering with higher antibiotics and methotrexate. Placenta is known to disintegrate by autolysis.

Standard hysterectomy procedure is started with identification of round ligament. A self-retaining retractor may be placed to improve visualisation. Round ligaments are clamped with Kocher's clamps, ligated and cut on both sides. Care is taken to see that tips of the clamps lies on an avascular plane of broad ligament so as to avoid unnecessary bleeding. With electrocautery the anterior leaf of broad ligament is opened and proceeded medially to the point where the vesicouterine peritoneum was dissected off the lower uterine segment to create the bladder flap. In postpartum hysterectomy the vesicouterine peritoneum is opened along with the anterior leaf of broad ligament and the bladder is then pushed away and down from the lower uterine segment. Posteriorly, the broad ligament is incised laterally and parallel to the infundibulopelvic ligament to expose the retroperitoneum. The loose areolar tissue is carefully dissected parallel to the course of the ureter so as to allow proper visualisation of the retroperitoneal space and the course of the ureter.

An avascular area is identified in the posterior leaf of the broad ligament and perforated with electrocautery. Straight Kocher's clamp is placed on the cornu of the uterus, the utero ovarian ligament which attaches the adnexa (tubes and ovary) to the uterus are included in this clamp. A second clamp is placed lateral to this clamp, avoiding ovarian tissue. The tissue between the medial and lateral clamps is divided, and the pedicles are ligated by a transfixing suture using 1-zero vicryl or chromic catgut. Double ligation may be done to reinforce the first ligature. The lateral clamp is then removed. The clamp on the uterine cornu is left in place for traction and to control back bleeding. This procedure is repeated on the other side also.

Next, the uterine arteries are identified and ligated. The uterine arteries are palpable, grossly enlarged due to the pregnancy. The parametrial tissue surrounding the uterine vessels is delicately "skeletonised" anteriorly until the uterine arteries are identified. Curved clamps (Heaney or Kocher's) are placed such that the curved end is perpendicular to the vessels at the level of internal os. Care should be taken to see that the uterine artery is clamped properly and entirely. Some prefer to use two clamps, but it is always better to use one to reduce the chances of ureteral injury. A straight clamp (Kocher's) may be applied on the medial aspect of the above clamp close to the uterus to prevent the back flow of blood from uterines when they are cut. The uterine artery is cut and ligated (double often) with 1-zero vicryl sutures. The suture is passed beyond the tips of the clamp and tied behind the clamp. A portion of the leaves of broad ligament is incorporated with the pedicle so as to prevent the retraction of the vessel. Alternatively, Heaney's ligature can be used to secure the pedicle. The curved clamp on the lateral aspect is removed. The procedure is repeated on the other side.

A second clamp may need to be placed medial to the previous pedicle moving down the parametrial tissue and hugging the cervix, which will allow ligation of any branches of the uterine artery not ligated with the first clamp.

Now decision is to be made whether to do a supracervical/subtotal hysterectomy or total hysterectomy. In emergency condition where the patient has bled a lot, further prolonging the surgical procedure is not suitable for her general condition; supracervical/subtotal hysterectomy is commonly done as a life-saving procedure. The uterus is amputated with a scalpel or cautery, cutting superiorly to the ligated uterine arteries proceeding medially and downward, thus allowing removal of an inverted cone of the cervix, which will facilitate approximation of the edges of the cervical stump regardless of the degree of dilation. Once amputated, the cervical stump can be approximated in an anterior-to-posterior fashion using interrupted figure-of-eight ligatures. Special care should be taken to avoid the bladder injury.

If the patient's conditions are favourable and when it is a planned procedure then total hysterectomy is done. But the problem here is identification of cervix. If the patient was in late stages of labour with cervix fully dilated and effaced it becomes difficult to identify it from vagina. Some surgeons prefer to "mark" the cervix, either by placing a ring forceps on the anterior lip of the cervix or placing a suture on the cervix. If total hysterectomy is decided then bladder has to be pushed further down. Extreme care should be taken as the bladder wall is extremely soft and friable and likely to get damaged. When the cervix is not dilated its level can be felt through the vaginal wall. The clamps are applied to the cardinal ligaments, cut and ligated. Sometimes, the uterosacral ligaments are quite prominent and may need to be individually clamped and ligated. Clamps need to be reapplied medial to the previous pedicle, and thus proceed downwards till the surgeon reaches the external os. Suture line approximating the uterine incision may be released now and the cervix can be palpated from within the uterus. Now the vagina is opened and cervix is amputated with curved scissors. Allis forceps can be used to maintain traction on the anterior, posterior, and lateral angles of the vaginal wall. The vaginal epithelium is very friable and must be handled gently.

Closure of vaginal cuff begins with supporting angle sutures that incorporate the lateral vaginal angles, the lower cardinal ligament pedicles, and the uterosacral pedicles. The vaginal cuff may be closed with continuous locking or interrupted sutures. Or the cuff may be left open putting continuous non-locking suture to the anterior and posterior cuff edges to secure hemostasis which allows drainage of any discharge until spontaneous reperitonealisation occurs.

Pelvis is irrigated with warm saline. All pedicles are inspected for any bleeding. Vaginal cuff must be inspected for any bleeding. In supracervical hystectomy, amputated cervical stump is inspected for any bleeding. Cystourthroscope can be done per operatively to exclude any bladder or ureteric injury. Indigocarmine dye can be injected intravenously to the patient. Both ureteric orifices are visualised. Gush of blue dye through the ureteric orifices confirm ureteral patency. Also staining of the operative site indicates bladder injury which needs to be identified and closed with 2-zero or 3-zero vicryl in two layers. Continuous bladder catheterisation is done for 7–10 days. In case of placenta, percreta there may be placental intrusion into the bladder wall. In such cases excision of that portion of the bladder wall with bladder wall reconstruction should be done by a urologist.

Abdomen is later closed after taking the count of instrument and mops.

Complications

a. Sepsis: Quite common. It can be in the pelvis, urinary tract, abdomen, or in the wound. Seroma, wound infection, cuff haematoma and cellulites, pelvic haematoma and abscess are often seen. It is due to excessive handling of the genital tract as it occurs in PPH, bleeding. Higher antibiotics have to be started before hand as the patient may quietly slip into septicaemia.
b. DIC: It is mainly due to excessive bleeding that has lead to hysterectomy or due to sepsis. Transfusion of blood, platelets, FFP, and cryoprecipitate is done.
c. Deep venous thrombosis: Thrombosis in pelvic veins and leg veins are likely to occur with the risk of pulmonary embolism. Early mobilisation, use of compression stockings will reduce the risk of thrombosis.
d. Bladder injury/ureteric injury: If not identified and repaired can lead to vesicovaginal fistula and ureterovaginal fistula.
e. Psychological impact of hysterectomy in young women has to be dealt by proper counselling and support.
f. Prolonged hospital stay.

TUBAL STERILISATION PROCEDURES

It is the procedure where the fallopian tubes are occluded so that the woman will not be able to conceive and become pregnant in the future. It is a permanent method of contraception normally done in women who feel that they have completed their family.

Approach: It can be done by minilaparotomy or along with caesarean section or by laparoscopic approach.

Timing: It can be done along with caesarean section as mentioned before or abortion (*concurrent*) or within 24–48 hours of normal delivery (*puerperal*) or any time after 3 months of delivery or abortion (*interval*). It is commonly done in the immediate postmenstrual period.

Anaesthesia: It can be done under general or spinal anaesthesia or local anaesthesia (1% lignocaine infilteration) with IV sedation (Injection Pethedine 50 mg + injection Phenergan 25 mg).

Informed consent of the couple is taken after proper counselling regarding the irreversibility of the procedure and also informing about the chances of failure (due to tubal recanalisation).

Procedure

Minilaparotomy

Patient is kept fasting for 6–8 hours. Abdomen is shaved. There is no compulsory bladder catheterisation. Patient is made to void urine just before the procedure.

Incision: When done in immediate postpartum period where the uterus is palpable below the umbilicus, the incision of ½"–¾" is made two fingers breadth below the fundal height; whereas in interval period, it is done two fingers breadth above the symphysis pubis. It can be midline, paramedian or transverse incision.

The abdomen is opened in layers as usual. Once the peritoneum is opened small specialised retractors are used to retract the incision while delivering the tube out.

The surgeon now introduces his index finger into the abdomen, goes behind the uterus, feels for the tubes and delivers it out hooking it with fingers. An instrument inserted through the vagina to lift the uterus would be useful especially in interval sterilisation to draw the tubes towards the incision. It is identified by the fimbrial end of the tube. It is held with Babcock's forceps at the junction of proximal and middle third portion **(Fig. 32-4)**.

Methods of tubal occlusion

- *Pomeroy tubal ligation:* Here part of the tube is elevated to create a loop or knuckle. An absorbable ligature (1/0 chromic catgut) is tied around the base of the elevated segment tightly, and the tubal segment (approx 1 cm) is cut out. The cut ends of the fallopian tube separate as the ligature dissolves. Within a few days, the peritoneum grows over and covers the cut ends of the tubal segments. It is the most commonly used method.
- *Madlener procedure:* Similar to the above procedure but here a loop of tube is elevated and crushed before ligation.
- *Parkland tubal ligation:* It involves tying two non-absorbable ligatures around the fallopian tube in its proximal to middle segment and then cutting out the tubal segment between the ligatures. The end result is similar to the Pomeroy method of tubal ligation.
- *Irving's tubal ligation:* Two ligatures are placed around the fallopian tube in its proximal to mid-segment and the tubal segment between the two ligatures is removed. Using blunt dissection, a tunnel is made within the substance of the uterine myometrium on its posterior aspect and the proximal tubal segment is pulled into this tunnel and sutured. And the distal tied end is buried in the substance of the broad ligament.
- *Fimbriectomy:* A portion of the fallopian tube closest to the ovary is removed, thereby eliminating the tubal ability to capture eggs and transfer them to the uterus.
- *Bipolar coagulation:* This method uses electrical current to cauterise sections of the fallopian tube, commonly used in laparoscopic female sterilisation.
- *Tubal clip:* It involves application of permanent clip to the tube (*Filshie Clip or Hulka Clip*) thereby blocking the transference of eggs from the ovary.
- *Tubal ring:* It involves application of a silastic band to the fallopian tubes.

The last three procedures are used in laparoscopic tubal ligation.

Tubal ligation is done on both sides. The resected tubal segment is sent for biopsy. The peritoneum is closed by purse string suture. The abdomen is closed in layers. The patient can be discharged in 24–48 hours.

Complications

- Preoperative—bladder injury, bowel injury, broad ligament haematoma, uterine perforation.
- Postoperative—sepsis, wound infection, haematoma, peritonitis.

Laparoscopic tubal ligation: Usually done as an outpatient procedure.

Anaesthesia: General anaesthesia or local (done in camp).

Position: Patient is placed in lithotomy position, with 15° Trendelenburg tilt. Both abdomen and vagina are cleaned with antiseptic solution. Uterine sound can be inserted to manipulate the uterus **(Fig. 32-5)**.

Procedure: Through a small skin incision of ½"below the umbilicus, Verres needle is inserted into the abdominal cavity at a 45° angulation, tip directed towards the pelvis. The abdomen is inflated with gas (carbon dioxide). The needle is removed and trocar with cannula is introduced through the incision by twisting movement. Laparoscope is introduced through the cannula. The pelvic organs are visualised. Through another small incision laterally placed either on left or right side another trocar with cannula is inserted. Through this cannula either bipolar forceps or *ring applicator* loaded with silastic ring is introduced. Ring applicator needs no sized 7 trocar as ring applicator is 7 number sized. The tube is grasped 2–3 cm from uterotubal junction. It is either cauterised with the bipolar till 1 cm of the tube blanches or the silastic ring is slipped to the base of the loop of tube that was picked up and drawn into the cylinder of applicator. The procedure is repeated on the other side. The tubes have to be visualised to see that the rings are placed properly and there is no bleeding. After confirming haemostasis laparoscope is removed. Abdomen is deflated and skin incisions are sutured.

Complications

- Bowel and bladder perforation.
- Vessel injury.
- Cardiorespiratory embarrassment.

SURGERIES FOR OVARIAN PATHOLOGY

Many ovarian tumours are cystic, but some cysts are not tumours and some tumours are not cysts.

Their simplified classification:

- *Benign:*
  - Functional cysts of the follicles and corpus luteum.
  - Benign serous or mucinous cystadenomas.
  - Dermoid cysts (teratomas)
  - Endometriotic cyst (chocolate cyst)
  - Unclassified benign cysts (simple paraovarian cysts).
- *Malignant:*
  - Malignant serous or mucinous cystadenocarcinomas.
  - Metastatic carcinomas (from the gut, or breast)
  - Burkitt's lymphoma
  - Other rarer tumours.

Pseudocysts are postinflammatory collections of fluid between adhesions in the pelvis, and are not true ovarian cysts; but the distinction is not always easy, even at operation.

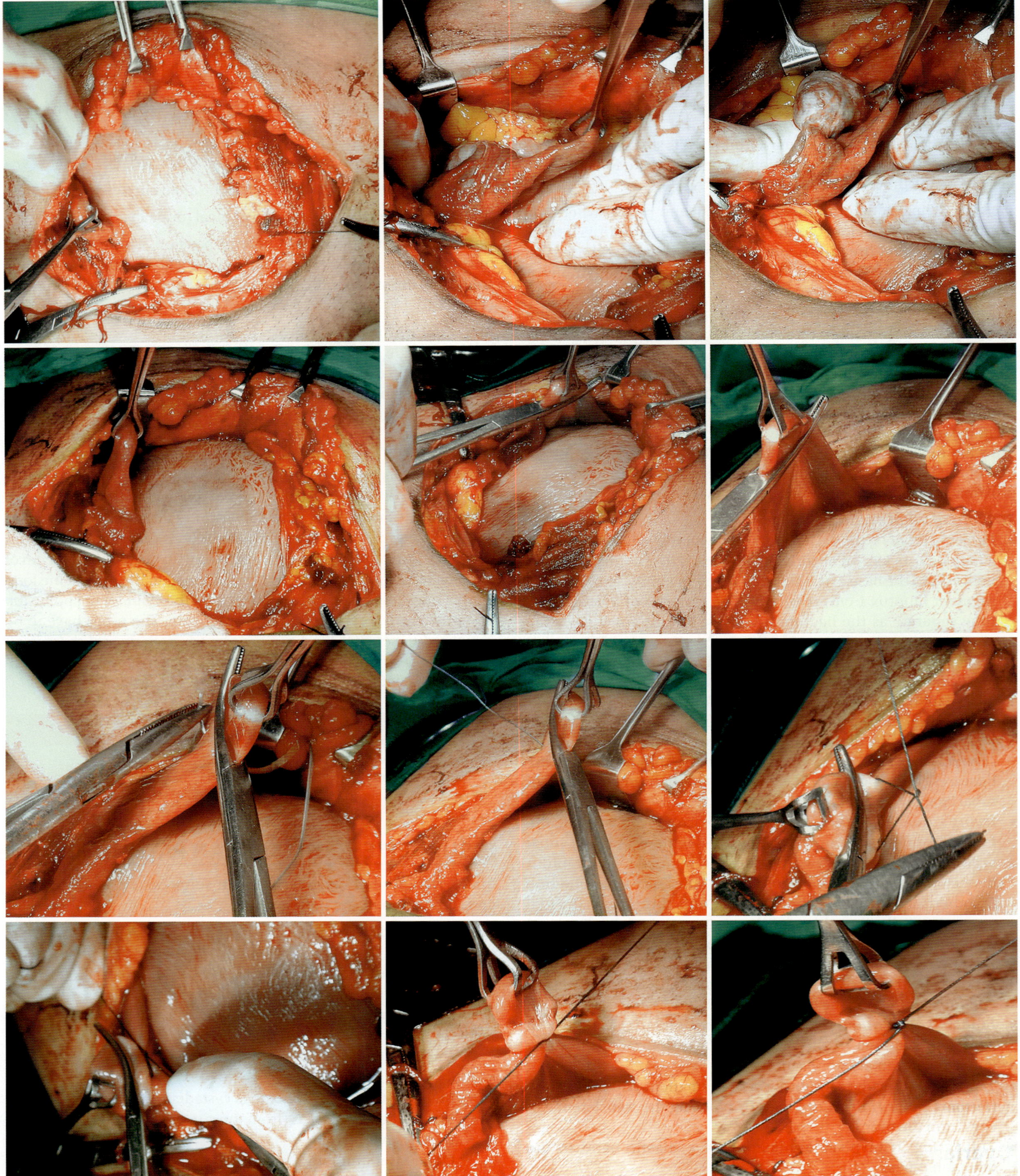

Figs. 32-4(1)

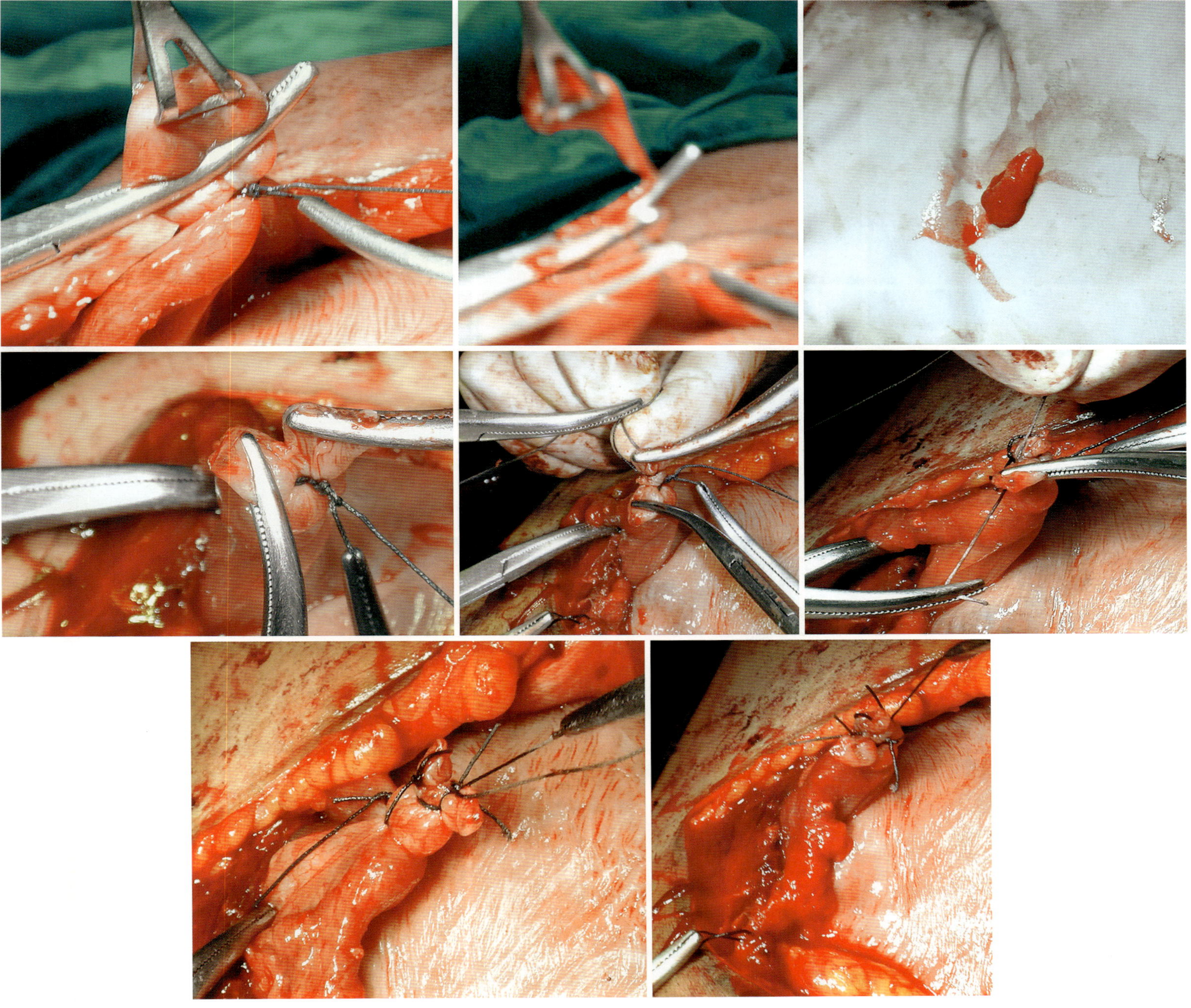

Figs. 32-4(2)

Figs. 32-4(1 and 2): Tubectomy is done during caesarean section after taking consent.

The *uterine adnexa* consist of the ovaries, the fallopian tubes, and the uterine ligaments and any pathology arising from these structures are referred to as *adnexal pathology*.

An adnexal mass may be noted in cases of acute abdomen and the differential diagnosis should include adnexal torsion, ruptured haemorrhagic cyst, degenerating leiomyomata, ectopic pregnancy, unruptured tuboovarian abscess.

Some of the surgeries performed in the ovaries are ovarian cystectomy, oophorectomy, ovarian drilling, salpingo-oophorectomy.

Ovarian Cystectomy

It is done in benign conditions where the cyst *only* is removed leaving behind the functional ovary in place. She needs its endocrine function, regardless of possible fertility. Of the benign cyst functional cyst, dermoid cyst and endometriotic cyst are commonly encountered in clinical practice.

Indication

Symptomatic cysts, cysts >6 cm size in premenopausal women/ >3 cm size in postmenopausal women not showing resolution in 2–3 months of close observation or failed to resolve with 2–3 cycles of oral contraceptive pills, cysts with ultrasonic features deviating from being functional cyst, and bilateral cysts are removed by cystectomy.

However cystectomy is not advisable in postmenopausal women with large cysts >10 cm size, complex cyst with multiloculation, thick septa and solid components, and cysts with elevated CA-125 levels.

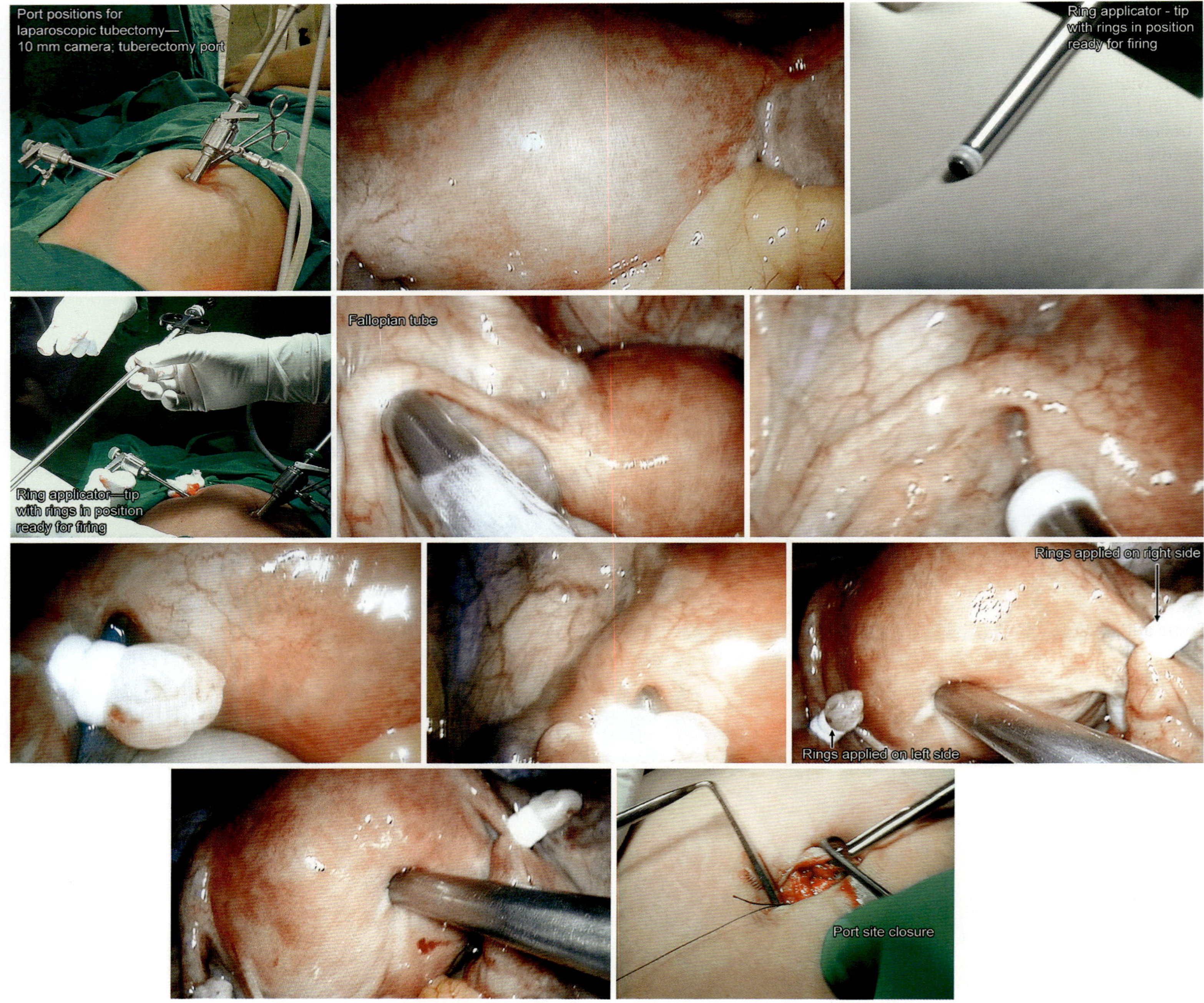

Fig. 32-5: Laparoscopic tubectomy/sterilisation.

Anaesthesia

General or spinal for laparotomy with cystectomy, general anaesthesia for laparoscopic cystectomy.

Position

Dorsal lithotomy for laparoscopic cystectomy as it allows the use of uterine manipulator; supine position for laparotomy.

The abdomen, perineum, and vagina are surgically prepared.

Technique of Cystectomy by Laparotomy

In postmenopausal age or above, it should be an infraumbilical midline incision for adnexal masses as the incidence of malignant disease is high in this age group and lower midline incision will give adequate access and exposure than the low transverse though it is cosmetically poor. Adequate exploration of the abdomen for a malignant ovarian process through a Pfannenstiel or transverse incision is difficult. A transverse incision or Pfannenstiel incision is adequate for younger patients in whom the chance of a malignant disease is quite low. If a malignant disease is encountered in this younger age group, the transverse or Pfannenstiel incision may be converted into inverted T incision.

After opening the peritoneum the abdomen is thoroughly explored. Any suspicious tissue in the upper abdomen (under surface of the diaphragm and surface of the liver) or along the aortic lymph nodes should be sent for a frozen section analysis. Ascites or any peritoneal deposits or papillary excrescences on ovarian surface are noted. In the presence of any of these features cystecomy is abandoned.

Uterus is pulled up towards the incision. Ovaries are indentified. Most ovarian cysts have few adhesions and can be easily drawn towards the incision. If adhesions are seen then it may be due to previous PID, malignant cyst in which the growth has already spread into the peritoneum, endometriotic/chocolate cyst, a cyst which has previously undergone torsion.

Cul-de-sac is packed with moist pack to prevent the pelvic contamination if there is a spill. The ovary is held with Babcock clamps placing on the ovarian ligament. An elliptical incision is made with a scalpel through the thin ovarian cortex of a benign cyst the end of the knife handle can be inserted and develop a plane between the cyst wall and the ovarian cortex. Alternatively, fine-needle electrocautery or small Metzenbaum scissors can be used to separate the cyst wall from the ovarian cortex. After the cyst wall has been completely separated from its adherent attachments to the thin ovarian cortex, it can be shelled out without rupture. If proper plane is got, shelling out the cyst will be without difficult except near the base which needs to be cut with cautery or scissors. However, because of the friability of the cyst wall, rupture can occur even with the gentlest technique. So instead of having accidental rupture which will uncontrollably soil the peritoneal cavity, it is better to aspirate the cyst before shelling out its capsule. Aspiration of cyst will also facilitate the removal of large cysts through small incision and also it eases to release the paraovarian adhesion before cystectomy **(Fig. 32-6)**.

After the cyst has been removed, the dead space can be obliterated with fine 5-zero non-reactive vertical mattress sutures or figure-of-eight sutures. The ovarian surface is then re-approximated with 5-zero fine subcortical running suture. Interrupted sutures may be placed if cortex is friable. Alternatively the redundant cortex can be removed and the dead space is obliterated with an internal closure taking care that suture material does not penetrate the ovarian cortex. This prevents ischaemia and adhesion formation. Some authors advocate leaving the ovary open after cystectomy.

Difficulties Encountered in Cystectomies

Extensive adhesions may be encountered in endometriotic cyst, post-inflammatory cyst where the ovary cannot be freely moved above the pelvis. Forceful attempt to pull the ovary may injure the bladder, rectum, ureter and lacerate the veins. Adhesions have to be released slowly with both sharp dissections with scissors or gently with hands. In endometriotic cyst the thick chocolate coloured fluid is aspirated and sucked out, the friable cyst wall is removed as much as possible. Haemostasis is achieved with diathermy. Post-inflammatory cyst is just aspirated and abdomen is closed giving her antibiotics. It is safer to leave a little cyst wall on her gut or the bladder, than to remove a little gut or bladder with the cyst wall.

Before closing the abdomen, it is always good to give a thorough peritoneal cavity wash with saline so as to wash out the spilled cyst content. Abdomen is closed in layer. Usually, no drain is required **(Fig. 32-7)**.

Complications

- Removal of large cyst may cause cardiorespiratory failure in immediate postoperative period.
- Supine hypotension syndrome while removal of large cyst due to its pressure over the veins, this can be prevented by giving lateral tilt during the surgery.
- Injury to bladder, ureter, bowel in presence of dense adhesions.
- Infertility due to adhesion.

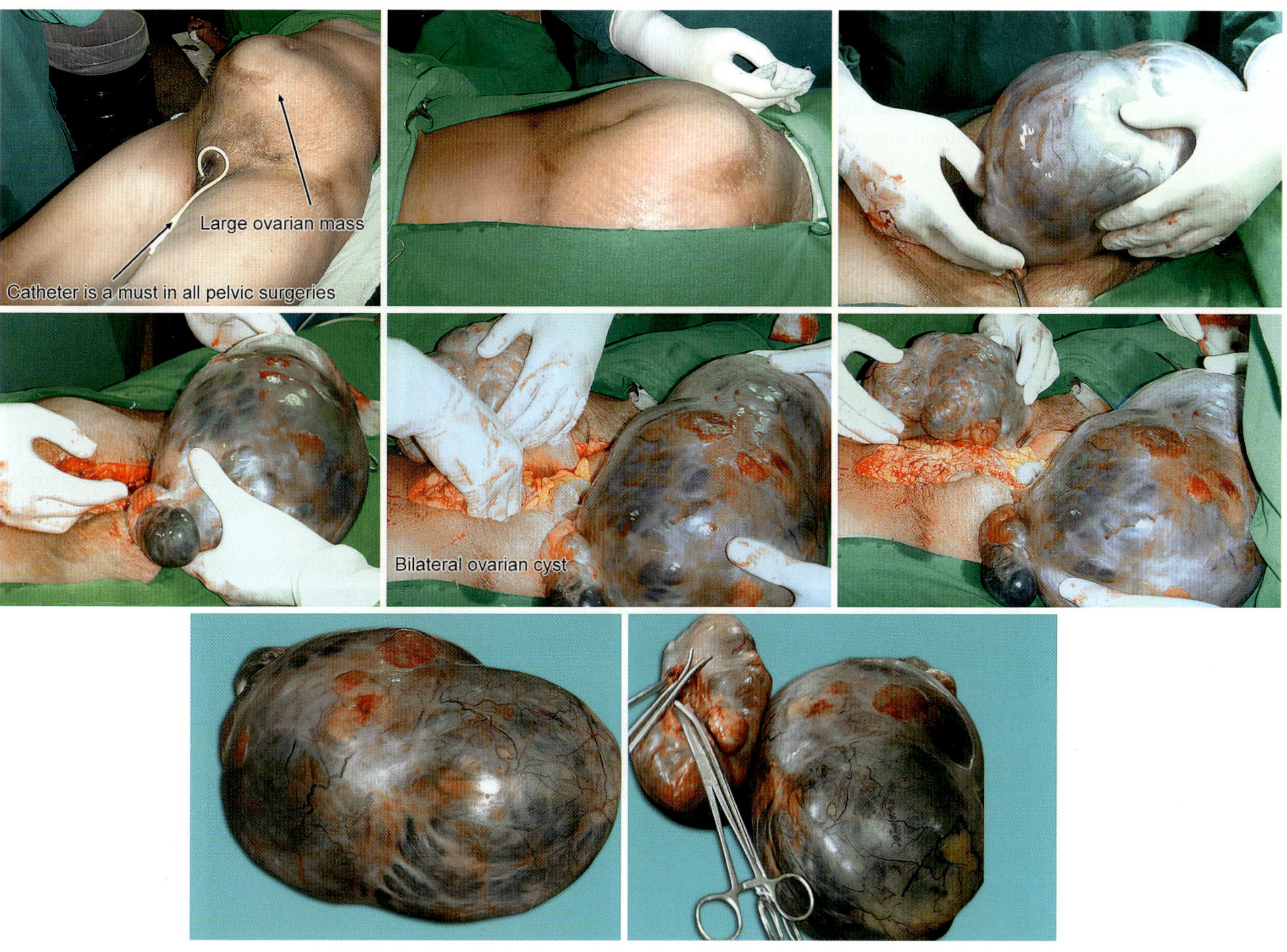

Fig. 32-6: Bilateral large ovarian cysts are removed through laparotomy.

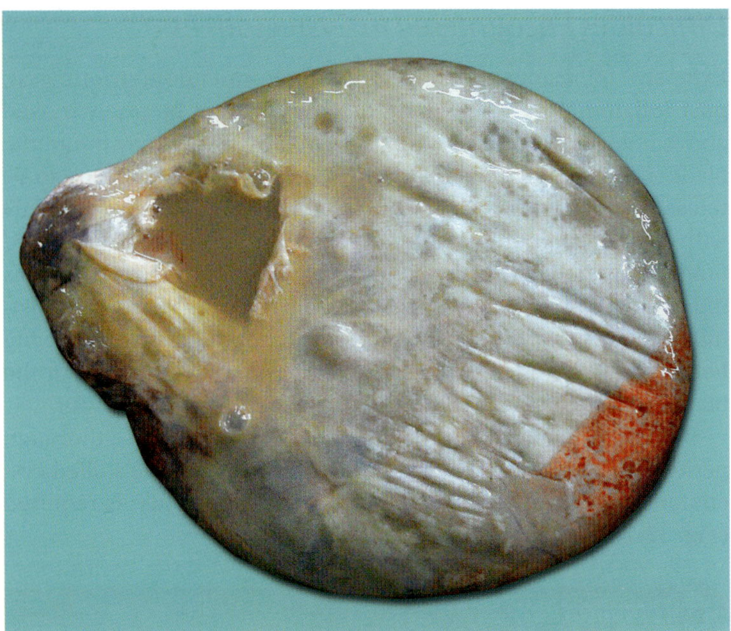

Fig. 32-7: Specimen of simple cyst of the ovary.

Laparoscopic Cystectomy

This is becoming very popular now as adhesions are less, so fertility will not be affected much. Postoperative recovery is faster. Endometriotic cysts are better tackled with laparoscopy than laparotomy.

Port site—periumbilical for telescope and camera. Two lateral port in the lower abdomen, one 5 mm another 10 mm. Additional ports can be used based on the requirement.

The ovarian capsule is incised with scissors or monopolar hook. The ovary is stabilised with a contralateral grasping forceps holding the suspensory ligament. The ovarian capsule is dissected/teased away from the cyst wall either by hydrodissection or a probe. Cyst is thus completely freed from the ovary. Bleeding points on the ovarian cortex is cauterised with bipolar forceps. The cyst sometimes ruptures while dissecting away from the ovarian capsule. The fluid can be aspirated and thorough wash to the pelvis is given later **(Figs. 32-8 and 32-9)**.

Alternatively in case of large cyst, it has to be aspirated by passing an 18-gauge needle through a trocar. Fluid is aspirated with 20 cc syringe or aspiration system. Fluid is sent for analysis. Pelvic wash is given. After draining the fluid, hole is made in the capsule of the ovary. The cyst wall is pulled away from the ovarian capsule. Contralateral traction is given with 5 mm grasping forceps. Complete capsule can be removed if the right plane is achieved. There may be some adhesions near the base which needs to be separated with monopolar hook or scissors. Resected area is thoroughly irrigated. Any bleeding points are coagulated with bipolar forceps. If stripping of the capsule cannot be achieved completely as in endometriosis, the residual part must be destroyed with laser or electrocautery. Suture of the margins are reserved for large cysts or when more than incision is done. This will restore the shape of the ovary thereby reducing adhesion **(Fig. 32-10)**.

The resected cyst wall is removed through 10 mm trocar. If the cyst is intact without rupture, a plastic bag may be inserted into the peritoneal cavity so that the cyst may be passed into it and retrieved though a small suprapubic incision or through an incision over the pouch of Douglas. Alternatively, the cyst when inside the bag can be aspirated and the size reduced so that it can be brought through the 10 mm trocar **(Fig. 32-11)**.

Oophorectomy

Oophorectomy is the surgical removal of an ovary or ovaries. Some call it also as *ovariectomy*, but this term has been traditionally used in basic science research describing the surgical removal of ovaries in laboratory animals.

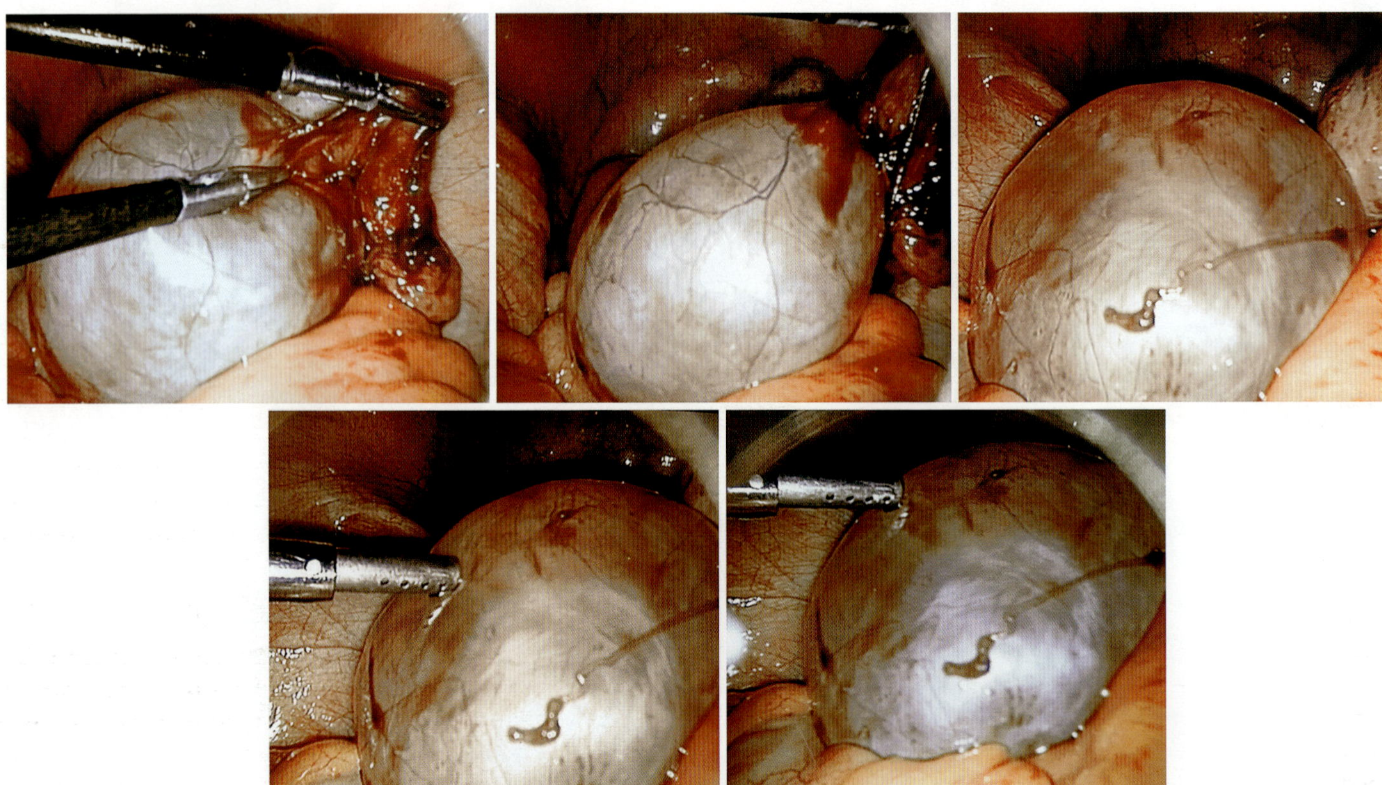

Fig. 32-8: Laparoscopic removal of simple cyst of the ovary.

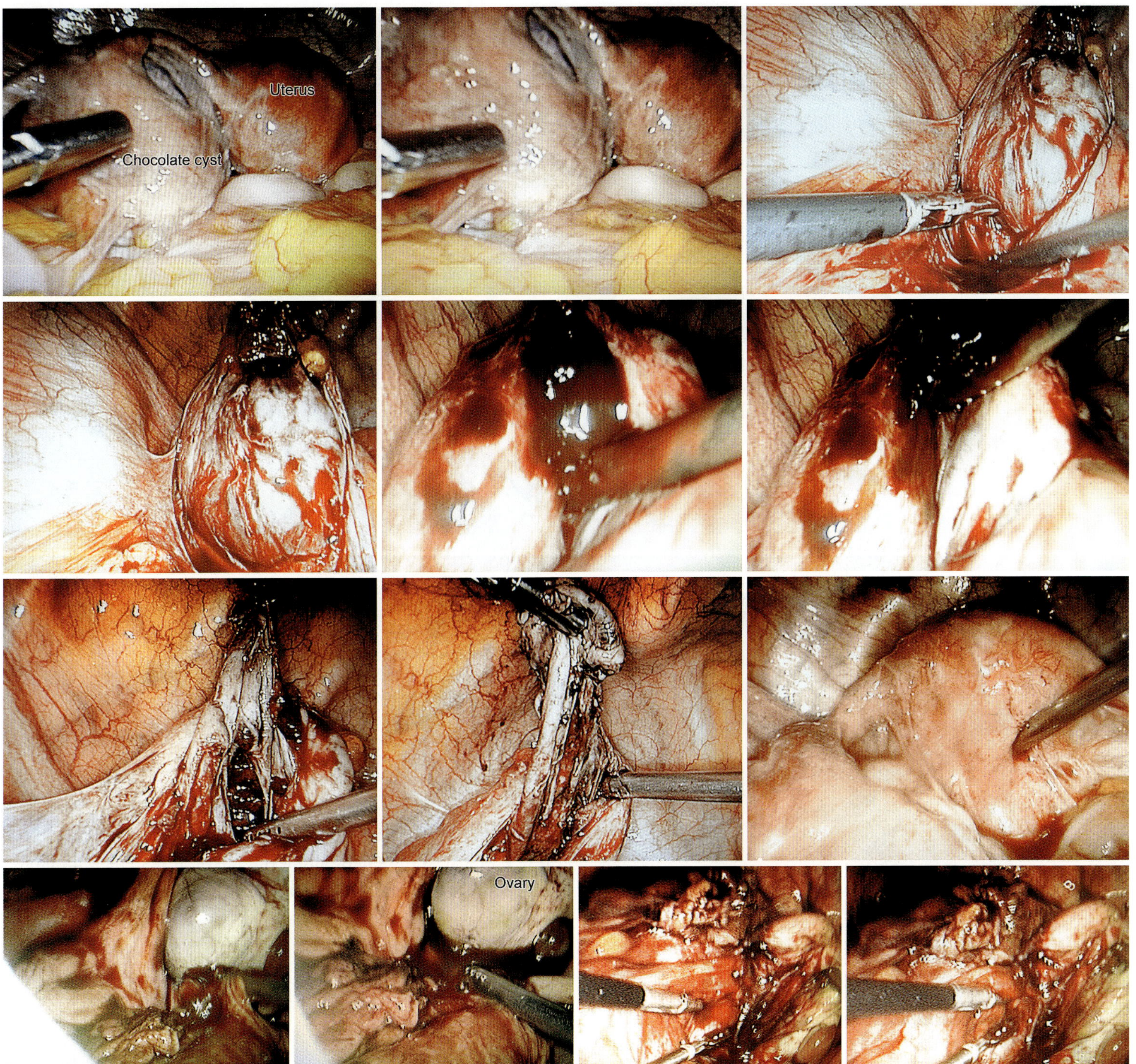

Fig. 32-9: Laparoscopic chocolate cyst removal.

Indications:

- Ovarian diseases—ovarian cyst, cancer
- Endometriosis
- As prophylaxis to reduce the chances of developing ovarian cancer or breast cancer
- In conjunction with removal of the uterus **(Fig. 32-12)**

Procedure:

Informed consent of the patient is a must before the ovary is removed.

Anaesthesia, exposure, positioning as in ovarian cystectomy.

The pedicle consists of the infundibulopelvic ligament and ovarian vessels, the ovarian ligament, and portion of the broad ligament. If the pedicle is wide clamp it with several clamps, taking bite not more than 2.5 cm in each of them. It will be less likely to slip if the pedicle is cut at some distance from each clamp. The pedicle in each clamp is transfixed with 1/0 vicryl sutures, taking care to avoid the plexus of veins when the needle is inserted. The stump is checked for any bleeding before cutting the ligatures short. Ovary thus removed is sent for biopsy. It is sometimes done on both sides **(Fig. 32-13)**.

Laparoscopic Oophorectomy

The ovary is stabilised with a grasping forceps over the ovarian ligament from contralateral port. The infundibulopelvic ligament is cauterised with bipolar forceps and cut with scissors. Alternatively harmonic scalpel or seal can be used. The ovarian ligament is cauterised and cut. The ovary can be retrieved using a plastic bag through 10 mm portal site.

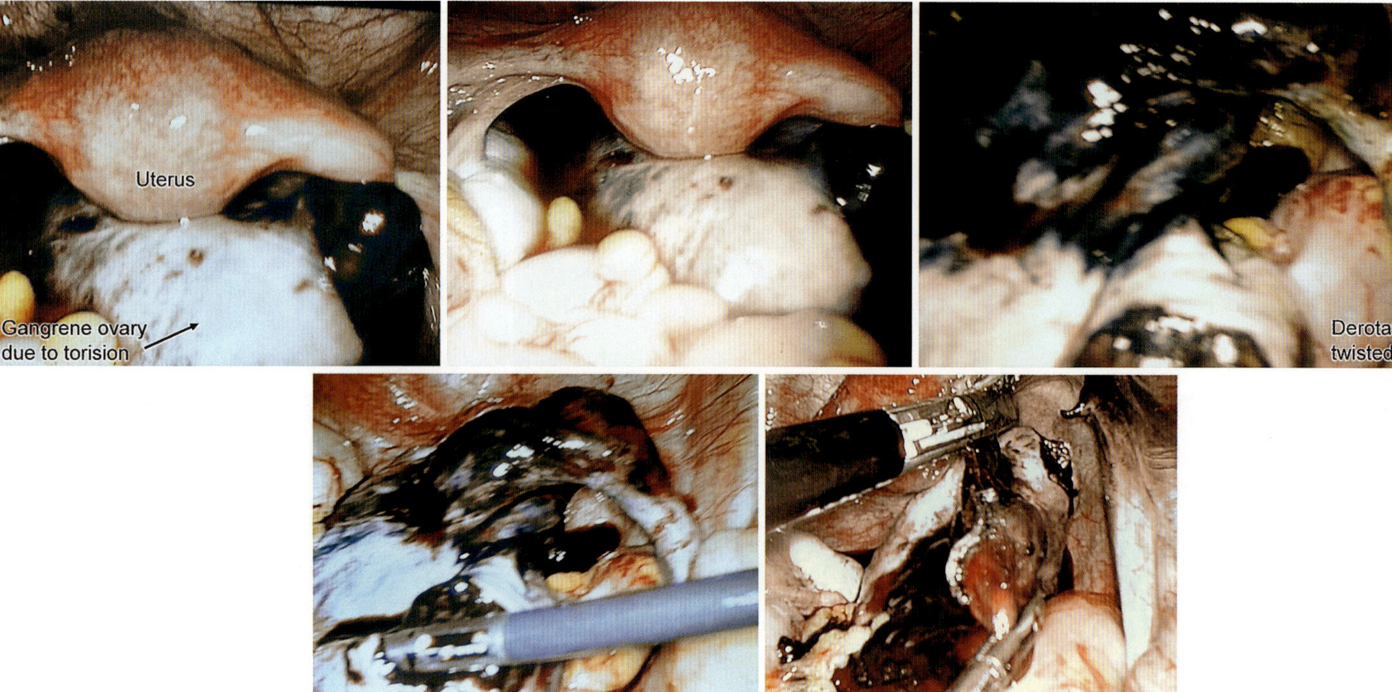

Fig. 32-10: Gangrene ovary due to torsion of ovarian cyst; it is removed through laparoscopy.

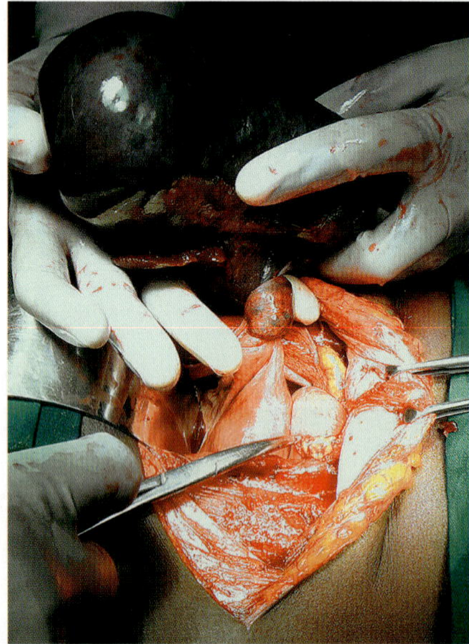

Fig. 32-11: Twisted ovarian cyst showing the twisted torsion pedicle.

Complications

- Greater risk of cardiovascular disease.
- Increased risk of osteoporosis and bone fractures.
- Significantly impairs sexual well-being.
- Libido loss, difficulty with sexual arousal, and vaginal dryness.
- Parkinsonism.
- Decline in psychological well-being.

Salpingo-oophorectomy

It is removal of tube with along the ovary. It may be a unilateral procedure or bilateral which is often combined with hysterectomy.

Indications:

- Benign adnexal mass
- Adnexal torsion
- Tubo-ovarian abscess and pelvic inflammatory disease.
- Ectopic pregnancy
- Endometriosis

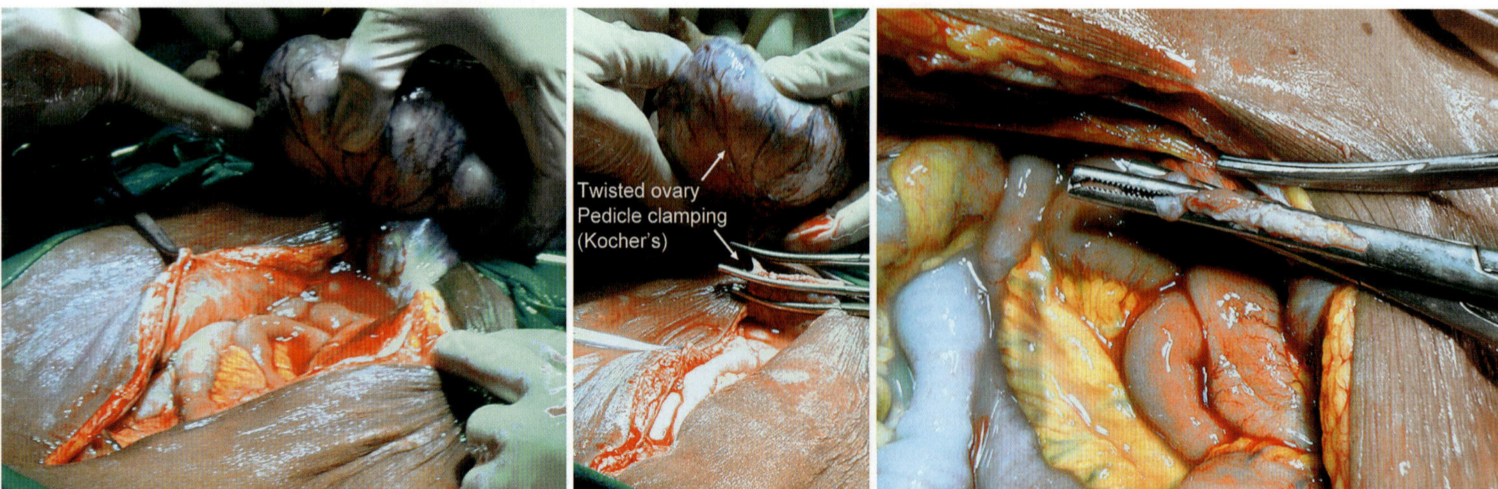

Fig. 32-12: Gangrene ovary with torsion of the cyst.

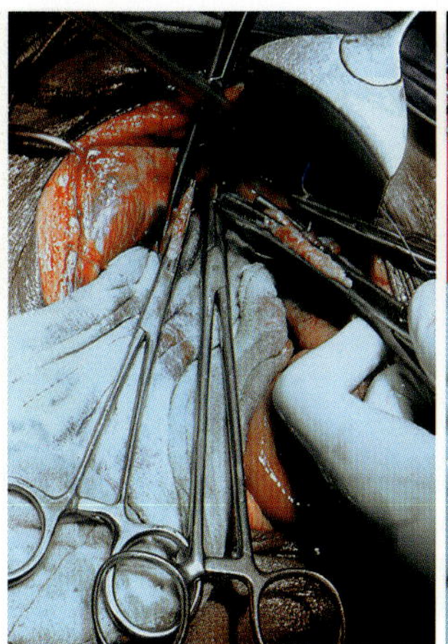
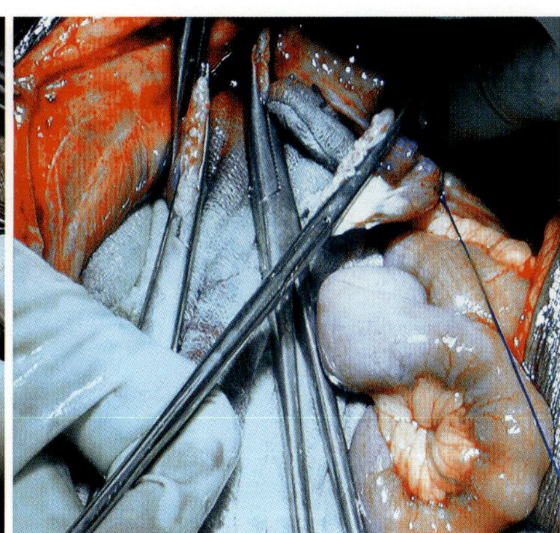
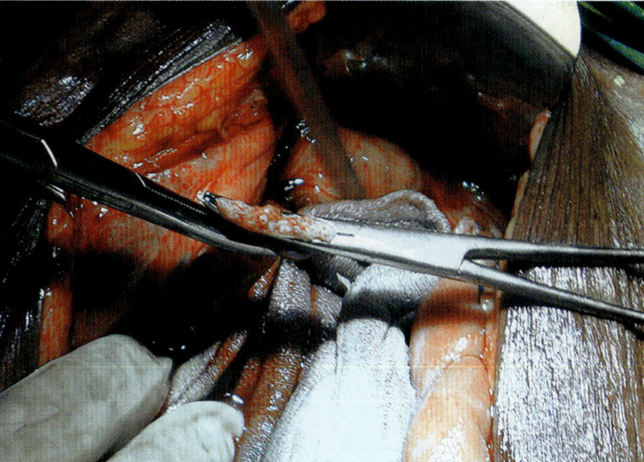

Fig. 32-13: Ovarian pedicle after removal of ovary.

- Removal of normal appearing ovaries and tubes at the time of hysterectomy for benign disease, to decrease the risk of development of ovarian pathology in future and so the need for any procedures.
- Malignancy—ovarian cancer, uterine cancer, or metastases to ovaries from a distant primary malignancy (gastrointestinal, breast, lung carcinoma)
- Removal of ovaries and tubes in women genetically susceptible to ovarian cancer.

Sometime, there may be extensive adhesions between tubes and ovary that it necessitates its removal with the ovary.

Procedure:
Approaching from below and behind, any adhesions between the ovary and broad ligament is carefully divided. Tube and ovary are raised and the infundibulopelvic ligament is identified. Ureter has to be identified before clamping the infundibulopelvic ligament so as to avoid injury to it. The IP ligament is clamped with 2 curved Kocher's clamp. It is cut between the two clamps. The pedicle is transfixed and ligated with 1-zero-or 2-zero vicryl suture. Next ovarian ligament and uterine end of the tube is together clamped, cut and ligated **(Figs. 32-14 and 32-15)**.

Complications

- Injury to ureter especially when there is severe adhesion as in endometriosis, PID.
- Injury to colon on left side while ligating the IP ligament.

MYOMECTOMY

Myomectomy is removal of myomas from the uterine wall. It may be intramural, subendometrial or subserosal. It causes infertility. Myomectomy is part of the treatment for infertility often.

Myoma can be removed either by open or laparoscopic method. Laparoscopic myomectomy needs more skill than laparoscopic hysterectomy.

Open Myomectomy

Bladder catheterisation is done. Patient with head down position is better to displace the bowel from the pelvis. It is done through Pfannenstiel incision. Site and size of the myomas should be assessed by preoperative imaging. Uterus is delivered/brought out of the abdominal wound. Often vasopressin injection into the uterus may be injected to reduce the bleeding; but its complications should be taken care of. Incision is made on the surface of the uterus directly on the myoma site. Myometrium is carefully separated using monopolar cautery or using no. 15 blade. Bleeding should be controlled. Well capsulated whitish yellow coloured myoma can be identified. Myoma screw is passed into the myoma which is manipulated to pull out the myoma off the uterine wound. Cautery, ligasure will also help from separating it from deeper plane. Once myoma is removed, bleeding points are fulgurated using bipolar cautery. Finger is inserted to confirm that endometrium is injured or not. If endometrium is injured, it is sutured with 2-zero vicryl sutures. Myometrium is also sutured using 2-zero sutures. Parametrium is sutured similarly **(Fig. 32-16)**.

Laparoscopic Myomectomy

Bladder catheterisation should be done. It is done under general anaesthesia with head down and lithotomy position. 10 mm supraumbilical camera port is placed; 10 mm working port on one side in the iliac fossa; another 5 mm on the opposite iliac fossa; one more 5 mm port on the right side above the earlier 5 mm port which is used for myoma 5 mm screw to pass. Incision is made on the uterus on the myoma site using monopolar cautery. Once glistening avascular myoma capsule is identified, laparoscopic myoma screw is inserted into the myoma. Using the screw myoma is manipulated gently, gradually and progressively to retrieve it from myoma bed in the uterine wall. Bleeders should be addressed using ligasure or harmonic scalpel or bipolar cautery. Uterine wall is sutured with intracorporeal suturing. Difficulty is identifying the endometrial tear and suturing it. If difficulty arises conversion should be done. Absolute haemostasis should be achieved.

HYSTERECTOMY

It is operative removal of the uterus. It is the most common gynaecological surgical procedure.

Indications

Benign condition	*Malignant condition*
♦ Dysfunctional uterine bleeding ♦ Fibroid and adenomyosis ♦ Bilateral ovarian cyst ♦ Postmenopausal bleeding ♦ Endometriosis ♦ Pelvic inflammatory disease ♦ Pelvic organ prolapse ♦ Obstetric causes like postpartum haemorrhage, rupture uterus, abnormal placentation	♦ Cervical intraepithelial neoplasia ♦ Cancer of endometrium, ovary, fallopian tube ♦ Gestational trophoblastic disease

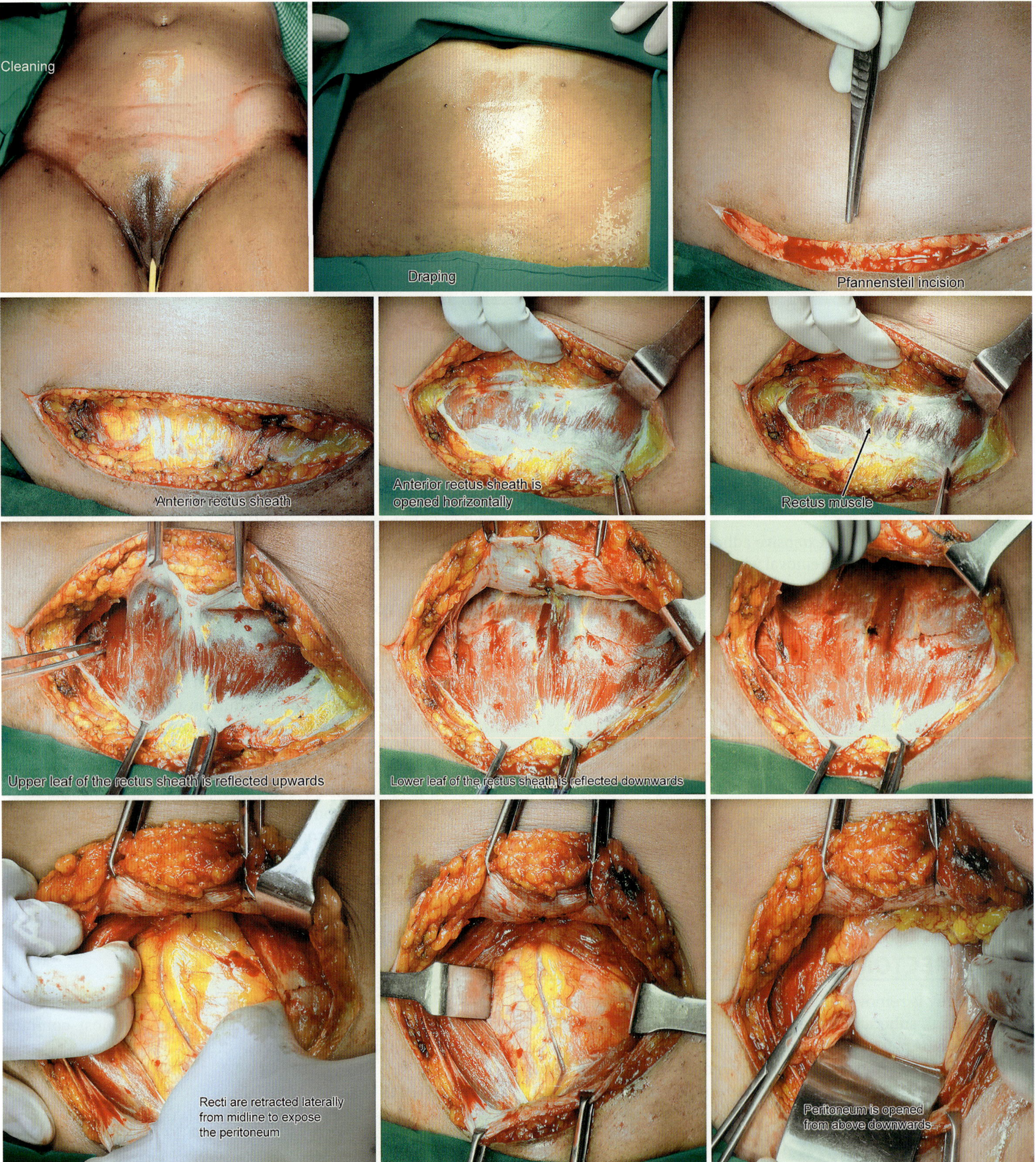
Cleaning
Draping
Pfannensteil incision
Anterior rectus sheath
Anterior rectus sheath is opened horizontally
Rectus muscle
Upper leaf of the rectus sheath is reflected upwards
Lower leaf of the rectus sheath is reflected downwards
Recti are retracted laterally from midline to expose the peritoneum
Peritoneum is opened from above downwards

Figs. 32-14(1)

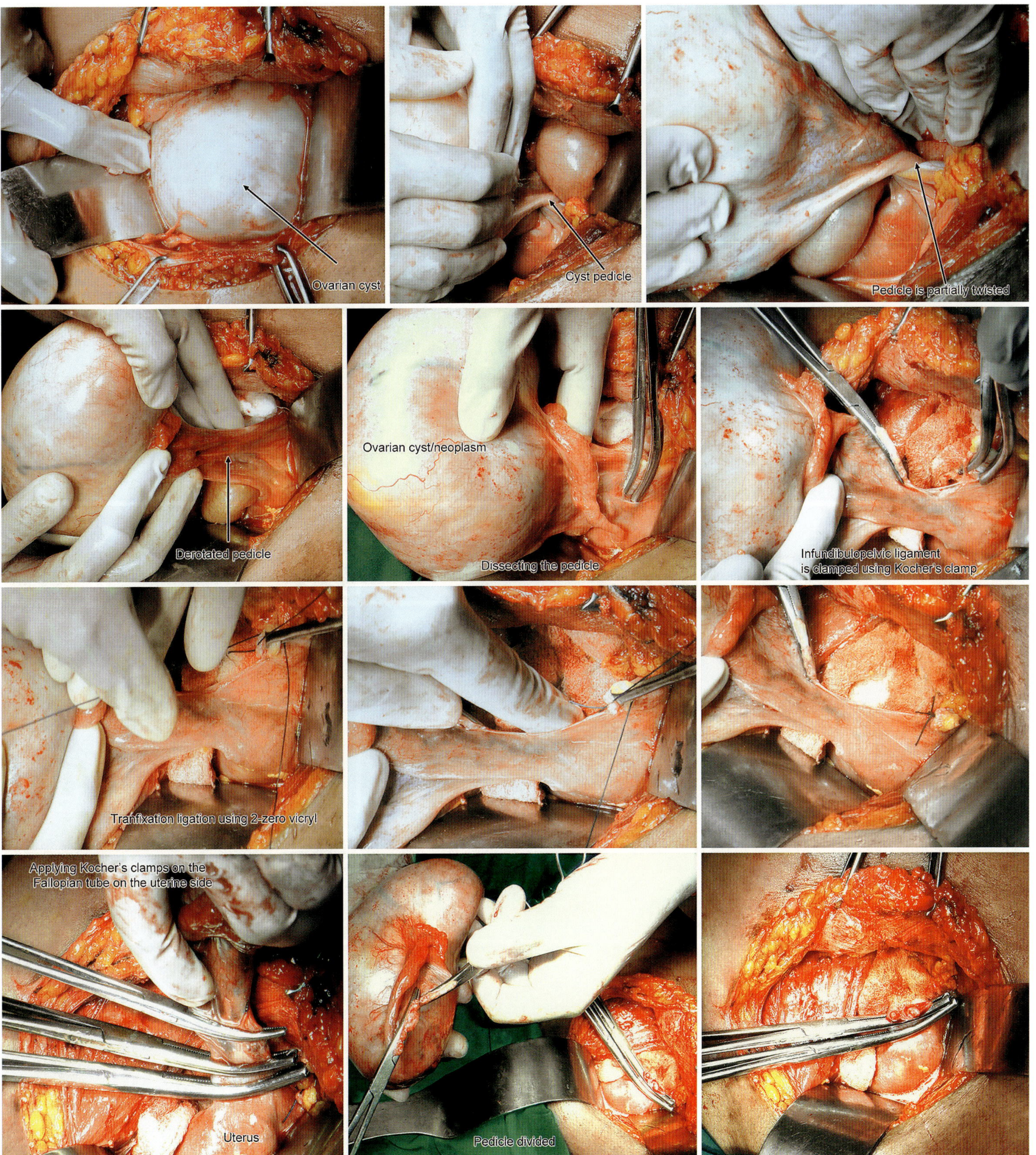
Ovarian cyst
Cyst pedicle
Pedicle is partially twisted
Derotated pedicle
Ovarian cyst/neoplasm
Dissecting the pedicle
Infundibulopelvic ligament
is clamped using Kocher's clamp
Tranfixation ligation using 2-zero vicryl
Applying Kocher's clamps on the
Fallopian tube on the uterine side
Uterus
Pedicle divided

Figs. 32-14(2)

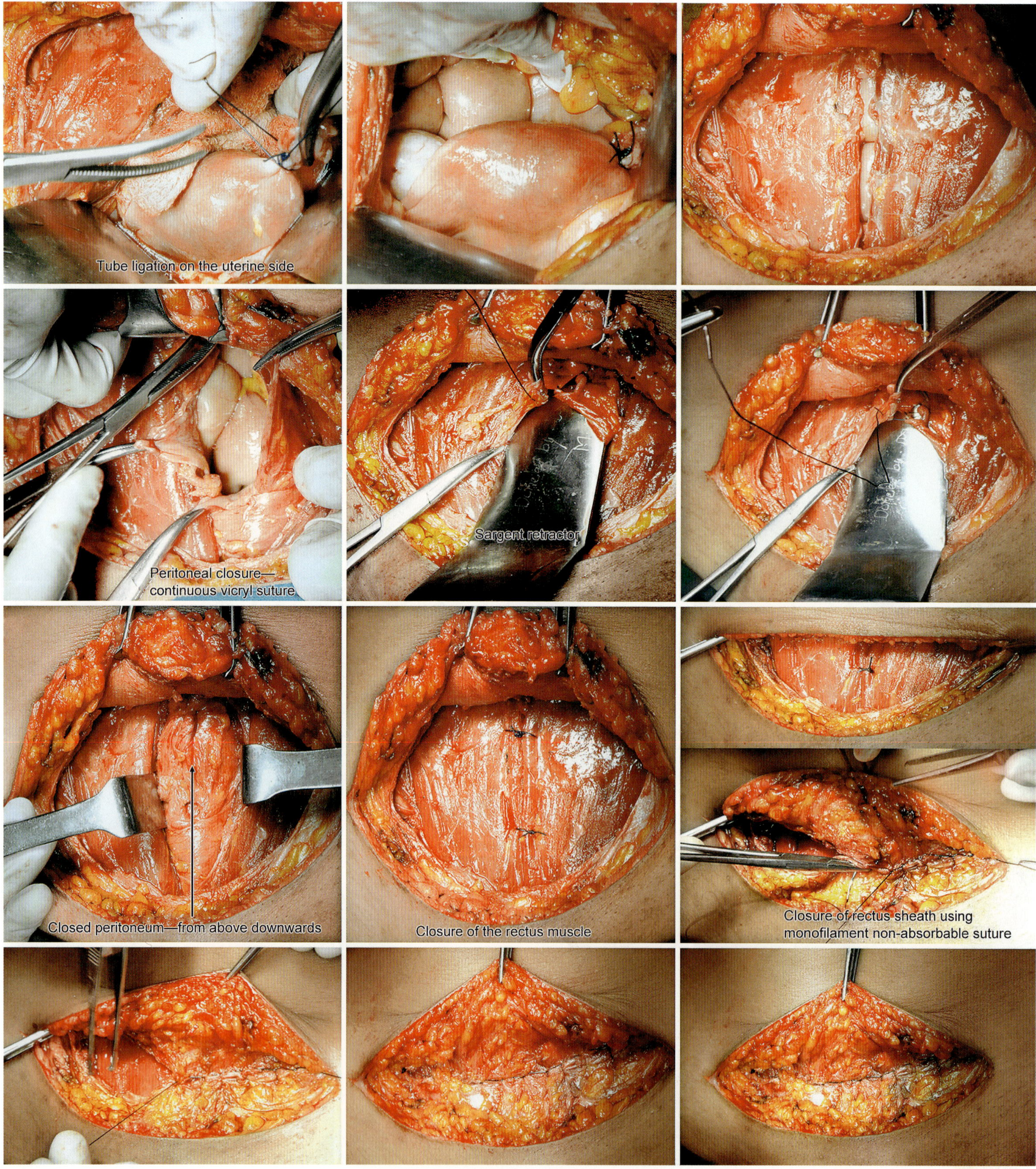
Tube ligation on the uterine side
Peritoneal closure—
continuous vicryl suture
Sargent retractor
Closed peritoneum—from above downwards
Closure of the rectus muscle
Closure of rectus sheath using
monofilament non-absorbable suture

Figs. 32-14(3)

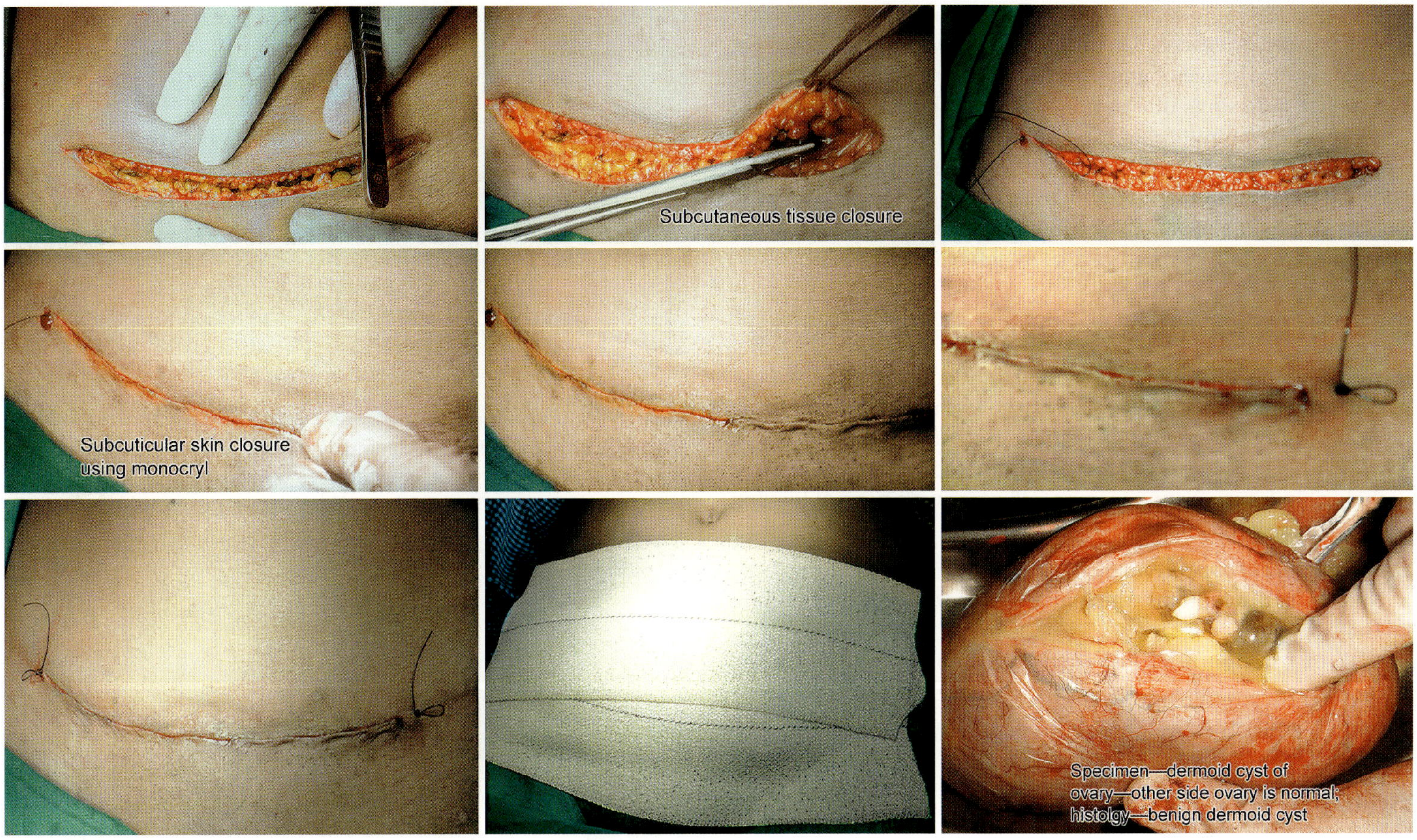

Figs. 32-14(4)

Figs. 32-14(1 to 4): Salpingo-oophorectomy for benign dermoid cyst of the ovary—technique.

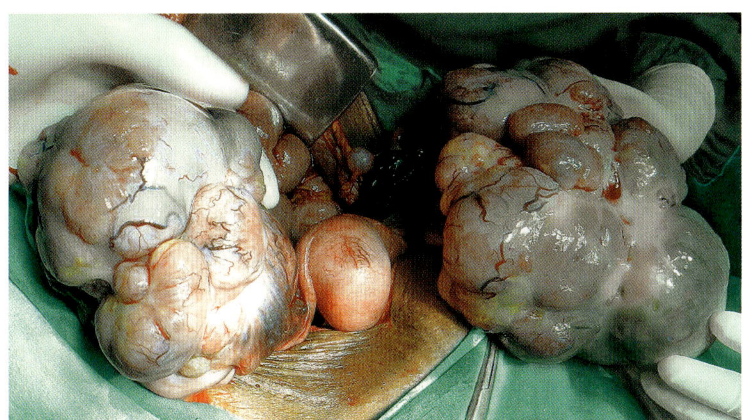

Fig. 32-15: Krukenberg tumour of the ovary.

Types

Total hysterectomy—uterine corpus with cervix removed.

Subtotal hysterectomy—only uterine corpus removed retaining the cervix.

Panhysterectomy—uterine corpus, cervix along with bilateral tubes and ovaries removed.

Radical hysterectomy—total hysterectomy, bilateral salpingo-oophorectomy, along with removal of parametrium, upper 1/3rd vagina and pelvic lymph nodes.

Routes of Removal

Uterus can be removed via abdominal, vaginal, or laparoscopic route.

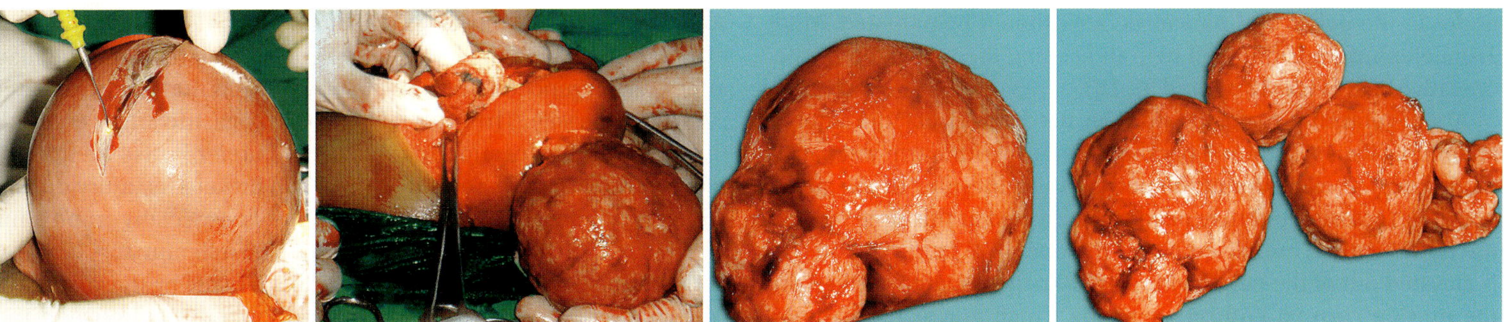

Fig. 32-16: Myomectomy—specimen—large and multiple.

Choice of this route depends on the uterine size, presence of pelvic pathology, uterine descent. Uterus up to 12–14 weeks size, with slight descent, with absence of any pelvic pathology like endometriosis, PID, pelvic adhesions due to previous surgeries, with absence of cervical hypertrophy/fibroid can be safely and effectively removed by vaginal route. Vaginal hysterectomy is less morbid and cost effective than abdominal hysterectomy. A diagnostic laparoscopy will clarify the situation and may allow the procedure to be converted to a laparoscopically assisted vaginal hysterectomy (LAVH).

Need of Oophorectomy During Hysterectomy

It is decided on the age of the patient, and gross structure of the ovary. *Prophylactic oophorectomy* is the term used for removing clinically normal ovaries, often done in postmenopausal women or in women aged >45 years to prevent the development of any ovarian pathology in future. Young women <45 years with normal looking ovaries can be left behind.

Disadvantages of oophorectomy:

- Menopausal symptoms which may be so severe that may require HRT.
- Risk of osteoporosis, atherosclerosis, coronary thrombosis increases.

Advantages: Risks of developing ovarian cancer, cysts are reduced.

Anaesthesia

It can be done under general/spinal anaesthesia. However, spinal anaesthesia is preferable for vaginal hysterectomy.

Abdominal Hysterectomy

Technique: The patient is placed in supine or modified lithotomy position with legs supported by the Allen universal stirrups. The latter position favours access to vagina. The vagina and perineum are cleaned with antiseptic solutions. Indwelling Foley catheter is inserted. A pelvic examination is routinely performed under anaesthesia. This examination helps to delineate the existing pathology and also in selection of the type of incision. The abdomen is then cleaned from the anterior thighs to the xiphoid with antiseptic solutions. Sterile drapes are applied.

Incision: Abdomen is opened either by a low transverse, Pfannenstiel (mostly preferred), or infraumbilical-midline/paramedian (when good exposure is required) incision.

Once inside the peritoneal cavity, the abdomen is explored and pelvic pathology is carefully evaluated. The surgeon should examine the appendix for any pathology. The upper abdominal organs, including liver, gallbladder, stomach, under surface diaphragm, and omentum should be palpated for any pathology. The retroperitoneal nodes in the pelvic and paraaortic area should be palpated. Mild Trendelenburg position will help in keeping the bowel out of the operative field **(Figs. 32-17 and 32-18)**.

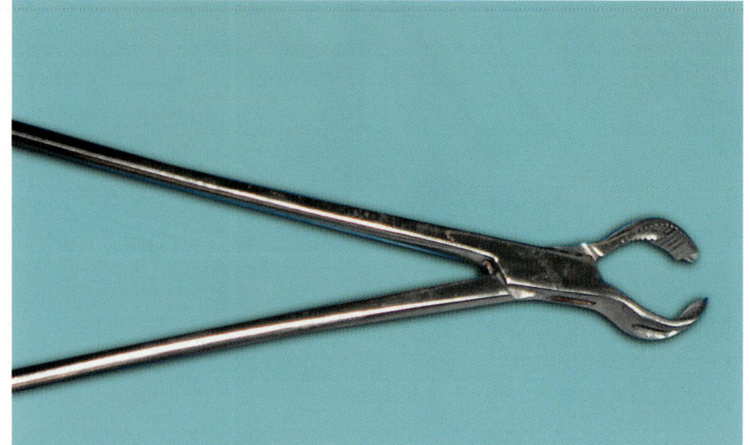

Fig. 32-17: Tissue forceps commonly used to hold the rectus sheath while raising the flap upwards.

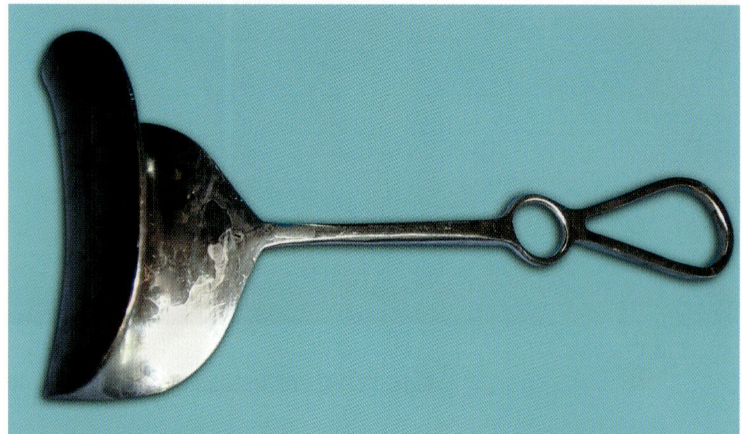

Fig. 32-18: Doyen's retractor is often used in pelvic surgeries.

A self-retaining retractor may be used to retract the lateral abdominal flaps. The bowel packed superiorly with warm wet packs to afford good exposure of the pelvis. Any adhesions of the small bowel or rectosigmoid may need to be divided at this time so that the bowel can be mobilised out of the operative field. The uterus is elevated out of the pelvis with pair of Kocher's clamp applied on the uterine cornual end on each side which grasps the isthmic portion of fallopian tubes and mesosalpinx. Bilateral clamps in this position will allow for elevation, traction, and rotation of the uterus. Uterine mobility is restricted in cases of extensive inflammatory disease, endometriosis, malignancy, or very large fibroids, but uterine mobility is satisfactory in most benign conditions. Bilateral tubes and ovaries are carefully examined for any pathology **(Fig. 32-19)**.

If the ovaries and tubes are healthy then *total hysterectomy* is done. The uterus is pulled to one side so that the opposite ovary and tubes are stretched and exposed. The round ligament is clamped midway with a pair of Kocher's clamp, divided and the clamps are removed after ligating with 1-zero vicryl sutures. This opens the retroperitoneal space, which is almost always a free space for blunt dissection, even in the patient with extensive tumour, inflammatory disease, or endometriosis. The loose areolar tissue of the retroperitoneum is divided with the index finger and the tip of the suction or the back of a tissue forceps. The external iliac artery on the medial surface of the psoas muscle is identified. Blunt dissection is done to expose superiorly to the level of the bifurcation of the common iliac artery. At this junction, the ureter always crosses the pelvic brim and is identified easily. The internal iliac or hypogastric artery entering the pelvis at this location, parallel to the ureter is also identified. Identification of ureter and its course will prevent its injury during clamping and ligating of pedicles. This is especially important when pelvic anatomy is distorted as in pelvic inflammatory disease, endometriosis and malignancy. A window is made by sharp or blunt way in the peritoneum beneath the fallopian tube between the uterus and ovary. A Kocher's clamp is used to clamp the tube and

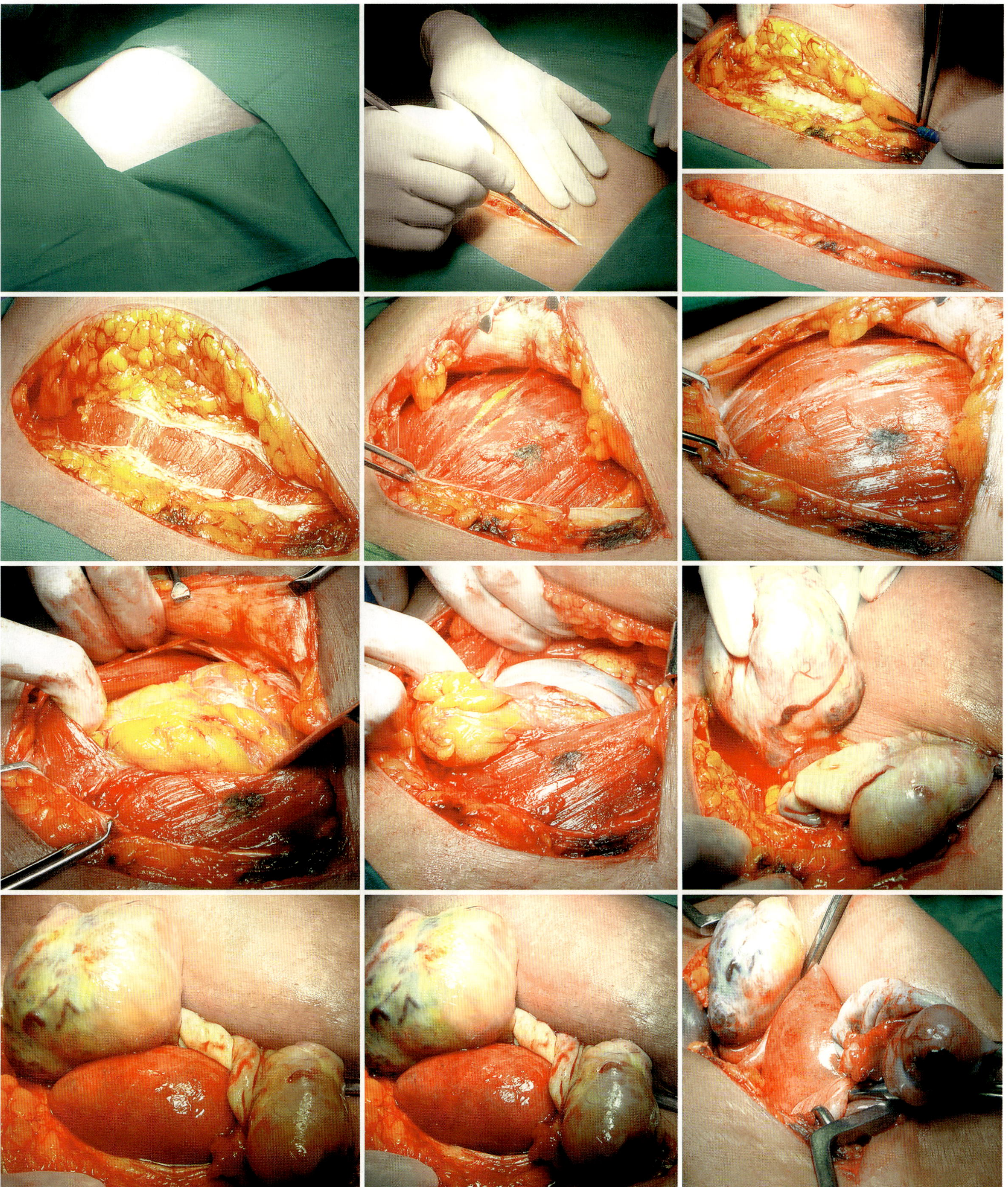

Figs. 32-19(1)

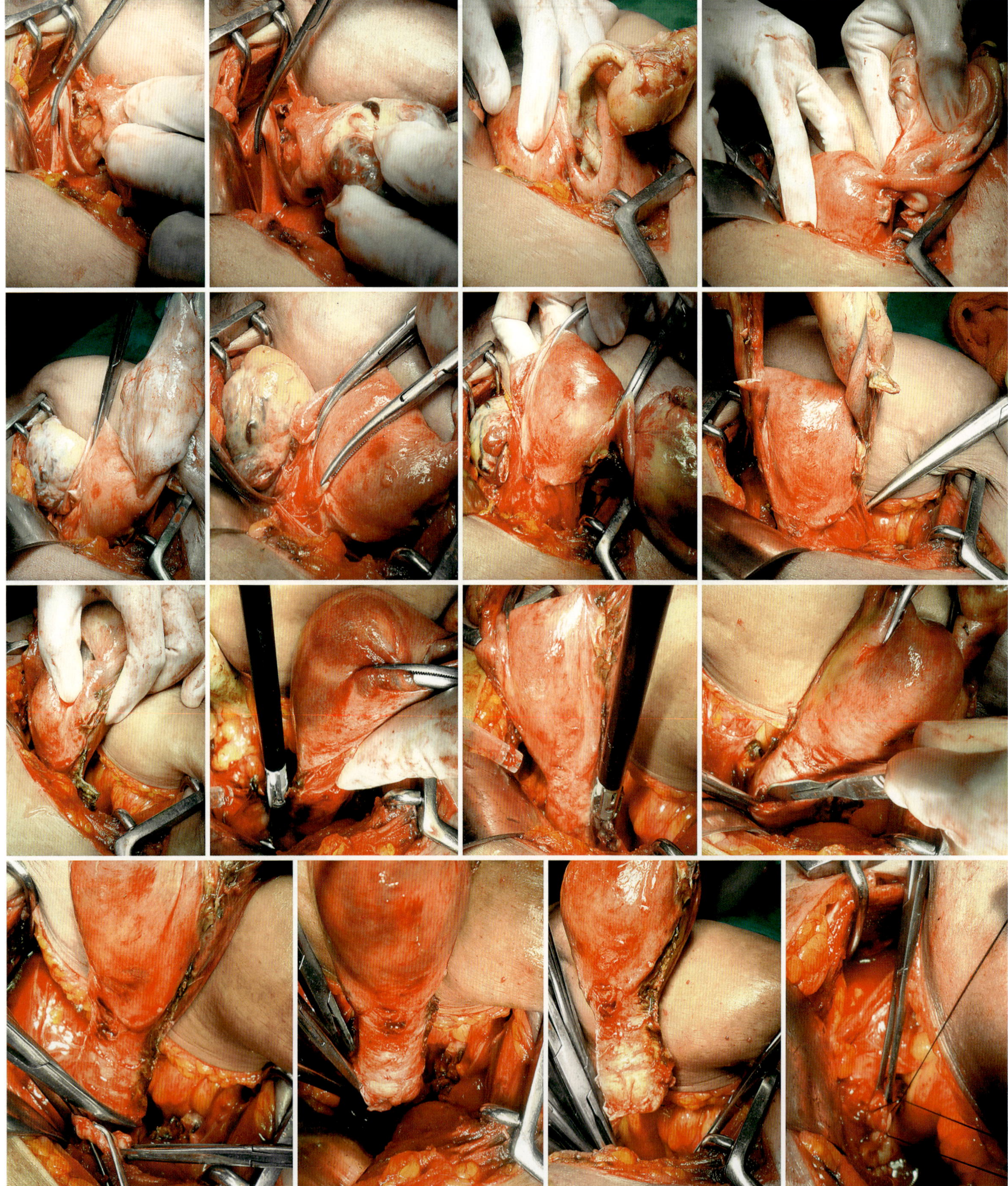

Figs. 32-19(2)

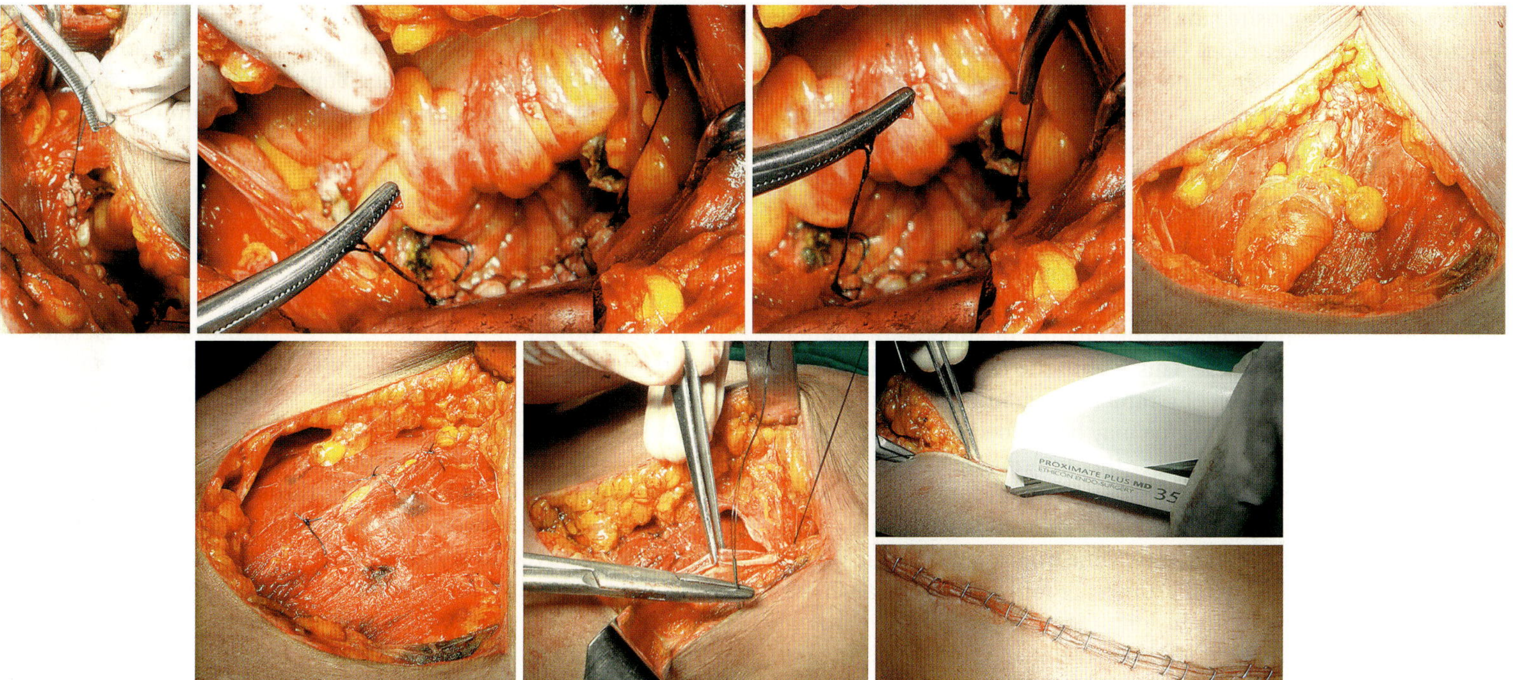

Figs. 32-19(3)

Figs. 32-19(1 to 3): Technique of open hysterectomy.

utero-ovarian ligament, its tip should lie in the window created in the peritoneum. The clamp that was initially placed at the corneal end of the uterus acts as a back clamp. The tube and utero-ovarian ligament are divided between the clamps and the pedicle is ligated twice. The procedure is repeated on the other side.

In *panhysterectomy* where the ovaries and tubes are to be removed, a hole in the peritoneum between the ureter and the ovarian vessels is made under direct vision. The ovarian vessels in the infundibulopelvic ligament are clamped with Kocher's clamp. A second back clamp is placed distally and the ovarian vessels are divided between the two clamps. Dissection done in the retroperitoneum will avoid the injury to ureter at this junction. The pedicles are transfixed and ligated with 1-zero vicryl sutures. The procedure is repeated on the other side also.

The uterus is now pulled upwards and backwards. Uterovesical fold of peritoneum is exposed and is divided with sharp scissors just inferior (5–10 mm) to its attachment to the lower uterine segment. At this junction peritoneum is usually mobile, and this peritoneal division is carried from one side round ligament to the other. An avascular plane of loose areolar tissue can be identified between the posterior bladder wall and the anterior cervix. By giving constant upwards traction on the uterus and peritoneal fold of the bladder, the bladder is dissected away from the cervix either by sharp dissection with scissors or by blunt dissection with a gauze held with an Allis forceps. Care should be taken to see that scissors should rest lightly on the fascia overlying the cervix and this dissection should take place over the cervix avoiding to go far laterally as one may encounter bleeding due to injury to uterine vessels. With the thumb of one hand in front and fingers of the other behind the uterus the extent of this bladder dissection below the cervix is determined. As the bladder is advanced below the cervix, the thumb in front and the fingers behind come into closer opposition as they now have only the vaginal wall between them. Posteriorly, it is not necessary to dissect the rectum off the posterior cul-de-sac; but if adherent and prevents good exposure, it should be dissected free slightly by blunt dissection after the uterine vessels have been divided. The posterior peritoneum between the uterosacral ligament beneath the cervix is incised. By blunt dissection with fingers in the avascular plane which exists between the rectum and posterior cervix/vagina, will push the rectum backwards away from the operative field.

Next step is a crucial step of hysterectomy which is the ligation of uterine vessels. Any improper ligation or slipping of ligatures will cause the vessels to retract and result in torrential bleeding. Blind catching of the vessels with a haemostat in an attempt to stop bleeding will likely to damage the ureter that traverse close by. Uterus is pulled sharply to one side, and the loose fatty tissue adjacent to the lateral lower uterine segment on the opposite side is dissected. The uterine artery is usually found immediately adjacent to the uterus at the level of the internal cervical os. Skeletonising the uterine artery and vein allows them to be clamped more accurately. Less adjacent tissue means a smaller vascular pedicle, which allows more precise and more secure ligation. However, excessive attempts to isolate the vessels may produce unnecessary bleeding. The exposed vessels are clamped with Heaney or Kocher's clamp adjacent to the uterus. The clamp must be applied at right angles to the vessels. A second clamp can be placed above the first for added safety. If the uterus is small, no back clamp is required. The uterine vessels are cut with scissors or a knife and the pedicle are doubly ligated with 1-zero vicryl sutures. The procedure is repeated on the opposite side.

It is once again made sure that the bladder anteriorly and the rectum posteriorly have been freed from the cervix. Giving upward traction on the uterus, the deeper portions of the broad ligament is exposed. By using a retractor bladder is retracted away and downwards and thereby pull the lower uterine segment away from the ureter. A straight Heaney or Kocher's clamp is now applied over the remaining portion of the broad ligament/parametrium close to the lateral portion of the cervix. Giving traction on the uterus towards opposite side, the cervix is freed from the parametrium with scissors. By staying close to the cervix the risk of damaging the ureter is minimised. The clamps are removed after transfixing and ligating the pedicles with 1/0 absorbable sutures. Procedure is repeated on the opposite side. Maintaining good exposure, one or two pedicles are tied on each side, and then the procedure is repeated on the opposite side until the level of the cervicovaginal junction has been reached. Once again, the bladder and rectum are checked and advanced if necessary to be sure that they are well clear off and the anterior and posterior vaginal walls are exposed. Haeney's clamps are then applied across the vagina below the cervix from either side, which should include the base of the cardinal ligaments laterally, the uterosacral ligament posteriorly, and anterior and posterior vaginal wall. With a knife or heavy, sharply angled scissors the vagina is divided above these clamps and below the cervix. This is closed technique of removing the cervix from the upper vagina which decreases the chance of spillage of vaginal contents into the abdomen. This technique decreases the risk of infection and the formation of symptomatic granulation tissue at the vaginal apex. Alternatively, vagina may be opened by a stab incision with a knife below the cervix over the anterior vaginal wall and is cut circumferentially under direct vision. Full thickness vaginal edge is held with Allis forceps. Uterus thus removed is placed in a tray. Gauze may be introduced into the vagina from above and the vagina is cleared of clots. The lateral clamps are removed after transfixing and ligating the pedicles. Inclusion of the uterosacral and cardinal ligament in this pedicle provides excellent support of the vaginal apex. The vagina is closed with interrupted sutures or continuous locking 1-zero vicryl sutures.

Pelvis is irrigated with warm saline; the pedicles are inspected carefully to be sure that haemostasis is achieved. Cautery or excessive suturing at the bladder base should be avoided as it may predispose fistula formation because of necrosis. Any bleeding areas at the uterine vessels or cardinal ligament should be grasped with an Allis clamp and resutured within the suture line. The pelvis is not reperitonealised. New mesothelium arises from the subperitoneal connective tissue cells and occurs simultaneously in all exposed areas independent of the size of the defect. Attempts to cover areas of peritoneal injury may lead to increased adhesion formation at the sites of reperitonealisation by preventing autolysis of early fibrinous attachment and introducing reactive responses to suture material. The packs and retractor are removed. The anterior peritoneum is closed with delayed absorbable suture to prevent the development of future incisional hernia. The abdomen is closed in the usual way.

Difficult Hysterectomy

Difficulties are encountered in severe pelvic endometriosis, PID, malignancies large myomas where the pelvic anatomy is distorted. Dense adhesions cause great restriction in uterine mobility. By sharp dissection with scissors and blunt dissection with hand the adhesions are to be released and proceeded. In large cervical myomas, the bladder may be pushed upwards into the abdomen which is likely to get injured while opening the peritoneal cavity. Often ureter may lie close to the myomas due to distortion of the anatomy. In cases of pelvic endometriosis or previous caesarean section, it may be difficult to separate and advance the bladder from the cervix. In some cases, adhesions are so extensive that an attempt to remove the cervix may cause trauma to bladder, rectum and ureter. In such cases, one may have to resort to *subtotal hysterectomy* **(Fig. 32-20)**.

The *technique of subtotal or supracervical abdominal hysterectomy* is similar to abdominal hysterectomy until the ligation and clamping of uterine vessels. Care should be taken to see that the bladder and rectum have been advanced far enough so that the cervix can be clearly visualised both anteriorly and posteriorly. Upward traction is given to the uterine fundus and with electrocautery the cervix is cut anteriorly just above the level of uterine artery ligation. A shallow V-shaped incision is made on both anterior and posterior aspect until the uterine fundus is excised. Figure-of-eight sutures are used to close the upper endocervix in a haemostatic fashion. The top of the cervix is checked for any bleeding, and this cervical stump may be covered by the bladder peritoneum to minimise the risk of adhesions **(Fig. 32-21)**.

Postoperative Care

Foley's catheter inserted for bladder drainage is removed after 24 hours. Patient is hydrated with IV fluids for 24–48 hours. Once the normal bowel movements gets resumed oral diet is started. Parenteral antibiotics given for 48 hours, later switched over to oral preparation. Analgesics to control pain, initially injection pethidine (50 mg) + phenargan (25 mg) later tramadol and paracetamol. Patient is motivated for early ambulation and respiratory exercise to avoid pneumonia and deep vein thrombosis. Skin suture are removed anywhere between 7th–10th postoperative day. If bilateral ovaries are removed in a young patient she may require hormone replacement therapy for certain period. Normal activities can be resumed in 2–3 weeks. Patient is advised to avoid lifting heavy weights and intercourse for 4–6 weeks. Driving and travelling can be resumed once the pain has completely reduced. Patient should consult the physician if there is any vaginal bleeding, fever, persistent nausea/vomiting, increase pain out of proportion to the postoperative period.

Complications of Hysterectomy

Intraoperative Complications

Ureteric injury: Common sites of ureteral injury during abdominal hysterectomy include the infundibulopelvic ligament where the ovarian vessels are ligated; the area of the uterine artery ligation and at the bladder base. It is wise to expose the ureter in the retroperitoneal space so that its injuries can be avoided. Despite proper precaution if there is a doubt of ureteric injury, *indigocarmine* dye is injected intravenously. Its spill through the ureteric orifices is seen either through cystoscopy or by making an incision over the dome of the bladder.

Bladder injury: Bladder may be unusually drawn up into the abdomen by large pelvic tumours, adhesions due to previous surgery leading to its injury while opening the peritoneum. Bladder may sometime be unusually adherent to the cervix due to previous caesarean section or pelvic endometriosis. So while advancing the bladder off the cervix or upper vagina its muscle fibres may get torn up. Apart from trigonal injuries bladder injury is repaired by 2 layer closure of continuous 3-zero vicryl sutures. Trigonal injuries are dealt by the urologist. Continuous bladder drainage by indwelling Foley's catheter for 7 days is done.

Haemorrhage: Often bleeding occurs from the slipping/loosening of ligatures from ovarian or uterine pedicles. Bleeding is also encountered near the bladder base. Blind application of haemostat should be avoided. Firm pressure is applied with a warm wet mop. By slowly releasing the pressure the bleeding vessel is identified, clamped and ligated with suture. Bleeding from small vessels can be cauterised with electrocautery. Bleeding from denuded surface can be controlled by pressure, or application of topical agents like thrombin/collagen.

Bowel injury: Bowel injuries do can occur when there are extensive adhesions in the pelvis due to endometriosis, malignancy, pelvic inflammatory disease. When the defects are small not involving the

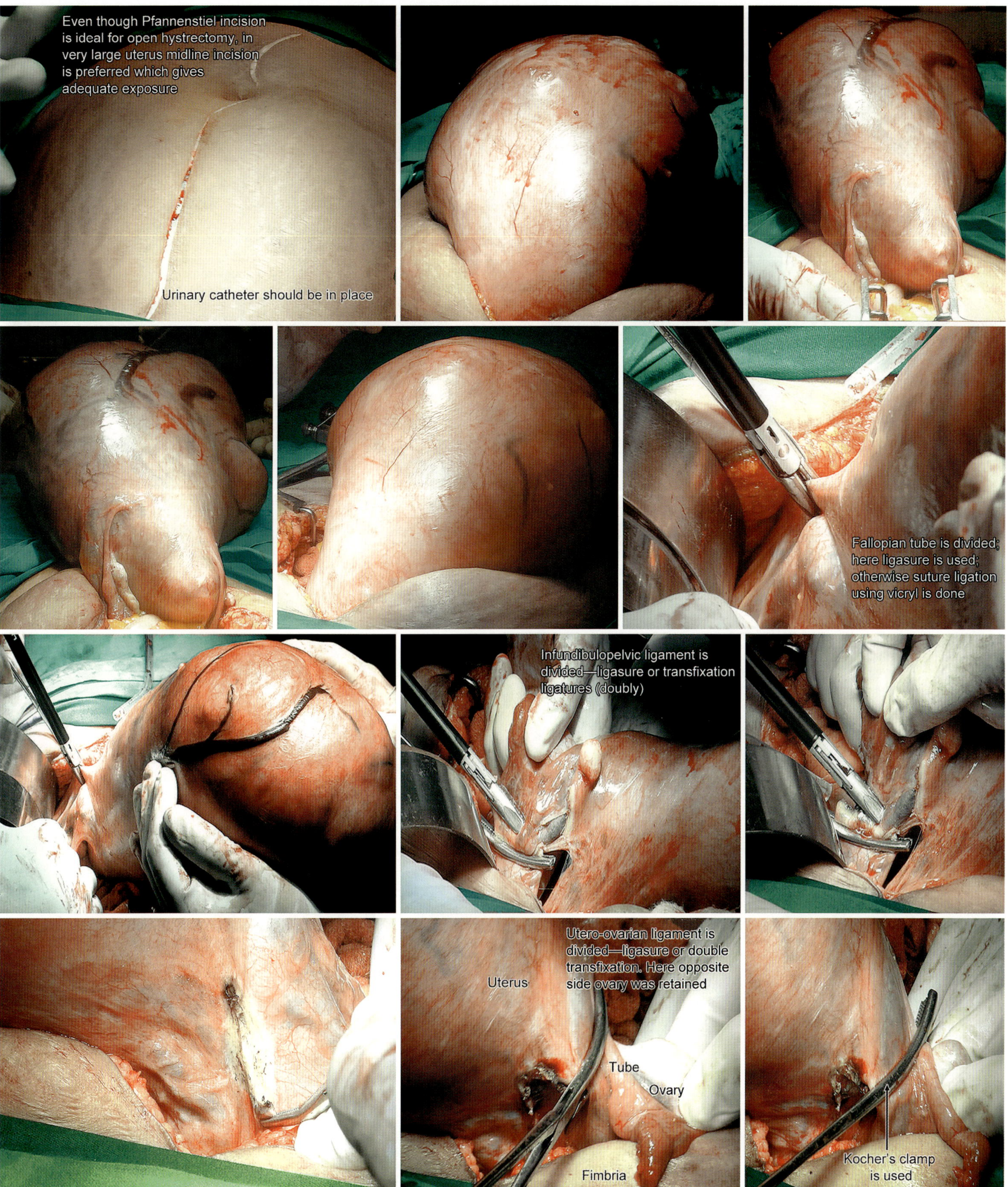
Even though Pfannenstiel incision is ideal for open hystrectomy, in very large uterus midline incision is preferred which gives adequate exposure
Urinary catheter should be in place
Fallopian tube is divided; here ligasure is used; otherwise suture ligation using vicryl is done
Infundibulopelvic ligament is divided—ligasure or transfixation ligatures (doubly)
Uterus
Utero-ovarian ligament is divided—ligasure or double transfixation. Here opposite side ovary was retained
Tube
Ovary
Fimbria
Kocher's clamp is used

Figs. 32-20(1)

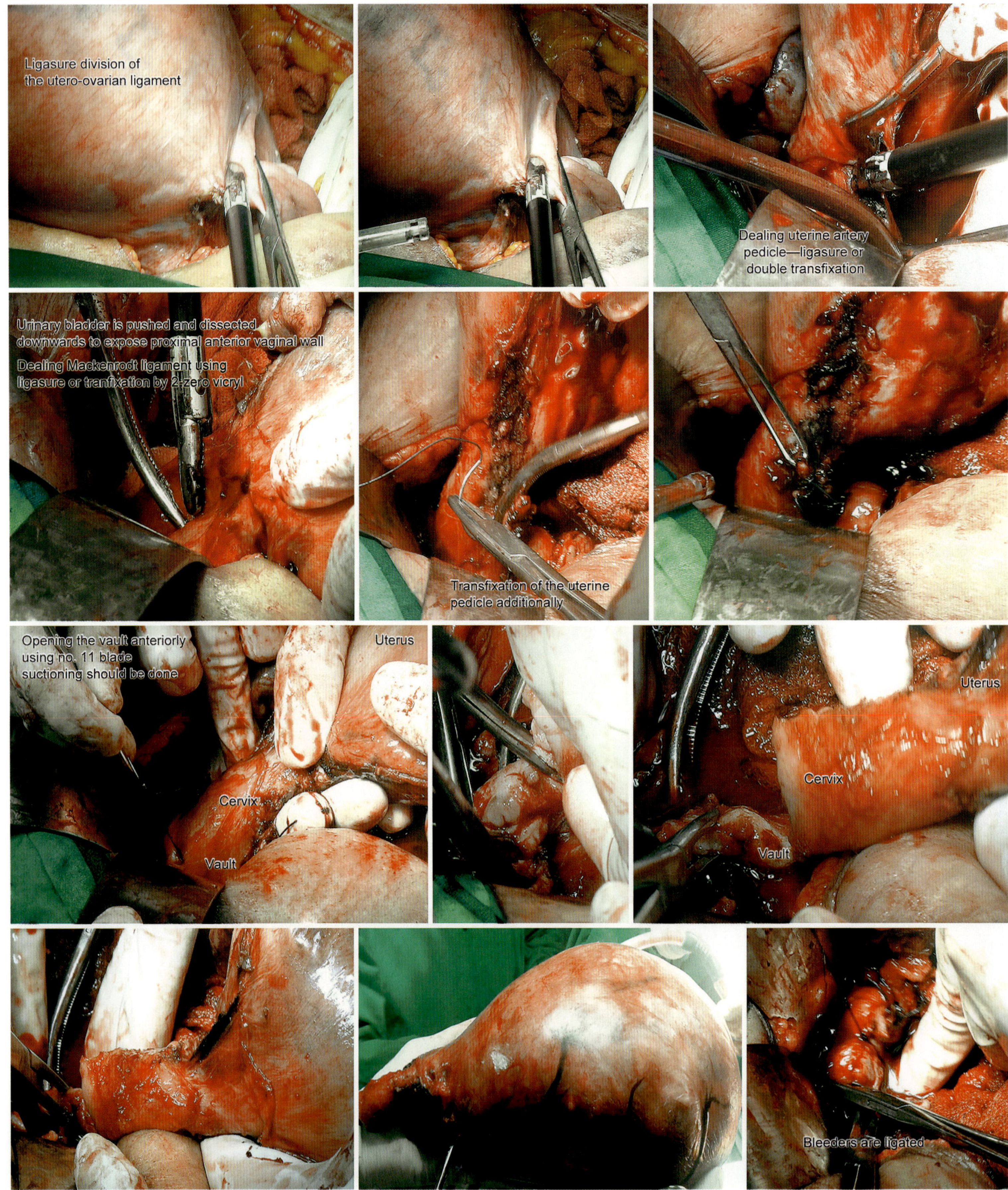
Ligasure division of
the utero-ovarian ligament
Dealing uterine artery
pedicle—ligasure or
double transfixation
Urinary bladder is pushed and dissected
downwards to expose proximal anterior vaginal wall
Dealing Mackenrodt ligament using
ligasure or tranfixation by 2-zero vicryl
Transfixation of the uterine
pedicle additionally
Opening the vault anteriorly
using no. 11 blade
suctioning should be done
Uterus
Cervix
Vault
Uterus
Cervix
Vault
Bleeders are ligated

Figs. 32-20(2)

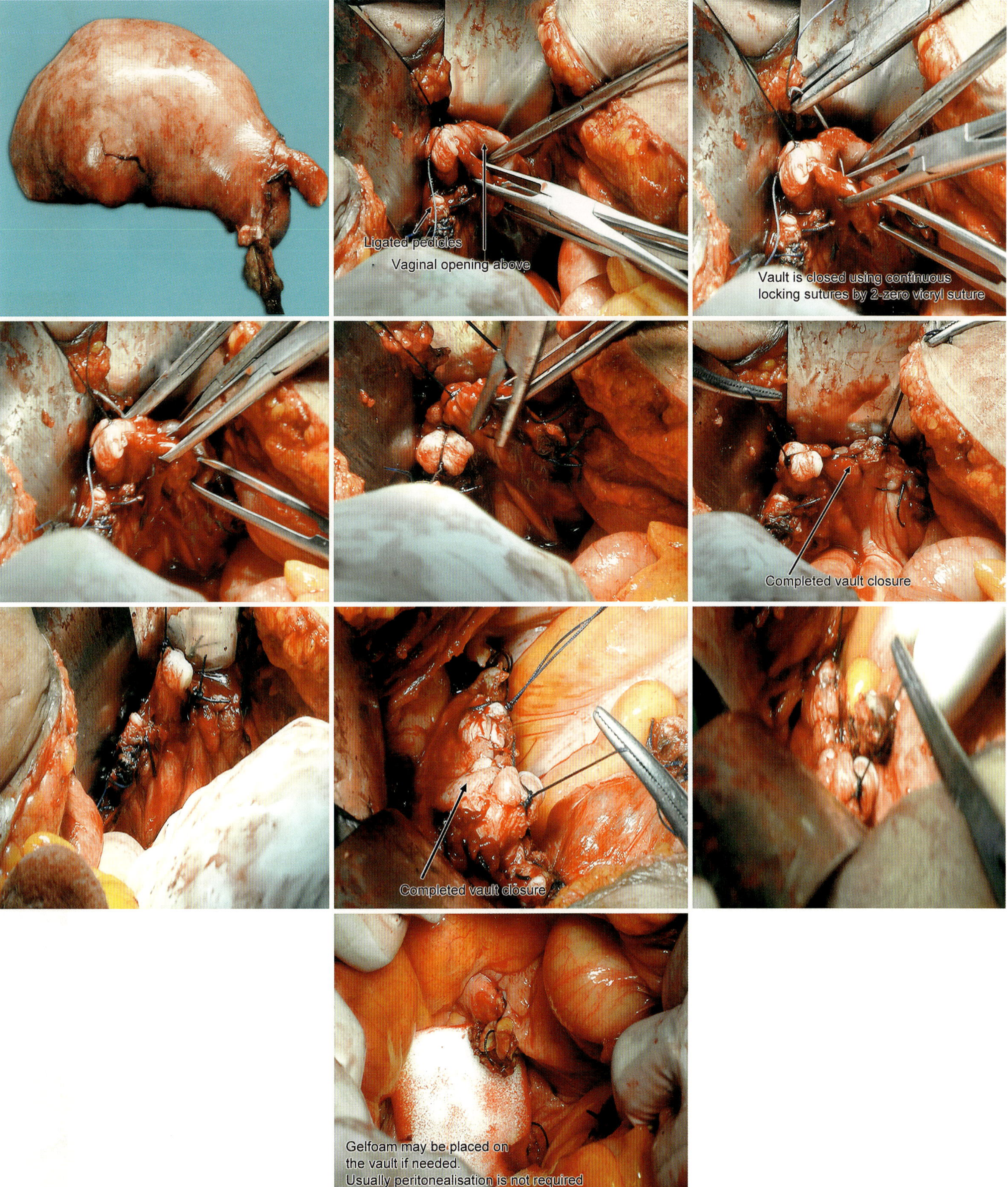

Figs. 32-20(3)

Figs. 32-20(1 to 3): Hysterectomy for a large uterine tumour through midline incision.

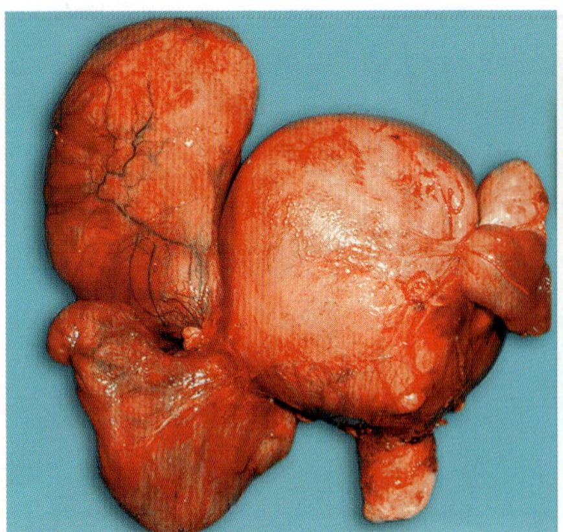
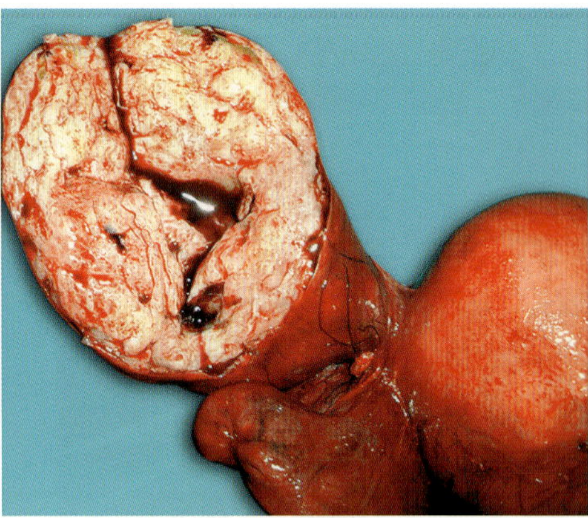
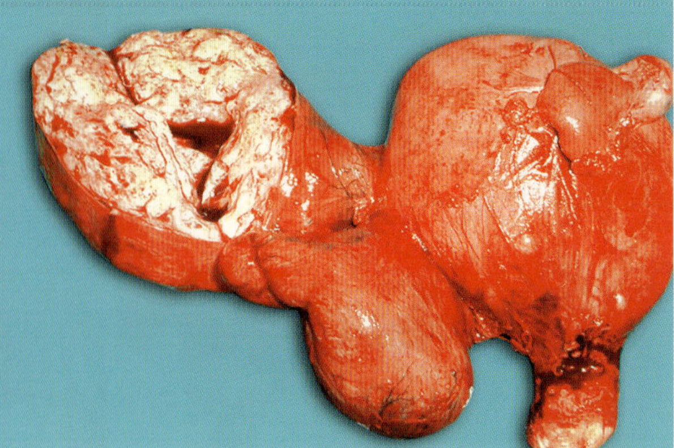

Fig. 32-21: Endometrial carcinoma specimen after hysterectomy.

mucosa in small bowel, it is closed with single layer of continuous/ interrupted 3-zero silk sutures in direction perpendicular to the intestinal lumen. If the defect is large than resection and anastomoses is done. In rectum and sigmoidal injuries, if the defect is small not involving the mucosa it can be closed in similar fashion to small bowel. Large defect involving the mucosa requires diversion colostomy along with primary repair.

Postoperative Complications

a. *Haemorrhage:* It is a serious postoperative complication. It may present with vaginal bleeding or change in vital signs like, tachycardia, pallor, tachypnoea, hypotension some with a palpable mass over the abdomen. Fluids are transfused. Blood transfusion should be done. When vitals are stable then the patient is shifted to operation theatre and examined for any bleeding from the vaginal vault. If it is from the raw vaginal edges one or two re-enforcing stitches over the vault will stop the bleeding. In the absence of any vaginal bleeding and the patient's vitals are not satisfactory, and then exploratory laparotomy is done keeping enough points of blood ready for transfusion. The bleeding vessel is identified and ligated. Sometimes, there may not be a intraperitoneal bleeding but from torn and retracted inferior epigastric vessels of the abdominal wall.
b. *Sepsis:* Infection may be at the wound site, intraperitoneal, urinary tract, vaginal vault, lungs. *Wound infection* is the most common form of sepsis. Anaemia, poor nutrition, preoperative sepsis, malignancy, ineffective haemostasis leading to haematoma are some of the predisposing factors. Infection may be superficial to the rectus sheath or may be deep to it involving all the layers. It may involve full length of incision or restricted to a small segment. When all the layers are involved the wound may disrupt suddenly leading to burst abdomen which needs to be treated as an emergency. Under anaesthesia resuturing is done. In case of superficial infection, it may lead to many discharging sinuses. The wound needs exploration under cover of higher antibiotics. Secondary suturing with deep mattress sutures using ethylon 2/0 is done which is removed only after 2 weeks. Mild superficial infection can be treated conservatively with antibiotics and regular dressing though it gives a bad scar.
   Fever in postoperative period can be due to urinary sepsis, pneumonia, bacteraemia, thrombophlebitis. Blood, urine are sent for culture. Chest X-ray is taken. Postoperative ultrasound will help to know any fluid collection in pelvis and abdominal cavity. Antibiotics are changed suitably. Sometimes, the collection may localise in pelvis forming a pelvic abscess which may need to be drained vaginally. By thrusting an artery forceps followed by finger through the vault will help to drain the pus from the pelvis.
   Peritonitis though rare, do can occur following bowel injury or due to retained foreign body like gauze/mops. Ultrasound abdomen or CT scan is done. Some patients may require relaparotomy if bowel injury or retained foreign body is suspected.
   Pneumonia: Quite common in elderly, obese ladies and those with history of chronic bronchitis. Postoperative respiratory exercises will help to prevent this.
c. *Oliguria/anuria:* In the presence of normal blood pressure, one should suspect ureteric ligation. Postoperative ultrasound will help to confirm this. Emergency nephrostomy may be done later, followed by exploration and reimplantation of the ureter.
d. *Paralytic ileus, intestinal obstruction:* Electrolyte imbalance, sepsis are known to cause paralytic ileus. Proper hydration, higher antibiotics, nasogastric aspiration with Ryles tube will help to restore the bowel function normally. Persistent vomiting with colicky pain should one be suspicious of intestinal obstruction. Occasionally, a loop of small bowel may get adherent to the vault. Laparotomy is done. Resection and end-to-end anastomosis is done.
e. *Thrombophlebitis and deep vein thrombosis*
f. *Pulmonary embolism*
g. *Early menopause:* Women who have undergone hysterectomy may experience menopause earlier than the average age of menopause (age 51). This may be due to an interruption in blood flow to the ovaries. Removal of ovaries also induces menopausal symptoms in the immediate postoperative period. Unless hormones replacement not started patient may develop severe symptoms that may affect the mental status.

Vaginal Hysterectomy

Indications: Common indications include abnormal or dysfunctional uterine bleeding, complex endometrial hyperplasia, leiomyoma (12–14 weeks size), adenomyosis, pelvic organ prolapse **(Fig. 32-22)**.

Prerequisites for vaginal hysterectomy:

- Good uterine mobility that can be demonstrated with valsalva manoeuvre
- Absence of adnexal pathology
- Pubic arch of 90° or greater with adequate vaginal canal, deep and wide posterior vaginal fornix will make the vaginal surgery easier to perform.

Proper selection of the patient is very important in vaginal hysterectomy.

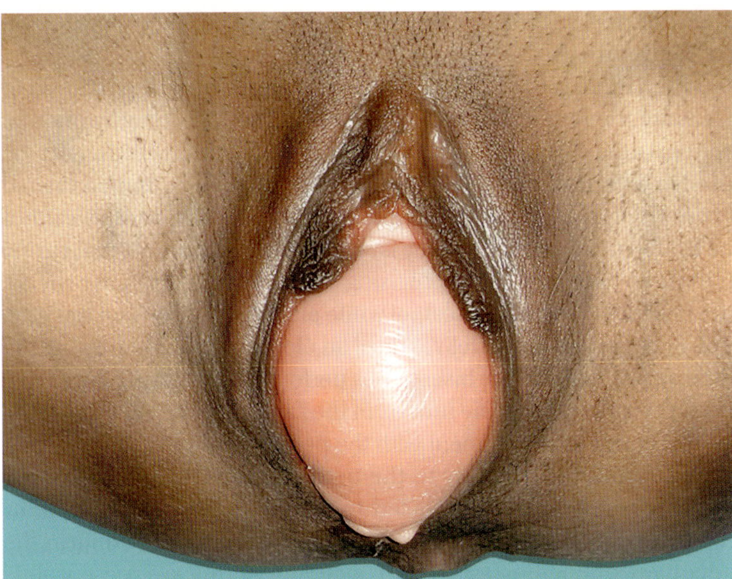

Fig. 32-22: Uterine prolapse.

Contraindications:
- Restricted uterine mobility
- Previous pelvic surgeries and caesarean section
- Severe endometriosis and pelvic inflammatory disease where there may be extensive pelvic adhesions
- Adnexal pathology—ovarian cysts and tumours, tumours of fallopian tubes
- Uterus enlarged beyond 12–14 weeks.
- Nulliparity
- Narrow pubic arch and narrow vaginal canal.

However, vaginal hysterectomy can be successfully done in nulliparous women and women who have undergone caesarean as long as adequate access for division of the uterosacral and cardinal ligaments is obtained by the surgeon and the uterus can be sufficiently mobilised to allow vaginal extraction. Even when the uterus is enlarged beyond 12–14 weeks vaginal hysterectomy can still be accomplished safely by means of morcellation, uterine bisection, wedge debulking, or intramyometrial coring techniques.

Benefits of vaginal hysterectomy over the abdominal: Morbidity of abdominal procedure like, wound infection and disruption, blood loss, intestinal obstruction, paralytic ileus, adhesions, deep vein thrombosis is less in vaginal hysterectomy. Postoperative pain and discomfort is less in vaginal hysterectomy, so need of less analgesia and early ambulation is possible. Duration of hospital stay is less. So more cost effective than the abdominal procedure.

Prior to vaginal procedure adnexa can be tackled by laparoscopy, thereby converting the hysterectomy into a vaginal procedure which would otherwise be an abdominal (LAVH).

Preoperative Preparation

For better postoperative healing of the vaginal vault, it is always advisable to give vaginal douche a day before and on the day of the surgery. This will help to clean the vaginal epithelium from any infection. The rectum is evacuated with an electrolyte purgative or fleet enema on the evening before surgery. Bowel cleansing evacuates solid stool from the rectum, reduces the bacterial load at the perineum, and reduces the incidence of postoperative ileus and constipation. Patient is kept fasting for 6–8 hours. Informed consent is taken.

Prophylactic broad-spectrum antibiotics are started before the surgery. The risk of postoperative infection can be reduced if antibiotics are given just before the surgery such that to be effective, the antibiotic must be in the tissue at the time of surgery.

Technique

Anaesthesia: It can be done under general, spinal or epidural anaesthesia. It depends on the condition and choice of the patient.

Positioning: The patient is positioned in the dorsal lithotomy position with the buttocks just over/well off the edge of the table. Type of stirrup used should take care to protect the vulnerable vascular, bony, and neurologic points of the lower limb. Use of adequate leg padding, avoiding marked flexion of the thigh, and avoiding pressure points, particularly laterally, where the peroneal nerve encircles the head of the fibula will prevent these injuries due to wrong positioning. In addition to this mild Trendelenburg (10–15°) positioning will help the surgeon to comfortably operate. Assistants need to stand inside the stirrups to see the operative field.

The vagina and perineum are cleansed with betadine or savlon lotion. In addition lavage of the vagina with saline will also help to reduce the postoperative infection. Bladder is drained with a metal catheter. The patient is then draped.

An examination under anaesthesia is now performed, in dorsal lithotomy position, to assess descent of the pelvic organs, respective defects, mobility, and uterine size. The final decision is made at this time as to whether the procedure can be done vaginally or abdominally.

A heavy speculum is placed into the posterior vagina. With a right-angle retractor anterior vagina is retracted and the cervix is visualised. The anterior and posterior lips of the cervix are grasped with a single- or double-toothed tenaculum/vulsellum forceps. Sounding the uterus now will help to confirm the suspected size and contour of the uterus.

Gentle traction over the cervix with the vulsellum is given in all directions so that the surgeon can visualise the cervicovaginal junction, the area where the initial incision has to be made. 0.5% lidocaine with 1:200,000 or a dilute solution of vasopressin may be injected into the paracervical tissue, the area around the uterosacral ligaments, the lower portion of the cardinal ligament, and the bladder pillars. This will help to decrease peroperative blood loss, and also to delineate the surgical planes. But the use of vasoconstrictive infiltration is not always necessary.

With adequate traction on the anterior and posterior lips of the cervix, a circumferential incision is made through the full thickness of vaginal epithelium at the cervicovaginal junction. Anteriorly, the junction is at where the vaginal rugae begin and the smooth cervical epithelium ends. As the incision is laid circumferentially, adequate counter-traction against the respective lateral vaginal wall will prove to be helpful. The full-thickness posterior vaginal mucosa is incised to meet the anterior incision. If this initial incision is made below the level of cervicovaginal junction close to the external os, a greater amount of dissection is needed to displace the vaginal mucosa and usually an increased amount of bleeding is encountered. And depth of the incision also should be adequate enough to involve only the full thickness of the vaginal mucosa, otherwise the dissection extends into the cervix leading to increased blood loss and technical difficulty. Now the vagina is dissected from the underlying tissue sharply with scissors or bluntly with the surgeon's sponge-covered finger. The bladder is dissected off the anterior lower uterine segment all the way up to the vesicouterine peritoneal fold. This step is frequently insufficiently performed for fear of entering the bladder.

Entry into the anterior cul-de-sac is difficult if this dissection is not sufficiently carried up to the vesicouterine peritoneal fold. The bladder is elevated with a right-angle retractor placed under the vaginal mucosa and bladder. Strong downward traction is applied on the cervix held by vulsellum. This manoeuvre aids in identifying the vesicouterine peritoneal fold which appears as a white transverse line across the lower uterine segment. It is grasped with forceps and incised with sharp curved scissors. The edge of this incision is held with artery forceps and a finger is inserted to explore the area so as to be sure that one is in the peritoneal cavity and not the bladder and also to identify any unsuspected pathologic condition that was not identified before. A right-angle retractor is placed into the peritoneal cavity underneath the finger. If the patient had a previous caesarean section, the scar of this procedure can be readily visualised and identified separately from the bladder. Sometimes, it is possible to dissect beneath the caesarean section scar to gain entry into the superior part of the vesicouterine space to identify the vesicouterine peritoneal fold.

With steep upward traction on the cervix, the cul-de-sac is exposed. Posterior vaginal cuff is retracted with forceps placing the peritoneum of the cul-de-sac on tension. The peritoneum of the cul-de-sac is incised with curved scissors. Care should be taken not to place this incision closer to the cervix in an attempt to prevent injury to the rectum, which results in retroperitoneal dissection ultimately pushing the peritoneum superiorly and posteriorly, thereby obscuring the identification of the peritoneum. Once the cul-de-sac is opened a finger inserted into the cul-de-sac and the area is explored for any unsuspected pathology. A right-angle retractor or weighted speculum is placed into the posterior cul-de-sac which will help to keep the rectum away from the operative site during the operation.

With the upward and lateral traction on cervix, a curved Heaney clamp is placed in the posterior cul-de-sac with one blade underneath the uterosacral ligament and the other over the uterosacral ligament, immediately lateral to the uterine cervix so that some carvical tissue is also included in this clamp. This prevents the possible ureteric damage during clamping of the uterosacral ligament. The uterosacral ligament is cut with curved scissors so that approximately 0.5 cm of tissue is distal to the clamp. A transfixion suture with 1-zero vicryl is placed at the tip of the clamp and tied. The procedure is repeated on the other side also. Next, the cardinal ligaments on both sides are identified, clamped, cut, and suture-ligated with 1-zero vicryl sutures in a manner similar to that previously described for the uterosacral ligaments.

Next the remaining portion of the broad ligament attached to the lower uterine segment containing the uterine artery is clamped, cut and suture ligated with 1-zero vicryl on both sides adjacent to the cervix. Use of a single clamp in the vaginal hysterectomy reduces the chance of ureteric damage.

The uterine fundus is now delivered out posteriorly by giving traction on the uterine fundus on the posterior aspect with tenaculum. By inserting fingers the utero-ovarian ligament is identified. Along with remaining portion of broad ligament and round ligament, it is clamped and cut. The pedicles are double-ligated, first with a suture tie and then with a suture ligature medial to the first tie. The fallopian tubes and ovaries are now inspected by drawing them into the operative field. If adnexa are to be removed, then the round ligaments should be clamped, cut and ligated separately. By applying traction on the utero-ovarian pedicle the ovary is drawn into the operative field with a Babcock clamp. A Heaney clamp is placed across the infundibulopelvic ligament, and the ovary and tube are excised. Even this pedicle is double ligated with a suture tie and a transfixation suture ligature.

When uterus size is big following techniques may be employed to facilitate the removal of the uterus—morcellation, intramyometrial coring, uterine bisection, and wedge debulking. Morcellation can be used in enlarged uterus, fixed uterus or when there is limited vaginal exposure. It should not be performed if the uterine arteries cannot be ligated or when malignancy is suspected. Intramyometrial coring is done by circumferentially incising the outer myometrium beneath the uterine serosa with a scalpel while placing the cervix on traction. The enlarged uterus is delivered as an elongated mass inverting the uterine fundus. Uterine bisection is performed by cutting the uterus from cervix to the uterine fundus in the sagittal plane.

The entire broad ligament with the pedicles from the tubo-ovarian round ligament anteriorly to the uetrosacral ligament posteriorly are exposed. Wet mop is placed in the peritoneal cavity to allow the surgeon to visualise the pedicles on both side and confirm the adequacy of haemostasis. If any bleeding points are present, it is ligated under direct vision.

Peritonealisation is done using a delayed absorbable suture beginning from anterior peritoneal edge. A continuous purse-string suture is applied beginning from 12 o'clock position proceeding in clockwise direction to incorporate the distal portion of the left upper pedicle and then the left uterosacral and cardinal ligaments. The suture then incorporates the posterior peritoneum as high as possible. The suture is then carried through the uterosacral and cardinal ligament on the patient's right side, and then through the right upper pedicle. This type of high peritoneal closure will help to prevent future enterocele formation.

The vaginal mucosa can be approximated either in a vertical or horizontal fashion, using either interrupted or continuous sutures. These sutures should involve the entire thickness of the vaginal epithelium, taking care not to take bite into the bladder anteriorly.

Vagina is packed with sterile gauze pack soaked with iodine solution. Bladder is catheterised for 24 hours. Both this pack and catheter is removed after 24 hours.

Postoperative care:

- Patient is kept nil oral for 12–24 hours as the intestinal mobility is sluggish.
- Hydration is maintained by IV fluids.
- Parenteral antibiotics for 24 hours followed by oral preparation. Analgesics may be required as there may be pelvic discomfort during the first 24–48 hours.
- Early ambulation will help to prevent DVT.

Complications

a. *Haemorrhage:* Bleeding may be from the vaginal cuff margin or from above from one of the pedicles. It may present as vaginal bleeding in the immediate postoperative period or retroperitoneal bleeding which may present with deterioration of vital signs with little amount of vaginal bleeding.
   Resuscitative measures should be undertaken. Haematocrit in the immediate postoperative period will give an idea of amount of blood loss. Ultrasound may sometimes be helpful if retroperitoneal/intraabdominal bleed is suspected. Blood transfusion is arranged. Patient is shifted to the theatre. Under anaesthesia vagina is inspected with proper light. If it seems to come from the cuff margins one or two re-enforcing stitches will stop the bleeding. If it appears to come from above, the vault stitches are opened and the bleeding pedicle is identified and ligated. Sometimes,

the bleeding vessel may get retracted and cannot be controlled from below. In that cases, laparotomy is done, bleeding vessel is identified if possible. If not then uni/bilateral anterior division of internal iliac artery ligation is done. Many retroperitoneal bleed stops on its own by tamponade effect forming a haematoma which eventually gets absorbed. Higher cover of antibiotics is put to prevent the infection of this haematoma.

b. *Sepsis:* In the form of pelvic infection is known to occur quite commonly after vaginal hysterectomy. Patient presents with fever, pain in lower abdomen and pelvis, tenderness in the vaginal cuff. Infection ranging from vaginal cuff cellulitis, pelvic cellulitis, pelvic abscess, infected pelvic haematoma, and adnexal abscess is known to occur. Usually pelvic cellulitis or vaginal cuff cellulitis gets controlled with combination of parenteral higher antibiotics. Pelvic abscess should be suspected when in spite of higher antibiotics the fever fails to come under control. Ultrasound helps in diagnosis. Vaginal cuff may need to be opened with an artery forceps and drain out the purulent material. Infected haematoma if present is drained. Once this is drained usually the sepsis gets controlled. Parenteral antibiotics are continued for another 24–48 hours after the temperature has come to normal **(Figs. 32-23 and 32-24)**.

Laparoscopic Hysterectomy

Laparoscopic hysterectomy is not an alternative to vaginal hysterectomy but for abdominal. Its main aim is to reduce the abdominal procedure which has higher morbidity in terms of intestinal adhesions, infection, blood loss, hospital stay, and postoperative pain.

Drawbacks

- Need of trained surgeons, and hospital staff.
- Equipment which are costly and difficult to maintain.
- Cost factor—not all patients can afford the procedure.

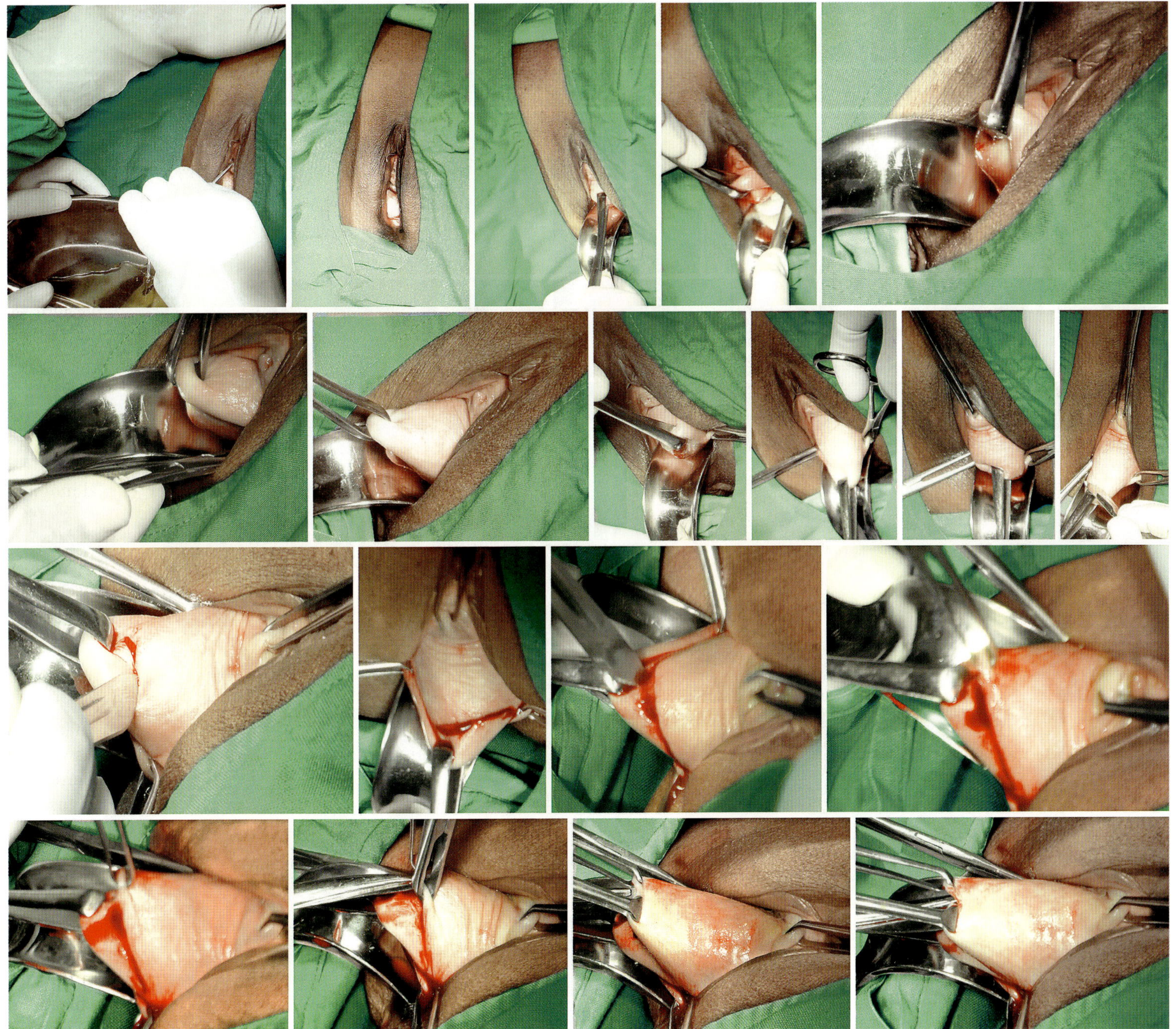

Figs. 32-23(1)

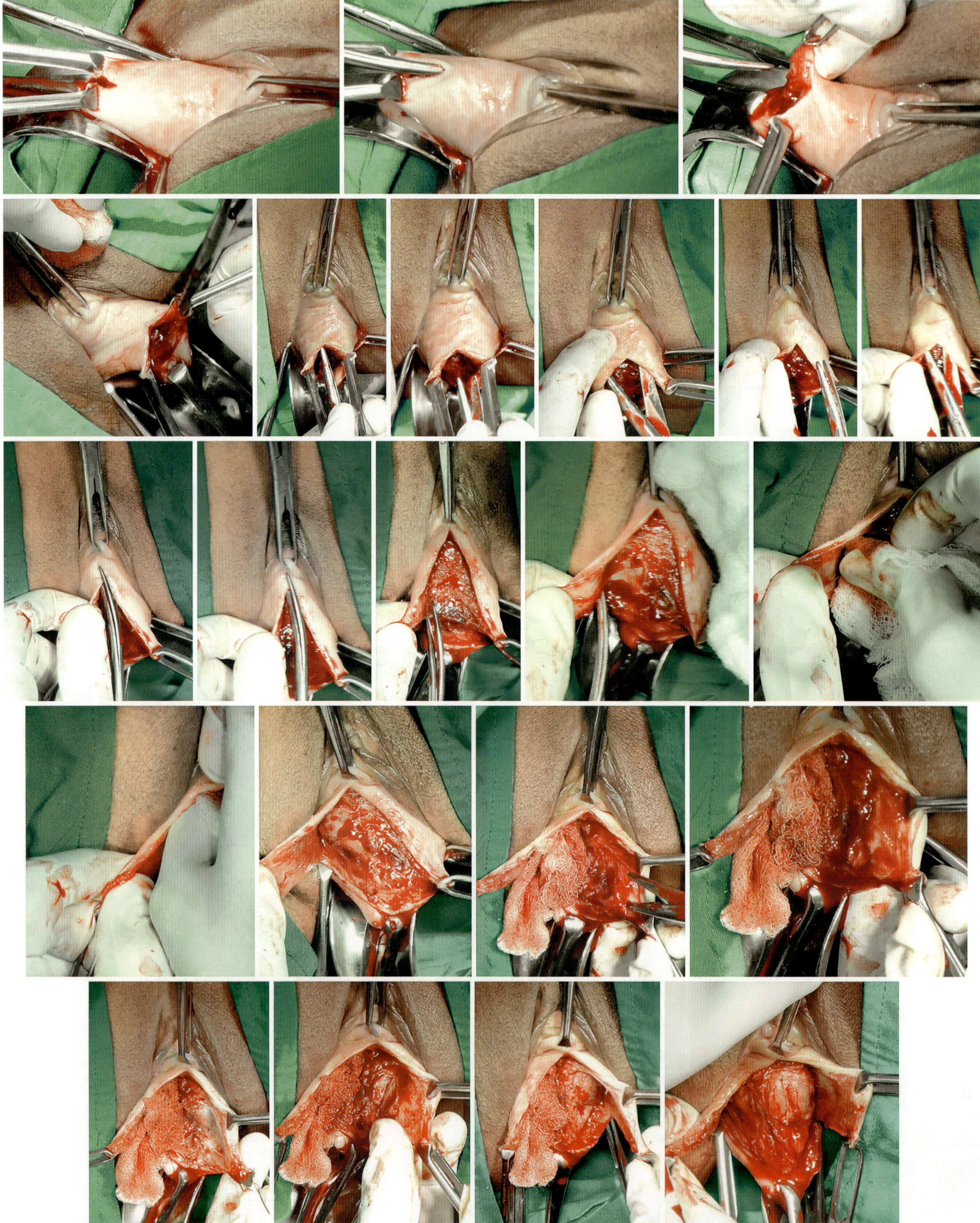

Figs. 32-23(2)

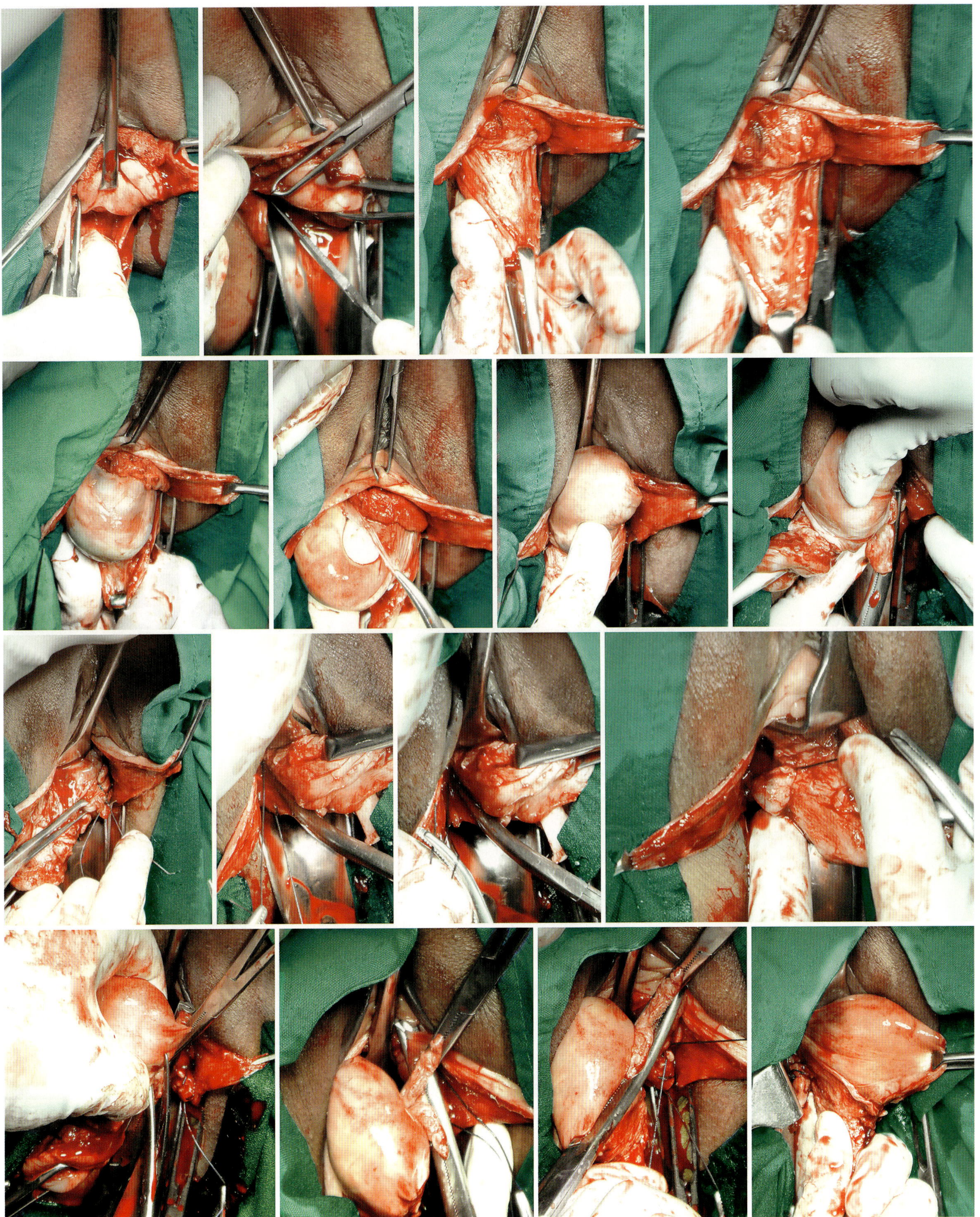

Figs. 32-23(3)

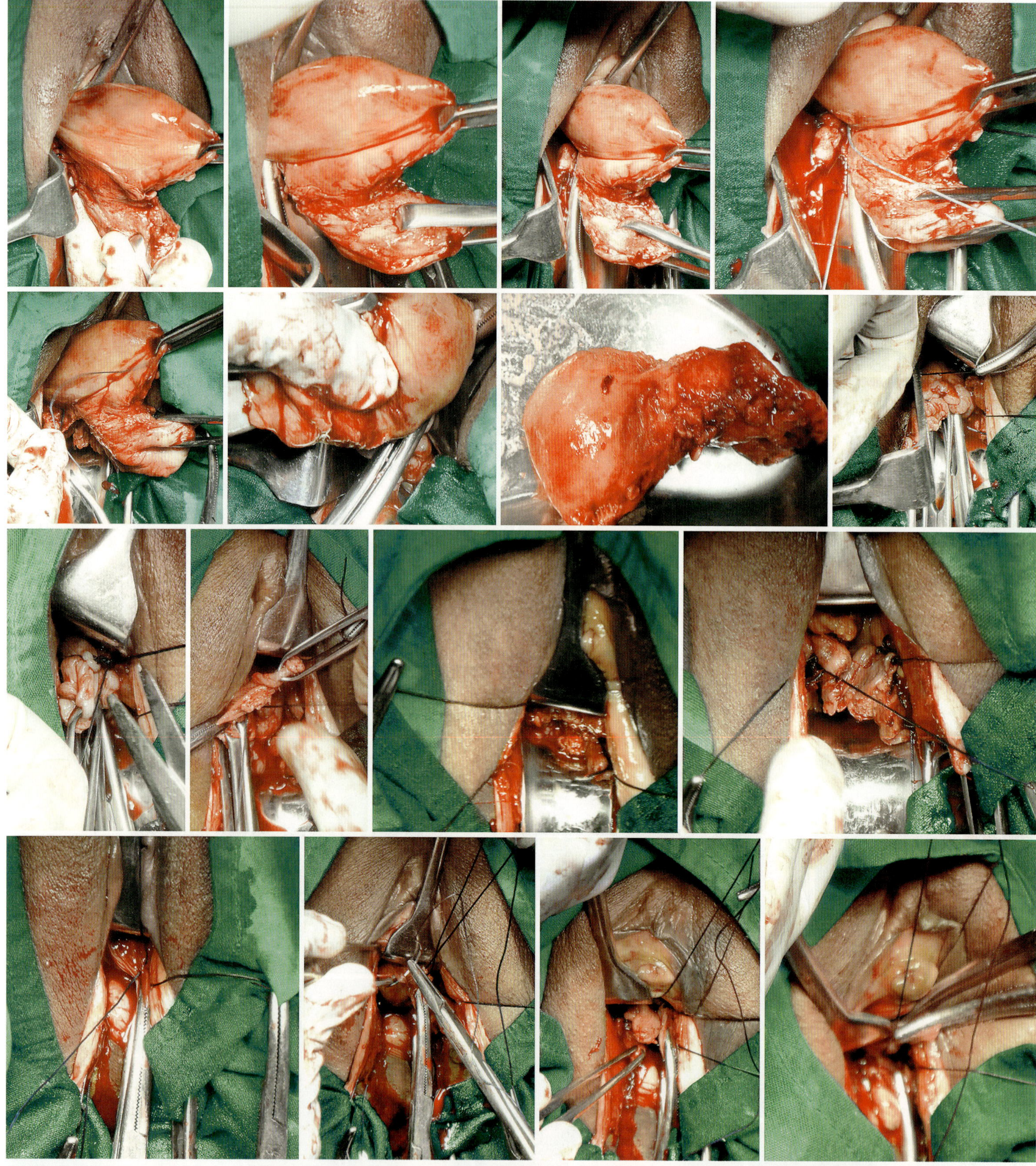

Figs. 32-23(4)

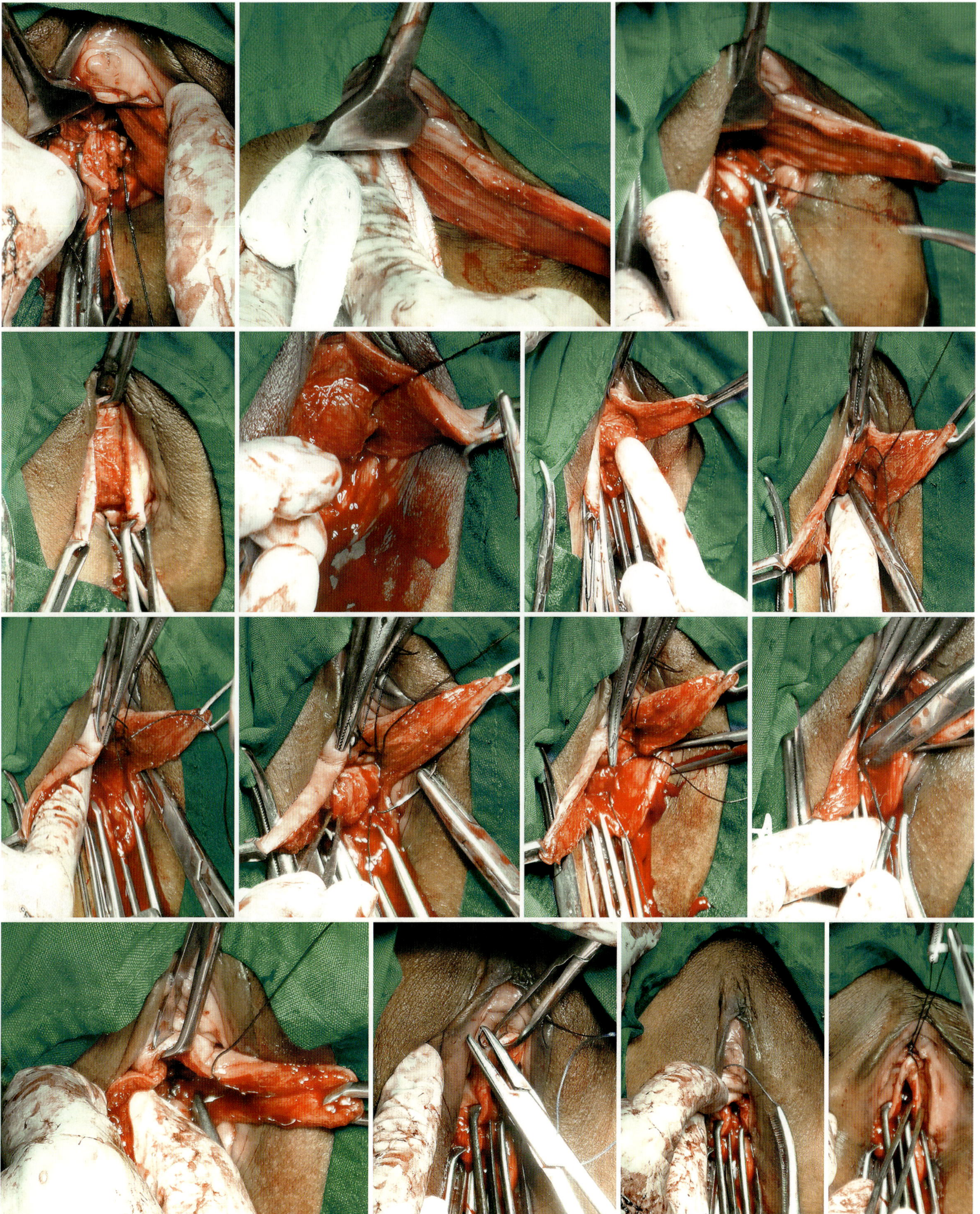

Figs. 32-23(5)

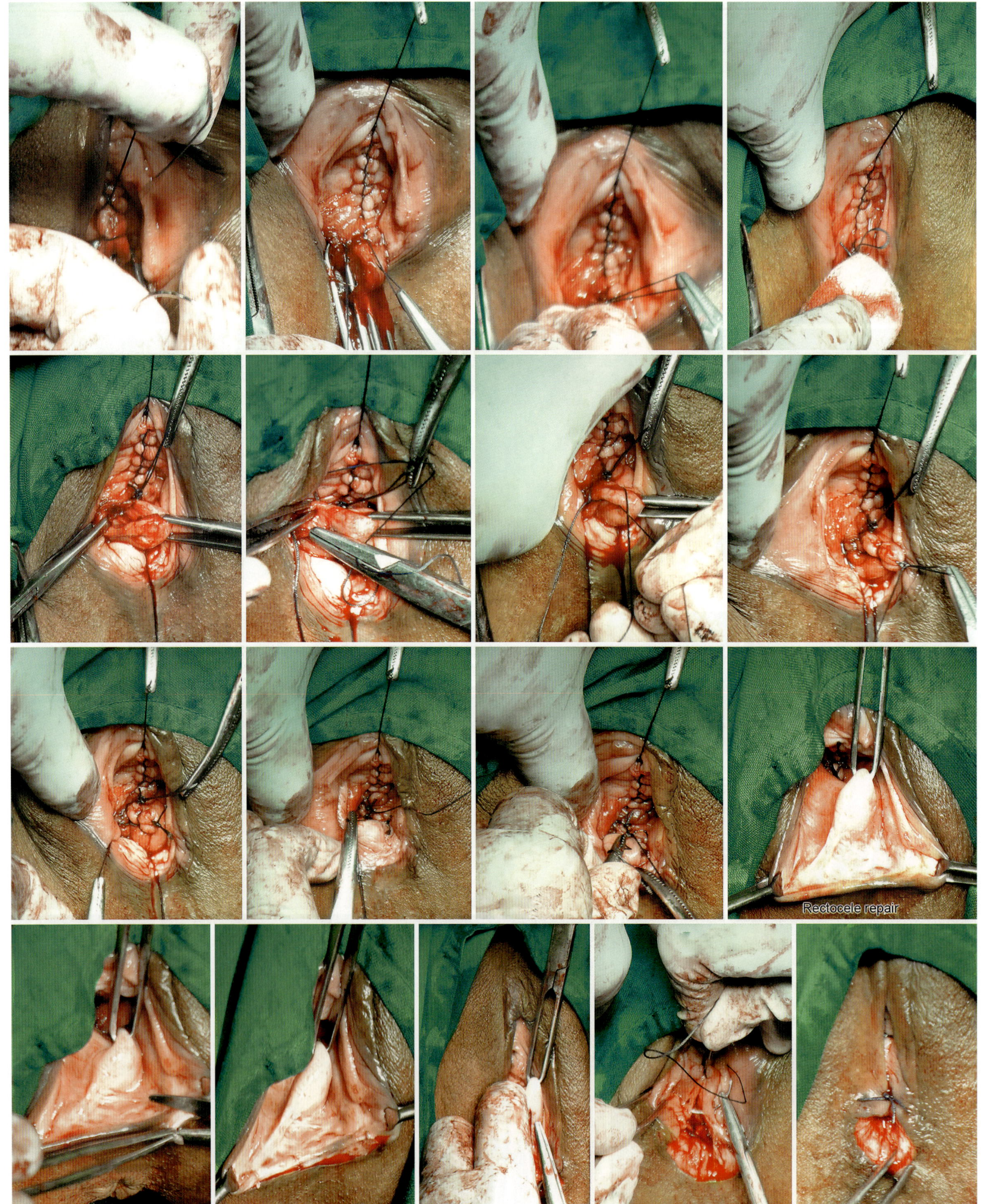

Figs. 32-23(6)

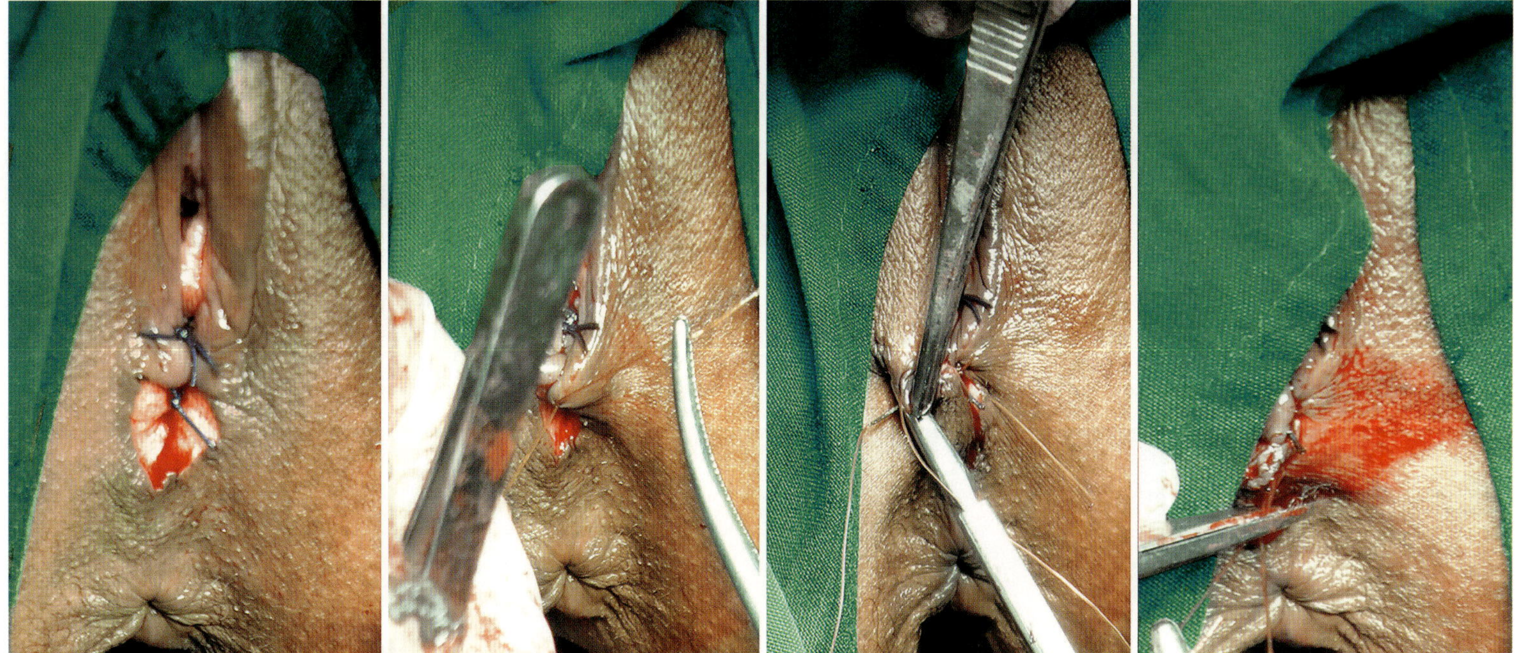

Figs. 32-23(7)

Figs. 32-23(1 to 7): Vaginal hysterectomy for uterine prolapse is technically demanding, skilled time consuming procedure. It is done under spinal anaesthesia in lithotomy position. After cleaning and draping, bladder is emptied using metal catheter. Cervix is held with vulsellum forceps. Anterior vaginal wall is incised like inverting 'T'. Anterior vaginal wall is separated carefully by blunt gauze and sharp scissor dissection to push the adherent bladder underneath upwards up to the urethral opening. Laterally is dissected adequately so as to make feasible to place Kocher's clamp. Peritoneum is opened both at uterovesical fold in front and uterovaginal fold behind. Fundus of the uterus is delivered out. Mackenrodt ligament, uterine pedicle and ovarian ligaments are serially ligated with transfixation carefully after applying Kocher's clamp and divided these structures. Usually 1- or 2-zero vicryl is used for transfixation ligatures. Uterus is removed. Peritoneum is closed with vicryl purse string sutures. Bladder is invaginated using purse string 2-zero vicryl sutures. Often polypropylene mesh may be placed to prevent recurrence of cystocele. Tied sutures of both Mackenrodt ligaments on both sides which were already kept long are passed through a needle and passed across the vaginal wall to continue with perineorrhaphy. Extra vault is carefully excised vertically. Vault (anterior vaginal wall) is sutured with 1-zero vicryl from above downwards as continuous locking sutures till the lower end. Suture passed across from the both side Mackenrodt ligaments are tied firmly on the vaginal wall. If rectocele is present, it is repaired. Horizontal incision is made on the posterior vaginal wall just above the skin margin; posterior vaginal wall is raised off the anterior rectal wall; care should be taken not to injure rectum; once this flap is elevated. Rectocele is repaired by placing interrupted sutures over pararectal tissues. 2/3 interrupted sutures are placed over the levator ani and tissues of perineal body; Rectum is pushed backwards when sutures are applied; posterior vaginal wall is excised adequately; remaining cut margin is resutured vertically using continuous vicryl suture to complete the rectocele repair. Foley's catheter is passed and kept in place for 5 days. vagina is packed with betadine soaked pack which is removed within 24 hours.

Types of Laparoscopic Surgery

- Laparoscopic-assisted vaginal hysterectomy (LAVH)
- Laparoscopic subtotal hysterectomy (LSH)
- Total laparoscopic hysterectomy (TLH)

Though laparoscopic supracervical hysterectomy (LSH) has been associated with a shorter operating time, decreased chances of visceral trauma, and less technical difficulty, however, some patients continue to have cyclical bleeding until menopause, and there is a small risk of developing cervical cancer in the retained cervix.

Preoperative Preparation

Routine tests including chest X-ray, ECG, ECHO is done. Patient kept fasting for 6–8 hours. Bowel is evacuated on the previous evening by enema. Prophylactic antibiotics are given. Informed consent taken. The chances of conversion to laparotomy is explained.

Preparation and Positioning

Patient is placed in a dorsal lithotomy position with pneumoboots. The arms are tucked by the sides and a foam mattress under the patient prevents the sliding during steep Trendelenburg position. Or the patient needs to be tied to the table to prevent from sliding. The table is kept in a lowest position. Monitor is placed directly facing the surgeon. Bladder is catheterised. Uterine manipulator is inserted after cleaning the perineum and vagina.

Instruments

- 10 mm telescope 0°/30°
- Video camera
- Light source—xenon source best
- Trocar—two 5 mm, three 10 mm
- 5 mm grasping forceps—toothed/plain
- Scissors
- Unipolar electrode
- Bipolar forceps and the electrical cable
- Suturing forceps
- Suction and irrigation system
- Optional—harmonic scalpel, ligasure, morcellator.

Technique

Primary trocar is inserted just below the umbilicus or above if the uterine size is big. It is inserted either by closed method with help of Veress needle or by open method by making a small incision near the umbilical margin and opening the peritoneum under vision. CO_2 gas is insufflated into the peritoneal cavity. Zero degree telescope

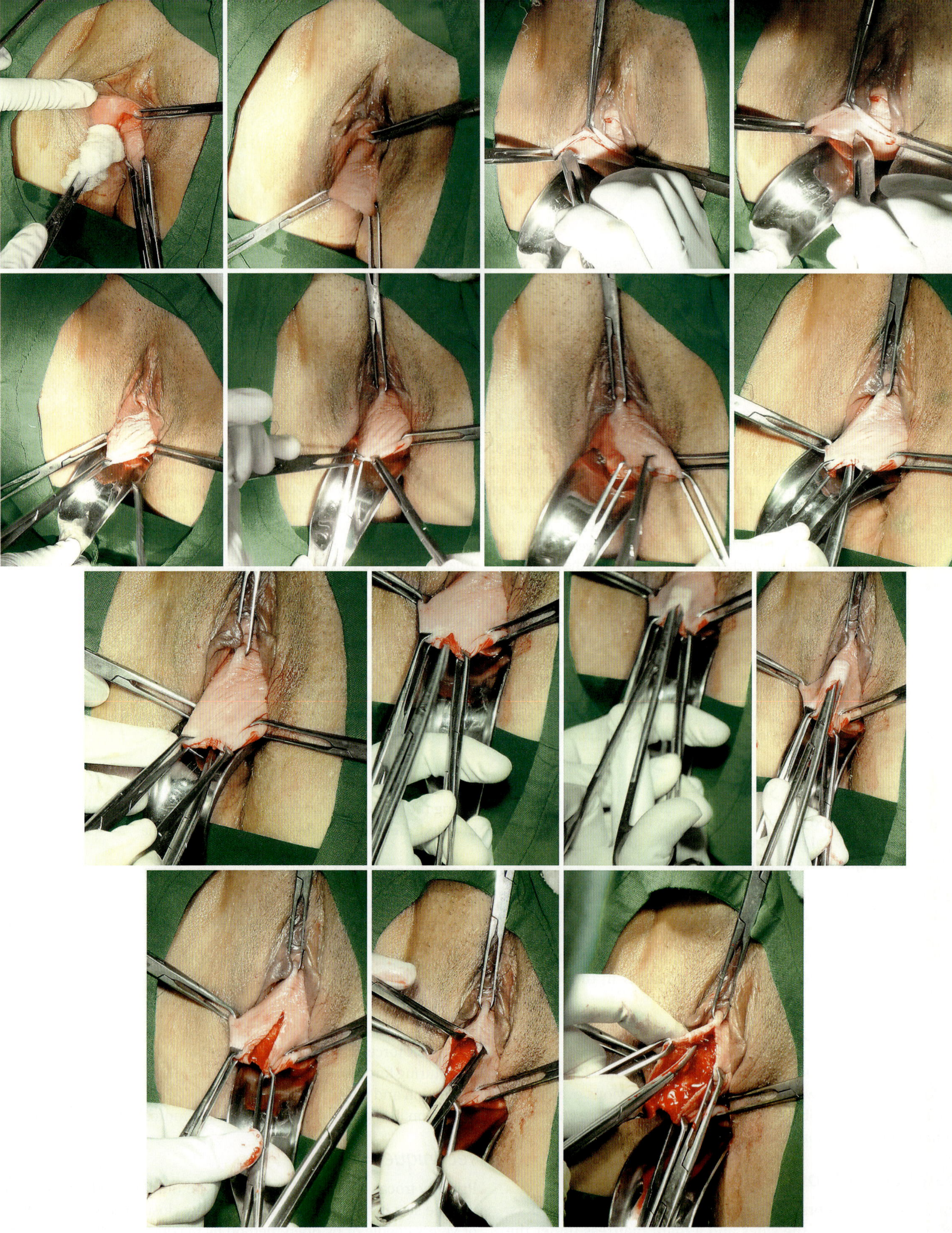

Figs. 32-24(1)

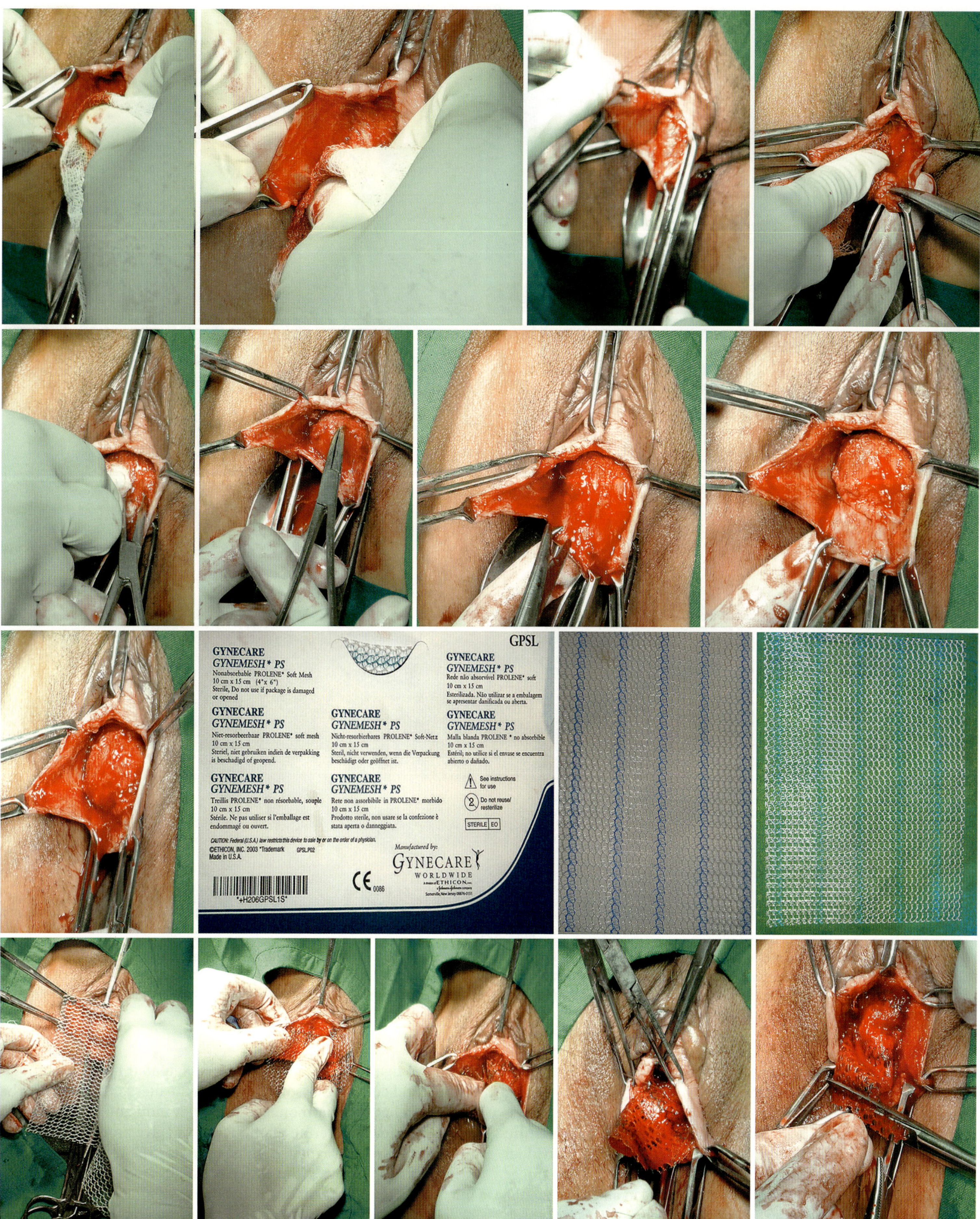
GPSL
GYNECARE
GYNEMESH* PS
Nonabsorbable PROLENE* Soft Mesh
10 cm x 15 cm (4"x 6")
Sterile, Do not use if package is damaged or opened
GYNECARE
GYNEMESH* PS
Rede não absorvível PROLENE* soft
10 cm x 15 cm
Esterilizada. Não utilizar se a embalagem se apresentar danificada ou aberta.
GYNECARE
GYNEMESH* PS
Niet-resorbeerbaar PROLENE* soft mesh
10 cm x 15 cm
Steriel, niet gebruiken indien de verpakking is beschadigd of geopend.
GYNECARE
GYNEMESH* PS
Nicht-resorbierbares PROLENE* Soft-Netz
10 cm x 15 cm
Steril, nicht verwenden, wenn die Verpackung beschädigt oder geöffnet ist.
GYNECARE
GYNEMESH* PS
Malla blanda PROLENE * no absorbible
10 cm x 15 cm
Estéril; no utilice si el envase se encuentra abierto o dañado.
GYNECARE
GYNEMESH* PS
Treillis PROLENE* non résorbable, souple
10 cm x 15 cm
Stérile. Ne pas utiliser si l'emballage est endommagé ou ouvert.
GYNECARE
GYNEMESH* PS
Rete non assorbibile in PROLENE* morbido
10 cm x 15 cm
Prodotto sterile, non usare se la confezione è stata aperta o danneggiata.
See instructions for use
Do not reuse/ restorilize
STERILE EO
CAUTION: Federal (U.S.A.) law restricts this device to sale by or on the order of a physician.
©ETHICON, INC. 2003 *Trademark GPSL.P02
Made in U.S.A.
Manufactured by:
GYNECARE
WORLDWIDE
ETHICON
+H206GPSL1S
CE 0086

Figs. 32-24(2)

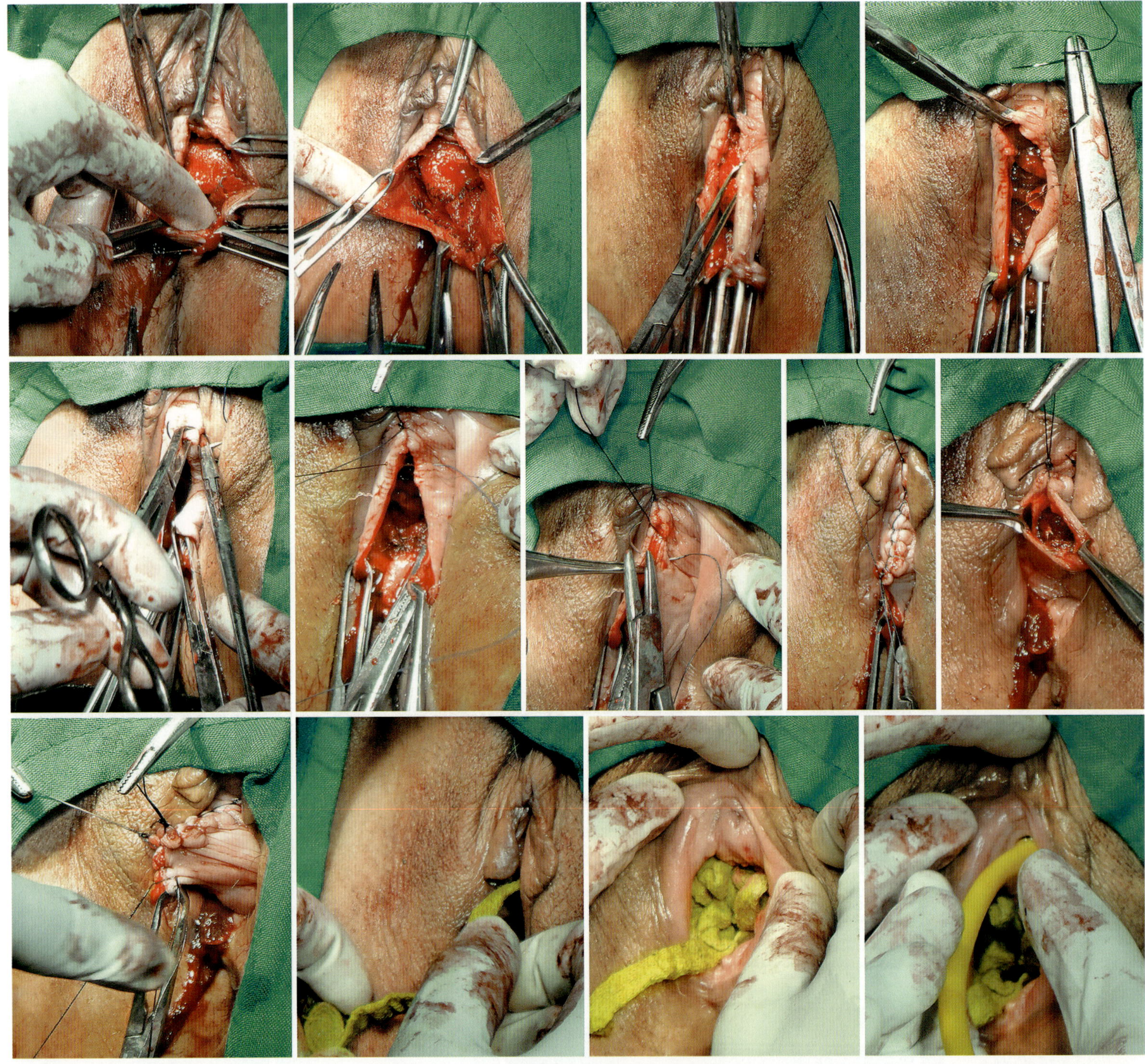

Figs. 32-24(3)

Figs. 32-24(1 to 3): Cystocele repair done by placing specialised polypropylene mesh under the anterior vaginal wall. After opening the anterior vaginal wall, urinary bladder is separated from the anterior vaginal wall laterally up to the pubic ramus. Mesh is placed snuggly over the bladder, the sides of which is anchored to the vaginal flaps near the pubic ramus. Vaginal flaps are trimmed. Excess trimming is avoided. Anterior vaginal flaps are closed with continuous locking sutures using no. 1 chromic catgut.

is inserted through this trocar. Whole of the abdomen and pelvic anatomy is visualised. Any visceral injury during trocar insertion is looked for. Liver, under surface of the diaphragm, paracolic gutters, appendix are visualised for any additional pathology. Now the number of working ports and their site is decided by the individual surgeon and the pelvic pathology. Two lateral ports for 5 mm trocar are inserted under vision 2 cm above and medial to anterior superior iliac spine. Care is taken to avoid injury to inferior epigastric vessel. One 10 mm port lateral to the rectus at the level of umbilicus is put on left side (surgeon side). Additional ports may be put depending on requirement of the surgeon.

Round ligament on both sides is coagulated first with bipolar forceps and cut with scissors, 3 cm from the uterus. This can also be done with ligasure/harmonic scalpel. Elevation and traction to the opposite side with uterine manipulator will give proper exposure of the pedicles to be coagulated. If the ovary is to be removed, ureter is identified at the pelvic brim which is usually easy on the right side, but may be more difficult on the left due to sigmoid colon. The ovary or fallopian tube is grasped from the contralateral side for proper exposure of the infundibulopelvic ligament. Infundibulopelvic ligament is coagulated with bipolar forceps/ligasure under vision and sectioned. It is better to coagulate the pedicle with bipolar before using harmonic scalpel. While coagulating care is taken to see that ureter and iliac vessels are far away from the coagulating instrument. The coagulation and ligation are then proceeded anteriorly to join the previously sectioned area of the round ligament. The procedure is repeated on the opposite side. If the ovaries are to be preserved then the utero-ovarian ligaments are coagulated close to the ovaries and sectioned. Special care is taken to desiccate the parametrial veins that run between the ovary and the round ligament as these can be quite tortuous and tend to bleed if left unattended.

The procedure can now be carried from vaginal route (LAVH). Vaginal route can also be proceeded after opening the uterovaginal pouch and pushing the bladder down.

At the junction where round ligament is sectioned, the leaves of the broad ligament is separated with a Maryland grasper. The anterior leaf of broad ligament is opened downwards and forwards towards the bladder on either side with monopolar hook. Uterovesical junction is identified, grasped and elevated with forceps, cut with scissors or monopolar hook. The bladder pillars are identified, cut with scissors thereby freeing and pushing the bladder off the lower uterine segment and cervix with a blunt suction probe. In patients with history of prior caesarean delivery, this area may be scarred and is important to stay relatively high on the uterus during the dissection. A re-evaluation of the route of dissection is advised if fat is encountered because the fat belongs to the bladder indicating that the dissection is moving too close to the bladder.

Due to variation in anatomy and the course of the uterine vessels, it is initially helpful to skeletonise them. With the uterine manipulator uterus is pushed cephalad and to opposite side which helps to move the uterine vessels away from the ureter. The ascending uterine vessels are coagulated with the bipolar forceps at the level of internal cervical os, staying above the rim of the cervical cup. When the bubbles stop coming from the vessel it means that the vessel is desiccated completely and is safe to transect with the scissors or harmonic scalpel. Uterine artery can also be coagulated and cut with ligasure. Uterosacral ligaments are desiccated and cut.

Disposable silicone tube of diameter of 45 mm or 35 mm is inserted into the vagina and is pushed upwards and forwards. This tube helps to stretch the cervicovaginal junction and helps in identifying the vaginal fornices. The outer end of the tube is covered with a cap thus helping to maintain the pneumoperitoneum. The uterine movements can be controlled with help of myoma screw inserted through 5 mm trocar. Colpotomy is done along the indentation of the vaginal tube, first anteriorly with monopolar hook or harmonic scalpel and extended laterally. The lateral angle of the vault may need to be coagulated with bipolar or ligasure as vaginal branches of uterine arteries are frequently encountered. Colpotomy is continued on posterior aspect. Thus uterus with cervix is separated. It can be drawn out through the vagina. If uterus is large it can be broken down with morcellator. Vaginal vault can be sutured laparoscopically or from the vagina. If vault suturing is done laparoscopically then pneumoperitoneum has to be maintained either by a wet mop placed in the vagina or placing the uterus drawn from the pelvis in the vagina. Vault is closed laparoscopically by 1-zero vicryl continuous sutures using needle holder forceps. With training and practice suturing by laparoscope would not be a difficult job **(Fig. 32-25)**.

Once the suturing is done mop from the vagina is removed. Pelvis is irrigated with saline. All pedicles are seen for any sign of bleeding. Once haemostasis is confirmed CO_2 gas insufflation is stopped. Trocars are removed under vision. Telescope is removed. Trocar site is closed with 2-zero vicryl sutures/Dermabond.

Patient is kept nil oral for 24 hours. Catheter can be removed in 24 hours. Antibiotics are continued for 5 days. Patient can be discharged from the hospital in 3–4 days.

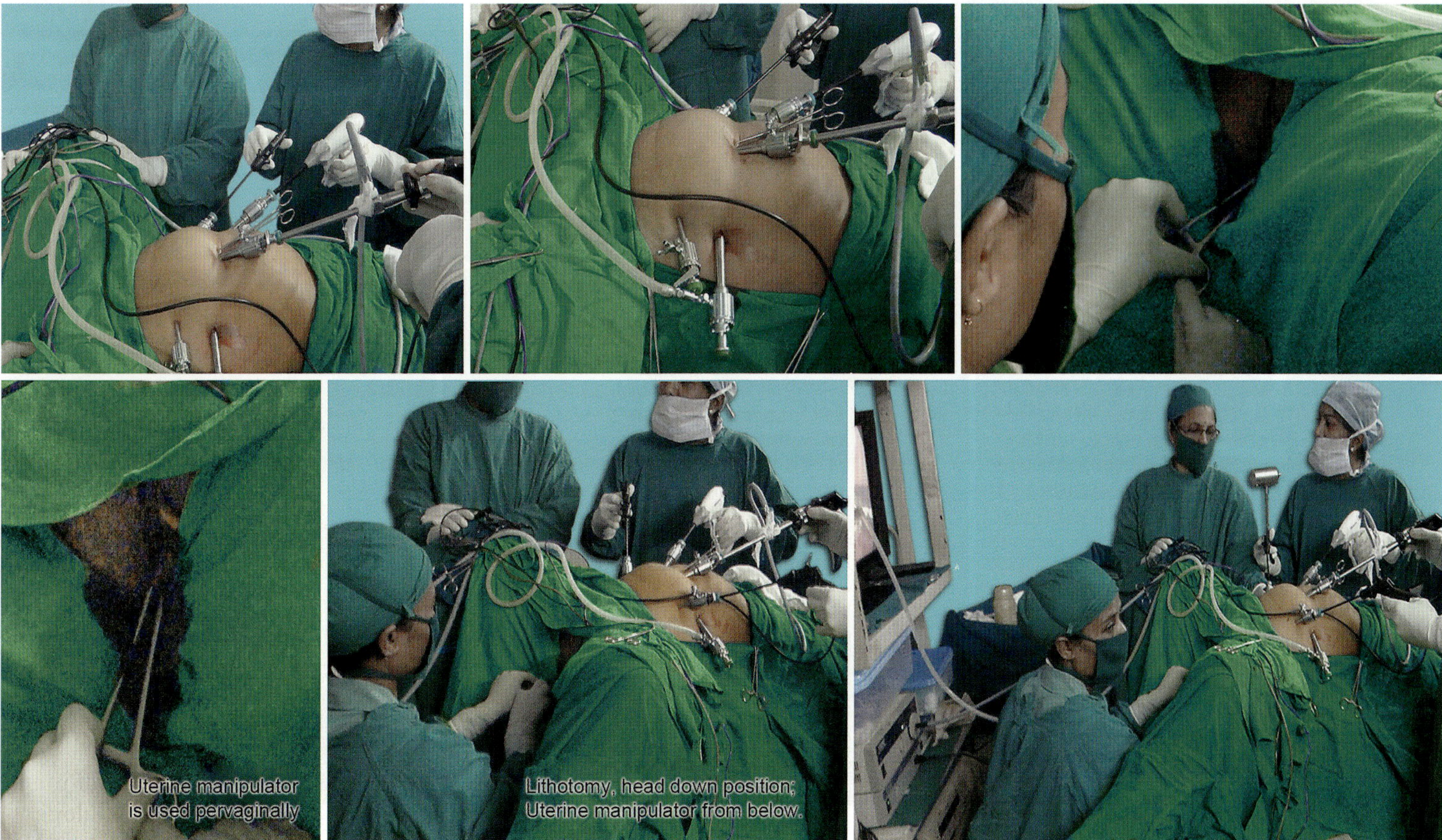

Figs. 32-25(1)

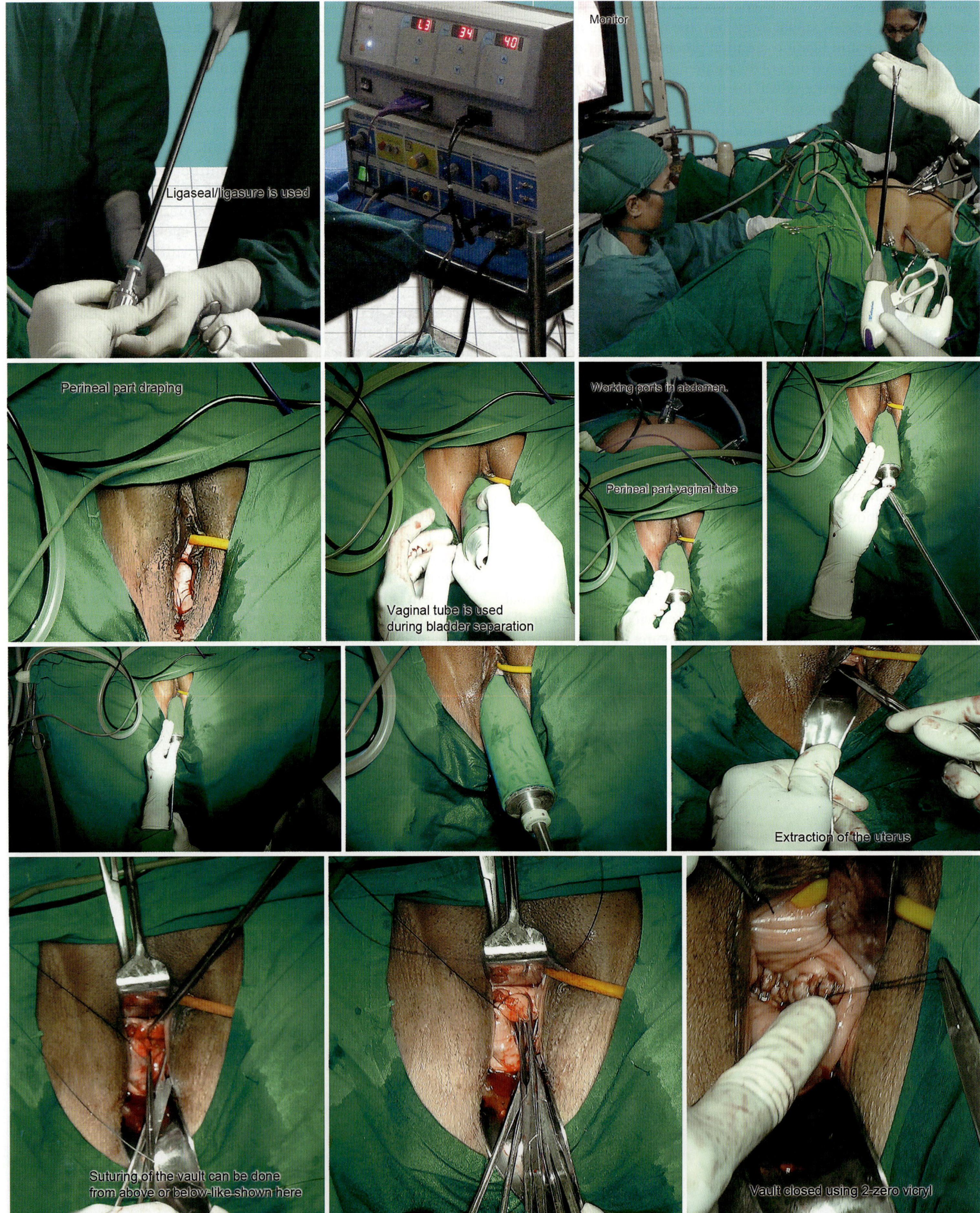
Ligaseal/ligasure is used
Monitor
Perineal part draping
Vaginal tube is used
during bladder separation
Working ports in abdomen.
Perineal part-vaginal tube
Extraction of the uterus
Suturing of the vault can be done
from above or below-like shown here
Vault closed using 2-zero vicryl

Figs. 32-25(2)

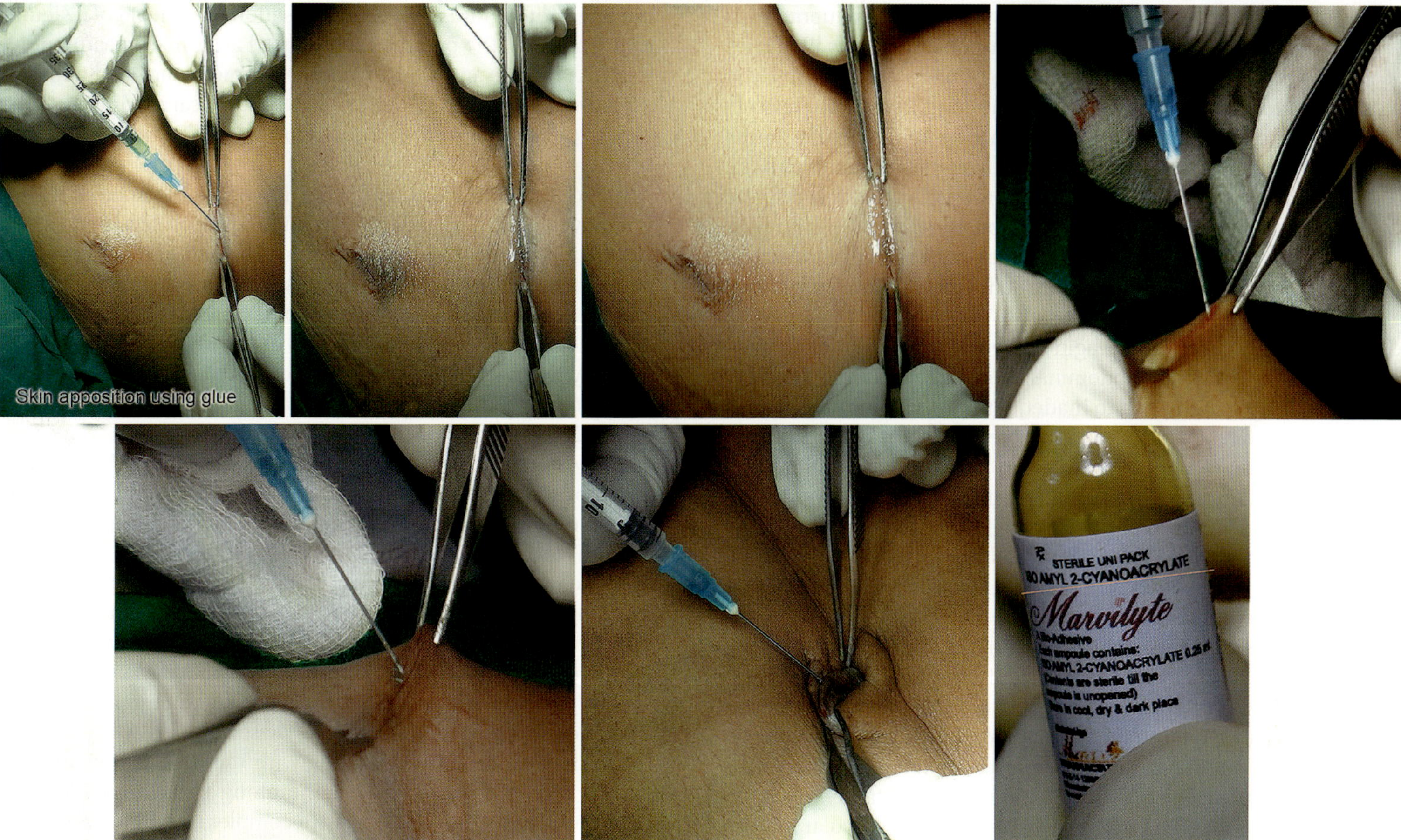

Figs. 32-25(3)

Figs. 32-25(1 to 3): External part of the laparoscopic hysterectomy—position, ports, vaginal tube and uterine manipulator.

Complications

a. *Injury to bladder:* Endometriosis, previous surgery, inexperience of surgeon, over distended bladder, and pelvic adhesions are proposed risk factors for bladder injury. Bladder injury can occur during insertion of trocar, especially in the suprapubic site piercing dome of the bladder; in base while separating the bladder off the cervix especially in patient who had previous caesarean section where adhesion are present between the bladder wall and cervix; or as the result of thermal energy. Fistula may result due to thermal injury. In suspected cases, the bladder is filled with methylene blue dye and observed for leakage of dye. Unrecognised cases present with abdominal discomfort and oliguria as cardinal sign. According to type, size, and localisation of injury, surgical management is planned via laparoscopy, laparotomy, or vaginal approach. Bladder can be repaired successfully by laparoscope or by laparotomy with 2 layer of 2-zero vicryl sutures.
b. *Ureteral injury:* Electrocautery (unipolar or bipolar) is the leading cause of laparoscopic iatrogenic ureteral injury. Injuries with loop suturing, trocars, laser devices, staples, and sharp dissection are also known. The 3 following locations carry the risk for ureteral injury during laparoscopic surgeries: at the pelvic brim, where the ureters lie beneath the insertions of the infundibulopelvic ligaments; deep ovarian fossa where the ureter passes; and the ureteral canal. Ureters are often injured while coagulating the uterine arteries, 4–5 cm above the uterovesical junction. Lack of precise recognition of the cervicovaginal margin and dissection too far down the vagina can injure the ureter 2 cm to 3 cm from the ureterovesical junction. Injuries may include transection, ligation, avulsion, crush injury, devascularisation, resection, fulguration, and perforation.
   Intraoperative methods for identifying ureteral injury:
   - 5 mL to 10 mL intravenous indigo carmine injection
   - Intraoperative ureteral catheterisation
   - Intravenous excretory urography
   - Dissection of the ureter.

   Intraperitoneal urine leak cannot be demonstrated in a coagulated or ligated ureter when tested intraoperatively. Absence of ureteral jet on cystoscopic examination reveals the problem clearly in such a case.

   Depending on the type of injury, patients may present in the early postoperative period or the presentation of thermal or laceration injuries may be delayed by several days or weeks. Postoperative presentation is variable and non-specific, such as acute pelvic pain, nausea, vomiting, malaise, and leakage of fluid though the trocar sites, abdominal distension, costovertebral angle tenderness, ileus, fever, peritonitis. X-ray of the abdomen may reveal a ground-glass appearance indicating fluid collection; CT scan reveals the presence of urine in the peritoneal cavity after intravenous injection of contrast medium.

   Repair by laparoscope can be done if recognised intra-operatively. If recognised in the early postoperative period passing double J-shaped stent allows spontaneous healing of focal ureteral injuries. But delayed recognition, and extensive damage may require laparotomy to perform an end-to-end anastomosis or ureteral re-implantation.
c. *Intestinal injury:* Nearly half of bowel injuries occur during trocar insertion and the rest occur during the operation. Entry-related

bowel injuries are mostly lacerations common in patients with previous laparotomies. Most of the intraoperative bowel injuries are thermal and is not diagnosed during surgery leading to delayed intervention which may be life-threatening. If intraoperatively unrecognised, patients present with non-specific complaints not exactly pointing to peritonitis, such as mild abdominal pain, fever, diarrhoea, and abdominal distension, further delaying the diagnosis. Late consequences may be generalised peritonitis, abscess formation, and septic shock. Intestinal obstruction though rare can occur when obstructive small-bowel adhesions develop to the vaginal apex.

d. *Haemorrhage:* Present as vaginal haemorrhage, retroperitoneal haemorrhage, and intraabdominal haemorrhage. Intraabdominal haemorrhage can be due to inadequate coagulation or excessive coagulation leading to charring and break off of the adjacent vessel wall. Bleeding can also occur due to trauma to abdominal wall vessels while trocar insertion. Injury to inferior epigastric vessel and less commonly muscular arteries are known to occur. They may present as continuous dripping of blood from the port during surgery or massive intraperitoneal bleed in postoperative period or abdominal wall haematoma which may get infected. Bleeding is controlled by tamponade or suturing. Sometimes may require exploration of the portal site to visualise the bleeding vessel and ligate it under vision. It is good practice to inspect all the trocar sites for any active bleeding before the laparoscope is finally withdrawn. Retroperitoneal major vascular injuries are related to the Veress needle, trocar, or energy source. It is trauma to aorta, vena cava, or, more commonly, the common iliac vessel. Major vascular injuries rarely remain unrecognised intraoperatively. Immediate laparotomy is done by midline incision and the vessel repair is done.
e. *Sepsis:* May present with wound infection especially of umbilical site, vault granuloma, pelvic cellulitis.
f. *Hernia:* It can occur at the trocar site. It is common in the extra-umbilical port of ≥10 mm size not adequately repaired. Bowel, omentum may get sucked into the portal site leading to intestinal obstruction. Laparotomy is needed for this. To minimise the risk of herniation, secondary trocars should be removed under supervision before the primary one, valves should be kept closed to prevent a sucking effect, 5 mm trocars should be preferred as much as possible and the trocar site should be correctly closed.
g. *Others problems related to pneumoperitoneum:* Subcutaneous emphysema, pneumomediastinum, and pneumothorax, gas embolism. All discussed in detail in the previous chapters.

Radical Hysterectomy

Indications: Radical hysterectomy is performed as a primary therapy for:

- Stage IB or IIA cancer of the cervix.
- Selected patients with stage IIb adenocarcinoma of endometrium (with gross cervical invasion)
- Upper vaginal carcinoma, uterine or cervical sarcomas, and other rare malignancies confined to the area of the cervix, uterus, and/or upper vagina.
- As a potential salvage therapy for women with cervical cancer who have been treated with irradiation and subsequently develop a small central pelvic recurrence or have a small central area of persistent disease.

Types of radical hysterectomy:

- *Type 1 hysterectomy is extrafascial, or simple hysterectomy* which involves removal of the cervix along with the uterine corpus, but does not require ureteral mobilisation or removal of a significant amount of the parametria. It is used as primary treatment for stage IA1 disease and after concurrent chemotherapy and radiation therapy for stage IB2 and bulky stage IIA cervical carcinoma.
- *Type 2 (modified) radical hysterectomy, or Wertheim operation,* involves more extensive dissection than the extrafascial hysterectomy where the central portion of the parametrial tissues is removed while minimising disruption of the ureteral and vesical vasculature. It involves removal of medial half of the uterosacral ligaments and the cardinal ligaments, ligation of the uterine artery just medial to the point where it crosses the ureter, removal of a 1–2 cm portion of the upper vagina along with pelvic and para-aortic lymphadenectomy. Here it does not involve dissection of the ureter from the vesicouterine ligament. It is done in stage IA2 cervical carcinoma.
- *Type 3 radical hysterectomy,* originally described by *Meigs,* aims at removal of parametrial tissue as much as possible. It involves transaction of the uterosacral ligaments near their origin from the sacrum, excision of the cardinal ligaments as widely as possible after the uterine artery is ligated at its origin where it branches off from the hypogastric artery, removal of a 2–3 cm portion of the upper vagina along with pelvic and para-aortic lymphadenectomy. Care is taken to preserve the superior vesical artery.
- *Type 4 hysterectomy* is seldom done, represents an extended radical hysterectomy. It involves complete dissection of the ureter from the vesicouterine ligament along with sacrifice of the superior vesical artery. 3/4th of the vagina along with the uterus and parametria are removed along with complete lymphadenectomy.
- *Type 5 hysterectomy* also has limited application. This procedure involves resection of involved portions of the bladder, distal ureter, rectum along with the uterus, parametria, adnexa, and pelvic lymph nodes. Subsequent ureteral reimplantation is done.

Preoperative preparations:

- Abdominal and pelvic CT scan/MRI helps to evaluate the pelvic disease, ureter and lymph nodes.
- Along with routine blood investigations patients should have a thorough evaluation to insure that there are no other major medical contraindications to surgery. ECG, ECHO, chest X-ray are done to rule out cardiac complications.
- As there is potential for blood loss in these patients, central venous access should be done by an anaesthetist and required amount of properly typed and cross-matched blood should be kept ready. Anaemic patients should receive preoperative blood transfusion.
- Prophylactic antibiotic, usually a first generation cephalosporin is started.
- Patients are asked to start liquid diet 24 hours before surgery. Bowel preparation is done with Peglec/exelyte.
- For thromboembolic prophylaxis subcutaneous injection of low molecular weight heparin is started prior to surgery and continued in the postoperative period.
- Sequential compression devices (SCDs) are placed on both lower limb immediately prior to surgery, and are left in place until the patient becomes ambulant.

Technique

The patient is placed in the modified dorsal supine lithotomy position (15° Trendelenburg). The urethral orifice, vaginal introitus, and anal orifice are all available for instrumentation in this position and a second assistant can stand at the foot of the table between the patient's legs. The thighs are elevated 15 to 20° relative to the abdomen as there will be less strain on the patient's lumbosacral spine in this position. Care is taken to avoid pressure on the peroneal nerves in the legs by giving cushions. The abdomen from the rib margin to the midthigh, perineum, and vagina are surgically prepared. The bladder is emptied with a Foley catheter. A thorough bimanual examination is always performed. This can be followed by cystoscopy or proctosigmoidoscopy.

An abdominal incision is made in the midline, extending around and 2–3 cm above the umbilicus and inferiorly up to the pubic symphysis. Self-retaining retractors are used to retract the muscle. Moist pack is placed beneath each arm of the self-retaining retractor to avoid excessive compression of the epigastric vessels that course beneath the rectus muscles and it is advisable to release the mechanical retractors at periodic intervals to improve circulation through the abdominal musculature.

Before starting the dissection in the pelvis, the entire abdominal cavity is carefully evaluated for evidence of metastatic disease. This includes superior and inferior surfaces of the liver and under surface of diaphragm, the celiac plexus, omentum, serosal surface of small and large bowel as well as the mesentery. The kidneys and the retroperitoneal space along the aorta and vena cava is palpated because these are the major sites of extrapelvic spread of cervical cancer. Pelvic and para-aortic/para-caval lymph nodes are palpated, and any enlarged or suspicious nodes are removed and sent for histopathology. If there is histopathologic evidence of unsuspected, metastatic tumour in a para-aortic lymph node, radical hysterectomy operation is abandoned. These patients are treated with concurrent chemotherapy and extended-field radiation therapy.

Intestines are packed in upper abdomen with moist packs. Uterus is held by Kelly Clamps applied at its corneal ends. The round ligament is clamped, cut, and ligated near the lateral pelvic wall. The anterior leaf of the broad ligament is incised inferiorly along the lateral pelvic wall for a distance of approximately 3 cm. The posterior leaf of the broad ligament is incised superiorly along the lateral pelvic wall to the level of the infundibulopelvic ligament. The infundibulopelvic ligament is clamped, cut, and doubly ligated at the lateral pelvic wall. Next the utero-ovarian ligament is clamped, cut, and ligated, and the tube and ovary are removed. The procedure is repeated on the other side.

The retroperitoneal space is approached along the lateral pelvic wall. The common iliac, external iliac, and internal iliac arteries and associated lymph nodal tissue are exposed. The ureter is identified. By placing two silk sutures in the adjacent medial peritoneum the ureter is pulled medially away from the iliac vessels. The base of the aorta is exposed. The lymph nodal tissue surrounding the common iliac, external iliac, and internal iliac arteries are all removed by sharp dissection from the bifurcation of the aorta to the inguinal ligament at the femoral canal. Care is taken to avoid bleeding from the middle sacral vessels as well as from the proximal part of the left external iliac vein, which courses through this retroperitoneal space. Only the loose areolar tissue and fascial sheath from the iliac vessels; should be removed avoiding trauma to the intima or wall of the vessels particularly the veins. The external iliac and common iliac arteries are retracted laterally, and lymph nodal tissue surrounding the common iliac, external iliac, and internal iliac veins are removed by sharp dissection. The genitofemoral nerve lying lateral to the external iliac vessels, should be preserved because damage to this nerve produces postoperative discomfort in the groin and medial aspect of the thigh. Lymph nodes from each of the major anatomic sites (i.e. common iliac, external iliac, internal iliac) is placed in separate containers, labeled accordingly and sent for histologic analysis. The external iliac artery and vein are retracted laterally by a vein retractor. All lymphatic tissues are removed from behind these vessels and from the obturator fossa by sharp dissection. Particular care is taken to avoid trauma to the obturator nerve and vessels. They are also labeled separately and sent for histology. The obturator nerve is identified and preserved. The uterine artery is identified as it comes off the anterior division of the internal iliac artery and is ligated and tied with 2-0 suture. All these procedure is repeated on the opposite side.

By blunt dissection, the pararectal space and paravesical spaces are exposed on both sides with the intervening web, which is the lateral extent of the cardinal ligament.

The paravesical space composed of loose connective tissue and fat is bounded by:

- Medially by the bladder and the retropubic space
- Laterally by the pelvic sidewall and obturator internus muscle
- Posteriorly by the cardinal ligament
- Anteriorly by the pubic symphysis
- Floor by the levator muscle
- Roof by the anterior leaf of the broad ligament that blends with the bladder peritoneum medially and the parietal peritoneum laterally.

The pararectal space is bounded by:

- Medially by the rectum
- Laterally by the hypogastric artery (the internal iliac artery)
- Posteriorly by the sacrum
- Anteriorly by the cardinal ligament.

The lateral aspect of the cardinal ligament containing the vascular web is clamped, cut, and ligated on both sides with 2-zero silk ties.

The distal stump of the transected uterine artery is traced entering the tunnel and it is related to the ureter within the tunnel where it crosses the ureter from lateral to medial side. The ureter is seen as it enters the tunnel. Two horizontal curved clamps are inserted beneath the roof of the tunnel over the ureter. The tissue in the roof of the tunnel which also consist the uterine artery and vein, is clamped, cut, and ligated. This dissection is undertaken on both sides. The ureter on both sides are rolled laterally out of the tunnel and dissected free from surrounding tissue lysing the flimsy adhesions between it and floor of the tunnel until its entrance into the bladder.

The bladder is dissected from the anterior vagina by sharp dissection. The uterus is retracted upward. The cul-de-sac peritoneum between the uterus and the rectum is incised. Retracting the uterus upwards, finger is inserted between the uterosacral ligaments, and the posterior wall of the vagina is dissected off the anterior rectal wall. Keeping the uterus under upward traction the upper portion of the uterosacral ligaments is clamped, cut and ligated on both sides. The lower portion of the uterosacral ligaments, containing the parasympathetic nerves to the bladder, is retained.

The anterior, posterior, and lateral attachments of the uterus and parametria have now been ligated. The paravaginal tissue on either side is clamped with Haeney's clamp, cut, and ligated with 1-zero vicryl sutures. The vagina should be transected approximately 3 cm below the cervix and the isolated bleeding sites on the vaginal cuff are ligated using 2-zero vicryl sutures. The vagina is closed with continuous interlocking 1-zero vicryl suture.

Abdomen is closed in layers after placing a closed suction drains in both retroperitoneal spaces. These drains are brought out through the anterior abdominal wall in each lower quadrant and are sutured to the skin.

Postoperative Complications

a. *Infectious and febrile morbidity:* It is the most common postoperative complication. Prophylactic use of broad-spectrum antibiotics reduces the frequency of this complication.
b. *Postoperative bleeding:* Most often they are self-limited and can be treated conservatively with close observation for haemodynamic instability and blood transfusions but sometimes may require re-exploration.
c. *Bladder dysfunction:* Due to interruption in the autonomic nerve supply to the bladder resulting from bilateral stripping of sacral nerves, excision of large portion of paracervical and paravaginal webs of retroperitoneal tissue and bilateral pelvic node dissection will damage the sympathetic fibres of the bladder. This results in transient hypertonia, gradually being replaced by hypotonia. Most patients get back the ability to void within 2–3 weeks; however, it may persist in approximately 5% of patients. In addition, a substantial number of patients develop persistent urinary incontinence postoperatively.
d. *Lymphocyst formation:* Results from interruption of efferent pelvic lymphatics leading to lymphedema, pelvic discomfort, and infection and also increase the frequency of deep venous thrombosis and pulmonary embolism. Lymphedema develops insidiously over time, occurs more frequently when pelvic lymphadenectomy is followed by radiation or groin node dissection. Similarly, lymphocyst formation can occur as a result of extensive pelvic lymphadenectomy. Lymphocyst may cause ureteral obstruction or presents as a pelvic mass. Percutaneous drainage under ultrasound guidance or surgery with marsupialisation may be necessary.
e. *Sexual dysfunction and surgical menopause:* Reduces the quality of life, can impose psychological problems.
f. *Vesicovaginal and ureterovaginal fistula:* Most dreaded and troublesome complication, results from ligation of the superior vesical artery and disruption of blood supply to the distal ureter. The need for postoperative radiotherapy will worsen this problem. Patient presents with fever, continuous dribbling of urine per vagina, sometimes with enlarged pelvic mass. To determine whether it is a vesicovaginal or ureterovaginal fistula, intravesical instillation of methylene blue followed by intravenous injection of indigo carmine is done and colour change in the swab placed in the vagina at high, mid, and low level is noted (*three swab test*). Alternatively, an intravenous pyelogram or computed tomography may help to locate the fistula. Most often uretero-vaginal fistula is located in the distal 1/3rd of ureter. Small vesicovaginal fistulas may heal spontaneously with prolonged bladder catheterisation; however, larger defects that fail to heal with conservative management needs surgical repair. Stenting is required for uretero-vaginal fistulas. If retrograde stent cannot be passed, then percutaneous nephrostomy with anterograde stenting is done. Repair of uretero-vaginal fistula is done after 3–6 months.
g. *Ureteric stricture*—can also occur after radical hysterectomy.

NERVE SPARING RADICAL HYSTERECTOMY

The classical radical hysterectomy is the primary treatment in cases of cervical cancer in the IA2-IIA FIGO stage. The basic assumption of classical radical hysterectomy is excision of the uterus with the vaginal cuff, parametria and pelvic lymphatic nodes and potentially para-aortic nodes. Full oncological radicality is obtained at the expense of the patient's fertility and complications related to the excision of a part of the lymphatic system and vegetative innervations. After classical radical hysterectomy patients develop a wide spectrum of undesired symptoms like inability of spontaneous urination, urine retention, decreased stream strength, urinary urgency, interrupted urination, feeling of incomplete bladder emptying after micturition, urinary incontinence, nocturia; all are due to damage to the autonomic innervation of pelvic organs. The improvement of the techniques of surgical treatment of cervical cancer should aim in limiting the early and late complications connected with the surgery, but without worsening the radicalness of the procedure. Within the last 15 years, an essential progress was made in recognition and understanding of anatomy of the autonomic nervous system within the pelvis. The concept of preserving vegetative nerves during the radical hysterectomy became a standard in many centres. The technique aimed at saving the vegetative innervation and individual adjustment of the surgical procedure so that there is improvement of the quality of life of patients after radical procedures.

The technique of radical hysterectomy which saves vegetative innervation developed in the second half of the 20th century, at first in Japan and then also in Europe and North America. The application of the nerve-sparing technique requires knowledge of the anatomy of the most important structures of the vegetative nervous system, that is, hypogastric nerve, lower pelvic splanchnic nerve and its cervical and bladder branches.

The pelvic nerve plexus consists of hypogastric nerves and pelvic splanchnic nerves, as well as sacral splanchnic nerves. The hypogastric nerves join the pelvic nerve plexus from the superior ventral side. The pelvic splanchnic nerves, originates from the ventral rami S2 to S4, join from the lateral dorsal side. To accomplish the conventional nerve-sparing procedure, the parametrium and paracolpium tissue should be transected just above the hypogastric nerves, allowing the pelvic nerve plexus to be preserved.

The rectum was resected beforehand to widely develop pararectal and presacral spaces. Then the sacral nerves (S1 to S4) is exposed at the anterior sacral foramina. This is the site of origin of the pelvic splanchnic nerves, which join the pelvic nerve plexus. Consequently, this identification helps in the complete exposure of the pelvic splanchnic nerves. After identifying the hypogastric nerves and pelvic splanchnic nerves, the pelvic nerve plexus and its vesical branches can easily be exposed. After developing the pararectal space, the hypogastric nerves can be observed easily along the lateral sides of the mesorectum. The lymph node tissue around the internal iliac region is removed completely, and then the S2 to S3 roots are identifiable beneath the fascia of the piriform muscle. The pelvic splanchnic nerves, which join the pelvic nerve plexus, are visible as visceral branches originating from S2 to S3 roots after meticulously removing the lymph node tissue around the cardinal ligament. After transecting the vessel part of the cardinal ligament, the pelvic nerve plexus can be exposed. When adipose tissue around the posterior part of the vesicouterine ligament is removed nerve plexus can be exposed. When adipose tissue around the posterior part of the vesicouterine ligament is removed completely, the vesical branches from the pelvic nerve plexus can be exposed as fibrous tissue connecting the pelvic nerve plexus with the bladder. At the point the uterosacral ligament and paracolpium tissue are transected, so the the radicality of the procedure is maintained. The uterosacral ligament and the paracolpium tissue are transected above the hypogastric nerves.

ROBOT ASSISTED LAPAROSCOPIC SURGERY IN GYNAECOLOGY

The da Vinci robotic system is the only FDA approved and commercially available robot in gynaecology, consists of three main components: the robotic cart, the vision cart, and the operating console. There are four robotic arms mounted on the robotic cart, which can be placed freely next to the patient. The robotic cart docked to the laparoscopic trocars on the patient's abdomen is connected to the operating console through a cable. There is 3-dimensional (3D) vision system in the da Vinci surgical system, in which double endoscopes generate two images resulting in the perception of a 3D image. The robotic arms with surgical instruments have three or four joints, which can reproduce the range of motion and dexterity of a surgeon's hand. Sitting at the surgical console, the surgeon performs the surgery by manipulating the controller in it. The movement is translated from the surgeon's fingers to the tip of the surgical instruments; thus during this process, the physiologic tremor is eliminated by the robotic system. The surgeon can conduct more precise surgical procedures. These instruments including the 3D vision system and endowrist allow the surgeon to conduct more precise surgical procedures during surgery with these instruments including the 3D vision system and endowrist.

Laparotomies in all patients with cervical or endometrial cancer have increased operative and postoperative morbidity. To reduce the surgical morbidity of laparotomies, robot-assisted laparoscopic surgery was introduced as an alternative surgical method in gynaecologic cancers. Robot-assisted laparoscopic type II/III radical hysterectomy is associated with a shortened hospital stay, few operative complications, acceptable lymph node yields, and acceptable operative times. Robotic staging surgery for endometrial carcinoma in obese women resulted in shorter operation times, shorter hospital stay, lower transfusion rate, and less frequent conversion to laparotomy when compared to laparoscopic staging.

Advantages of Robotic surgery: 3-dimensional view, wrist like motion of the robotic arm and ergonomically comfortable position for the surgeon offer significant technical ease in performing complicated surgical procedures, including suturing and tying of knots by the surgeon, providing a familiar environment similar to that of the laparotomic approach.

Disadvantage: High cost of robotic surgery is the main weak point, which prevents robotic surgery from spreading worldwide. Absence of tactile feedback of robotic arms, requirement of larger ports for robotic surgery compared to conventional laparoscopic staging surgery are the other disadvantages. The need of placement of a large sized port, more than 8-mm in diameter for robotic surgery, larger than that of laparoscopic surgery, causes aggravated postoperative pain , poor cosmetic results and additionally risk of trocar site hernia.

FEASIBILITY OF SINGLE PORT LAPAROSCOPIC SURGERY

The principle concept of single port laparoscopic surgery (SPLS) is to place all of the laparoscopic working ports through the same incision. However, this results in hand collisions out of the abdomen and clashing of instruments within the abdomen. Various devices are been designed to overcome the technical challenges for SPLS. Those devices include laparoscopic ports designed to apply multiple instruments through a single incision, flexible/long endoscopes and articulating/variable length instruments.

SPLS is considered a feasible approach for hysterectomy and oophorectomy in gynaecology. In the field of gynaecologic oncology, SPLS may be applied to adnexal surgery in patients with adnexal tumours, prophylactic oophorectomy in patients with high risk of developing ovarian cancer, and hysterectomy in patients with preinvasive cervical neoplasia or microinvasive cervical cancer.

Advantages: (1) Operative complications-related trocar insertion such as epigastric vessel injury, visceral organ herniation, wound infection, and visceral organ damage might be reduced by eliminating the need of ancillary ports. (2) Postoperative pain resulting from skin incision and trocar penetration of muscle and fascia might be reduced. (3) Cosmetic result may be better. (4) In cases of adnexectomy, resected specimens can be easily extracted through the larger umbilical incision of the SPLS than that of conventional laparoscopy.

Disadvantages: Clashing of laparoscopic instruments and limited vision of in-line view are potential disadvantages of SPLS. These cause longer operative times and longer learning curves clashing of laparoscopic instruments and limited vision of in-line view is potential disadvantages of SPLS. These weaknesses which cause longer operative times and longer learning curves might be major obstacles for the popularity of SPLS.

If technical challenges are overcome in laparoscopic instruments, then, more complicated procedures in gynaecologic oncology, such as radical hysterectomy and comprehensive endometrial cancer staging surgery might be conducted with SPLS in the near future.

REPAIR OF GENITOURINARY FISTULAS

Types of Genital Fistulas

a. *Ureters*—ureterovaginal, ureterocervical, ureterouterine
b. *Bladder*—vesicovaginal (high, mid, low), vesicocervical, vesicouterine
c. *Urethra*—urethrovaginal.

Investigation

Per speculum examination: Most fistula can be easily seen by perspeculum examination after instilling the bladder with dilute methylene blue especially VVF. Continuous trickling of urine from the vagina is seen. Vaginitis and vulvitis may be present due to constant dribbling of urine.

Fluid creatinine estimation and simultaneous comparison with serum creatinine is done. If the fluid creatinine is many times more than the serum creatinine, then the fluid is nothing else but urine because only the kidney has the capacity to concentrate creatinine to a high level.

Moir's three swab test: Three swabs are placed in the vagina at three levels. Bladder is filled with dilute methylene blue. Patient is made to walk for 10–15 minutes. If the lower most swabs get wet and stained blue, it is incontinence per urethra. If the middle swab gets wet and stained blue it is due to VVF. If the uppermost swabs get wet but not stained blue it is uretero-vaginal fistula.

Cystoscopy—helps to identify the level of fistula, its relation to the ureter, number of fistula. It is of limited use in large fistula as it is difficult to distend the bladder. In these cases the bladder can be distended with air/CO_2.

Intravenous urogram—helps to identify the level of fistula. If this fails then retrograde pyelography is done.

Spiral CT scan—reveals renal and ureteric anatomy, abscess, fluid collection.

Ureterovaginal Fistula

Invariably the distal 1/3rd ureter is involved.

Sites of ureteral injuries:

- At or just below the pelvic brim, dorsal to the infundibulopelvic ligament.
- Along the course of the ureter in lateral pelvic wall above the uterosacral ligament.
- At the base of the broad ligament where the uterine artery crosses the ureter from lateral to medial side.
- As the ureter passes in the tunnel in Mackenrodt's ligament
- In the intramural portion of the bladder.

Nature of injury:

- Trauma to the vascular sheath leading to ischaemia—damage to the adventitia should be avoided as much as possible during dissection of ureter.
- Ligature incorporation.
- Segmental resection.
- Thermal injury—though the mean distance of thermal damage with most of the instruments is approximately 2 mm, it may be as much as 5 mm.
- Injury by staplers in laparoscopic surgery.

Though abdominal hysterectomy for conditions like endometriosis, pelvic inflammatory disease, ovarian tumours is the commonest cause it is known to occur in radical hysterectomy, caesarean hysterectomy. The best way to prevent ureteric fistula is its identification in the retroperitoneal space and trace its course from pelvic brim to the bladder. Blind application of clamps over the bleeding uterine vessels should be avoided. Judicial usage of thermal current near the ureter will help to avoid thermal injury. As the pelvic part of ureter receives blood supply from lateral aspect, dissection and mobilisation is carried out from medial aspect so as to avoid devascularisation injury.

Repair

In the immediate postoperative period, repair is not attempted. Ureteric stenting with J stent is done. Indwelling catheter is placed. Only when there is infected urinoma or in generalised sepsis measures are taken to divert the urine from the kidney like percutaneous nephrostomy so to protect the kidney function. Small fistula often heals spontaneously. If fails to heal then after 3–6 months once the tissue oedema subsides ureteral resection and re-implantation is done. The ureter is transected above the healthy site and re-implanted into the posterior aspect of the bladder. If the ureter cannot be reached to the bladder without tension then *psoas hitch* is done. The entire ventral surface of the bladder is freed from its areolar attachment in the retropubic space. On the anterior wall of the bladder, a curved incision is put. This incision is put at 90° to the direction desired to elongate the bladder. Two fingers are inserted into the posterosuperior portion of the bladder. A pliable bladder can be extended to reach the psoas tendon across the iliac vessels to reach the transected proximal end of ureter. The posterior surface of the bladder is anchored to the psoas tendon by interrupted absorbable sutures. These sutures are attached to the bladder wall without entering the bladder lumen. The transected ureter is implanted into the posterior aspect of the bladder dome, some distance from the trigone so as to minimise any potential stenosis or injury to the contralateral ureteral orifice. The ureter is stented, and the bladder is closed in two layers at right angles to the way it was opened. A drain is placed near the ureteroneocystostomy which is to removed in the 2 to 3 days once it is certain that there is no leak. The bladder is drained for 10 days and ureteral stent is removed after 6 weeks.

Vesicovaginal Fistula

Bladder trauma commonly occurs during hysterectomy and caesarean section while dissecting the bladder off the cervix and vagina. Failure to identify the bladder injury, thermal injury, suture placement through the bladder and vaginal wall while closing the vaginal cuff, ischaemic necrosis of the bladder wall due to prolonged pressure of the foetal head in 2nd stage of labour, forceps delivery of the baby are the common cause of vesicovaginal fistula.

Treatment

Once the fistula has occurred, it is wise to wait for 3–6 months. Indwelling catheter antibiotics are put to subside the infection and oedema. Small fistulas <3 mm may heal spontaneously during this waiting period. Meanwhile local condition is improved with vaginal estrogen cream; zinc oxide cream for ammoniacal dermatitis. Small fistulas can be tried to close with fibrin sealants.

a. *Vaginal repair*

Patient is placed in lithotomy position. Fistula is exposed properly. This may demand an extended episiotomy especially for high fistulas near the vault. Foleys is passed across the fistula. Bulb inflated and the fistula is given mild traction below.

- *Flap-splitting technique:* In this technique, the vaginal epithelium is incised circumferentially around the fistula and widely dissected from the underlying endopelvic fascia for a distance of about 2 cm. the tract is left unresected, the bladder is closed, tension-free, in 2 layers with 3-zero or 4-zero vicryl—first layer includes the full thickness of vaginal skin previously left intact at the fistula tract, along with the partial thickness of the bladder wall, and second layer involves closure in the muscularis placed perpendicular to the prior suture line. Martius bulbocavernosus flap can be advanced near the fistula for vasularisation. The surgery is completed with the vaginal closure over the bladder defect.
- *The Latzko procedure:* It is an excellent procedure for correcting small posthysterectomy fistulae at the vaginal apex with adequate vaginal length. A circumferential incision is made around the fistula. Vaginal epithelium is stripped from the anterior and posterior fascia at least 2.5 cm in all directions around the fistula tract. The fistula is not excised. The vesical edges of the fistula are not denuded. The pubovesical fascia is closed in two layers, and vaginal epithelium is closed using interrupted sutures. The walls have a natural tendency to fall together and are easily approximated without tension. The vaginal wall in contact with the bladder becomes the posterior vesical wall and which eventually gets re-epithelialised with transitional epithelium. Indwelling catheter is placed to prevent undue filling of bladder and tension over the stitches.

b. *O'conor's abdominal repair*

Indications for abdominal approach:

- The need for concomitant abdominal surgery, such as augmentation cystoplasty and ureteral reimplantation
- Adequate vaginal exposure of the fistula not possible
- VVF involving the ureters, bowel, or other intra-abdominal structures
- Involvement of the VVF with ureteric orifices.

By midline/Pfannenstiel incision laparotomy is done. After entering the peritoneal cavity, the posterior wall of the bladder is dissected free as much as possible. Incision made on the posterior wall of the bladder is extended down to the level of the fistula. Stay sutures may be placed along the incision for every few centimeters to permit traction so as to aid in exposure and dissection. Location of fistula and its relation to the ureteric orifice is identified. If necessary ureteral catheters may be placed. The fistula tract, scarred and necrotic tissue are resected. The posterior wall of the bladder is dissected from the underlying endopelvic fascia and vagina. The bladder and vagina are closed separately. The bladder is closed in 2 layers of 3-zero vicryl suture in continuous fashion beginning from the apex. First layer includes the mucosa and full thickness bladder wall, second layer involves the seromuscular layer inverting the first. Bladder is drained by a suprapubic catheter removed after 2–3 weeks and transurethral catheter removed after 4–5 days.

c. ***Bladder mucosal autologous grafts***

By laparotomy, cystotomy is done and bladder mucosa is denuded circumferentially near the fistula site for a distance of 1 cm. The fistula tract and vaginal wall are left undisturbed. At the edge of the anterior cystotomy margin, a free bladder mucosal graft is dissected sharply from underlying muscularis layer. This mucosal graft is then secured with interrupted 4-0 vicryl sutures over the fistulous tract. These sutures are placed into the superficial muscularis at a distance of 2–3 cm. The bladder is closed in 2 layers. A transurethral catheter is used for 4–5 days. A suprapubic Malecot catheter is placed for 2–3 weeks.

Rectovaginal Fistula Repair

It is the abnormal communication between rectum and anal canal. Though obstetric trauma is the commonest cause, carcinoma cervix invading the posterior vaginal wall tuberculosis, radiotherapy induced are other causes.

Foul smelling discharge or faeces though the vagina is the presentation. Fistula may *below* just above the anal sphincter or *high* up near the vault.

Investigation

- *Contrast study*—using a contrast material a vaginogram or a barium enema is done to identify a fistula located in the upper rectum.
- *Computerised tomography (CT) scan*—of abdomen and pelvis helps to locate a fistula and determine its cause.
- *Magnetic resonance imaging (MRI)*—can show the location of a fistula, as well as involvement of pelvic organs or the presence of a tumor. MR fistulogram can be more useful.

Preparation

Complete mechanical bowel preparation is essential for the repair of rectovaginal fistula (RVF). Diversion colostomy is essential in high fistula, radiation-induced fistulas and in recurrent/failed repair of RVF. Vagina is prepared with antiseptic solution. Preoperative higher antibiotics are started.

Technique

Patient is put in lithotomy position. Vaginal mucosa is incised circumferentially round the fistula. The vaginal flap is raised all round the fistula. Extreme care is taken to see that the bowel mucosa is adequately mobilised and the devitalised, scarred, or avascular portions of the mucosa is been excised. After adequate mobilisation of the intestinal mucosa, its edges are sutured in an inverting fashion with interrupted 3-zero vicryl sutures. A second layer of closure involving the perirectal fascia and sometimes even levator ani muscle is done. To improve the vascularity of the area bulbocavernosus flap may be drawn into the area. A longitudinal incision down the labia majora is done through the pad of fat until the bulbocavernosus muscle is exposed. After its dissection, it is transected above its insertion into the perineal body, leaving its blood supply from the pudendal artery intact. A tunnel approximately 3 cm wide is created from inside the vaginal canal and the bulbocavernosus muscle is drawn through this tunnel underneath the labia minora. It is placed over the repaired area and is sutured over the perirectal fascia with interrupted 3-zero vicryl sutures. The vaginal mucosa and the labial skin are sutured with 2-zero vicryl sutures. Stool softeners are given for 3–6 months.

However higher fistulas cannot be dealt satisfactorily through vagina and may require open abdominal approach. After dissecting the rectovaginal septum, the fistula is divided, and the rectum and vagina are closed primarily without bowel resection. Omentum may be interposed in between to separate the suture lines. This is useful when the fistula is not large and the tissues available for closure are healthy. But when tissues are unhealthy because of irradiation, inflammation, or neoplasm, unless the abnormal tissues are resected this type of repair is likely to fail. Functional anal sphincters are preserved whenever possible by use of a low anterior resection, and coloanal anastomosis.

TRANSOBTURATOR TAPE (TOT) FOR STRESS URINARY INCONTINENCE

Under spinal anaesthesia, in lithotomy position, Foley's catheterisation is done. A point is marked on the outer aspect of the labia majora which is a point of intersection of an imaginary horizontal line passing to the clitoris and vertical line passing through the adductor longus tendon. Suburethral anterior vaginal wall flap is raised for 2 cm by making a vertical incision. Dissection upwards and laterally is carried out as far near the pubic ramus. A stab incision is made on the marked point on the outer aspect of the labia majora (vertical incision). Through this small incision specialised curved stout trocar which is having an opening (helical trocar) is inserted under guidance over the pubic bone and then to pass under and around the pubic bone across the obturator membrane so as to enter its tip into the anterior vagina adjacent and under the flap created; through the eye at its tip polypropylene tape (strip of lengthy mesh) is fed and gradually withdrawn to bring the tape out through the incision on the skin. Helical trocars are different for right and left side. Similar procedure is repeated on the opposite side to pass another end of the tape (mesh strip) to the opposite side labia majora incision. One should confirm that tape should fit only snugly neither too tight nor too loose. Ends of the mesh tape are buried under the skin (both sides) and skin is closed on both sides. Anterior vaginal wall incision is closed using chromic catgut. Urinary catheter is kept for 2 days.

Problems

Injury to bladder, obturator vessels, mesh displacement, failure of the procedure, it is a blind procedure. It is considered to be safe in spite of the fact that it is blind **(Fig. 32-26)**.

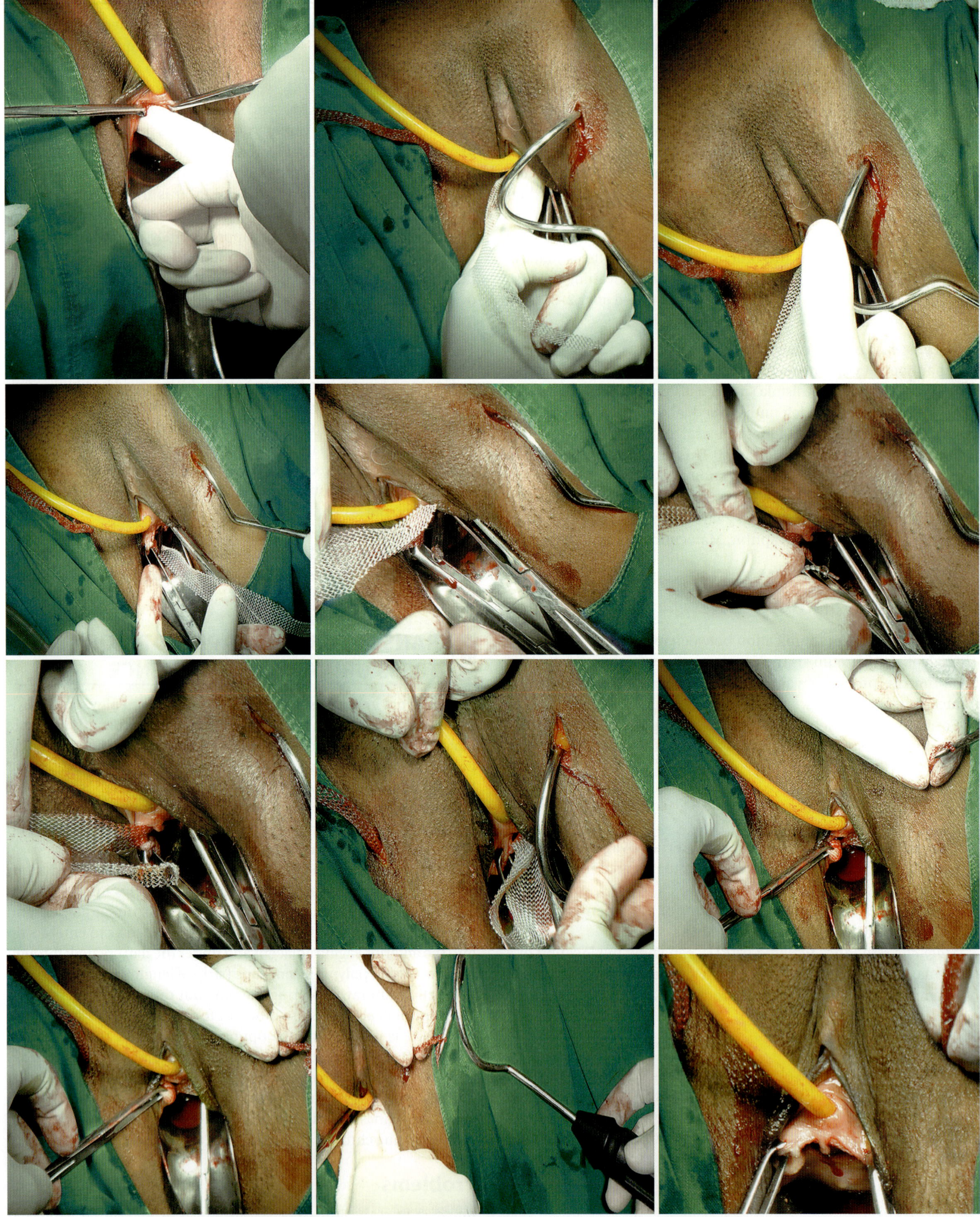

Figs. 32-26(1)

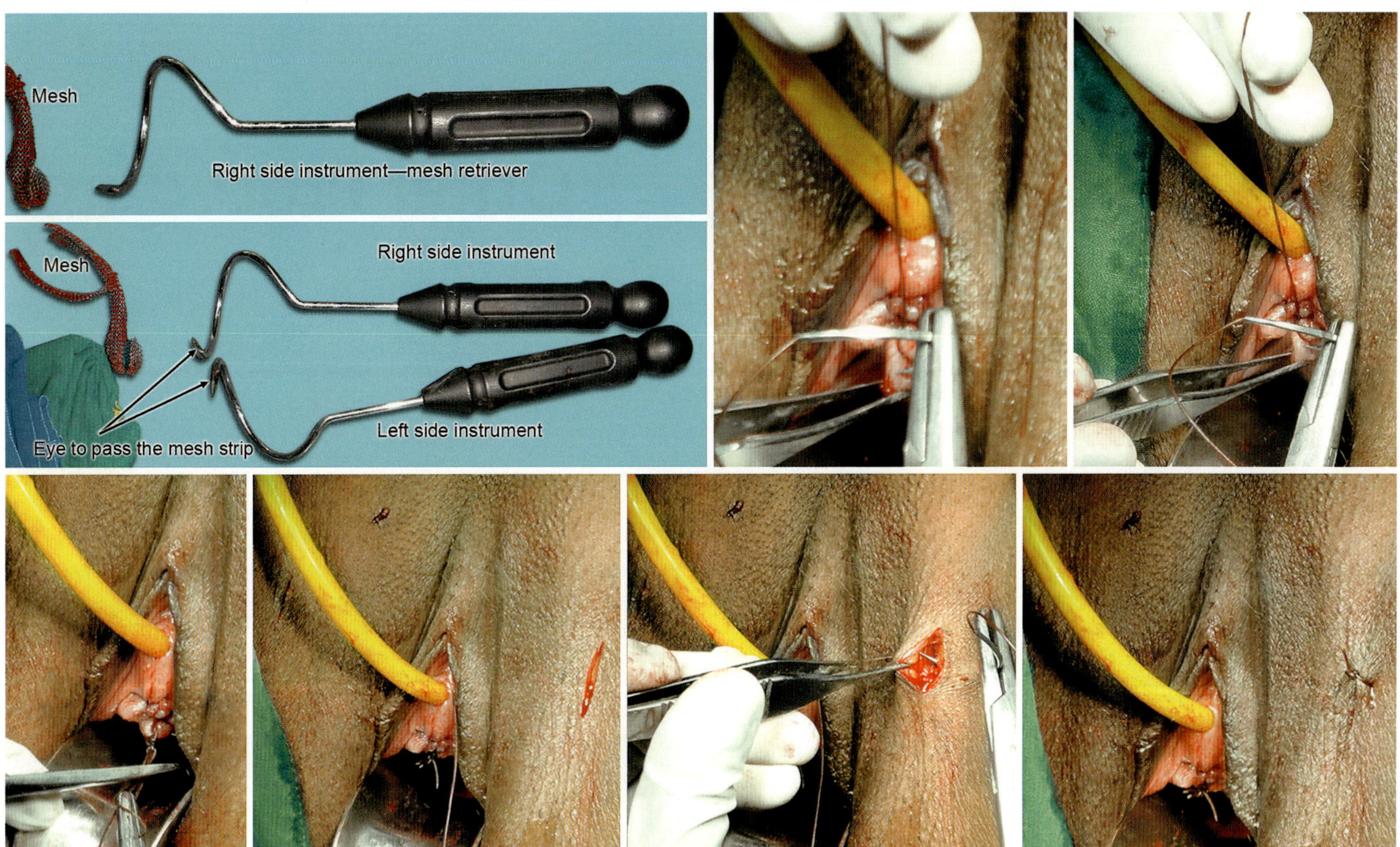

Figs. 32-26(2)

Figs. 32-26(1 and 2): Technique of transobturator tape (TOT) placement for stress urinary incontinence.

33 CHAPTER

Other Procedures

ROBOTIC SURGERY

Word—*Robota (Czech)* means for compulsory labour. First robot was deviced by Leonard da Vinci. Surgical robot is powered computer-controlled manipulator with artificial sensing that can be reprogrammed to move and position tools to carry out a range of surgical works. Initially da Vinci robot is developed from defense advanced research project agency (DARPA) for military research of remote battlefield surgery. Cholecystectomy was performed remotely via telesurgery from 300 miles away. Intuitive surgery created in 1999 after acquiring military patent rights from military. First robotic prostatectomy was performed in 2001 **(Fig. 33-1)**.

There are three parts in robotic system:

- Surgeon's console
- Patient's cart
- Optical cart.

As the surgeon manipulates the remote control unit, movements of the surgeon is translated to robotic arms. Each robotic arm contains multiple appendages connected by joints. The 'hand' of the robot holds interchangeable surgical instruments that can be moved in a manner similar to wrist of human. Scaled, filtered, translated movements are achieved without hand dominance. In laparoscopy, it is surgeon's hand, team work and proper instruments, tremor at the working end is always present; camera is controlled by camera surgeon not operator whereas in robotic surgery camera is controlled by operator. Endowrist moves 360° at all angles, makes dissection and suturing perfect **(Fig. 33-2)**.

Special features are: Binocular stereoscopic 3D vision with stability of camera; increased dexterity because of endoinstrumentation; high density camera with 15X magnification; easy dissection; quick intracorporeal suturing and knotting; precise technique; surgeon sits comfortably and operate with arms rested; adequate ergonomics with equal tremor less movements of right and left arms; multitasking instrumentations; harmonic robotic arm; three arms with 3D HD robotic camera arm with 4th arm robot for retraction; patient friendly as well as surgeon friendly.

Advantages: It is less painful; less blood loss; fast recovery; needs short hospital stay; small incision; cosmetically accepted; better outcome.

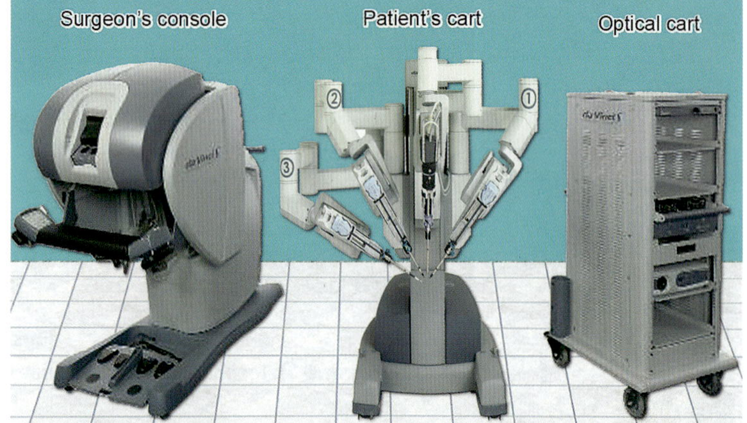

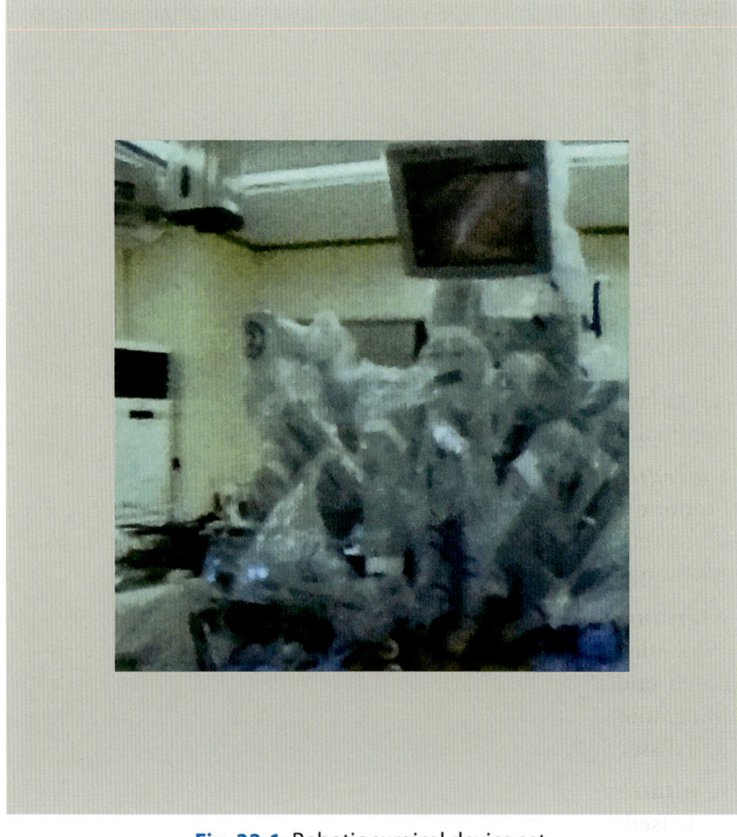

Fig. 33-1: Robotic surgical device set.

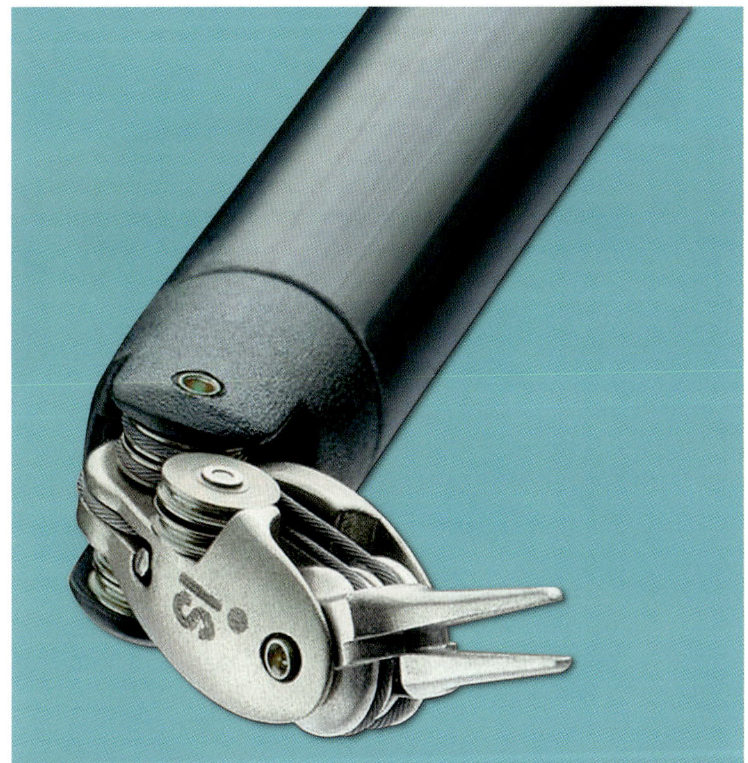

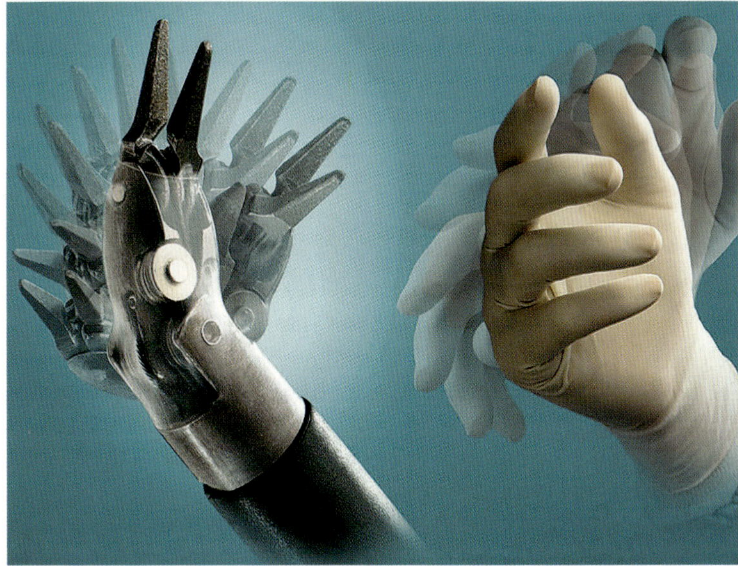

Fig. 33-2: Robotic endowrist which moves in all angles—360º.

Robot facilitates the performance of most complex procedures with minimally invasive high standard techniques.

Procedure done: All procedures done through laparoscopy can be done through robotic surgery. Nephrectomy, prostatectomy, hysterectomy, oesophageal surgeries; thyroid surgeries; oropharyngeal surgeries.

Learning curve: Surgical simulator to learn the robotic surgery is available—as red dragon/blue dragon. This skill simulator can teach endowrist manipulation, cameras and clutching; 4th arm integration; system settings; needle control and driving; energy use and dissection **(Fig. 33-3)**.

Limitations: Absence of tactile feedback, fixed patient position; increased cost to patient.

Future: Present set has got following features—monopolar/bipolar/advanced bipolar energy; harmonic; advanced grasper; laser.

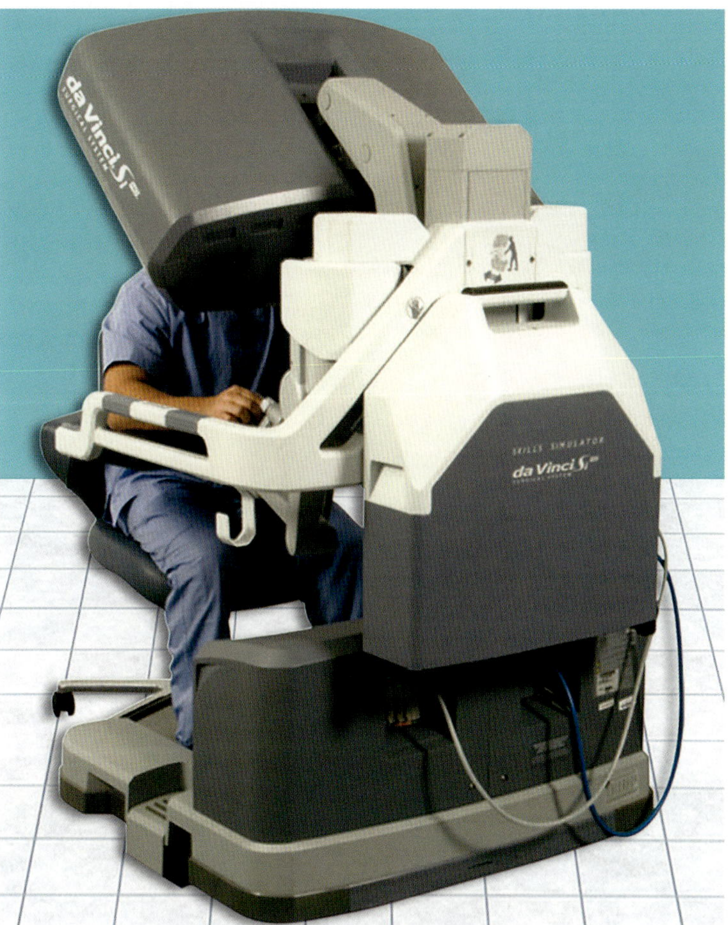

Fig. 33-3: Robotic skill simulator.

Future set will have linear cutter, seal, suction irrigation, drill, etc. Endowrist one vessel single use 8 mm diameter sealer with compact snake wrist is designed to seal and cut up to 7 mm diameter vessels. Image guidance fluorescence, lymph node mapping are newer one. Firefly fluorescence imaging of da Vinci identified real time anatomy using near infrared guidance which enhances visualisation of the critical vasculature like of mesentery, permits real time perfusion of the bowel prior to resection mainly in colon.

Advanced single port robotic set is the future. Single port very flexible robotic arm with snake like robots are possible in coming days **(Figs. 33-4 to 33-6)**.

Robotic scrub nurse as a helper robot in changing instruments like a scrub nurse.

LIPOSUCTION

Liposuction, also known as *lipoplasty* ("fat modelling"), *liposculpture suction lipectomy* ("suction-assisted fat removal") is a cosmetic surgery operation that removes fat from many different sites on the human body. Areas affected can range from the abdomen, thighs and buttocks, to the neck, backs of the arms.

Several factors limit the amount of fat that can be safely removed in one session. Finally, the operating surgeon and the patient make the decision. There are negative aspects to removing too much fat. Unusual "lumpiness" and/or "dents" in the skin can be seen in those patients "over-suctioned". The more fat removed, the higher the surgical risk.

Liposuction may be performed under general, regional ("tumescent"), or local anaesthesia. The safety depends on the

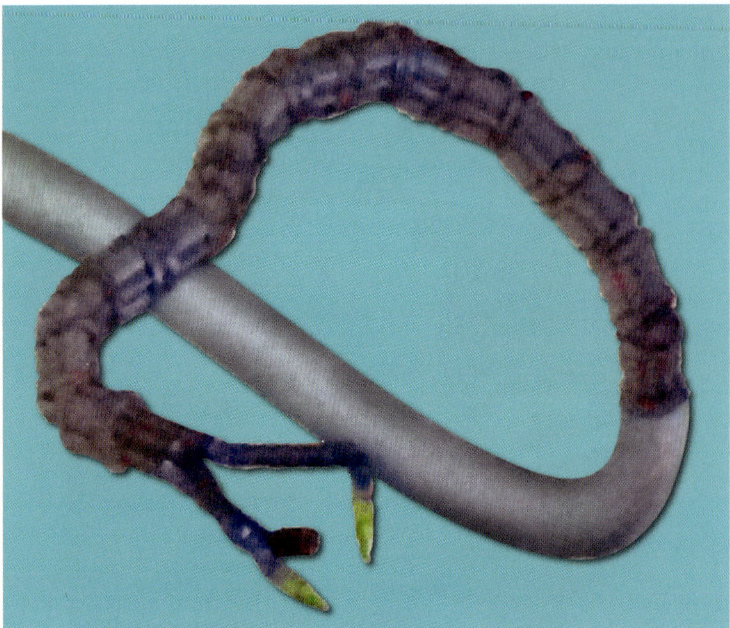

Fig. 33-4: Robotic flexible system.

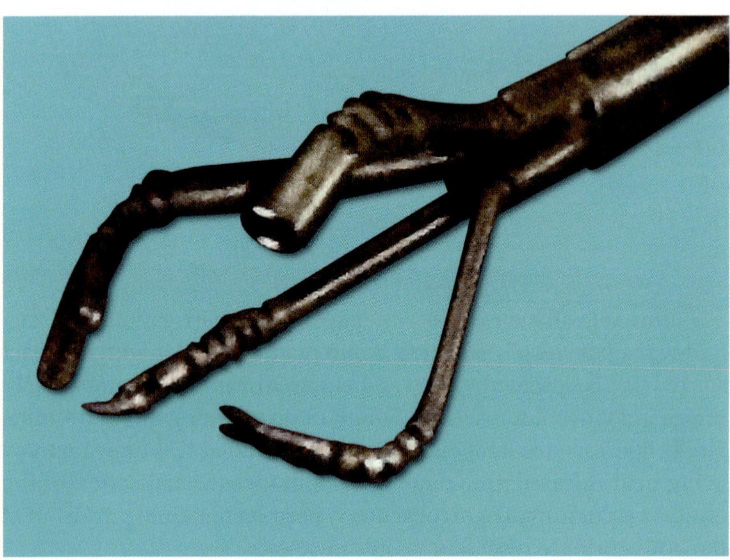

Fig. 33-5: Robotic SILS port.

amount of tissue removed, the choice of anaesthetic and the patient's general condition. Fit patient, patients who have stopped smoking for many months are ideal candidates for this contour correction surgery.

Technique was first performed by a French surgeon, Charles Dujarier. In 1926, a French model underwent contour surgery of leg by Charles Dujarier to later develop gangrene of the leg was a tragic story. This was the oldest history about contour surgery. In 1960, curettage surgery was proposed with variable results and morbidity. Again a French surgeon, Dr Yves-Gerard Illouz, in 1982 originated a method of suction-assisted lipolysis after infusing fluid into tissues using blunt cannulas and high-vacuum suction—Illouz method. In 1985, Klein and Lillis described the "tumescent anaesthesia", a regional technique which with high volumes of fluid containing local anaesthetic with intravenous sedation. High volume of fluid and potential toxicity of xylocaine tumescent technique later changed to low volume "super wet" tumescence. In the late 1990s, ultrasound was introduced to facilitate the fat removal by first liquefying the

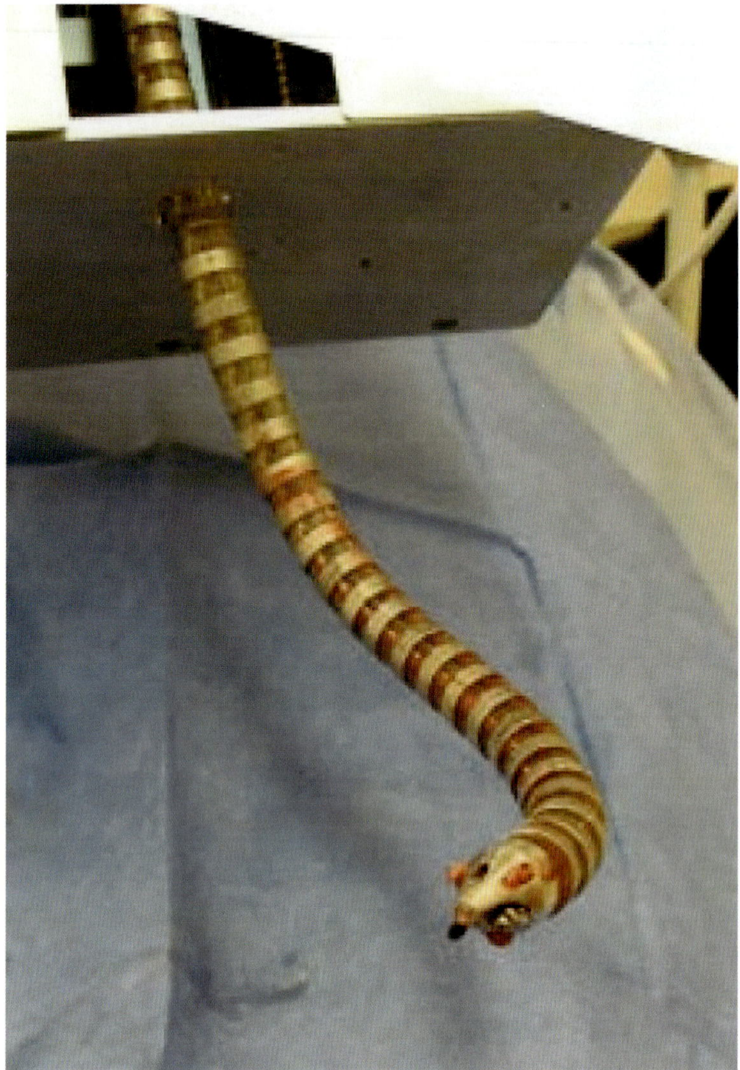

Fig. 33-6: Robotic snake instrument.

fat using ultrasonic energy. But it showed more complications. Laser thermal lipolysis is modern technology. Whatever the type is used, it is the surgeon's skill finally matters for adequate liposuction to create normal contour without complications.

Diabetes, cardiac illness is the relative risks for liposuction.

Principles

To remove the right amount of fat; to cause the least disturbance of other tissue, such as blood vessels; to keep the person's fluid balance normal.

Sites Where Liposuction is Done

Abdomen; hips; outer and or inner thigh; flanks; back; inner knee; upper arm; submental/chin; gynecomastia in males.

Preparation

Anticoagulants should be avoided for 2 weeks. Preoperative antibiotics are needed. Cardiac evaluation, respirator exercises are given.

Technique

Power-assisted liposuction cannula is often used nowadays.

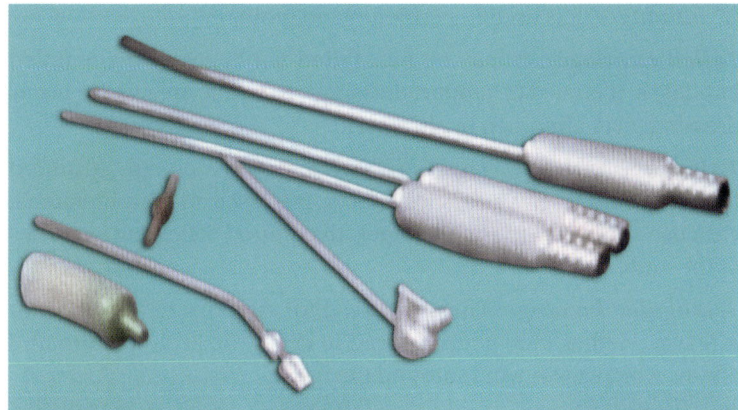

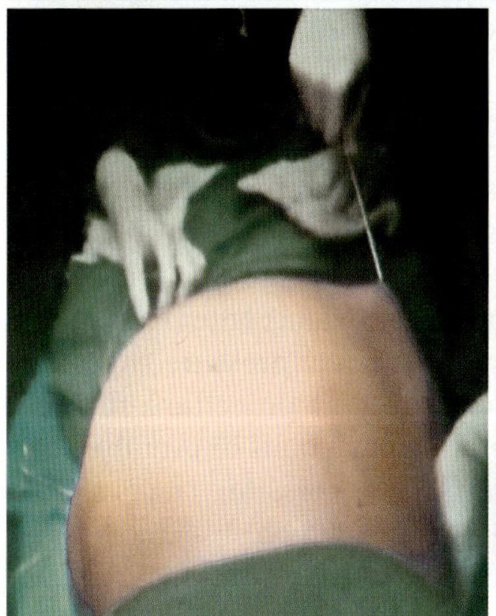

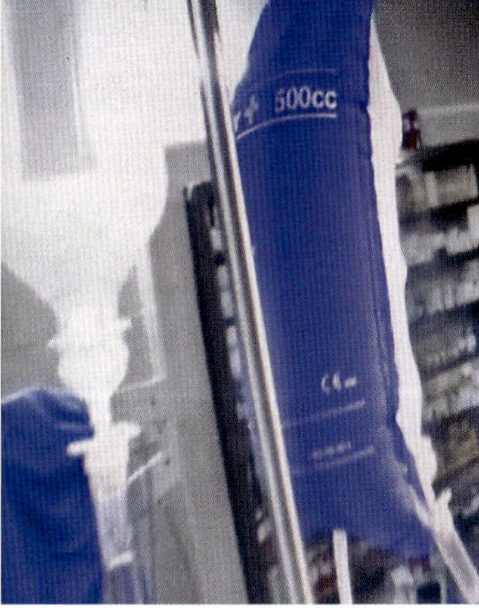

Fig. 33-7: Liposuction technique and device.

Fat is removed through a cannula and a suction device. Liposuction technique depends on the amount of fluid injection and the mechanism by which the cannula functions. The surgeon creates forwards and backwards motion, carefully through the fat layer, breaking up the fat cells and drawing them out of the body by suction. The patient will feel only a scraping or rasping sensation from the cannula movement. During liposuction, multiple small puncture wounds are made for inserting the cannula that can vary in size depending on the technique **(Fig. 33-7)**.

Ultrasound-assisted liposuction is useful for working on more fibrous areas, like the upper back or male breast area. It takes longer time; but with less blood loss.

Water-assisted liposuction is done by using a thin fan-shaped water beam, which loosens the structure of the fat tissue, so that it can be removed by a special cannula. During the liposuction, the water is continually added and almost immediately aspirated via the same cannula. It utilises less infiltration solution and oedema is less in this.

Postoperative Management

A compression garment which can easily be removed by the patient is worn for four weeks, this garment must have elasticity. Analgesics may be needed. Patient can go for work in 1–2 weeks.

Side-effects

Bruising which is painful; swelling; scars; pain in the abdominal wall; numbness in the abdomen which will subside in few weeks; post-operative weight gain; restricted mobility due to abdominal binder; pain, inflammation.

Complications

Allergic reaction to medications or material used during surgery. Infection: any time the body is incised or punctured, bacteria can get in and cause an infection. Damage to the skin: most surgeons work on the deeper levels of fat, so as to avoid wounding the skin any more than they must for the insertion of the cannula. Sometimes the cannula can damage tissue beneath the skin. Skin necrosis can occur rarely; and adjacent skin falls off in the necrotic area. Injury to internal organ during puncture of the abdominal wall can occur; such as the intestines during abdominal liposuction. Contour irregularities can occur. Thromboembolism and fat embolisation can develop occasionally. Burns due to friction of the cannula can occur. Xylocaine toxicity presenting as tingling and numbness and eventually seizures, followed by unconsciousness and respiratory or cardiac arrest. Fluid imbalance as fat contains a lot of fluid and is removed in liposuction, and also the surgeon injects fluid for the procedure, a very large amount for tumescent liposuction, fluid imbalance can set in. This could happen afterwards, after the patient is at home. If too much fluid remains in the body, the heart, lungs and kidneys could be badly affected.

DRESSINGS

They are the materials used to cover wounds, ulcers to provide support and to encourage healing.

Advantages

It covers the wound and so prevents further contamination. It gives comfort to the patient.

Disadvantages

It may get soaked. It may delay the epithelial layer formation.

Types

Dry dressings: It is used in clean, sutured operated wound. It is not changed at regular intervals.

Wet dressings: It is used in ulcers and wounds. Dressings are made wet by using jelly or Sofra-Tulle sheets.

Components of Dressing

Inner contact layer: It is non-absorbent and only allows secretion to pass into the absorbent layer. It does not allow penetration of granulation tissue. It is usually kept wet. Either mesh gauze or Sofra-Tulle is used.

Intermediate absorbent layer made up of cotton which absorbs the secretions.

Outer layer as supportive is made up of gauze.

Dressings are fixed to the place by: Bandages; plasters; dynoplast; crepe bandages; depending on the condition and amount of discharge from the wound/ulcer, it is changed as required—twice a day/once a day/once in two days. Small dressings are done without anaesthesia. Large areas like burn wounds or dressing in children require general anaesthesia.

BANDAGES

Technique of bandaging is called as ***dysmergia***.

Indications

To reduce the swelling like in lymphoedema; to keep dressings in position; to support splint; to stop bleeding/oozing.

Types of Bandages

Roller bandages: It is a continuous roll of material, which is rolled over the part to cover the area. It is used in limbs.

It is available in different lengths and widths—1 inch, 2 inches, 4 inches or 6 inches. It is used in different ways.

- ***Circular turns:*** Continuous rolls placed over the same place.
- ***Spiral turns:*** After the initial turn of the bandage, it ascends proximally overlapping the distal 2/3rd of the previous turn.
- ***Reverse spiral turn:*** Here each spiral turn is reversed in opposite direction so as to attain uniform pressure. It is used in limbs and areas which end as cones.
- ***Figure eight turn:*** It is used in knee, elbow, wrist, ankle and for clavicle.
- ***Recurrent turn:*** It is used in head and amputation stump. Here initially circular rolls are made and over that half turns are made to cover other parts of the area required.
- ***Spica bandage:*** It has got ascending and descending turns, with each turn overlap and cross each other. It is used in hip, groin, shoulder, breast or thumb. *Spica means eye of a bean.*

'T' bandages: It is used in perineum and groin.

Tailed bandages: It may be four tailed bandages or many tailed bandages. It is used to support dressings on a wide area like in burns dressing, over abdomen or chest wall.

Tubular bandages: These are stockings which are unrolled over the limb to give pressure effects. It is used in lymphoedema, varicose veins and in the postoperative period following surgeries of the limb.

Triangular bandage: These are used for supporting the elbow or forearm. Here a wide gauze is used to cover the arm, forearm and elbow, which again winds around the neck.

Cravat bandages: It is a folded type of triangular bandage, which is used as sling around the neck, when elbow requires to be rested.

Principles of Bandaging

Bandage is applied to the part from distal to proximal end. Proper positioning of the limb is a must before bandaging. After initial few circular turns, the required type of bandaging is then done. Bandage is unrolled outwards. During bandaging, latter turn should overlap 2/3rd of earlier turn. Firm, adequate pressure should be used during bandaging. After completing the procedure, the knot should not lie over the area or over the bony points or over the back. It should not cause venous or arterial compression. Digits should be left open and circulation in the digits should be observed for.

Size of bandages used at different places are: Finger/toe—one inch; Arm—two and half inches; Leg—four inches; Thigh—six inches; Trunk—six inches; Head—four inches.

Index

Page numbers followed by *f* refer to figure, *fc* refer to flowchart, and *t* refer to table.

A

B

C

D

E

F

G

H

J

K

L

M

N

O

P

Q

R

S

T

U

V